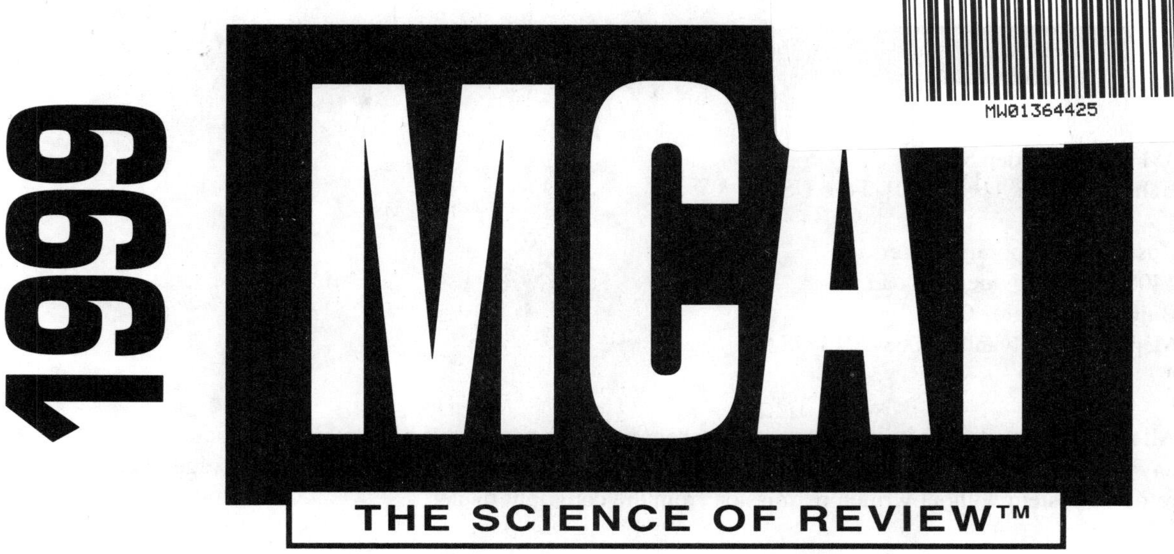

Complete Preparation for the Medical College Admission Test

AFTAB S. HASSAN, Ph.D.

Contributing Authors

Dorothy H. Air, Ph.D.
R. Gerald Bass, Ph.D.
Glen A. Bauer, M.A.
Angelica Braestrup, M.A.
Charles M. Bump, Ph.D.
Mary E. Duafala, M.S., M.B.A.
Martin R. Feldman, Ph.D.
James L. Flowers, M.D., M.P.H.
Richard K. Hill, Ph.D.
Evelyn Jackson, Ph.D.
Frank Kessler, M.A.
Jack Lochhead, Ed.D.
Carol Banks Setter, Ph.D.
S. William Whitson, Ph.D.

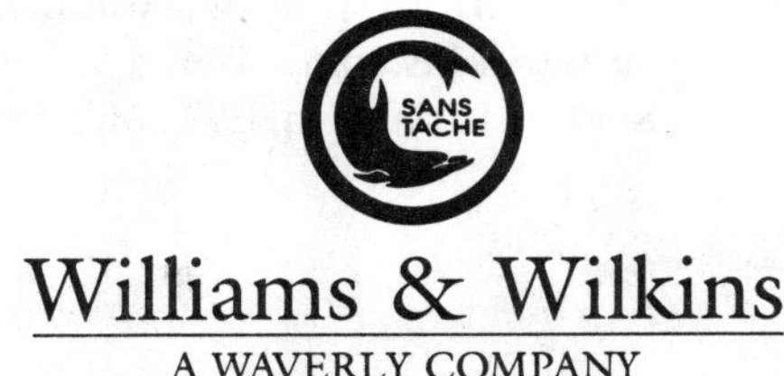

Williams & Wilkins
A WAVERLY COMPANY

BALTIMORE • PHILADELPHIA • LONDON • PARIS • BANGKOK
BUENOS AIRES • HONG KONG • MUNICH • SYDNEY • TOKYO • WROCLAW

351 West Camden Street
Baltimore, Maryland 21201-2436 USA

Rose Tree Corporate Center
1400 North Providence Road
Building II, Suite 5025
Media, Pennsylvania 19063-2043 USA

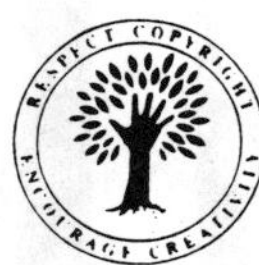

Printed in the United States of America

Library of Congress Cataloging-in-Publication Data

ISBN: 0–683–30522–0

The publishers have made every effort to trace the copyright holders for borrowed material. If they have inadvertently overlooked any, they will be pleased to make the necessary arrangements at the first opportunity.

To purchase additional copies of this book, call our customer service department at **(800)638-0672** or fax orders to **(800) 447-8438.** For other book services, including chapter reprints and large quantity sales, ask for the Special Sales department.

Canadian customers should call **(800) 665-1148,** or fax **(800) 665-0103.** For all other calls originating outside of the United States, please call **(410) 528-4223** or fax us at **(410) 528-8550.**
E-mail address: MCATPREP@WWILKINS.COM

Visit Williams & Wilkins on the Internet: **http://www.wwilkins.com** or contact our customer service department at **custserv@wwilkins.com**. Williams & Wilkins customer service representatives are available from 8:30 am to 6:00 pm, EST, Monday through Friday, for telephone access.

98 99 00
1 2 3 4 5 6 7 8 9 10

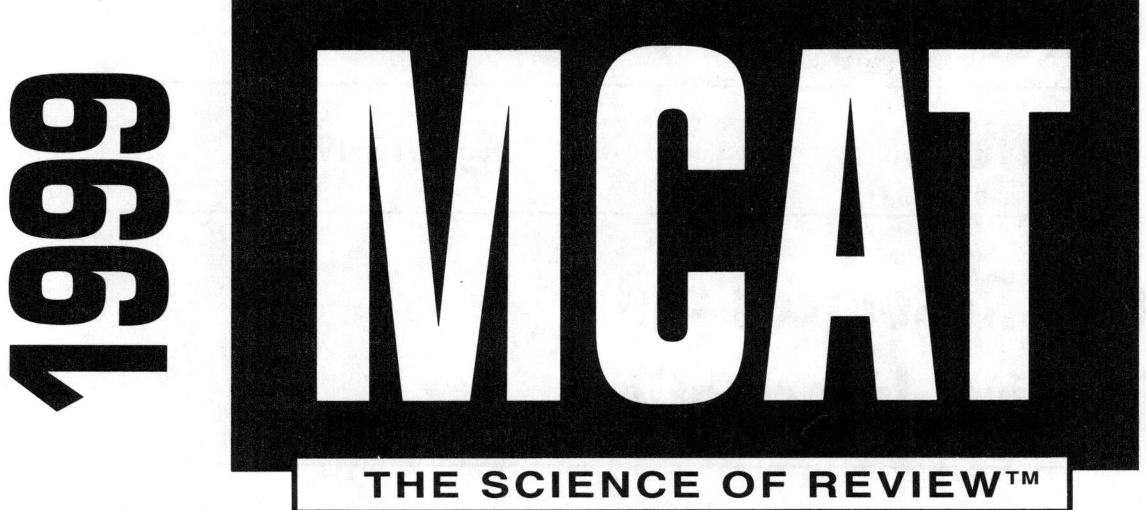

Complete Preparation for the Medical College Admission Test

Test Dates

April 18, 1998 | **August 15, 1998**

Selected Resources for Pre-Medical Information

Williams & Wilkins
Science of Review Hotline
1-800-634-4365
E-mail: mcatprep@wwilkins.com

Association of American Medical Colleges
2450 N Street, NW
Washington, D.C. 20037
(202) 828-0416

MCAT Program Office
P.O. Box 4056
Iowa City, IA 52243
(319) 337-1357

Afrinatino, Inc.
1000 Ewing Road
Coraopolis, PA 15108
http://iweb4u.com/afrinatino

Student National Medical Association, Inc.
National Office
1012 Tenth Street, NW
Washington, DC 20001
(800) 636-SMNA
E-mail: SMNA@SMART.NET

Columbia Review-Intensive MCAT Preparation-Courses
220 Madison Avenue
San Francisco, CA 94134
(800) 300-PREP or (415) 337-2009

The Journal of Pre-Med Studies
P.O. Box 3029
Garden City, NY 11531
(516) 873-0626
E-mail: JMSFJEFF4@aol.com

Selected Internet Sites

Williams & Wilkins Homepage
http://www.wwilkins.com

AAMC Newsletter
http://www.aamc.org/events/aamcstat/aamcnews.htm

Welcome to Premedical.com
http://www.premedical.com

American Medical Student Association
http://www.amsa.org/

The Pre-Med and Medical Information
http://www.efn.org/~brideb/Deb/medstuff/Medstuff.html

World Wide Web for Premeds
http://www.washcoll.edu/WC.HTML/academics/resources/premed.html

Pre Med Internet Resources
http://www.sc.edu/library/sciences/premed/html

The Pre Med Major
http://ww2.globalvision.net/admissions/pops/premed.html

UCI Chemistry/ Instruction/ Online Resources/ Pre-Med
http://chem.ps.uci.edu/instructions/premed.html

Finding Pre-Med Information
http://www.fas.harvard.edu/~cabref/premed.html

MCAT Mania
http://mail.utep.edu/~lfloyd/hmome.html

Applying to Med School
http://www.geocities.com/Athens/7103/apply.html

The Pre-Med Zone
http://www.netside.net/~hochstim/index.html

Premed.Edu Hunter Pre-Med
http://www.spacelab.net/~premed/

Medical Servers
http://www.columbia.edu/cu/gspremed/med.html

Premed@jhu
http://jhunix.hcf.jhu.edu/~scheel/aed/v_two/v2for2top.html

Brad's Premed Resource Center
http://rio.atlantic.net/~xyz/premed.html

Alpha Epsilon Delta
http://www.utexas.edu/students/aed/

Students who have recently taken the MCAT had these comments:

I took the MCAT in April of 1996 as a senior undergraduate student at Brown University. I was fortunate in that I only had to take the exam once. I believe the most important thing to remember about taking the MCAT is that this exam is not necessarily about one's ability to retain tons of scientific information, it is about one's ability to solve problems logically. This does not mean you don't have to study if you are a good problem solver, it means memorizing facts and formulas should only be the beginning of your studying; spend enormous amounts of time taking the exams again and again. Try taking the exam in a crowded place to see if you can concentrate. Most importantly, remember it is only an exam. If you do not do well the first time, you can try again. Yes this is one of the more important exams you will have to take in your life, but keep everything in perspective. Good Luck!!!

Stephanie Davis

I needed to quickly relearn and synthesize the information. I felt overwhelmed about the amount of material I had to know. It frightened me and made me feel inadequate at times. However, I had a goal and I was going to accomplish that goal. Rather than getting stuck on a small point, I would try to understand major concepts, theories, and rules. It is important to understand the big picture. Also, I found it beneficial to take practice tests. I wish I had more time to take these tests and do an actual simulation. I would recommend that everyone take at least one full blown simulation and several other practice tests (including the writing sections). If I could go back and do it all over, I definitely would take more practice tests.

After taking the MCAT, I remember feeling relieved and accomplished. I had just completed something that I had invested lots of time, energy, and money into. However, I also had a great feeling of anxiety: did I do a certain problem correctly, did I write concise, to the point, and legibly, what are my scores going to be, and will my scores be good enough to get me into school. Though the MCAT tests some basic core science, I find it to be more of a test of endurance, dedication, and test taking strategies. The day my scores came, I didn't want to open the envelope. I was so relieved when I saw I did well enough to get into school. Preparation for the MCAT helped me fine tune my study habits and taught me ways to learn, memorize, and enhance test taking skills. As a medical student, I currently use many of these techniques. Overall, the MCAT helped me to prepare to be an efficient student.

Craig Flinders

The MCAT is not a true measure of intelligence. In fact, I believe everyone who meets the prerequisites for medical school has been exposed to the necessary concepts to do well on the test. Perhaps a more accurate description of the MCAT would include an element of desire. The desire and commitment to become a doctor. Like medical school, the MCAT requires time, repetition, and sacrifice. Think of the MCAT as measure of your own personal commitment to the profession. The MCAT serves as a device to test your desire.

David Skolnick

I consider the MCAT to be a "catch 22"situation for most students. To answer all the questions, one needs to read very quickly. But if one reads very quickly, one is unlikely to answer the questions correctly. I found this to be a very difficult balance to achieve. The test day itself was stressful (since so much was at stake) and a great deal longer than I had expected sincethe test preparation manuals that I used did not account for breaks when indicating how long the test day was to be. The day was so long that one of the proctors fell asleep and actually snored. I found this to be immensely distracting. The room itself was comfortable and otherwise facilitated test-taking. I underestimated how much material was to be covered on the MCAT. I started to study for the test only four weeks beforehand and was, I felt, not thoroughly prepared. I consider the need to memorize a sizable number of physics formulas for the MCAT to be an unnecessary waste of time. Application, I believe, is more important than memorization and the physical sciences portion of the test should efficiently reflect this but does not. After taking the MCAT I felt as if I had spent 4 years in undergraduate school without learning a single thing. While taking the test I became very frustrated during the Physical Sciences and the Biological Sciences sections, the two I felt were most important. It seemed as if there were so many things on the test that I didn't know or couldn't remember. I was especially discouraged by the Physical Sciences section; so discouraged that I considered having my scores deleted after the lunch period. I thought that I had done horrible and I was concerned about admissions committees seeing a bad score. After finishing the test, I went home feeling very discouraged and disappointed. I felt that I had known so many more things when I took the practice tests and studied from the MCAT preparation books that I had purchased. I didn't feel any better about the test until my test scores came back. They turned out a lot better than I thought they would. It wasn't until then that I realized that I knew a lot of the things on the MCAT. It only seemed like I didn't because I was focusing only on the questions that I wasn't comfortable with and forgetting about the ones that I knew.

Brian Pollock

I hated taking the MCAT. Preparation for it was exhausting and drained my self-confidence. I felt as if the undergraduate science courses I had taken were inadequate in preparing me for this experience. I do not know how anyone could perform well on the rest without having taken some kind of preparatory course. The anxiety alone, associated with one's performance can be crippling on the day of the examination. I felt I would never take a more important test , or one that would have such an impact on the path I prayed my life would follow. The only positive thing I can now say, is that I'm here and all the hard work, tears and self-doubt were worth it to get here.

Ilysa Diamond

Do You Really Want High Scores on the MCAT?

If your answer is "yes," you should be better prepared! The following illustrations highlight four specific tools that you need to score high on the MCAT. Use these tools frequently during your school year.

FOUR ESSENTIAL MCAT TOOLS

A. Developing Active Learning Habits
B. Developing Verbal Reasoning Abilities
C. Developing Problem-Solving Abilities
D. Reviewing MCAT Sciences

Once you understand the "four essential tools," read Appendix A to analyze closely the structure of MCAT passages. Now you are ready to start with Chapter 1.

A. DEVELOPING ACTIVE LEARNING HABITS

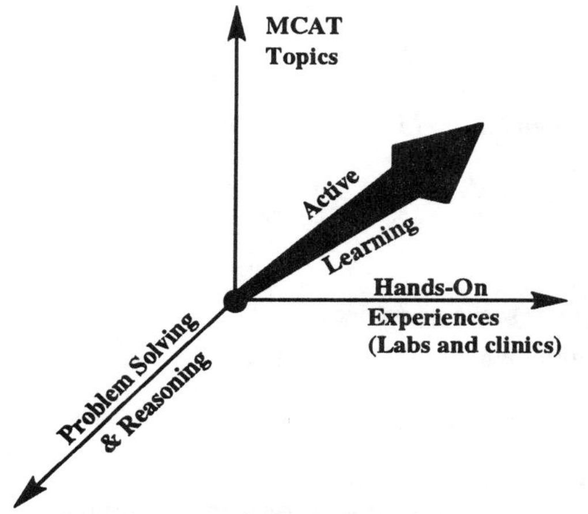

Components of Active Learning

Active learning results in reviewing MCAT topics for better understanding and retention using problem-solving, reasoning, and hands-on experiences (labs, clinics). Collaborative problem-solving efforts result in better perception of difficult concepts and in application of critical thinking skills to preclinical situations. Active learning principles can help you learn MCAT concepts more efficiently and retain them longer.

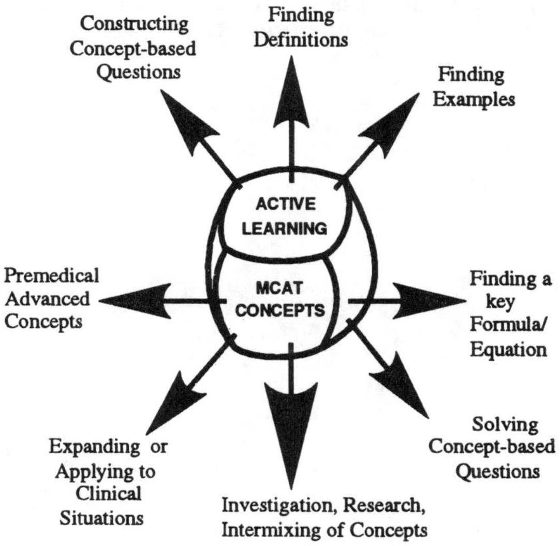

Elements for Active Learning of MCAT Concepts

B. DEVELOPING VERBAL REASONING ABILITIES

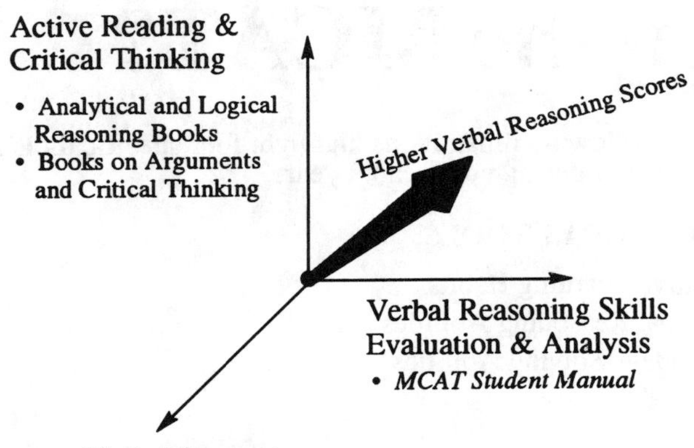

Higher verbal reasoning scores are achieved by:

1) active reading and critical thinking
2) verbal reasoning skills mastery and application
3) working with verbal reasoning practice problems

Suggested resource books and materials are shown in the diagram. Most of these resources are listed in Chapter 3.

Resources to Achieve Higher Verbal Reasoning Scores

Example of How Verbal Reasoning Skills Are Analyzed

1. Components of Major Verbal Reasoning Skill

"Application" consists of:

- Use understanding or interpretation of a passage to solve a problem.
- Interpret a hypothetical situation outside the immediate scope of the passage.

2. Definition and Components of MCAT Verbal Reasoning Skill III.D

Determine the implications of conclusions or results for real-world situations.
Step I: Understand the operational meaning of "implications of conclusions" and "implications of results."
Step II: Learn *how* to determine the implications of conclusions or implications of results.
Step III: Learn *how* to connect the implications in Steps I and II to real-world situations in actual passages.
Step IV: The process of application is now complete because projections of earlier conclusions have been made for solving problems beyond or outside the scope of the given passage.

C. DEVELOPING PROBLEM-SOLVING ABILITIES

NO published review book or MCAT prep course provides students with a complete problem-solving model for individual, self-managed learning except *Complete Preparation for the MCAT.* In Chapter 4, the problem-solving model is a set of building blocks required to solve *any* MCAT problem. The MCAT student should master the components of this problem-solving model. The student needs to understand the problem as it is **given** in the **test item stem** (the actual statement of the problem without the four responses). This problem **assumes** that . . . . Why? You must find one answer using a probability matrix; for example, most probable, least probable, somewhat probable, equally probable, highly probable.

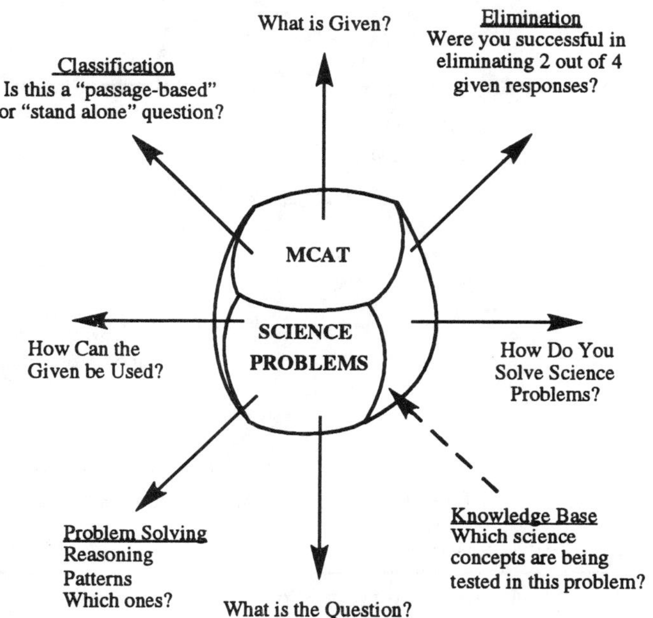

How do you solve MCAT science problems?

D. REVIEWING MCAT SCIENCES

The MCAT problem-solving format in the physical and biological sciences *requires* you to learn intermixed concepts. A concept learned in biology may be used or extrapolated to apply to a clinical instrument. In your science review, you may find up to 1,000 concepts in physical sciences and 1,000 concepts in biological sciences. Review Chapter 7 to explore active learning of some advanced concepts, e.g., operons, freeze-fracture micrographs. Explore what different components fit together to form physical sciences and biological sciences concepts for the MCAT.

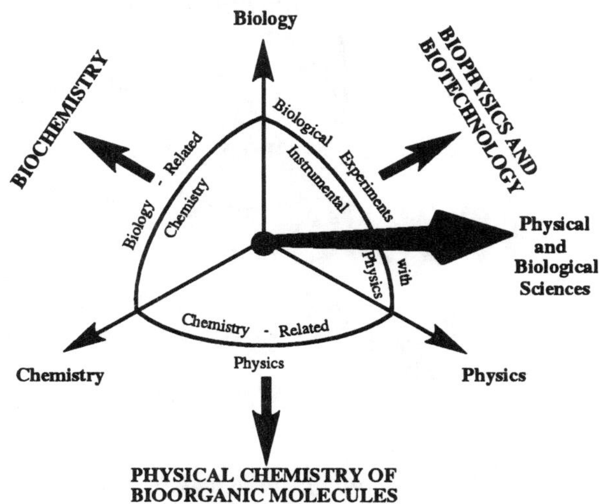

Composition of MCAT Sciences (Biology, Chemistry, and Physics)

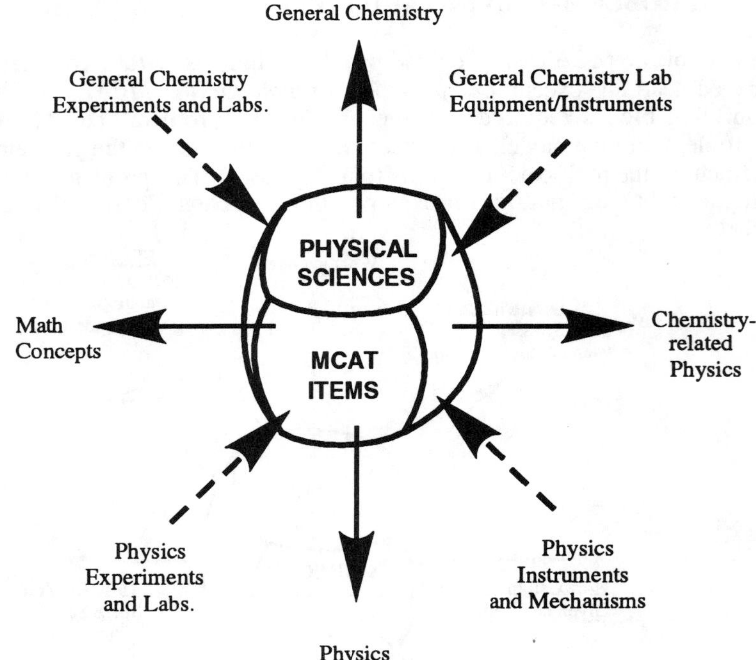

Composition of Physical Sciences Items

Refer to Appendix A for "Interpretation of MCAT Passages" on the actual MCAT.

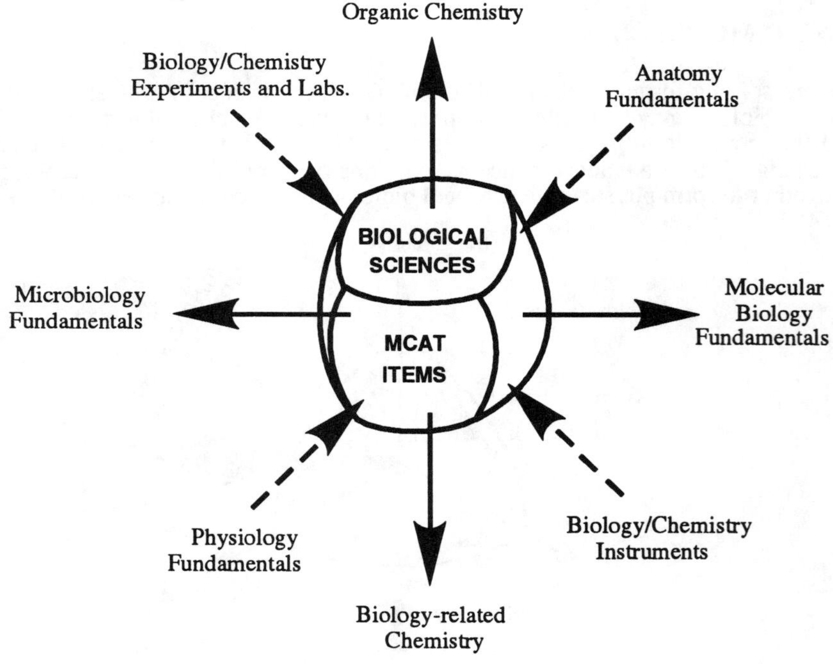

Composition of Biological Sciences Items

WHY THIS BOOK IS CALLED *COMPLETE PREPARATION FOR THE MCAT*

This is the only book that provides you with:

- a **complete** directory of study skills, problem-solving skills, writing skills, verbal reasoning skills, and test-taking strategies
- a **complete** problem-solving model linked to nine patterns in reasoning
- a **complete** model to review physical and biological sciences, including:
  - introduction to the *major topics* found in the MCAT
  - information and focused review of *subtopics* found in the most widely used texts
  - quick review questions on each *subtopic*
  - discussion of answers linked to the *review questions*
  - premedical advanced concepts relevant to *major topics*
  - suggested books for extended review of *advanced concepts*
- an **advanced** section in verbal reasoning and critical thinking, including:
  - structure of an argument
  - evaluating arguments
  - linking verbal reasoning to evaluation of scientific information
  - special techniques for marking passages in your textbooks/class notes
  - preparing mind maps to master new information
- a **complete** updated mathematics concepts review
- a **complete** analysis of passages by content and by type, as shown in the examples below:

AAMC Topics		Content	Type
XVII.B, XIII	PS	Electromagnetic rail gun	→ Instrumental problem-solving passages
VIII.B, D, E	PS	Two chemists analyze reaction pathways	→ Descriptive persuasive argument passages
XIV.B, XVII.B	PS	Harmonic oscillator, magnetic dipoles	→ Experimental research study passages
I.A, XII.B	BS	Photosynthesis, Calvin cycle	→ Graphical description research study passages
X.C, I.B, II.B	BS	Binary fission reproduction co-stimulation	→ Experimental problem-solving passages
XIII.D, A; XIV.C	BS	Alkylation of carbanion	→ Experimental persuasive argument passages
XVI.A, V.B	PS	Gasoline separation, glass fibers	→ Instrumental research study passages

- This is the *only* book that tells you how test items are designed, how distractors are included, what basic steps are needed to check your solution to the item using estimation, and much more. . . .

HOW TO SCORE HIGH ON THE MCAT USING *COMPLETE PREPARATION FOR THE MCAT:*

This checklist gives you a quick self-knowledge appraisal about taking the MCAT. Respond to each question carefully. Answer "*not sure*" if there is a doubt in your mind. Do **not** guess! Check (✓) one response per item.

Survey Item	**Yes**	**No**	**Not sure**
1. Do you know how to study and prepare for the MCAT?			
2. Do you have books or handouts that give you specific directions on how to prepare for the MCAT?			
3. Are you aware that medical instruments, college labs, and experimental medical research are included in passages on the MCAT?			
4. Do you know how to minimize your review time and maximize your long-term memory?			
5. Do you know how to extract MCAT science passages from your textbooks, lecture notes, and laboratory reports?			
6. Do you know how to learn and apply specific MCAT concepts?			

Survey Item	Yes	No	Not sure
7. Do you understand the elements that make up a good MCAT test item or problem?			
8. Do you use an MCAT problem-solving model for every science course you have taken ?			
9. Do you know that specific mathematics concepts and skills, e.g., estimation and approximation, are needed on the MCAT?			
10. Do you understand that verbal reasoning is a tool to use in reading scientific journals?			
11. Do you know how to link concepts in various sciences, e.g., Biology (transport in specialized eukaryotic cells) and Physics (using lasers to detect flow of hormones in tissues)?			
12. Do you know the difference between signal words and trigger words?			
13. Do you know the structure of arguments and how to evaluate them?			
14. Do you know relevant study strategies and references to find the difference between Ruff degradation and Fischer Synthesis or DNA sequences and DNA synthesizer?			
15. Are you aware of 10 test-taking strategies that you can use on the MCAT?			
16. Do you know how to differentiate among text-based, text-linked and text-extension items?			
17. Do you know how to interpret the nature of passages published in the MCAT booklets by AAMC?			

REFERENCES FOR ITEMS TO WHICH YOU ANSWERED *"NO"* OR *"NOT SURE"*

1. Chapter 2, "Skills Development and Review Strategies," *Complete Preparation for the MCAT.*
2. AAMC Practice Tests I, II, and III and Practice Item Booklets.
3. *MCAT Student Manual,* published by AAMC (1993 printing).
4. Chapter 2, "Skills Development and Review Strategies," *Complete Preparation for the MCAT.*
5. Chapter 4, "Introduction to Problem Solving in the Physical and Biological Sciences," *Complete Preparation for the MCAT.*
6. Chapter 2, "Skills Development and Review Strategies," *Complete Preparation for the MCAT.*
7. Chapter 8, "Test-Taking Strategies and Practice Passages," *Complete Preparation for the MCAT.*
8. Chapter 4, "Introduction to Problem Solving in the Physical and Biological Sciences," *Complete Preparation for the MCAT.*
9. Chapter 5, "Problem Solving in the Physical Sciences," *Complete Preparation for the MCAT.*
10. Chapter 3, "Verbal Reasoning," and Chapter 4, "Introduction to Problem Solving in the Physical and Biological Sciences," *Complete Preparation for the MCAT.*
11. Chapter 2, "Skills Development and Review Strategies," *Complete Preparation for the MCAT.*
12. Chapter 3, "Verbal Reasoning," *Complete Preparation for the MCAT.*
13. Chapter 3, "Verbal Reasoning," *Complete Preparation for the MCAT.*
14. Chapter 7, "Problem Solving in the Biological Sciences," *Complete Preparation for the MCAT.*
15. Chapter 8, "Test-Taking Strategies and Practice Passages," *Complete Preparation for the MCAT.*
16. Chapter 8, "Test-Taking Strategies and Practice Passages," *Complete Preparation for the MCAT.*
17. Chapter 8, "Test-Taking Strategies and Practice Passages," *Complete Preparation for the MCAT.*

CONTENTS

List of Figures *xvi*
Preface *xx*
About the Authors *xxi*

Chapter 1: **Organization and Use of *Complete Preparation for the MCAT***
Sec 1.1 MCAT Specifications **1-1**
1.2 MCAT Publications and Registration **1-2**
1.3 Organization of *Complete Preparation for the MCAT* **1-2**
1.4 How to Use the Schematic Layout of this Book **1-3**

Chapter 2: **Skills Development and Review Strategies**
Sec. 2.1 MCAT: A Test of Analytical and Integrative Skills **2-1**
2.2 Strategies for Skills Enhancement **2-4**
2.3 Reading Comprehension Skills for Scientific Text **2-18**
2.4 Steps for Conducting an Effective MCAT Science Review **2-30**

Chapter 3: **Verbal Reasoning**
Sec. 3.1 Verbal Reasoning and Critical Thinking **3-1**
3.2 Reading Comprehension and Critical Thinking **3-2**
3.3 Argument Analysis **3-7**
3.4 Changing Reading Behaviors **3-10**
3.5 References **3-35**

Chapter 4: **Introduction to Problem Solving in the Physical and Biological Sciences**
Sec. 4.1 Problem Solving Connected With Science Knowledge **4-1**
4.2 Mathematics Concepts for MCAT Sciences **4-20**
1 Basic Arithmetic Operations **4-25**
2 Estimating Square Roots of Common Numbers **4-31**
3 Simplifying Algebraic Equations **4-33**
4 Proportional Analysis of Algebraic Equations **4-34**
5 Percentage Increase or Decrease **4-36**
6 Exponentials **4-38**
7 Scientific Notation **4-41**
8 Logarithms **4-42**
9 Cartesian or Rectangular Coordinate System **4-50**
10 Graphic Representation of Functions **4-52**
11 Slope or Rate of Change **4-53**
12 Graphic Interpretation of Functions **4-58**
13 Quadratic Equations **4-68**
14 Simultaneous Equations **4-69**
15 Introduction to Trigonometric Functions **4-70**
16 Characteristics of 30°, 45°, 60° Right Triangles **4-72**
17 Inverse Trigonometric Functions **4-73**
18 Vector Operations and Rules **4-76**
19 Using Metric and British Unit Systems **4-80**
20 Experimental Error: 1) Relative Magnitude, 2) Propagation **4-82**
21 Approximation and Estimations **4-86**
22 Permutations, Combinations and Probability **4-91**
4.3 Data Analysis in Physical/Biological Sciences **4-106**
23 Reading Data Tables **4-107**
24 Graphs and Data Tables **4-108**
25 Interpretation of Equations **4-109**
26 Other Modes for Displaying Data **4-110**
27 Determining Inherent Trends and Relationships in Data **4-113**
28 Statistical Data Analysis **4-114**
29 Calculating Expected Value or Average **4-116**
30 Variation or Dispersion Around Average **4-118**
31 Graphical Interpolation **4-120**
32 Problem Solving Using Data Analysis Techniques **4-120**

4.4 Practice Problems in Data Analysis and Reasoning **4-123**
4.5 Mathematics Definitions **4-138**
4.6 References **4-142**

Chapter 5: Problem Solving in the Physical Sciences*
Sec. 5.1 Electronic Structure of the Atom **5-8**
5.2 The Periodic Table **5-14**
5.3 Chemical Bonding **5-21**
5.4 Stoichiometry **5-29**
5.5 Electrochemistry **5-33**
5.6 Quantitative Chemistry: Compounds and Chemical Reactions **5-46**
5.7 Solution Chemistry **5-58**
5.8 Acids and Bases **5-65**
5.9 Phases and Phase Equilibria **5-76**
5.10 Gas Properties **5-83**
5.11 Solid and Fluid Properties **5-91**
5.12 Thermodynamics and Thermochemistry **5-101**
5.13 Rate Processes in Chemical Reactions—Kinetics and Equilibrium **5-118**
5.14 Force and Motion, Gravitation **5-127**
5.15 Work and Energy **5-133**
5.16 Translational Motion **5-138**
5.17 Equilibrium and Momentum **5-146**
5.18 Electrostatics and Electromagnetism **5-151**
5.19 Electric Circuits **5-161**
5.20 Wave Characteristics and Periodic Motion **5-174**
5.21 Sound **5-184**
5.22 Light and Geometrical Optics **5-191**
5.23 Nuclear and Atomic Structure **5-206**
5.24 References **5-214**

Chapter 6: The MCAT Writing Sample
Sec. 6.1 Writing Skills and Communication **6-1**
6.2 Writing Skills Assessment **6-1**
6.3 Getting Started **6-3**
6.4 Writing for the MCAT **6-4**
6.5 Practice Essays **6-8**
6.6 Practice Essay with Examples **6-9**
6.7 Scoring the MCAT Essay **6-19**
6.8 References **6-19**

Chapter 7: Problem Solving in the Biological Sciences*
Sec. 7.1 Molecular Structure of Organic Compounds **7-9**
7.2 Bioorganic Molecules **7-18**
7.3 DNA and RNA (Molecular Biology) **7-35**
7.4 Protein Synthesis (Molecular Biology) **7-39**
7.5 Prokaryotic and Eukaryotic Cells (Microbiology) **7-43**
7.6 Enzymes (Molecular Biology) **7-56**
7.7 Cellular Metabolism (Molecular Biology) **7-61**
7.8 Reproductive System **7-68**
7.9 Developmental Mechanisms (Embryology) **7-77**
7.10 Genetics and Evolution **7-82**
7.11 Nervous System **7-104**
7.12 Endocrine System **7-113**
7.13 Circulatory System **7-120**
7.14 Lymphatic and Immune Systems **7-129**
7.15 Digestive System **7-133**
7.16 Excretory System **7-140**
7.17 Muscle System **7-146**
7.18 Skeletal System **7-152**

7.19 Respiratory and Skin Systems **7-157**
7.20 Hydrocarbons **7-164**
7.21 Alcohols, Aldehydes and Ketones (Oxygen-Containing Compounds) **7-190**
7.22 Carboxylic Acids and Derivatives, Ethers and Phenols (Oxygen-Containing Compounds) **7-206**
7.23 Amines (Nitrogen-Containing Compounds) **7-219**
7.24 Separations and Purifications **7-224**
7.25 Use of Spectroscopy in Structural Identification **7-234**
7.26 References **7-246**

Chapter 8: Test-Taking Strategies and Practice Passages
Sec. 8.1: Using Logic to Improve Test-Taking Skills **8-1**
8.2 Studying Definitions During MCAT Review **8-4**
8.3 Using Question Analysis to Improve Performance **8-4**
8.4 Using Error Analysis to Improve Test Performance **8-7**
8.5 Determining Your MCAT Test-Taking Speed **8-12**
8.6 Learning to Cope with Initial Stress **8-13**
8.7 Using Intuition, Not Guesswork **8-14**
8.8 Planning Three Weeks Before the Test **8-14**
8.9 Planning the Last Week Before the Test **8-15**
8.10 Planning the Test Day **8-16**
8.11 Practice Exercises with Passages and Test Items **8-17**

Appendix A: An Interpretation of Passages from AAMC Practice Tests and Materials
A.1 Introduction **A-1**
A.2 AAMC Publications Currently Available **A-1**
A.2.1 Problem Solving and Passage Interpretation According to the AAMC Video **A-2**
A.2.2 Experimental and Medical Equipment According to the AAMC Video **A-2**
A.2.3 Writing Sample According to the AAMC Video **A-3**
A.2.4 Verbal Reasoning Strategies According to the AAMC Video **A-3**
A.3 What is an MCAT Scientific Passage **A-3**
A.3.1 Understanding the Nature of MCAT Scientific Passages **A-4**
A.3.2 Frequency Analysis of Passage Content (AAMC Practice Materials) **A-5**
A.3.2.1 Passage Format and Types **A-5**
A.3.2.2 Passage Related Comments According to AAMC **A-6**
A.3.2.3 Scientific Content-Related Comments According to AAMC **A-6**
A.3.2.4 Total Number of AAMC Items and Passages **A-7**
A.4 Functional Classification of AAMC Science Passages **A-8**
A.5 Observations and Conclusions Concerning Scientific Passages **A-13**
A.6 MCAT Bibliography cited in AAMC Publications and Materials **A-14**

*Note: A more detailed content locator can be found at the beginning of chapters 5 and 7.

LIST OF FIGURES

Chapter 1:		**Organization and Use of** ***Complete Preparation for the MCAT***
Fig.	1.1	MCAT Testing Specifications **1-1**
Chapter 4:		**Introduction to Problem Solving in the Physical and Biological Sciences**
Fig.	4.1	Application of the Problem Solving Model to the MCAT **4-18**
	4.2(a)	Linear Variation **4-34**
	4.2(b)	Non-linear/hyperbolic Variation **4-34**
	4.3(a)	Common Geometric Shapes **4-48**
	4.3(b)	Physical Characteristics of Astronomical Bodies **4-49**
	4.4	Cartesian Coordinate System **4-51**
	4.5(a)	Definition of Slope for I) Straight and II) Curved lines **4-53**
	4.5(b)	Sign Convention and Magnitude of Slope **4-55**
	4.5(c)	Maximum and Minimum Points on a Curve **4-56**
	4.5(d)	Types of Inflection Points **4-57**
	4.6(a)	Slope and Intercept of Straight Lines **4-59**
	4.6(b)	Hyperbolic Functions **4-59**
	4.6(c)	Parabolic Functions **4-60**
	4.6(d)	Segmental Analysis of Slope (three segments) **4-60**
	4.6(e)	Segmental Analysis of Slope (five segments) **4-60**
	4.6(f)	Exponential Functions **4-61**
	4.6(g)	Semi-log Axes **4-62**
	4.7(a)	Similar Triangles **4-70**
	4.7(b)	Right Triangles **4-70**
	4.7(c)	Graphical Representation of Trigonometric Functions **4-71**
	4.8	Three Special Right Triangles **4-72**
	4.9(a)	Definition Sketch for a Vector **4-76**
	4.9(b)	Addition of Vectors **4-76**
	4.9(c)	Subtraction of Vectors **4-76**
	4.9(d)	Demonstration of Right-hand Rule for Vectors **4-77**
	4.9(e)	Orthogonal Components of a Vector **4-77**
	4.9(f)	Orthogonal Components of Multiple Vectors **4-77**
	4.10(a)	Data Table Showing Four Variables **4-107**
	4.10(b)	Histogram Showing Frequency Analysis **4-107**
	4.10(c)	Pie Chart **4-108**
	4.11(a)	Graph 1 **4-108**
	4.11(b)	Graph 2 **4-108**
	4.11(c)	Graph 3 **4-108**
	4.11(d)	Graph 4 **4-108**
	4.12(a)	Pie Graph **4-110**
	4.12(b)	Histogram Types **4-111**
	4.12(c)	Grouped Data Graph **4-111**
	4.12(d)	Before and After Graphs **4-112**
	4.13(a)	I) Scatter Plots for Data II) Continuous Line Graph **4-113**
	4.13(b)	Approximate Curve Fitting for a Scatter Plot **4-113**
	4.13(c)	I) Raw Data Plot II) Broken Line Graph III) Smooth Curve **4-114**
	4.14	Histograms Showing Mean, Median, and Mode **4-117**
	4.15	Histograms Showing Dispersion of Data Around the Mean **4-118**
	4.16	Graphic Interpolation **4-120**
Chapter 5:		**Problem Solving in the Physical Sciences**
Sec.	5.1	Example of the Quantum Number Relationships **5-9**
	5.2	A Way of Remembering the Sequence of Filling of Orbitals **5-10**
	5.3	Hund's Rule **5-10**
	5.4	Orbitals **5-10**
	5.5	The Periodic Chart/Table **5-15**
	5.6	Hybrid Bonding Orbitals **5-22**
	5.7	Sigma and Pi Bonds **5-22**

5.8 Comparison of MO and Valence Bond Approaches **5-23**
5.9 Hydrogen Bonding **5-24**
5.10 Titration Curves **5-67**
5.11 Kinetic Energy of Molecules **5-77**
5.12(a) Phase Diagrams: Water **5-77**
5.12(b) Carbon Dioxide **5-77**
5.13 Effect of Solutes on BP and FP **5-78**
5.14(a) Tensile Stress **5-91**
5.14(b) Compressive Stress **5-91**
5.14(c) Shear Stress **5-92**
5.15 Illustration of the Concept of Density **5-93**
5.16 Buoyancy **5-94**
5.17 Hydrostatic Pressure **5-94**
5.18 Concept of Mass Flux/Bernoulli's Equation **5-95**
5.19 Illustrations of Laminar Flow and Turbulent Flow **5-96**
5.20 Heat Conduction **5-104**
5.21 A Reaction Coordinate **5-118**
5.22 Course of a Reaction **5-119**
5.23 Frictional Forces related to Normal Forces **5-128**
5.24 Inclined Plane **5-128**
5.25 Motion on an Incline I **5-129**
5.26 Motion on an Incline II **5-129**
5.27 Translational Motion Parameters **5-138**
5.28 Projectile Motion **5-140**
5.29 Torque (Rotational Moment) **5-146**
5.30 Illustration of Coulomb's Law **5-151**
5.31 Electric Field Lines **5-152**
5.32 Electrical Potential **5-152**
5.33 Dipoles **5-153**
5.34 Electromotive Force **5-161**
5.35 Capacitor without Dielectric **5-163**
5.36 Capacitor with Dielectric **5-163**
5.37 EMF or Alternating Voltage Curve **5-164**
5.38 Vector Triangle Relating Resistance, Reactance, and Impedance **5-165**
5.39(a) Transverse Wave **5-174**
5.39(b) Longitudinal Wave **5-174**
5.40 Characteristics of Waves **5-175**
5.41 Maximal Constructive Interference **5-175**
5.42 Maximal Destructive Interference **5-175**
5.43 Schematic for ΔL **5-176**
5.44 Standing Waves **5-176**
5.45(a) Simple Harmonic Motion **5-176**
5.45(b) Simple Harmonic Motion (Oscillator) **5-176**
5.45(c) Simple Harmonic Motion (Pendulum) **5-176**
5.46(a) Long Waves **5-177**
5.46(b) Short Waves **5-177**
5.47 The Human Ear **5-185**
5.48 Audible Sound Intensities **5-185**
5.49 The Human Eye **5-192**
5.50(a) Myopia **5-192**
5.50(b) Hypermetropia **5-192**
5.51 Reflection by Spherical Mirrors **5-193**
5.52(a) Refraction through Convex Lens **5-194**
5.52(b) Reflection from Concave Mirrors **5-195**
5.53 Refraction **5-195**
5.54 Lens **5-196**
5.55 Binding Energy Diagram **5-207**
5.56 Stability of Atoms **5-207**
5.57 Absorption and Emission Spectra **5-208**
5.58 Fluorescent Emission **5-209**

Chapter 7: Problem Solving in the Biological Sciences

Sec. 7.1 Isomer Comparisons **7-9**
7.2 Enantiomers **7-10**
7.3 Absolute Configurations **7-11**
7.4 Fischer Projections and Their Absolute Configurations **7-11**
7.5 Relative Configurations and Carbohydrates **7-12**
7.6 Diasteriomer, Enantiomer Interrelationship **7-13**
7.7 Meso Compounds **7-13**
7.8 Chiral Stereoisomer Reactions I **7-14**
7.9 Chiral Stereoisomer Reactions II **7-14**
7.10 Peptide Bond Characteristics **7-21**
7.11 Peptide Illustration **7-21**
7.12 Hydrolysis of a Peptide Bond **7-21**
7.13 Relation of Nucleotides, Nucleosides, and Nucleic Acids **7-35**
7.14 Components of Nucleotides **7-35**
7.15 Base Pairing **7-36**
7.16 Semiconservative Replication **7-36**
7.17 Activation of Amino Acid (AA) by Activating Enzyme (AE) **7-40**
7.18 Protein Synthesis on Ribosome (Translation) **7-42**
7.19 Typical Prokaryote, Eukaryote and Bacteriophage **7-45**
7.20 Fluid Mosaic Membrane Model **7-47**
7.21 Rigid Membrane Model **7-47**
7.22 Typical Virus **7-49**
7.23 Several Common Viruses **7-49**
7.24 Life Cycle of a Typical Fungus **7-50**
7.25 Enzyme and Substrate Model **7-57**
7.26 Relative Rates of Substrate Reactions **7-59**
7.27 Catalytic Inhibitors **7-60**
7.28 Glycolysis **7-63**
7.29 Glycolysis, Gluconeogenesis, Glycogenesis **7-64**
7.30 Citric Acid Cycle **7-64**
7.31 Electron Transport Chain **7-65**
7.32 Oxidative Phosphorylation **7-65**
7.33 Female Reproductive System **7-68**
7.34 Male Reproductive System **7-69**
7.35 Gametogenesis in Females **7-69**
7.36 Gametogenesis in Males **7-70**
7.37 Mitosis **7-71**
7.38 Meiosis **7-72**
7.39 Menstrual Cycle **7-72**
7.40 Early Development of Frog Embryo (Embryogenesis) **7-78**
7.41 Mendel's Law: Crossing-over; Recombination; Gamete Formation **7-84**
7.42 Chromosomal Aberrations **7-84**
7.43 Autosomal and Sex Chromosomes: Phenotype Expressions **7-85**
7.44 Pedigree Terminology **7-86**
7.45 Dominant Pedigree **7-86**
7.46 Recessive Pedigree **7-86**
7.47 Sex-Linked Pedigree **7-86**
7.48 Gamete Formation by Example **7-87**
7.49 Punnet Square With One Trait **7-87**
7.50 Punnet Square With Two Traits **7-87**
7.51 Genotypic Frequencies **7-87**
7.52(a) Neuron (Type I) **7-105**
7.52(b) Neuron (Type II) **7-105**
7.53 Various Potentials of a Nerve **7-106**
7.54(a) Sagittal Section of Brain and Spinal Cord **7-107**
7.54(b) Brain (Lateral View) **7-107**
7.55 Spinal Cord **7-107**
7.56 Chart of CNS Organization **7-107**
7.57 Feedback Loops **7-117**

7.58 Fundamental Principles of Blood Circulation **7-120**
7.59 Schematic of the Circulatory System **7-121**
7.60 Capillary Fluid Exchange **7-123**
7.61(a) Closed Capillary **7-123**
7.61(b) Fenestrated Capillary **7-123**
7.61(c) Discontinuous Capillary **7-123**
7.62 Hemoglobin-Oxygen Saturation Curve **7-124**
7.63(a) Lymphatics **7-130**
7.63(b) Lymph Node Schematic **7-130**
7.63(c) Basic Structure of an Antibody Molecule **7-131**
7.64 Intestinal Lining **7-134**
7.65 Structure of the Digestive System **7-135**
7.66 Lipids **7-136**
7.67(a) Kidney **7-142**
7.67(b) Excretory System **7-142**
7.67(c) Microscopic View of the Nephron **7-142**
7.67(d) Schematic of Function of a Nephron **7-143**
7.68 Phases of Muscle Contraction **7-147**
7.69 Formation of Lactate **7-147**
7.70 Components of a Sarcomere (Skeletal Muscle) **7-148**
7.71 Attachments of a Muscle **7-149**
7.72 Long Bone **7-153**
7.73 Bone Cross Section **7-153**
7.74 Human Skeleton **7-154**
7.75 Respiratory System: Bronchiole and Alveoli **7-158**
7.76 Respiratory Epithelium (specialized eukaryotic cells) **7-159**
7.77 Typical Spirogram **7-159**
7.78 Human Skin and Epidermis **7-160**
7.79 Stability of Carbocations **7-174**
7.80 Separation of Benzoic Acid, Toluene, Phenol, and Aniline by Solvent Extraction **7-225**
7.81 A Typical Gas Chromatograph **7-226**
7.82 tlc Separation of a Three Component Mixture **7-227**
7.83 Silica Gel Interaction with Fluorene and Fluorenone **7-228**
7.84 Column Chromatographic Separation of Fluorene and Fluorenone **7-228**
7.85 Liquid and Vapor Composition of an Ideal Two Component Mixture as a Function of Temperature **7-229**
7.86 Distillation of Ethyl Acetate and Toluene **7-230**
7.87 Variation of Temperature with Volume during the Distillation of Ethyl Acetate and Toluene **7-230**
7.88 Vibrational Modes of Carbon Dioxide **7-234**
7.89 Magnetically Different Protons **7-236**
7.90 [18]-annulene Showing Shielding and De-shielding **7-237**
7.91 PMR Spectrum of Cumene **7-238**
7.92 PMR Spectrum of Ethylbenzene **7-239**
7.93 Potential Structures for Sample Spectroscopy Problem **7-242**

PREFACE TO THE 1999 EDITION

Welcome to the 1999 edition of *Complete Preparation for the MCAT,* which is published by Williams & Wilkins. Williams & Wilkins is a world-wide leader in medical publishing, offering thousands of publications to keep medical students and professionals informed, educated, and prepared throughout their careers. With the purchase of your first Science of Review product, you join a long tradition of excellence. We are the experts in presenting medical information. No other test preparation company has this focus or expertise. Simply put, we know what you need for success on the MCAT, throughout your years in medical school, and in your medical career.

The 1999 edition is a culmination of our efforts to produce a **self-managed MCAT study program**. This edition now includes advanced concepts from medical and premedical curricula. Problem-solving practice using passage-based problems is a special feature of this edition. Appendix A is a research report that interprets MCAT passages and their content.

The text of *Complete Preparation for the MCAT,* formerly known as The Betz Guide, is passaged based. Information passages in this book, such as the paragraphs within each subsection, present material similar to that found in college textbooks. Questions associated with each section are organized at an increasing level of difficulty: straightforward review questions are followed by questions requiring problem-solving skills. The review questions demand a clear knowledge of the concepts presented, whereas the problem-solving questions, which are now more prevalent in the test, require a greater ability to analyze, synthesize and make judgments based on information given or on knowledge acquired elsewhere.

The Advanced Concepts subsection in the sciences is a special feature of this edition. It was added to inform students about current medical research, medical instrumentation, and experimental sciences. The Advanced Concepts checklists include medical terms, procedures, and scientific models not covered in regular college courses. Familiarity with the concepts will add to your information about medical experimentation and scientific instruments currently used in medicine.

Acknowledgments

As we go to press, our sincere appreciation is extended to all our authors and reviewers, and to the many students and advisors who provided steady feedback over the years. Their contributions have made the 1999 edition the most thorough independent study program available to the MCAT student. The Science of Review team evaluated the basis for the 1999 edition and has created a book that gives students the most extensive information available to them about the current examination. Our authors and editors have a special vision, conviction, and commitment to students that are reflected in the pages of this edition. This edition reflects fundamental, comprehensive, and systematic changes to the older editions, saving the best of the old and adding new problem-based lessons and learning materials.

We extend special appreciation to our research team headed by Aftab S. Hassan, MCAT science specialist, who carried on for S. William Whitson in transforming the book to reflect the changes brought about by the new MCAT. These authors and reviewers have added immeasurably to the quality of the work: Dorothy H. Air, Frank Allegra, Robert G. Bass, Glen Bauer, Angelica Braestrup, Charles M. Bump, Mary E. Duafala, Martin R. Feldman, Richard K. Hill, Evelyn Jackson, Frank Kessler, Jack Lochhead, Carol Banks Setter, and Rawatmal Surana, M.D.

Acknowledgment is hereby made to James L. Flowers, M.D., M.P.H., author of an original manuscript for MCAT review, which forms a portion of the science review.

We acknowledge the excellent proofreading and manuscript evaluation by Holly Wagner and Brian Chou. We heartily acknowledge the tireless work of Susan Kimmer for her editorial support in manuscript preparation, and particularly for her skilled technical support in preparing the visual displays. Last, but not least, we express our gratitude to Deborah Fredericks Zimmer, Wendy Stetter, and Jeanne Angel for their steady hands in keeping all required support services in place.

Editor

ABOUT THE CONTRIBUTING AUTHORS

Dorothy H. Air

Ph.D., Speech-Language Pathology and Special Education, University of Cincinnati. Dr. Air is Assistant Dean for Student Affairs at the University of Cincinnati College of Medicine, with major responsibility for student development programs. Serves as lecturer in both medical school and residency training programs. Director for nationally recognized continuing education programs in communication disorders and has several years' experience in cognitive retraining and teaching of undergraduate and graduate-level students. Joint effort with Dr. Setter has produced an innovative program in developing critical thinking skills at medical school level.

Robert G. Bass

Ph.D., Organic Chemistry, University of Virginia, Charlottesville. Dr. Bass is professor of chemistry at Virginia Commonwealth University with research interests in polymer and organic chemistry and related areas. He was postdoctoral Research Fellow at the University of Virginia, and has served as Visiting Associate Professor at UV and the Medical College of Virginia. He was a research chemist for E. I. DuPont de Nemours Co., Inc., in Richmond.

Glen A. Bauer

M.A., completed 3 years of doctoral studies (A.B.D.) at Wayne State University, Detroit. Mr. Bauer is currently the associate professor of mathematics and computer science at the Lawrence Technological University, Southfield, Michigan. He is actively involved with the MCAT program for Test Preparation Services, Inc. He is also a volunteer softball coach for Novi Parks and Recreation department.

Angelica Braestrup

B.A., Magna cum laude in English and philosophy and course work completed for M.A. in English, Georgetown University. Ms. Braestrup was consultant to Ventures in Education, Inc. She specializes in design and development of curricula, programs, and material for analytical thinking, reading, and problem solving, test-taking and study strategies and writing for all levels, high school through graduate. She has worked with the Educational Testing Service, the University of California School of Medicine at Irvine, the Charles R. Drew University of Medicine and Science, and Georgetown University.

Charles M. Bump

Ph.D., Organic Chemistry, Pennsylvania State University. Dr. Bump is associate professor of chemistry at Hampton University. Research interests range from synthesis of porphyrins to Friedel-Crafts–type reactions in room-temperature molten salts. He is an active member of the premedical advisory committee and the advisory committee of the University's Center for Teaching Excellence.

Mary E. Duafala

B.S., Pharmacy, University of Pittsburgh; M.S., Clinical Hospital Pharmacy, The Ohio State University; M.B.A., Rutgers, The State University of New Jersey. Ms. Duafala is an independent medical communications consultant. Her areas of specialization include infectious diseases, immunology, biotechnology, formulary management, and cost containment. Previously, Ms. Duafala was the Associate Director of Pharmacy, Memorial Sloan-Kettering Cancer Center.

Martin R. Feldman

Ph.D., Organic Chemistry, University of California, Los Angeles. Dr. Feldman is professor of chemistry, Howard University. Research interests are physical organic chemistry: mechanism of electron transfer reactions of organic compounds with transition metal ions. Postdoctoral experiences include visiting scientist to Kings College, University of London, England; National Science Foundation Science Faculty Fellow, University of California, Irvine; Smithsonian Faculty Fellow, National Museum of American History. Research grants received from American Chemical Society, National Science Foundation, National Institutes of Health.

James L. Flowers

M.D., M.P.H.; earned his medical degree at Harvard Medical School, Boston, Massachusetts. His internship and residency were in Internal Medicine. Presently he combines his private medical practice with teaching and writing. In addition, Dr. Flowers has a medically related approved patent on Capsagel and several patents pending approval. While at Harvard Medical School, he wrote the original text of *A Complete Preparation for the MCAT,* which has since been revised and supplemented by other contributing authors.

Aftab S. Hassan

Ph.D., Doctorate Water Resources and Hydraulics, Columbia Pacific University (UCLA program); doctoral scientist in Ocean, Coastal and Environmental Engineering, George Washington University. Dr. Hassan is an educational specialist in the health and life sciences and has strongly supported active learning and problem based teaching through his extensive teaching experience. Dr. Hassan also specializes in hydrodynamics, pollutant transport and coastal engineering. He was formerly affiliated with George Washington University School of Engineering and Applied Science, and with Georgetown University, Department of Community and Family Medicine. He has been actively involved in MCAT and DAT teaching for students at Georgetown University, Washington, D.C., and Charles R. Drew University of Medicine and Science, Los Angeles, California. In addition, he has given active learning workshops including physician assistant programs, for approximately twenty other schools across the U.S. He has taught, tutored, and advised premedical, medical and engineering students for over 22 years. He has worked with several editions of this book since 1984 and is currently a major author for several chapters in this book.

Richard K. Hill

Ph.D., Chemistry, Harvard University. Dr. Hill is acting head and professor, Chemistry Department, University of Georgia. Research interests in synthesis and stereochemistry of organic natural products, stereochemistry and mechanism of enzyme catalysis and related areas. Has served as professional consultant to major corporations, NIH Medicinal Chemistry Study Section, Senior Fulbright-Hays Program for chemistry fellows, and Petroleum Research Fund.

Evelyn M. Jackson

Ph.D., Education/Reading, Southern Illinois University at Carbondale (SIU-C). Dr. Jackson, Associate Professor of Medical Education, teaches courses in reading/writing and study skills in the Medical Education Preparatory Program (MEDPREP) at SIU-C's School of Medicine. Serves as academic advisor for MEDPREP students and study skills advisor for freshmen medical students.

Frank Kessler

B.A., history, Eastern Michigan University. Formerly, Assistant Professor in history at Virginia State University, Petersburg. Mr. Kessler entered graduate studies program in American history at the University of North Carolina. Currently reading instructor at the Academic Learning Skills Center, UNC-Chapel Hill.

Jack Lochhead

Ed.D., Educational Research and Statistics, University of Massachusetts. Dr. Lochhead is director of the Scientific Reasoning Research Institute, Hasbrouck Laboratory, and Assistant Dean, University of Massachusetts. Consultant to Ventures in Education, Inc. Received numerous grants from National Science Foundation for investigation/development of instructional materials in scientific problem solving. Cooperative project with Dr. Arthur Whimbey has resulted in two books, *Problem Solving and Comprehension* and *Beyond Problem Solving and Comprehension*.

Carol Banks Setter

Ph.D., Curriculum and Instructional Theory and Design and Educational Administration, Miami University in Educational Leadership. Dr. Setter is adjunct assistant professor at the University of Cincinnati College of Medicine, working with student development programs in the Office of Student Affairs. Certified instructor in reading, English and speech, teaching at the undergraduate and graduate levels. Has developed programs in gifted education, problem solving and media design. Joint author with Dr. Air of program for developing critical thinking skills at medical school level.

S. William Whitson

Ph.D., Anatomy, University of Arkansas Medical School. Postdoctoral Fellow, anatomy and radiology, University of Utah College of Medicine. Dr. Whitson is full professor, Department of Biomedical Sciences, School of Dental Medicine, Southern Illinois University. Recently completed duties as visiting scientist, Naval Medical Research Institute, Bethesda; also was visiting scientist, Laboratory of Biological Structure, National Institute of Dental Research. Research interests in many aspects of bone formation, including cell growth, effects of vitamins and related areas.

Chapter 1:

Organization and Use of

"A Complete Preparation for the MCAT"

1.1 MCAT SPECIFICATIONS

The Medical College Admission Test (MCAT) is a day-long test divided into a morning session and an afternoon session (see Fig. 1.1). The morning session includes the subtests in Verbal Reasoning and Physical Sciences. The afternoon session includes the Writing Sample (two essays) and Biological Sciences. According to the *MCAT Student Manual*, the test day approximates this schedule:

Section	Number of Questions	Time in Minutes
Verbal Reasoning	65	85
- 10-minute break		
Physical Sciences	77	100
- 60-minute lunch break		
Writing Sample	2	60
-10-minute break		
Biological Sciences	77	100

Fig. 1.1 - MCAT Testing Specifications

Verbal Reasoning, the first MCAT test of the day, includes 65 questions based on nine reading passages, each 500 to 600 words long. Each passage has six to ten multiple-choice questions in the humanities, social sciences, and areas of the natural sciences not tested in the Physical and Biological Sciences subtests. Since all questions are based on information in the passages, test questions do not require any outside knowledge of topics. You are not tested for subject mastery in the problems that follow the passages. (See Chapter 3.)

Physical Sciences is the second morning test. It includes 77 questions (62 of which are based on passages, each about 250 words long) and 15 additional questions independent of any passage and of each other. This subtest measures comprehensive scientific understanding and reasoning skills in general chemistry and physics. There are about ten problem sets, each having from four to eight questions based on the passage. The emphasis is not on memorization of facts, but on problem-solving skills and knowledge of basic science concepts in physics and physics-related chemistry. You are also asked to demonstrate your ability to interpret information and solve problems based on tables, charts, graphs and figures. Skills tested may include analyzing and interpreting data, identifying trends and relationships basic to data, determining prior or background knowledge important to the information, and selecting the best means of portraying the data or information. (See Chapter 5.)

Writing Sample, the first MCAT test given in the afternoon, consists of two essay topics. You will be expected to compose an essay for both topics within one hour (30 minutes each). Formerly an experimental test, it is now part of the MCAT scores with an alphabetic grade. Communication skills are important for the medical profession and increased concern has been shown for the deficiency in writing skills among entering medical students. The writing exercise allows examinees the opportunity to demonstrate evidence of their writing and analytical skills and their ability to develop and present ideas. (See Chapter 6.)

Biological Sciences, the last test of the day, has the same number and type of questions and passages as the Physical Sciences test. This test measures scientific understanding and reasoning skills in biology and organic chemistry. The emphasis on basic knowledge of concepts and problem solving skills parallels that in the Physical Sciences test. (See Chapter 7.)

1.2 AAMC MCAT PUBLICATIONS AND REGISTRATION

Publications. Information about the MCAT is found in publications written by the Association of American Medical Colleges (AAMC). These can be purchased from Betz Publishing Company, Inc., or obtained directly from AAMC. Call or write to:

Betz Publishing Company, Inc.
P.O. Box 1745
Rockville MD 20849
(800) 634-4365 (toll free)
Fax: (301) 340-0253

Association of American Medical Colleges
Attn: Membership and Publication Orders
2450 N Street NW
Washington DC 20037-1123
(202) 828-0416
Fax: (202) 828–1123

Registration. Information about registration, administration, and MCAT scoring may be obtained from Betz Publishing Company, your premedical advisor, your career guidance office, or:

MCAT Program Office
P.O Box 4056
Iowa City, IA 52243
(319) 337-1357

The actual MCAT scores are only available from the MCAT Program office.

Information about the American Medical College Application Service (AMCAS) may be obtained from:

AMCAS
Association of American Medical Colleges
Section for Student Services
2450 N Street NW
Washington, DC 20037-1126
(202) 828-0600

If you need to send any correspondence through an express or courier service, address it to:

MCAT Program Office
P.O. Box 4056
Iowa City, IA 52243
(319) 337–1357

1.3 ORGANIZATION OF *A Complete Preparation for the MCAT*

A Complete Preparation for the MCAT provides a concise and thorough review of both premedical subjects and the skills tested by the MCAT. Full review in science is organized to integrate physics with general chemistry and biology with organic chemistry. This book addresses the requirements of the MCAT by stressing the development of special skills essential to reading, mathematics and writing.

Chapter 2 provides "Review Strategies and Skills Development" in order to begin an actual self-managed MCAT review. Analysis and integration of content and skills for sample MCAT topics is fully explored. It presents visual learning and reasoning skills which are vital for a critical thinker. Specific time management, note-taking and reading comprehension strategies are explained to make you an independent active learner.

"Verbal Reasoning," chapter 3 of this book, is a unique active reading guide for the MCAT student. It provides you with eight specific critical thinking and reading comprehension rules supplemented with a short section on argument analysis and evaluation. It also includes twelve passages taken from a variety of sources in the humanities, social sciences and the natural sciences followed by MCAT-type verbal reasoning questions.

"Introduction to Problem Solving in the Physical and Biological Sciences," chapter 4, is a stand-alone unit for students who need practice in various types of *problem solving*. In the first part, a fully operational reasoning and problem-solving model is given which is applied to several hundred quantitative reasoning problems. In the second part, the mathematics concepts required for the MCAT sciences are fully covered.

"Problem Solving in the Physical Sciences," chapter 5, is a curriculum-based review of physics, general chemistry and chemistry-related physics topics found in the MCAT. The MCAT content outline is fully covered in this chapter, although the sequence of material has been modified. In this book the physical sciences are presented in a logical sequence and related topics are grouped coherently. Chapter 5 reflects the use of actual scientific passages to teach content learned in college. However, this material should in no way be construed as the only material to be presented in the exam, nor should it be inferred that the exam will include all the material discussed here. The format of the science questions contained within the MCAT are of two types: 1) a series of questions based upon a brief passage (problem-solving questions) and 2) independent questions. The problems and explanations found at the end of each section in both chapter 5 and 7 are a mixture of these two science question types, and they provide a thorough review of content for the two science subtests of the MCAT.

"The MCAT Writing Sample," chapter 6, demonstrates communication through writing. Instruction in the development of appropriate skills is presented lucidly. Emphasis is placed on the requirements for developing essays under timed conditions. Chapter 6 offers practical writing experience and criteria by which your writing may be evaluated. This approach allows you to organize your writing in a more systematic way so that your ideas come across clearly through your writing. Examples of actual student writing are included to illustrate different levels of writing skills.

"Problem Solving in the Biological Sciences," chapter 7, is a curriculum-based review of biology, and organic chemistry and biology-related chemistry topics found in the MCAT. In addition, special premedical materials are presented as "advanced concepts" to acquaint you with medical terminology used in MCAT passages. As in chapter 5, the content of this chapter is in accordance with the MCAT content outline, but the sequence and grouping of topics is changed to facilitate logical learning.

The "Test-Taking Strategies and Practice Passages" in chapter 8 display the use of appropriate logic and definitional information to improve test-taking skills. Actual application of these skills to test-items is illustrated throughout this chapter. This chapter also includes systematic strategies to use in taking tests. Error analysis is introduced and additional practice reading exercises are given to encourage you to apply the skills taught in the chapter.

1.4 HOW TO USE THE SCHEMATIC LAYOUT OF THIS BOOK

The schematic layout on the inside cover of this book shows all chapters at a glance and the usual order in which to review them. The way you use this book will depend upon your prior experience with the MCAT and your current needs. Suggestions are given both for first-time users of this book and for persons who have experience with earlier editions.

I. If you are **using this book for the first time**, consider following steps 1 through 7 below.
   1. Review chapter 2 with emphasis on MCAT resources, study plans, and learning more about specific components of the MCAT.
   2. Skim chapters 3, 4 and 6 to become acquainted with verbal reasoning, problem solving and writing as presented in the MCAT.
   3. Skim appendix A to correlate textbook-based science knowledge to the actual MCAT science content according to official materials.
   4. Skim chapters 5 and 7 to help you recognize the science review components in physical and biological sciences. Understand how each topic is presented as an independent learning unit.
   5. Start a formal review of the entire book beginning with chapter 3; then proceed through chapters 4 and 6.
   6. Study and practice the materials in chapters 5 and 7 according to your needs. The topic sections and subsections in both chapters are directly linked to the MCAT content outline. Refer frequently to chapter 2 as a guide to develop a good study schedule and to reinforce newly learned study skills.
   7. Use chapter 8 after completing a few months of MCAT study or after taking a practice test such as the practice test included with the MCAT Student Manual.

II. If you have **prepared for the MCAT before**, follow steps 8 through 12 below.
   8. Review chapter 2 with the focus on overcoming your weaknesses. Devise a comprehensive study plan before reviewing the other chapters.
   9. Use this book with specific goals in mind. For example, if you have difficulty with verbal reasoning review chapter 3 and appendix A. Apply what you have learned in chapter 3 to specific passages in chapter 8. Concentrate on verbal reasoning errors and how to correct them.
   10. Use this book to learn about advanced concepts, which are usually found at the end of each section in chapter 7. Integrate information from the advanced concepts with the comprehensive problem solving model in chapter 4. This will provide advanced biological sciences material in order to handle the difficult sections on the MCAT. Integrate chapter 4 with chapter 5, appendix A and chapter 8 if you are weak in physical sciences; integrate chapter 4 with chapter 7, appendix A and chapter 8 if you are weak in biological sciences.
   11. Use this strategy to close the gaps in your science knowledge or problem solving skills as required.
   12. Review verbal reasoning in chapter 3 to improve your knowledge of argument and how arguments are tested for soundness, relevance, and cogency.

The schematic layout and steps 1 through 12 above will help you develop a self-managed study outline. At this stage we recommend that you go to the inside back cover of this book and introduce yourself to *MCAT: The Betz Package*. In case you need a copy of the Betz Personal MCAT Prep Planner, write to us at P.O. Box 1745, Rockville, MD 20849-9947 or use the business reply mail card (Send me free information) in the back of this book.

Chapter 2.

Skills Development and Review Strategies

2.1 MCAT: A TEST OF ANALYTICAL AND INTEGRATIVE SKILLS

The Medical College Admission Test is designed to help medical schools choose the best possible candidates. In addition to testing science knowledge in a problem-solving format, the MCAT measures students' skills in areas that have been identified as fundamental to success in medical school. The most successful medical students tend to be those who can effectively analyze and synthesize (integrate) large amounts of theoretical and research-related information.

Most college students focus on the analytical stage of learning. They do this by taking notes on important points in class and by underlining and marking text while reading. Few students, however, consciously use synthesis (integration) to help in mastering information, i.e., connecting class notes in physics to class notes in chemistry.

Analysis is an important part of the learning process. Students often try to learn difficult material by reducing it to its most simplified form. Learning is more difficult when done in small compartmentalized bits. Instead it appears that effective learning involves integrated webs of information. The more connections that are made, the easier it is to add and retain new pieces of information. If you are in the habit of keeping what you learn in biology, chemistry, and physics separate from each other, and separate from what you see and understand about the world around you, then you probably want to reconsider your strategies for learning. One of your goals in preparing for the MCAT is to work consciously to integrate or make connections between content topics.

Synthesis is this ability to combine or unify individual pieces of information into a meaningful whole. Synthesizing what you learn occurs when you summarize what you read, are able to explain the solution to a problem in your own words, or suddenly realize that what you learned in biology today is simply another way of saying what you learned in organic chemistry last week. The most prepared premedical students are those who make the connection between the physical and biological sciences, seeing them as different pieces as they relate to the complete picture. For example, understanding the structure and functions of the lungs includes physical, chemical and biological characteristics of lungs.

How does all of this relate to the MCAT? Your level of content mastery in the physical and biological sciences will be tested in the MCAT. You will be required to use your skills in analytical reading, critical thinking, and scientific reasoning. These skills are like tools in a toolbox. As you prepare for the MCAT you need to be able to use them all, and it is better to do so consciously than by accident. Before a formal review of MCAT topics content, work to improve your study skills. Learn the best and most efficient ways to use these tools or study skills.

Because many students acquire their skills in a sporadic way, they are often unprepared for the MCAT. With proper preparation using the study skills recommended in this chapter, you will be able to prepare for the MCAT while you also build the foundation necessary for success in medical school.

The information that follows has been written to help you accomplish two goals: 1) to organize a systematic preparation program, and 2) to develop analytical and synthetic verbal reasoning and problem-solving skills that will be tested in the MCAT.

2.1.1 Skills Assessment Inventory

The Skills Assessment Inventory lists the kinds of study skills that will translate into medical school success. Do you have the needed skills? Given your success in school so far, you may quickly answer "yes." But it is easy to take your study skills for granted. Despite your previous successes, medical school represents a new level of academic rigor that most students have not yet experienced. The inefficiencies of study habits that may not have created problems at an undergraduate level suddenly become key issues in medical school survival.

Before launching into a plan for specific MCAT preparation, take time to assess your typical study strategies. Note that the key word here is typical. In preparing to take the MCAT, students often take preparation courses or read preparation guides for advice on effective study strategies. These strategies then become part of their preparation approach for MCAT. They do not always represent a typical approach to medical course work. As a result, an MCAT score derived from these conditions may be misleading as a predictor of success in medical school.

Using the Skills Assessment Inventory below, evaluate your habits critically. As you read this book you will have a better idea of the skills you want to continue to refine and those that you need to develop. Use this inventory at the beginning of your preparation. It will serve as a model to evaluate your strengths and weaknesses and help you to set your goals for improvement.

Study Skills:	**I do**	**I do not**
Break time into manageable units to increase productivity.	_____	_____
Pace study to allow adequate time for reviewing and memorizing.	_____	_____
Memorize only after understanding information.	_____	_____
Reinforce information through timely repetition at intervals ranging from the same day to several weeks later.	_____	_____
Use organized system for learning new vocabulary words.	_____	_____

Note-taking Skills:	**I do**	**I do not**
Listen for speaker's organizational structure during lecture.	_____	_____
Take own notes during lecture.	_____	_____
Identify central ideas in textbook passages.	_____	_____
Use a system that shows the relationship among facts rather than a list of facts.	_____	_____
Vary the format of taking notes according to the content of the material.	_____	_____
Consolidate information taken from several sources into a master set of notes.	_____	_____
Consistently update and summarize the information learned.	_____	_____

Problem-solving Skills:	**I do**	**I do not**
Determine the intent of a problem and the accompanying passage.	_____	_____
Identify components of a problem.	_____	_____
Clarify unfamiliar or vague terms.	_____	_____
Consider multiple paths to problem solution.	_____	_____
Distinguish fact from opinion and claims from arguments in the passage.	_____	_____
Attempt to reason through a problem, even when uncertain.	_____	_____
Apply a systematic reasoning process through entire problem.	_____	_____
Rely on reasoning rather than feelings and/or impressions.	_____	_____
Determine similarities and differences among concepts and details.	_____	_____

Select appropriate data to be used in problem solution.	______	______
Draw diagrams, when appropriate, to clarify ideas.	______	______
Test answers for relevancy to a problem.	______	______
Integrate new information in a problem with previous knowledge from the passage.	______	______
Establish relationships across subjects as well as within.	______	______

Test-taking Skills:	**I do**	**I do not**
Try to predict test questions while studying.	______	______
Read test instructions carefully.	______	______
Read questions carefully and identify key terms.	______	______
Attempt to define key terms in a question before working through the question.	______	______
Determine the intent of the test question without over-interpretation.	______	______
Evaluate all information before choosing an answer.	______	______
Use a problem-solving strategy rather than guessing when uncertain of an answer.	______	______
Apply consistent logic to answer choice options within a test question.	______	______

Now take a moment to review your answer patterns and record your observations in the spaces below. Where are your strengths and weaknesses? As you work with this book, you will want to pay particular attention to those suggestions that address your weaknesses. As you make changes in your approach, however, take care not to lose track of your areas of strength and instead take advantage of them.

Strengths

____

____

____

____

____

____

Weaknesses

____

____

____

____

____

____

Goals

____

____

____

____

____

____

NOTE: Study skills, including note-taking skills, are explained in this chapter. Problem-solving skills are covered in chapter 4 and test-taking skills are in chapter 8. Appendix A at the back of the book includes a complete section on passage interpretation and presents a critical summary of the MCAT practice tests and materials from the Association of American Medical Colleges.

2.2 STRATEGIES FOR SKILLS ENHANCEMENT

The best background for taking the MCAT is good preparation in high school and college. But even if this is lacking, a well-planned review can improve your performance on the test. It is perhaps best to view MCAT preparation time as an opportunity to master those skills and concepts that you failed to master previously but which are essential parts of the solid foundation you will need as a medical student and as a practicing doctor. This section presents strategies of time management, note-taking, and mapping that will enhance the background you bring to your preparation for the test. Beginning with time management, the skills enhancement strategies presented in this section apply to preparation for all sections of the test. Suggestions for managing your preparation time immediately prior to the test and for the test day itself appear later in chapter 8.

2.2.1 Scheduling and Time Management

Daily and Weekly Schedules

A realistic, well-planned schedule provides appropriate study time that will help correct the natural tendency to avoid what you do not like. If there is a subject you do not enjoy or one that you find most difficult, plan to study that subject first. Begin by scheduling each day with a checklist called "Things To Do Today," the more detailed the better. Before going to bed, check off what you actually finished or even list them as "Things Done Today." Make sure that topics not reviewed on one day are reviewed the next day. This should give you a gauge of how realistically you have planned your time. Keep these daily charts with you until the MCAT is over.

To develop your schedule for each day, use the course content outline found in the *MCAT Student Manual* as your guide to study topics. Block out available time for MCAT study and list as precisely as you can what you plan to study during each session. Wherever possible, connect your lecture or laboratory class time with your MCAT preparation. If you take organic chemistry, for example, review your class notes for the MCAT while you study for the class. The two activities can be mutually beneficial. (Remember that many biological sciences questions in the MCAT will integrate laboratory experience with lecture material, e.g., NMR spectroscopy labs, titration labs, preparation of buffer solutions, etc.)

Tackle the more difficult tasks when you have the most energy. You will not only do a better job, but you will also benefit by gaining a feeling of accomplishment. Avoid burnout by taking short breaks, but coordinate your breaks to coincide with the completion of the goal you set for that scheduled study period. Work with a clock in front of you. Notice the time you begin and the time you normally take a break. A break can be both *conscious* or *unconscious*. Getting coffee is an example of a conscious break; reading a page or more without knowing what you read constitutes an unconscious break.

Even if time is theoretically available, do not schedule a twelve-hour MCAT preparation day. Six to eight hours of study time is enough. Do not schedule study later than 11 p.m., even though you may consider yourself to be a "night person." You learn best when you are fresh and, of course, the MCAT is not given at night. The schedule that follows shows you one way in which you might divide your review time into productive segments for a typical three-hour review session.

15 minutes: Review salient features of older content (learned before).
15 minutes: Review and use important concepts from older content (learned before).
60 minutes: Study and master new skills (to be learned today).
60 minutes: Evaluate and learn new content (to be learned today).
30 minutes: Remember and use older skills (mastered before).

Practice for Verbal Reasoning. If you are not ready for sleep after 11 p.m., or if you still have free time, plan to practice verbal reasoning skills by reading debate-oriented articles such as those found in *USA Today*, *Wall Street Journal*, *The New York Times*, *Scientific American* or other well-written articles in newspapers or magazines such as *Science*, *The Washington Post*, *Journal of American Medical Association* and other medically based journals. This helps to balance your study time as well as to give you important practice in developing critical thinking and understanding. Of all the areas tested by the MCAT, remember that verbal reasoning will probably be the slowest to improve.

Schedule reading practice to overcome this problem, knowing that the best way to improve your reading abilities is to read actively and to read more both in terms of time spent and in the variety of scientific and technical materials and lab reports available. Foregoing television during your MCAT preparation time increases the time available for reading and other study, working to your benefit in verbal reasoning.

Weekly Schedule Worksheets. After establishing your goals and your agenda, determine the amount of time required for your review. Create a detailed weekly schedule for your MCAT review by using the charts below. Begin by planning for a productive week by identifying your present and future obligations as well as other activities that impact upon planning your time. Hold yourself accountable for any schedule you make. Periodically identify periods of time where there is waste. If at the end of a day you have to ask yourself where the time went, chances are that you probably did not use your time efficiently.

CHART FOR PLANNING FOR A PRODUCTIVE WEEK

CURRENT OBLIGATIONS

Academic

Personal

Social

ADDITIONAL ACTIVITIES

Academic (MCAT)

Personal

Social

IDEAL SCHEDULE

Future Deadlines

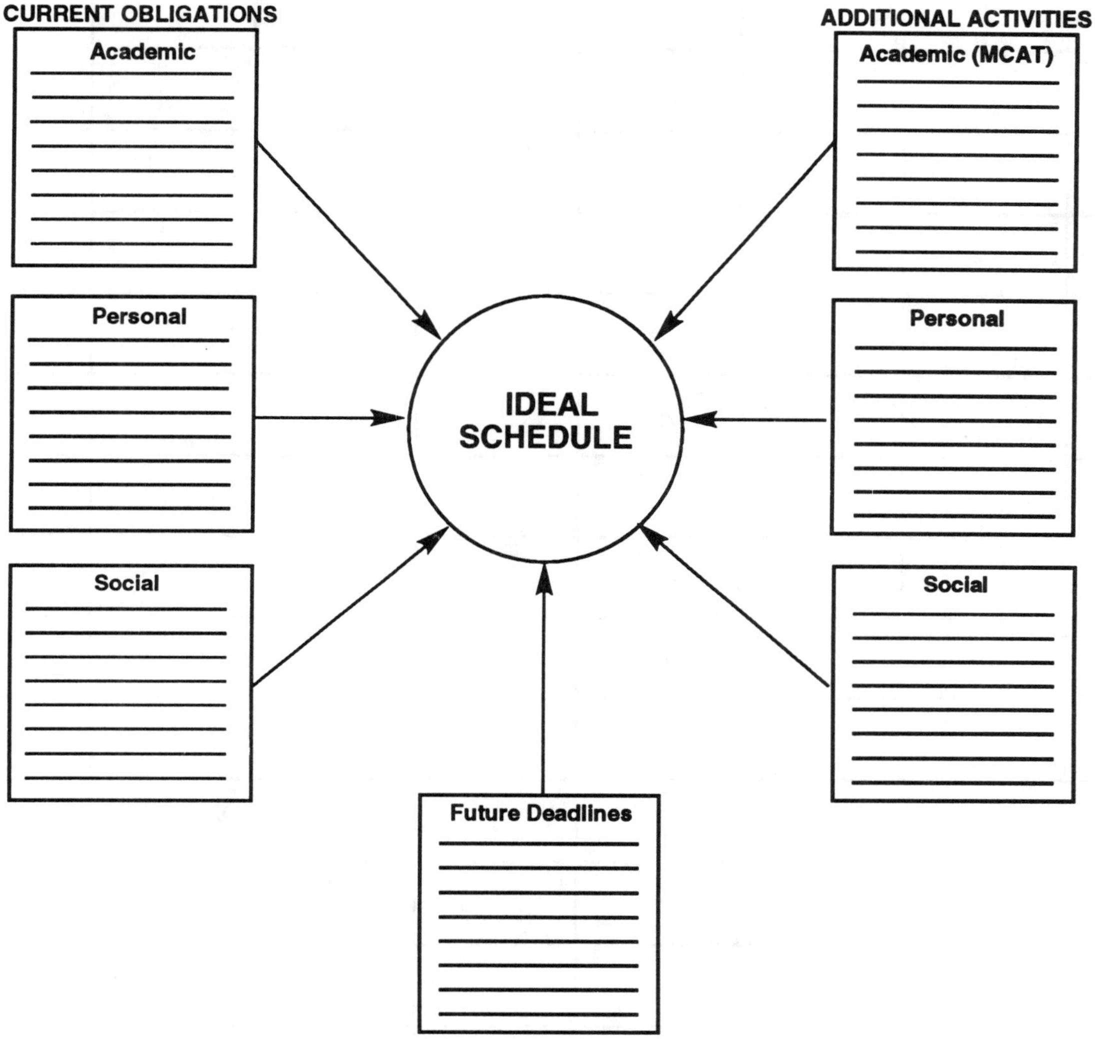

The most common complaint of a premedical student is, "Where do I get the spare time to prepare for the MCAT?" A good study schedule is one that lets you set priorities based on your requirements. Strongly recommended for learning time management skills is an excellent book, *Plan for Success: An Organizing Guide for Prehealth Professions Students,* written by Charles E. Kozoll. This book is published by the National Association of Advisors for the Health Professions, P.O. Box 5017, Station A, Champaign, IL 61820, and may be purchased from them or directly from Betz Publishing Company.

WORKSHEET FOR CONSTRUCTING A PERSONAL WEEKLY SCHEDULE

Using the daily "Things To Do" lists and the previous worksheet, develop a realistic weekly schedule. Use a separate sheet for each week.

PERSONAL SCHEDULE: WEEK ________							
HOUR	**Monday**	**Tuesday**	**Wednesday**	**Thursday**	**Friday**	**Saturday**	**Sunday**
7:00							
8:00							
9:00							
10:00							
11:00							
12:00							
1:00							
2:00							
3:00							
4:00							
5:00							
6:00							
7:00							
8:00							
9:00							
10:00							
11:00							
12:00							

Environmental Considerations

Your learning environment has a considerable impact upon your study productivity. There may be rare individuals who are able to learn at any time and in any place, but in order for most of us to be productive, our study environment must be conducive to learning. In planning a study location, consider the following:

Comfort. Find a place that will be comfortable enough to let you concentrate, but not so comfortable that you will be nodding off to sleep after 15 minutes.

Distractions. Choose a place that is free of the most tempting distractions. Remember that whenever you stop for any reason, you must also spend time getting started again. This can equal much wasted time. Be honest with yourself in choosing a study location. If you know you have trouble ending a conversation when the phone rings, then forward your calls, use an answering machine or don't study near a telephone.

Lighting. Proper lighting seems so obvious, yet is so often overlooked. Poor lighting leads to fatigue and fatigue encourages to burnout.

Set a goal to develop a disciplined approach to study with maximum concentration and minimum environmental distraction. Use the following study environment assessment chart to evaluate your current study environment and plan for modifications that will improve it.

CHART FOR ASSESSMENT OF STUDY ENVIRONMENT

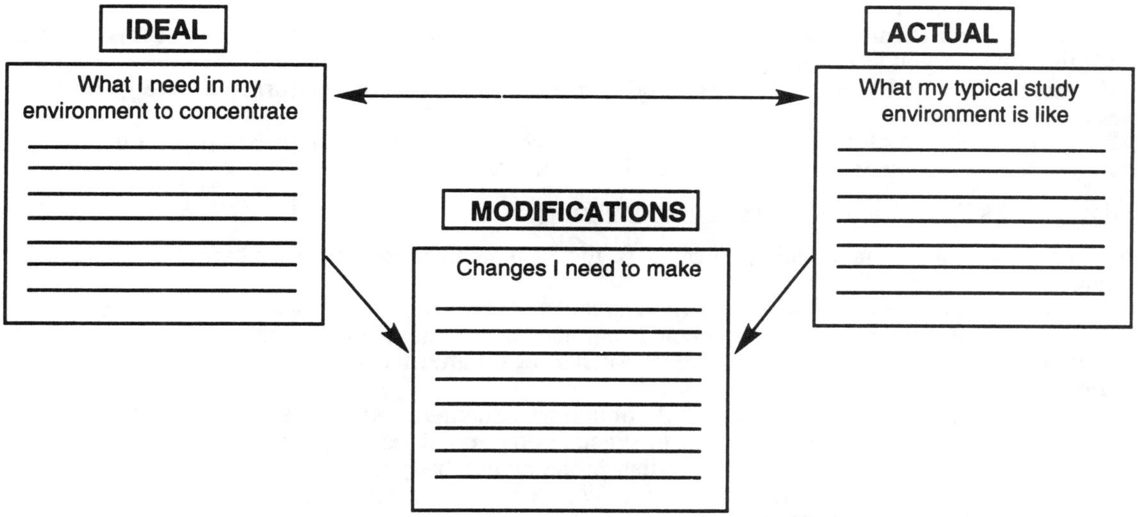

IDEAL

What I need in my environment to concentrate

____

____

____

____

____

____

____

ACTUAL

What my typical study environment is like

____

____

____

____

____

____

____

MODIFICATIONS

Changes I need to make

____

____

____

____

____

____

____

____

Study Partners

Explaining difficult material to someone else is a good way to make sure you understand what you read and memorize. Look for study partners who are strong in areas where you are weak and whose weaknesses complement your strengths. When your study partner is having difficulty, you can act as listener. It is the job of the critical listener to make sure that what the speaker says is accurate, complete, precise, and to the point. Working with others provides a check that is less punitive than waiting to test your knowledge on the exam day itself. Finally, have textbooks, reference materials and course objectives handy to redress any differences of opinion about facts or interpretations.

Developing Your Powers Of Concentration

The MCAT requires more than five hours of concentrated work, including problem solving that involves knowledge and perception, and another hour of expressing yourself through writing. You may need to work on your ability to apply yourself without a break for an entire morning. This can be unexpectedly difficult because the MCAT tests your problem-solving abilities. The problem-solving aspects of the test can increase as time passes and your concentration can decrease.

Correlating *A Complete Preparation For The MCAT* With The *MCAT Student Manual*

Your MCAT review using *A Complete Preparation For The MCAT* provides what the MCAT requires, but you must continually refer to the table of contents and to the content outlines in the *MCAT Student Manual* to stay on track. Your use of the practice materials in *A Complete Preparation For The MCAT* should be guided by the focus provided from the *MCAT Student Manual.* To enhance the effectiveness of your study program, try to answer the following questions as your MCAT review progresses:

1. Have you worked chapters 3 and 4, the comprehension and problem-solving skills chapters, to prepare you to review the physical and biological sciences in chapters 5 and 7? Practice and refine the skills first, then attempt the review.
2. Are you regularly referring to the table of contents in *A Complete Preparation for the MCAT*, cross-checking it with the content outlines in the *MCAT Student Manual* and the other practice tests and materials from AAMC? Make conscious connections between them.
3. Do you continuously review the MCAT content outlines and look for relationships across disciplines within the outlines? An example would be "work and energy" (physical sciences) related to "enzymes" (biological sciences).
4. By topic and concept, are you able to connect your review to various textbooks, journals, class notes, medical books, science labs and experiments? **All** are sources of text and problems.

Self-Managed Study Program Resources [available from Betz Publishing Company]

- *MCAT Practice Test 1* (AAMC). Use it as a pretest to discover your weaknesses.
- *MCAT Student Manual* (AAMC). Use it with *A Complete Preparation for the MCAT* to develop a systematic review of concepts from the content outlines.
- *MCAT Practice Items* (two booklets from AAMC) Use them with *A Complete Prep. . .* to test yourself in applying the concepts you have learned.
- *MCAT Practice Test 2* (AAMC). Use it as a midterm test to evaluate your performance and gauge your progress.
- *MCAT Practice Test 3* (AAMC). Use it as a post-test to check your final level of preparation for the MCAT.
- Chapter 8 of this book. Use it as a resource for reviewing test-taking skills.

Strengthening Your Skills In Reading, Mathematics and Writing

1. Review the 24 verbal reasoning skills (chapter 3), the 32 mathematics concepts (chapter 4), and the 10 reasoning patterns (chapter 4).
2. Practice one verbal reasoning skill and one mathematics concept on a daily basis. Spend about an hour on each. If you finish the list, start over again and continue throughout your entire review.
3. Work with one reasoning pattern a day (chapter 4); start again after the 10 reasoning patterns have been completed.
4. To refine your verbal and mathematical skills obtain a challenging book in a subject such as microbiology or physiology. Assuming you want to practice one verbal skill, one mathematics concept and one reasoning pattern, first study the renal system in the human body, then read the chapter, and finally apply each of the verbal and mathematical skills. For example, for verbal skill 1: distinguish between supported and unsupported claims; for mathematics concept 1: compare the components of graphs and diagrams using percentages; and for reasoning pattern 1: use analogical/associative reasoning.
5. Continuing with the example above, read the chapters on the renal system from a physiology book and from *A Complete Prep . . .* and see if you can use the skill/concept/pattern matrix in the following ways:

   - to understand components of renal system—organs, tissues, etc.;
   - to understand chemicals in plasma, urine and filtrate;
   - to understand filtration fraction, tubular transport, renal clearance, etc.;
   - to learn what the common kidney diseases are and what causes them;
   - to trace the path of a particle as it enters the renal system; list which organs it traverses before it is excreted as urine.
   - to try to relate what you have learned in the physiology book to various diagrams and concepts described in *A Complete Prep. . .* ;
   - to answer review questions in *A Complete Prep. . .* to evaluate your understanding of the renal system.

6. For any of the exercises, summarize what you have learned in small written passages to practice your writing skills.

If you wish to increase your concentration, the first step is to begin with an honest self-assessment. The second step is to improve your concentration by legitimizing your breaks. It is important that you take conscious breaks. Give yourself permission to stop when you have had enough. Remember that without that permission, your brain will take a break anyway, only you won't always be aware of what you missed. If you can only concentrate for fifteen minutes at a time, then fifteen minutes is the base-line from which you will build. (And you need not regret it either. Current cultural influences may have contributed to shortening the concentration time span.)

Step three is to build your concentration slowly. If you start with fifteen minutes, work toward a twenty-minute stretch, then twenty-five minutes, etc.

Finally, the fourth step is self-awareness. What subjects are the hardest for you to concentrate on? What time of your day is best for concentration? Worst? Does the kind of food you eat affect your concentration? How about background noise or lack of it? Does stress in school, in your job, or in personal relationships affect your concentration? Does your working place or study area affect your concentration? Use your self-awareness to circumvent the negatives that drain on your powers of concentration.

Concentration requires both endurance and discipline to correct for the variables. It may help to consciously limit the time you spend on some subject. Avoid open-ended study sessions, the kind where you say "I'm going to work on this organic chemistry until I've finished it, all night if I have to." Open-ended study sessions give permission to daydream. Tell yourself instead, "I have exactly one and one-half hours to finish this organic chemistry. If it isn't finished by then, too bad." At the end of one and one-half hours, stop. While limitless sessions tend to encourage a lack of focus, limiting the time in advance encourages you to concentrate harder.

Building Discipline

You must be as disciplined as you study for the MCAT as you will need to be in taking it. For example, many students don't like organic chemistry. If this is true, you may be in no hurry to study organic chemistry and, on the test itself, you may find that your are in no hurry to get to that portion of the test, either. As a result, you may spend a longer time in working over the biology questions in the Biological Sciences (since you feel more comfortable about them), and defer the organic chemistry questions to the point that you do not leave yourself enough time to cover all questions. A disciplined approach learned through your study skills practice can be most beneficial to you during the actual testing sessions.

Using Test Items

When working test items, practice on only a small number at one time (one verbal reasoning passage and its follow-up questions, or ten test items in any of the other areas). To improve, you need to be able to analyze your errors. This requires you to remember the reasoning you used as you worked the problem.

To analyze your errors, use the answer key first. Only use the problem solutions section as a last resort and to check yourself after you are able to explain the keyed response. Once you have decided why the keyed response is correct, then check your reasoning against the problem solutions section.

Keep a written record of your errors, even if only by making a check mark (√) next to the corresponding topic in the outline printed in the *MCAT Student Manual*. Your errors can be classified in a number of ways. For example, specific content errors (e.g., genetics problems in the biological sciences) and specific question format errors (e.g., multiple-choice) can give you trouble. This "error journal" will help you use your time most efficiently, since you will know where you most need to review or develop more successful strategies for answering the questions. Study chapter 8 to learn how to set up your "error journal."

As you work problems, note where the test emphasis lies. Once again the outline in the *MCAT Student Manual* will help. For example, you may find that genetics is an important topic, so time spent on reviewing Mendelian genetics and application of the Hardy-Weinberg principle will repay the effort; conversely, you do not need to take a course just so you can answer a single obscure question from a topic that only appears once. Appendix A provides a comprehensive list of references used in the AAMC tests and other practice materials.

2.2.2 Note-taking

Extracting and Recording Information

As you begin your study process for the MCAT, you may find that there are specific areas in which you need to do a fairly intensive review of content, including the construction of notes to synthesize information. In order to help you accomplish this task, consider further development of your note-taking skills. Effective note-taking methods may also be useful in your current course work to maximize your retention of information and increase the efficiency of time invested in review.

The process of note-taking is two-fold: extract information from a source (e.g., newspaper, textbook, lab report) and record it efficiently for easier recall. You then have the challenge of organizing the information that you have collected over a number of years and reducing it to a manageable unit that still contains important principles and concepts.

Reorganizing your notes on a regular basis improves your information extraction skills. The concepts you learned earlier can be rephrased and presented with your inner understandings. This makes you more confident with managing large volumes of notes and books.

Relational maps provide a graphic image of certain concepts, processes, experiments and solutions to complex problems. Your mastery of "extracting" information integrated with relational maps will provide good review material as you go along. (See section 2.2.3 below.)

Using the Cornell Method of Note-taking

There are three note-taking methods that are practical for MCAT preparation. The Cornell method is recommended for lecture notes, while relational maps and Venn diagrams, discussed below in section 2.2.3, can be used to synthesize lecture and text notes.

The Cornell method of note-taking (adapted here with permission from Walter J. Pauk of Cornell University) is a way of recording lecture notes in a manner that allows for subsequent analysis and reduction of the information. In order to practice this method, you will need lined, loose-leaf paper that has a line drawn down the page approximately three inches from the left margin. (In most university bookstores you can also purchase paper ruled with three-inch margins.) Listed below are steps that summarize the method:

During a lecture, seminar or meeting with your study partner:

- Record the speaker's purpose, which is usually presented during opening comments.
- Write down an informal outline of the overview presented in the introduction.
- Record your lecture notes in the column on the right side of your paper. You do not need to write whole sentences, but try to select and record the important concepts or details.
- Write only on the right hand pages of your notebook. The facing pages can be used for adding notes from the textbook in order to combine and integrate information.
- Draw illustrative diagrams and record examples. They not only serve as clarifications to the topic, but they can also provide quick review to determine if you remember a process or cycle. Be sure that you label relevant parts.
- Record the lecturer's comments about content to be covered in the next lecture.
- Make sure the information you have is accurate and makes sense.

After the lecture:

- Complete notes:
  - Fill in and complete sections of notes that are unclear. You may need to check with your instructor, a classmate, or use a reference book if additional information or clarification is needed.
- Reduce notes:
  - Use the left margin of your note-taking page for key words that represent important vocabulary, main ideas, and associated details.
- Analyze notes:
  - Determine which parts of the lecture contain primary information versus elaboration of text. Are there details in the textbook that you must also consider to understand the topic?
  - Review the overview outline presented during the introduction. Are there uncovered areas which you are responsible for? Make a "learning issues" list and research the topics on your own.
- Review notes on a regular basis:
  - Cover up the right-hand column and, using the cues in the left-hand column, try to recall information suggested by your cues.
  - Note that whole sentences do not need to be written in your left-hand column. The left-hand column in the handwritten notes that follow may be further abbreviated as "receptive versus expressive language?," "sequence of language behaviors," "receptive development," etc.

After you have practiced writing Cornell notes a few times, you will find that you become much more adept at looking for classifications and groupings of concepts. You will also find that taking notes in the conventional manner, where information is embedded, will seem cumbersome and awkward.

The Cornell note-taking method is also quite useful for textbook reviews, especially when you use the headings as organizers. Because it organizes and highlights important information, this method can also be used for identifying material that must be memorized later. Following is a list of steps to construct MCAT notes from various resources.

STEPS FOR CONSTRUCTING MCAT NOTES FROM SCIENTIFIC JOURNALS, TEXTBOOKS AND CLASSNOTES:

- Whenever you read an article in a scientific journal or a magazine, always read the first paragraph and stop. Close the journal and extrapolate as to what is the author's primary purpose or hypothesis in writing this article. See if you can predict any scientific conclusions that the author will probably make.

- Open textbooks or classnotes to sections that relate to the article. Is there any hidden connection between the journal article and your textbooks? Become an active learner by comparing classnotes, textbooks and research articles to understand applications of MCAT concepts.

- Now return to the second paragraph and read the journal article to the end. Write down in short sentences what MCAT concepts were covered in the article. Check your college textbooks and classnotes to see if you learned these concepts in class. Make notes on any new concepts or skills used.

- If you find scientific theories, hypotheses or scientific terms that have not been covered before in your studies, record them in the corresponding sections of *A Complete Preparation for the MCAT* for future review.

- Keep all your notes in an "MCAT Concepts notebook" for repeated review. Discover your reading flaws and determine how you can improve your "MCAT concept extraction" skills in future reading of other scientific articles.

Now read through the following Cornell notes. On one page, essential information has been extracted from the notes and provided in the left margin. On the second page, the basic information has been presented. Try summarizing the important points in the margin space provided. Especially look for cause and effect relationships as well as comparisons and contrasts.

These notes are taken from Jane W. Kessler, *Psychopathology of Childhood*, second edition, copyright 1988, pp. 144-145. Adapted by permission of Prentice-Hall, Inc., Englewood Cliffs, NJ.

	Receptive Language Development
How is receptive language similar to + different from expressive language?	1. Spoken words only understood if accompanied by tone, gesture or context EXAMPLE: Word "hot" ignored if not accompanied by negative commanding voice
Describe the sequence of language behaviors.	2. Stages (Infant to 2) a. baby - recognizes cue words that precede routine events b. end of 1st year - child responds to words such as "give me" - but may not truly understand words
What principles could describe receptive development?	c. Child learns to pair auditory discrimination with predictable outcome d. Child begins to connect sounds with objects rather than actions e. Child learns to discriminate between object + uses
Speculate: what might cause language delay?	EXAMPLES: Year 1 - all objects treated the same Year 2 - object usage is discriminated - fork for eating, ball for throwing
Give 2 examples to illustrate parallel process: a. b.	3. Parallel process between recognition of objects and uses compared to discrimination of words and recollection of associations with activities and objects.

4. Use of meaningful words
   a. Child points out parts of own body (sequential fashion)
   b. Child can identify body parts on self or others
   c. Child can identify parts on doll (18 months)
   d. Child can identify parts on 2-dimensional representation (2 yrs.)

Expressive Language Development
1. Components of language
   a. playing with sounds
   b. pre-linguistic signals or cries that child tries to make and sustain

2. Important Research
   a. Anna Freud (WW II)—infants raised in residential nurseries were normal under 1, but verbally backward by 2, indicating vocalization stimulated by different influences in 1st + 2nd years
   b. Snow (1984)—identified 2 principles of language acquisition
      i—adults interpret child behaviors as attempts to communicate—even when there is no explicit intention
      ii—Children search for relationship between objects, persons and events in the world and the behavior of caretaker.

Note-taking Summary

Regardless of the note-taking system you are using, there are a number of techniques that can be used to optimize your performance.

- Date all notes and number the pages.
- Write in erasable ink. Lectures written in pencil can smudge over time and lose clarity. By contrast, erasable ink is easier to read and corrections can still be made.
- Look up vocabulary that is not fully defined.
- Try to determine the organizational patterns used to develop the material, since these patterns are essential both to Cornell notes and relational maps.
- Use timesavers such as mnemonics, standard abbreviations, simplified indented format, and your own shorthand style. Beware, however, of inventing abbreviations that you may not be able to read when reviewing at a later time.
- Keep notes on similar topics together. This avoids wasting study time in search of related bits of information. Use a loose-leaf notebook. Incorporate your handouts into the relevant lecture materials.
- Maintain active behavior by consistently predicting what will come next.
- Try to keep facts and opinions separate.
- When formulas are used, solve problems using derivations as well as the basic formula.
- When examples are worked by the professor, record all steps of the explanation.
- To reduce internal distractions, avoid daydreaming, doodling, and writing notes to yourself on other topics.
- Review your notes within 24 hours. This is very important since it reinforces short-term memory. As mentioned in the memory section, distributed practice is a very effective way to increase long-term memory.

2.2.3 Visual Imaging or Mapping

One limitation to the Cornell note-taking method that you may encounter in preparing for the MCAT is that it does not reveal the relative weighting of ideas in a passage or reveal the relationships between them. One method that allows you to integrate information effectively is relational or semantic mapping. These maps represent concepts and details in a visual format that synthesizes and reduces information into meaningful groups.

It is important to keep maps flexible. Information can be developed in linear or circular patterns, but maps are most effective when they reflect the same organizational patterns as the text or lecture notes.

Mind Mapping

A mind map traces and records ideas as you carefully read a passage. It is a schematic chart of your observations as you work through the passage. It also leads you back to the right location in a passage when you must answer the questions that follow. Mind maps are useful in extracting basic detail and arranging it for later use.

A mind map lets you develop a strong control right from the start and traces major ideas as you scan or read them. It is also a tool to develop a layout for an entire passage. Try to construct a mind map for articles that you read. Soon you will be able to draw such maps quickly and accurately. Although the mind map shown opposite was constructed for a passage on connective tissue that appears later in this chapter, it is included here as an example of semantic map construction.

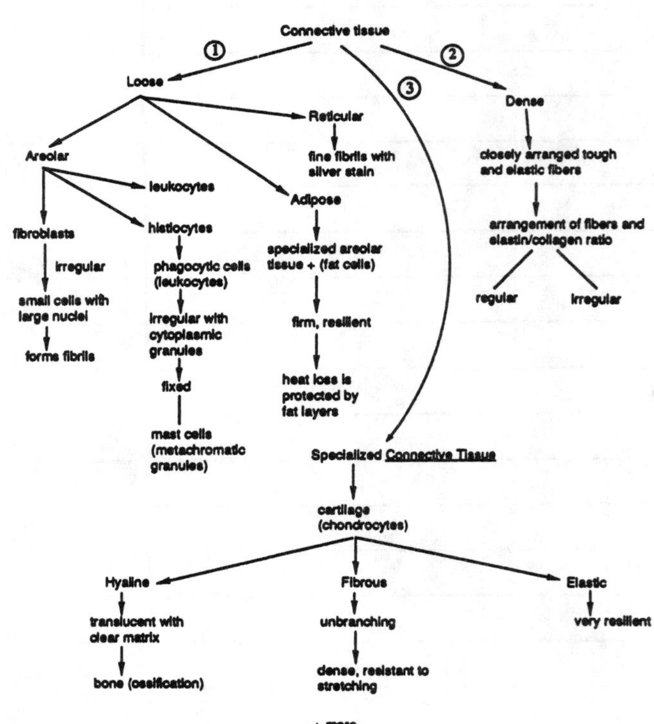

Relational Maps

There are six types of relational maps:

Type I:	Comparison and contrast
Type II:	Linear (parts to whole)
Type III:	Structure or function
Type IV:	Process
Type V:	Complex cause and effect
Type VI:	Venn association diagram

TYPE I: COMPARISON AND CONTRAST

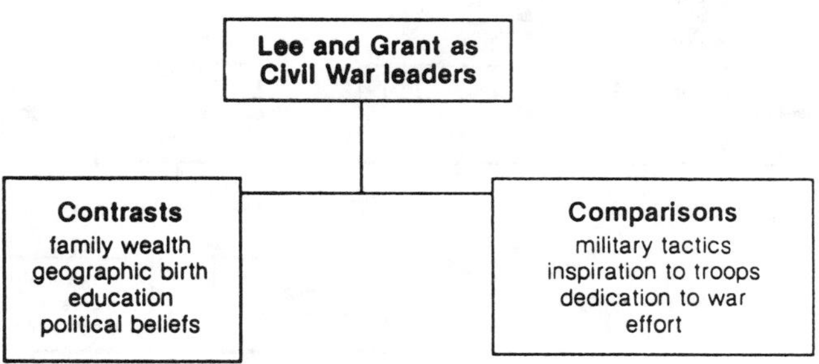

TYPE II: LINEAR (PARTS TO WHOLE)

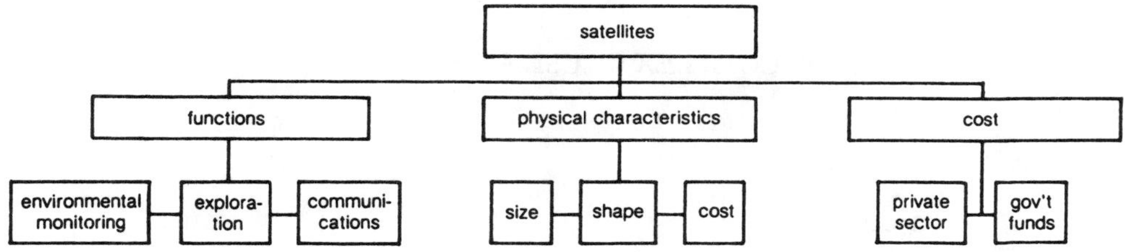

TYPE III: STRUCTURE OR FUNCTION

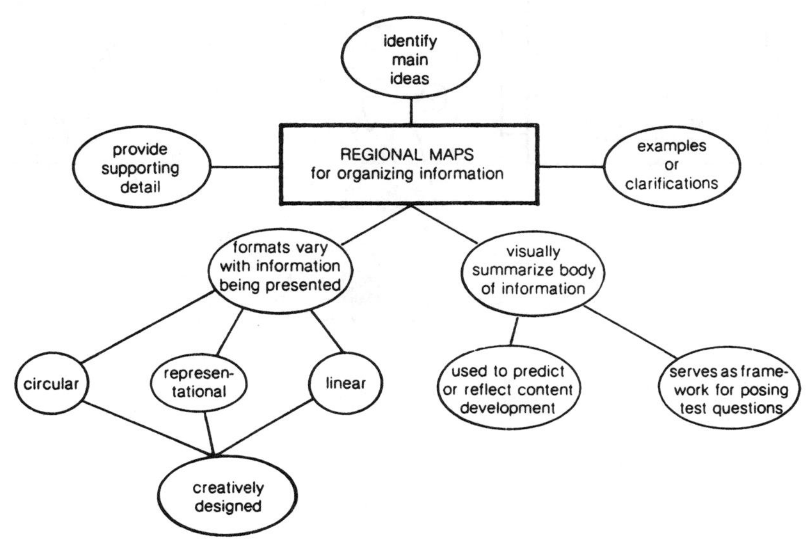

TYPE IV: PROCESS

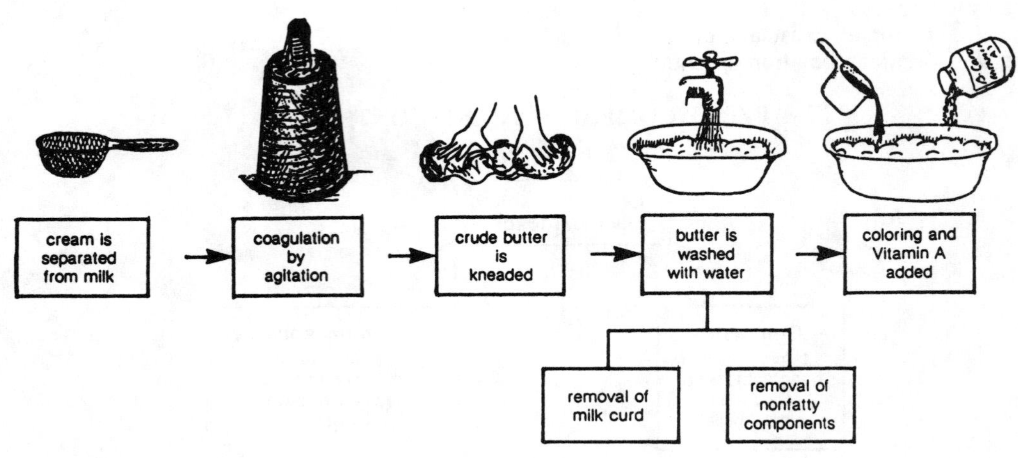

TYPE V: COMPLEX CAUSE AND EFFECT

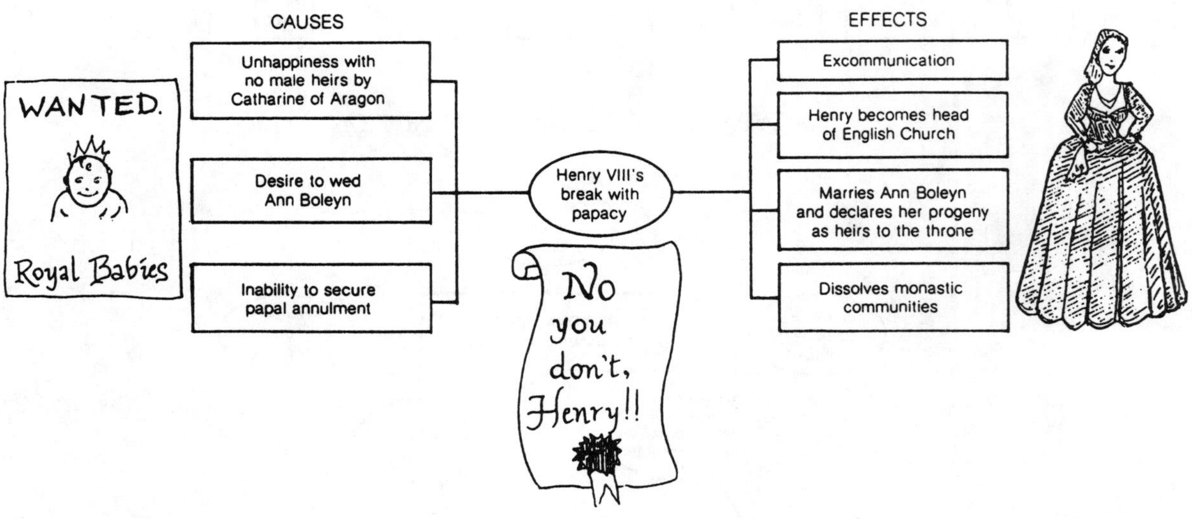

TYPE VI: VENN ASSOCIATION DIAGRAM

Venn or association diagrams are especially important in dealing with concepts that emphasize differences, such as *some* and *all* as well as *what should be* and *what should not be* included in analyzing information. Venn diagrams are used to visually represent statements as well as concepts.

Consider the following illustration:

Example: The statement "All roses are red," can be diagrammed as follows:
- things that are red
- roses (all red)
- things that are red, but are not roses

"All roses are red." = 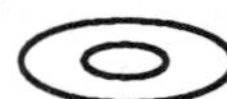

In a Venn or association diagram, a circle entirely contained within another circle means that all the members of the inner group belong in the outer group as well. In the diagram representing "All roses are red," the inner circle denotes *roses* (and all of them are red) and the outer circle denotes *things that are red*. The space inside the larger circle (but outside the smaller *roses* circle) represents all those things that are red but are not roses. (Note: Look only at the relationship given in the statement. For the purpose of this diagram, it does not matter that in real life not all roses are red.)

Example: The statement "*Some* roses are red," can be diagrammed as follows:
- roses
- red things

"Some roses are red." = 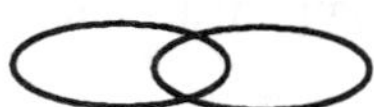

If you look at the lines of the circles, you can see the relationship between red things and roses, only some of which are red. But if you look at the spaces rather than the lines, you see the relationships between three categories:
- roses that are not red (the space on the left)
- *some* roses that are red (the space in the middle)
- red things that are not roses (the space on the right)

Example: The statement "*No* roses are red," can also be diagrammed as follows:
- roses (none of which are red)
- red things (which include no roses)

"No roses are red." = 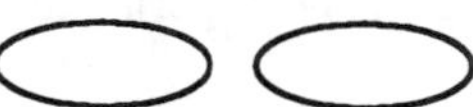

Mapping tips for reading. Scan the chapter, noting headings and graphs, and read the summary.

- Do not underline or highlight as you read. Since you have not read the topic, you will be unable to sort the main ideas from the details. Additionally, when you continually stop reading to underline, it breaks memory into small pieces, making it more difficult to construct larger concepts.
- Place checkmarks in the margin next to important ideas and keep reading until you come to a natural break. Then go back and decide what should be underlined or noted in the margin.

Mapping tips for MCAT review. State your main idea. It works best to identify the topic within a brief sentence so that you can accurately recall the central focus of the topic.

- Develop a visual schemata to represent the main ideas of the topic.
- Determine the relationship between ideas (i.e., time order, comparison and contrast, cause and effect, etc.) and designate them on your map.
- Add details to your map to complete your understanding of the topic. Note facts that need to be memorized.
- Use the size of headings to indicate structure. Your Cornell notes will give you vital data on determining which parts of the material are background compared to essential information.
- Be creative. Remember the goal of the map is to provide visual memory. Add illustrations, pictures, symbols, and other visual images that will distinguish this map from others. Consider encasing the image in the object that it represents, such as the heart.
- Add color. You may want to have separate branches in different colors so that you can more easily trace ideas from memory.
- Summarize main points at the bottom of the page. This can be an effective tool for synthesizing and condensing author's main points.

2.2.4 Understanding Instruments and Experiments

The following section on instruments and experiments should be included as exercises in your review and linked to your study of the physical and biological sciences in chapters 5 and 7.

Study Skills for Scientific Instruments

Questions containing references to scientific instrumentation appear on the MCAT. Activities are suggested here that will enhance your understanding of highly technical instruments and procedures.

1. Learn how to read a complex sketch or drawing (look at the size, position, shape and name of each part).
2. Draw a representative schematic of an instrument showing its structure and function.
3. Relate principles of biology, chemistry or physics to an explanation of the instrument drawn in 2 above.
4. Interpret the functions of the instrument from its description.
5. Connect the application of an instrument to medical technology, e.g., its use in a laboratory or a hospital.
6. Compare possible sources of breakdown to the smooth working of the instrument.
7. Find scales of measurement and range; precision, accuracy, and precautions (if any) from manufacturer's label or instructions.
8. Compare and contrast the separate parts of an instrument and the role each one plays in its operation.

Components of a Scientific Experiment

There are usually ten components to the laboratory report of a scientific experiment. Some MCAT passages are followed by tabulated observations but give only a few of the listed components in the passage. Students should know the list of components well enough to know when some are missing from MCAT passages and why they are important for answering the test questions. (Components shown with an asterisk [*] are usually provided, while the others are not.)

1. Purpose or scope of the experiment.
2.* Introduction and background material.
3. Equipment, instruments and chemicals list.
4. Sequential set-up and skills in the overall procedure.
5.* Procedural sketch or schematic of experiment.
6.* Data sheet and observations.
7.* Calculations and results including graphs.
8. Precautions observed during experiment.
9. Comments (usually something new you have observed that is different from what is in the textbook or laboratory manual) including sources of errors.
10. Open questions and problems to be solved by the experiment.

2.3 READING COMPREHENSION SKILLS FOR SCIENTIFIC TEXT

Comprehension means that you retain enough information from reading to make connections. While the ability to comprehend what you read depends somewhat on your reading speed, your concentration, and your interest in the subject matter, difficulty with a reading passage usually stems from problems with content (new information) and vocabulary.

Broaden Your Reading Base

The MCAT requires you to read, organize and analyze new information from a broad reading base. New information can come from lectures and notes or sources can include medical research reports, magazine and journal articles or newspapers such as *The New York Times*. For practice you can find other sources of new information at the library. Make a habit of reading regularly to broaden your reading base from sources like those that follow:

- *The New York Times* (daily newspaper)
- *Scientific American* (monthly magazine)
- *Discover* (monthly magazine)
- *American Scientist* (bimonthly magazine by Sigma Xi)
- *The New England Journal of Medicine* (weekly journal)
- *Encyclopedia Britannica*
- *U.S.A. Today* (daily newspaper)

Develop Your Vocabulary

A strong vocabulary is a useful tool in decoding MCAT passages and test items. Vocabulary expansion should be an active part of your MCAT preparation, especially if you sometimes use words that you cannot define. Construct a vocabulary notebook. Record daily any new words you encounter and as a regular part of your study approach, ask yourself the meaning of even the most routinely used terms. As an example, consider the following puzzle:

> There is a square, man-made lake with a tree at each corner. How can you double the area of the lake, still keeping it square, without disturbing the trees?

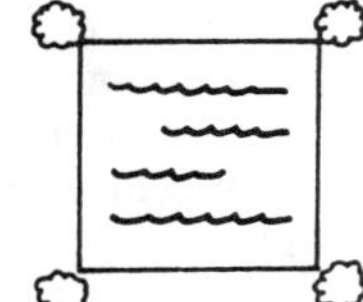

Invariably, the first answer is, "Dig the lake deeper." If you thought this, too, you have insufficiently comprehended the distinction between "area" and "volume"—a definition problem—and this difficulty might adversely affect your solutions to physics problems. Review basic definitions, even of those terms you use quite regularly, and enter them in your notebook. (The answer to this problem is at the end of the section.)

The ability to define indicates a specific rather than a global or diffuse understanding of terms. Definitional knowledge is important to your performance on the MCAT because it provides you with a broad base of information to use in problem-solving during the test. Definitional knowledge in science includes knowing not only how to formulate a definition, but also determining the essential characteristics of the term, i.e., function, location, structure, example, etc. You must be able to manipulate definitions backwards and forwards, since a question may be posed from definition to term or from term to definition. Working with proper resources will help you build definitional knowledge. Students preparing for the MCAT should routinely use resources such as a good general dictionary, a medical dictionary, a glossary of medical terminology, and thesauri in biology, physics and chemistry.

In addition to working with the right resources, you should develop a systematic approach for learning new definitions. For efficient learning, definitions should be memorized as groups of words that belong together. If you look up "synapse" in a biology thesaurus, you will notice that the definition of synapse contains several other technical words (neuron, axon, dendrite, effector organ, etc.). All of these terms belong together and are found at your fingertips in the section on the nervous system.

You will find that learning a term as part of a matrix of related terms helps in correctly answering multiple-choice test items. For example, if the term "synapse" appears in a question stem, the correct answer choice is likely to include one of the other terms (axon, neuron, dendrite, etc.) that belongs with it. In addition, you know that the term "synapse" belongs under the general heading "nervous system." The organization of the thesaurus is a reminder of that. If "synapse" appears in the question stem, we would not expect the correct answer choice to come from the endocrine system. Classification and sorting of large amounts of information becomes easier when definitions are used.

Consider the following problem:

> A person touching a hot item immediately pulls his/her hand away from that object.
> This is an example of:
>
> A. irritability.
> B. a feedback loop.
> C. conscious nervous control.
> D. a reflex arc.

Most students eliminate A and C, but then they have to think about B and D. However, if you studied with the biology thesaurus, you know that B, a feedback loop, is found in the section on the endocrine system and would not apply, whereas answer D, a reflex arc, is a term found in the section on the nervous system and, therefore, is the best answer choice.

Note that both the right answer and the most likely distractor came from two systems that are often paired together in textbooks. The endocrine system and the nervous system are the two systems that modulate, integrate, and control the activities of the body, and test-makers know that students often confuse the details of these two systems. Always review your material with the test-makers in mind.

Studying from a page of connected words in the biology thesaurus helps in synthesizing facts around a core (or central topic) similar to a reading passage. Deliberately working towards such a synthesis will improve your understanding, problem-solving ability, and most fundamentally your ability to retain a great deal of information. Remember to consider the total concept as well as the details when distinguishing between the almost-right answer and the correct answer in problem-solving.

In working with definitions, there is a tendency to focus only on technical terms. However, general vocabulary is also important to performance in verbal reasoning and in the physical and biological sciences sections of the MCAT. At the most basic level, you need a broad, generalized reading vocabulary. If you do not read extensively outside assigned texts, or if your scores on the verbal portions of the SAT and ACT examinations were low, you might want to assess and review your basic reading vocabulary. Even if you do command a strong reading vocabulary, you will still need to focus on the uses of definitions for the MCAT. Scientific writing is replete with definitions embedded in sentence and paragraph structure to establish precisely what a word means in the context in which it appears.

The importance of definitions is stressed because students too often are hampered by their neglect of mastering terminology. Not only can you improve your score on the MCAT by building definitional knowledge, but in your first year of medical school you will be better prepared to handle all the new terms that typically overwhelm many students. In learning definitions of important terms, there are two types of definitions to consider: defining by synonym and defining by genus.

Defining by synonym. Can you define "pleasant"? If your answer was "agreeable" or "nice" you were defining by synonym. It is useful to think about synonyms, both to assist your memory and to offer more versatility in solving problems.

Scientists attempt to use words very precisely, almost mathematically. They want one term to have one meaning. As a result science teachers often tell students that scientific terms have little or no correspondence to the same words used in ordinary life, or even in other disciplines. Sometimes, of course, this is true. However, in general, the scientific word often does have a relationship to ordinary English usage that is found in the etymology. For this and other reasons, a glossary of medical terminology is recommended.

In understanding and remembering precise scientific meaning, it may be useful to work from the common meaning. Consider, for example, "intercostal muscles." Partridge's *A Short Etymological Dictionary of Modern English Origins* shows that "costal" and "coastal" are related terms, so "intercostal" would appear to mean "between the coasts" or "between the ribs." Similarly, in the biological term "parallel evolution", the word "parallel" has a relationship to "parallel" as it is used in geometry as well as to the parallel bars used in gymnastics.

Making connections, or synthesizing and cross-referencing language and ideas will aid your understanding, memory, flexibility, and application of words to solving MCAT problems. It will especially help you to analyze passages and develop connections between topics in the passage, such as "interstitial fluids" and "hormones." This will link the physics of fluids to diffusion of hormones in various biological entities such as tissues or organs.

Defining by genus. The most usual definition in science is one by genus and difference. Consider the definition of "northwest" as "a point on the compass equidistant between north and west." The first part, "a point on the compass", tells you its genus. The second part, "equidistant between north and west", tells you in what way this particular point is different from others in its genus. Similarly, if you define "heart", you would want to give its genus as "a major organ of the body", as well as its difference, which in biology tends to be its location and functions.

Definitions have been important from the very beginning of recorded history. Indeed, the power of naming was the first power God gave to Adam in the Garden of Eden. A definition was at the heart of the riddle Oedipus solved to save Thebes from the Sphinx. The Sphinx was, according to Edith Hamilton in *Mythology*, "a fearsome creature shaped like a winged lion" (genus), "but with the breast and face of a woman" (difference). The Sphinx asked Oedipus, "What creature goes on four feet in the morning, on two at noonday, on three in the evening?" Had he failed the test, the Sphinx would have killed Oedipus, as she had killed many contestants before him. In the riddle, the Sphinx gave Oedipus the definitional information, and he was required to supply the term, just as many test items give the definitions and require the students to find the term.

Since definitional test items can be played both ways, it is a good idea to build the habit of keeping definitions on index cards with the term on one side and the definition on the other. Practice thinking both from term to definition and from definition to term.

Here is the answer to the "Man-made Lake" problem above:

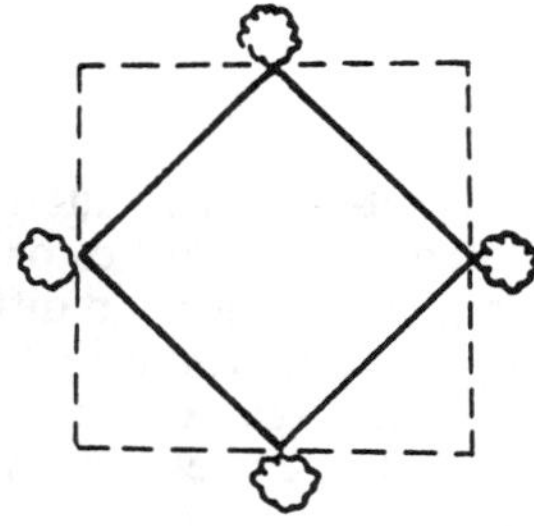

Apply Analytical Reasoning

Analytical reasoning can help you to become a more discriminating reader of all forms of information. It is an approach to reading that consists of breaking a complex passage into short understandable pieces, as one would break a sentence into short, more readable phrases. The following reading comprehension tools are useful in analyzing any new information that you encounter.

1. Find the central idea
2. Identify cause and effect statements
3. Develop interrelationships in the text, including chronological mapping
4. Recognize comparison-contrast shifts
5. Uncover assumptions: - direct or stated
   - indirect or unstated.
6. Determine conclusions: - direct or obvious
   - indirect or implied.
7. Locate errors in reading and determine how to avoid them

Recognize Passage Types

You should be able to identify standard passage types that typically appear in verbal reasoning and scientific information passages on exams. Knowing the method of passage development will prepare you for the types of questions that follow. Once you identify the main ideas of the paragraphs in the passage, analyze the way these ideas are linked. This skill relates directly to the organization of ideas discussed under relational maps in the note-taking section (2.2.3). You need to know what pattern is being used to organize the given information. (Note: real-world MCAT passages may have more than one pattern.)

Cause and effect. In this pattern, there is a causal relationship between two or more events. In other words, **A** leads to **B,** or **B** is the result of **A**. Since cause and effect cannot occur simultaneously, you may perceive a sequence of ideas or a chronological order. When working with this pattern be sure that **B** is truly an outcome of **A** and not just an event that comes after **A**.

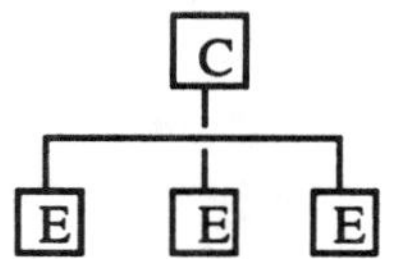

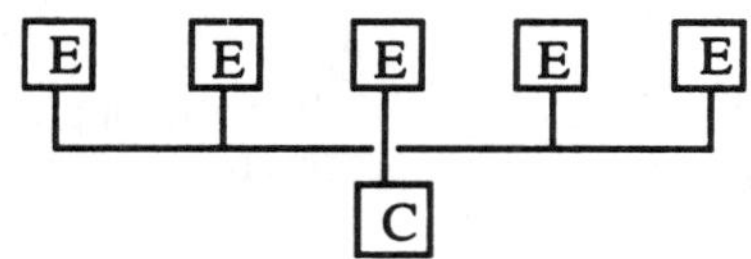

Test questions may be worded:

- Damage to the cornea could cause an impairment in which of the following?
- Cancer of the pancreas usually results in consequences for which secondary areas?

Classification. The writer presents a subject by identifying its category. A system of organization is used to represent groups with varying characteristics. This could be based upon demographics, phyla, behavioral traits, family trees, etc. This pattern is somewhat different from simple listing where items are only named. In classification questions the categories are frequently named, but in order to determine the correct answer you must consider whether the information provided fits into a designated group.

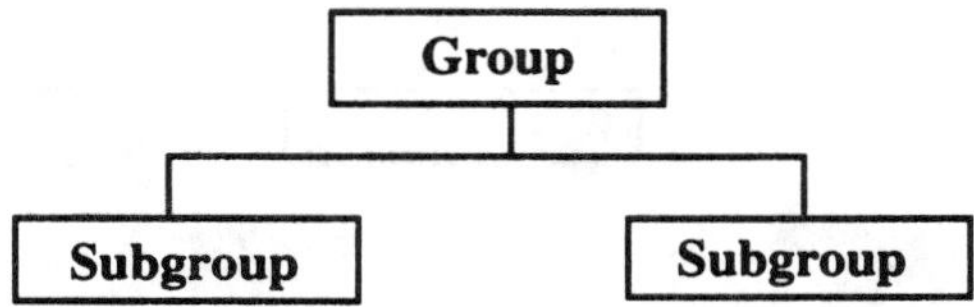

Test questions may be worded:

- The census figures indicate that the homeless and those beneath the poverty level make up what percent of the total population?
- Which of the following statements best describes the writer's concept of the doctor-patient relationship?

Comparison and Contrast—In this pattern, the writer presents two or more subjects for discussion. These subjects may be compared for similarities or contrasted for differences. Some authors may use a combination pattern that includes both similarities and differences. Comparisons and contrasts are usually organized in one of two ways: subject by subject (where first one topic or person is presented and then another), or alternating pattern (in which a feature is discussed first relative to one subject then to the other). As you work through test questions, identify not only those questions that have a direct or stated comparison or contrast, but those that ask you for an inferred relationship.

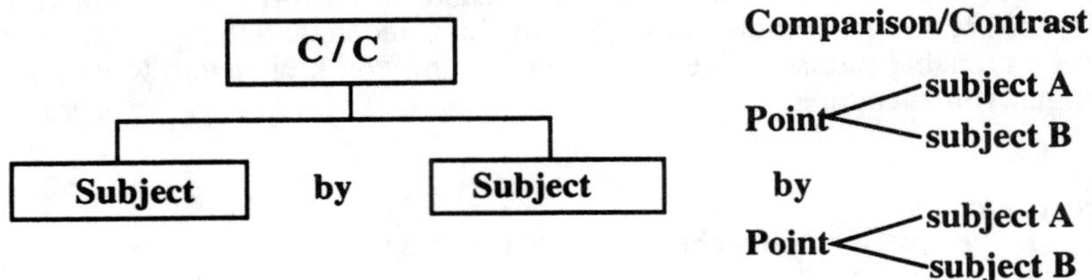

Test questions may be worded:

- How did Triconodon differ from other mammals living 150 million years ago?
- The proof that Shakespeare and Marlowe were not the same individual is represented by which of the following?

Word Usage. A concept or a word is explained by identifying the general class in which it belongs and specific features that distinguish it from others in its class. Within test formats, word usage questions are frequently used to evaluate whether students understand the precise word. Sometimes words can have different meanings and may vary with authors and context. Test items are often constructed around these words since students may choose a typical usage that does not match the context if they have not read the passage carefully.

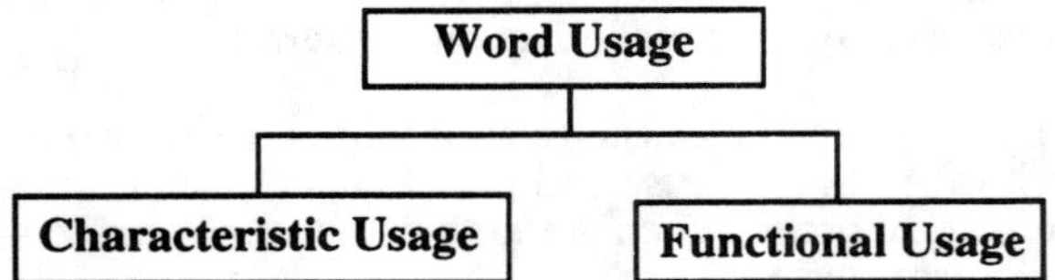

Test questions may be worded:

- Which of the following best describes a glomerulus?
- According to the text, a "proselytizer" is what?

Process. The primary emphasis of this pattern is to explain how something functions, works, or evolves. It usually presents an orderly or prescribed series of steps or operations that lead to a result or product. In some usages, it can be similar to cause and effect in that it may occur as a chain where the result of one step becomes the cause of another. On test questions, carefully identify the steps indicated, but also watch for a step skipped.

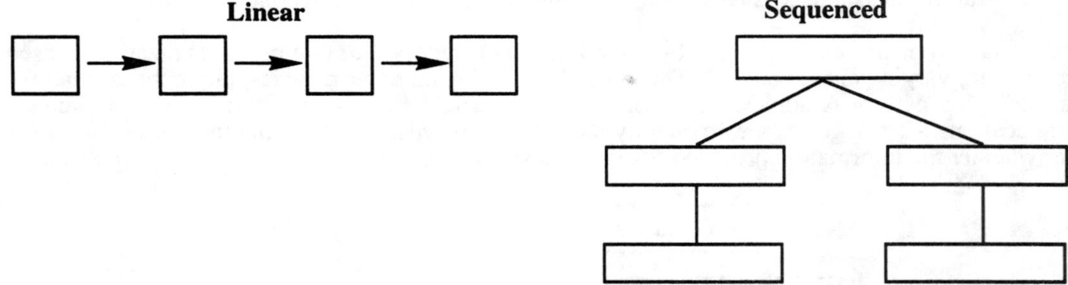

Test questions may be worded:

- Which of the following sequences was not identified by the author as relating to decision-making?
- In diplomatic negotiations relating to release of Americans held prisoners in Iran, the author considered which step by President Carter to have the most influential effect in their eventual release?

Reasons. This pattern is most frequently used when an author has an opinion or an assumption and wants to validate it by giving the basis or underlying logical justification of his/her position. Similarly, the author may have a conclusion and want to establish the reasons or verification for why it should be believed. This pattern is frequently used in explaining an opinion or presenting an argument. As you work with test questions you may notice that often more than one option that could be a correct reason is tested. However, you are asked to identify the BEST reason for an action or belief. (Note 1-2-3-4 sequence; reasons are usually prioritized.)

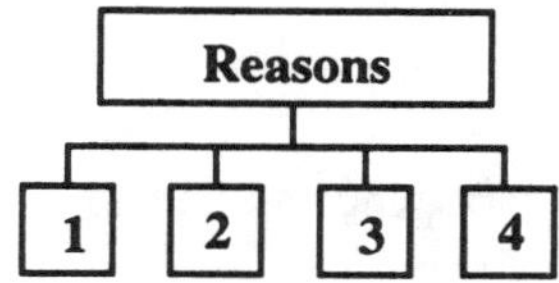

Test questions may be worded:

- The justification for excluding atherosclerotic heart disease as a contributing factor in the patient's disorientation is based upon which of the following?
- The primary factor documenting that ulceration is often followed by thrombosis is based upon which observation?

Spatial or Geographic. When a writer organizes data using maps, charts, diagrams, outlines, etc., the purpose is to help the reader visualize or see relationships. Often this pattern can be used to summarize information, such as when a large volume of quantitative information is presented. When working with passages that contain spatial or geographic references, it is helpful to sketch a quick diagram of your own that shows the relationships among the parts before you begin answering the questions.

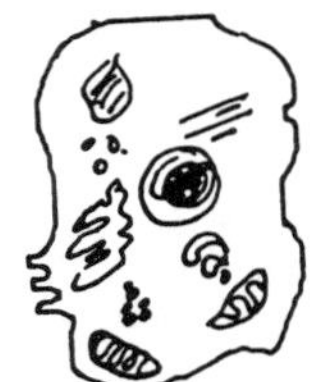

Parts of a Cell

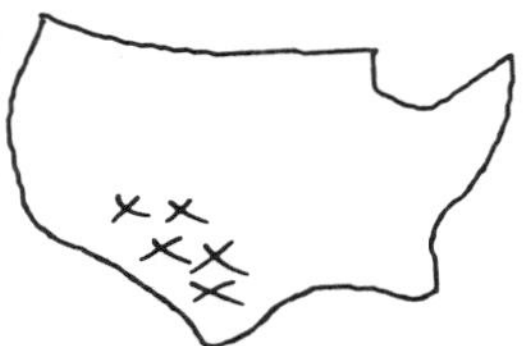

Deposits of Oil Reserves

Test questions may be worded:

- The San Andreas fault lies beneath which highly populated cities?
- In his march to Russia, Hitler moved his troops through which country?

Time Order. This organizational pattern is used when a writer needs to sequence events or provide a step-by-step description. It is frequently used in giving directions. Time period can be variable, i.e., from millenniums to milliseconds. In working with this pattern on test questions, determine that events did occur in the order presented.

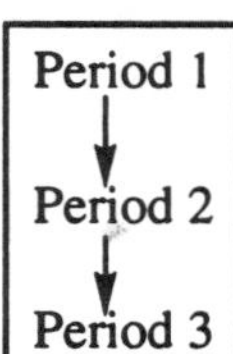

Test questions may be worded:

- Hepplewhite furniture was designed in which period of early English cabinetmaking?
- Which of the following body systems is most developed during the third trimester of pregnancy?

The above patterns might seem like a lot to remember, but with practice the reading of main ideas and selection of patterns of organization become almost ritual. You will see other applications of this information in chapter 6, "The MCAT Writing Sample."

Reading and Writing Practice: Do not concentrate exclusively on science review. Set aside time each day to include reading and writing practice as well. Practicing your reading and writing can be like daily warm-up exercises, or they can serve as "breaks" between your science studies. Remember, this is not an examination of basic science knowledge only. It is a passage-based science test and your verbal reasoning and writing skills will be equally tested.

Practice Your Skills

This is an appropriate time for you to experience a typical MCAT passage containing "new information" as it is described at the beginning of section 2.3. As you read the passage, you should actively mark up your passage to highlight important points. Use your reading comprehension skills, including definition awareness, analytical reasoning, and visual imagery. This is a classification type passage similar in format and style to passages in the MCAT. Consider the following techniques during this reading exercise:

1. Skim the passage for approximately 30 seconds. Decide what the passage is about.
2. Read the questions for clues to the type of questions asked.
3. Take 3 to 5 minutes to read the passage.
4. Answer the questions that follow.

Connective Tissue: General Characteristics and Functions

Connective tissue allows movement and provides support. In this tissue there is an abundance of intercellular material called matrix, which is variable in type and amount and is one of the main sources of difference between the types of connective tissue. It consists of various fibers embedded in a ground substance.

Loose Connective Tissue

The fibers of loose connective tissue are not tightly woven. The tissue, filling space between and penetrating into the organs, is of three types: areolar, adipose, and reticular.

Areolar Tissue. The most widely distributed connective tissue is pliable and crossed by many delicate threads; yet, the tissue resists tearing and is somewhat elastic. Areolar tissue contains fibroblasts, histiocytes (macrophages), leukocytes, and mast cells.

Fibroblasts are small, flattened, somewhat irregular cells with large nuclei and reduced cytoplasm. The term fibroblast refers to the ability of a cell to form fibrils. Fibroblasts are active in repair of injury. It is generally believed that suprarenal steroids inhibit and growth hormones stimulate fibroblastic activity. **Histiocytes** are phagocytic cells similar to **leukocytes** in blood; however, they perform phagocytic activity outside the vascular system. The histiocyte is irregular in shape and contains cytoplasmic granules. The cell is often stationary (or "fixed"). **Mast cells**, located adjacent to small blood vessels, are round or polygonal in shape and possess a cytoplasm filled with metachromatic granules. Mast cells function in the manufacture of heparin (an anticoagulant) and histamine (an inflammatory substance responsible for changes in allergic tissue). Depression in mast cell activity results from the administration of cortisol to patients. Areolar tissue is the basic supporting substance around organs, muscles, blood vessels, and nerves forming the delicate membranes around the brain and spinal cord and comprising the superficial fascia, or sheet of connective tissue, found deep in the skin.

Adipose Tissue. Adipose tissue is specialized areolar tissue with fat-containing cells. The fat or lipid cell, like other cells, has a nucleus, endoplasmic reticulum, cell membrane, mitochondria, and one or more fat droplets. Adipose tissue acts as a firm yet resilient packing around and between organs, bundles of muscle fibers, nerves, and supporting blood vessels. Since fat is a poor conductor of heat, adipose tissue protects the body from excessive heat loss or excessive rises in temperature.

Reticular Tissue. Reticular fibers consist of finely branching fibrils taking a silver stain as observed under the microscope. The primary cell of the reticular fiber is the reticular cell. Reticular fibers form the framework of the liver, lymphoid organs, and bone marrow.

Dense Connective Tissue

Dense connective tissue is composed of closely arranged tough collagenous and elastic fiber. It can be classified according to the arrangement of the fibers and the proportion of elastin and collagen present. Examples of dense connective tissue having a regular arrangement of fibers are tendons, aponeuroses, and ligaments. Examples of dense connective tissue having an irregular arrangement of fibers are fasciae, capsules, and muscle sheaths.

Specialized Connective Tissue

Cartilage. Cartilage has a firm matrix consisting of protein and mucopolysaccharides. Cells of cartilage, called **chondrocytes,** are large and rounded with spherical nuclei. Collagenous and elastic fibers are embedded in the matrix, increasing the elastic and resistive properties of this tissue. The three types of cartilage are hyaline, fibrous, and elastic.

In utero, **hyaline cartilage**, the precursor of much of the skeletal system, is translucent with a clear matrix caused by abundant collagenous fibers (not visible as such) and cells scattered throughout the matrix. Hyaline cartilage is gradually replaced by bone in many parts of the body through the process of ossification; however, some remains as a covering on the articular surfaces. The hyaline costal cartilages attach the anterior ends of the upper seven pairs of ribs to the sternum. The trachea and bronchi are kept open by incomplete rings of surrounding hyaline cartilage. This type of cartilage is also found in the nose.

Fibrous cartilage contains dense masses of unbranching, collagenous fibers lying in the matrix. Cells of fibrous cartilage are present in rows between bundles of the matrix. Fibrocartilage is dense and resistant to stretching; it is less flexible and less resilient than hyaline cartilage. Fibrous cartilage, interposed between the vertebrae in the spinal column, is also present in the symphysis pubis, permitting a minimal range of movement.

Elastic cartilage, which is more resilient than either the hyaline or the fibrous type because of a predominance of elastic fibers impregnated in its ground substance, is found in the auricle of the external ear, the auditory tube, the epiglottis, and portions of the larynx.

Bone is a firm tissue formed by impregnation of the intercellular material with inorganic salts. It is living tissue supplied by blood vessels and nerves and is constantly being remodeled. The two common types are **compact,** forming the dense outer layer, and **cancellous**, forming the inner lighter tissue of the shaft of a long bone.

The **dentin** of teeth is closely related to bone. The crown of the tooth is covered by enamel, the hardest substance in the body. Enamel is secreted onto the dentin by the epithelial cells of the enamel organ before the teeth are extruded through the gums. Dentin resembles bone but is harder and denser.

Blood and Hematopoietic Tissue. Marrow is the blood-forming (hematopoietic) tissue located in the shafts of the bones. The red blood cells (erythrocytes) and most white blood cells (leukocytes) originate in the capillary sinusoids of bone marrow. Some leukocytes are formed in the lymphoid organs.

Blood is a fluid tissue circulating through the body, carrying nutrients to cells, and removing waste products.

Lymphoid tissue is found in the lymph nodes, thymus, spleen, tonsils, and adenoids. The germinal centers of lymph tissue produce plasma cells and lymphocytes. Lymphoid tissues function in antibody production.

Connective tissues perform many functions, including support and nourishment for other tissues, packing material in the spaces between organs, and defense for the body by digestion and absorption of foreign material.

Reticuloendothelial system. Connective tissue cells, carrying on the process of phagocytosis, are frequently referred to as the reticuloendothelial system. The cells ingest solid particles similar to the manner in which an amoeba takes in nourishment. Three types of phagocytic cells belong to this classification; reticuloendothelial cells lining the liver (Kupffer's cells), spleen, and bone marrow; macrophages, termed tissue histiocytes or "resting-wandering" cells; and microglia, located in the central nervous system. The reticuloendothelial system is a strong line of defense against infection.

Synovial Membranes. Synovial membranes line the cavities of the freely moving joints and form tendon sheaths and bursae.

In order to better understand passage-based problems, answer the following questions for yourself before moving to the pre-marked passage below.

(a)	How long is this passage? (answer in number of words)	___ no. of words
(b)	How much time did it take to read the passage?	___ no. of minutes
(c)	What is the main idea conveyed in the passage?	______________
(d)	Did you mark up the passage to extract information?	___ yes ___ no
(e)	Do you remember 20 new or difficult terms? (do not re-read passage)	___ yes ___ no
(g)	Which parts of the passage were most difficult?	______________
(h)	Is there irrelevant information in the passage?	___ yes ___ no

The marked up passage that follows illustrates active reading. Its important points are marked by underlines, circles and other relevant notations. Compare your mark-up of the passage above with the sample mark-up below. How accurate were you in marking the various key points?

Connective Tissue: General Characteristics and Functions

Connective tissue allows movement and provides support. In this tissue there is an abundance of intercellular material called matrix, which is variable in type and amount and is one of the main sources of difference between the types of connective tissue. It consists of various fibers embedded in a ground substance.

Loose Connective Tissue

The fibers of loose connective tissue are not tightly woven. The tissue, filling space between and penetrating into the organs, is of three types: areolar, adipose, and reticular.

Areolar Tissue. The most widely distributed connective tissue is pliable and crossed by many delicate threads; yet, the tissue resists tearing and is somewhat elastic. Areolar tissue contains fibroblasts, histiocytes (macrophages), leukocytes, and mast cells.

Fibroblasts are small, flattened, somewhat irregular cells with large nuclei and reduced cytoplasm. The term fibroblast refers to the ability of a cell to form fibrils. Fibroblasts are active in repair of injury. It is generally believed that suprarenal steroids inhibit and growth hormones stimulate fibroblastic activity. **Histiocytes** are phagocytic cells similar to **leukocytes** in blood; however, they perform phagocytic activity outside the vascular system. The histiocyte is irregular in shape and contains cytoplasmic granules. The cell is often stationary (or "fixed"). **Mast cells**, located adjacent to small blood vessels, are round or polygonal in shape and possess a cytoplasm filled with metachromatic granules. Mast cells function in the manufacture of heparin (an anticoagulant) and histamine (an inflammatory substance responsible for changes in allergic tissue). Depression in mast cell activity results from the administration of cortisol to patients. Areolar tissue is the basic supporting substance around organs, muscles, blood vessels, and nerves forming the delicate membranes around the brain and spinal cord and comprising the superficial fascia, or sheet of connective tissue, found deep in the skin.

Adipose Tissue. Adipose tissue is specialized areolar tissue with fat-containing cells. The fat or lipid cell, like other cells, has a nucleus, endoplasmic reticulum, cell membrane, mitochondria, and one or more fat droplets. Adipose tissue acts as a firm yet resilient packing around and between organs, bundles of muscle fibers, nerves, and supporting blood vessels. Since fat is a poor conductor of heat, adipose tissue protects the body from excessive heat loss or excessive rises in temperature.

Reticular Tissue. Reticular fibers consist of finely branching fibrils taking a silver stain as observed under the microscope. The primary cell of the reticular fiber is the reticular cell. Reticular fibers form the framework of the liver, lymphoid organs, and bone marrow.

Dense Connective Tissue

Dense connective tissue is composed of closely arranged tough collagenous and elastic fiber. It can be classified according to the arrangement of the fibers and the proportion of elastin and collagen present. Examples of dense connective tissue having a regular arrangement of fibers are tendons, aponeuroses, and ligaments. Examples of dense connective tissue having an irregular arrangement of fibers are fasciae, capsules, and muscle sheaths.

Specialized Connective Tissue

Cartilage. Cartilage has a firm matrix consisting of protein and mucopolysaccharides. Cells of cartilage, called **chondrocytes**, are large and rounded with spherical nuclei. Collagenous and elastic fibers are embedded in the matrix, increasing the elastic and resistive properties of this tissue. The three types of cartilage are hyaline, fibrous, and elastic.

In utero, **hyaline cartilage**, the precursor of much of the skeletal system, is translucent with a clear matrix caused by abundant collagenous fibers (not visible as such) and cells scattered throughout the matrix. Hyaline cartilage is gradually replaced by bone in many parts of the body through the process of ossification; however, some remains as a covering on the articular surfaces. The hyaline costal cartilages attach the anterior ends of the upper seven pairs of ribs to the sternum. The trachea and bronchi are kept open by incomplete rings of surrounding hyaline cartilage. This type of cartilage is also found in the nose.

Fibrous cartilage contains dense masses of unbranching, collagenous fibers lying in the matrix. Cells of fibrous cartilage are present in rows between bundles of the matrix. Fibrocartilage is dense and resistant to stretching; it is less flexible and less resilient than hyaline cartilage. Fibrous cartilage, interposed between the vertebrae in the spinal column, is also present in the symphysis pubis, permitting a minimal range of movement.

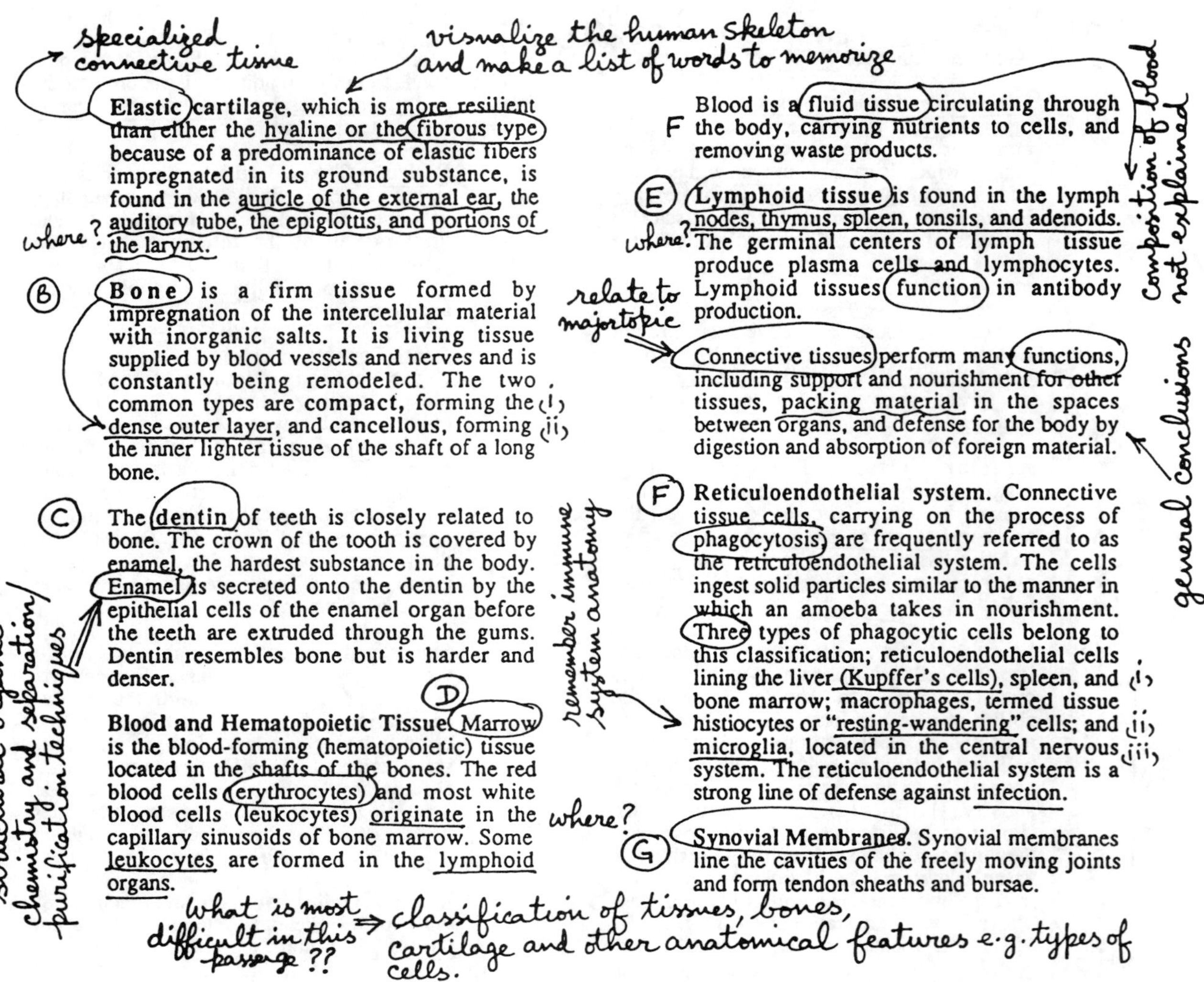

Elastic cartilage, which is more resilient than either the hyaline or the fibrous type because of a predominance of elastic fibers impregnated in its ground substance, is found in the auricle of the external ear, the auditory tube, the epiglottis, and portions of the larynx.

Bone is a firm tissue formed by impregnation of the intercellular material with inorganic salts. It is living tissue supplied by blood vessels and nerves and is constantly being remodeled. The two common types are compact, forming the dense outer layer, and cancellous, forming the inner lighter tissue of the shaft of a long bone.

The dentin of teeth is closely related to bone. The crown of the tooth is covered by enamel, the hardest substance in the body. Enamel is secreted onto the dentin by the epithelial cells of the enamel organ before the teeth are extruded through the gums. Dentin resembles bone but is harder and denser.

Blood and Hematopoietic Tissue. Marrow is the blood-forming (hematopoietic) tissue located in the shafts of the bones. The red blood cells (erythrocytes) and most white blood cells (leukocytes) originate in the capillary sinusoids of bone marrow. Some leukocytes are formed in the lymphoid organs.

Blood is a fluid tissue circulating through the body, carrying nutrients to cells, and removing waste products.

Lymphoid tissue is found in the lymph nodes, thymus, spleen, tonsils, and adenoids. The germinal centers of lymph tissue produce plasma cells and lymphocytes. Lymphoid tissues function in antibody production.

Connective tissues perform many functions, including support and nourishment for other tissues, packing material in the spaces between organs, and defense for the body by digestion and absorption of foreign material.

Reticuloendothelial system. Connective tissue cells, carrying on the process of phagocytosis are frequently referred to as the reticuloendothelial system. The cells ingest solid particles similar to the manner in which an amoeba takes in nourishment. Three types of phagocytic cells belong to this classification; reticuloendothelial cells lining the liver (Kupffer's cells), spleen, and bone marrow; macrophages, termed tissue histiocytes or "resting-wandering" cells; and microglia, located in the central nervous system. The reticuloendothelial system is a strong line of defense against infection.

Synovial Membranes. Synovial membranes line the cavities of the freely moving joints and form tendon sheaths and bursae.

Answers to questions (a) through (h):

(a) This passage consists of around 500 words (average the number of words per line and multiply by the number of lines). Knowing the passage length enables you to estimate your working time and adjust your speed.

(b) You should spend no more than 5 minutes reading this kind of passage. Furthermore, passage reading time should be only **half** the time spent reading and answering the questions.

(c) If you made a mind map you know the passage is about structure, function and types of connective tissue. The mind map is also a visual index to the passage that helps identify items for later reference.

(d) This is reinforcement to mark the passage for details. Use long arrows or leaders to connect terms that repeat in the passage, e.g., arrows connecting the use of words such as fibroblasts and histiocytes.

(e) Use your mind map to find 20 terms, including: loose tissue, dense tissue, areolar, adipose, reticular, fibroblasts, fibrils, histiocytes, cytoplasmic granules, mast-cells, metachromatic granules, hyaline, ossification, cartilage, chondrocytes, fibrous cartilage, elastic cartilage, elastin/collagen ratio, phagocytic cells, leukocytes, resilient, etc. Add any new terms to your vocabulary notebook. A sample mind map for this passage follows below.

(f) You should be able to write one or two paragraphs based on your marked-up passage and mind map. A summary repeats important things in a passage and impr oves your short-term memory of its content.

(g) The most difficult part of a passage has the most details. A solution to mastering the details is in making a mind map, which will help you to remember the details because they are written down.

(h) Information that you do not use to answer questions is unused information, but do not consider it irrelevant. Irrelevant information is usually limited in such passages (textbook or encyclopedia information).

DEVELOP A "MIND MAP" AS YOUR EYES TRAVEL FROM BEGINNING TO END OF THIS PASSAGE

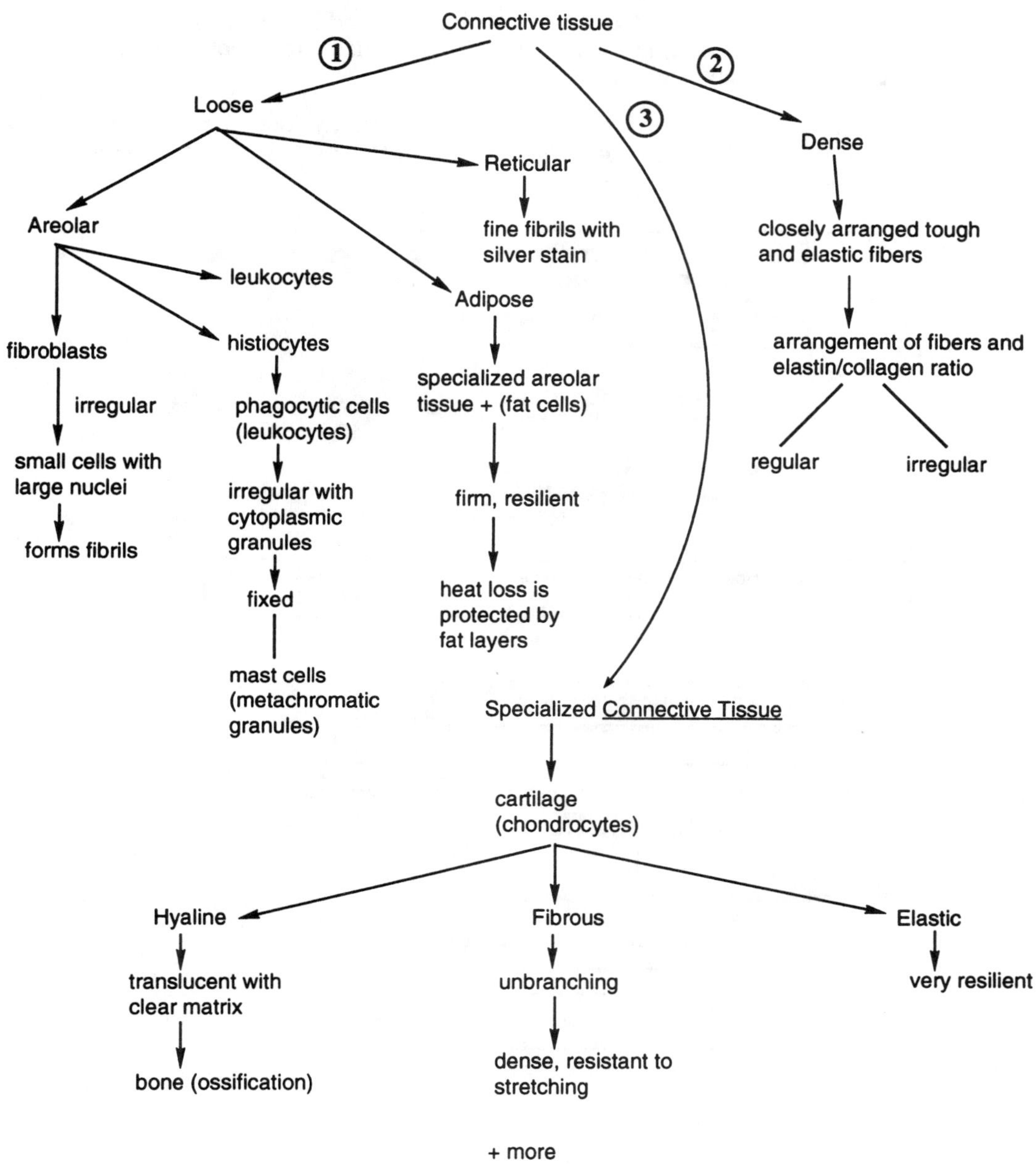

2.4 STEPS FOR CONDUCTING AN EFFECTIVE MCAT SCIENCE REVIEW

Conducting a major review over an area as broad as the MCAT physical and biological sciences can be an intimidating process. But with an organized review approach, you can utilize your time more wisely, cover more information, and learn more effectively.

There are four key elements in a systematic review: environmental considerations, preliminary planning, content review, and practice for maximum effectiveness. Let us consider each of these points in greater detail, referring to section 2.2.1 for environmental considerations.

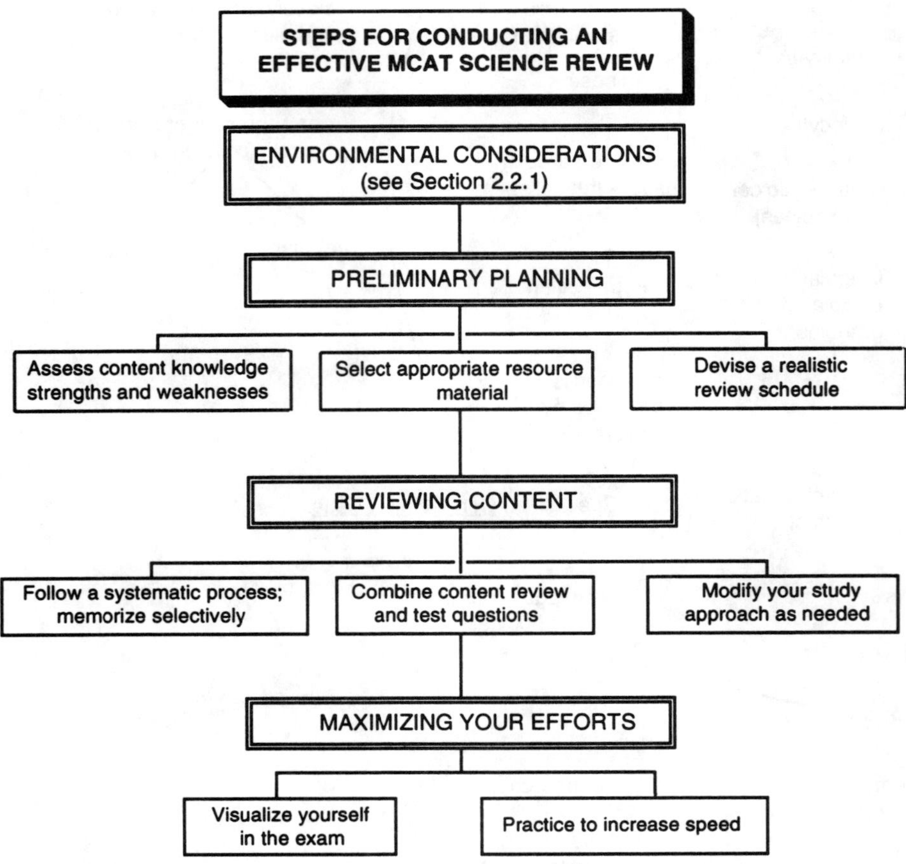

2.4.1 Preliminary Planning

Getting started is the hardest part of preparing for a comprehensive science review. Careful planning, however, can smooth the way and allow you to progress in the most efficient and effective manner. There are three areas to consider in the planning stages.

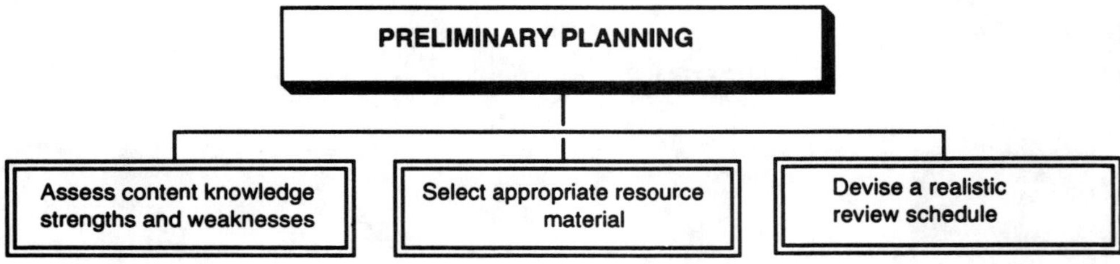

Assess Content Knowledge Strengths and Weaknesses

Start your review by determining the scope of the task and by assessing your strengths and weaknesses in relevant content areas. Obtain the *MCAT Student Manual* and the published MCAT test packages from either the AAMC or Betz Publishing Company. Used properly these materials will guide you in evaluating your strengths and weaknesses against the content areas named.

Select Appropriate Resource Material

Select carefully when you choose the resource materials to use for content review. Your primary resources should be those materials with which you are already familiar. New books or materials often have a different style and/or organization. This takes time to get used to and slows you down. If you are familiar with several resource books, use the one that provides the most comprehensive coverage of the subject. If the book you choose is generally complete in most sections but weak in a particular area, use another resource to supplement this topic and then go back to your original resource. Do not jump back and forth among a large number of study materials because your review will become disjointed.

Devise a Realistic Review Schedule

You already know the importance of preparation, but you probably have some concerns about how you can incorporate additional time into your schedule for MCAT review. Since time cannot be expanded, the only alternative is to use it efficiently. The following are suggestions for maximizing the use of your time.

Establish an Agenda. Determine exactly what it is that you need to accomplish in a given period of time. Itemize the areas you need to review. Then segment the whole into parts to make your job more manageable and bring greater organization to your process.

Set Goals. Once you have identified the areas to be reviewed, set goals for each area. Your review will be more focused if you write out exactly what you want to accomplish. Use the following worksheet to construct an outline of your goals, adding as many more pages as you need to complete the task. Be sure to compare your goals and sub-goals with the subjects covered in this book and the *MCAT Student Manual* to be sure you are concentrating on relevant topics.

SAMPLE WORKSHEET FOR SETTING REVIEW GOALS
(study the example first)

Topic: Molecular Biology

Major Goal: Review of Enzymes

Sub-goals: General function and importance in catalyzing biochemical reactions
Basic principles of enzyme specificity
Enzyme cofactors
Feedback inhibition

Topic: ______________________________

Major Goal:
____

Sub-goals: ______________________________
____
____
____

Topic: ______________________________

Major Goal:
____

Sub-goals: ______________________________
____
____
____

2.4.2 Reviewing Content

Now you are ready to begin your science review. The following suggestions are made to help you in your overall MCAT preparation as you work with this book, *A Complete Preparation for the MCAT.* Since the test is both long and difficult, you will want to do everything possible to ensure that you only have to take it once.

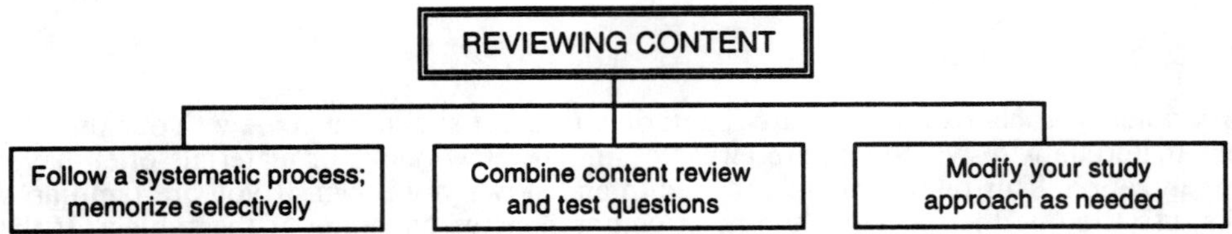

Follow a Systematic Process

As you develop your review approach, there are two guiding points to keep in mind in order to be effective: 1) incorporation of highly active learning strategies, and 2) timely and varied repetition.

Since frequent exposure to content is one of the most important factors in long-term retention, your study approach should not only include a plan for initial learning, but for repetition as well. However, not all review approaches are as effective as others. Although many students rely on multiple re-readings to review, this is one of the least effective approaches. Each time you re-read, the act becomes more and more passive as your eyes begin to see words your brain no longer processes. Re-reading everything is also time-consuming, making this a very impractical approach when large volumes of information must be covered. Another problem is that you tend not to distribute your time according to where you need it most, but you re-read all information equally whether you know it well or not. A focused approach to reviewing will help you to conform to your test preparation schedule deadlines and also to review with your own special goals in mind:

A FOCUSED REVIEW APPROACH

1. As you study, do not leave gaps in your information base when you are studying with the assumption that somehow it will all become clear later on.

2. To review a topic, first determine what you remember instead of going immediately to a text or notes.

   Hint: Start with a blank sheet of paper and brainstorm on the topic for five to ten minutes. What main subdivisions of the topic do you recall? Write them down on your paper. (A good format is to use relational mapping, which is explained in section 2.2.3.) Now look at the logical divisions of the topic that you have written down and jot down as much detail as you can remember. Even if you think you have not remembered very much, push yourself to put down as much as you can. Now evaluate your relative strengths and weaknesses on the topic.

   What did you find? Chances are that you remembered a lot of information in some areas, a modest amount in others, and very little in the remaining areas. However, you will have accomplished a great deal by going through the exercise. This highly active process helps you to achieve a high level of concentration very quickly so that you avoid wasting a lot of time getting warmed up. You also will know how to best distribute your time, since you will be able to identify those areas needing only a quick review and those that require more time.

3. Selectively re-read according to your content strengths and weaknesses. In areas where your recall of information was good, skim over the information in the book or your notes to confirm accuracy and to make sure you did not forget something important. Slow down and read more carefully in places where your recall was incomplete. You will find that any re-reading you do at this point tends to go much faster. Selective re-reading after brainstorming tends to be a much more active process since you are actively looking for specific information to fill in the gaps on your map.

4. Periodically, stop reading and summarize what you have just read. Talk to yourself and actually put into words what you think is important. Include a statement of the main idea as well as relevant details which develop the main idea. If information is missing in the notes you jotted down while brainstorming, add it to your notes at this time.

5. To confirm your understanding and to consider the information from a different perspective, try to predict test questions you think a professor might ask and then try to answer them.

6. During the next day spend 5-10 minutes reviewing the topic again by quickly trying to reconstruct your notes from memory. Since the literature shows that the greatest loss of learned information occurs during the first 24 hours, repetition of the previous day's information at this time is very important. If you do not include this step, when you finally come back to review you will find yourself in the position of having to rebuild a significant portion of your foundation.

7. On weekends, try to summarize what was important from the week. If you keep to this schedule, your review will go very quickly because information you studied during the week is still fresh in your mind.

Memorize Selectively

In general, our ability to memorize information is very poor compared with other societies and other times. This is partly because we rely heavily on the written word to accumulate information gradually. Thus the science courses you took before college were supposed to build a foundation for those you took in college. And now both are supposed to provide a foundation for medical school.

Early review should concentrate on the conceptual understanding of a topic and its component parts. Developing the conceptual framework of understanding encourages long-term memory retention. For example, learning the functions and what goes on at each step of the circulatory system is a long-term memory task. Drawing it or explaining it to another person helps you to synthesize information and provides an additional avenue for reinforcement.

Routinely memorize important points at periodic intervals to enhance your ability to retrieve specific information. However, do not try to do this at the same time that you are also trying to gain a basic conceptual understanding. Memorizing should come only after you have achieved understanding of the concepts. You develop long-term memory by focusing on conceptualization, not on memorizing details.

Distinguishing Short-term from Long-term Memory Tasks. In the cumulative information model of how memory works, there is an assumed distinction made between long-term memory and short-term memory. An example of a short-term memory task might be remembering a doctor's appointment. Once you have kept the appointment, you "erase" the date and time. Anything that you intentionally memorize, perhaps because you have a test the next day, tends to be stored in your short-term memory and gets erased after the test just as the medical appointment is erased.

The point to remember here is that rote memorization is a short-term memory technique, while long-term memory is based on understanding what it is you have read or learned. You retain the information you really understood when you took biology in high school. The understanding formed the foundation for subsequent learning. But you also probably memorized areas of high school biology that you didn't really understand. This helped you pass the tests, but did not create a strong foundation for subsequent learning. A better approach to learning biology would be to learn biological concepts. If you *understand* as you learn, the information stays with you longer. The best way to know you have done this is to explain the topic to someone who knows enough about the subject matter to act as a critical listener (see "Study Partners," 2.2.1).

Research shows that unless you review what you have read or heard before you go to sleep at night, you will have forgotten more than 90 percent of it twenty-four hours later. High school is set up to take advantage of this because most classes are held every day. But when you go to college, classes come every other day or with an even longer time between sessions. To improve your retention, you need to review your class notes every night before you go to sleep, or tell a friend about your class over lunch. If you are preparing for the MCAT, the same principle applies. Unless you review what you have gone over for that day, you will not remember it. The study preparation time for the MCAT will have been largely wasted unless you build immediate review time into your schedule. You may want to combine your chart of "things done during the day" with review of "things you have learned today."

Remember also that constant use contributes to long-term memory. Your chemistry teacher knows a great deal about chemistry and has a remarkable amount of information that he or she can talk about easily without referring to notes or books. This is partly because your chemistry teacher thinks about and works with chemistry every day. If he or she didn't think about it at all for a while, a great deal of information would fade. While preparing for the MCAT, think about various subject areas each day.

Learning the circulatory system well is a long-term memory task; it requires you to understand what happens at each step as the blood enters and leaves the heart. As you discuss or draw it, explaining it to your study partner, you will be storing it in your long-term memory. You may also go to the physiology and anatomy labs and carefully examine models of animal organs such as the heart and kidneys. You may have the opportunity to observe and feel actual organs, holding each one under a water faucet where you can observe the flow of water through each organ and observe its texture. If you visit a drugstore and look at the labels of prescription and non-prescription drugs, it may help to remember chemical names, symbols, and units of measurement for chemical compounds. This will give you a real-life exposure to chemicals and a basic preparation in stoichiometry. For example, what are the ingredients in aspirin? Can you draw the molecules of the ingredients? Using many different approaches to understanding a topic helps you retain the details as well as reinforce the concepts. You will improve your long-term memory by explaining biological concepts, by repeating your lessons or review material, by observation and by making drawings.

Repetition and drawing are keys to long-term learning, as is anything that encourages retention of visual images. An example in a difficult subject like organic chemistry might be that three-dimensional perception may be improved by buying plastic model molecules and observing changes in structure by changing atoms or groups with these organic molecular structures. Using visual props in this way, you can actually observe and correct the kinds of mistakes you make in organic chemistry.

Short-term Memory Tip. Short-term memory items are used and then forgotten, unlike long-term memory which you develop by focusing on conceptualization and not on memorizing details. Three months before the test, do not waste your time memorizing seldom-used equations or short-term information such as a comparison of smooth, skeletal, and cardiac muscles. When working items that require short-term memory information, solve the problem with the information in front of you. During the last few days of your study time and just before taking the MCAT, commit to memory what you have identified as short-term memory tasks and on the test day itself take a few minutes after the exam begins to write out some of those short-term items in the margins of the test booklet so that you have them to use without having to hold them in your memory.

Combine Content Review and Test Questions

Making time in your study routine for practice test questions is an excellent way to evaluate and reinforce learning. Practice questions provide you with additional exposure to the subject matter and enhance long-term retention. Much can also be learned from test questions, which encourage you to consider the information from a different perspective and which can be an effective indicator of study problems. An analysis of your error pattern may indicate specific patterns of weaknesses. For example, you may find that your error analysis identified questions reflecting deficits in the areas of broad concepts, details, and/or relationships. An additional benefit of working with test questions is that you receive feedback on your study effectiveness early enough to be able to do something about it.

Try to formulate MCAT-type questions while you study or read. Develop four response choices to each test question you write, considering what is false or the exception as well as what is true. This is especially important when the text provides a concept and one or two examples. The examples are important for understanding but not for memorizing because the test maker is unlikely to use those precise examples in a test item. Rather the test maker will check to see if you can understand "new" examples by applying your understanding of those you were given in textbooks or in class.

As you work through test questions, you may identify and review topics that were not listed on your goal sheet. Take time to address these topics if you find your information base is weak. Also consider the pattern of your content weaknesses. If you have determined that you are studying disproportionately between basic concepts and details, modify your strategies to obtain better balance. You may want to do additional practice questions to monitor your progress as you make changes.

Modify Your Study Approach as Needed

Modify your study approach for the MCAT by performing the following tasks, which require both analytical and synthetic reasoning:

1. **Divide major topics into subtopics--**Example: divide a major topic in molecular biology into subtopics, e.g., enzymes divided into enzyme structure, enzyme function, enzyme activity, etc.

2. **Divide subtopics into study units called concepts--**Example: divide enzyme structure into concepts, e.g., substrate specificity, stereospecificity, geometric specificity, coenzymes, etc.

3. **Divide each concept into learning components--**Example: separate the concept of stereospecificity into learning components, e.g., definition of stereospecificity, examples of stereospecificity, sketch illustrating chiral stereospecificity, experimental basis of stereospecificity, application of stereospecificity to biochemical reactions.

4. **Connect concepts in one subject to concepts in another to create interdisciplinary concepts.--** Example: once you have divided a major topic into learning components (steps 1-3) the interdisciplinary concepts can then be created. For example, you have divided reaction rates of chemical reaction into activation energy, reaction rate law, temperature dependence of reaction rate (general chemistry). Following that, combine concepts in task 2 with these general chemistry concepts, e.g., reaction rate law for coenzymes, activation energy and substrate specificity of chymotrypsin, sterospecificity, and temperature dependence of chymotrypsin, etc.

5. **Integrate interdisciplinary concepts.--**Example: task 4 illustrated how biology and general chemistry concepts are synthesized. These in turn should be studied in the context of verbal reasoning (passage evaluation, passage type and format, appraising strength of evidence from an experiment), mathematics concepts (graphs for reaction rate law, balancing molecular reactions for coenzymes, determining equilibrium constants from kinetic data, determining catalytic efficiency), and studying and analyzing experimental and instrumental investigations in mini-passages (X-ray studies, research reports on bisubstrate mechanisms and types, etc.).

THE ANALYTICAL PROCESS CHART

Return to your worksheets on setting review goals. Check to be sure your goals cover mixed content. Your review must reflect the interconnection of subjects because this is the way it will be presented to you in the MCAT. The Analytical Process Chart below shows interrelated subject matter at all levels, from undergraduate courses to the MCAT content outline topics. Note that the Chart includes mapping techniques, which are to be used in deciphering passages, and math techniques, which are to be used in solving problems.

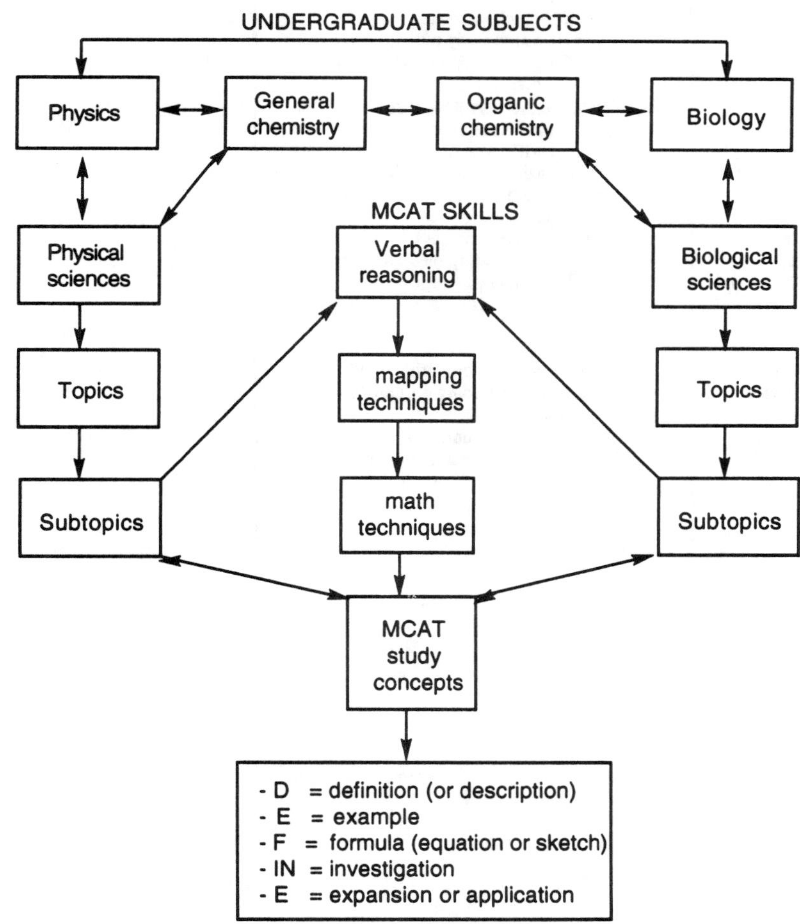

The main point is to examine how one subject can be related to others in order to study within a conceptual framework. Relationships of this kind should be evident in the review goals you set. (Review goal worksheets were developed earlier in this chapter.) As you read research reports and journals during your review, there may be instances where by chance you discover a connection between two concepts. Show these relationships in your review goals and search out other areas where you have not yet made logical connections. An example of

EXAMPLE OF THE ANALYTICAL PROCESS

General Chemistry Topics

1. Stoichiometry

1 a Ability to work with chemical formulas, chemical reactions, and resulting equations and to balance them.

1 b The ability to understand moles and their intersection with chemical formulas and equations.

1 c Memorizing the process and learning transformation of electronic structures (outer shell electrons) into oxidation numbers or valency numbers.

1 d The ability to perform stoichiometry calculations with speed and accuracy.

1 e The ability to apply and extend concepts learned in stoichiometry to one or several experimental situations, with emphasis on compare/contrast relationships among experiments.

1 f The ability to discover, determine, and use chemical relationships between interacting elements and their products as chemical compounds in a chemical reaction.

2. Rate Processes in Chemical Reactions

2 a The ability to determine several rates of chemical reactions in relation to several levels of completion.

2 b The learning of various concepts related to equilibrium states of a chemical reaction and its relation to rates of chemical reactions, including (a) for preferred reaction, determination of limiting conditions (physical and chemical), and (b) for unpreferred reactions, determination of limiting conditions (physical and chemical).

2 c A complete, in depth conceptualization of kinetically controlled or thermodynamically controlled reactions.

2 d Complete linkage to experimental/theoretical biological situations, such as metabolic pathways using enzyme as catalysts.

2 e Application of kinetics and equilibrium concepts to various types of chemical reactions.

Verbal Reasoning

1. Evaluation (accuracy, consistency, relevance, or reliability)
2. Application (Solve problems and interpret hypothetical situations)

Passage Format and Classification

1. Information Passages
   a. Source: Textbook or journal articles
   b. Structure: Assume background knowledge
      - New information
      - New *uses* of information
2. Problem solving passages
   a. Source: Chemistry or physics situations (descriptive)
   b. Structure: Probable causes of situations
      - Events
      - Phenomena
      - Problem-solving methods
3. Research study passages
   a. Source: Research studies (NIH, lab reports, etc)
   b. Structure: Background rationale (whole or part)
      - Research methods
      - Research study results
      - Understanding of underlying research
4. Persuasive argument passages
   a. Source: Newspaper articles, Scientific American magazine/Discover magazine
   b. Structure: Checking for validity of persuasive arguments
      - Looking at pieces of evidence
      - Understanding methodologies
      - Interpretation of particular perspectives on products

Mathematics Concepts

1. The ability to perform arithmetic calculations, including proportion, ratio percentage
2. The use of metric units, the ability to balance equations containing physical units

Biology Topics

Microbiology (topics)

1. Understand viral structures relating to
   a. nucleic acid and protein components
   b. bacteriophage structure
   c. size of viral structures in comparison to bacteria and eukaryotic cells
   d. phage and animal virus life cycles
2. To understand the structural types of fungi
   a. prokaryotic cells
   b. bacteria
3. To understand the structural types of fungi
4. To understand the life history of fungi
5. To learn the physiologic functions of
   a. common viral diseases in animals
   b. prokaryotic cells
   c. bacteria
   d. bacteriophage
   e. fungi
6. Applications of modern microbiology instruments techniques used in research and experimentation.

Exercise. During your review try to make connections between topics (use the content topic outline in the *MCAT Student Manual*). Examples are:

- bonding and hydrocarbons
- wave characteristics and periodic motion in fluids and solids
- equilibrium and momentum of biological molecules
- microbiology of the nervous and endocrine systems
- use of spectroscopy in structural identification of acids and bases.

Exercise. Use analysis to understand the relationship of topics across disciplines. Analysis will help you to reduce your science review to the smaller functional learning units or MCAT study concepts. The mnemonic D-E-F-I N-E includes components that can be used to review an MCAT concept. In the example below, the clue D-E-F-I N-E is applied to the topic 'molarity.' Construct other such exercises for yourself.

D = definition	Define 'molarity' and its relation to concentration measurement.
E = example	Prepare a 0.5 M solution for NaCl (or HCl or NaOH) and determine the pH value of the solution. Can you apply this concept to a real-world situation, experiment or instrument?
F = formula	Is there a formula to find molarity, an equation for molarity, and can you draw molarity on a volume diagram? Yes, molarity is defined as moles/liter; it can also be drawn.
IN = investigation	Investigate concept in detail; compare and contrast molarity, molality, pH, normality, etc.
E = expansion	Expand the topic to other science subjects. Apply the concept of molarity to titration problems. Review acids, bases and salts. Learn how to link physics with chemistry.

THE SYNTHETIC PROCESS CHART

During the analytical process you divided MCAT topics into skills and concepts. Now is the time to combine them across disciplines as this chart suggests. A key to symbols follows this chart.

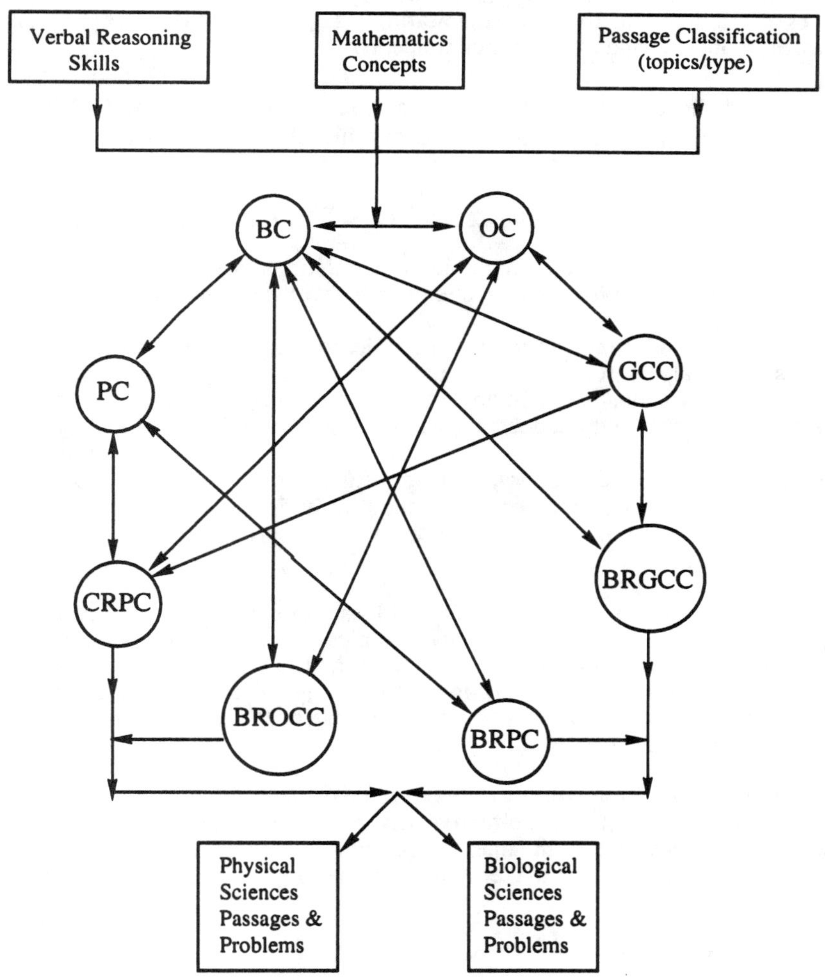

You will need to refer to descriptions of the skills and topic areas shown on the chart. Sources of these descriptions are given below. Note that no sources are available for cross-discipline science concepts. These you develop yourself from information available primarily in the *MCAT Student Manual*.

SYMBOL	TOPIC	SOURCE
-	Verbal Reasoning Skills	*MCAT Student Manual*
-	Mathematics Concepts	*MCAT Student Manual.*
-	Passage Classification, by topics or format	*MCAT Student Manual* and Appendix A
PC	Physics concepts	*MCAT Student Manual*
GCC	General Chemistry concepts	*MCAT Student Manual*
BC	Biology concepts	*MCAT Student Manual*
OCC	Organic Chemistry concepts	*MCAT Student Manual*
CrPC	Chemistry-related Physics concepts	student develops list
BrPC	Biology-related Physics concepts	student develops list
BrGCC	Biology-related General Chemistry concepts	student develops list

EXAMPLE OF THE SYNTHETIC PROCESS

The synthetic process recombines information disclosed in the analytic process. Referring to the lists on page 2-36 above, understand how review of combined topics should enable you answer the following questions.

BIOLOGY TOPICS: Microbiology

1. Have your read and understood a persuasive argument passage or article and evaluated it for accuracy, consistency, or reliability? Assume an article uses various AIDS-related viral studies and conceptualizes the kinetic or thermodynamic control studies to develop an AIDS vaccine. Were special laser microscopic studies carried out in the experimentation? **Topics:** verbal reasoning skills, biology-related general chemistry concepts and mathematics concepts.

2. Do you understand the chemical structure of a special HB2-γ virus and how the chemical structure affects its life cycle? **Topics:** biology-related organic chemistry concepts and passage classification concepts.

GENERAL CHEMISTRY TOPICS: Stoichiometry and Rate Processes in Chemical Reactions

3. Can you quickly and accurately do stoichiometry calculations of kinetically controlled or thermodynamically controlled reactions? **Topics:** general chemistry concepts and mathematics concepts.

4. Can you apply and extend concepts learned in stoichiometry to one or several experimental situations using enzymes as catalysts for metabolic pathways, with special emphasis on comparison-contrast relationships among various experiments? **Topics:** biology-related general chemistry concepts, biology-related organic chemistry concepts, passage classification and verbal reasoning skills.

More Examples of the Synthetic Process. During your review try to mix topics such as "bonding and hydrocarbons," "wave characteristics and periodic motion in fluids and solids," "equilibrium and momentum of biological molecules," "microbiology of the nervous and endocrine systems" and "use of spectroscopy in structural identification of acids and bases."

The content topic outline in the *MCAT Student Manual* lists 9 topics in general chemistry, 11 topics in physics, 20 topics in physical sciences, 12 topics in biology, 6 topics in organic chemistry, and 18 topics in biological sciences. Theoretically there are approximately 703 combinations possible to make mixed-subject passages. Texts in biochemistry, biophysics, microbiology, physiology, histology and pharmacology will give you practice in reading advanced passages. As you read be aware of the basic science (biology, chemistry and/or physics) that is fundamental to the passages.

Finally, as you progress toward the MCAT, always refer to the content topic outline in the *MCAT Student Manual* to guide your review. For greatest effectiveness, remember to employ timely and varied repetition and highly active learning strategies such as the ones suggested in this section. Use the Synthetic Process Chart as a final clue to the many ways you or a test maker may combine subject matter and skills testing for a good review and a fair exam.

2.4.3 Maximizing Your Efforts

After you have constructed and implemented a review plan, there is one final stage left in your preparation—PRACTICE. The more practicing you do, the more confident and better equipped you will be to do well on the test. Consider the following as you work on this stage:

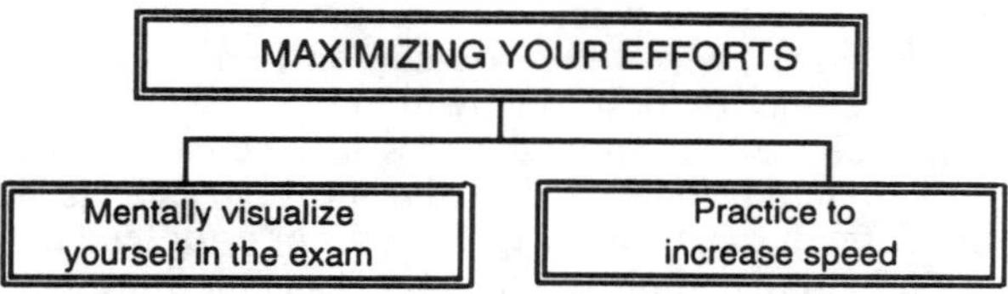

Mentally Visualize Yourself in the Examination

You want to be comfortably relaxed when you take the MCAT. The best preparation plan may fall flat if anxiety takes hold and reduces your ability to think logically. Anxiety is often the by-product of worrying about the unknown. By conditioning yourself to the idea of successfully taking the examination, you will be better able to control your anxiety. Deliberately think positive thoughts. You have reason to do so! You have taken all the prerequisite courses. You have done a systematic review of relevant content areas. In addition, you have worked to develop the test-taking skills that will allow you to be in control. In other words, YOU ARE READY. Thinking about the familiarity of the typical classroom setting should give you some reassurance. Picture yourself receiving your test booklet and opening it. Again this is a very familiar experience. You have done this many times before.

Finally, visualize yourself actually taking the test. You have had a lot of practice taking tests in your courses and your MCAT preparation has involved working with many test questions. If there is one thing that you have experience with, it is answering test questions. What do you think the MCAT questions will be like? Compare your perceptions with the models and exercises included in this manual. As you visualize yourself taking the test, do not dwell on how difficult the questions might be. Rather try to keep your thinking in perspective by reminding yourself that there will be a range of difficulty as on any other test. Some questions will be easier, some more challenging but manageable and only a percentage will be truly difficult.

Most worries are about the test itself. However, as you try to visualize yourself in the exam, are there any other concerns that come to mind? Do you find yourself worrying about the temperature of the room, or getting hungry, etc.? If you identify something specific, then develop a plan ahead of time to eliminate the problem.

Walk through this scenario frequently until thinking about the test finally feels comfortable.

Practice to Increase Speed

In the earlier section on reviewing content, it was suggested that you divide your time between content review and working with test questions. As you work with test questions concentrate not only on content, but also on your problem-solving strategies as well. When your approach is solid and starts to feel comfortable, begin to add time constraints as a variable. If you are particularly slow, you may want to try to increase your speed in gradual steps. Start out at a speed that feels just slightly faster than normal and each day push yourself to work a little faster than before. You should record the time spent in the early practice stages, but not impose a time limit. Once you know how long it takes to complete a unit or a passage-question set, begin to work within specified time limits.

Keep track of your progress as you increase your speed. Use a clock to monitor the time used to answer each question. Do not rely only on your own perception of whether or not you are working faster. If your accuracy decreases as you speed up, slow down and practice longer at that speed. As your accuracy stabilizes, begin again to gradually increase your speed.

Look for Patterns of Error. Remember that student errors will be evenly spread across all the alternate answers in a test maker's ideal multiple-choice item. This means that each distractor ideally represents typical student errors. To complicate matters, we each tend to have patterns of errors that we repeat over and over unless an intervention strategy is introduced.

When you make an error, note whether you say to yourself, "I always have trouble with Boyle's law" (or whatever causes you difficulty). Such an admission is usually followed with a rationalization, "It's not that I don't know it, it's just that the test items confuse me." We often tend to confuse recognition with knowing or understanding. If you cannot explain a concept clearly to someone who knows it well and who thus would know how accurately your reasoning is, you really do not know the concept. Use graphic or mapping skills to better understand any concept you tend to forget.

The first step in correcting error patterns is to recognize when they occur. The second step is to develop a mnemonic or memory device. Apply your device every time you see an item in the category you have identified. For example, it may help you to remember Boyle's law by thinking of your car. As you step on the accelerator, the piston goes down and as the volume decreases, the pressure increases. You can even draw a picture in the margin of the test booklet to remind yourself. But the message here is that if you need a mnemonic, you must apply it every time the difficult topic comes up. Patterns of error tend to be well developed and they do not lend themselves to correction by rote memorization alone. Chapter 8 presents the error journal model to use when you work with test items. The following chart gives you a list of reasoning patterns associated with integrated premed skills. Try to analyze your error patterns on problems that you solved incorrectly. Correlate your error patterns, reasoning skills and typical integrated premed skills.

Tips on Linking Reasoning Patterns to Integrated Premed Skills	
WHY? **WHAT?** **WHEN?**	Look for physiological interpretation or functional reasoning (partly visual, partly conceptual and partly relational) Example: system to system connections such as renal-to-nervous (CSF-to-distal tubule).
HOW? **WHAT IF?**	Understand various components of a biochemical or biophysical process (partly sequential, partly analytical and partly conditional) Example: renaturing and denaturing of DNA based on iterative kinetics, including newest research methods.
WHERE? **WHAT?**	Look for word roots before anatomical memorization or locational understanding (mostly visual, partly word roots and definitions) Example: learning differences between decidua parietalis, decidua basalis and decidua capsularis.
HOW? **HOW MANY?** **WHAT IF?**	Investigate mechanical reasoning or inside working (mostly putting parts of a mechanism together, operational reasoning, partly linking all possible permutations) Example: parts and operation of an electromagnetic rail gun. MCAT instruments or mechanical devices may be REAL or HYPOTHETICAL. You should know PROCEDURES to operate EQUIPMENT without catastrophe.
WHAT IF? **HOW?** **WHERE?** **WHEN?**	Correlate investigations (partly lab experience; partly decision making: Hypothesis, Conclusions, Assumptions, Objectives, Data Presentation techniques; partly comparative and proportional reasoning) Example: Tooth decay due to soft drinks.

Chapter 3

Verbal Reasoning

3.1 VERBAL REASONING AND CRITICAL THINKING

The format of the MCAT is designed to assist medical schools in selecting candidates who have breadth and flexibility in their thinking and who exhibit competent analytic skills within the demands of longer, more complex materials. While the earlier MCAT used a reading subtest to evaluate comprehension skills, the current test samples those skills but with two primary differences: nine prose passages are selected from the humanities, social sciences, and natural sciences, and the reasoning skills tested focus on higher level comprehension, which is frequently referred to as critical thinking skills.

Since the MCAT is designed to assess levels of critical thinking, it will not only test factual knowledge, but will examine how well you handle inference and argument. It also will test your ability to comprehend, evaluate, apply and incorporate new information. This chapter presents the most widely used MCAT verbal reasoning question formats, as well as some variations found in medical school examinations. This broad-based approach is provided through a range of practice examples in order to help you develop critical thinking skills .

MCAT verbal reasoning passages range in length from 500 to 600 words, accompanied by 6 to 10 questions each based on information in the passage. According to the *MCAT Student Manual*, passages may be selected from a range of subjects in 26 major fields. Since the range of information is potentially so broad, you are not expected to have a detailed knowledge of the subjects. Instead it is expected that your reading and related skills are developed enough to produce the answers to questions from the information given. A familiarity with the vocabulary of different disciplines can be most helpful to you now, which suggests the need for you to continue to read from a diverse number of sources. Many such sources are suggested in this book.

There are patterns in reasoning that you may not be using consciously, but which can be learned to your advantage for the MCAT and beyond. This chapter and the following problem solving chapter (chapter 4) present those patterns in the form of study materials and exercises that can help you build more effective analytical reasoning skills. Your study may be as detailed as you choose, since the information in this book covers nearly all of the critical thinking skills you will need, both for the MCAT and for your classwork. Reasoning patterns and exercises of many types are included in both of these chapters.

3.1.1 Verbal Reasoning Skills Assessment

The information you gather from using this inventory will be helpful in showing how well you have developed your skills in verbal reasoning and it can act as a basis for setting your goals for improvement.

Basic Reading Skills:	**I do**	**I do not**
Establish the purpose of the information.	_____	_____
Scan information for sense of organization.	_____	_____
Understand main concepts after reading information one time.	_____	_____
Determine details relevant to the development of the main idea.	_____	_____
Identify the organizational pattern.	_____	_____

Critical Thinking Skills:	**I do**	**I do not**
Identify relationships among the facts.	_____	_____
Prioritize relevant information.	_____	_____

	I do	I do not
Apply information to new situations.	_____	_____
Determine relevant interpretations.	_____	_____
Infer from given information.	_____	_____
Differentiate premises from conclusions in arguments.	_____	_____
Draw logical conclusions	_____	_____
Evaluate strength of conclusions.	_____	_____

3.2 READING COMPREHENSION AND CRITICAL THINKING

Some readers may consider skipping over this section. It may be that after spending years reading for your education and enjoyment you feel you can gain little in a few pages on reading improvement in a book like this. In some respects, this may be true since reading is a skill you practice over a long period of time. However, there are two important aspects to consider relative to your background in reading and your achievement on the MCAT:

1. Has your practice of reading skills led to a standard that ensures your success in medical school?
2. Can practice that is directed to reading and critical thinking improve academic performance?

In addressing these issues, first review your answers in the Verbal Reasoning Skills Assessment. Did you find yourself thinking "I sometimes do that" or "I should do that"? If so, then you may find that your comprehension skills are vulnerable in the MCAT Verbal Reasoning test.

Another equally important issue is whether practice in reading and critical thinking skills can be improved and result in subsequent improvement of academic performance. There is evidence to support the idea that positive changes occur when students learn strategies to improve the way they think about concepts and ideas. Reading can serve as an important vehicle for practicing thinking skills.

3.2.1 Reading Like a Detective

Thinking about your reading skills, it may be useful to consider this familiar process from a new perspective. A reader is very much like a detective involved in cracking an important case. What attributes do you bring to your task? Curiosity? Observation? Guidelines and procedures? To be an effective reader, you need to develop the same types of skills as a detective and practice them until you feel competent.

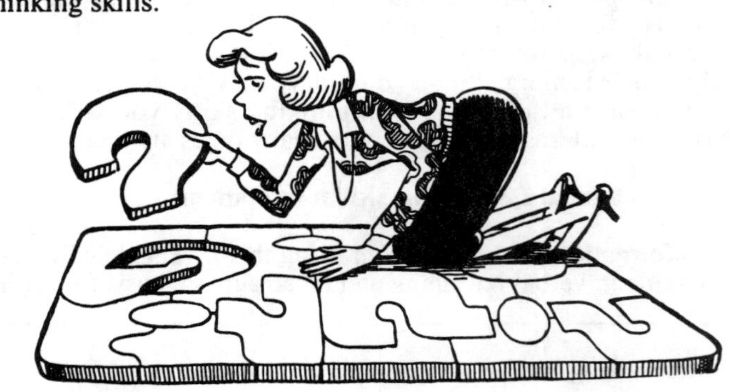

A common error to guard against in taking the MCAT is reading too quickly and answering questions based upon incomplete knowledge. You may be tempted to rush through the passages and then grab at responses that have superficial relativity. If you were to operate this way as a detective, you might find that the pieces of information you obtained were randomly gathered and compiled in a haphazard manner. This would lead to hasty and premature conclusions founded on what feels right rather than on established facts. If a suspect were indicted by evidence gathered with this approach, the case would probably be thrown out of court and your ego badly bruised by the district attorney for failing to consider all of the evidence. In order to make a stronger case, a detective should uncover the relevant information hidden in all the pieces of evidence. Information that was not relevant would systematically be put aside or discarded so as not to confuse the issue.

To avoid bruised egos and shoddy investigation, restrain your impulse to jump to a conclusion without full study of the evidence (whether you are working the MCAT or a detective case). Study the techniques of good investigation and apply them to the reading process. You should note a much improved comprehension and evaluation ability, knowing how to apply your knowledge while incorporating new information. This meets the objectives of the MCAT Verbal Reasoning test.

Consider how as a detective you might approach a case. You enter the crime scene and immediately scan the surroundings. Why? Probably to establish early impressions and appraise the situation. You are also looking for anything unusual that might be of further importance in the investigation.

After a cursory inspection, your first question may be, "What has happened here?" The purpose or motive underlying the crime will determine the selection of investigative tools used to solve the case. For example, investigating computer theft for the purpose of altering and destroying records could necessitate much different strategies than those used in solving a kidnapping case.

It would be unlikely for a good detective to overlook any truly obvious clues: a fired weapon on the floor, a smashed window, or a broken lock. While others in a flurry of activity start with details, such as combing the carpet for hair samples or checking the windows for fingerprints, you concentrate your attention on broadly surveying the scene for obvious clues that might lead to solving the case. Once the basic clues of the crime are uncovered, you move quickly into selecting the method to use for further investigation. This step necessitates a reliance on details as well as established evidence, but you must also piece together the pattern of events that lead to a conclusion.

Finally, you test the premises and conclusions used in solving the case to determine if the conclusions drawn are relevant, compelling, and provide a logical interpretation of information gathered from many sources. Throughout the investigation you continue to work in an organized and efficient manner.

In somewhat the same way as a detective approaches the clues in a case, the requirements of the MCAT encourage you to follow sequential steps in your approach to reading passages.

3.2.2 Steps for Active Reading

RULE #1: SURVEY THE PASSAGE

In the same way that a detective surveys the scene and becomes actively involved, you should scan a reading passage noting its length, whether tables or graphs are included, presence or absence of a summary, and unusual vocabulary. This does not take long, but it does provide a reference point for beginning to assemble the passage clues.

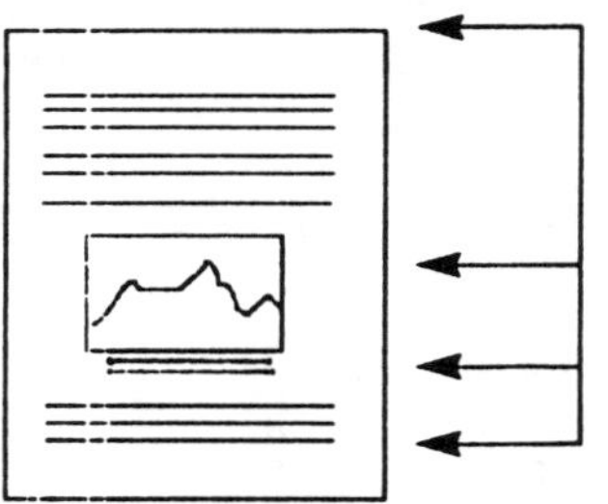

* Note passage length.
* Check for conclusion.
* Scan graphics and read legends

RULE #2: DETERMINE THE PURPOSE

Following your initial survey, estimate the purpose of the passage. In the MCAT passages, you may find that the purpose is to inform, to present an opinion, or to present a controversial view or idea. Usually, a quick check of the first and last paragraphs will indicate the purpose of the passage. Based on a closer reading of the passage, however, you may later need to refine your earlier observations.

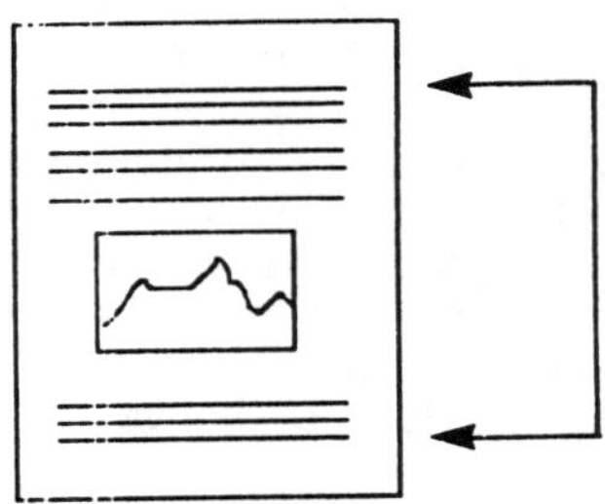

* Check for the purpose.

RULE #3: IDENTIFY THE MAIN IDEA

Unless you are reading dialogue, virtually every paragraph you read on the MCAT will have a "smoking gun"—a clue so central to the passage that it cannot be ignored. You can be sure that the writers of MCAT test questions are going to want to know if you read in enough depth to understand the fundamental elements of the passage. They may use various formats, as in "Which of the following phrases best describes the central idea of the passage?" or "The main topic of this passage is . . ." or "The author's primary emphasis is upon . . . ." But as you can observe, each of these questions implies that you are able to identify the main idea when it is embedded in text.

How do you practice this skill? Try the following: First, use the checkmark system while reading and look in the obvious places. The author will usually place the main idea in the following locations: beginning of the paragraph, ending of the paragraph, or middle of the paragraph. Second, after you read the paragraph or passage, it is easier to pull out these important foundational pieces if you say to yourself, "What is the most important thing I need to remember?"

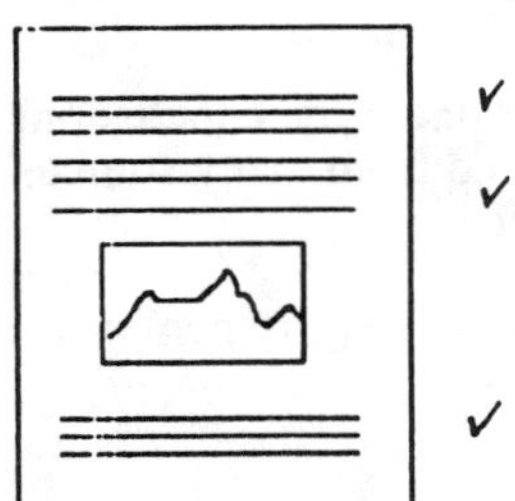

* Use checkmark system

* Watch for placement of main ideas in paragraphs.

RULE #4: LOOK FOR THE WRITER'S METHOD

Determining the method of passage development is frequently neglected by students during their examination preparation, but nearly always included by test constructors. It is essential, once you have identified the main ideas of the paragraphs, to analyze the manner in which these ideas are linked together. (This skill relates directly to the discussion under relational maps in the note-taking section.) On the test don't try to skip directly from identifying the main idea to the questions. It may leave you without preparation for the variety of test questions that are based on understanding the connections among ideas. Instead, you may want to consider which pattern is being used to organize the information.

Reviewing the discussion in chapter 2, there are passage format patterns that most typically arise on tests. You should now be able to identify them quickly. They are:

- Cause and effect
- Classification
- Comparison and contrast
- Word usage (definition)
- Process
- Reasons
- Spatial or geographic
- Time order

RULE #5: UNDERSTAND VERBAL CLUES IN PASSAGES

A key requirement for the MCAT Verbal Reasoning section is to adjust your reading skills to the varied conventions of writing in fields outside the natural sciences. Unlike typical science readings, data are unlikely to appear in the way you are accustomed to seeing them. In fact, you will rarely encounter numerical data in the MCAT Verbal Reasoning section. A fact to a chemist or a biologist is not necessarily the same as a fact to a literary critic, political scientist or historian. Your job as test taker is to be flexible in your reading approach. As you read, account for differences in the vocabulary used in the writing of experts in a wide variety of fields.

The new MCAT requires you to understand passages in humanities, social sciences, and natural sciences—not an easy task. It will require you to comprehend quickly what subject the passage exposes, what position (if any) the author takes on the subject, and what the implications are of the author's point of view. You may not agree with arguments presented by the author, but you need to avoid the temptation of superimposing or adding your own point of view into the passage (either based on your prior knowledge or personal convictions). You must differentiate how the <u>author</u> thinks about a subject and how you connect it to various test items.

Another difficult task is to deal with nuance and ambiguity while you sort through unfamiliar information. Remember that your objective is to answer questions about the passage. Unlike the scientific reading you do in traditional college courses, here you are not trying to understand and remember the material for a future test. You can always refer back to the passage. <u>Do not</u> spend time memorizing lists, names, or other kinds of specifics from the passage. If a question calls for detailed information, look back at the passage and retrieve it. Rather than remembering details, try to get an overall sense of how the author presents and organizes information. A key to the author's organization can often be found in language clues such as signal words.

Signal Words. Signal words are often basic to an understanding of structure, which in turn helps you to comprehend the author's ideas. Signal words help you predict what you will read. As you read the passages, circle or underline words or phrases like those that follow.

<u>Words that indicate a continuous thought</u>: also, first, besides, next, furthermore, then, in addition (to), one reason, likewise, another reason, similarly, for example, moreover, for instance.

<u>Words that indicate a shift in direction (usually opposite)</u>: although, on the contrary, but, otherwise, despite, rather, however, whereas, in spite of, yet, on the other hand, nevertheless.

<u>Words that may signal a list or pattern</u>: many, a few, much, a number of, several, most, another, besides, also, furthermore, too, in addition; one, two, three, etc.

<u>Words that may signal material in order of importance</u>: next; first, second, etc.; then, soon, later, after, finally, subsequently, at last, ultimately, begins, ends, more and most, less and least, worse and worst, better and best.

<u>Words that may signal ideas compared or contrasted</u>: Comparisons—like, as, again, still, likewise, same, similarly. Differences: but, on the other hand, however, on the contrary, rather, in comparison, different, in contrast, instead.

<u>Words that may signal cause-and-effect relationships</u>: because, since, therefore, consequently, so, effects, brought about, is the outcome of, determines, if, then, results, affects, resulted in, as a result (of), for this reason, leads to, thus, either/or.

[Adapted from Shirley Quinn and Susan F. Irvings, *Active Reading*, © 1986 by Houghton Mifflin Co., Boston.]

Trigger Words. Trigger words are another set of clues to help you understand the shades of meaning found in specific words that distinguish the definite (deductive) from the conditional (inductive).

It is vital for you to be sensitive to the nuance of word usage in the MCAT reading passages. By changing a single word, the entire meaning of a passage can be dramatically changed or an otherwise acceptable answer choice can be disqualified. This is particularly true with answer choices that are similar in meaning. Many of the more difficult questions will ask you to determine what the author "suggests" or "implies." With these kinds of questions you must use your judgment, meaning you must evaluate on the basis of the author's argument.

The key to recognizing "best" answers often lies in cues from what we call trigger words. Rather than expending great amounts of energy on comprehending all the information contained in the passage, look for trigger words and circle or underline them. These words may help resolve questions that are ambiguous. For instance, there is a major difference between the statements "I will come" and "I may come." If we were to quantify the phrase "may come," we would look to the general context in which the statement was made and decide upon a likelihood of 25 to 90 percent. But if we see "will come," there is no likelihood—100 percent is the only possibility. "Will" is definite and "may" is conditional and ambiguous.

You can add to the following list. The words themselves are not to be memorized but are here to give you the sense of definite and conditional meaning.

<u>Definite (deductive)</u>	<u>Conditional (inductive)</u>
shows, establishes, proves, confirms, concludes	suggests
always	usually, most
never	often, occasionally, largely
none	rarely
all, any	some, most, prevalent, principally, extensive
same	similar, typical
only	usually
will	can, might, probably
is	seems
every, each	most, usually
constant	normally, primarily
essential, indispensable, necessary	significant, usually

These suggestions are not intended to be applied mechanically. Because you will find some passages more comprehensible than others, these suggestions are given for the following reasons:

- to help you sort through the information presented in a reading passage,
- to identify the key ideas, which includes identification of thesis,
- to recognize where an argument may switch in direction, and,
- to enable you to quickly refer back to the passage to answer questions.

According to the *MCAT Student Manual,* passages may be selected from any of the following 26 major fields: anthropology, archaeology, architecture, art and art history, astronomy, botany, business, computer science, dance, ecology, economics, ethics, geology, government, history, literary criticism, meteorology, music, natural history, philosophy, political science, psychology, religion, sociology, technology and theatre. Given the range of possible subjects that the test designers have, do not be surprised by what you see. Don't panic if the subject of nineteenth century European art (about which you may know very little) appears on the test. What you need to do is identify the author's purpose in the passage and answer questions based on passage information; whether or not you have a deep understanding of nineteenth century European art is emphatically not at issue.

RULE #6: IDENTIFY AND EVALUATE THE WRITER'S ARGUMENTS

What are the writer's arguments regarding a point of view expressed in the passage? While argument analysis is explained in greater detail in section 3.3, you can judge the soundness of the arguments against the following:

- generalizing from limited experience
- begging the question
- avoiding the question
- arguing against the person rather than the issue
- setting up a false dichotomy, etc.

RULE #7: ASSESS CREDIBILITY OF THE EVIDENCE

In the detective analogy, an important step was assessing conclusions drawn against information collected and inferences made. Similarly, it is very important to include this step in reading analysis. Both the detective and the reader must constantly ask whether the evidence gathered and the conclusions made are both logical and truthful. Without these vital skills of critical thinking, many serious errors could be made due to judgments based upon incomplete or false assumptions.

RULE #8: LOOK FOR THE VERBAL REASONING SKILL IN THE ITEM STEM

In order to answer questions efficiently, identify which verbal skill is being tested. The list of 24 verbal skills from the MCAT are your main resource here. Refer to them often to gain the experience you need. Understanding the skill behind the test item will provide a quick clue to its answer. Following is a list of verbal reasoning skills to be used in item analysis. This list is adapted from the *MCAT Student Manual*, page 12.

VERBAL REASONING SKILLS

	STATEMENT OF SKILL	SKILL PERFORMANCE AREA
1.	Identify thesis.	Comprehension
2.	Identify reasons to support thesis.	Comprehension
3.	Identify background knowledge.	Comprehension
4.	Determine meaning of significant vocabulary.	Comprehension
5.	Identify assumptions (stated or unstated).	Comprehension
6.	Judge credibility of source.	Evaluation
7.	Identify a general theory or model.	Application
8.	Recognize a paraphrase of complex information.	Comprehension
9.	Identify comparative relationships.	Comprehension
10.	Recognize questions of clarification.	Comprehension
11.	Judge soundness of an argument or a reasoning step.	Evaluation
12.	Predict result based on content and specific facts.	Application
13.	Judge if reasons lead to a given conclusion.	Evaluation
14.	Use information to solve problem.	Application
15.	Identify probable cause of event or result.	Application
16.	Recognize scope of application of hypotheses and conclusions.	Application
17.	Appraise strength of the evidence.	Evaluation

VERBAL REASONING SKILLS
(Continued)

	STATEMENT OF SKILL	SKILL PERFORMANCE AREA
18.	Distinguish between supported and unsupported claims.	Evaluation
19.	Judge relevant information related to argument.	Evaluation
20.	Determine implications of conclusions or results.	Application
21.	Recognize alternative hypotheses or solutions.	New information
22.	Determine how to modify conclusions to incorporate new information.	New information
23.	Judge the effect of new evidence on conclusions.	New information
24.	Recognize methods or results that challenge given models, hypotheses or theories.	New information

3.3 ARGUMENT ANALYSIS

3.3.1 Understanding Arguments

The MCAT includes passages that involve argument analysis. For that reason it is beneficial to review the structure of logical thinking. The term "argument" is not meant in the sense of a conflict with winners and losers. Rather, it is a reasoning process based upon elements of logic. Arguments consist of statements that are called propositions. These propositions can be either true or false. The structure of the argument is comprised of a set of propositions that can be used as premises or conclusions.

Here is an example of an argument:

Poodles do not shed.	Proposition #1
Joan's dog is a poodle.	Proposition #2
----------	----------
Therefore, Joan's dog does not shed.	Conclusion

You can see from the example that the first two propositions serve as premises leading to a conclusion. Signal words can help you to discriminate premises from conclusions. Premises might be indicated by words such as *in addition to, and, because, but, since,* and *for that reason.* Conclusions may be indicated by *therefore, thus, as a result, consequently,* and *finally.*

At times in a passage you may sense a gap between the premise and the conclusion. In these cases, there may be an unexpressed premise: "Sue's third set must have won the tennis match." Clearly, there is an underlying assumption that must be identified.

Stated premise:	Sue won the third set.
(Unstated premise:	If a three-set tennis match goes into the final set, the winner of the set will win the match.)
----------	----------
Conclusion:	Sue won the match.

As you work through longer examples, it is important to differentiate the premise and premise support from the conclusion. Consider the following:

<u>Argument 1</u>: Some coaches and administrators say that athletic shoe companies, through promotional deals with coaches, are exerting too much influence on college sports. Therefore, promotional endorsements should be eliminated.

<u>Argument 2</u>: Some coaches and administrators say that athletic shoe companies, through promotional deals with coaches, are exerting too much influence on college sports. In some cases, coaches' connections with these companies are inappropriately determining a student's choice of school. Therefore, promotional endorsements should be eliminated.

As you can observe in the first example, there is a linkage between the influence of promotional deals with coaches and the conclusion that these arrangements should be ended. In the second example, there is specific support for the premise, which is that the relationship between the coaches and promotional contracts is affecting a student's choice of school due to financial inducement. In evaluating premises leading to a conclusion, it is important to separate premises from premise support. You can then judge the strength of support given as additional evidence.

While considering the way in which arguments are constructed, keep in mind that there are two general patterns. Inductive thinking begins with specifics, which in combination lead to a general conclusion. By contrast, deductive thinking begins with a conclusion and the supporting evidence must be constructed. For example, a scientist may assemble his observations about life and derive a general conclusion. (Columbus did not fall off the edge of the world, therefore, the earth must be round.) Similarly, an attorney knows the general charge or conclusions made about his client, and must construct an explanation of innocence.

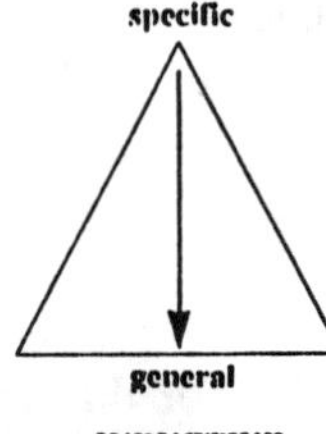

INDUCTIVE

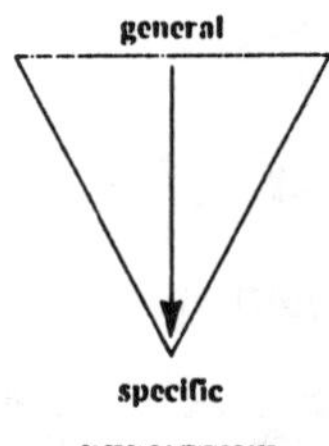

DEDUCTIVE

While reading MCAT verbal reasoning passages, judge the method of logic development. If you recognize the pattern of organization, it will help you predict the questions to follow. Since the verbal reasoning passages are in the form of argument, you need to determine how well prepared you are to understand argument. Of course, the MCAT passages are accompanied by multiple-choice questions so you also need to determine how well prepared you are to answer questions about the content of arguments. A third component of your preparation assessment should be to ask yourself how well prepared you are to answer questions about arguments in a given time frame. Following is a brief explanation of argument that may help to orient you to the MCAT verbal reasoning passages.

3.3.2 Structure of Arguments

In an argument, a writer takes a position on an issue and provides support for the position in an effort to persuade the reader. Thus the concept of argument is straightforward. The position the writer takes, however, may be called a claim, thesis, proposition, assertion or conclusion. The claim may be explicitly stated or implied. If stated, it may be found in the beginning, middle, or end of the argument. There are three broad categories of claims: fact, value and policy. Writers often clue their readers by prefacing their claims with words and phrases before the author's position is presented, for example:

therefore	then
hence	it follows
so	in summary
thus	as a result
consequently	proving/suggesting that

To substantiate a position, writers offer examples, definitions, descriptions, comparisons, contrasts, classifications and/or statements of cause and effect relationship. These writing devices are referred to as premises, backing, appeals, evidence, reasons, data, support or opinion. A number of words provide clues that substantiate an author's position, for example:

because	given that
for	as shown by
since	in the first place
if	whereas

Usually claim and support for the claim constitute an argument. A writer may, and often does, provide more information for the reader's consideration. An argument may be strengthened by the writer acknowledging that there is another side to the issue. In effect, s/he is giving the counterargument, rebuttal, or opposing viewpoint. Assumptions, generalizations or warrants underlie the writer's position and may or may not be included in the argument.

Writers reason both inductively and deductively in the course of persuading the reader. The process of reasoning dictates the form and direction of the argument and each requires a different evaluation approach. If you are studying argument as a form of discourse, one of your goals is to be able to evaluate arguments. You learn to examine the components of the argument and test the inevitability of the conclusion in a deductive argument and the probability of the conclusion in an inductive argument. Below is a discussion about detecting fallacies, which forms the basis for evaluating arguments.

3.3.3 Detecting Fallacies

The discussion above reviewed the structure of arguments as well as the reasoning processes they employ. When the premises are true and the reasoning process is accurate, then the argument is considered valid. However, this is not always the case. Observe the difference in the following examples:

Fallacy of Premise:	All men can cook. John is a man. Therefore, John can cook.
Fallacy of Logic:	Many mothers have a nurturing instinct. Betty is a mother. Betty must have a nurturing instinct.

As the examples illustrate, fallacies can occur either in the structure of the argument (whether the premises and conclusions are true) or in the reasoning process itself. Also fallacies can be identified within single sentences or within the context of passages.

There are many types of fallacies identified by authors writing in the field of critical thinking. For the purpose of studying for the MCAT, ten fallacies have been selected for review here. They are:

1. Appeal to authority: Use of an inappropriate authority figure to give credibility.
2. Appeal to tradition: Support based upon long-held beliefs and notions, rather than upon facts held about a topic.
3. Argument from analogy: An analogy in which there are not enough points of similarity or difference to substantiate a comparison.
4. Begging the question: Circular argument in which the premise and the conclusion contain the same information.
5. Either-or: Forced choice where other alternatives are possible.
6. Equivocation: Intentionally vague language.
7. Hasty generalization: Conclusions drawn from insufficient information.
8. Non sequitur: Irrelevant premise used as a basis for a conclusion.
9. Semantical ambiguity: Words used with multiple-meanings or in an unclear manner.
10. Slippery slope: One event precipitously leading to others.

3.3.4 Evaluating Arguments

In the process of evaluating an argument, you have to ascertain whether the writer did or did not use fallacious reasoning while trying to persuade the reader. For the MCAT you will not have to name any fallacies. However, you may be asked to consider a line of reasoning that would weaken an argument. You could evaluate each option by asking yourself whether the statement is ambiguous, introduces irrelevant information, or whether it presumes too much. Note that this discussion of argument evaluation is not sufficient for enabling you to function in a logic or rhetoric course. The description of argument provided here is to orient you to the passages you will read on the MCAT.

MCAT verbal reasoning passages are selections from published works. You will find a citation at the end of each one that tells you who wrote the passage, in what year and for which audience. Don't ignore this information. Your understanding of the passage—and your ability to evaluate the argument put forth by its author—can be enhanced by knowing when the passage was published and who was writing for whom. Once an argument is identified in an MCAT verbal reasoning passage, the following is a list of steps to take in evaluating it.

1. Evaluate factual and inferential claims.
2. Test to see if the argument is valid or invalid.
3. Check whether the premises and/or conclusions are true or false.
4. Differentiate between sound and unsound, cogent and not cogent, in evaluating an argument.
5. Classify an argument as deductive or inductive and test the claims of the author's argument as:

Deductive Arguments	Inductive Arguments
1. Valid and sound	1. Strong and cogent
2. Valid but unsound	2. Strong but not cogent
3. Invalid (unsound)	3. Weak (not cogent)

3.4 CHANGING READING BEHAVIORS

Your biggest problem in taking the MCAT is the possibility of resorting to old habits under pressure of time and uncertainty. Therefore, if you are to improve your reading and verbal reasoning skills with the certainty that they will be natural to you on the day of the test, you must develop and practice an approach that is both comfortable and adaptable. Practice often well in advance of the MCAT so that you can concentrate on the passages you confront rather than on the process. In your practice, emphasize the transference of skills learned when practicing different types of content-related passages. Finally, the remainder of this chapter is devoted to practice exercises. You can come back to them more than once.

3.4.1 Practice Exercises

Before beginning the practice exercises, quickly look back over this chapter and refresh your memory on the patterns of reasoning and the process recommended for critical thinking. You may also find the chapter on test-taking skills useful. From this information, you should be able to determine the personal skills that you want to develop in order to improve and to synthesize approaches that are most effective for the MCAT.

TIPS FOR BECOMING A CRITICAL READER:

- Read at least two pieces of lengthy and complex materials each week.
- Treat reading as an analytical exercise.
- Watch the tone of the passage or the author's attitude toward a particular idea.
- Detect implied or expressed assumptions involved in an argument or a specific chain of reasoning.
- Recognize how resolutions to conflicting facts or arguments are made.

VERBAL REASONING PASSAGES

Below are verbal reasoning passages in MCAT format. They provide exercises in critical thinking and reasoning skills, based on the list of 24 skills on page 12 of the *MCAT Student Manual.* In certain passages there is less than the 6 to 10 questions usually found with each passage. For those passages, space is provided for you to construct questions of your own. This is an excellent way to improve passage analysis and develop the understanding of critical thinking skills required for the MCAT.

Passage #1 (Questions 1–6)

There are many paradoxes about the nuclear age in which we live. Recognizing them is an important first step on the road to resolving them. The Neanderthal had little patience with paradoxes, puzzles, and games. If he recognized them at all, he either bulled his way through or promptly forgot. Homo Sapiens, on the other hand, had always been intrigued by such logical problems; in fact, paradoxes have often been the steppingstones to his highest achievements in philosophy and science. Here are a few of the paradoxes of the world today.

Paradox I. The greater the destructive capacity of the weapons in our hands, the less most people seem to worry about it. I have heard it estimated by a physicist friend of mine that if all the destructive energy in nuclear weapons now stockpiled were to be transformed into 10 million tons of TNT and so forth—and if then it were to be spread evenly over the surface of our country, we would all be wading around nearly up to our ankles in dynamite! Be that as it may, it is certainly true that never before in human history have so few been able to destroy so many and so much in so little time. Yet how many people are as worried about this as they are about the next raise or about what the fellow next door thinks of them? How many intellectuals have fully committed themselves to working on this problem, which surely by all odds is the most significant of all times? How much effort have our mass media given to the search for fresh alternatives to war? Let one madman loose on the streets of our town, and we form citizens' posses; but let hundreds of millions of tons of destruction hang over our heads, and we couldn't be less concerned, apparently.

Paradox II. While feverishly engaged in a nuclear arms race, both sides express peaceful intentions and fervently hope that these weapons will never be used. I believe that these hopes and intentions are sincere, on both sides. Nobody wants a nuclear war. Yet roughly half the national budgets of the two polar powers go into military preparations—that is, into producing things no one expects ever to use. The Russians resume testing, and we condemn them for polluting the air with radioactive fallout. And then, with almost the same breath, we claim we must also resume testing in the atmosphere, to keep ahead in the arms race and thereby defend ourselves. Surely future generations will look back upon these grim years as the Age of Unreason.

Paradox III. The more nations spend for what they call "Defense," the less real security their people have. Who will deny that over the past ten years we have been steadily increasing our expenditures for weapons? And who will deny that now we are really less safe, less secure, less defended than ever before in our national history? The reason for this is to be found in a basic fact about military technology in a nuclear age. This is the fact that offensive capability has completely outstripped defensive capability. Policy-makers are fond of talking about great defensive "shields" or "umbrellas," but these defenses are more in men's minds than their weapons. Defense in this nuclear age adds up to more than mutual fear.

Paradox IV. The greater a nation's military power, the less seems to be its freedom of initiative in foreign policy. Witness the squashing of the Suez situation, the attempts on all sides to neutralize Laos, the Soviet backdown in the Congo, or the ambivalence of the mighty American elephant in dealing with the little Cuban mouse. Quite apart from fears of retaliation, the mere possession of nuclear weapons has a sobering, restraining effect. For rational men, at least, possession of power brings along with it a sense of responsibility. And so we find this nuclear age characterized by a Great Freeze on initiative in foreign policy.

1. The author's primary contention is that:

   A. there are many paradoxes in the nuclear age.
   B. the spending on defensive weapons is equal to the spending on offensive weapons.
   C. Neanderthal man had little understanding of puzzles.
   D. spending on national defense provides security.

2. The author states that the greater the military power:

   A. the greater is the ability to defend one's self from aggression.
   B. the greater is the need to develop more sophisticated weaponry.
   C. the less flexible is the area of foreign policy.
   D. the less flexible is the area of foreign aid.

3. The author believes that in the nuclear arms race:

   A. nations respond only to perceived threat.
   B. the Russians break arms agreements more than the U.S.
   C. more than half of the national budgets for the polar powers has been used for military preparation.
   D. the polar power countries have not acted in a reasonable manner.

4. According to the passage, which of the following statements is true?

   I. Nations in the nuclear age often act in an irrational manner.
   II. The behaviors of nations can be compared to the behaviors of individuals.
   III. Nuclear science has brought about the age of missiles and bombs.

   A. I, II, and III
   B. I and II
   C. I only
   D. II and III

5. A current day example, such as an arms accord agreement between the U.S. and the Soviet Union to reduce nuclear and chemical weapons while permitting underground nuclear testing, would:

   A. strengthen the author's position.
   B. weaken the author's position.
   C. neither strengthen nor weaken the author's position.
   D. eliminate Paradox II and Paradox IV.

6. In the statement, "Defense in this nuclear age adds up to more than mutual fear," the author implies:

   A. countries have a mutual distrust for each other.
   B. defense is costly to the countries involved.
   C. defense is not based upon nuclear fear.
   D. defense is more complex than economic or political realities.

Passage #2 (Questions 7–11)

The archaeological dig on the Hanson Trust site by Southwark Bridge in London has found an entrance to the original Globe. How far past the entrance it will be possible for archaeologists and theatre historians to go will depend in large part on what judgment the British government makes about the value that the site may have. The dig has confirmed what was always suspected, that nearly half of the theatre's original site is under Southwark Bridge Road, and most of what has survived subsequent rebuilding is under the row of late eighteenth-century houses, until recently offices for the brewery which owned the site, now known as Anchor Terrace. The level of the cellar floors in Anchor Terrace is about three feet above the grade level where a cross section of the Globe's remains might be found, so there is a good chance that in the end more than forty percent of the Globe's original circuit could be excavated. But Anchor Terrace has a preservation order on it, and it already leans some way from the vertical. Heavy digging in its cellarage might imperil the building, not to mention the archaeologists, and digging up Southwark Bridge Road would certainly have a distinct effect on London's traffic-flow; thus the question of whether to dig for the rest of the Globe becomes complicated and political.

The exploratory dig by the Museum of London team of archaeologists has found a lot more that just the theatre's precise location and a small slice of its perimeter walls. Essentially, what the dig has found is a stair turret. This means a great deal to the scholars who have been trying to work out what its structure was just from the pieces of paper that comprised all the evidence previously available. Wenceslas Hollar's drawing of the second Globe, from which his "Long View" was made, shows a building about one hundred feet in outside diameter, with two stair turrets for access to the galleries opposite the stage, located more or less on the east-northeast and north-northeast flanks of a seemingly round structure. What the initial dig seems to have turned up is the foundations of the stair turret on the east-northeast side and sections of the related foundations...

The existence of the stair turret is important not just for its design details but because it differentiates the Globe from the Rose and confirms the conjecture that admission to the Globe was markedly different from the system of admission built into the earlier playhouses. References in contemporary accounts indicate that the Rose and the Theatre had an entry system like that described by William Lambarde in 1596, where audiences "first pa(id) one pennie at the gate, another at the entrie of the Scaffold, and the thirde for a quiet standing." Admission in the early playhouses was first by a gate into the yard, where the "gatherer" collected the first penny. Those who wanted a seat and a roof over their heads paid a second and sometimes a third charge to get into the galleries. Access into these galleries was internal. It went from the yard, most likely by steps like those marked "ingressus" in De Witt's drawing of the Swan....

The Globe opened as the first players' co-operative, with the leading sharers, Shakespeare included, taking yard income as players and gallery money as landlords. Separate gatherers for the different sorts of income may not have been necessary. Possibly the introduction of the stair turrets, if it was an innovation at the Globe, came as a development out of the new system of financial management at the new theatre. But it would be safer to be more pragmatic. By cutting out the gangways needed for internal access up each gallery bay, stair turrets did allow more seating space.

Andrew Gurr, "Notes: A First Doorway into the Globe," *Shakespeare Quarterly*, 41 (Spring 1990): 98–100. Reprinted by permission.

7. The Globe Theatre lies under which of the following:

   I. Southwark Bridge Road
   II. 18th century houses
   III. the Museum of London

   A. I only
   B. I and II
   C. II and III
   D. I and III

8. The author implies that a major benefit of finding the location of the stair turret was that it:

   A. allowed for better measurement of the Globe.
   B. helped identify the original structure of the first Globe Theatre.
   C. helped archaeologists uncover the other turrets.
   D. permitted interpretations on audience payment procedures.

9. According to paragraph three, which of the following had similar entry systems?

   I. Rose
   II. Globe
   III. Theatre

   A. I only
   B. I and II
   C. II and III
   D. I and III

10. The author states that the finding of the turret primarily indicates:

   A. the Globe had more seating capability than previously estimated.
   B. the Globe was built like the Swan.
   C. there were financial payment innovations.
   D. those who entered had to pay three times.

11. True statements regarding further excavation of the Globe include which of the following:

   A. Political/economic issues outweigh the archaeological benefits.
   B. Further excavation will be determined by whether or not it will jeopardize the Anchor Terrace.
   C. The government does not support further excavation.
   D. Making the decision to excavate will not be easily resolved.

Passage #3 (Questions 12–15)

The conventional interpretation of the (Cuban) missile crisis has changed dramatically over the past decade. For many years, it had been argued that the Kennedy administration's handling of the crisis—its ability to calibrate the level of tension and thus to strike just the right balance between firmness and flexibility—had demonstrated that there was a kind of art of crisis management. But by 1987 it had become clear that the standard interpretation had changed. The argument now was that crises between nuclear powers are inherently unmanageable. The missile crisis, it was claimed, was a good deal more dangerous than people had realized. There were so many things that did go wrong, and so many more that could have gone wrong, especially once military action had begun, that the crisis could very easily have gotten out of hand.

This was certainly the view of certain key officials of the Kennedy administration who gathered on a number of occasions to look back and reflect on the crisis. Former Secretary of Defense Robert S. McNamara, for example, argued repeatedly that no one can with any confidence predict how events in a nuclear crisis would unfold, especially if military force is actually used. The way a crisis runs its course would be dominated by such factors as "misinformation, miscalculation, misjudgment and human fallibility." It was therefore "not possible," he said, "to manage a crisis in the nuclear age," in the sense of being able to exercise strong control over how the confrontation works itself out. For McGeorge Bundy, President Kennedy's national security adviser in 1962, the missile crisis appeared in retrospect not as an exercise in successful crisis management; it looked more like a "battle of blunders," and had resulted mainly from a kind of communication failure: "With more foresighted and better informed governments, more able to communicate with each other openly and honestly, the Cuban missile crisis need never have happened." The same sorts of arguments were made by other commentators on the crisis—by Raymond Garthoff, for example, and by Daniel Ellsberg and Seymour Hersh. Greiner here takes a similar line. He speaks, for example, of the Soviets losing "control over military decision-making in Cuba." The dangers inherent in such a situation, he says, were not really understood, and only at the last minute did Khrushchev realize "how close both sides had come to the brink of war."

This new interpretation did not take shape as people tried to come to terms with the new evidence on the crisis that became available over the past decade. Indeed, that evidence should have had the opposite effect. The most important point to emerge from these new sources was that President Kennedy was much more willing to compromise on the issue of the Jupiter missiles in Turkey than had previously been thought. This implied that there was more of a "cushion," more room for diplomatic settlement, and less risk than had earlier been assumed.

This was, however, only the most important of many new findings that pointed—or should have pointed—to the basic conclusion that the risks were not as great as people had thought.

12. In paragraph three, the author refers to "these new sources." To whom is he referring?

- **A.** The commentators listed in paragraph two
- **B.** President Kennedy's presidential papers
- **C.** Khrushchev's memoirs
- **D.** Members of President Kennedy's administration

13. If it were found with release of new documents under the Freedom of Information Act that President Kennedy had been warned of defective firing mechanisms in the missiles in Turkey, what effect would this new insight have upon the author's argument?

- **A.** Would strengthen the author's argument
- **B.** Would weaken the author's argument
- **C.** Would neither strengthen nor weaken the author's argument
- **D.** Would challenge the Freedom of Information Act

14. What does the passage suggest about the current unity of President Kennedy's former administration officials?

- **A.** They have only recently concurred with each other since there has been significant disagreement between them over the years.
- **B.** They have changed their minds over time.
- **C.** They have not had an opportunity to talk with each other about the crisis until recently.
- **D.** They were restrained by the government from discussing the events leading to and during the crisis.

15. In the author's conclusion that the Cuban missile crisis was not as risky as previously assumed, he is basing this observation upon:

- **A.** an analysis of the United States' military strike force.
- **B.** the comments of George McBundy, President Kennedy's national security advisor.
- **C.** reanalysis of President Kennedy's range of options.
- **D.** President Kennedy's skill in crisis management.

Write a question with four responses based on the passage. Base your question on information not used in items above. Use a separate piece of paper, following the format suggested above.

Passage #4 (Questions 16–21)

I passed all the other courses that I took at my university, but I could never pass botany. This was because all botany students had to spend several hours a week in a laboratory looking through a microscope at plant cells, and I could never see through a microscope. I never once saw a cell through a microscope. This used to enrage my instructor. He would wander around the laboratory pleased with the progress all the students were making in drawing the involved, and so I am told, interesting structure of flower cells, until he came to me. I would just be standing there. "I can't see anything," I would say. He would begin patiently enough, explaining how anybody can see through a microscope, but he would always end up in a fury, claiming that I could too see through a microscope but just pretended that I couldn't. "It takes away from the beauty of flowers anyway," I used to tell him. "We are not concerned with beauty in this course," he would say. "We are concerned solely with what I may call the *mechanics* of flars." "Well," I'd say, "I can't see anything." "Try it just once again," he'd say, and I would put my eye to the microscope and see nothing at all, except now and again a nebulous milky substance—a phenomenon of maladjustment. You were supposed to see a vivid, restless clockwork of sharply defined plant cells. "I see what looks like a lot of milk," I would tell him. This he claimed, was the result of my not having adjusted the microscope properly, so he would readjust it for me, or rather, for himself. And I would look again and see milk.

I finally took a deferred pass, as they called it, and waited a year and tried again. (You had to pass one of the biological sciences or you couldn't graduate.) The professor had come back from vacation brown as a berry, bright-eyed and eager to explain cell-structure again to his classes. "Well," he said to me, cheerily, when we met in the first laboratory hour of the semester, "we're going to see cells this time, aren't we?" "Yes, sir," I said. Students to the right of me and to the left of me and in front of me were seeing cells; what's more, they were quietly drawing pictures of them in their notebooks. Of course, I didn't see anything.

"We'll try it," the professor said to me grimly, "with every adjustment of the microscope known to man. As God is my witness, I'll arrange this glass so that you see cells through it or I'll give up teaching. In twenty two years of botany, I—" He cut off abruptly for he was beginning to quiver all over, like Lionel Barrymore, and he genuinely wished to hold onto his temper; his scenes with me had taken a great deal out of him.

So we tried it with every adjustment of the microscope known to man. With only one of them did I see anything but blackness or the familiar lacteal opacity, and that time I say, to my pleasure and amazement, a variegated constellation of flecks, specks, and dots. These I hastily drew. The instructor noting my activity, came back from an adjoining desk, a smile on his lips and his eyebrows high in hope. He looked at my cell drawing. "What's that?" he demanded, with a hint of a squeal in his voice. "That's what I saw," I said. "You didn't, you didn't, you **didn't!**" he screamed, losing control of his temper instantly, and he bent over and squinted into the microscope. His head snapped up. "That's your eye!" he shouted. "You've fixed the lens so that it reflects! You've drawn your eye!"

16. The author states that the reason he was taking the botany course was because:

A. he was a premedical student.
B. he needed it to graduate.
C. he wanted to see the structure of cells.
D. it was required of science majors.

17. Based on the passage, it could be inferred that the professor's attitude toward the author was:

I. encouraging.
II. disbelieving.
III. instructive.

A. I
B. I and II
C. II and III
D. All of the above

18. The phrase "lacteal opacity" in paragraph four means:

A. milky color.
B. differentiated shadows.
C. distinct shapes.
D. darkness.

19. In considering the example provided by the author, the probable outcome of this episode is:

A. the author failed the course.
B. the professor gave him another chance.
C. the student learned from his errors.
D. the student passed by "faking" it.

20. The primary reason the author had difficulty with the microscope probably was due to:

A. the fact that he didn't try.
B. a faulty instrument.
C. poor instruction.
D. the professor adjusting it to his own eyes.

21. The tone of this passage could best be described as:

A. self-congratulatory.
B. irony.
C. degrading.
D. critical.

Passage #5 (Questions 22–27)

Among intelligence, police, and military agencies, there exists no agreement on the definition of *terrorism*. Some parameters need to be delineated and it obviously would be highly desirable if these parameters could be universally accepted. Clearly, this is unrealistic, given the attachment of those doing the defining to their particular views on this emotionally charged and highly political issue.

However, while a definitive description of terrorism might be politically useful, it would not change the nature or gravity of the threat, nor should it affect the way in which our government responds to terrorism.

Over 30 different government agencies are involved in the war against terrorism. Each one perceives and interprets the phenomenon differently. "Think tanks" and the new flock of private terrorist experts exacerbate the problem by adding different biases.

U.S. government definitions have only one commonality. They dismiss the root cause theory, which has been expressed by Yassir Arafat: "Nobody is a terrorist who stands for a just cause." The government does not accept that terrorism—the commission of terrorist acts—is justifiable if used to remedy political or social injustices or for any other reason. Therefore, terrorism cannot subsist as part of a "just" war.

The 1986 Public Report of the Vice President's Task Force on Combatting Terrorism was supposed to be the definitive document regarding international terrorism and the U.S. role in combatting it. The high-level panel of experts who prepared the report defined terrorism as the unlawful use or threat of violence against persons or property to further political or social objectives. Terrorism is generally intended to intimidate or coerce a government, individuals or groups to modify their behavior or politics.

Already the report's definition is outdated, if ever it was valid. (Whose law applies—American, Soviet, Iranian, etc.?) *Violence*, the focal point of this definition, excludes nonviolent acts or passive resistance as well as many actions that are logically considered self-defense. Many actions of terrorists have been destructive and fearsome without being violent. Witness the recent "computer viruses" injected into the Defense Department computer system as one example of the devastating effect a terrorist could have on our nation's infrastructure and ability to defend itself. Rather than taking people hostage, such terrorists hold integral and vulnerable systems hostage. Other nonviolent actions could terrorize populations by disrupting communication or transportation systems. For example, residents of New York could consider stoppage of rush hour traffic to be a terrorist act. Trucks or other barriers placed on all streets leading out of New York City would disrupt and terrorize the lives of millions without physically harming anyone. The spectrum of nonviolent acts is limited only by the imagination of the perpetrators.

The third aspect of the report's definition, that terrorism is to "further political or social objectives," is also too limiting. There are many categories of terrorism that are not motivated by political or social objectives. Narcoterrorism, perpetrated by narcotics traffickers, may be aimed at reducing the threat of competition or capture. Many left-wing European terrorists of the late 1960s were driven by their personal inadequacies and the need to increase the level of fear and anarchy in their victims, believing that they would have no impact on the society at large.

As further evidence that terrorism cannot be defined only by motive, much of contemporary American terrorism, such as narcoterrorism and extortion rings, is devoted to personal economic gain. Terrorist objectives range from divine orders to retribution to no logical reason at all. Some "loony tunes" and "mad-men," as President Reagan labeled them, perpetrate terrorist activities for reasons alien to the rational mind. Jerrold Post writes that some people commit these acts solely for the inner catharsis they feel—terror for terror's sake. Just as the rapist's act may be motivated by the desire for some gratification other than sexual, the terrorist may act out of inner motivations not related to any stated political or social objective, although he generally asserts one.

James Prince, "Is There a Role for Intelligence in Combatting Terrorism?", *Conflict*, 9:3, (1989): 302–303.

22. Without a definition of terrorism, the author states that:

A. combatting it should be held in check until nations agree.
B. a task force should be convened to expand the existing definition.
C. legal prosecution is not valid against terrorists.
D. governments should go forward based upon existing policies.

23. When the author states that the United States dismisses the root cause, he means terrorism:

A. has no viable reason for existence.
B. can exist for a just cause.
C. is outdated.
D. is agreed upon by other countries.

24. According to the author's point of view, the definition of the Vice President's Task Force on Combatting Terrorism:

I. became valid in 1986.
II. may never have been valid.
III. was politically motivated.

A. I only
B. I and II
C. II only
D. II and III

25. According to the Task Force definition, which of the following would be EXCLUDED from the definition?

I. A deliberate black-out of a major metropolitan area
II. The downing of a military aircraft
III. Scrambling of the air controllers' interactions with pilots

A. I only
B. I and II
C. II only
D. I and III

26. If the United States sent troops to assist Cambodia in combatting a drug cartel, how might the author define such action?

A. State terrorism
B. A justifiable act
C. Furthering a social objective
D. An irrational act

27. J. Post believes that terrorists are motivated by:

A. a desire to hold society responsible for its actions.
B. a need to free themselves from sin or guilt.
C. the desire to stimulate competition.
D. acts of desperation.

Passage #6 (Questions 28–31)

Who would dare change the arms of God on the first day of creation? Michelangelo. First he scribed outlines for God's arms into wet plaster with quick strokes of a sharp tool. Then he abandoned those outlines in a flash of brushstrokes. He painted God's left arm so it swept directly overhead, made that arm plunge a divine hand into the turbulent light and wrenched it from the darkness.

The Sistine Chapel quivers still with the aftershocks of Michelangelo's daring now even more as nine years of careful cleaning and restoration by Vatican experts come to an end. They have been separating darkness—the accumulated grime of nearly five centuries—from Michelangelo's light. It is a light to amaze the eye and blind the soul.

Yet what a reluctant light it was, for the artist who was cajoled and harassed, forced really, into completing one of the crowning masterpieces of Western civilization.

By age 33 Michelangelo had already made his reputation as a sculptor equal to any ancient Greek or Roman. His marble "Pieta," the crucified Christ lifeless across the knees of a Mary forever young and innocent, transcended grief. His giant "David" glowered fiercer than any Goliath.

Now he had a commission from Pope Julius II to make for him a tomb of sculptures so elaborate and so huge as to confound the imagination. Julius, however, first insisted that Michelangelo paint the ceiling of the Pope's own Sistine Chapel.

Michelangelo did not want the Sistine job he began in 1508. Though trained to the brush, he had painted infrequently. Julius, whose fame came from enlarging the papal domain by the sword, bullied him like a drill sergeant, once hitting him with a cane, once threatening to throw him off the scaffold. The artist grumbled constantly, asking for release, signed his letters: "Michelangelo, sculptor."....

The artist was desperate to quit the commission: the Pope was adamant that he continue. The work did not go well at first, partly from inexperience. The fresco of the Flood was soon hazed over by "mildew," the result perhaps of mixing too much water in the surface plaster, or *intonaco*. Michelangelo complained to the Pope:

"Indeed I told your Holiness that this is not my art; what I have done is spoiled." Julius did not relent; Michelangelo must *make* it his art.

The restorer's credo is like the physician's: First, do no harm. The treatment is to lift layers of Rome's dust, sooty grease from burning candle tallow, and other substances—even the residue of Greek wine used as a cleaning solvent some 275 years ago. All have obscured Michelangelo's Promethean work.

Worst of all were varnishes made of animal glues. Applied in various centuries to brighten the darkening surface, they did so for a time. Then each deteriorated and turned the ceiling darker than before.

Despite its dingy appearance, most of the fresco remained in good condition. The technique of painting on fresh plaster was its own best protection. In the hours after Michelangelo painted, the day's application of fresco dried. As it did, the pigments were chemically bonded in a hardening layer of calcium carbonate. The various glues and gums of centuries did not penetrate the hard carbonate shell.

The glues have, however, shrunk and puckered, and in spots scabs of glue have fallen away, pulling pigment with them. This slow destruction by glue pox, rather than some large and immediate threat, has been the Vatican's principal motivation for cleaning the ceiling now. Water damage from roof leaks since plugged has also infiltrated dissolved salts to the surface, stains that cannot be removed as easily as ordinary grime.

The restoration plan calls for examination of each section of fresco with scientific instruments and assessment of the results with human judgment. Then under exacting procedures, the gentlest effective solvent is applied to overlying grime and both are rinsed away. It seems a nearly magical process to watch.

David Jeffrey, "A Renaissance for Michelangelo," *National Geographic*, 176 (December 1989): 688, 696, 699. Reprinted by permission.

28. According to the passage, the relationship between Pope Julius II and Michelangelo could be described as:

A. tempestuous.
B. collegial.
C. defamatory.
D. ecclesiastical.

29. It can be inferred from the passage that Michelangelo signed his name with the word "sculptor" because:

A. he wanted to begin the tomb of sculptures for the Pope.
B. he wished to annoy the Pope.
C. he wanted to get permission to finish his sculpture "David."
D. he saw it as a way to annoy Pope Pius II.

30. A church in England had a painted ceiling which had darkened with time. As the restorers attempted to lift the grime, the paint also was lifted off. The probable difference between this ceiling and the one in the Sistine Chapel is that:

A. the varnishes were made of animal glue.
B. paint was not applied to fresh plaster.
C. the ceiling had glue pox.
D. the solvent was not rinsed away.

31. The author infers that Michelangelo's artistic process included:

A. copying his designs from preliminary plans onto the ceiling.
B. the use of outline drawing with artisans filling in detail.
C. creative changes as he worked.
D. meticulous detail with fresco added as a stabilizer.

Write a question with four responses based on the passage. Base your question on information not used in items above. Use a separate piece of paper, following the format suggested above.

Passage #7 (Questions 32–36)

Although every planet in our solar system, with the possible exception of Mercury, has an atmosphere, the earth's atmosphere is probably the only one that is composed entirely of nitrogen and oxygen. Mars and Venus have atmospheres composed mostly of carbon dioxide, while Jupiter's and Saturn's atmospheres contain mostly hydrogen, helium, and compounds of hydrogen, such as methane and ammonia. The origin of the earth's particular kind of atmosphere is still the subject of much speculation. However, one thing seems fairly certain—when the earth was formed five billion years ago, it was probably too hot to retain any atmosphere that it may have had to begin with. This is because high temperature implies high molecular speeds. What keeps the moving gas molecules from escaping from a planet is gravitational attraction, which depends on the mass of the bodies. Thus, small, hot planets such as Mercury can hold only the most massive molecules. The release of gases from the earth's interior is generally thought to be the process that produced our atmosphere. Most of the lighter gases produced in this way have since been lost, but the earth is massive enough and cool enough at the present time to retain the thin envelope of gases that remain. The atmospheres of extremely massive planets such as Jupiter and Saturn are probably much the same today as they were at the time of their origin.

At the outer limits of the earth's atmosphere, a slow seepage of molecules to outer space continues. At levels above 600 km, the gases are thin enough and hot enough so that some of the lighter, faster molecules can escape the gravitational pull of the earth. Because the upward escape velocity required for a particle to escape from the earth is quite high—about 11.3 km/s (compared to 2.4 km/s for the much smaller moon)—only the very light gases, such as hydrogen and helium, can leave the earth at a significant rate.

At the beginning of Earth's existence, the original atmosphere was probably composed chiefly of a mixture of methane (CH_4) and ammonia (NH_3), which are even now important constituents in the atmospheres of Jupiter, Saturn, Uranus, and Neptune. It is fairly certain that the first atmosphere was devoid of free oxygen.

According to one theory, the earth's present atmosphere did not evolve until much of the original one had been driven off and the earth had started to cool. This new atmosphere was created when gases that had been dissolved in the molten rock bubbled out of the surface, a process called outgassing. As cooling continued, the water vapor condensed to form the great oceans. The liquid water gradually absorbed most of the atmosphere's carbon dioxide, thus leaving nitrogen as the predominant gas. The oxygen in our atmosphere is believed to have appeared only after primitive plant life developed (about three billion years ago?) and began acting on carbon dioxide through photosynthesis to form oxygen. The concentration of oxygen in the atmosphere probably increased very slowly at the outset, since much of the oxygen was consumed in the oxidation of the earth's surface materials, and the present level was probably not reached until a few hundred million years ago.

32. Gas molecules which escape the Earth's atmosphere include:

A. fast moving molecules.
B. slow moving molecules.
C. lightweight gases.
D. heavyweight gases.

33. In the first phase of the Earth's development, the Earth's atmosphere was a direct result of:

A. release of gases from inside the planet.
B. the ratio of oxygen and carbon dioxide.
C. weak gravitational force on heavy molecules.
D. the retention of gases within the planet.

34. If the Earth were subject to global warming, which of the following would occur?

I. Gas molecules would move faster.
II. Lighter gases would escape at a greater rate.
III. Gravitational force would be less upon the lighter molecules.

A. I and II
B. II only
C. I and III
D. All of the above

35. The second and third stages of the Earth's atmosphere are characterized by which of the following:

I. a vacuum created by lack of oxygen.
II. carbon dioxide being broken down by photosynthesis.
III. the cooling of water vapor to form the seas.

A. I and II
B. II only
C. II and III
D. All of the above

36. What is the ratio comparing the age of the Earth to the length of time oxygen has been in enough quantity to sustain life (assume the Earth began to support life 2 billion years ago)?

A. 5:2
B. 2:50
C. 50:2
D. Not determinable by the passage

Write a question with four responses based on the passage. Base your question on information not used in items above. Use a separate piece of paper, following the format suggested above.

Passage #8 (Questions 37–41)

For two centuries, federal, state, and local governments have worked together in constantly changing patterns.... The challenge is to assure that each level of government retains the freedom and authority it needs to carry out its own responsibilities well, without unnecessary limits and constraints.

The Supreme Court's recent decisions have made it clear that little protection is provided for the states under the 10th Amendment. The Court has suggested that the states must seek to limit federal power through the political process, rather than relying on the limitation included in the initial delegation of powers to the federal government....

While the simplest answer is the model established 200 years ago—for the states to convene a constitutional convention to renew the commitment to power shared between states and the federal government—current fear of a runaway convention has forced the states to rely on the Congress to voluntarily give up powers it has centralized on the national level. History makes it clear, however, that power is rarely given up voluntarily.

The impact of this problem is now more acute as a result of *South Carolina vs Baker.* In that case, the Court repealed the last vestiges of intergovernmental tax immunity and reinforced its intent to remove itself from defining clear lines between state and federal authority.

For this reason, the governors are convinced that a measured, practical constitutional solution to the federalism issue is needed—a solution that restores the state's ability to initiate constitutional change without being stymied by the threat of the perceived problem associated with a convention, a solution that assures the people of a continued say in the decisions about the basic structure of the nation and the appropriate roles of each level of government.

Such a solution is clearly possible within the current intergovernmental structure. As the Governors' Task Force on Federalism noted, "The Constitution envisioned that amendments could be initiated by both federal government and the states. However, the fear of a 'runaway' convention has effectively closed the door to state-initiated amendments. Until recently, the 10th Amendment was thought to protect the states and localities from an uncontrolled expansion of federal power through legislation and regulatory action." Now, however, the Supreme Court has effectively removed that protection, and the Congress is free to act without constitutional constraints. Furthermore, the concern over a constitutional convention has blunted the balancing capacity originally provided in the Constitution.

Therefore, the governors have called on the Congress to restore the intended states' ability to initiate amendments. Congress can do this by referring to the states a constitutional amendment that would create a more practical route under Article V for states to initiate amendments to the Constitution.

Under this approach, two-thirds of the states could pass memorials that seek the addition of a specific constitutional amendment. Unlike the petitions for a constitutional convention that must be served on the Congress, these memorials would be filed with every state. When the necessary 34 states are reached, the proposing states would appoint representatives to a Committee on Style to reconcile the details of the language of the various memorials. When a majority of the states represented on the Committee of Style approve the proposed amendment, it would be submitted to the Congress. A two-thirds vote by both houses within the next congressional session would be necessary to stop the amendment from going back to the states for ratification. If the Congress did not vote by two-thirds to stop the amendment, it would be submitted to the states for ratification by the required three-fourths. This reasonable, measured approach can restore the balance of power without any radical alteration of the structure, process or specific responsibilities exercised today.

John Sununu, "The Spirit of Federalism: Restoring the Balance." *The Journal of State Government,* 62:1 (January/February 1989): 26–27.

37. The passage indicates that the Supreme Court has suggested to the states that an appropriate way to limit federal power is to:

A. wait for the federal government to voluntarily transfer power.
B. use the political process.
C. stand upon the limitation in the initial delegation of powers.
D. sue the federal government for breach of contract.

38. The importance of the *South Carolina vs Baker* decision is that it:

A. emphasized states' rights.
B. emphasized the federal government's supremacy over states.
C. decreased the role of the Supreme Court as a mediator between the states and the federal government on issues of authority.
D. mandated tax immunity for the state of South Carolina.

39. The author implies that neither the states nor the government want to risk a constitutional convention. The most likely reason is:

A. too many issues will be addressed which do not deal with the limitation of the federal government's role.
B. the states feel that the Supreme Court will take a stand against them.
C. the 10th Amendment will be enforced to limit states' powers.
D. the states fear if they use the convention to confront the issue, the federal government might find a way to block future uses.

40. The most fundamental right that the states wish to have protected is the authority to:

A. initiate amendments to the constitution.
B. ratify decisions made by the congress by 3/4ths majority.
C. repeal the 10th Amendment.
D. have representatives on the Committee of Style.

41. If it were found that the President chose new members for the Supreme Court who had been recorded as promoting the powers of central government, what effect would this have on the states' rights issue?

A. No effect since the Supreme Court has limited power over state governments.
B. No effect since previous views of Supreme Court Justices have no effect on future cases.
C. Possible effect in that the Supreme Court Justices may have preconceived opinions limiting the role of the states.
D. Possible effect in that the Supreme Court Justices may wish to initiate an arbitration system between the states and the federal government.

Passage #9 (Questions 42–45)

What do crabs, sea urchins, earthworms, malaria parasites and corals have in common? In fact, these very diverse groups share very little, apart from the fact they all lack a backbone. Of the 1,071,000 or so known species of animals about 1,029,300 are invertebrate, that is, over 95 percent are animals without backbones. Invertebrates make up the bulk of animals, measured both in terms of numbers of species recognized and numbers of individuals. Some invertebrates, like garden snails and earthworms, are conspicuous and familiar animals, while others, although abundant, pass unnoticed by most people.

Invertebrate body forms range in size from the lowly microscopic *Amoeba*, which may be just one micrometer in diameter, to the Giant squid, 18m (59 ft) in length, a ratio of 1:18,000,000. They include life forms as diverse as the Desert locust and the sea anemones. They inhabit all regions of the globe, and all habitats, from the ocean abyss to the air. Life almost certainly originated in the seas, and virtually all the major invertebrate groups (phyla) have marine representatives. Somewhat fewer (almost 14 phyla) have conquered fresh water. Fewer still (about 5 phyla) live on land and of these only the jointed-limbed groups (arthropods) have mastered the air and really dry places. Most numerous among arthropods are the uniramians (e.g., insects, millipedes, centipedes) and the chelicerates (e.g., scorpions, spiders, ticks, mites).

Many invertebrates, like slugs (whether of the garden or sea), are free living; others, such as barnacles, are attached to the substrate throughout their adult life; yet others live as parasites in or on the bodies of plants or other animals. Some invertebrates are of great commercial significance, either as direct food for man (e.g., prawns and oysters), or as food for man's exploitable reserves (e.g., the planktonic copepods on which herring feed). Others (e.g., earthworms) are much appreciated because they improve the soil for agriculture. Many invertebrates live as parasites, either in man himself or in the bodies of domestic animals and plants, where great damage may be wrought, and so are of great medical or agricultural importance.

This great diversity of form and life-style in animals has led zoologists to sort out, or classify, animals according to type and evolutionary connections. To be certain that they are speaking of the same animals, they give each species a unique scientific name (e.g., *Lumbricus terrestri,* the Common earthworm). Every species is classified into one of the major groups, or phyla. A phylum comprises all those animals which are thought to have a common evolutionary origin. According to their understanding of the probable evolutionary processes involved, zoologists may recognize some 39 animal phyla. With one exception, they are made up exclusively of invertebrate animals. The phylum Chordata includes all animals with a hollow dorsal nerve cord. Nearly all—including fishes, amphibians, reptiles, birds—have a backbone, but some are invertebrate, such as the sea squirt.

The technical classification that zoologists employ leads from the most primitive and simple animal types to the most complex and advanced. In order to achieve some form of system, various levels of organization are recognized which give clear distinctions between phyla. The most fundamental of these lies in the number of cells in the body. A cell is the smallest functional unit of an animal, governed by its own nucleus which contains genetic material, known as DNA.

Keith Banister and Andrew Campbell, eds., *The Encyclopedia of Aquatic Life,* New York: Facts on File Publications, 1985, 148–49. Reproduced by permission of Equinox (Oxford) Limited.

42. The main idea of this passage can be summed up best by which of the following statements?

- **A.** There are many more invertebrates than are known to most of us.
- **B.** Invertebrates are considerably more diverse than they are similar.
- **C.** Invertebrates vary greatly in size and place of habitation.
- **D.** Zoologists have created a classification system to keep track of invertebrates.

43. If a new invertebrate were to be discovered, it would most likely:

- **A.** have ancestors which could be traced back to the sea.
- **B.** be a uniramian.
- **C.** live in the sea.
- **D.** be microscopic in size.

44. According to this article, the most important factor in classifying animal types is:

- **A.** DNA.
- **B.** presence or absence of a backbone.
- **C.** complexity of the nervous system.
- **D.** number of cells.

45. Based upon the passage, one could assume that:

- **A.** barnacles are parasites.
- **B.** some parasites are of commercial significance.
- **C.** the invertebrates which provide agricultural benefits are not the same ones as those which find hosts in people and animals.
- **D.** free living vertebrates are more ecologically beneficial than those which attach themselves to the substrate.

Write a question with four responses based on the passage. Base your question on information not used in items above. Use a separate piece of paper, following the format suggested above.

Now write a second question with four responses based on the passage. Base your question on information not used in items above. Use a separate piece of paper, following the format suggested above.

Passage #10 (Questions 46 –50)

The performing arts are a source of pleasure most of the time for the actor and often for the audience. The fortuitous disclosure of the *Reward System of the Brain* by James Olds and Peter Milner at McGill University at the end of the 1950s followed by the discovery of the brain's capacity to synthesize a wide variety of hormones, contributed to give new significance to the question of pleasure in performance.

In 1956, James Olds was surprised by laboratory rats who could be led to gratify their hunger, thirst and sexual drive by self-stimulation of their brains with electricity. He called 'pleasure centres' the local centres in the brain which he thought underlay 'motivation' (Olds, 1956). Today neurophysiologists prefer to use the expression 'reward system of the brain', and consider that these centres in the human brain belong to a system of pathways that appear to play a vital role in the guidance of behaviour, and more precisely in learning, memory, emotion and perhaps drug addiction (Waukier and Rolls, 1976; F.E. Bloom, 1988).

The physical phenomenon of thrills—tingling sensations—illustrates the biological aspect of pleasure in theatre and dance. It appears among subjects exposed to emotionally arousing stimuli and has been described in the artistic context (Avram Goldstein, 1980). According to the data, the items most frequently able to cause thrills are musical passages (96 percent), in the second position are 'a scene in a movie, play, ballet, or book' (92 percent).

In a preliminary test, the experimenter found that thrills were attenuated with naloxone (an opiate receptor antagonist) in some subjects. Mood and 'feeling' are probably dependent on the activity of the brain monoamines and endogenous morphins (opiate-like substances, several of which have 'euphoriant' properties) which are involved in reward effects (Amalric, 1987; Bloom, 1988).

It is tempting to see a performance as a kind of neurohormonal reward autostimulation. This hypothesis has yet to be confirmed through experiments. What is certain is that a relation exists between the psychic exaltation of the actor—professional or not—and his/her capacity to resist pain in the case of an accident on stage. This fact makes us think about endogenous opioids, like beta-endorphin, which block pain sensitivity, or at least pain experience, as has been observed among 'motivated' wounded people.

Furthermore, intense satisfaction in performing or in being involved in a performance even when the performance is aesthetically mediocre, suggests that this kind of situation offers physiological and psychological 'rewards', the effects of which succeed in silencing the critical sense of the subjects. The classical depressive state of actors who cannot perform seems to be close to withdrawal symptoms in drug dependence. The benefit of performing healing rituals (such as Gnaoua's *Lila* in Morocco) is certainly underlied by the increase of endogenous opioids in the performer's brain. What can we say about the wild ecstasy of political, religious, and military spectacles?

Jean Marie Pradier, "Towards a Biological Theory of the Body," *New Theatre Quarterly*, vol. 6 (February 1990):p. 92. Reprinted with the permission of Cambridge University Press.

46. The study by Olds in the 1950's was significant because:

A. it showed that rats could gratify their basic needs by self-stimulation of their brains with electricity.
B. it showed that drug addiction and memory have a common neurological pathway.
C. it laid a foundation for the development of a better understanding of physical response to pleasurable stimuli.
D. it provided a thorough understanding of how the body responds to pleasure in performance.

47. According to more contemporary neuro-physiologists, the reward system of the brain would best be described as:

A. an expansion of the pleasure centre.
B. a structure which plays an important role in the body's pleasure response to a performance.
C. a structure which plays a peripheral role in the guidance of behavior.
D. none of the above.

48. Information provided in the passage supports the following statement(s) respective to the perception of pain:

I. Euphoria can affect the perception of pain.
II. There may be a similarity in the underlying mechanism involved in pain perception between 'motivated' wounded people and an injured actor.
III. Endogenous opioids have been shown to have a pain-blocking effect for actors who have been injured on stage and can continue to perform.

A. I only
B. I and II
C. II only
D. II and III

49. Based upon this passage, which of the following would be expected to elicit a pleasure response?

A. An undistinguished performance of a Shakespearean play
B. Soldiers marching in formation
C. A Broadway performance of *Phantom of the Opera.*
D. All of the above

50. The author makes the point that an artistic performance:

A. produces a biological response that is different from that produced by other stimuli.
B. stimulates a stronger pleasure response on the part of the audience than the actor.
C. must be of high quality to elicit a strong pleasure response.
D. stimulates more than just the senses.

Write a question with four responses based on the passage. Base your question on information not used in items above. Use a separate piece of paper, following the format suggested above.

Passage #11 (Questions 51–56)

Feathers, together with adaptations of muscles, heart, bones, and lungs, make birds the most efficient of flying machines. Feathers have many advantages. They are light. They are regularly replaced when worn, lost, or damaged. Each is individually attached to a muscle for greater maneuverability. Feathers enable birds to ride effortlessly on the wind, to travel faster than 100 miles per hour, to hover and fly backwards, to fly more than 48 hours without resting, and to migrate thousands of miles a year. No bird does all of these things, but feathers make them all possible. Swifts, for example, are such accomplished aerialists that they feed, drink, bathe, court, and even mate while flying. In addition to flying at the great speeds (80 miles per hour and faster) that have given them their name, swifts sometimes spend the night on the wing a few thousand feet above the ground.

The shape of the wings and tail tells us that at a glance how specialized a bird is for flight. Some of the fastest fliers—falcons and swallows, for example—have long pointed wings and long narrow tails. This streamlined profile creates the least resistance as the bird moves through the air. The Peregrine Falcon, diving after prey, has been clocked at 175 miles per hour. The broader wings and tail of slower fliers, such as vultures, eagles, and storks, catch every movement of air so these birds can soar and wheel high in the sky. Birds such as pheasants and grouse, which seldom fly, have short rounded wings that provide quick lift but little sustaining power. Their leg muscles are much more developed than those used in flight. Because the hardest working muscles are nourished by more capillaries and are therefore darker, earthbound birds like chickens and turkeys have "dark meat" in their legs and "white meat" in their breasts. In most birds the breast muscles form the dark meat.

The bird's skeleton, a marvel of flight engineering, fuses lightness with strength. Most birds do not have a bone like the one in humans that separates the nasal cavity from the mouth—one of the many adaptations that keep flying weight to a minimum. Their skulls are usually paper thin. The heads of woodpeckers, however, are specially reinforced to absorb the constant stress of hammering trees. Many powerful fliers are equipped with hollow bones, which are filled with air sacs to increase buoyancy. The skeleton of the frigatebird, a soarer with a seven-foot wingspan, weighs only four ounces—less than its feathers. Hollow bones are stronger than solid bones of the same weight because they bend more easily and the air inside them absorbs shocks. Longer wing bones are reinforced with struts, a device also found in airplanes.

Strong fliers have proportionately larger hearts that pump blood more rapidly than those of nonfliers, weak fliers, and soaring birds. When hovering, a hummingbird beats its wings about 50 times a second, with its heart pulsing 1,200 times a minute. The lungs, aided by air sacs in the bones and other cavities—even the toes—supply oxygen needed for flight. The reproductive system also enhances aerodynamic efficiency; the testes of male birds expand in size and weight only during the brief season they are producing sperm.

Roger F. Pasquier, "The Diversity of Birdlife," in *The Wonder of Birds,* Washington, D.C.: National Geographic Society, 1983, 38–39. Reprinted by permission.

51. According to the passage, one might conclude that the most important point about feathers is that they:

A. appear to be more important than muscles, heart, bones, and lungs in adaptation for flying.
B. allow for a great deal of versatility in possible types of flying feats but are not solely responsible for what a bird actually can do.
C. are responsible for maneuverability.
D. lessen air resistance.

52. One can infer from the phrase "make birds the most efficient of flying machines" that:

A. natural features are more efficient than manufactured ones.
B. airplanes have been structured after birds.
C. a bird's parts function in a mechanical way.
D. none of the above.

53. All of the following statements are true EXCEPT:

A. Peregrine Falcons probably have long, pointed wings and a long, narrow tail.
B. Broad wings and tail allow for greater height than long pointed wings and tails.
C. Length of wings affects duration.
D. Storks have wider wings with highly developed leg muscles.

54. Based upon heart size, one could infer that:

I. a swift would be proportionately larger than a frigatebird.
II. a hummingbird would be proportionately larger than a swift.
III. a grouse would be proportionately equal to a turkey.

A. I only
B. I and II
C. II only
D. I and III

55. Based upon the information presented on bone structure, one might conclude that:

I. the bone structure of most birds weighs proportionately less than that of humans.
II. the bone structure of Peregrine Falcons is hollow.
III. the bone structure of powerful fliers has air sacs which increase buoyancy and decrease speed.

A. I only
B. I and II
C. II only
D. All of the above

56. Which of the following facts is/are true?

A. Hummingbirds have very fast heart beats compared to many other birds.
B. Air sacs can be found in the toes of some birds.
C. A bird's skeleton is compared to flight engineering.
D. All of the above.

Passage #12 (Questions 57–61)

The tape handling system (of a tape recorder) consists of two hubs that hold the tape supply reel and a take-up reel plus the machinery necessary to pull the tape past the heads. The drive mechanism typically comprises a constant-speed motor coupled by a rubber friction drive wheel to a *capstan,* which moves the tape. The motor shaft can drive various-size wheels, hereby offering differing tape speeds....

Early tape machines fed tape through the recorder from one reel to a second reel. For the purposes of convenience, tape deck manufacturers developed cartridges to eliminate the need for an independent take-up reel. The first tape cartridge contained a single reel on which the tape was spooled in an endless loop. The tape was fed to the heads from the inside of the reel and back onto the reel from the outside. This caused the tape to slide over itself as the reel turned and thus early cartridges frequently stopped because a layer of tape stuck to the next layer of tape and wound itself too tightly. These problems were lessened by the development of lubricants....

Current cartridges, called *cassettes*, use two reels but the entire mechanism is encased in a single shell of plastic, eliminating the inconvenience of open reel-to-reel tapes. The costs of the convenience of cartridges are that, in making smaller cartridges, manufacturers are using thinner tape...and running the tape at slower speeds, which has implications for frequency response, head construction, quality of the transport mechanism, and quality of recording....

The quality of a tape recorder is a function of the mechanical or electrical design in its construction. In general, electrical devices are less variable in recording and reproduction quality than mechanical devices so that the more expensive the tape machine, the more likely it is to use electrical rather than mechanical components in its design where there is a choice between the two.

In those machines that might be considered for home use or for other less critical applications, the components of operation are entirely mechanical. The capstan is driven by a belt stretched between a stepped motor pulley with several different sizes and a similar stepped motor pulley on the capstan itself. The speed of the tape can be changed by moving the belt from one set of pulleys on the motor and capstan to another set that has a different size ratio and hence a different ratio between motor speed and capstan speed. When the play button is pressed, the pinch roller is moved against the tape by a system of levers to drive the tape. The rewind and fast forward functions are also mechanically controlled by a system of gears and pulleys so that the motor can also drive the take-up and supply reels.

More expensive machines use an electromechanical system. In this case the activation of a push-button energizes devices called *solenoids.* A solenoid is an electromagnet and an attached rod that can perform mechanical operations by being attracted or repelled by the electromagnet.

The advantage of solenoid operation is twofold. First, the button needs a much lighter touch because no mechanical function is being performed. The electrical system energizes only the solenoid, and the solenoid itself may be adjusted to determine the distance over which some mechanical linkage moves. Second, solenoid operation allows all of the functions of the tape recorder to be remotely controlled; the operator needs only a set of push-buttons that are electrically connected to solenoids that, in turn, control the mechanical movements of the tape parts.

Jack F. Curtis and Martin C. Schultz, *Basic Laboratory Instrumentation for Speech and Hearing.* Boston: Little, Brown and Co., 1986, 150–52. Reprinted by permission.

57. According to the passage, it is explicitly stated that early tape machines:

A. utilized one reel which fed the tape to the heads from the inside of the reel and a second reel which received the tape as it fed onto it from the outside.
B. did not perform as well as cassette models.
C. used a constant-speed motor, rubber friction drive wheel, and capstan.
D. did none of the above.

58. Based upon the information in the passage, one can infer that:

I. convenience was the driving force for the development of cartridges.
II. development of the early cartridge solved some problems and created other problems.
III. people prefer mechanical components over electrical.

A. I only
B. I and II only
C. II and III
D. All of the above

59. According to the facts presented, in a mechanical machine:

A. speed of the tape depends on the ratio between motor speed and capstan speed.
B. when the machine is on play, levers press against the tape and move it along.
C. mechanical action is achieved by an electromagnet and attached rod.
D. the capstan is driven by a single stepped motor pulley.

60. The key difference between an electromechanical system and a mechanical system is that in the electromechanical system:

A. there is a more expensive solenoid component.
B. the solenoid allows all functions to be remotely controlled.
C. mechanical action is achieved by an electromagnet and attached rod.
D. solenoids eliminate the need for mechanical operations.

61. Based upon this passage, one can conclude which of the following?

A. The best quality machine is probably beyond the reach of the average person.
B. The level of quality provided by the most expensive equipment is most likely not needed for typical home use.
C. There is an inverse relationship between level of technology and cost.
D. **A** and **B** are correct.

3.4.3 ANSWERS TO EXERCISES

3.4.3.1 Answer Key

Passage #1	1. A	2. C	3. D	4. C	5. A	6. D
Passage #2	7. B	8. D	9. D	10. A	11. D	
Passage #3	12. D	13. B	14. B	15. C		
Passage #4	16. B	17. D	18. A	19. A	20. D	21. B
Passage #5	22. D	23. A	24. C	25. D	26. C	27. B
Passage #6	28. A	29. B	30. B	31. C		
Passage #7	32. A	33. A	34. D	35. C	36. A	
Passage #8	37. B	38. C	39. A	40. A	41. C	
Passage #9	42. B	43. A	44. D	45. C		
Passage #10	46. C	47. B	48. B	49. D	50. D	
Passage #11	51. B	52. A	53. D	54. D	55. A	56. D
Passage #12	57. D	58. B	59. A	60. C	61. D	

3.4.3.2 Expanded Answer Summary

Passage #1 (Explanations)

This passage discusses a series of predicaments, which the author calls paradoxes, related to the current war-making capabilities of the great powers. The core of the argument is that rational humans have created a so-called defense system that is essentially irrational.

1. **A** **B** is not stated in the passage, while **D** is false. **C** is a correct statement but is not the primary emphasis.

2. **C** Stated as Paradox IV, **D** is not stated in the passage. **A** is incorrect and **B** refers to a "need" to develop weaponry when it is indicated that weapons are now stockpiled.

3. **D** The Age of Unreason is discussed in Paradox II. The almost right answer is **C**, but the article states that it is "roughly half" instead of "more than half."

4. **C** **II** and **III** are not discussed.

5. **A** The example provides a paradox with two irreconcilable actions which fits into the author's view.

6. **D** **A** and **B** are correct, but are not comprehensive enough for the meaning of the quotation. **C** is incorrect. **D** addresses both economic and political concerns, thus is closer to the meaning of the quote.

Passage #2 (Explanations)

What is the central theme of this passage? Write a short statement describing the main idea of the passage.

7. **B** Choices **I** and **II** are stated in paragraph two. The Museum of London is conducting the dig.

8. **D** **B** is not mentioned. **A** is probably true, but is not the major point of significance. **C** is false since further excavation has not proceeded. The answer is in the last paragraph.

9. **D** Lambarde wrote of how the Rose and the Theatre were alike, findings that are now being refuted. See paragraph three.

10. A **A** and **C** are the closest answers, but the author prioritizes their relationship in the last sentence of paragraph four.

11. D **A, B,** and **C** are not indicated by the passage. **D** is most closely stated in paragraph one.

Passage #3 (Explanations)

Write a short statement describing the central idea of this passage.

12. D The "new sources" refer to officials in Kennedy's administration as they reveal insights on the international climate that provided the background to Kennedy's decision-making process.

13. B If the Jupiter missiles were found to be defective, then that lessened Kennedy's options which would weaken the author's argument that he had additional alternatives through the use of missiles.

14. B The passage uses terms such as "look back and reflect" and "in retrospect." When these terms are combined with a change in the standard interpretation of the crisis, it would indicate that the officials' views have altered with time. **A** and **D** are not indicated by the passage and **C** is negated by sentence one in paragraph two.

15. C. **A** is not discussed. **B** and **C** are negated by the article. Paragraph three indicates that President Kennedy had more "cushion" than had previously been thought.

Passage #4 (Explanations)

In this passage the author, through the use of irony and self-deprecation, explains how he was totally frustrated in attempts to use a microscope. He also provides a rather vivid picture of the frustration he caused his professor.

16. B Stated in paragraph two.

17. D At various points in the story, he exhibited all three behaviors.

18. A Since he indicates it is familiar "lacteal opacity", it could have been answered from context that it was the milky color mentioned earlier.

19. A Since he had failed before, and there was no improvement during this course, the probability is great that he will fail again.

20. D At the end of paragraph one, the author states that the professor adjusted the microscope for his own eyes.

21. B The ending is ironical in that he can finally see an image, but the image is an unexpected one.

Passage #5 (Explanations)

This passage provides an explanation of the difficulties experienced by policy-makers in defining terrorism. The bulk of the passage provides examples to debunk a government report. The passage does not provide a solution to the definitional problem.

22. D **A, B,** and **C** are not discussed. **D** is implied in paragraph two.

23. A **C** and **D** are incorrect. Paragraph four states that the U.S. does not accept the Arafat "root cause" definition.

24. C Stated in paragraph five.

25. D Paragraph five indicates that the definition did not provide for "nonviolent acts or passive resistance." **I** and **III** met those conditions.

26. C The passage indicates that there is need for an international definition, but it does not indicate that the U.S. (or any other country) can operate on sovereign soil.

27. B The author refers to the "inner catharsis" terrorists feel—which is freedom from guilt.

Passage #6 (Explanations)

Write a short statement describing the central idea of this passage.

28. A The passage indicates that Michelangelo and the Pope had a very stormy relationship with the Pope hitting Michelangelo and threatening to throw him from the scaffold. There is no indication that they were colleagues, religiously similar, or libeled each other to others.

29. B **A** might be true, but is not the primary reason. **C** is wrong since the sculpture was already completed. **D** uses an incorrect name for the Pope. The passage indicates that Michelangelo grumbled constantly, asking to be released from painting the Sistine Chapel. Signing his name as "sculptor" was an example of the bickering between him and the Pope over art and was most likely meant to be provoking or annoying.

30. B This question asks for a difference. **B** is different in that Michelangelo painted onto fresh plaster which sealed the color.

31. C **A** is incorrect since he altered his designs as he worked. **B** is not discussed. **D** is backwards since the passage indicated that he painted onto fresco. In the first paragraph, Michelangelo sketches and adapts as he designs.

Passage #7 (Explanations)

This passage appears to be excerpted from a text on meteorology. Consequently it does not offer an argument but rather describes a theory of how the earth developed an atmosphere. The process of how the atmosphere evolved is at the core of the passage.

32. A The molecules must be fast enough to exceed a speed of 11.3 km/s (paragraph two). These include light as well as heavy gas molecules.

33. A Answer in paragraph one and in paragraph three because the gases bubbled to the surface.

34. D **I, II,** and **III** are correct.

35. C **I** is not stated. **II** and **III** are stated in paragraph three.

36. A Paragraph one indicates the Earth's age is 5 billion years old. If there were enough oxygen to sustain life 2 billion years ago, then the ratio would be 5:2.

Passage #8 (Explanations)

Write a short statement describing the central idea of this passage.

37. B This question involves detail which is explicitly answered in paragraph two.

38. C Paragraph four states that the Supreme Court will "remove itself from defining the clear lines between state and federal authority."

39. A **B** is incorrect since the Supreme Court would not be involved with the convention. **C** is incorrect since the states would favor the 10th Amendment. **D** is not discussed or indicated. **A** is the most logical answer since a "runaway" convention could not be controlled by the states.

40. A This question involves detail and is found in paragraph 7.

41. C **D** is not indicated in the passage. **A** is incorrect since the Supreme Court does have jurisdiction over the states (as an example of South Carolina vs Baker). **B** is incorrect since Supreme Court Justices are chosen in part based upon their views. **C** is the most likely answer in that their opinions and former rulings would probably effect the directions of their decisions.

Passage #9 (Explanations)

Write a short statement describing the central idea of this passage.

42. B While **A** is a correct idea, it is too broad and lacks the specific focus of the idea that is developed. Information in **C** is too narrow since diversity other than size and habitation is discussed. **D** is incorrect, since the need for a classification system is a result of the main idea which is expressed in **B**.

43. A Paragraph two states that virtually all major invertebrate groups have marine representatives, so it would be most likely that a newly discovered invertebrate would also have ancestors which could be traced from the sea. All other choices have an implied lower frequency.

44. D DNA is discussed only relative to the definition of a cell, so **A** is wrong. While **B** and **C** might be factors used in classifying animals, the last paragraph states organization based upon number of cells is the most fundamental factor considered.

45. C Paragraph three states that barnacles attach to the substrate, making **A** incorrect. There is no mention of commercial importance to parasites, negating **B. D** is incorrect because no comparison of value between free living and attached invertebrates is provided. **C** is the correct answer. The last two sentences in paragraph three indicate that invertebrates which improve the soil and those which are parasites in humans and animals are two separate groups, since one is described in a positive and the other in a negative context.

Passage #10 (Explanations)

This passage discusses theoretical explanations on what happens physiologically in the human body when it experiences pleasure. The author argues that experimental data is suggestive but not definitive.

46. C **A** is too limited because, while the study itself was about rats, the importance of that study to this passage relates to how the information set the stage for trying to understand human response to pleasurable stimuli. **B** is wrong because it was today's neuropsychologists who noted neurological pathways involved in guiding behavior. Paragraph one indicates that Olds' study was only a stepping stone in trying to understand response to pleasurable stimuli which supports **C** and negates **D.**

47. B There is an inference that these two terms are referring to the same thing, with no mention of the concept of expansion which makes **A** wrong. **C** is wrong because the reward system is thought to have a more direct role. The first sentence in paragraph three confirms **B.**

48. B Psychic exaltation has been shown to affect one's ability to resist pain, making Statement **I** correct. The last sentence in paragraph five implies a comparison between "motivated" wounded people and injured actors, but it is speculative about the role of endogenous opioids. This provides support for Statement **II** but not for Statement **III.**

49. D All statements are correct. All have an element of performing and/or healing effect. The last paragraph indicates that quality is not an issue.

50. D **A** is incorrect because information is not provided about whether the response is unique to artistic performance. The first sentence negates **B**. The last paragraph negates **C** by stating that quality is not an issue and that there are other types of rewards. The second paragraph indicates that imagination and emotional excitation as well as the senses are stimulated, making **D** the correct answer.

Passage #11 (Explanations)

In this passage the author discusses factors important to the flight of birds. He details the effect of feathers, musculature, organs, and skeleton on aerodynamic lift. The passage primarily gives descriptive information with focus on efficiency of flight.

51. B **A** is incorrect because sentence one in the first paragraph indicates that all five things are important, and it does not indicate level of importance of each. **C** is wrong since the muscle attachments are important in maneuverability. Wing shape affects air resistance making **D** incorrect. Support for **B** is found in that other factors which play a role in what a bird is capable of doing are discussed as well as in the statement indicating that not all birds do all things.

52. A No specific comparisons are made to airplanes, leaving no support for **B**. Emphasis is on natural features of the bird and no mention is made of functioning in a mechanical way, eliminating **C. A** is correct because sentence one provides a list of natural features and involves an implied comparison with machines.

53. **D** A is correct based on long-pointed wings and long, narrow tails (streamlining) being important for speed, and Peregrine Falcons have been clocked at 175 miles per hour. Sentence five in paragraph two confirms **B. C** is correct since paragraph two makes reference to the fact that some birds have short rounded wings which give them quick lift but limited sustaining power. **D** is incorrect because storks are slower, but soaring fliers, and highly developed leg muscles would indicate it were more of a land bird.

54. **D** This answer requires putting several pieces of information together. The first sentence of the last paragraph contains information about which type of bird has the larger heart. One must go back to the passage to determine which category each bird fits.

55. **A** Lightness of bone structure is stressed in paragraph three, and birds do not have the bone separating the nasal cavity from the mouth cavity as do humans. Peregrine Falcons cannot be assumed to have hollow ones since paragraph three says "many" and "not all" powerful fliers have hollow bones. Air sacs were associated with buoyancy in the third paragraph, but there was no mention of effect on speed.

56. **D** This question tests your attention to detail. All of the above are directly stated in the passage.

Passage #12 (Explanations)

This passage describes the development and functioning of tape recorders. The author's purpose is primarily to describe the working of electronic machines or mechanical equipment. Some judgments about the relative efficiency of different types of equipment are also included.

57 **D** **A** is wrong since feeding the tape from the inside of one reel to the outside of a second reel refers to the first tape cartridge. **B** is not explicitly stated. **C** is wrong since these details refer to tape handling systems now. **D** is the correct answer.

58. **B** Paragraph two, sentence two supports Statement **I**. Statement **II** is supported in that the first cartridges eliminated the need for an independent take-up reel but had the problem of sticking tape. While people buy mechanical equipment for home use because of cost, there is no discussion of preference, so Statement **III** is wrong.

59. **A** The answer to this question depends on your understanding of the details. These are presented in paragraph five.

60. **C** The answer involves identifying the structural difference between the two machines. Information in paragraph six indicates **C** as the correct answer. According to the passage, electromechanical systems are more expensive, but the cost of parts is not broken out, ruling out **A**. **B** is cited as a benefit but not as the key difference. **D** is wrong since solenoids are responsible for the mechanical operations; it does not eliminate them.

61. **D** **A** is a correct statement. This involves considering that the most expensive machines provide the best quality and yet people buy mechanical equipment for the home. If the cost were within the average range, one might assume that more people would opt for better quality. **B** is also correct since the first sentence of paragraph five implies home use is less critical and mechanical operation provides adequate performance. The opposite is true of Statement **C.**

3.5 REFERENCES

A Concise Introduction to Logic, 4th ed. 1991. Patrick Hurley. Belmont, CA: Wadsworth Publishing Co.

Active Reading in the Arts and Sciences. 1991. Shirley Quinn and Susan Irvings. Boston: Allyn and Bacon, Inc.

Managing Your Reading, 1987. Phyllis A. Miller. Littleton, CO: Reading Development Resources.

Reading for Results, 1987. Laraine E. Flemming. Boston: Houghton Mifflin Co.

Reading Enhancement and Development, 1992. Rhonda Holt Atkinson and Debbie Guice Longman. St. Paul: West Publishing Co., College and School Division.

Building Thinking Skills, 1984. Howard and Sandra Black. 4 volumes. Pacific Grove, CA: Midwest Publications Co., Inc.

QUEST: Academic Skills Program, 1973. Ruth Cohen, et al. San Diego: Harcourt Brace Jovanovich.

Literary Tales: Inside Stories to Literature for Critical Reading and Thinking, 1980. Dan Dramer. Providence: Jamestown Publications, Inc.

Reading Faster: A Drill Book, 10th printing, 1983. Edward B. Fry. Cambridge, England: Cambridge University Press.

Improve Your Reading Ability, 4th ed., 1983. Arthur W. Heilman. Columbus: Merrill Publishing Co.

Chapter 4:

Introduction to Problem Solving in the Physical and Biological Sciences

Scientific problem solving is a culmination of verbal reasoning, organized approach and higher level reasoning patterns blended into a strong problem solving model. Premedical sciences require special attention in developing connections between given information and problem structure before applying the problem solving model. This chapter attempts to provide fundamental cognitive strengths to prepare for scientific problem solving in the MCAT. The chapter is divided into three parts: reasoning patterns and a problem solving model; an applied review of MCAT Mathematics Concepts; selected data analysis passages with practice problems.

Scientific problem solving comes by regular and extensive practice on premedical problems. While you develop competency in Sections 4.1 and 4.2, begin practice problems in Section 4.3 right away. Work as many problems as you can right up to the day before the test. Getting answers is only part of the drill; it is the various ways in which the same problem should be solved over and over again that is also important. Passage-based science problems on the new MCAT provided in this chapter should be solved using the new problem solving model.

In this chapter you will study the different types of skills and strategies needed to solve passage-based science problems found in the MCAT.

4.1 PROBLEM SOLVING CONNECTED WITH SCIENCE KNOWLEDGE

A major effort in your review for the MCAT will be mastery of knowledge areas of the physical and biological sciences. Some elements of effective problem solving can be practiced as you study for premedical course work and as you prepare for the MCAT. These are:

(a) Acquire scientific knowledge in a conceptual form.

- Example: Understand the physical meaning of activation energy and relate the activation energy concept to a chemical reaction.

(b) Develop reasoning skills and apply them to each acquired concept.

- Example: compare activation energy diagram of a chemical or an organic compound to the energy conservation principle as applied to an amusement park roller coaster.

(c) Read scientific journals, encyclopedias and medically related research reports to develop extraction and application skills.

- Example: use an activation energy diagram of a histamine or other vasodilator to compare the effects of a vasoconstrictor. Materials of this type will improve your evaluation and application techniques. It will help you to understand the limitations and assumptions in a scientific study and know whether the arguments in a report or book are persuasive enough to generalize.

(d) Analyze and understand graphic data to check the components of a graph.

- Example: obtain the titration curve of a histamine from lab notes or research material to determine its pK_a and its physiological effects on the digestive system. Note: try to understand the trend represented in the graph and formulate a conclusion, rule or functional relation from the graph.

(e) Synthesize reasoning skills, science knowledge, and mathematics concepts to solve problems.

- Example: understand the interaction of activation energy to the time-release mechanism when seeking information about time-release capsules for an allergy patient taking time-release antihistamines. Learn how to use a problem-solving model to simplify and solve the problem.

There is no part of the new MCAT that causes students more concern than the inclusion of problem solving within the context of the sciences. Yet if you were not interested in solving medical problems, you would not be trying to enter medical school. Problem solving can be difficult and frustrating, but it is also exciting, satisfying and fun. Try to view problem solving as a competitive game: you against the test-maker. Pick an image of this contest that strengthens your resolve to win. You might think of the question writer as a villain to be vanquished, a disease to be conquered, or a puzzler to be out-foxed. Remember that the rules of this game have been defined by the test-maker and that your task is to win working within those rules whether or not you like them.

4.1.1 Problem Solving Using Textbooks and Scientific Journals

Problem solving always requires background knowledge. Some knowledge will come from what you have already learned in your college courses and some will be given to you in the charts or reading passages that precede the problem statement. The new MCAT includes physical sciences passages and biological sciences passages. These passages should not surprise you or hinder you from recalling and applying your science knowledge. An approach like the one below will serve you well if you apply it to each passage:

o Where is this passage taken from (book, laboratory research report, or encyclopedia)?
o Which branch(es) of science (one or more) are revealed in this passage?
o What topics does the passage discuss in detail?
o What is given in the passage about a topic?
o What is it about the topic that is <u>not</u> given in the passage. Why not?

In the new MCAT the premedical science passages before each set of problems come from a variety of sources. These include college textbooks (chemistry, physics, microbiology, introductory physiology, biochemistry), scientific publications (medicine, genetic engineering, bioinstrumentation), and research reports (National Institutes of Health, *Journal of the American Medical Association, New England Journal of Medicine).*

To understand the various types of passages used in the MCAT, you should refer to Appendix A in this book, which also lists the publications that are likely sources of science passages. While your college courses teach the background knowledge required for problem solving, scientific journals and books display the form and content of the premedical material that the MCAT passages are based upon. If you have difficulty in reviewing scientific journals or your science textbooks, return to Chapter 2 for more practice in advanced study skills; also, the reasoning patterns described in section 4.1.2 below will help you hone reasoning in the acquisition of knowledge.

Another important resource in textbooks and journals is the graphic representation of scientific data. Most research publications and some medical books present scientific data in compact representations that may require considerable effort to convert to a form useful in problem solving. A frequently used form of data presentation is the continuous line graph representing a functional relation. The task is to identify the functional relation and check its validity, e.g., viscosity versus temperature, nitrogen concentration versus volume (exhalation), growth rate of psychrophiles versus temperature and myogram (force versus time) of a typical muscle. The best methods for making sense out of graphs, tables and functional equations are rarely taught in school. Section 4.2 provides all the Math concepts for MCAT Sciences. Section 4.3 presents the techniques of numerical interpretation and concludes with a comprehensive review of all the standard techniques of data analysis that may be needed in the MCAT.

4.1.2 Reasoning Skills

You need a solid foundation from college to take you into medical school, and the MCAT attempts to test your level of mastery. That is, on a specific topic such as optics, do you really understand or have you merely memorized what you need in order to pass? Applying something you learned in one way, can you solve a problem that is unlike anything you have seen before? In your own words, can you explain a concept to a colleague who is having trouble understanding it? If you find yourself saying: "I know that material, but I just can't put it into words" you know you have not mastered the information.

The MCAT is designed to help medical schools choose the best possible candidates. The best students tend to be those who can effectively and efficiently analyze information and then integrate it (synthesis). Thus academic learning can be thought of as having two steps: analysis and synthesis.

Content mastery can be tested by asking you to use skills developed throughout your academic life in analytical reading, logical reasoning, quantitative reasoning, perceptual reasoning and problem solving. These skills are like tools in a toolbox. For efficiency and effectiveness, you need to be able to use them all, and it is better to do so consciously than to fumble around in a hit-or-miss fashion.

A conscious awareness of reasoning skills can improve your understanding of the material you study and result in improved test performance. As you read this section, concentrate on the similarities and differences in the patterns. Anticipate how test questions could be formulated to assess particular reasoning skills and how passages leading to the test items are structured around different patterns in reasoning.

ANALYTICAL REASONING

Analysis involves breaking something down into its component parts. This is as true of reading analysis as it is of chemical analysis. Analysis involves identifying primary and secondary pieces of information and then, by reasoning, determining the relationship between them. Learn how to separate relevant and irrelevant pieces of information provided.

For example, you are practicing analysis as you take notes in class. You are selecting the main points (the primary information) and the supporting details. At the same time, by means of an outline, you are indicating the relationship between the two. Underlining can also be a tool for analyzing text if used appropriately. The good student reads first and then selectively underlines key words. At the same time he or she makes notes in the margin or uses numbers to indicate the relationship of one piece of information to another and, especially, how both relate to the whole. Constructing Venn diagrams or relational maps is a graphic analytical tool to read complex passages (refer to the Visual Imaging section, 2.2.3, for an explanation of Venn diagrams).

If analysis involves identifying key nouns as indicators of primary and secondary information, reasoning often requires a focus on words that are important in the sorting process. The careless or hurried reader may overlook qualifying words such as *always*, *some*, *for example*, *most likely*, *probably*, *however*, *consequently*, *as a result of*, *or*, etc.. These words should serve as warning signals. As you read practice passages, circle qualifying words and think about what they are telling you.

Analytical Reasoning Exercises

Exercise 1: Four doctors—Harry, Louise, Kate and Bob—collect automobiles. Among them are owned 20 cars of which 12 are vintage. Harry has three new cars and Louise has the same number of vintage autos. Louise has 1 more car than Harry, who has 5. Kate has three more vintage cars than new ones and the same number of new ones as Bob. How many vintage cars does Bob have?

Exercise 2: Make a Venn Diagram to illustrate the relationship between the following words:

• mothers • daughters • grandmothers • aunts

(This is not an easy relationship to diagram. As a hint, start with mothers and daughters only, and remember that any circle that is contained within another circle means that all its members belong to both groups. When you have that relationship represented by Venn diagrams, add a circle for grandmother. Then add aunts.)

As with any skill, it is important to practice the process of visually representing and summarizing concepts. While relational maps condense and integrate classroom information, they can also be used on the MCAT as a "sorting" tool to organize and analyze content.

Exercise 3: Read the following biological sciences passage and develop a relational map.

"The eye is a layer of photoreceptor cells and associated neurons packaged within a fibrous, rubber-like protective globe that is transparent in front. The eyeball is almost spherical in shape, about 2.5 centimeters in diameter, with three concentric coats or tunics surrounding the refractive media. These coats are the fibrous coat, the vascular coat, and the nervous coat.

The fibrous tunic is the outermost coat and consists of the sclera and the cornea. The sclera, meaning 'hard,' is a tough, white supporting tunic. It covers the posterior five-sixths of the eye. The cornea, meaning 'horny,' covers the anterior one-sixth and is continuous with the sclera. The radius of the cornea is less than that of the sclera—that is, it has a greater curvature, so it bulges somewhat. In addition to transmitting light, the cornea also is a refractive medium and focuses the light rays.

The middle coat, or vascular tunic, is divided into the iris, the ciliary body, and the choroid. The iris forms a diaphragm between the cornea and the lens and is like a curtain with a central perforation—the pupil. The diameter of the pupil may be altered by the muscles in the iris that are oriented in two directions. One set of muscles pulls the iris back toward the ciliary body to dilate the pupil. The other muscle draws the iris down around the front of the lens to constrict the pupil. The color of the iris is largely a function of the amount of pigment within. The ciliary body is ring-shaped with protrusions or folds on the internal surface that are responsible for the secretion of aqueous humor. The choroid, chiefly composed of blood vessels and pigment, lines the posterior part of the sclera. This vascular, highly pigmented layer absorbs the light and prevents scattering.

The innermost coat, or tunic, is the retina which is the light-sensitive layer of the eye. It consists of several layers of cell bodies and fibers. One of these layers, called rods and cones, is photoreceptor neurons. The rods are highly sensitive to light and insensitive to color, whereas the cones are sensitive to color and provide the highest visual acuity."

Make sure your map contains the following elements:

- main concept in modified sentence form
- organizational pattern
- details represented relative to main idea
- summary statement

Exercise 4: Read the biological sciences passage below and construct a Venn diagram.

Review of Carbohydrates

Carbohydrates have the general formula $C_n(H_2O)_m$ where *n* and *m* are whole numbers. Monosaccharides are the basic units of carbohydrates. They are classified by the number of carbons they contain, i.e. *hexoses* (C_6), *pentoses* (C_5), etc. Hexoses and pentoses exist in predominantly ring forms called *pyranoses* (six-membered rings) or *furanoses* (five-membered rings) in equilibrium with the open-chain forms. Ring forms are hemiacetals; open-chain forms are polyhydroxyl aldehydes. In the ring forms, alpha or betaanomers are possible. The pyranoses exist in the stable chain conformation with most, if not all, of the hydroxyls in equatorial positions. When two monosaccharides differ by the configuration of one hydroxyl group, they are called *epimers*. If *n* is the number of asymmetric carbons, then 2^n is the number of optical isomers (based on open-chain).

Hexoses usually have n=4, and pentoses usually have n=3. Sugars are given a relative configuration on the basis of the orientation of the next-to-last carbon's hydroxyl group as compared to D-glyceraldehyde. Most naturally occurring sugars have the D configuration. A *ketose* is a carbohydrate with a ketone group; and *aldose* has an aldehyde group.

Monosaccharides join together to form *disaccharides.* The new bond is called a *glycosidic* bond and is between the hemiacetal carbon and an hydroxyl group of the other sugar; water is released when the bond is formed. Hydrolysis (breaking) of the bond requires water. The glycosidic bond is an acetal grouping. *Sucrose* (common sugar) is made of glucose and fructose. *Lactose* (milk sugar) is made of galactose and glucose. *Maltose* (alpha-1,4 bond) is made of two glucose units and is an hydrolysis product of starch or glycogen. *Cellobiose* (beta-1,4 bond) is also made of two glucoses, and it is the breakdown product of the cellulose.

Polysaccharides are many monosaccharides joined by glycosidic bonds; they may be branched also. *Starch* (plant energy storage), *glycogen* (animal short-term energy storage), and *cellulose* (plant structural component) are all made from glucose. Cellulose has beta-1,4 bonds not found in the other two. Starch and glycogen both have alpha-1,4 bonds but differ in the frequency and position of branch points (alpha-1, 6 bond).

Insulin is a polymer of fructose.

Using the information above, make an association diagram using the following words: carbohydrates, monosaccharides, disaccharides, starch, lactose, glucose, polysaccharides, fructose, sucrose, maltose, cellobiose, glycogen, and cellulose.

Exercise 5: Here are three more exercises. The more you practice, the more proficient you will become. First decide what information belongs in the diagram to help you remember the concept. Then, be as careful and precise as possible. Check especially what each space represents. These exercises may be done along with your reading of related sections in Chapter 7.

(a) Draw a Venn diagram illustrating the characteristics of eukaryotic cells and prokaryotic cells.

(b) Draw Venn diagrams that illustrate the relationship between isomers, stereoisomers, and enantiomers.

(c) Draw Venn diagrams to illustrate the relationship between diastereomers and meso compounds.

Remember, problem areas present opportunities for learning. Use your textbook or other resources to clarify any word or term that is difficult for you.

SYNTHETIC REASONING

If all reasoning were analytical, we would understand only how pieces are derived from the whole. With synthetic reasoning, the opposite process occurs; individual pieces are recombined in a way to form a larger integrated piece. For example, take 3 individual slices of apple pie and 3 individual slices of peach pie to form a complete or whole apple-peach pie (6 slices).

One example of synthetic reasoning is when you construct summaries or relational maps. Another is when you explain the relevant information covered in a lecture to a classmate. Both of these activities are involved in constructing meanings from a body of information. The MCAT, in particular, is interested in your ability to synthesize facts from various subjects to construct new possibilities, e.g., in the way that human physiology may be seen in light of what you have learned in physics, chemistry, biology, and math. Synthetic reasoning often involves creativity in reviewing ways to integrate content information and constructing frameworks.

Another word for synthetic reasoning would be "integrated reasoning", e.g., biology of the bone involves studying the bone matrix at a cellular level; physics of the bone studies stress, forces on bones, elasticity of bones, etc. Integration of biology and physics results in the biophysics of the bone.

It is a reflection of synthetic reasoning when science disciplines are combined as subtest names in the MCAT. The Physical Sciences subtest contains physics and general chemistry; Biological Sciences subtest contains biology and organic chemistry. The problems presented in the MCAT, especially the passage-based problems, require integration of concepts and principles from across science disciplines; for example, a study of the viscosity of bone marrow, or the measurement of human blood characteristics using Doppler/ultrasonic instrumentation. Students should master the process of combining topics from all the natural sciences to gain proficiency in synthetic reasoning.

Synthetic Reasoning Exercises

Exercise 6: Complete this sequence and describe the pattern it follows.
1000 1500 1450 1950 1900 2400 2350 _____ _____ _____

Exercise 7: Complete the following sequence and explain how it is formed:
12, -6, 3, -1.5, ___, ___, ___

Exercise 8: Derive a rule concerning the sum of a fraction and its reciprocal.

Exercise 9: **A** travels 20 miles a day; **B** starts 3 days later and travels 8 miles the first day, 12 the second, and so on, in arithmetical progression. In how many days will **B** overtake **A**?

ASSOCIATIVE/ANALOGICAL REASONING

Associative or analogical reasoning enables a transfer of concepts from one subject to another using the principle of similarity, such as learning biology principles within a physics framework. As an example, consider how does the movement of blood inside veins and arteries relate to the concept of fluid flow in physics?

Analogical reasoning utilizes associations in a particular way. In analogical reasoning, an easily understood concept is compared to something more difficult in order to develop better understanding. Analogy is often a creative tool used by scientists. The structure of DNA, for example, is often presented as a visual analogy of two snakes coiled around each other.

The terms used for this form of reasoning—analogical, associative—are important since by definition they imply a linkage between key words. They are useful in establishing connections, analyzing similar situations and are powerful tools in memorization. For example, if you wanted to remember Boyle's law, you might associate it with the action of pushing on the accelerator while driving a car. In Boyle's law, pressure is inversely proportional to volume. When you push down on the accelerator, you are decreasing the volume and increasing the pressure in the piston. Conversely, when you let up on the accelerator, the volume in the piston increases and the pressure decreases.

In many textbook charts and tables the data included are examples of associations. Charts and tables should be studied for the relationships between given information, but constructing your own associations is a powerful exercise for clarifying your reasoning and assisting in your memorization. Develop analogies between laboratory experiments and theoretical knowledge of theories, principles, and laws.

Analogical Reasoning Exercise:

Exercise 10: The number 60 is to 10 as ___ is to ___

A. 120, 20
B. 20, 5
C. 150, 100
D. 5, 20

Exercise 11: Acorn is to oak as ___ is to ___

A. nut, crack
B. cone, hemlock spruce
C. squirrel, nut
D. spruce, cone

Exercise 12: Hand is to shoulder as ___ is to ___

A. foot, hip
B. head, neck
C. toes, finger
D. toes, foot

COMPARATIVE REASONING

Associative reasoning leads naturally to comparison and contrast. We tend to compare things that are similar in some ways, yet dissimilar in others. No one bothers to compare an orange and a truck, but one would compare and/or contrast smooth and skeletal muscles or afferent and efferent nerves. When reading how two things are different, remember that they are being contrasted because they also have similarities.

In order to distinguish adequately between similarities and differences, it is necessary to organize information so that these distinctions are discernible. For example, as every test-maker knows, it is easy to confuse the functions of the liver with those of the spleen. A table of comparison and contrast, between electrochemical and electrolytic cells, is presented in the section on electrochemistry. Constructing comparison and contrast tables speeds up your review and makes it more detailed.

Comparative Reasoning Exercises:

Exercise 13: Compare and contrast the two figures below. How are they similar; how are they different? List ten similarities and ten differences.

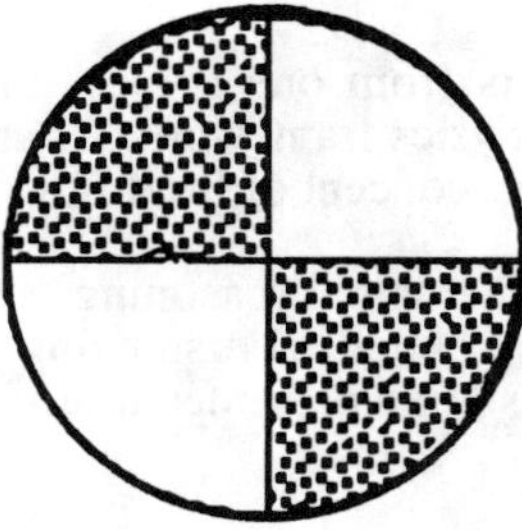

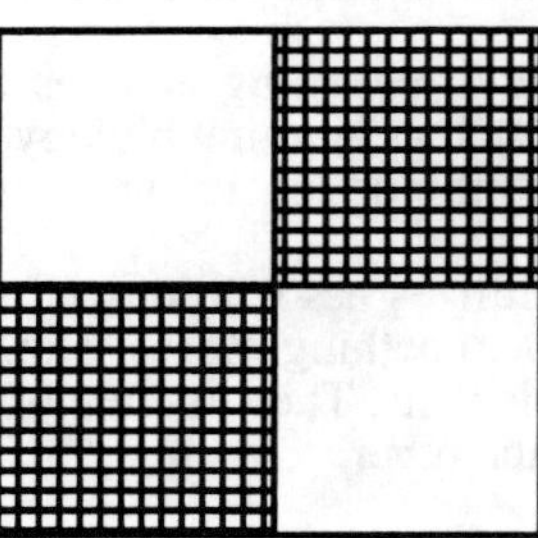

Exercise 14: For the following comparison-contrast exercises, list aspects that are shared or are not shared and make a yes/no list for each. Then check your list against information in your text book or other references.

(a) Electrolytic, galvanic, and concentration cells.
(b) Heterozygous and homozygous genes.
(c) Period and group for the atomic table.
(d) Entropy and enthalpy.
(e) Capacitors and resistors.

INTUITIVE REASONING

Intuitive reasoning (also called creative or abstract reasoning) is a creative use of the imagination to solve problems. The subject is rarely mentioned in the classroom because we know neither how to teach it nor how to test it. Basically, a creative imagination makes an intuitive leap (often unasked for and instantaneous) that was not logically apparent. Thus a doctor might have a preliminary diagnosis that is then systematically and carefully checked with further questions, examinations, tests, etc. The scientist who discovered the way stars age did so by making an intuitive connection between aging stars and humans.

If you would like to develop your creativity further, you might work some of the exercises in Edwards' *Drawing On the Right Side of the Brain*. Also, Vitale's *Unicorns are Real: A Right-Brained Approach to Learning* includes information about individual learning styles.

Intuitive Reasoning Exercises:

Exercise 15: The electric knife and electric spoon exist. How could an electric fork be used?

Exercise 16: How long would it take to skateboard from Seattle to Maine?

Exercise 17: You are a passenger on a train. How could you calculate its speed? Repeat this problem for a subway and an airplane.

Exercise 18: Prove that light travels in straight lines without using any equipment.

VISUAL REASONING

There is experimental evidence that very young infants can reason visually—well before they have acquired language. Although the ability to reason visually is the key to solving many science problems, some students find they have neglected their visual reasoning skills (perhaps they attended a school without windows or possibly watched too much television).

Use your visual reasoning skills to help solve physics problems such as those concerned with the flow of water through pipes of different diameters. (As a doctor, you will be concerned with the flow of liquids through the "pipes" of living beings.) Picture a first floor apartment and a sixth floor apartment in the same building. Which apartment is likely to have better water pressure in the shower? Why? Which apartment is likely to have the better bathtub drainage? Why? How could you improve water pressure or drainage?

Visual reasoning involves the process of representing concepts in such a way that relationships become apparent. For example, in geometry, the parts of the problem must often be sketched so that the relationships are evident. On the MCAT, the ability to reason visually is an important key to solving many problems both in the science and verbal reasoning sections. Often a quick diagram or sketch to yourself can be an important tool to establishing relationships.

Visual Reasoning Exercises

Notice that in addition to picturing objects you must also be able to imagine how they move.

Exercise 19: A box is set on a series of rollers with a circumference of 3 feet. The rollers lie on level ground. If the box is pushed causing the rollers to make one revolution, how far does the box travel with respect to the ground? (Assume no slippage occurs.)

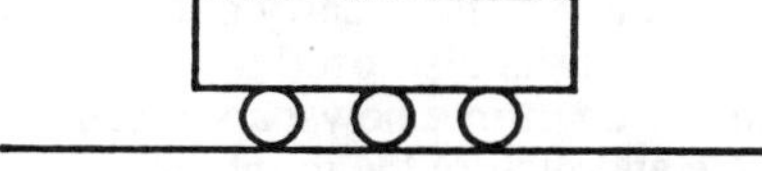

Exercise 20: In the following science exercises draw a schematic or a clear sketch which demonstrates your mastery of the concept:

(a) Visualize the Doppler effect. Can you explain in one sentence what causes it?

(b) Draw the molecules of epimers and anomers to help you conceptualize them in your mind. (Use straight lines.)

(c) Sketch the filtration process that takes place in the glomerulus and nephron of a human kidney.

Exercise 21: Describe the trace of corner **A** as the illustrated square turns end-over-end along level ground.

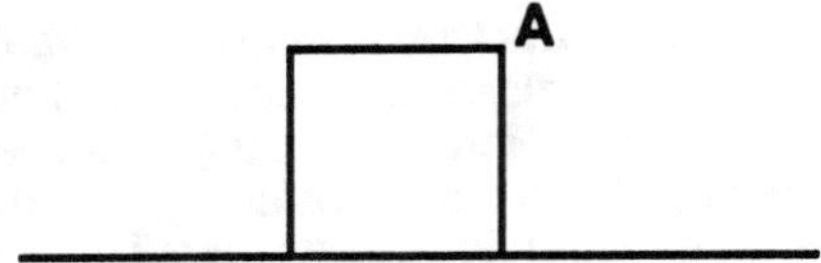

LOGICAL REASONING

Logical reasoning provides a systematic means for testing or proving a hypothesis or conclusion. Because it is concerned with proof, logical reasoning is a way of thinking that is associated with the development of science and scientific method. Conclusions can be valid or invalid and come in three degrees of certainty: hypothesis, conclusion suggested, and conclusion confirmed. In addition to understanding the rules of formal logic, it is also important to know fallacies of reasoning since they can pinpoint errors in thinking patterns. See Chapter 3 to reinforce your understanding of logical arguments and their evaluation.

There are many books available that provide the formal rules of logic and exercises to practice them. We recommend that you use these books to improve your logical reasoning ability. One recommended text is S. Morris Engel's *With Good Reason: An Introduction to Informal Fallacies.*

Logical Reasoning Exercises

Exercise 22: If some teacups are olimunds and all olimunds have handles,

A. do all teacups have handles?
B. do some teacups have handles?

Exercise 23: Make a Venn drawing showing the following relationships:

A. all apples are brown
B. no brothers are crazy
C. some colas are diet

Exercise 24: The town clerk of Mudville needs to mail license renewal notices to all residents who own one or more dogs and to all gun owners. Using these statistics, how many people must be contacted?

A. Gun owners	500
B. Dog owners	850
C. Gun owners with dogs	350

QUANTITATIVE REASONING

Quantitative reasoning involves choosing a reasonable mathematical method to begin to solve a problem. It involves identifying the known from the unknown and applying the information to a mathematical process or formula. It might also involve estimating and judging the appropriateness of an answer. For example, in solving for the leg of a right triangle, all answers could be eliminated which are longer than the hypotenuse.

Quantitative skills are used when you quickly and precisely carry out mathematical operations in your head. For example, multiply 41 x 41. Quantitative reasoning is also used to translate words to numbers and numbers to words. For example, looking only at a graph or chart in a newspaper, can you tell what the accompanying story is about? Conversely, can you read the article and picture the graph or chart? (For more examples and additional practice, refer to section 4.2 on "Mathematics Concepts for MCAT Sciences.")

The new MCAT tests your quantitative reasoning indirectly through mathematical problems in physical and biological sciences. The application of mathematics concepts to problem solving is required and mastery of these concepts is essential. In this chapter, the MCAT mathematics review is organized by concept and each concept is followed by conceptual examples and exercises.

Quantitative Reasoning Exercises

Exercise 25: Distribute $3 among Tom, Dick, and Harry so that Tom and Dick shall each have twice as much as Harry.

Exercise 26: Arrange in order of magnitude: 9 times the square root of 3, 6 times the square root of 7, 5 times the square root of 10.

Exercise 27: Which statement is correct?

A. $.7/7 > 7/.7$
B. $.7/7 = 7/.7$
C. $.7/7 < 7/.7$

Exercise 28: A technician counts a quantity of syringes which he knows is between 50 and 60. When he counts them three at a time there are 2 left over; when he counts them 5 at a time there are 4 left over. How many are there in all?

Exercise 29: Which is greater, *m* x *m* + *m* or *m* cubed + 1, given *m* is positive.

PROPORTIONAL REASONING

Proportional reasoning is often used to measure changes in one variable relative to changes in another, as in problems applying Boyle's law. It may also be used to solve problems in physics and chemistry, such as velocity of moving particles, acid-base concentrations, etc. The MCAT may utilize proportional reasoning on the science sections, as with velocity and concentration problems. It may also be apparent in questions relating to population tables and charts.

Proportional reasoning is very important to both physical and biological sciences and, therefore, worth additional emphasis. It can be contrasted with additive reasoning in which one asks, "What do I add to (or subtract from) x in order to get y?" In proportional reasoning one asks, "What do I multiply x by to get y?" The easiest method to find this unknown is to divide y by x; if these numbers are in a constant proportion the result will be a constant number no matter which set of (x,y) pairs we pick. For example, the length of the circumference (C) of a circle is in direct proportion to the length of that circle's diameter (D). If we divide the circumference by the diameter we will always get the number pi. (There is no one number that you can add to the diameter that will always yield the circumference.) In proportional problems we often leave out the constant and equate two pairs of numbers: $C_1/D_1 = C_2/D_2$.

The fact that both these ratios are equal to pi is what makes it possible to equate them.

It is useful to have a visual image of the proportion. There should be two quantities, one usually larger than the other and a factor (constant number) that will tell you how much to inflate the smaller to get the larger.

Proportional Reasoning Exercises

Exercise 30: Two numbers are in the ratio 3:4. The ratio of their sum to the sum of their squares is 7:50. Find the two numbers.

Exercise 31: The speeds (or rates) of a bicycle and a tricycle are in the ratio of 5:4. In a one-mile race, the tricycle had a half-minute head start but was beaten by 1/10 mile. Find the rate of each.

4.1.3 SOLUTIONS TO EXERCISES

Analytical Reasoning

1. For this type of problem it is useful to make a table. The table below shows information that is given directly for the problem.

		new	vintage	total
Harry		3		5
Louise			3	5 + 1
Kate		n	n + 3	
Bob	n	?		
			12	20

Next, work with the rows and columns to figure the missing elements.

	new	vintage	total
Harry	3		5
Louise	3	3	5 + 1
Kate	n	n + 3	
Bob	n	?	
	8	12	20

It is clear that n = 1, hence Kate has 5 cars; therefore Bob must have 4 cars of which only 1 is new. Bob owns 3 vintage cars.

2. In the left-hand drawing, the outer circle is "daughters" because all mothers are daughters, but daughters are not necessarily mothers. The space between the circles becomes "daughters who are not mothers." In the right-hand drawing, all mothers and grandmothers are daughters and all grandmothers are mothers. While all aunts are daughters, the drawing shows some aunts are grandmothers and mothers.

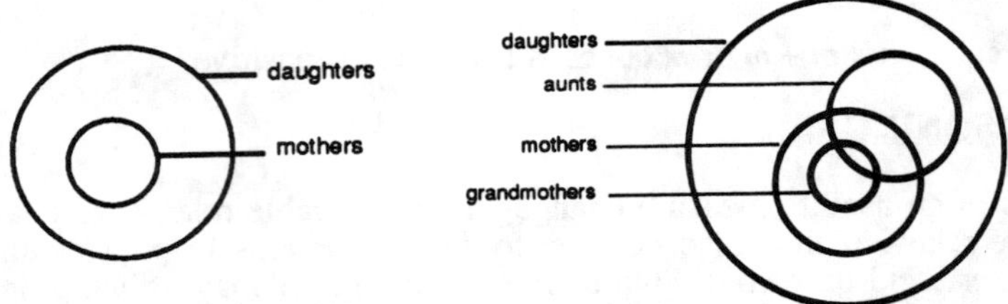

3. Instructions for this exercise include a statement of the main idea, which is physical description; the organizational pattern, which is spatial; and representation of details relative to the main idea, which is in drawing the parts of the eye. The summary statement is "physical characteristics and functions."

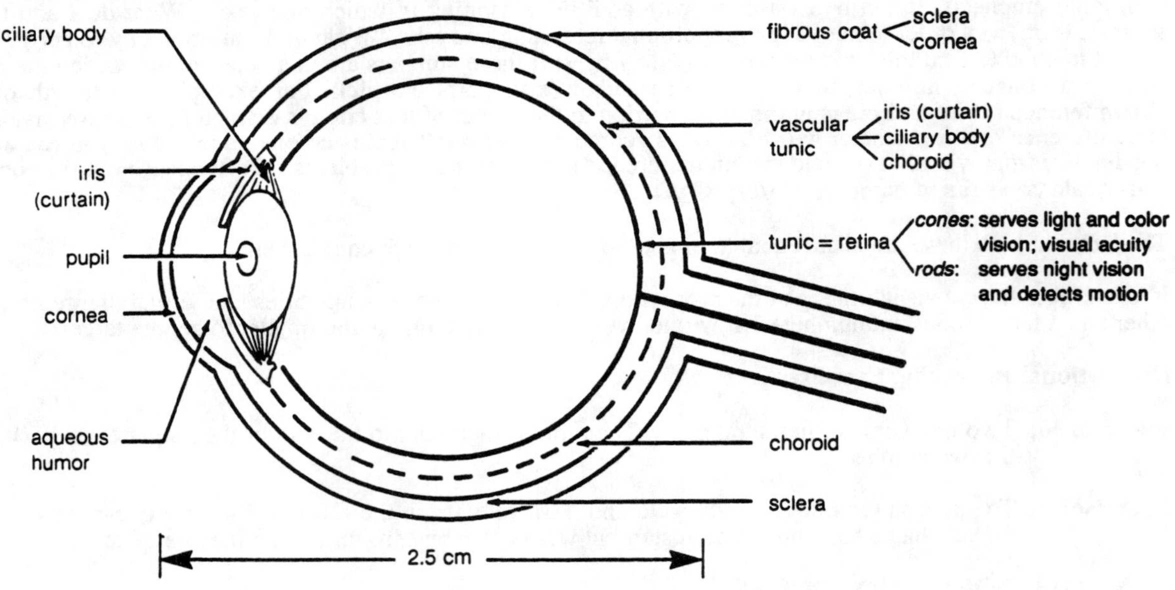

4.

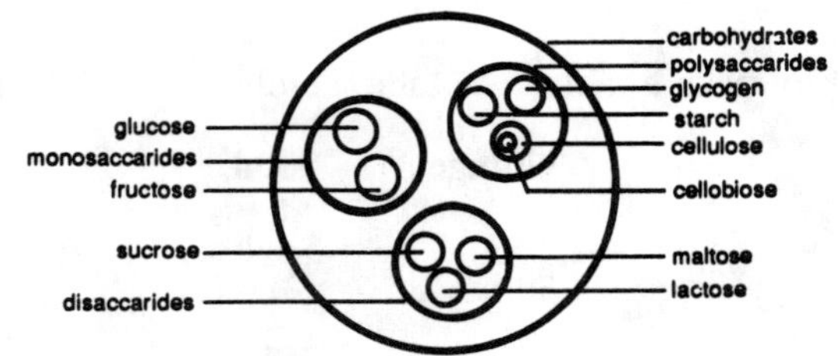

5. These exercises should be done using Chapter 7. Use the knowledge in Chapter 7 to construct Venn diagrams.

Synthetic Reasoning

6. The additive jumps are: 500, -50, 500, -50, 500, -50. The next elements will be: 2850, 2800, 3300.

7. Additive changes don't seem to work; try multiplicative. The sign keeps changing so try a negative number; the size keeps reducing, so try a fraction. The factor is - 1/2. The next three elements are: 3/4, - 3/8, 3/16.

8. What is the sum of 1/x + x? Try some examples.

1/2 + 2 = 2 and 1/2 = 5/2 = (4 + 1)/2
1/3 + 3 = 3 and 1/3 = 10/3 = (9 + 1)/3
1/4 + 4 = 4 and 1/4 = 17/4 = (16 + 1)/4
1/x + x = $(x^2 + 1)/x$

9. Drawing a diagram may be useful. **B** will overtake **A** after 13 days or 260 miles.

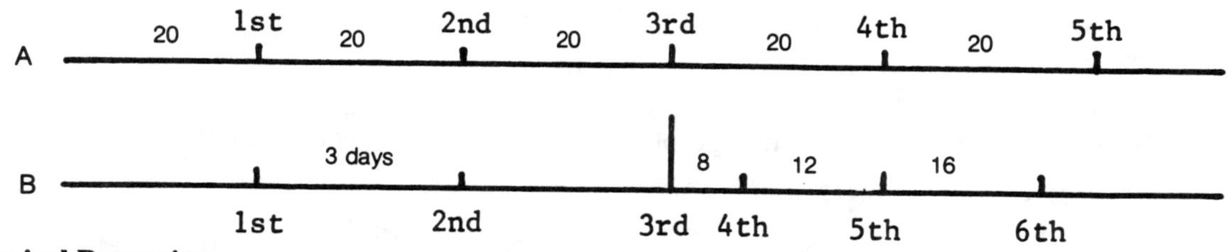

Analogical Reasoning

10. The simplest operations that get us from 60 to 10 and 120 to 20 are to divide by 6.

11. Acorns are the fruit of an oak; cones are the fruit of a hemlock spruce.

12. The hand is at the end of the limb that starts at the shoulder; the foot is at the end of the limb that starts at the hip.

Comparative Reasoning

13.
- Both figures are divided into quarters with half of the area shaded.
- The left figure is round while the right figure is square.
- The first and third quadrants of the right figure are shaded, while on the left figure these quadrants are clear...., etc.

14. The comparison-contrast exercises should be done using the text in Chapters 5 and 7.

Intuitive/Creative or Abstract Reasoning

15. Electric fork problem. Answers will vary depending on how an electric spoon and knife are used by you.

16. Estimate the distance, perhaps 4,000 miles. Try to think how far one can skateboard in an hour, remembering that some roads may not be as easy to skateboard on. It is probably quicker than a fast walk, maybe 6 miles per hour. If you cover 40 miles per day it will take 100 days.

17. For the train, measure how many seconds between the telephone poles, and then estimate the spacing of the poles. For the subway it is much harder to find a repetitive object with an even spacing that you can estimate, but there may be one if you look for it. For the plane, you may be able to use the wing edge to measure how long it takes to cross a field, but estimating the field size could prove difficult. If you cannot see the ground, the problem is much harder; you might find the average speed for the trip using the flight time and estimating the distance using the map in the flight magazine.

18. The phenomenon that "light travels in straight lines" can be demonstrated by holding a book in front of a light source. No equipment is allowed, though! Watch sunrise and sunset and how sun rays filter in straight paths through branches of trees. On a partially sunny day the sun rays travel through clouds in straight lines.

Visual Reasoning

19. This may require that you actually try the problem with a model. The box will move forward one circumference with respect to the roller and the roller will move forward one circumference with respect to the ground. The box therefore moves two circumferences by 6 feet.

20. Use your knowledge in Chapters 5 and 7 to construct these diagrams.

21.

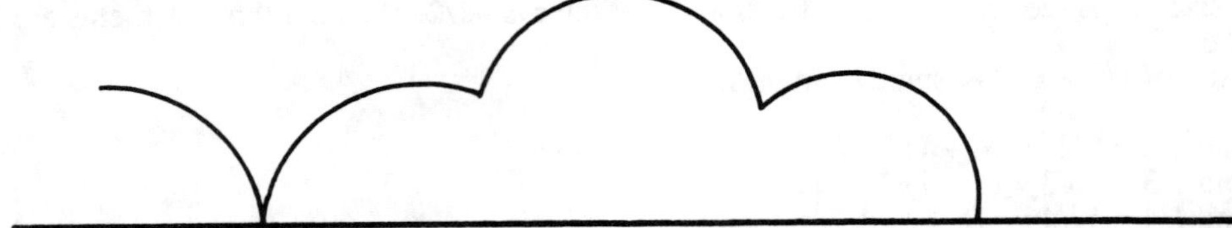

Logical Reasoning

22. A. maybe, if all these teacups are olimunds.
    B. yes

23. A. Apples = A, Brown objects = B   B. Brothers = B, Crazy people = C   C. Colas = C, Diet drinks = D

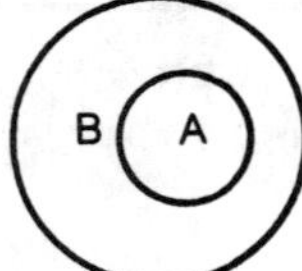

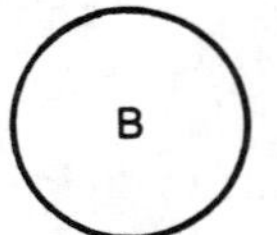

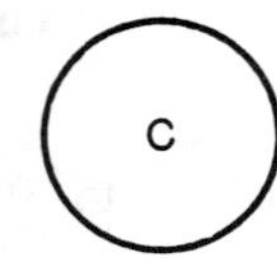

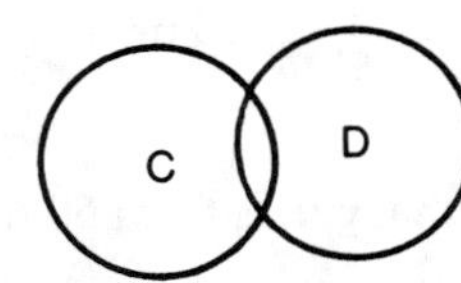

24. A Venn diagram may be useful. Answer: 1000 people.

Quantitative Reasoning

25. Tom gets 2x, Dick gets 2x, and Harry gets x:
    2x + 2x + x = \$3.00 (or 5x = \$3.00) and x = .60
    [Tom = \$1.20, Dick = \$1.20, Harry = \$.60]

26. To arrange these numbers in order: $9\sqrt{3}$, $6\sqrt{7}$, $5\sqrt{10}$, one can square each number to remove the square roots, as in: 81 x 3 = 243, 25 x10 = 250, 36 x 7 = 252.

27. C

28. The given information is: $3x + 2 = 5y + 4$
    or, $x = (5y + 2) \div 3$.

We also know that 3x + 2 must fall between 50 and 60 and therefore x must be less than 20. Try values for y that might generate such an x.

Begin by choosing values of y, which when multiplied by 5 yield a number between 50 and 60. The first such number is 10, which does not work in the equation above. The next number-11-yields an answer of 59 (5y + 4), which is also equal to 3x + 2 when x = 19.

29. Make a table:

m	m x m + m	m x m x m + 1
1	2	2
2	6	9
3	12	28
4	20	65

$m^3 + 1$ is larger for values of m larger than 1

Proportional Reasoning

30. Two numbers that are in the ratio of 3:4 are 3x and 4x. The rest of the problem says that:

$(3x + 4x)/(9x^2 + 16x^2) = 7/50$

$7x/25x^2 = 7/25x = 7/50$; hence, $x = 2$

The two numbers are 6 and 8.

31.

	Distance	Rate	Time
Bicycle	1	(5/4)R	t - 1/2
Tricycle	9/10	R	t

Distance = Rate x Time
Therefore, Rate = $\frac{\text{Distance}}{\text{Time}}$

Bicycle:
Tricycle:
$$\frac{5}{4} = \frac{\frac{1}{t - 1/2}}{\frac{9/10}{t}} \qquad \begin{matrix} \left(\frac{\text{Distance}}{\text{Time}} \text{ for bicycle}\right) \\ \left(\frac{\text{Distance}}{\text{Time}} \text{ for tricycle}\right) \end{matrix}$$

t = 9/2 minutes (the time the tricycle spends racing)

Tricycle rate: $\frac{9/10}{t} = \frac{9/10}{9/2} = \frac{9}{10} \cdot \frac{2}{9} = \frac{1}{5}$

Bicycle rate: $\frac{5}{4} R = \frac{5}{4} \cdot \frac{1}{5} = \frac{1}{4}$ mile/min.

Problems 25-31 were selected from a standard high school algebra book that was in use over 100 years ago.

4.1.4 EXERCISES IN INTEGRATED REASONING

No problem can involve only one kind of reasoning, nor is it possible to solve a problem using only reasoning and no facts. The MCAT problems are designed to see how well you can coordinate several different kinds of reasoning while working with the knowledge you gained from your undergraduate science courses. Try to identify the types of reasoning you use in solving the wheelchair and ladder problems that follow:

Wheelchair

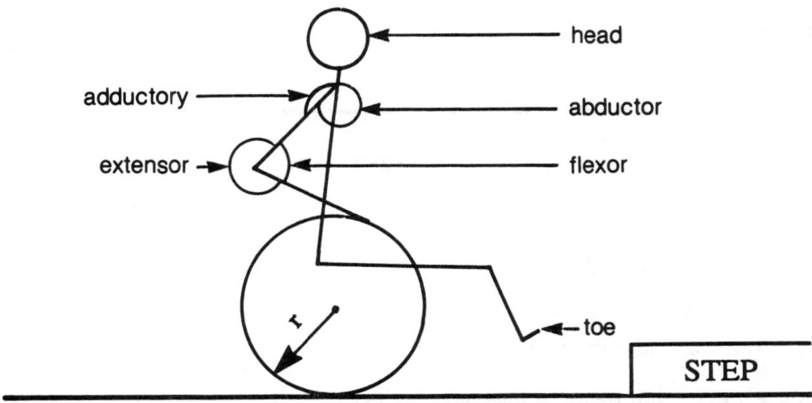

1. Which pattern of muscle activity will have the effect of moving the wheelchair forward?

A. Stimulate the extensor and abductor, inhibit the flexor and adductor
B. Stimulate the abductor and adductor, inhibit the flexor and extensor
C. Inhibit the flexor and abductor, stimulate the extensor and adductor
D. Inhibit the extensor and abductor, stimulate the flexor and adductor

2. The maximum technical advantage is found in:

A. the adductor or the abductor.
B. the flexor or the adductor.
C. the extensor.
D. the wheel.

3. In the diagram above, the force applied to the wheel is directed along a tangent to the wheel at an angle of about 45 degrees in the horizontal. In which of the following directions could the force be applied to obtain an equally efficient or a more efficient effect? There may be more than one correct answer.

A. Tangential to the wheel applied closer to the hub
B. Tangential to the wheel applied horizontally
C. Any horizontal force whether or not it is tangential
D. A force applied at 30 degrees to the horizontal plane

4. When the wheelchair reaches the step indicated in the diagram the extra force needed will be

A. W (the weight of the chair and the occupant)
B. W/r (W divided by the radius of the wheel)
C. W/2pr
D. W/2

5. The wheelchair comes to a smooth up-ramp with railing which it can negotiate without having the wheels slip. Will more force need to be applied pulling on the railings or pushing on the top rim of the wheel?

A. More on the railings
B. More on the wheels
C. The same on each
D. Depends on the slope of the ramp

6. The ladder in the diagram starts to swing out to the left. In order to return to the house, which of the following actions should the man take? More than one way may be correct.

A. Swing his arms clockwise
B. Swing his arms counter-clockwise
C. Lean forward
D. Lean backward

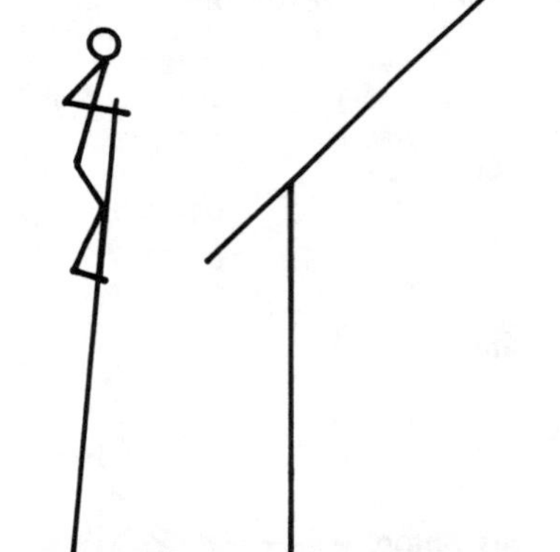

7. The man will have less leeway in time to react if (indicate all correct responses):

A. the ladder is long.
B. the ladder is short.
C. he recently had two shots of alcoholic beverages.
D. he is over 40 years old.

8. As the ladder continues to swing left (indicate all correct responses):

A. the man's heart rate will increase and he will begin to lose heat rapidly.
B. the man's vision will blur.
C. the man's angular momentum will be conserved.
D. the concentration of CO_2 in his exhaled breath will decrease.

4.1.5 Solutions to Exercises in Integrated Reasoning

Wheelchair Problems

1. **A** Extensor increases the angle at joint, abductor moves bone away toward midline

2. **D** All muscles work at a fractional mechanical advantage

3. **B** Tangential to the wheel applied at rim

4. **D** The wheel will act as a lever of length 2r with the weight concentrated at its center

5. **A** You can think of the wheel as a lever or consider the distance through which the forces are applied. When the rail is pulled, the force is applied through the same distance as the chair moves. But when pushing on the rim of the wheel, the force is applied through twice the distance as the chair moves. This is not easy to see. One revolution of the wheel produces a forward movement of one revolution. The point of force application at the top of the wheel moves forward both by the forward motion of the entire chair and by the rotation of the wheel.

Ladder problems

6. **B** and **D** (if ladder swings to right), or **A** and **C** (if ladder swings to left). The counter torques (due to swinging of arms and leaning) should resist the torque of the falling ladder. Note: Center of mass of the man and ladder, and friction between ladder and ground should be considered in your analysis.

7. **B, C,** and **D** The period of swing decreases with length: therefore, the longer the ladder the longer it will take the ladder to move, giving the man more time to respond. Age and alcohol both increase human reaction times making it much harder to respond in time.

8. **A, C,** and **D** The fright response includes an increased heart rate, sharper vision, faster blood flow, increased rate of breathing. Faster blood flow and rapid movement through the air would increase heat loss. Faster breathing without strenuous exercise would decrease the concentration of CO_2 in each breath.

4.1.6 MODEL FOR PASSAGE-BASED PROBLEM SOLVING

Technically, you need only one year of college biology, a year of general chemistry, a year of organic chemistry, and a year of physics to prepare yourself in the sciences for the MCAT and for medical school. This means that from the MCAT test-maker's point of view, the science content of the MCAT is limited by definition with emphasis increased on reasoning skills required in scientific passage-based problems.

Passage-based problems in the new MCAT frequently contain material that is likely to be unfamiliar or unexpected. Familiar knowledge may be cast in unusual circumstances or combined with knowledge from a different discipline. You may need to apply both biology and physics in answering a single question. To build your confidence in solving passage-based science problems in the MCAT, you will need to work with the unfamiliar and the unexpected, with unusual research studies, and with the demands of combined or separate disciplines. In the remainder of this section, we will systematically help you construct your own approach to conquering these challenges.

Many students develop these problem solving skills in a hit-or-miss fashion because most schools teach these skills in a random or unorganized way. This section helps you develop your problem solving skills and gives you practice and confidence in answering science problems questions within a conscious problem-solving framework. When doing science problems be precise and work quickly. Be sure you fully understand each problem; read carefully and think actively. You must recall facts, but you should be able to apply scientific concepts. The more precisely you can apply these concepts, the greater is your mastery of the information.

You are advised to read section 3.3 on "Argument Analysis", the chart on Page 4-143 (Passage Types) and Appendix A (pages A-10, A-11, A-12) to understand the background of the problem solving model.

Problem Solving Model

This problem solving model should guide you to solve almost any physical and biological science problem on the MCAT. This model has been tried on a host of audiences—including students, assistant faculty, counselors, and other health professions candidates. You are urged to really understand this model and develop confidence by using it over and over again.

STEP I: Complete Understanding by Reading: What is Given?

This step includes a full understanding and total comprehension of the passage and the accompanying problem. The step may be subdivided into:

Substep 1-- Passage interpretation by content
- Include recall of related concepts, ask questions to yourself as you read the passage.

Substep 2-- Passage interpretation with stress on data presented or given, graphs, diagrams or designs
- Watch for every graphic detail.

Substep 3-- Passage interpretation to understand research procedures or experimental findings
- Look for most probable causes, discovering underlying cause-effect relationships and developing familiarity with new information.

Substep 4-- Comprehension of relationships among several variables or methods.
- Helps you choose a better problem solving method or strategy.

Substep 5-- Learning how to comprehend new technical terms in medicine
- Make certain that **no** assumptions are made about their meaning; instead, constantly try to find their contextual meaning by association with problems.

Substep 6-- Trying to investigate the source of the passage (journal, textbook, or other source) in relation to why was the passage written.
- Gives you clues to separate the relevant and irrelevant information.

Substep 7-- The above substeps lead you to the following question, "What is given in the passage and in the problem?"
- Detailed understanding and comprehension eventually help you to dissect all the given information.

STEP II: Preparing Perceptive Model of Given Information: How Can the Given be Used?

This step is creative and requires a higher level of concentration. It involves organization and assembling of pertinent information. It really helps you draw a rough sketch or a flow diagram from the given. Graphical extraction from the given is easier to use than textual information. The following substeps will help you keep your attention focused on:

Substep 1-- Use similar situations to draw a simple sketch.
- Use analogical, analytical, and logical reasoning methods to help you mentally see the given information

Substep 2-- Reread some sections or parts of the passage slowly
- Underline or circle cues linking you to already known concepts and sketch what you see (a mental picture is acceptable but a rough picture on paper is more convenient to use). This substep will help you remove the doubts about superficial familiarity with the passage.

STEP III: Understanding the Problem: What is the Question?

This step is critical before you solve the problem. Ask yourself, "What question is really being asked?" The following substeps will help you:

Substep 1-- Try to condense the question as much as possible, to really comprehend the nature of the question.
- Check to see if the question is complete and directly stated. A word of caution! Do not try to rephrase the question according to a simpler or easier version that you have seen before.
- Do not assume or pretend that if you can answer a simpler question, you also know this problem equally well. In order to test you, the test-maker may have considered the simpler option and included a response to check your precision in understanding the question.

Substep 2-- **The limitations and assumptions inherent in the question stem should be isolated and examined.**

- The process of elimination used to delete wrong answers (from the four multiple-choice responses) will prove to be successful if the limitations of the question are properly examined.

STEP IV: Finding the Appropriate Problem Solving Method: How Do You Solve It?

This step is time consuming because it integrates the earlier steps of given information, the perceptual model and the nature of the question asked. You could waste time in this step if you do not know which way to go. It is important to mention here that MCAT problems are not mechanical—you should <u>not</u> plug any numbers in any equation unless you are sure. Each calculation that you carry out uses up precious time. It is always worthwhile to break a complex or long problem into simpler and easily manageable units. A few fundamental approaches are suggested to help you pick up the right one. The new MCAT problems do require a mixture of approaches to solve various parts of a problem. Do <u>not</u> be discouraged if the answer is not obvious. You should not sacrifice a systematic approach in problem solving for any other short cuts. Use the following approaches as you need them:

(1) You should apply already-learned concepts to fill in the gaps from information provided in the passage. Only use principles, definitions, equations, theories and laws to fill in the gaps. Information given in problems should be integrated with the passage.

(2) You should apply the newly-learned concepts from the passage as and when appropriate after a thorough understanding.

(3) When working with mathematic problems watch for consistency in units and conventions, and always start from the given data (see Step II).

(4) Use all the relevant facts, <u>only</u>.

(5) Do not erase or write over your calculations. Performing mathematical operations in small spaces can be a frustrating experience. Write carefully and clearly.

(6) Do not expect formulas and equations (except the *MCAT Student Manual formulas*) to be provided during the test. You have to learn to memorize important formulas.

(7) Use proportional reasoning as and when required to compare various options.

(8) Evaluate designs, methods, phenomena and their effects in a logical and systematic way. Do not get persuaded by the writer's arguments if you discover technical flaws or problems. These problems may <u>not</u> require any mathematical operations to solve, only analytical/logical reasoning will suffice.

(9) You should also use integrated reasoning in looking at pieces of evidence, parts of instruments, steps in procedures and various actions in phenomena. You should evaluate and interpret particular perspectives including technical views and opinions of scientists.

(10) Always try to get the answer in the form presented, especially in data analysis problems. Organize and interpret your data so it is directly linked to the format of the answers presented.

(11) You should learn how to test the four responses against your answer and make sure to follow basic logic.

(12) Pick up various strategies and approaches to solve the problem in any order as long as they are well connected and sequential in solving the problem.

STEP V: Evaluating the Solution Given and Your Solution: Is Your Solution Accurate?

All the above steps will prove meaningless if you did not obtain an accurate solution. Hasty calculations or reading may lead to an incorrect response. Always try to check your solution against the responses. You should be able to go back if the answers do not relate (between your solution and the given solution). Check each response as an argument and see if it is valid. Do not sacrifice accuracy at any cost (including speed or reasonable guessing). Unreasonable answers should be thoroughly cross-examined by using another solution method. Your previous knowledge in the subject will provide you with a "ball park" estimate to lead you in the right direction.

Step VI: Evaluate Your Experience with Passage-Based Problems: What Did You Learn?

This is not a step you can take on the actual MCAT, but it is good exercise for your practice items and should be an integral part of your review process. Problem solving comes by experience and experience is gained by problem solving. The following questions should be asked for each practice exercise:

(1) Was the passage difficult? If so, Why?
(2) Was the problem difficult? If so, Why?
(3) Were the four responses hard to understand? If so, Why?

In the following sections an application of the problem solving model is given. Examples at the end will help you understand how to use this model in various situations.

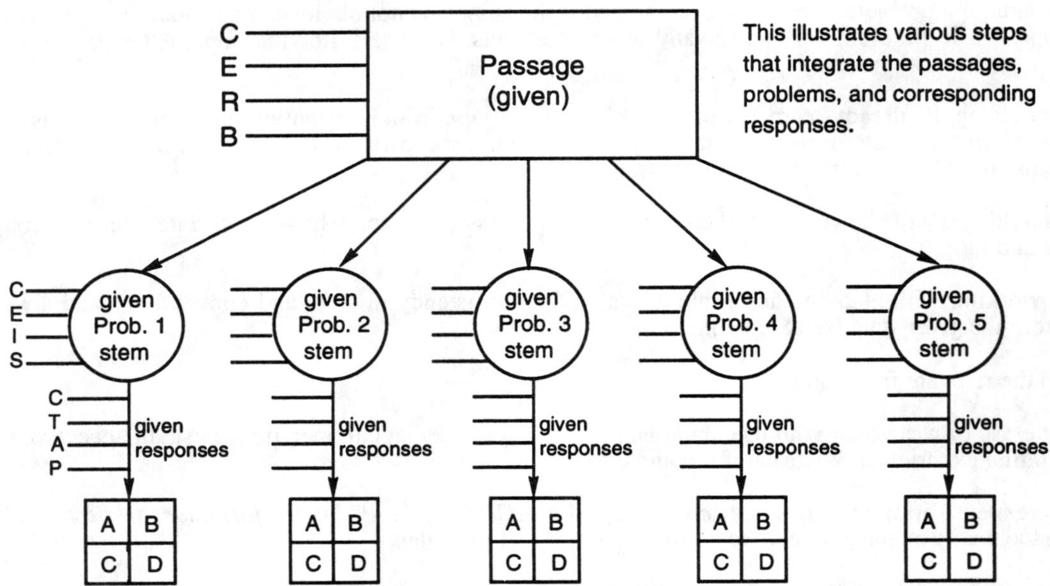

Fig. 4.1— Application of the Problem Solving Model to the MCAT

1) **C** = Comprehension of given information in the passage, problems, and responses
2) **I** = Any new information provided to problems from the passage and the problems
3) **E** = Evaluation of given information
4) **B** = Bringing knowledge-based concepts from various disciplines into the passage and trying to make sense
5) **R** = Understanding the direct or hidden relationship or link between the passages and the problems
6) **S** = Solving problems using one of several available methods
7) **T** = Testing and checking each response as a possible solution
8) **A** = Application of elimination procedures to cross out irrelevant information
9) **P** = Picking up the "best response", not "almost correct" response

4.1.7 HOW TO REVIEW SCIENCES USING THE PROBLEM SOLVING MODEL

The following provides the practice you need to move from theory to real problems. Do the following example problems NOW and complete them before you read further in the chapter. As you work the problems, write out ALL the steps and draw diagrams to help you.

Example 1 (Subjective Problem)

To test your mastery of the nervous and endocrine systems, try the following, referring to textbooks only when you need help:

(a) **LIST** the major structures of the nervous system in a way that is clear to a reader (e.g., there should be some order to your list and a drawing or diagram will help.)
(b) **DESCRIBE** the characteristics of the major structures (location and functions).

(c) **DEFINE** the parts of the nervous system. (If you were given a definition, could you name the part?)
(d) **DESCRIBE** basic nerve cell structures.
(e) **DISCUSS** the concept of action potential.
(f) **LIST** the endocrine glands and describe the characteristics of each.
(g) **DISCUSS** the effects of hormonal products on target tissues.
(h) **DISCUSS** how the feedback loop works.

Since the endocrine and nervous systems are paired in most texts, test-makers find it natural to write comparison-contrast test items. Can you compare and contrast different parts of the endocrine and nervous systems?

When you complete the exercise above, check your work in the biological sciences, Chapter 7 of this book, and review the nervous and endocrine systems. Is there anything you missed or do not fully understand? If there is something that still seems unclear, consult a textbook (preferably one you have not used before) and work to clarify the concept. Or ask a professor or fellow student for help. Now is the time to master what may have been imperfectly learned before. A thorough approach will pay off in the MCAT and, more importantly, in medical school where the pressure of time frequently prevents review or clarification of previously learned materials.

Example 2 (Objective Problem)

Mirages are considered as optical illusions. What causes a mirage? Is it reflection, refraction, diffraction or polarization of light? Hot air rises because it is lighter. A mirage is caused by refraction of light rays passing through various heated layers of air (all having different densities). In order to perform experiments on optical illusions and to understand solar and lunar eclipses, a man 2 m tall stands 3 m from an intense source of light at the level of his feet. The man's shadow appears on a wall 15 m from the source of light. How tall is the shadow?

A. 6 m
B. 10 m
C. 12.5 m
D. 17.5 m

In the problem, if you recognize that you had two similar triangles, solving the problem becomes easy because you can carefully make a ratio according to the rule that allows you to compare similar triangles: $3/15 = 2/x$. You should also note that extra or irrelevant information was given as a distractor.

We underlined the word *carefully* in the paragraph above because the test-maker, who knows that some students will do this step carelessly, has included a distractor that fits. For example, if your answer was 6, you probably put 12 in place of the 15 in the ratio.

Many students don't have the patience or confidence to work through all the steps to solve the problem; they take short-cuts and make errors. For example, some students draw the picture accurately and then try to solve for the hypoteneuse—a complicated and time-consuming task that fails to yield the correct answer although, once again, the test-maker has included a distractor that fits.

The third step, solving the problem, is elementary only if you have correctly completed the first two steps. This problem is not especially difficult either in content or mathematics, but in order to solve it correctly you must think carefully and be precise. These are the qualities of a good problem solver. If you think about it, these are the qualities we want in our doctors as well. The sketches below give you examples of a poorly proportioned sketch vs. one that is well-proportioned. Reflect on the significance of the two sketches in terms of information provided.

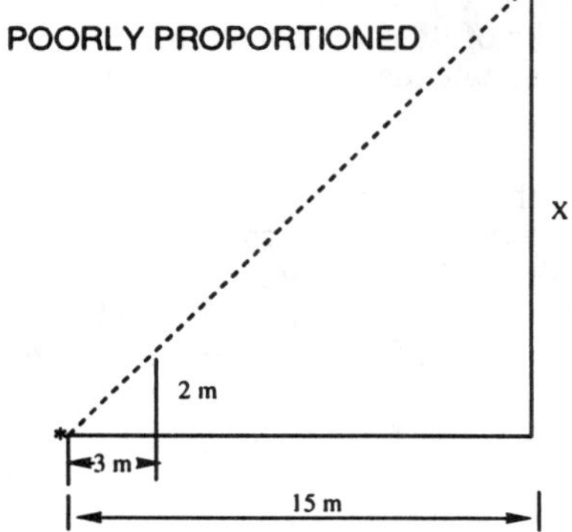

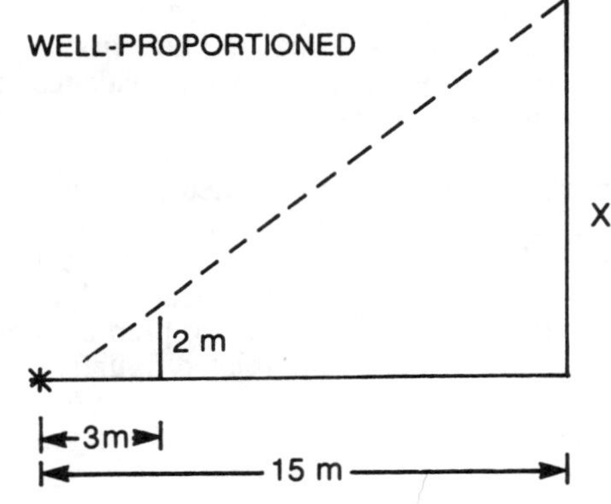

4.1.8 SUGGESTED READING TO MASTER PROBLEM SOLVING

Cognitive Maps (Novack and Gowin, 1985) and *Mind Maps* (Buzan, 1983) are two other approaches to organizing data and providing a visual aid to your memory. If you do not have a strongly visual memory you may find the techniques described in *Knowledge as Design* (Perkins, 1986) to be useful. Whether or not your mind is visual, the techniques described in this book are ones no student should ignore, especially for tasks that require a deep understanding of complex bodies of information.

If you are concerned about developing your memory, *The Complete Problem Solver* (Hayes, 1989) contains an extensive chapter describing techniques that have proven effective. These will probably take you some time to learn and master, but if you put in the time and effort they can significantly increase your ability to retain and recall several different kinds of information.

In addition to diagramming, a conscious awareness of reasoning skills is essential to achieving peak performance in problem solving. Begin by reviewing the material in the "Patterns in Reasoning" section. Eight types of reasoning are described: analytic, synthetic, associative/analogical, comparative, visual, logical, quantitative and proportional.

For additional practice in problem solving, Whimbey and Lochhead's *Problem Solving and Comprehension* and *Beyond Problem Solving and Comprehension* provide hundreds of suitable problems as well as worked examples that illustrate useful techniques. Additional problems can be found in the manuals designed to prepare students for the SAT (Scholastic Aptitude Test), LSAT (Law School Admission Test) and GRE (Graduate Record Examination.) Some of these manuals are available from Betz Publishing Company.

4.2 MATHEMATICS CONCEPTS FOR MCAT SCIENCES

The mathematics review that follows is included here as an important reference. It should be sampled selectively as you find the need for specific material in it.

4.2.1 The Role of Mathematical Skills for Medical Students and Physicians

Historically, collection of medical data can be traced back to 1854, when Florence Nightingale started keeping records of health care systems. She recognized that reliable data on the incidence of preventable deaths made compelling arguments for reform. She was a pioneer in the uses of social statistics in the medical profession. In today's society the medical student also relies increasingly on modern technology in the form of computerized medical instrumentation. For both medical researchers and practicing physicians, such instruments have vastly increased the ability to gather and manipulate large volumes of quantitative data. Having this information at their disposal, medical professionals must be able to analyze data critically. Modern medical instrumentation and research depends on proficiency in mathematics skills.

A wide variety of situations exist in which medical students and physicians must be able to deal effectively with quantitative information. For example, it is necessary to analyze data pertaining to research and development. Analyzing data or quantitative information includes "looking" at a quantity of numerals and "extracting" useful or pertinent information for later use. Physicians must be able to evaluate data on new diagnostic instruments and on new or experimental drugs that are the result of clinical research. It is imperative that they should be able to interpret such data in order to determine the precision of medical instruments and the sensitivity of drugs, among other things, to determine correct dosages from clinical data.

Physicians must also be able to make 'risk vs. benefit' judgments on the basis of quantitative information, such as in the decision, relative to patient age, to use mammography as a detector of breast cancer in women. In this example, in order to be able to maximize the benefits and minimize the the risks of its use, physicians must be able somehow to match data on the age group prevalence of breast cancer against data that show mammography as predisposing its recipients to breast cancer.

As these examples show, physicians and medical students must be skilled in the use and interpretation of all specialized types of quantitative information. Premedical students are tested on mathematical skills in the physical and biological sciences subtests of the Medical College Admission Test. The skills tested include the ability to estimate, to calculate quickly and accurately, to recognize and analyze inaccuracies in data and look for possible sources of error in information, to predict numerical outcomes from given facts and figures, and to understand the use of graphs, tables and related figures.

4.2.1.1 How Mathematics Concepts and Skills Are Tested on the MCAT

There is no actual mathematics subtest in the MCAT. Instead, the applied knowledge of mathematics is tested indirectly in the subtests.

Knowing **how** to compute is not enough for MCAT preparation. Emphasis should be placed on approach or method of attack, on calculation or quick evaluation, on interpretation or critical analysis, and finally, on speed or time-wiseness. [Remember, calculators are not allowed.]

The MCAT is designed to appraise the following:

1. Can you **perform** calculations mentally or manually under pressure of time?
2. Can you **reason** proportionally when comparing two sets of information?
3. Can you **remember and use** basic formulas learned in plane geometry (Pythagorean theorem, areas and volumes of common figures and shapes)?
4. Can you **convert** units from one system to the other using scientific notation? Can you **convert** percentages to fractions?
5. Can you **use** definitions of trigonometric functions and their relationships?
6. Can you **understand** the concepts of exponentials, logarithms, reciprocals, semi-log and log-log graphs?
7. Can you **calculate** the probability of an event?
8. Can you **add and subtract** vectors?
9. Can you **conceptualize** arithmetical mean, standard deviation, statistical correlation, and relative error analysis of experimental data?
10. Can you **identify, explain** and **predict** mathematical trends in continuous line graphs?
11. Can you **determine** the underlying equation or function in a line graph or a mathematical plot?

4.2.1.2 Problem Types in Physical and Biological Sciences Subtests

Mathematics is an integral part of the problem-solving aspects that are tested in the MCAT physical and biological sciences subtests. These problems are designed and structured to diagnose certain skills, as follows:

- Problems involving **integration** of several principles applied to a medical situation (synthetic reasoning).
- Problems involving **separation** of relevant and irrelevant information, deriving and predicting new information (analytical reasoning).
- Problems involving **detailed information** (raw data) given in a tabular or a graphical format to be **interpreted** by the student without a calculator (quick mathematical interpretation).
- Problems **describing** research methodology, experimental methodology, complex organization of types of information collected from natural sciences, social sciences, and medically related topics (analytical reading and reasoning).
- Problems involving **compare/contrast** proficiency to recognize similarity and differences between two sets of information such as "statistical summary" (proportional and logical reasoning).
- Problems involving tables of **scrambled data** that need an appropriate format including sorting with the eye, classification and interpretation (mathematical interpretation).
- Problems involving **multiple image graphs** to study correlations, rates of change or slope, discovering and explaining inconsistent trends using simple mental/manual arithmetic (perceptive proportional reasoning).
- Problems involving **actual data** which may lead to deceptive empirical trends and relationships leading to erroneous conclusions if not well analyzed (predictive reasoning).

- Problems involving **detection** of an underlying assumption, finding and filling gaps in information given and forming valid "information-based" conclusions (analytical reading and reasoning).

- Problems involving **testing of reliability** of information for precision, accuracy and validity over long time spans: predicting values in the future (predictive reasoning).

- Problems involving **simple arithmetic** skills such as quick addition, converting numerical data into percentages or fractions, approximating to get the right answer (learning how to approximate).

- Problems involving **sensitivity testing** of a given equation by changing one variable at a time in relation to another variable.

- Problems using **components of graphs, figures and diagrams** to identify and compare various segments (analytical reasoning).

Familiarize yourself with the topics given in the list above and locate them in this text. These are the topics you should concentrate your practice on. Resolve to test yourself by solving each problem that appears difficult to you.

4.2.1.3 MATHEMATICS DIAGNOSTIC TEST

The Mathematics Diagnostic Test should be taken without a calculator. Answer each question as quickly as you can and record your answer. If your test score is less than 75 points, further review and practice are essential. The High-speed Math Refresher, which follows in section 4.2.2, is included for that purpose. It will help you to reinforce your lost calculating skills and make your MCAT preparation more fruitful.

Total time allowed for the this diagnostic test (problems 1-4) should not exceed 30 minutes. Score your test carefully when you are finished. Additional space in the right-hand margin is available for calculations.

1. Change each of the following numbers to the percent form:

(a) .25 = 25% (b) $.33\overline{3}$ = (c) 1.65 =

(d) .05 = (e) .005 = (f) 3 =

(g) 1.065 = (h) 1.2 = (i) $3\frac{1}{2}$ =

(j) .16 = (k) 2.05 = (l) .008 =

(m) 10 = (n) .0036 = (o) $1\frac{1}{4}$ =

(p) .90 = (q) .005 = (r) .7 =

(s) .025 = (t) $1\frac{1}{2}$ =

2. Change each of the following percents to the decimal form:

(a) 2% = .02 (b) 200% = (c) .5% =

(d) $\frac{1}{4}$% = (e) 1.6% = (f) 1.5% =

(g) 16% = (h) 25% = (i) 300% =

(j) $16\frac{1}{2}$% = (k) .05% = (l) $32\frac{1}{2}$% =

(m) 9% = (n) $4\frac{1}{2}$% = (o) 568% =

(p) $\frac{1}{2}$% = (q) 23.2% = (r) .56% =

(s) 1.7% = (t) 115% =

3. Change each of the following percents to a fraction or a mixed number:

(a)	$25\% = \frac{1}{4}$	(b)	$16\frac{2}{3}\% =$	(c)	$12\frac{1}{2}\% =$
(d)	$11\frac{1}{9}\% =$	(e)	$108\frac{1}{3}\% =$	(f)	$20\% =$
(g)	$5\% =$	(h)	$3\frac{1}{2}\% =$	(i)	$30\% =$
(j)	$125\% =$	(k)	$15\% =$	(l)	$83\frac{1}{3}\% =$
(m)	$60\% =$	(n)	$17\% =$	(o)	$.22\% =$
(p)	$6\% =$	(q)	$\frac{2}{5}\% =$	(r)	$38\% =$
(s)	$46\% =$	(t)	$375\% =$		

4. Change each of the following fractions or mixed numbers to the percent form:

(a)	$\frac{3}{8} = 37.5\%$	(b)	$\frac{5}{6} =$	(c)	$\frac{1}{12} =$
(d)	$\frac{3}{9} =$	(e)	$\frac{2}{5} =$	(f)	$\frac{5}{12} =$
(g)	$\frac{1}{30} =$	(h)	$\frac{1}{25} =$	(i)	$\frac{1}{2} =$
(j)	$\frac{3}{4} =$	(k)	$\frac{7}{8} =$	(l)	$3\frac{3}{4} =$
(m)	$\frac{1}{6} =$	(n)	$\frac{2}{3} =$	(o)	$\frac{2}{16} =$
(p)	$\frac{4}{32} =$	(q)	$1\frac{2}{5} =$	(r)	$\frac{5}{9} =$
(s)	$1\frac{1}{3} =$	(t)	$20\frac{1}{2} =$		

4.2.1.4 Answers to the Mathematics Diagnostic Test

1.

(a)	25%	(b)	$33\frac{1}{3}\%$	(c)	165%	(d)	5%
(e)	.5% or $\frac{1}{2}\%$	(f)	300%	(g)	106.5% or $106\frac{1}{2}\%$	(h)	120%
(i)	350%	(j)	16%	(k)	205%	(l)	.8%
(m)	1000%	(n)	.36%	(o)	125%	(p)	90%
(q)	$\frac{1}{2}\%$	(r)	70%	(s)	$2\frac{1}{2}\%$ or 2.5%	(t)	150%

2.

(a)	.02	(b)	2.00	(c)	.005	(d)	.0025
(e)	.016	(f)	.015	(g)	.16	(h)	.25
(i)	3.00	(j)	.165	(k)	.0005	(l)	.325
(m)	.09	(n)	.045	(o)	5.68	(p)	.005
(q)	.232	(r)	.0056	(s)	.017	(t)	1.15

3.

(a)	$\frac{1}{4}$	(b)	$\frac{1}{6}$	(c)	$\frac{1}{8}$	(d)	$\frac{1}{9}$
(e)	$1\frac{1}{12}$	(f)	$\frac{1}{5}$	(g)	$\frac{1}{20}$	(h)	$\frac{7}{200}$
(i)	$\frac{3}{10}$	(j)	$1\frac{1}{4}$	(k)	$\frac{3}{20}$	(l)	$\frac{5}{6}$
(m)	$\frac{3}{5}$	(n)	$\frac{17}{100}$	(o)	$\frac{11}{5000}$	(p)	$\frac{3}{50}$
(q)	$\frac{1}{250}$	(r)	$\frac{19}{50}$	(s)	$\frac{23}{50}$	(t)	$3\frac{3}{4}$

4. Answers to Problem 4 (a-t) can easily be obtained by using a calculator once you have finished the test. This will give you enough practice to make up your own problems and solve them.

4.2.1.5 Score Interpretation

Each problem has 20 parts (a-t). Assign one point for each correct answer. The highest score possible is 4(20) = 80 points. You may diagnose your score by using the following chart:

Score Obtained	Interpretation
75 - 80	excellent
70 - 74	good
60 - 69	satisfactory

If your score is less than 60, your math *skills and speed* are poor. Don't feel discouraged. To improve your math speed and accuracy, structure your practice in mathematics with special emphasis on 4.2.2 (The High-Speed Math Refresher). You may have to practice materials similar to those in section 4.2.2 for several weeks until you have mastered them. Practice all the problems with a clock in front of you. The actual MCAT is an instrument that checks your problem solving ability to calculate *quickly and precisely*. Use this guide to prepare for things you may have forgotten because of insufficient recent practice.

4.2.2 THE HIGH-SPEED MATH REFRESHER—*Time and Precision*

This section has been provided for the student who desires to review fundamental yet possibly forgotten concepts in basic mathematics. Mastery of this section can be acquired fairly easily by repeated practice on similar problems. [Once again, no calculators.]

This section will teach you topics with emphasis on background MCAT concepts and skills, and clues on how to acquire them. Time and precision are the key words for MCAT quantitative problems. It is difficult to calculate accurately with time constraints unless well prepared. But even well-prepared students, in preparation for various subtests in the MCAT, will benefit from some of the quick math skills given in this section .

Arithmetic is a Science, Calculation an Art

Science is mostly knowledge; art, such as moving a paintbrush on canvas, the professional strokes of tennis, golf and baseball, is a skill. Repeated practice on fundamental skills make them seem automatic. An example of the fundamental skill of calculation at the level of a typical MCAT student is having the knowledge you need to determine that 67 multiplied by 25 equals 1,675 and being able to do so mentally or manually in about five seconds. Without that level of skill you may not be adept at the art of calculation as it is required for the MCAT.

Genuine skill in calculation may be acquired by anyone of average intelligence, regardless of educational background. This section will lead you by easy steps to a point where you can possess really exceptional calculating ability. The key to learning from this section is the ability to hold and manipulate figures in your head. This ability can be developed by an understanding of "number sense," which is the ability to recognize the relationships that exist between numbers considered as quantities in terms of their relationship with each other.

Example:

Using different methods, solve the multiplication problem: 67 x 25:

Long Method

```
   67
 x 25
  335
+134
1,675
```

Vertical multiplication
(10 seconds)

Horizontal Algebraic Method

67 x 25 = (70 - 3)(20 + 5)
= 1400 - 60 - 15 + 350
= 1750 - 75 = 1,675

Algebraic multiplication
(8 seconds)

If you know the multiplication table for 25, you could solve this problem with double digit multiplication in 5 seconds.

```
67 x 25 =   6
          x 25        7
           150      x 25
           - - -  ←   175    [carry over to the places shown]
          1,675
```

The quickest method sometimes is a combination of the above methods.

$$67 \times 25 = (70 - 3)25$$
$$= 1750 - 75 = 1675$$

Study the following materials at your own pace and review them daily until you have mastered them.

MCAT MATHEMATICS CONCEPT 1: Basic Arithmetic Operations

Adding by Pairs

Instead of adding one vertical column, learn how to add a **pair** of digits in a vertical column. You might make a few mistakes, but eventually you will get to be good at it. For extra practice, add your monthly checking account statement when you receive it from the bank or add your grocery receipt. ***Do all of these additions mentally.***

Exercise A

Adding Single Columns by Pairs

Add the following columns of figures. Taking successive double-digit numbers one at a time, add from the top down beginning with "51":

1.	2.	3.	4.	5.	6.	7.	8.
51	42	12	34	12	43	58	74
30	53	73	12	81	61	48	48
96	43	32	97	11	38	62	65
24	79	12	19	39	36	49	74
25	87	81	69	43	37	47	71
75	76	11	94	10	33	92	49
48	92	44	83	85	38	34	47
49	52	84	68	99	87	52	35
93	45	70	38	29	62	98	63
80	38	40	46	14	96	87	67
13	18	92	17	95	95	34	84
58	63	67	57	10	44	84	45
88	22	56	66	74			
86	21	16	64	31			
20	47	37	89	77			
99	91	55	92	74			
59	15	27	60	28			
65	78	54	23	84			
1,059							

9.	10.	11.	12.	13.	14.	15.
87	99	14	39	68	63	84
85	84	12	68	55	62	99
91	96	26	23	52	62	36
76	77	29	37	34	63	73
85	87	24	47	69	89	74
82	96	24	35	56	59	56
69	93	18	98	46	67	82
58	21	37	29	67	92	89
49	69	98	85	53	42	68
74	47	36	91	37	64	53
28	89	29	48	64	97	59
95	53	49	96	59	24	84

Answer and Solution to Problem 1

Add 51 and 30 to get 81, then add 81 to 96 to obtain 177, then add 177 to 24 to obtain 201, then add 201 to 25 to obtain 226, then add 226 to 75 to obtain 301, then add 301 to 48 to obtain 349, then add 349 to 49 to obtain 398, then add 398 to 93 to obtain 491, then add 491 to 80 to obtain 571, then add 571 to 13 to obtain 584, then add 584 to 58 to obtain 642, then add 642 to 88 to obtain 730, then add 730 to 86 to obtain 816, then add 816 to

20 to obtain 836, then add 836 to 99 to obtain 935, then add 935 to 59 to obtain 994, then add 994 to 65 to finally get 1059.

The other problems can be solved in the same way to get the answers given below. Each problem should take about 10 seconds.

Answers to Problems 2 through 15

(2) 962	(3) 863	(4) 1028	(5) 896	(6) 670
(7) 745	(8) 722	(9) 879	(10) 911	(11) 396
(12) 696	(13) 660	(14) 784	(15) 857	

Exercise B

Adding Single Columns by Pairs. Add From the Bottom Up.

1.	2.	3.	4.
$ 698504.99	$ 457012.91	$ 662533.75	$ 473105.74
845643.09	820823.58	380277.80	141593.51
761979.28	622529.46	847236.82	111290.63
401349.83	715303.47	735356.57	897350.49
740614.80	159363.96	236569.58	379128.68
553930.31	380272.36	862061.71	966221.52
896554.52	268195.94	178735.81	644107.29
975160.67	789234.47	464385.34	104004.99
417337.75	773286.20	425919.44	266722.95
882110.35	425922.98	789249.94	987983.35
116448.16	669001.18	395497.48	183216.92
477406.66	502733.07	194426.67	295788.92
801415.93	906396.55	129066.12	336353.75
340939.01	301831.11	464347.56	578389.73
380272.36	820889.83	316085.34	740638.09
656958.68	548620.61	499498.27	236540.11
882152.17	874185.10	776980.14	159383.58
401304.99	761944.26	518437.35	729128.36

This exercise might seem impossible at first, but with the ability to hold and manipulate figures in your head it can be done by learning how to add two digits upwards (adding by pairs of digits). Ideally, each exercise should take about 40 seconds.

Answers to Problems 1 through 4

(1) Start by adding 99 to 17 which is 116, add 116 to 68 to obtain 184, add 184 to 36 to obtain 220 and so on. There are eight vertical columns, which means there are four pairs of two-digit columns. The answer is $11,230,083.55.

(2) $10,797,547.04

(3) $8,876,665.69

(4) $8,230,948.61

Factors of Common Numbers

This table showing factors of numbers should be reviewed from time to time and used frequently for multiplication problems. Remember that a prime number cannot be divided by any number but itself or the number one. Formally, a *prime* is an integer greater than one that has exactly two distinct positive integer divisors.

2	=	prime	35	=	5 x 7	68	=	2 x 2 x 17
3	=	prime	36	=	2 x 2 x 3 x 3	69	=	3 x 23
4	=	2 x 2	37	=	prime	70	=	2 x 5 x 7
5	=	prime	38	=	2 x 19	71	=	prime
6	=	2 x 3	39	=	3 x 13	72	=	2 x 2 x 2 x 3 x 3
7	=	prime	40	=	2 x 2 x 2 x 5	73	=	prime
8	=	2 x 2 x 2	41	=	prime	74	=	2 x 37
9	=	3 x 3	42	=	2 x 3 x 7	75	=	3 x 5 x 5
10	=	2 x 5	43	=	prime	76	=	2 x 2 x 19
11	=	prime	44	=	2 x 2 x 11	77	=	7 x 11
12	=	2 x 3 x 2	45	=	3 x 3 x 5	78	=	2 x 3 x 13
13	=	prime	46	=	2 x 23	79	=	prime
14	=	2 x 7	47	=	prime	80	=	2 x 2 x 2 x 2 x 5
15	=	3 x 5	48	=	2 x 2 x 2 x 2 x 3	81	=	3 x 3 x 3 x 3
16	=	2 x 2 x 2 x 2	49	=	7 x 7	82	=	2 x 41
17	=	prime	50	=	2 x 5 x 5	83	=	prime
18	=	2 x 3 x 3	51	=	3 x 17	84	=	2 x 2 x 3 x 7
19	=	prime	52	=	2 x 2 x 13	85	=	5 x 17
20	=	2 x 2 x 5	53	=	prime	86	=	2 x 43
21	=	3 x 7	54	=	2 x 3 x 3 x 3	87	=	3 x 29
22	=	2 x 11	55	=	5 x 11	88	=	2 x 2 x 2 x 11
23	=	prime	56	=	2 x 2 x 2 x 7	89	=	prime
24	=	2 x 2 x 2 x 3	57	=	3 x 19	90	=	2 x 3 x 3 x 5
25	=	5 x 5	58	=	2 x 29	91	=	7 x 13
26	=	2 x 13	59	=	prime	92	=	2 x 2 x 23
27	=	3 x 3 x 3	60	=	2 x 2 x 3 x 5	93	=	3 x 31
28	=	2 x 2 x 7	61	=	prime	94	=	2 x 47
29	=	prime	62	=	2 x 31	95	=	5 x 19
30	=	2 x 3 x 5	63	=	3 x 3 x 7	96	=	2 x 2 x 2 x 2 x 2 x 3
31	=	prime	64	=	2 x 2 x 2 x 2 x 2 x 2	97	=	prime
32	=	2 x 2 x 2 x 2 x 2	65	=	5 x 13	98	=	2 x 7 x 7
33	=	3 x 11	66	=	2 x 3 x 11	99	=	3 x 3 x 11
34	=	2 x 17	67	=	prime	100	=	2 x 2 x 5 x 5

Continue to expand this list to 1000 by regularly adding new numbers.

Factors of 1000 = 2 x 500 = 2 x 2 x 250
= 2 x 2 x 2 x 125
= 2 x 2 x 2 x 5 x 25
= 2 x 2 x 2 x 5 x 5 x 5

Review of the foregoing factors table should help you in learning how to multiply horizontally on a straight line.

Exercise A

Multiplying Three Digits by One

Mentally multiply the following:

1. 141 x 6
2. 252 x 6
3. 363 x 6
4. 484 x 6
5. 585 x 6
6. 696 x 6
7. 767 x 6
8. 851 x 6
9. 962 x 6
10. 173 x 6
11. 293 x 6
12. 395 x 6
13. 446 x 6
14. 568 x 6
15. 661 x 6
16. 772 x 6
17. 849 x 6
18. 884 x 6
19. 145 x 6
20. 256 x 6

Exercise B

Multiplying Three Digits by One

Mentally multiply the following:

1. 131 x 7	8. 838 x 7	15. 637 x 7
2. 242 x 7	9. 951 x 7	16. 748 x 7
3. 383 x 7	10. 152 x 7	17. 861 x 7
4. 464 x 7	11. 263 x 7	18. 962 x 7
5. 575 x 7	12. 384 x 7	19. 189 x 7
6. 676 x 7	13. 485 x 7	20. 284 x 7
7. 797 x 7	14. 596 x 7	

Exercise C

Multiplying Three Digits by One

Mentally multiply the following:

1. 141 x 8	8. 858 x 8	15. 666 x 8
2. 252 x 8	9. 969 x 8	16. 777 x 8
3. 383 x 8	10. 181 x 8	17. 868 x 8
4. 474 x 8	11. 282 x 8	18. 999 x 8
5. 575 x 8	12. 343 x 8	19. 761 x 8
6. 696 x 8	13. 444 x 8	20. 652 x 8
7. 767 x 8	14. 555 x 8	

Answers to Exercises A, B, C

Exercise A:

(1) 141 x 6 = 846, multiply 6 by 1 to get 6, then 14 x 6 = 84, hence the answer is 846.

(2) 1512	(3) 2178	(4) 2904	(5) 3510	(6) 4176
(7) 4602	(8) 5106	(9) 5772	(10) 1038	(11) 1758
(12) 2370	(13) 2676	(14) 3408	(15) 3966	(16) 4632
(17) 5094	(18) 5304	(19) 870	(20) 1536	

Exercise B:

(1) 917	(2) 1694	(3) 2681	(4) 3248	(5) 4025	(6) 4732	(7) 5579
(8) 5866	(9) 6657	(10) 1064	(11) 1841	(12) 2688	(13) 3395	(14) 4172
(15) 4459	(16) 5236	(17) 6027	(18) 6734	(19) 1323	(20) 1988	

Exercise C:

(1) 1128	(2) 2016	(3) 3064	(4) 3792	(5) 4600	(6) 5568	(7) 6136
(8) 6864	(9) 7752	(10) 1448	(11) 2256	(12) 2744	(13) 3552	(14) 4440
(15) 5328	(16) 6216	(17) 6944	(18) 7992	(19) 6088	(20) 5216	

Divisibility Rules

These rules and examples that follow will enhance your ability to divide quickly.

A NUMBER IS DIVISIBLE BY:	IF:
2	it **ends** in 0, 2, 4, 6, or 8.
3	the **total** of its digits is divisible by 3 (example 1).
4	the number formed by the **last two** digits is divisible by 4 (example 2).
5	if it **ends** in 0 or 5.
6	if it is divisible by 2 and 3 (use the rules for both and see example 3).

7	(no simple rule)
8	the number formed by the **last three** digits is divisible by 8 (example 4).
9	the **total** of its digits is divisible by 9 (example 5).

Example 1.
Is 126 divisible by 3? Total of digits = 9. Since 9 is divisible by 3, 126 is divisible by 3.

Example 2.
Is 1,748 divisible by 4? Since 48 is divisible by 4 then 1,748 is divisible by 4.

Example 3.
Is 186 divisible by 6? Since 186 ends in 6, it is divisible by 2. Total of digits = 15. Since 15 is divisible by 3, 186 is divisible by 3. 186 is divisible by 2 and 3; therefore, it is divisible by 6.

Example 4.
Is 2,488 divisible by 8? Since 488 is divisible by 8, then 2,488 is divisible by 8.

Example 5.
Is 2,853 divisible by 9? Total of digits = 18. Since 18 is divisible by 9, then 2,853 is divisible by 9.

Problem 1.
4,620 is divisible by which of the following numbers: 2,3,4,5,6,7,8,9?

Problem 2.
13,131 is divisible by which of the following numbers: 2,3,4,5,6,7,8,9?

Answers to Divisibility Problems

1. 2,3,4,5,6,7

2 - the number is even
3 - the digits total 12, which is divisible by 3
4 - the number formed by the last two digits, 20, is divisible by 4
5 - the number ends in 0
6 - the number is divisible by 2 and 3
7 - divide 4,620 by 7 and you get 660
8 - the number formed by the last three digits, 620, is not divisible by 8
9 - the total of the digits is 12, which is not divisible by 9

2. 3,9

2 - the number is not even
3 - the digits total 9, which is divisible by 3
4 - the number is not even
5 - the number does not end in 0 or 5
6 - the number is not even
7 - divide and you will see that there is a remainder, hence not divisible
8 - the number is not even
9 - the digits total 9, which is divisible by 9

More Mental Multiplication and Division Problems

Exercise A: Mental Multiplication

Mentally multiply the following:

1. 46 x 71	8. 48 x 77	15. 46 x 77
2. 58 x 72	9. 56 x 71	16. 56 x 76
3. 66 x 73	10. 66 x 72	17. 66 x 71
4. 76 x 74	11. 76 x 73	18. 76 x 72
5. 88 x 75	12. 86 x 74	19. 86 x 73
6. 96 x 76	13. 96 x 75	20. 96 x 74
7. 36 x 77	14. 36 x 76	

Exercise B: Mental Division

Mentally divide the following:

1. 5338 ÷ 772	8. 3606 ÷ 485	15. 5954 ÷ 666
2. 5393 ÷ 883	9. 4518 ÷ 596	16. 5887 ÷ 647
3. 6001 ÷ 994	10. 4711 ÷ 637	17. 7123 ÷ 758
4. 908 ÷ 145	11. 2284 ÷ 282	18. 8221 ÷ 869
5. 1576 ÷ 256	12. 3183 ÷ 393	19. 9257 ÷ 973
6. 1859 ÷ 263	13. 3956 ÷ 444	20. 1721 ÷ 184
7. 2736 ÷ 374	14. 4795 ÷ 555	

Exercise C: Mental Multiplication

Mentally multiply the following:

1. 47 x 79	8. 47 x 87	15. 47 x 86
2. 57 x 81	9. 57 x 79	16. 57 x 87
3. 67 x 82	10. 67 x 81	17. 67 x 79
4. 77 x 83	11. 77 x 82	18. 77 x 81
5. 87 x 84	12. 87 x 83	19. 87 x 82
6. 97 x 85	13. 97 x 84	20. 97 x 83
7. 37 x 86	14. 37 x 85	

Answers to Exercises A, B, C

Exercise A:

(1) 46 x 71 = 46 (70 + 1)
= 3220 + 46 = 3266

(2) 4176 (3) 4818 (4) 5624 (5) 6600 (6) 7296 (7) 2772 (8) 3696
(9) 3976 (10) 4752 (11) 5548 (12) 6364 (13) 7200 (14) 2736 (15) 3542
(16) 4256 (17) 4686 (18) 5472 (19) 6278 (20) 7104

Exercise B:

(1) 5338 ÷ 772: in order to divide mentally or manually, first try to divide the first digit of the numerator (5) by the first digit of the denominator (7), and it is not possible. Next try to divide 53 by 7; it works, but 772 is closer to 800 than 700 and the answer (5404) is too high. Try again with 6: the answer (4632) leaves a remainder (706) or 706 ÷ 772. For the decimal, 7 goes into 70 ten times, but 772 is nearer to 800, so try one less which is 9. Manual division yields 6.9 as well.

(1) Answer: 6 remainder 706, or 6.9 when done manually.
(2) 6r95 (3) 6r37 (4) 6r38 (5) 6r40 (6) 7r18 (7) 7r118 (8) 7r211
(9) 7r346 (10) 7r252 (11) 8r28 (12) 8r39 (13) 8r404 (14) 8r355 (15) 8r626
(16) 9r64 (17) 9r301 (18) 9r400 (19) 9r500 (20) 9r65

Exercise C:

(1) 47 x 79 = 47 (80 - 1) = 3760 - 47 = 3713
(2) 4617 (3) 5494 (4) 6391 (5) 7308 (6) 8245 (7) 3182 (8) 4089
(9) 4503 (10) 5427 (11) 6314 (12) 7221 (13) 8148 (14) 3145 (15) 4042
(16) 4959 (17) 5293 (18) 6237 (19) 7134 (20) 8051

MCAT MATHEMATICS CONCEPT 2: Estimating Square Roots of Common Numbers

The square roots of whole numbers from 1 to 100 are floating point decimal numbers. In the table that follows, they are rounded **to the nearest hundredth**. For example, the table has these entries:

Number	Square Root	
17	4.12	(rounded from 4.123106...)

$(4.123)^2 = 16.999$ which is very close to 17.

When the square root entry has a "0" in the thousandths place, the "0" can be ignored. For example:

$\sqrt{22} = 4.690$ (or simply 4.69)

When using the table, one can round the square root entries even further. For example:

Round the entry below **to the nearest hundredth**:

$\sqrt{31} = 5.57$ (from 5.568)

Round the entry below **to the nearest tenth**:

$\sqrt{95} = 9.7$ (from 9.74)

The table can also be used to find a close approximation to the square roots of decimal numbers from 1 to 100. To do so, simply round to the nearest whole number and use its square root from the table. For example:

$\sqrt{12.8}$ is very close to $\sqrt{13}$ or 3.61

$\sqrt{84.36}$ is very close to $\sqrt{84}$ or 9.17

Note: When rounding to the nearest whole number, one occasionally gets a whole number that is a perfect square. As in the example below, use the whole number (5) as an approximation of the square root of the decimal number (25.33). For example:

$\sqrt{25.33}$ is very close to $\sqrt{25}$ or 5.

Square Roots of Whole Numbers From 1 to 100

Number	Square Root	Number	Square Root	Number	Square Root	Number	Square Root
1	1.00	30	5.48	59	7.68	88	9.38
2	1.41	31	5.57	60	7.75	89	9.43
3	1.73	32	5.66	61	7.81	90	9.49
4	2.00	33	5.74	62	7.87	91	9.54
5	2.24	34	5.83	63	7.94	92	9.59
6	2.45	35	5.92	64	8.00	93	9.64
7	2.65	36	6.00	65	8.06	94	9.70
8	2.83	37	6.08	66	8.12	95	9.75
9	3.00	38	6.16	67	8.19	96	9.80
10	3.16	39	6.24	68	8.25	97	9.85
11	3.32	40	6.32	69	8.31	98	9.90
12	3.46	41	6.40	70	8.37	99	9.95
13	3.61	42	6.48	71	8.43	100	10.00
14	3.74	43	6.56	72	8.49		
15	3.87	44	6.63	73	8.54		
16	4.00	45	6.71	74	8.60		
17	4.12	46	6.78	75	8.66		
18	4.24	47	6.86	76	8.72		
19	4.36	48	6.93	77	8.77		
20	4.47	49	7.00	78	8.83		
21	4.58	50	7.07	79	8.89		
22	4.69	51	7.14	80	8.94		
23	4.80	52	7.21	81	9.00		
24	4.90	53	7.28	82	9.06		
25	5.00	54	7.35	83	9.11		
26	5.10	55	7.42	84	9.17		
27	5.20	56	7.48	85	9.22		
28	5.29	57	7.55	86	9.27		
29	5.39	58	7.62	87	9.33		

Note:
When you do not remember a square root, guess and check. The square root of 640 must be between 20 and 30; guess 25, 25 x 25 = 625 (too small), 26 x 26 = 676 (too large), 25.5 x 25.5 = 650 (too large), 25.4 x 25.4 = 645 (too large), 25.3 x 25.3 = 640.1 (close enough). Notice that 640 = 6.4 x 100 ($\sqrt{640} = \sqrt{6.4} \times 10$).

4.2.3 Arrangement of Topics to Review Algebra, Geometry, and Trigonometry

The knowledge of mathematics outlined in the *MCAT Student Manual* (pages 30,31) has been used as a reference in the selection and organization of the review material. The topics covered here have been designed to provide a concise yet adequate preparation for the mathematics that appears on the MCAT physical and biological sciences.

Topics that are not necessarily required for the MCAT are included only when they are considered conceptually useful. If the review of any topic seems insufficient for your needs, try to find a more comprehensive and detailed treatment of the topic in textbooks and other sources (see section 4.6).

But before you begin, make sure that your basic skills, as outlined in section 4.2.2 (The High-Speed Math Refresher), are strong.

Following is a list of topics to review math. They are not necessarily in order:

- **Algebra**
  - Simplification and solution of algebraic equations involving fractions, logs, and radical signs (covered in this guide).
  - Radical algebra, scientific notation, exponential and logarithm expressions with basic laws (covered in this guide).
  - Ratio and proportion as applied to quantitative physical and biological sciences problems. Introduction to **"principle of proportionality"** with problems involving direct and inverse relations (covered in this guide).

- **Numeric/Data Transformations**
  - Intuitive feel of numeric/alphabetic series and pattern recognition.
  - Dimensional analysis involving units of quantities in a long formula. Transferring and calculating variables in a specific physics/chemistry formula.

- **Permutations, Combinations, Probability**
  - Arrangements, combinations and logic problems involving genetics and chemistry. Basic probability and fundamental statistics (covered in this guide).

- **Plane/Solid Geometry, Trigonometry, Analytic Geometry of Lines, Curves and Graphs**
  - Review of plane and solid geometry formulas including areas and volumes of regular figures.
  - Slope and intercept of a line and a curve. Basic use of y = mx + b in math problems. Slope of a quadratic function. Slopes and intercepts of exponential and composite functions.
  - Trigonometric functions; analysis, uses, definitions, and graphs. Relation of trigonometric functions to vector algebra. Definition and use of vector components, vector resultant.
  - Reading and drawing graphs with linear, log-log and semi-log axes. Concept of limits of a function on a graph. To understand inherent trends in continuous line graphs.

The organization of the review material below is based on definitions or concepts, examples, and practice problems. For each topic, the main emphasis is on examples followed by practice problems in order to test comprehension immediately. The solutions to these practice problems are at the end of each section.

4.2.3.1 Algebra Concepts

A basic knowledge of algebra that covers solving simple equations, quadratic equations, and manipulating formulas is required for the MCAT.

Basic Definitions

- A **variable** is a symbol that, without further definition, can stand for any number or an unknown quantity.
- A **constant** is a symbol (or number) that has a fixed value.
- An **expression** is any combination of variables and constants connected by arithmetic symbols, e.g., $3x + 7 - 2/x$.
- An **equation** expresses the equality or balance between different expressions. It is satisfied by certain values of the variables.

MCAT MATHEMATICS CONCEPT 3: Simplifying algebraic equations

An **algebraic equation** is an algebraic expression in which one variable usually amounts to the isolation of the "**unknown quantity**" or variable on one side of the equation. Any operation, except multiplication or division by zero, can be used to achieve this "isolation" as long as it is done to both sides of the equation. More generally, the basic rule for solving equations is that whatever is done to one side must be done to the other side so that the equality of the sides is not affected. It is like a weighing scale with two balanced sides or pans.

Order of Operations

Before considering some examples of solving equations, first it is important to recall that, when manipulating an expression (whether or not it is part of an equation), the order of operations is as follows:

(1) parentheses

(2) powers or exponents

(3) multiplication and division (whichever comes first from the left)

(4) addition and subtraction (whichever comes first from the left)

Example 1.

Solve for a: $4a + 5 = 13$

$4a + 5 - 5 = 13 - 5$

$4a = 8$

$\frac{4a}{4} = \frac{8}{4}$

$a = 2$

Example 2.

Solve for m: $\frac{10}{m} - 8 = \frac{5}{3}$

$\frac{10}{m}(3m) - 8(3m) = \frac{5}{3}(3m)$

$30 - 24m = 5m$

$30 = 29m$

$m = \frac{30}{29}$

Example 3.

Solve for c: $3c^2 = 75d^4$

$c^2 = 25d^4$

$\sqrt{c^2} = \sqrt{25d^4}$

$c = \pm 5d^2$

Example 4.

Solve for q: $3[(q+2)^2 - 4q] = 2q^2 + 13$

$3[(q + 2)(q + 2) - 4q] = 2q^2 + 13$

$3[q^2 + 4q + 4 - 4q] = 2q^2 + 13$

$3q^2 + 12 = 2q^2 + 13$

$q^2 = 1$

$q = \pm 1$

Problem 1.

Solve for a: $s(a - p) + q = ta + r^2$

Problem 2.

Solve for d: $\frac{1}{d - 2} + \frac{2}{d + 3} = \frac{4}{d - 2}$

Problem 3.
Solve for x: $3(4x - 2[1 - (x + 5) + 3]) = 13x + 19$

MCAT MATHEMATICS CONCEPT 4: Proportional analysis of algebraic equations

Some problems will be solvable by recognizing that the quantities in question are directly or inversely proportional to each other. Two variables, x and y, are **directly proportional** if their ratio has a constant value, a:

$$\frac{y}{x} = a \quad \text{or} \quad y = ax.$$

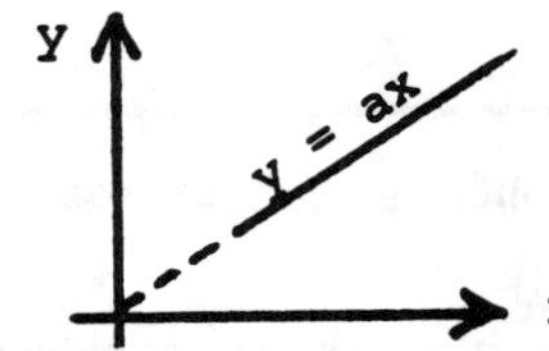

Fig. 4.2a—Linear variation

Consequently, for any distinct values of x, x_1, and x_2, there are corresponding values of y, y_1, and y_2, such that:

$$\frac{y_1}{x_1} = \frac{y_2}{x_2}. \qquad \text{(x, y directly proportional)}$$

If we know three of the terms in this proportion, then we can always determine the fourth term.

Example 5.
If two moles of compound A react with 5 moles of compound B to form 3 moles of compound C, then how many moles of A are required to react completely with 7 moles of B?

In a chemical reaction, the quantities of reactants/products are directly proportional. (Why?)

Let $x_1 = 2$ moles of A and $y_1 = 5$ moles of B.

Then, x_2 = number of moles of A and $y_2 = 7$ moles of B such that:

$$\frac{5}{2} = \frac{7}{x_2}; \; x_2 = 2.8 \text{ moles of A.}$$

Problem 4.
In Example 5, how many moles of C are formed?

Two variables, x and y, are **inversely proportional** if their product has a constant value, b:

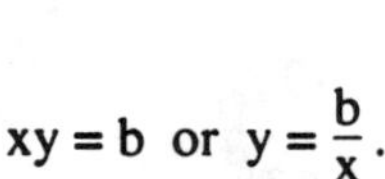

$$xy = b \quad \text{or} \quad y = \frac{b}{x}.$$

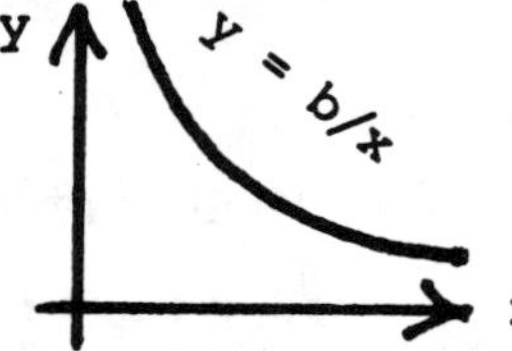

Fig. 4.2b—Non-linear /hyperbolic variation

Consequently, for any distinct values of x, x_1, and x_2, there are corresponding values of y, y_1, and y_2, such that:

$$x_1y_1 = x_2y_2 \quad \text{or} \quad \frac{y_1}{x_2} = \frac{y_2}{x_1} \qquad \text{(x,y inversely proportional)}$$

If we know three of the terms in this equation,

$$x_1y_1 = x_2y_2$$

then we can always determine the fourth term.

Example 6.

A car traveling at x mph takes 5 hours to go from city A to city B. Traveling at x - 15 mph, the car makes the return trip in six and two-thirds hours. What was the speed of the car on the return trip?

Since displacement = (speed)(time), d = vt, speed and time are inversely proportional for a constant displacement. Let $v_1 = x$ mph and $t_1 = 5$ hours; $v_2 = x - 15$ mph and $t_2 = 6\frac{2}{3}$ hours $= \frac{20}{3}$ hours. Then:

$$5x = (x - 15)\frac{20}{3}$$

$$15x = 20x - 300$$

$$5x = 300$$

$$x = 60\ ;\ v_2 = x - 15 = 45 \text{ mph.}$$

Problem 5.

Before an engine tune-up, a car with a gas consumption rate of r gallons/mile can go 400 miles on a full tank of gas. After a tune-up, the same car has a gas consumption rate of r - .01 gallons/mile and can go 500 miles on a full tank of gas. What was the gas consumption rate of the car before it had an engine tune-up?

Problem 6.

The ideal-gas law for 1 mole of any gas is PV = RT. Thus, two different macroscopic states of a mole of a particular gas are respectively described by

$$P_1V_1 = RT_1 \text{ and } P_2V_2 = RT_2.$$

Write an equation that shows the relationship between these two states. According to this equation, the pressure P is inversely proportional to what quantity?

An important application of proportionality is to use it to find proportional changes in variables that occur when other related variables change. This is called "sensitivity analysis" and is an important part of the MCAT on all subjects being tested. It teaches how to think proportionally.

Example 7.

The equation for the electric field E of a point charge q at a distance r from the point charge is $E = k\frac{q}{r^2}$ where k is a constant.

If the charge is doubled and the distance from the charge is halved, how much is the field changed?

It is worth noting that E is directly proportional to q and inversely proportional to r^2 (**not** r!!!)

(1) Define the fields before and after the changes respectively as:

$$E_1 = k\frac{q_1}{r_1^2}, \quad E_2 = k\frac{q_2}{r_2^2}.$$

(2) Consider the ratio E_2/E_1, which is equivalent to determining E_2 in terms of E_1, this being the desired result:

$$\frac{E_2}{E_1} = \frac{k\frac{q_2}{r_2^2}}{k\frac{q_1}{r_1^2}} = \frac{q_2}{q_1} \cdot \frac{r_1^2}{r_2^2}.$$

(3) Observe that the changes in q and r can be written as:

$$q_2 = 2q_1 \text{ and } r_2 = r_1/2.$$

(4) Substitute these expressions for q_2 and r_2 into the ratio E_2/E_1 to get the desired result:

$$\frac{E_2}{E_1} = \frac{2q_1}{q_1} \cdot \frac{r_1^2}{\frac{r_1^2}{4}} = 8 \text{ or } E_2 = 8E_1.$$

The final field E_2 is eight times the original field E_1.

Important Conclusion:

- If **only** the charge is doubled, then the field is doubled;
- If **only** the distance is halved, then the field is 2(2) = 4 times the original field;
- If the charge is doubled **and** the distance is halved, then the field is 2(4) = 8 times the original value.

The key point here is just to **remember that everything that does not change will cancel out,** e.g., *k* in the example above: when considering the ratio of the value of the "solved for" variable, after any changes in the other variables, to its value before these changes, e.g., E_2/E_1 in the example above.

Problem 7.
The force holding an object of mass m on a circular path is

$$F = m\frac{v^2}{r}$$

Where v = its speed and r = the radius of the circular path. How much is the force on this object changed if the radius r is reduced to a third of its original value and its speed v is halved? If the original force was 14 newtons, what is the new force on the object?

MCAT MATHEMATICS CONCEPT 5: Percentages Increase or Decrease

A percentage is just an alternative way of representing a fraction or ratio. The statement "x is P percent (P%) of y" means that:

$$x = \frac{P}{100} \cdot y \text{ or, equivalently, } P = \frac{x}{y} \cdot 100$$

Important: A percentage is a fraction with a denominator of 100, e.g., a nickel is 5% of a dollar.

Percentages are typically used to express the fractional part that one quantity is of another; for example, if there are 16 women in a class of 25 students, then alternatively one can say that P = (16/25)(100) = 64% of the students in the class are women. Percentages are also used to express a change in a quantity in terms of its percent increase or decrease. By definition, if x_2 is the result when x_1 is increased by P%, then:

$$x_2 = x_1 + \frac{P}{100} \cdot x_1 = x_1 \cdot \left(1 + \frac{P}{100}\right);$$

if x_2 is the result when x_1 is decreased by P%, then:

$$x_2 = x_1 - \frac{P}{100} \cdot x_1 = x_1 \cdot \left(1 - \frac{P}{100}\right).$$

It is important to note that in both of these definitions the change in the variable is expressed as a percentage of its original value (x_1), not its final value (x_2).

Example 8.
What is the percent increase or decrease in a quantity x when its value is: a) doubled, b) halved, c) reduced by a third, d) reduced to a third of its original value, and e) reduced to a fifth of its original value?

(a) $x_2 = 2x_1$; $2x_1 = x_1\left(1 + \frac{P}{100}\right)$ P = 100% increase

(b) $x_2 = \frac{1}{2}x_1$; $\frac{1}{2}x_1 = x_1\left(1 - \frac{P}{100}\right)$ P = 50% decrease

(c) $x_2 = \frac{2}{3}x_1$; $\frac{2}{3}x_1 = x_1\left(1 - \frac{P}{100}\right)$ P = $33\frac{1}{3}$% decrease

(d) $x_2 = \frac{1}{3}x_1$; $\frac{1}{3}x_1 = x_1\left(1 - \frac{P}{100}\right)$ P = $66\frac{2}{3}$% decrease

(e) $x_2 = \frac{1}{5}x_1$; $\frac{1}{5}x_1 = x_1\left(1 - \frac{P}{100}\right)$ P = 80% decrease

Problem 8.

In 1984, a particular item A cost $2,500. In 1986, the price of A rose 20% due to scarcity while in early 1987 there was 10% increase in the price of A over its 1986 price. At the end of 1987, A was put on sale with a 30% decrease in price. What was the sale price of A?

Solutions to Algebra Problems

(1) $a = \frac{r^2 + sp - q}{s - t}$; $s(a - p) + q = ta + r^2$

$sa - sp + q = ta + r^2$

$a(s - t) = r^2 + sp - q$

$a = \frac{r^2 + sp - q}{s - t}$

(2) d = -13 ; $\frac{1}{d-2} + \frac{2}{d+3} = \frac{4}{d-2}$ [Multiply through by (d-2)(d+3)]

$d + 3 + 2(d - 2) = 4(d + 3)$

$3d - 1 = 4d + 12$

$d = -13$

(3) $x = \frac{13}{5}$; $3(4x - 2[1 - (x + 5) + 3]) = 13x + 19$

$3[4x - 2(4 - x - 5)] = 13x + 19$

$3(4x + 2x + 2) = 13x + 19$

$18x + 6 = 13x + 19$

$x = \frac{13}{5}$

(4) $C = \frac{21}{5}$ moles Let $x_1 = 5$ moles of B and $y_1 = 3$ moles of C;

then $x_2 = 7$ moles of B and y_2 = number of moles of C.

Since B and C are directly proportional:

$\frac{y_2}{7} = \frac{3}{5}$; $y_2 = \frac{21}{5}$ moles of C

(5) r = .05 gallons/mile

From the problem, xy = a, where:

x = gas consumption rate (gallons/mile),

y = number of miles that the car can go on a full tank of gas,

a = number of gallons in full tank of gas (constant).

Thus, x and y are inversely proportional with $x_1 = r$, $y_1 = 400$, $x_2 = r - .01$, and $y_2 = 500$;

$r(400) = (r - .01)500$

$400r = 500r - 5$

$r = .05$ gallons/mile

(6) $\frac{P_1V_1}{T_1} = \frac{P_2V_2}{T_2}; \frac{V}{T}$

$P_1V_1 = RT_1$ and $P_2V_2 = RT_2$ can be rewritten as: $\frac{P_1V_1}{T_1} = R$ and $\frac{P_2V_2}{T_2} = R$.

Therefore, the two states are related by:

$$\frac{P_1V_1}{T_1} = \frac{P_2V_2}{T_2}.$$

From the definition of inversely proportional variables, if P is one of the variables, then the other variable is V/T.

(7) $F_2 = \frac{3}{4}F_1$; $F_2 = 10.5$ newtons

$$\text{Let } F_1 = m\frac{(v_1)^2}{r_1},\ F_2 = m\frac{(v_2)^2}{r_2},$$

$$\text{then } \frac{F_2}{F_1} = \frac{(v_2)^2}{(v_1)^2} \cdot \frac{r_1}{r_2}$$

$$r_2 = \frac{1}{3}r_1 \text{ and } v_2 = \frac{1}{2}v_1$$

$$\frac{F_2}{F_1} = \frac{(v_1/2)^2}{(v_1)^2} \qquad \frac{r_1}{\frac{1}{3}r_1} = \frac{\frac{1}{4}}{\frac{1}{3}} = \frac{3}{4} \text{ or } F_2 = \frac{3}{4}F_1$$

If $F_1 = 14$ newtons, then $F_2 = \frac{3}{4}(14) = 10.5$ newtons.

(8) Sale price (1987) = $2,310

1984: cost of A	= $2,500
1986: cost of A	= $2,500 + $\frac{20}{100}$ • $2,500
	= $3,000
1987: cost of A	= $3,000 + $\frac{10}{100}$ • $3,000
	= $3,300
Sale price (1987)	= $3,300 - $\frac{30}{100}$ • $3,300
	= $2,310

MCAT MATHEMATICS CONCEPT 6: Exponentials

The simplest use of exponentials is as a shorthand way of symbolizing a repeated multiplication of a number by itself, e.g., $10^3 = 10 \cdot 10 \cdot 10$, where 10^3 is the exponential expression for this repeated multiplication of 10 by itself. Obviously, 10^3 is also another way of expressing the number 1,000. In general, for

$$y = x^n = x \cdot x \cdot x \ldots x \leftarrow n \text{ factors of } x$$

Above, x^n is defined as an exponential form of y, x as the base, and n as the exponent. In this definition, x can be any number except zero and n is a positive integer. Starting from this definition, we can develop rules for arithmetic operations with exponentials and also generalize the definition of the exponential form so that the exponent can be any real number, not just a positive integer.

Rules for Exponentials
In the discussion below are ten rules for using exponentials; following at the end of this section the "Chart of Rules in Exponential Algebra" is given for your use in solving problems.

Using the definition for exponentials given earlier, the three basic rules for arithmetic operations with exponentials are:

(1) $x^m \cdot x^n = x^{m+n}$

(2) $\frac{x^m}{x^n} = x^{m-n}$ — m,n are positive integers; $x \neq 0$

(3) $(x^m)^n = x^{mn}$

(Note that the addition/subtraction of exponentials is deferred until the discussion of scientific notation below.)
By manipulating these basic exponent rules, we can now show:

(4) $x^0 = 1$; $x^0 = x^{n-n} = \frac{x^n}{x^n} = 1$

(5) $x^{-m} = \frac{1}{x^m}$; $x^{-m} = x^{0-m} = \frac{x^0}{x^m} = \frac{1}{x^m}$

Example 1.
Evaluate each expression:

(a) $\frac{10^2 \cdot 10^3}{10^{15}} = 10^{2+3-15} = 10^{-10}$

(b) $\left(\frac{3^6 \cdot 3^3 \cdot 9}{3^0 \cdot 3^4}\right)^2 = (3^{6+3+2-0-4})^2 = (3^7)^2 = 3^{7 \cdot 2} = 3^{14}$

(c) $\left(\frac{1}{4}\right)^{-2} = \frac{1}{\left(\frac{1}{4}\right)^2} = \frac{1}{\frac{1}{16}} = 16$

Problem 1.
Evaluate each expression:

(a) $\frac{4^4 \cdot 4^8}{4^5}$

(b) $\left(\frac{6^4}{6^2}\right)^3 \cdot 6^{-5}$

(c) $(7^4)^0$

Continuing the present discussion of exponentials, so far it has been restricted to integral exponents; however, it can be extended to include non-integral (any real number) exponents. First, it can be seen that a radical is just a fractional exponent:

(6) $x^{1/n} = \sqrt[n]{x}$; $(\sqrt[n]{x})^n = x$ (by definition)

$(x^m)^n = x$ (by letting $x^m = \sqrt[n]{x}$)

$x^{mn} = x^1$

thus $mn = 1$; $m = \frac{1}{n}$

It therefore follows in a straightforward manner that:

(7) $x^{m/n} = (\sqrt[n]{x})^m = \sqrt[n]{x^m}$

(8) $x^{-m/n} = \frac{1}{x^{m/n}} = \frac{1}{\sqrt[n]{x^m}} = \frac{1}{(\sqrt[n]{x})^m}$

(Note that m, n at this point are still positive integers.)

In these last two exponent rules we have an exponent m/n that can be any rational number (recall that any rational number can be written as a fraction of two integers). Moreover, since any irrational number can be approximated by a rational number, we can define:

$$y = x^p$$

where the base x is any number except zero and the exponent p is any real number. If p is not an integer, it represents the combined operations of an integral exponent m and an nth root on the number x where p equals (exactly or approximately if it is irrational) m/n. In other words, the three basic exponent rules above apply for m, n = real numbers, not just positive integers. Finally, observe that:

(9) $(x \cdot y)^n = x^n \cdot y^n$
(10) $(x/y)^n = x^n/y^n$

Example 2.
Find the value of each expression:

(a) $8^{4/3} = \sqrt[3]{8^4} = (4{,}096)^{1/3} = 16$

$$= \left(\sqrt[3]{8}\right)^4 = 2^4 = 16$$

(b) $(289x)^{3/2} = (289^3)^{1/2}\, x^{3/2}$

$$= (289^{1/2})^3\, x^{3/2} = 17^3 \cdot x^{3/2} = 4913x^{3/2}$$

(c) $\dfrac{8^6 \cdot 8^3 \cdot \sqrt[3]{8}}{8^{5/3} \cdot 8^7} = 8^{6 + 3 + 1/3 - 5/3 - 7}$

$$= 8^{2/3} = (8^{1/3})^2 = 2^2 = 4$$

Problem 2.
Find the value of each expression:

(a) $216^{4/3}$

(b) $256^{3/4}$

(c) $\dfrac{\sqrt{ab} \cdot \sqrt[4]{a^3 \cdot b^3}}{\sqrt[3]{a^2 \cdot b^2}}$

(d) $\left(\frac{3}{5}\right)^8 \left(\frac{9}{25}\right)^3$

Use the following chart in solving problems:

Chart of Rules in Exponential Algebra

(1)	$x^m \cdot x^n$	$= x^{m+n}$	$3^2 \cdot 3^3 = 3^{2+3} = 243$
(2)	$\dfrac{x^m}{x^n}$	$= x^{m-n}$	$\dfrac{3^2}{3^3} = 3^{2-3} = 3^{-1} = \dfrac{1}{3}$
(3)	$(x^m)^n$	$= x^{mn}$	$(3^2)^3 = 3^6 = 729$
(4)	x^0	$= 1$	$3^0 = 1$

(x is any real positive number)

(5) $x^{-m} = \frac{1}{x^m}$ $\qquad 3^{-2} = \frac{1}{3^2} = \frac{1}{9}$

(6) $x^{1/n} = \sqrt[n]{x}$ $\qquad 3^{1/2} = \sqrt[2]{3} = \sqrt{3}$

It is customary to ignore the 2 in $\sqrt[2]{3}$. The figure $\sqrt{3}$ represents the square root of 3.

(7) $x^{m/n} = (\sqrt[n]{x})^m = \sqrt[n]{x^m}$ $\qquad 3^{2/3} = (\sqrt[3]{3})^2 = \sqrt[3]{9}$

(The figure $\sqrt[3]{9}$ represents the cube root of 9.)

(8) $x^{-m/n} = \frac{1}{x^{m/n}} = \frac{1}{\sqrt[n]{x^m}} = \frac{1}{(\sqrt[n]{x})^m}$

$3^{-2/3} = (\sqrt[3]{3})^{-2} \qquad = \sqrt[3]{\frac{1}{3^2}} = \sqrt[3]{\frac{1}{9}}$

(9) $(x \cdot y)^n = x^n \cdot y^n$ $\qquad (3 \cdot 4)^3 = 3^3 \cdot 4^3 = 27 \cdot 64 = 1728$

(10) $\left(\frac{x}{y}\right)^n = \frac{x^n}{y^n}$ $\qquad \left(\frac{3}{4}\right)^3 = \frac{3^3}{4^3} = \frac{27}{64}$

MCAT MATHEMATICS CONCEPT 7: Scientific Notation

Scientific notation is a convenient method for writing large and small numbers using powers of ten; it is essentially an application of exponentials. A number is said to be in standard scientific notation when it is written in the form:

$X = a \times 10^m$

where a is between 1 and 10 and m is an integral exponent.

Example 3a.

2 9 9 8 0 0 0 0 0 0 0 cm/sec = 2.998×10^{10} cm/sec

Example 4a.

0. 0 0 1 2 3 4 = 1.234×10^{-3}

Depending on what is most convenient, standard scientific notation does not always have to be used, e.g., in the two examples above the numbers could also have been rewritten as:

Example 3b.

2. 998 x 10^{10} cm/sec = 0.2998 x 10^{11} cm/sec
2 .9 98 x 10^{10} cm/sec = 29.98 x 10^{9} cm/sec

Example 4b.

1. 234 x 10^{-3} = 0.1234 x 10^{-2}
1. 2 34 x 10^{-3} = 12.34 x 10^{-4}

It should be observed in these two examples that when the decimal point is moved one place to the left, the power of ten increases by 1, and that when the decimal point is moved one place to the right, the power of ten decreases by 1. The arithmetic operations for numbers written in scientific notation are:

Addition/subtraction: to add and subtract numbers in scientific notation, the numbers must be in terms of the same power of 10.

Example 5.
$3 \times 10^3 + 4 \times 10^3 = 7 \times 10^3$

Example 6.
$3 \times 10^3 + 4 \times 10^4 = 0.3 \times 10^4 + 4 \times 10^4 = 4.3 \times 10^4$

Multiplication: $(a \times 10^m)(b \times 10^n) = (ab) \times 10^{m+n}$

Division: $\dfrac{a \times 10^m}{b \times 10^n} = \left(\dfrac{a}{b}\right) \times 10^{m-n}$

Exponents: $(a \times 10^m)^n = (a^n) \times 10^{mn}$

Example 7.
$(6.6\times10^{12})(1.1\times10^{-3}) = (6.6)(1.1)\times10^{12-3} = 7.26 \times 10^9$

Example 8.
$\dfrac{1.8\times10^7}{7.2\times10^{-10}} = \dfrac{18\times10^6}{7.2\times10^{-10}} = \left(\dfrac{18}{7.2}\right) \times 10^{6-(-10)} = 2.5 \times 10^{16}$

Example 9.
$(1.2\times10^3)^3 = (1.2)^3 \times 10^{3\cdot3} = 1.728 \times 10^9$

Problem 3.
Put in terms of standard scientific notation:

(a) 3430000

(b) 0.000000000824

Problem 4.
Find the value of each expression (in standard scientific notation):

(a) $\dfrac{(4\times10^{16})(7\times10^{-5})}{3.455 \times 10^4 - 3.427 \times 10^4}$

(b) $\dfrac{7\times10^7 - 2.8\times10^6}{10^{-7} + 1.24 \times 10^{-6} - 1.02 \times 10^{-6}}$

(c) $[(6 \times 10^4)(9 \times 10^3)(4 \times 10^{-1})]^{1/3}$

MCAT MATHEMATICS CONCEPT 8: Logarithms

We already saw in the discussion of exponentials above that:

- $x^m \cdot x^n = x^{m+n}$
- $\dfrac{x^m}{x^n} = x^{m-n}$
- $(x^m)^n = x^{mn}$
- $x^0 = 1$
- $x^{-m} = \dfrac{1}{x^m}$

where x is any number except zero and m, n are any real numbers. Logarithms arise when one considers that, by assuming a particular base x, these exponent rules could be rewritten in terms of the exponents only. We define the logarithm of a number M as the power (exponent) m to which a base x must be raised to give the number M; that is:

if $M = x^m$, then m = logarithm of M with respect to the base x and is usually written $m = \log_x M$;

if $N = x^n$, then $n = \log_x N$, etc.

By their definition, logarithms are simply exponents; more explicitly:

$X^{\log_X M} = M$ [take the log (base X) of both sides of this equation and it becomes obvious]

$\log X^{\log_x M} = \log_x M$

Example 10.
Write each expression in its equivalent logarithmic form:

(a) If $8^3 = 512$, then $\log_8 512 = 3$

(b) If $10^{4.6990} = 50{,}000$, then $\log_{10} 50{,}000 = 4.6990$

(c) If $2^{-2} = 1/4$, then $\log_2(1/4) = -2$

Example 11.
Find the value of x:

(a) $\log_2 32 = x \rightarrow 2^x = 32$; $x = 5$

(b) $\log_5 1 = x \rightarrow 5^x = 1$; $x = 0$

(c) $\log_m (m^{10}) = x \rightarrow m^x = m^{10}$; $x = 10$

(d) $2^{\log_2 3} = x \rightarrow \log_2 3 = \log_2 x$; $x = 3$

(e) $4^{\log_4 16} = x \rightarrow \log_4 16 = \log_4 x$; $x = 16$

Problem 5.
Find the value of x:

(a) $\log_4 \left(\frac{1}{16}\right) = x$

(b) $\log_{z^2} (Z^b) = x$

(c) $\log_x 1 = 0$

(d) $5^{\log_5 625} = x$

(e) $4^{\log_2 16} = x$

Rules of Logarithms

Using logarithms, the five rules for exponentials can now be rewritten as:

Rule 1: $\log_x M + \log_x N = \log_x (MN)$

Rule 2: $\log_x M - \log_x N = \log_x \left(\frac{M}{N}\right)$

Rule 3: $\log_x (M^n) = n(\log_x M)$

Rule 4: $\log_x 1 = 0$

Rule 5: $\log_x \left(\frac{1}{M}\right) = \log_x (M^{-1}) = -\log_x M$

It should be remembered that $\log_{10} M$ is usually just written as log M.

Example 12.
If log 2 = 0.3010 and log 3 = 0.4774, then:

(a) $\log 6 = \log (2 \cdot 3) = \log 2 + \log 3 = 0.3010 + 0.4774 = 0.7784$

(b) $\log 5 = \log\left(\frac{10}{2}\right) = \log 10 - \log 2 = 1 - 0.3010 = 0.6990$

(c) $\log 8 = \log (2^3) = 3(\log 2) = 3(0.3010) = 0.9030$

(d) $\log 60 = \log (2 \cdot 3 \cdot 10) = \log 2 + \log 3 + \log 10 =$
$0.3010 + 0.4774 + 1 = 1.7784$

Example 13.
Solve for x: $2\log x = \log a + \log b - \log c$

$$\log x^2 = \log\left(\frac{ab}{c}\right)$$

$$x^2 = \frac{ab}{c}$$

$$x = \sqrt{\frac{ab}{c}}$$

Problem 6.
Express as a single logarithm:

(a) $\log M^2 + 7\log N - \frac{1}{3}\log P$

(b) $\log\sqrt{x^5} - 3\log \sqrt[4]{x} + \log x^3$

Problem 7.
Solve for x:

(a) $\log_9 (x+1) = \frac{1}{2}$

(b) $3\log x = 2\log a + 3\log b + 4\log c - 5\log d$

The two most common bases used for logarithms are 10 (common logarithms) and e (natural logarithms). In a sense, common logarithms are an extension of scientific notation in terms of the fact that the coefficient of the power of ten (which is between 1 and 10) is also written as a power of ten. Thus, the number in question is written completely as an exponential using the base 10; consider:

$$y = a \times 10^b \qquad \text{(define } a = 10^c\text{)}$$

$$= 10^c \times 10^b = 10^{c+b}$$

$$\log y = c + b$$

where *c* is defined as the mantissa and *b* as the characteristic. Before calculators, common logarithms were an important tool for solving problems; however, calculators have largely replaced their use in solving problems. You cannot use calculators on the MCAT; consequently, **learning common logarithms is essential for solving science problems**. Conceptually, they are still important for topics such as pH, sound intensity, exponential decay and growth problems. The base of natural logarithms, *e*, is an irrational number that is approximately equal to 2.71828. Natural logarithms and the base *e* play an important part in many scientific problems, e.g., exponential growth and decay. Since only a basic understanding of logarithms is needed for the MCAT, further discussion of them, or problems involving them, is not necessary. Use these basic principles to work on advanced science problems on your own.

Solutions to Exponentials, Scientific Notation, and Logarithm Problems

(1a) 4^7 $\quad \frac{4^4 \cdot 4^8}{4^5} = 4^{4+8-5} = 4^7$

(1b) 6 $\quad \left(\frac{6^4}{6^2}\right) \cdot 6^{-5} = (6^2)^3 \cdot 6^{-5} = 6^{6-5} = 6$

(1c) 1 $\quad (7^4)^0 = 1$; recall $x^0 = 1$

(2a) 1296 $\quad 216^{4/3} = \left(\sqrt[3]{216^4}\right) = 6^4 = 1296$

$= 216^1 \cdot \left(\sqrt[3]{216}\right) = 216 \cdot 6 = 1296$

(2b) 64 $\quad 256^{3/4} = (256^{1/4})^3 = 4^3 = 64$

(2c) $(ab)^{7/12}$ $\quad \frac{\sqrt{ab} \cdot \sqrt[4]{a^3b^3}}{\sqrt[3]{a^2b^2}} = \frac{(ab)^{1/2}(ab)^{3/4}}{(ab)^{2/3}}$

$= (ab)^{1/2 + 3/4 - 2/3} = (ab)^{6/12 + 9/12 - 8/12} = (ab)^{7/12}$

(2d) $\frac{25}{9}$ $\quad \left(\frac{3}{5}\right)^8 \left(\frac{9}{25}\right)^3 = \frac{3^{-8}}{5^{-8}} \cdot \frac{3^6}{5^6} = \frac{3^{-2}}{5^{-2}} = \frac{5^2}{3^2} = \frac{25}{9}$

(3a) 3.43×10^6

(3b) 8.24×10^{-10}

(4a) 10^{10} $\quad \frac{(4\text{x}10^{16})(7\text{x}10^{-5})}{3.455\text{x}10^4 - 3.427\text{x}10^4} = \frac{28\text{x}10^{11}}{.028\text{x}10^4} = \frac{28\text{x}10^{11}}{28\text{x}10^1} = 10^{10}$

(4b) $2.1\text{x}10^{14}$ $\quad \frac{7\text{x}10^7 - 2.8\text{x}10^6}{10^{-7} + 1.24\text{x}10^{-6} - 10.2\text{x}10^7}$

$= \frac{70\text{x}10^6 - 2.8\text{x}10^6}{1\text{x}10^{-7} + 12.4\text{x}10^{-7} - 10.2\text{x}10^{-7}}$

$= \frac{67.2\text{x}10^6}{3.2\text{x}10^{-7}} = \left(\frac{67.2}{3.2}\right) \text{x } 10^{6-(-7)} = 21\text{x}10^{13}$

$= 2.1\text{x}10^{14}$

(4c) $6\text{x}10^2$ $\quad [(6\text{x}10^4)(9\text{x}10^3)(4\text{x}10^{-1})]^{1/3}$

$= [(6\text{x}9\text{x}4) \text{ x } 10^{4+3-1}]^{1/3}$

$= (216\text{x}10^6)^{1/3} = (216)^{1/3} \text{ x } 10^{6 \cdot 1/3} = 6\text{x}10^2$

(5a) $x = -2$ $\quad \log_4\left(\frac{1}{16}\right) = x \rightarrow \quad 4^x = \frac{1}{16}$; $x = -2$

(5b) $x = \frac{b}{2}$ $\quad \log_{z^2}(Z^b) = x \rightarrow \quad Z^{2x} = Z^b$; $b = 2x \rightarrow x = \frac{b}{2}$

(5c) x = any real number except zero

$$\log_x 1 = 0 \rightarrow x^0 = 1$$

(5d) x = 625

$$5^{\log_5 625} = x \rightarrow \quad \log_5 625 = \log_5 x \rightarrow x = 625$$

(5e) x = 256

$$4^{\log_2 16} = x$$

$$4^4 = x \rightarrow \quad x = 256$$

(6a) $\log\left(\frac{M^2N^7}{\sqrt[3]{P}}\right)$

$$\log M^2 + 7\log N - \frac{1}{3}\log P$$

$$= \log M^2 + \log N^7 - \log \sqrt[3]{P} = \log\left(\frac{M^2N^7}{\sqrt[3]{P}}\right)$$

(6b) $\frac{19}{4}\log x$

$$\log \sqrt{x^5} - 3\log \sqrt[4]{x} + \log x^3$$

$$= \log x^{5/2} - \log x^{3/4} + \log x^3$$

$$= \frac{5}{2}\log x - \frac{3}{4}\log x + 3\log x$$

$$= \left(\frac{5}{2} - \frac{3}{4} + 3\right)\log x = \frac{19}{4}\log x = \log x^{19/4}$$

(7a) x = 2

$$\log_9(x + 1) = \frac{1}{2} \quad \rightarrow \quad x + 1 = 9^{1/2} = 3$$

$$= 2$$

(7b) $x = \sqrt[3]{\frac{a^2b^3c^4}{d^5}}$

$$3\log x = 2\log a + 3\log b + 4\log c - 5\log d$$

$$\log x = \frac{1}{3}(\log a^2 + \log b^3 + \log c^4 - \log d^5)$$

$$\log x = \log\left(\frac{a^2b^3c^4}{d^5}\right)^{1/3}$$

$$x = \sqrt[3]{\frac{a^2b^3c^4}{d^5}}$$

4.2.3.2 Analytic Geometry

The knowledge of analytic geometry required for the MCAT is focused primarily on the interpretation of information presented in a graphical format, e.g., determining slopes of lines and curves, finding intercepts, and determining "equations" for experimental curves.

It is also emphasized in the *MCAT Student Manual* that the premedical student should be able to **remember and use** important, basic formulas to calculate areas and volumes. The reason for emphasizing areas and volumes of figures is to assure that the premedical student understands how to determine cross-sectional areas of any human artery or vein, volume of blood pumped by the heart, volume of head and brain, total surface area of the body, finding area of a cast, finding volume of air/oxygen capacity of lungs, and many other calculations pertaining to the human body. It should be added here, that the geometry formulas that follow will be useful in the physical and biological sciences subtests.

Regarding memorization, the *MCAT Student Manual* does not stress it, but there are advantages:
- memorizing a formula facilitates your problem-solving ability and enables you to work faster
- it improves your mental proportional reasoning ability
- it increases your confidence to know the formulas you will be using.

You are encouraged to refresh your memory of basic formulas!

Review of Plane Geometry

Following is a chart of commonly used geometry formulas. Learn to apply them to ordinary geometry problems.

Commonly Used Geometry Formulas

TRIANGLE

perimeter = $S_1 + S_2 + S_3$, $b = S_3$
area = 1/2 base x height = $(1/2)hS_3$

SQUARE

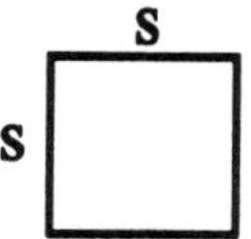

perimeter = 4S
area = S x S or S^2

RECTANGLE

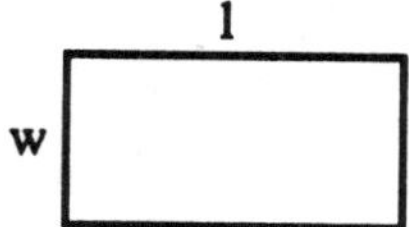

perimeter = 2(l+w) or 2l + 2w
area = lw

PARALLELOGRAM

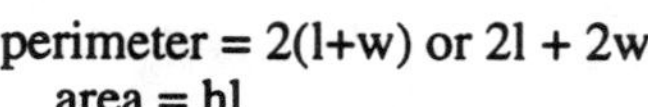

perimeter = 2(l+w) or 2l + 2w
area = hl

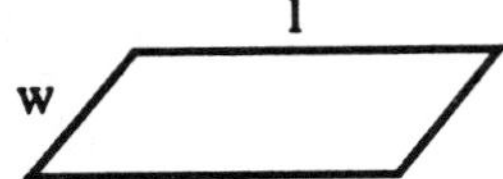

TRAPEZOID

perimeter = $b_1+b_2+S_1+S_2$
area = $h\left(\frac{b_1+b_2}{2}\right)$

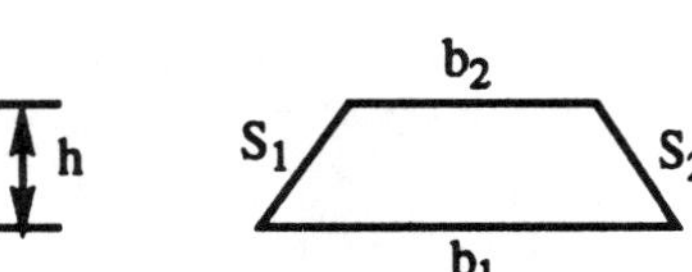

[Hint: draw a diagonal and find the area by summing the areas of the two triangles.]

CIRCLE

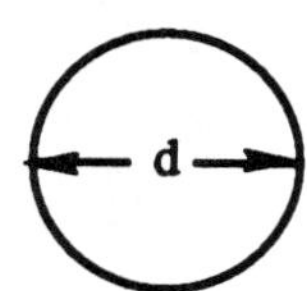

circumference = $2\pi r$ or πd
area = πr^2
[note: r = d/2]

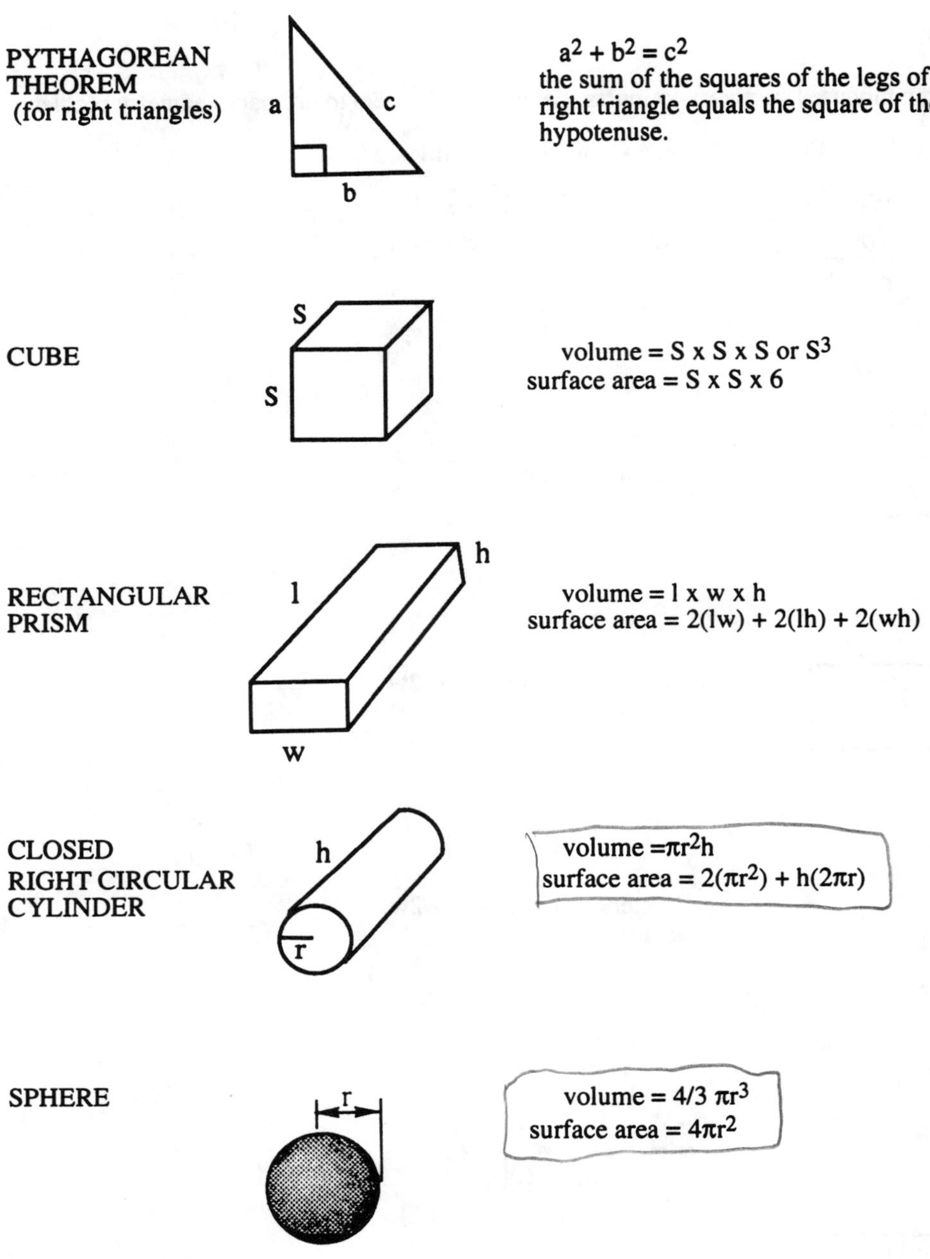

Fig. 4.3a—Common Geometric Shapes

An application of these formulas is found by using the following charts of astronomical data. The charts, and the questions that follow them, should be studied and used with the geometry formulas. Astronomical charts may appear on various subtests of the MCAT. Do not memorize these charts, just familiarize yourself with the principles.

	Sun	Moon
mass	4. 4 x 10^{30} lb	1.63 x 10^{23} lb
radius	4.32 x 10^{5} mi	1080 mi
average gravitational accleration	896.00 ft/sec^2	5.30 ft/sec^2
escape velocity	388.00 mi/sec	1.50 mi/sec
axial rotation period	25.40 days	27.30 days
average density	89.20 lb/ft^3	208.00 lb/ft^3

	Mercury	Venus	Earth	Mars	Jupiter	Neptune	Pluto
Period of Rotation About Sun	88 days	224.7 days	365.26 days	687 days	4,333 days	60,180 days	90,730 days
Equatorial Radius	1500 mi	3850 mi	3963 mi	2110 mi	44,370 mi	13,900 mi	1850 mi
Mass	.071x10^{25}lb	1.1x10^{25} lb	1.82x10^{25} lb	.14x10^{25} lb	420x10^{25} lb	22.7x10^{25} lb	1.2x10^{25} lb
Mean Density	330 lb/ft^3	306 lb/ft^3	340 lb/ft^3	247 lb/ft^3	81 lb/ft^3	144 lb/ft^3	250 lb/ft^3
Mean Surface Grav-itational Acceleration	12 ft/sec^2	28 ft/sec^2	32.2 ft/sec^2	12.5 ft/sec^2	85 ft/sec^2	49 ft/sec^2	26 ft/sec^2
Escape Velocity	2.6 mi/sec	6.3 mi/sec	7.0 mi/sec	3.1 mi/sec	38 mi/sec	16 mi/sec	6 mi/sec
Period of Rotation About Axis	88 days	30 days	23.93 hr	24.61 hr	9.84 hr	15.7 hr	16 hr
Orbital Speed	29.8 mi/sec	21.8 mi/sec	18.5 mi/sec	15 mi/sec	8.12 mi/sec	3.38 mi/sec	2.95 mi/sec

Fig. 4.3b—Physical Characterisics of Astronomical Bodies

Use the foregoing charts to solve the following problems and any others you may choose to make up for your own practice:

(1) What is the volume of the moon?

(2) What is the equatorial circumference of Jupiter?

(3) Which planet is denser, Mercury or Neptune?

(4) What is the ratio of the volume of Pluto to the volume of the sun?

(5) Which planet has the highest surface rotational speed? the lowest rotational speed?

(6) What is the escape velocity of an object from the sun?

(7) What is the surface area of Jupiter in relation to the surface area of Venus?

(8) Compare the surface area of the Earth to the surface area of your room. Use identical units.

(9) Which one is the greatest? the least?
(a) area of a circle with radius = 2 ft.
(b) surface area of a cylinder with radius = 1 ft ; height = 6 inches (without top and bottom).
(c) The area of a parallelogram with base = 1 ft and height = 2 ft.
(d) The area of a triangle with base = 4 ft and height = 4.5 ft.
(e) The area of a trapezoid with bases of 2 ft and 3 ft respectively and height of 1.25 ft.

These problems are direct applications of the geometry formulas given earlier. Finish the problems, check your answers below, and then proceed to the graphical analytic geometry section that follows.

(1) $V = (4/3)\pi R^3 = 5.27 \bullet 10^9 \text{ (miles)}^3$

(2) $C = 2\pi R = 278{,}643.6$ miles

(3) Mercury

(4) $V_{pluto}/V_{sun} = [(4/3)\pi R_p^3] / [(4/3)\pi R_s^3] = (1850 / 4.32 \bullet 10^5)^3$
$= (428.24)^3 \bullet 10^{-15} \quad = 78.5 \bullet 10^{-9}$

(5) Rotational speed at the surface (rotations/hour) x circumference

Rotational Speed (miles/hour)		
Mercury	4.46	lowest
Venus	33.60	
Earth	1037.00	
Mars	538.40	
Jupiter	28,317.00	highest
Neptune	5,560.00	
Pluto	726.50	

(6) 388 miles/sec.

(7) $A_j/A_v = 4\pi R_j^2/4\pi R_v^2 = (44370/3850)^2 = 132.76$

(8) $A_{earth} = 4\pi R^2 = 4\pi(3963)^2 = 4\pi(3963 \text{ x } 5280)^2 = 4\pi(20924640)^2 = 5.5\text{x}10^{15}$ sq.ft.

A_{room} = 2(length x width) + 2(length x height) + 2(width x height)

[Find the area of your room by measuring it, then compare it to the surface area of the Earth.]

(9) (a) $\pi R^2 = 12.56 \text{ ft}^2$ (greatest)

(b) $2\pi Rh = 2\pi(1)(1/2) = 3.14 \text{ ft}^2$

(c) $bh = 2(1) = 2 \text{ ft}^2$ (least)

(d) $(1/2)bh = (1/2)(4)(4.5) = 9 \text{ ft}^2$

(e) $(1/2)(2+3)1.25 = 3.125 \text{ ft}^2$

MCAT MATHEMATICS CONCEPT 9: Cartesian or Rectangular Coordinate System

All graphical representations of data and functions are based on some sort of coordinate system. Even bar graphs (histograms) and pie graphs have an implicit coordinate system in their construction. By far the most commonly used graphs are based on the rectangular (Cartesian) coordinate system that consists of two perpendicular axes, each representing a variable:

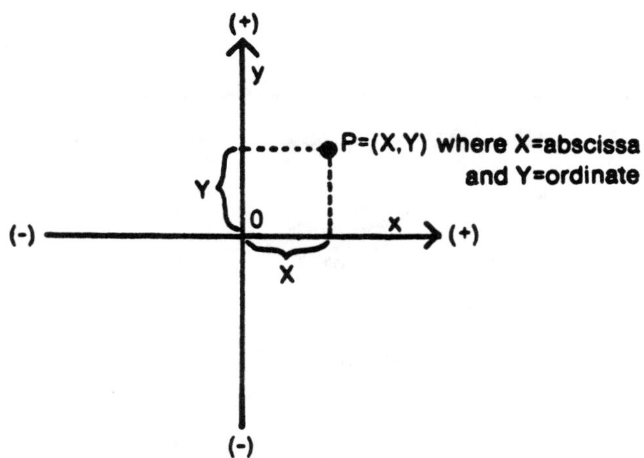

Fig. 4.4—Cartesian Coordinate System

The intersection of the two axes in the Cartesian plane is called the origin (O). The origin splits each axis into two segments that respectively represent positive and negative values of that axis' variable. The standard positive and negative segments of each axis are labelled on the graph above; this is also shown by the arrows that indicate the directions of positive change for each axis' variable. Each point in the Cartesian plane is represented by a pair of coordinates (called an ordered pair), each of which represents a displacement from the origin along one of the axes [e.g., the point P = (x,y) on the graph above and the origin O = (0,0)].

The first coordinate in the ordered pair is defined as the abscissa or the independent coordinate; the second coordinate is defined as the ordinate or the dependent coordinate. As is commonly done for discussion purposes, the abscissa will be labelled by x and the ordinate by y unless otherwise specified. With these coordinate labels, the Cartesian plane can be referred to as the xy-plane. Depending on the data or function being graphed, all or part of the xy-plane is used. In discussing the relation between the two variables being graphed, it may or may not be possible or necessary to say that one variable is independent while the other is dependent. In general, when dealing with data, an independent variable is one whose values are predetermined by the experimenter; the dependent variable is then determined for each of the values of the independent variable (hence it is "dependent" upon them). When dealing with functions, if "y is a function of x," then x is the independent variable on the x-axis and the dependent variable on the y-axis. Why?

What are Graphs?

Graphs are constructed by plotting values of one variable against the corresponding values of a second variable, i.e., by plotting a set of ordered pairs, as determined by experiments, by equations, or by some other known relationship between them.

Example 1.
An experimenter determines the following pairs of values for two related variables, x and y:

x	-2	+3	+4	+5	+6
y	-6	-4	+16	+18	+10

Plotting these points and connecting them by straight line segments, the graph is:

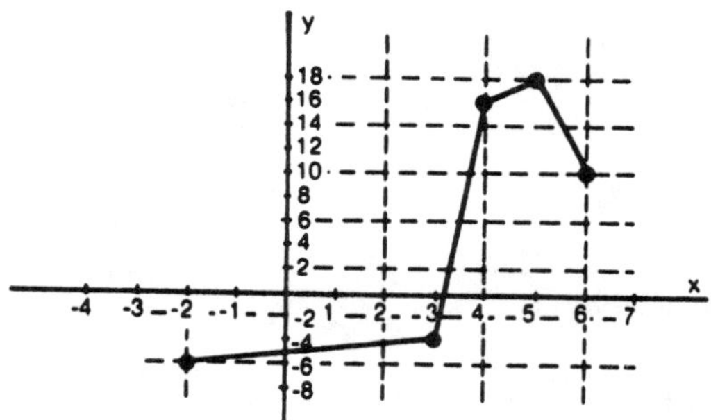

MCAT MATHEMATICS CONCEPT 10: Graphic representation of functions

Example 1.

Graph $y = \frac{a}{1+x}$ for $x \geq 0$: (reciprocal function)

Assume $a > 0$.

Using this function, possible pairs of values for x and y are:

x	0	1	3	7
y	a	$\frac{a}{2}$	$\frac{a}{4}$	$\frac{a}{8}$

Graphing these points and connecting them by a curve to graphically represent

$y = \frac{a}{1+x}$ for $x \geq 0$:

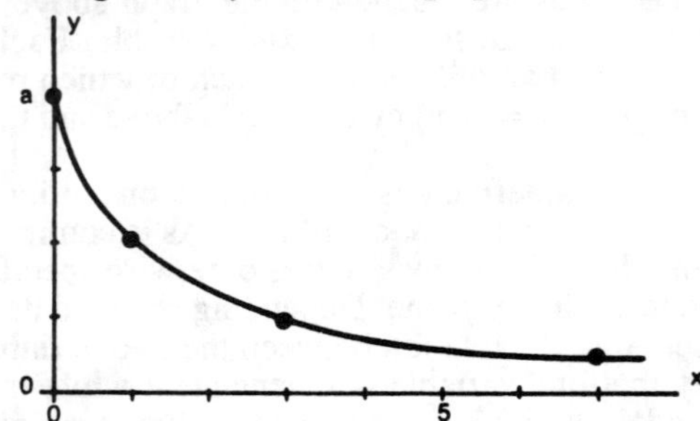

Example 2.

Graph the relationship between two variables, x and y, which are defined in terms of a third variable, t, as:

$y = 3t + 1$; $x = 2t$ (three variable equation)

Using these functions to get ordered pairs for (x,y):

t	-1	0	1	2	3
x	-2	0	2	4	6
y	-2	1	4	7	10

The graph is:

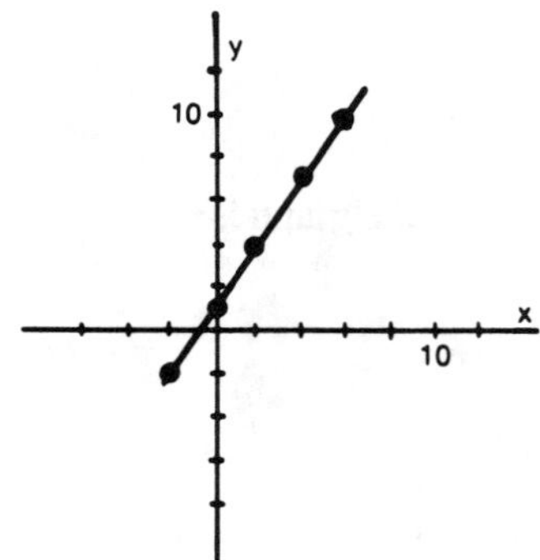

Note that this graph can also be algebraically represented by

$$y = \frac{3}{2}x + 1.$$

Problem 1.

Graph $y = \frac{5x}{1 + x}$

for $x \geq 0$ after first identifying the ordered pairs for x = 0, 1, 4, 9. As x gets very large, what value does y approach?

MCAT MATHEMATICS CONCEPT 11: Slope or rate of change

Probably the most important parameter in interpreting the relationship between the two variables in a graph is the slope. The slope of the line segment between two points is defined as the ratio of the change in the ordinate to the change in the abscissa:

$$\text{slope} = \frac{\text{change in ordinate}}{\text{change in abscissa}} = \frac{\Delta y}{\Delta x} = \frac{\text{Rise}}{\text{Run}} = \frac{\text{change in dependent variable}}{\text{change in independent variable}}$$

A slope exists at every point on a smooth graph whether it is a straight line or a curved line. For each point on a graph, the slope is the rate of change (positive or negative) in the ordinate with respect to the change in the abscissa. It may be constant as for straight lines or portions of curves that are straight, or it may be constantly changing as for curved lines. In practice, the slope is calculated as follows:

I) For straight lines:

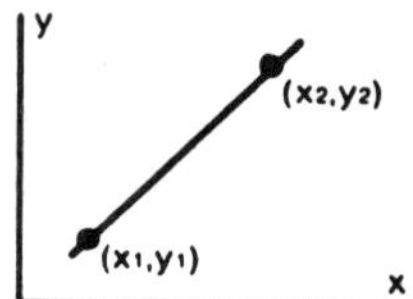

$$\text{slope} = m = \frac{y_2 - y_1}{x_2 - x_1} = \frac{\Delta y}{\Delta x} = \text{constant}$$

II) For curved lines:

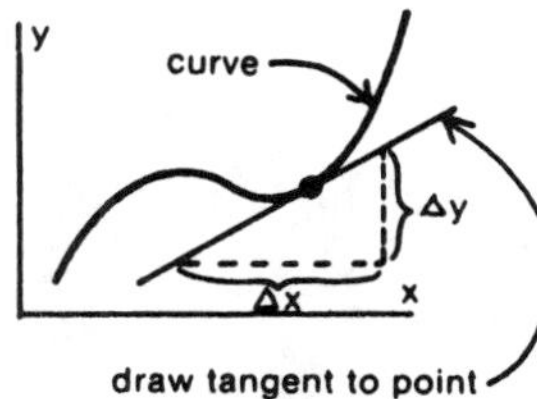

measure Δx,Δy for any two points on tangent

$$\text{slope} = m = \frac{\Delta y}{\Delta x} \pi \text{ constant (changes along the curve)}$$

Fig. 4.5.a — Definition of Slope for I) Straight and II) Curved lines

Example 1.

Calculate the slope of the line graphed below:

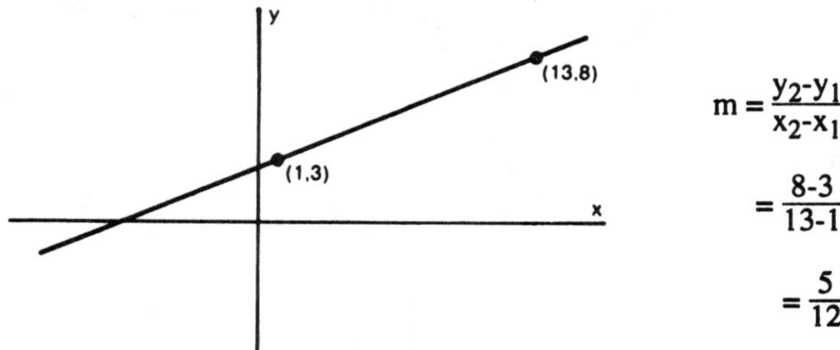

$$m = \frac{y_2 - y_1}{x_2 - x_1}$$

$$= \frac{8-3}{13-1}$$

$$= \frac{5}{12}$$

Problem 2.
Calculate the slope of the line graphed below (use the two points indicated):

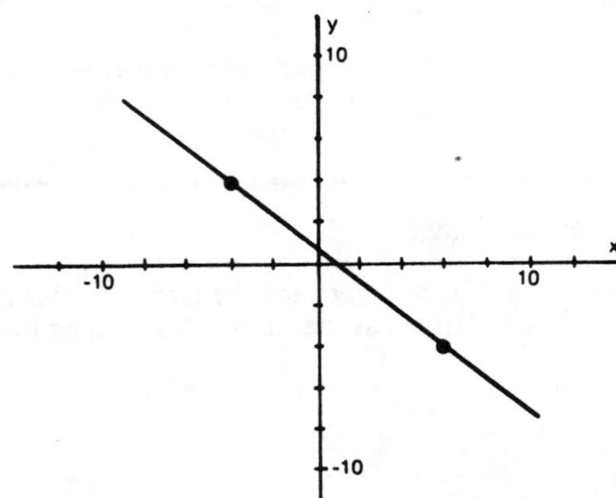

Having defined the slope, a review of its possible signs, relative magnitudes, and extreme values is worthwhile:

(I) positive slope; $\frac{\Delta y}{\Delta x} > 0$:

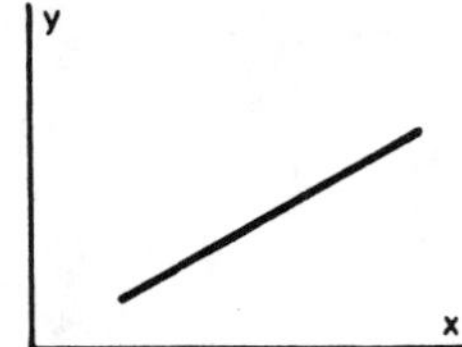

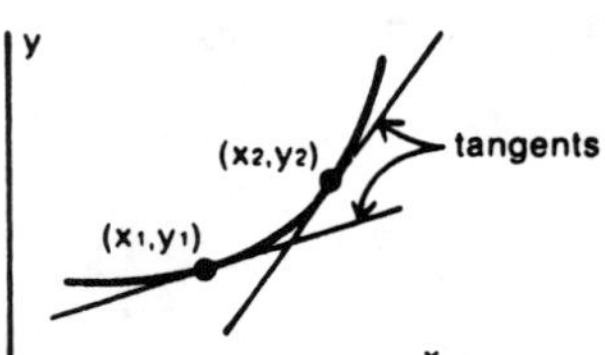

As x increases, y increases, and vice versa. Note in the graph on the right that the slope at (x_2,y_2) is greater than the slope at (x_1,y_1).

(II) negative slope; $\frac{\Delta y}{\Delta x} < 0$:

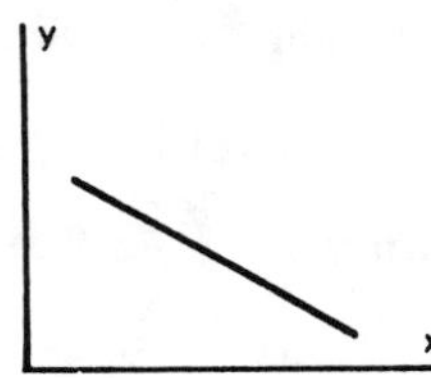

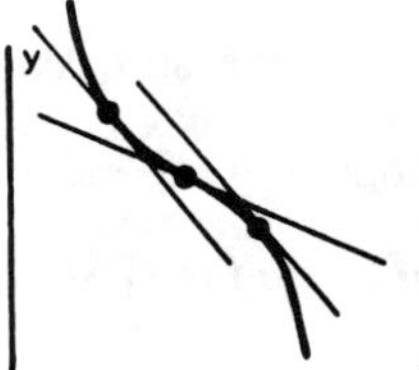

As x increases, y decreases, and vice versa. In the right-hand side graph, the slopes at the three points shown have negative values as indicated by their tangents.

(III) zero slope; $\frac{\Delta y}{\Delta x} = 0$:

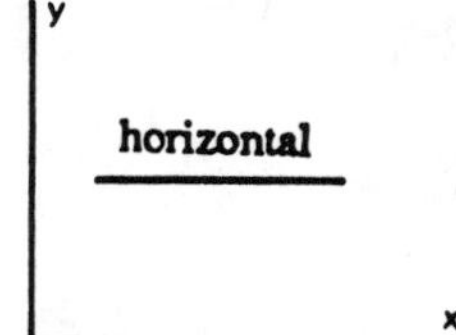

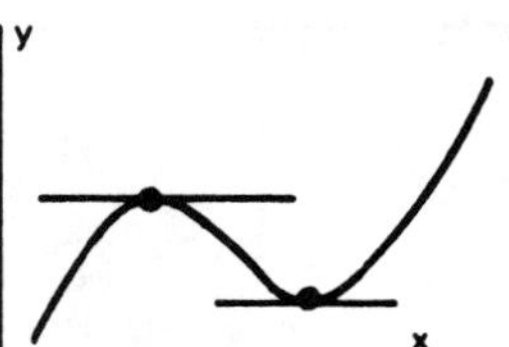

As x changes, there is no change in y, i.e.,

$$\frac{\Delta y}{\Delta x} = \frac{0}{\Delta x} = 0.$$

In the right-hand side graph, tangents are at points of zero slope.

(IV) infinite slope; $\frac{\Delta y}{\Delta x} = \pm\infty$ or $\frac{\Delta y}{\Delta x} = \pm\infty$ at finite value(s) of x:

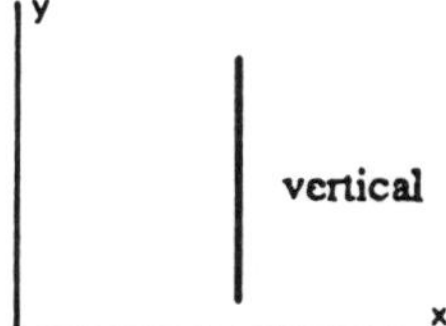

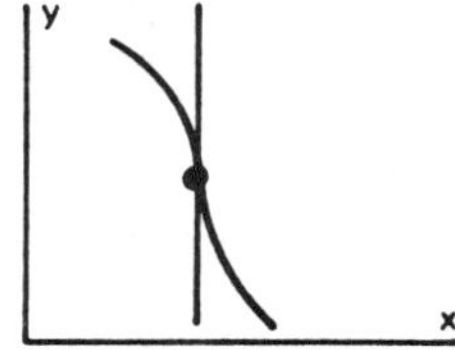

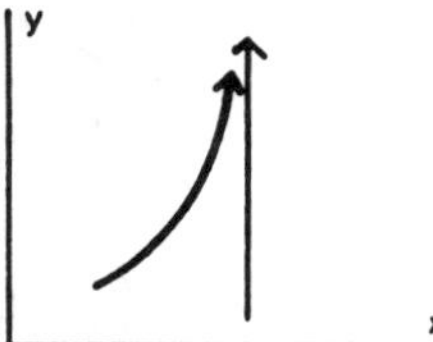

As y changes, there is no change in the value of x, i.e.,

$$\frac{\Delta y}{\Delta x} = \frac{\Delta y}{0} = \pm\infty$$

(actually $\frac{\Delta y}{0}$ is undefined, or more accurately $\lim_{\Delta x \to 0} \frac{\Delta y}{\Delta x} = \pm\infty$.)

In the center graph, the tangent is at a point where the slope becomes infinite. In the graph on the right, as the curve approaches the vertical line (an asymptote), its slope becomes infinite.

(V) large slope versus small slope:

Since vertical lines have slopes = ± ∞ and horizontal lines have slopes = 0, the more vertical the line, the larger the magnitude of the slope:

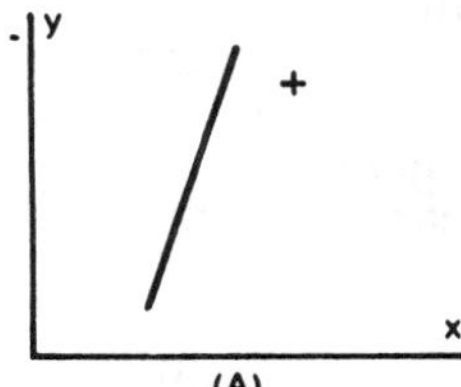

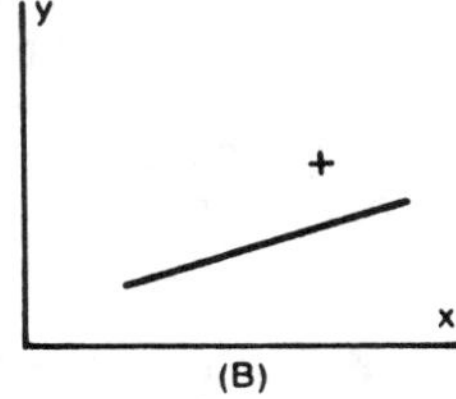

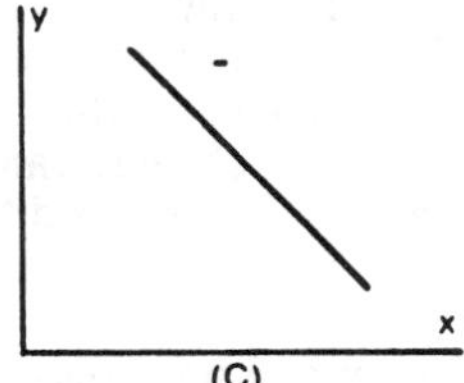

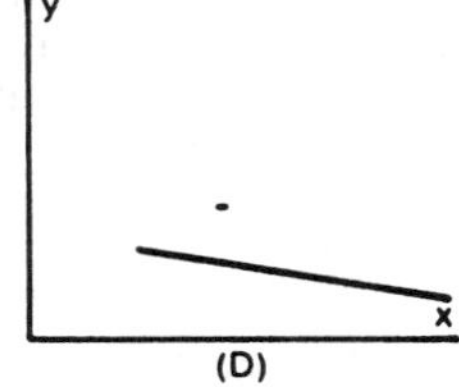

Magnitudes of slopes in A and C are greater than those of slopes in B and D respectively.

Fig. 4.5b—Sign Convention and Magnitude of Slope

Problem 3.
Calculate the slopes of lines 1 and 2. Which line has the slope of greater magnitude?

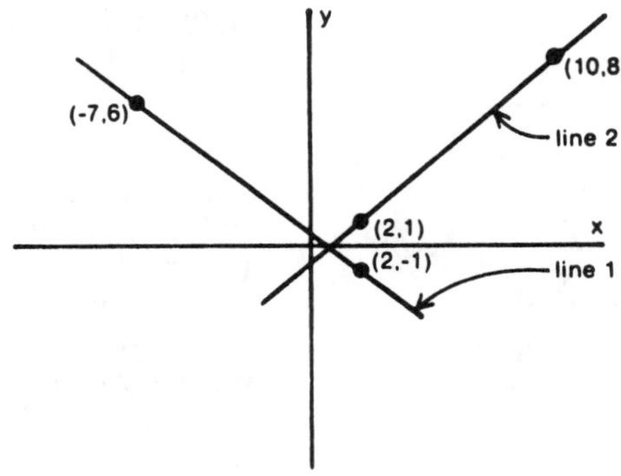

Problem 4.
At which of the three points indicated on the graph below is the slope the greatest?

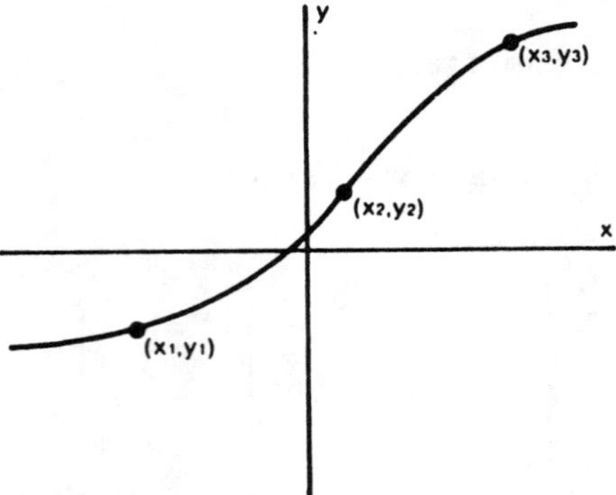

Maximum, Minimum and Inflection Points

Often, the relation between two variables will have local maximum point(s) and/or minimum point(s) which appear on graphs as:

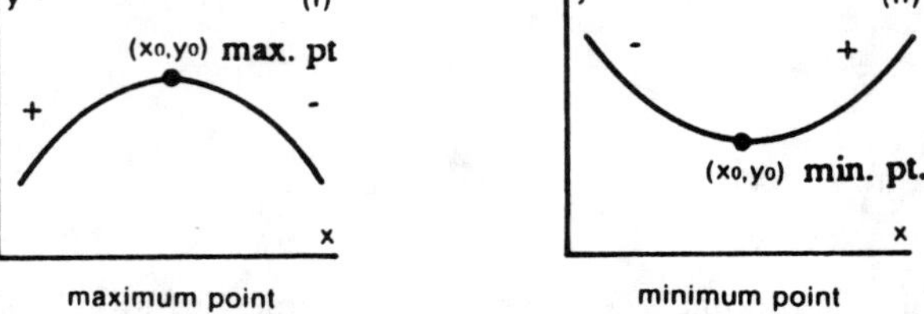

Fig. 4.5.c—Maximum and Minimum Points on a Curve

These curves are characterized by a critical point (x_0,y_0) at which the slope of the graph is zero and at which the slopes for points on one side of it have the opposite sign of the slopes for the points on the other side of it. In other words, as one moves along the curve, the slope decreases in magnitude as the critical point is approached until it is zero at the critical point; it then takes on the opposite sign on the other side of the critical point. [Observe in graphs I (maximum) and II (minimum) that the slopes to the left of (x_0,y_0) are respectively positive and negative, and that to the right of (x_0,y_0) they are respectively negative and positive.] For many problems in biology and medicine where they occur, curves with maximum and/or minimum points imply that for y there exist optimal (depending on how this is defined) ranges of x (about each maximum or minimum point). Maximum and minimum points were initially referred to as "local" above because there may exist many such points on a graph.

Inflection points are similar to maximum and minimum points because they can represent a significant point for the relation between the two variables graphed. Inflection points are points on a graph where the slope, **not the graph itself**, has a local maximum or minimum value. Unlike at maximum/minimum points, at an inflection point the sign of the slope does **not** change. Nevertheless, the slope at an inflection point can be zero. The four graphs below show types of inflection points; in each graph the inflection point is labelled by (x_0,y_0):

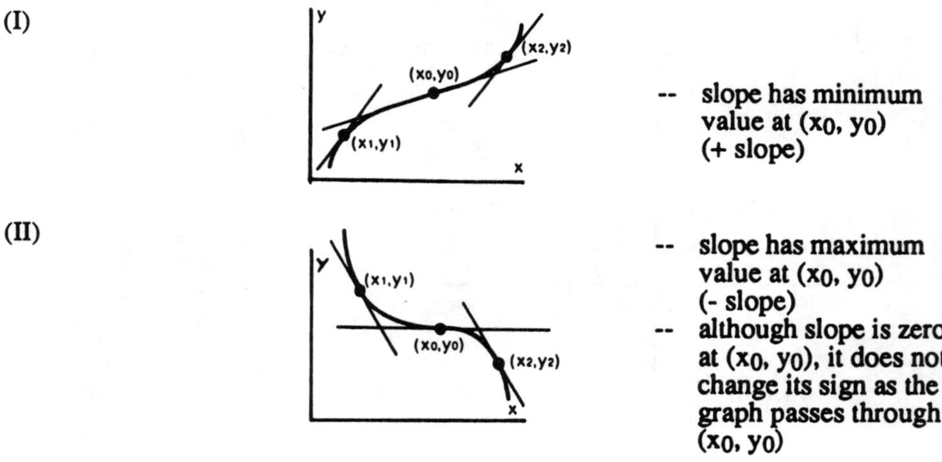

(III)

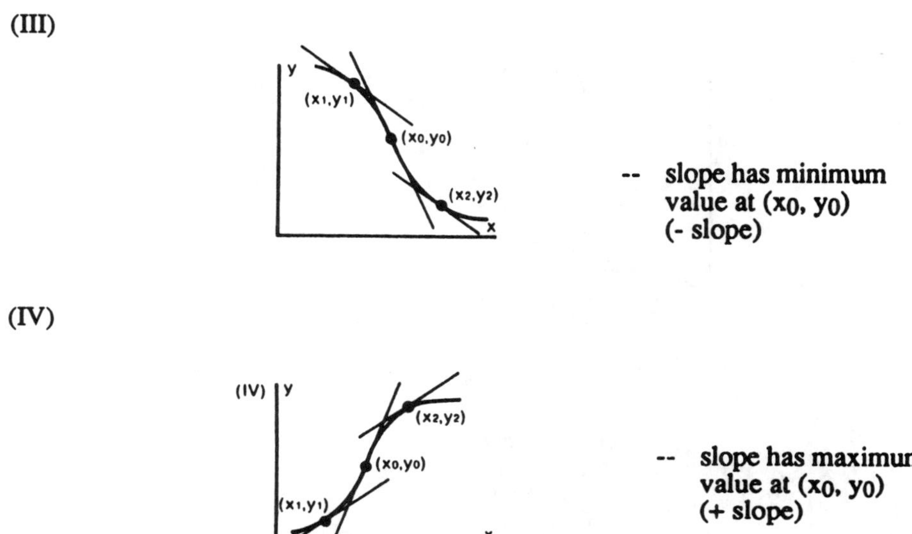

-- **slope has minimum value at (x_0, y_0) (- slope)**

(IV)

-- **slope has maximum value at (x_0, y_0) (+ slope)**

Fig. 4.5.d—Types of Inflection Points

In the four graphs above, each of the curves has been simplified to the extent that it has just an inflection point. A general curve may have maximum, minimum, and inflection points. As it turns out, between a pair of "adjacent" maximum and minimum points, there must be an inflection point.

When interpreting a graph, one can analyze both how y varies with x and how the slope, $\Delta y/\Delta x$, varies with x. In other words, the quantity of greatest interest on a graph can be the slope itself; if this is so, inflection points may be particularly significant.

Problem 5.
For inflection point graph (I) above, construct a graph for how $\Delta y/\Delta x$ varies with x.

Problem 6.
Which points, if any, are: maximum points? minimum points? inflection points?

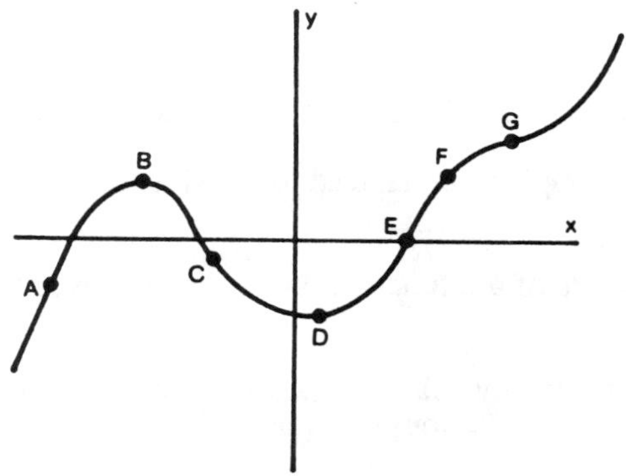

Area Under the Graph

If the quantity represented on the vertical axis is considered to vary as a function of the quantity measured on the horizontal axis, and if the product of these two quantities has meaning (e.g. distance = (speed)(time)), then the area under the graph also represents an important quantity. This area (called A) represents the continuous product of these variables over the interval shown on the horizontal axis. An example is the best way to illustrate how 'A' might be used.

Example 1.

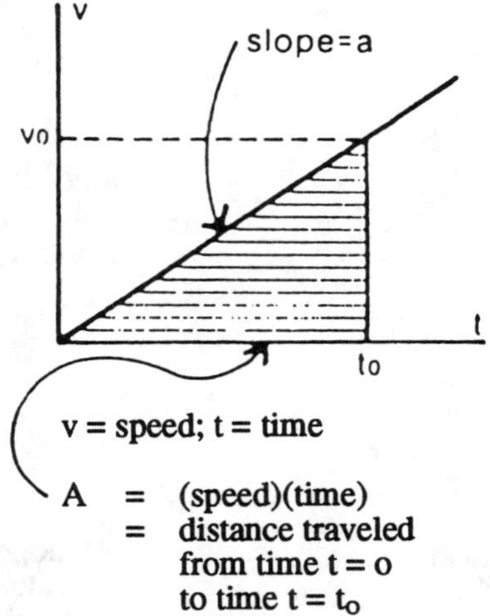

To check this, note that since v is constantly increasing with t, the acceleration is constant; so v = at.

The area of the triangle for a particular time $t_0 = (v_0 t_0)/2 = (at_0^2)/2$.

This is the distance formula for uniform acceleration: $s = (at^2)/2$. (Recall that $s = vt_0$ holds only when v is constant or an average value over the time between t = 0 and $t = t_0$.)

The area under the graph, A, and the slope, Dy/Dx, are related in the sense that the ordinate in a graph describes how fast A is changing in the same way that the slope describes how fast the ordinate is changing. In Example 5, the ordinate v describes how fast s is changing in the same way that the slope = a describes how fast v is changing. In practice, **the slope at a particular point on a graph is a much more important quantity than the corresponding area under the graph**, A, in interpreting the information in the graph. However, A should be kept in mind when analyzing a graph, especially when the product of the variables represented on the axes has meaning in terms of representing a third variable.

MCAT MATHEMATICS CONCEPT 12: Graphic interpretation of functions

The interpretation of a second or higher degree function represented by the graph should involve the following steps:

(1) Carefully analyze each axis as to:
 (a) what variable it represents;
 (b) the units (scale) used and the range of values on both axes.

(2) Estimate the overall shape of the graph. Can that lead to classification of linear, hyperbolic, or parabolic functions? (see below).

(3) Estimate the slope at various points of the function. Is the slope constant or changing? Is the slope the quantity of greatest interest?

(4) If the slope is changing, are there any maximum, minimum, or inflection points? If so, is their identification critical to answering the questions being asked?

(5) Estimate the area under the graph only for specific situations.

Basic Functions and Corresponding Graphs:

The purpose of interpreting a function is to determine whether a mathematical connection or relationship exists between the two variables in it. Commonly encountered graphs and their functional interpretations are reviewed below. The graphs selected for discussion are ones that tend to recur in medicine and biology and that have well-known interpretations of the relations between the variables in them. No new topics are covered; using the material discussed above, these graphs are basically examples of interpretation of the quadratic or exponential functions.

Linear functions:

The simplest type of graph is the linear (straight line) graph used to represent linear functions. Any straight line can be described by the equation $y = mx + b$ where x (usually the abscissa) and y (usually the ordinate) are the two variables, m is the slope of the line, and b is the y-intercept (the value of y when $x = 0$). As observed earlier, for any two points (x_1,y_1) and (x_2,y_2) on a straight line:

$$m = \frac{y_2 - y_1}{x_2 - x_1} = \frac{\Delta y}{\Delta x}.$$

Thus, observe that Δy is directly proportional to Δx; observe also that y is directly proportional to x when $b = 0$. Examples of linear graphs are:

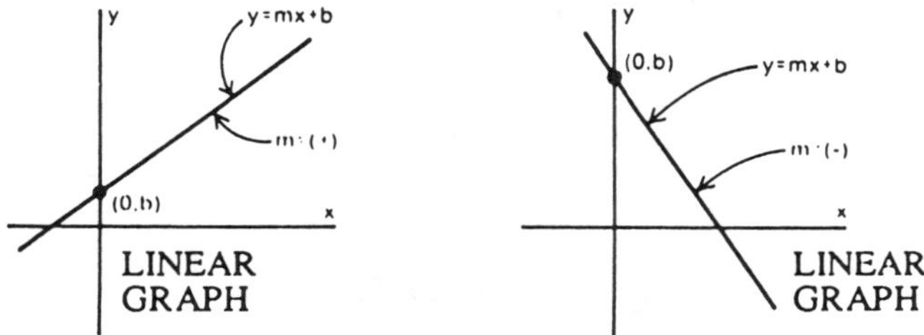

Fig. 4.6.a—Slope and Intercept of Straight Lines

Note that when the slope is negative, x increases as y decreases and vice versa. However, in this case, y and x are **not** inversely proportional (see next function considered) in which case they would be related in a non-linear manner. The basic interpretation for linear functions is that there is a constant relationship (as given by the slope) between x and y.

Hyperbolic functions:

A hyperbolic function results when two variables, x and y, are inversely proportional: "xy = a" where "a" is a constant. Examples of hyperbolic graphs are:

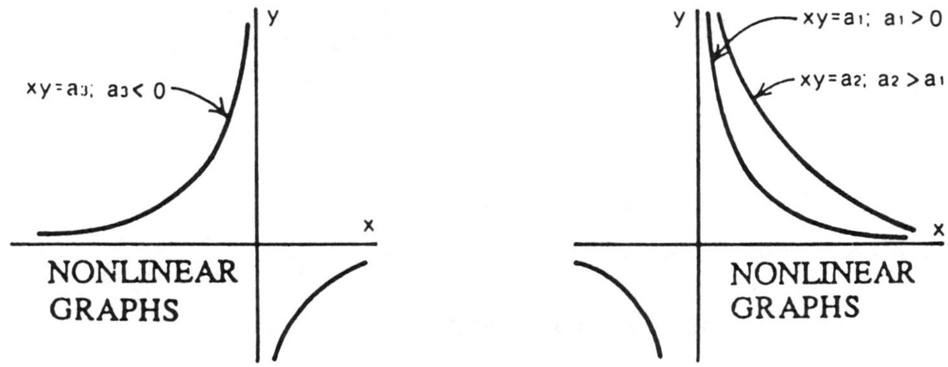

Fig. 4.6b—Hyperbolic Functions

Observe that because $xy = a$ is a non-linear relation for x and y, the slope is different at every point in a hyperbolic graph. Note also that hyperbolic graphs approach but never reach the x- and y-axes; consequently, the x- and y-axes are called the asymptotes in these graphs.

Parabolic functions:

In the xy-plane, a general parabola can usually be described algebraically by $y = ax^2 + bx + c$ or $x = my^2 + ny + p$ where a, b, c, m, n, and p are constants. Three parabolic functions of interest are shown below in three separate graphs:

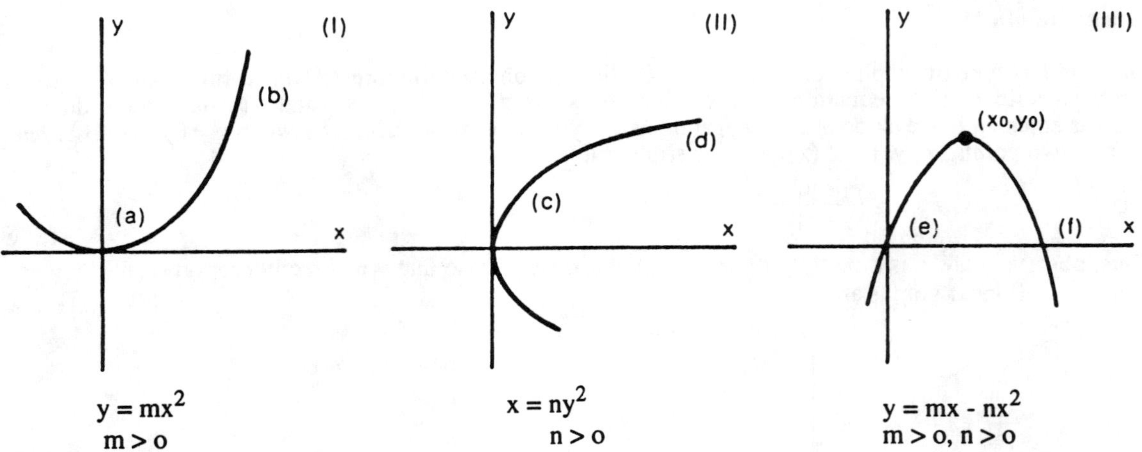

Fig. 4.6c—Parabolic Functions

The present discussion of these three functions is restricted to three graphs with positive values of x and y. Graph I shows an initially nearly flat slope (region a) that rapidly becomes large (region b). For graph II, the opposite interpretation ensues. Initially, there is a large slope (region c) that soon gives way to a larger region (region d) where the slope is flatter. Graph III shows an initially high positive slope (region e) which decreases to zero at a maximum point (x_0,y_0) and then becomes negative, increasingly so as the x-axis is approached (region f). Note that the slopes at (b), (e), and (f) are not of infinite magnitude and also that the slope at (d) is not zero.

Special functions in biological sciences.

The following curve is common in many biochemical situations:

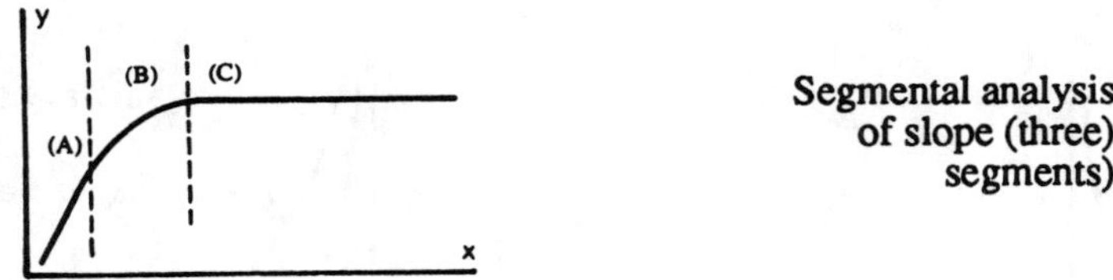

Fig. 4.6d—Segmental Analysis of Slope (three segments)

$y = \frac{ax}{b+x}$; a, b = positive constants.

The limit x << b implies that $y = ax/(b+x) \approx ax/b$ (region A), while the limit x >> b implies that $y = ax/(b + x) \cong a$ (region C).

Another graph found in many situations, such as population growth (biology), is the sigmoid or s-shaped curve:

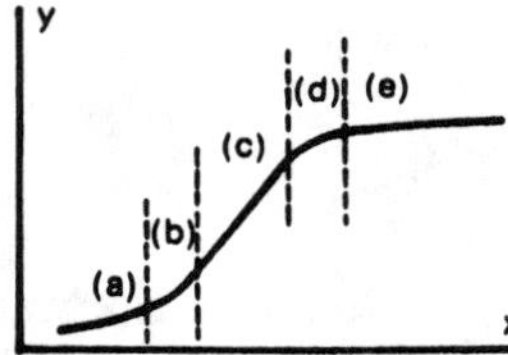

Fig. 4.6.e—Segmental Analysis of Slope (five segments)

It can be divided into five phases (or less):

(1) an initial latent phase of small positive slope (region a),
(2) an accelerative phase of rapidly increasing slope (region b),
(3) a phase of fairly constant high positive slope (region c) and note that there is an inflection point where the slope reaches its maximum value in this region,
(4) a decelerative phase of rapidly decreasing slope (region d), and
(5) a phase of essentially zero slope (region e). In general, these curves represent situations in which a latency phase (region a) exists before a phase of rapid changes in y for a given change in x (region c), the latter phase being followed by a phase of saturation of the system with x (region e).

Exponential functions:

Exponential relations between variables are common. Exponential curves are shown in figures I, II and III. All graphs assume A > 0.

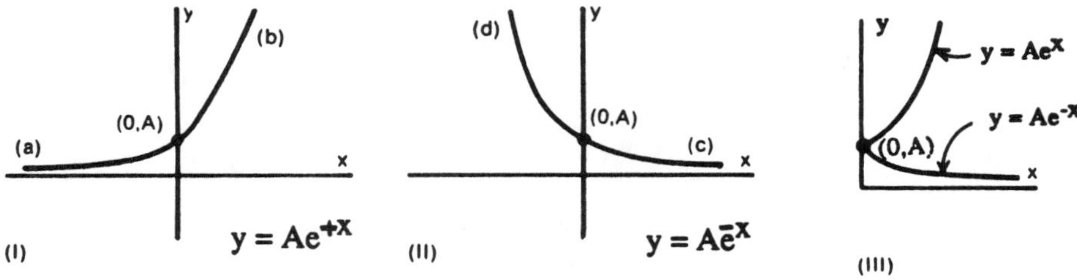

Fig. 4.6.f—Exponential Functions

The regions (a) and (c) approach the x-axis as an asymptote. The regions (b) and (d) approach no asymptote, but increase very rapidly with ever increasing slopes. Often one is interested in only positive values of x for exponential functions (see graph III). Graph I shows exponential growth while graph II shows exponential decay. All three graphs have y-intercepts at (0,A). These functions are useful in solving radioactivity decay problems and carbon dating.

Problem 7.
A linear graph can be algebraically described by the equation 8x-6y = 18. Write it in slope-intercept form and, then graph it, labelling the slope and y-intercept.

Problem 8.
An experimenter collects data on the pressure (p) versus the volume (V) of 1 mole of ideal gas A at a constant temperature T_1 (sample 1 in the graph below). He repeats the experiment with a 2 mole sample of gas A at a constant temperature T_2 and plots its data (sample 2 in the graph below). What are the relative magnitudes of T_1 and T_2?

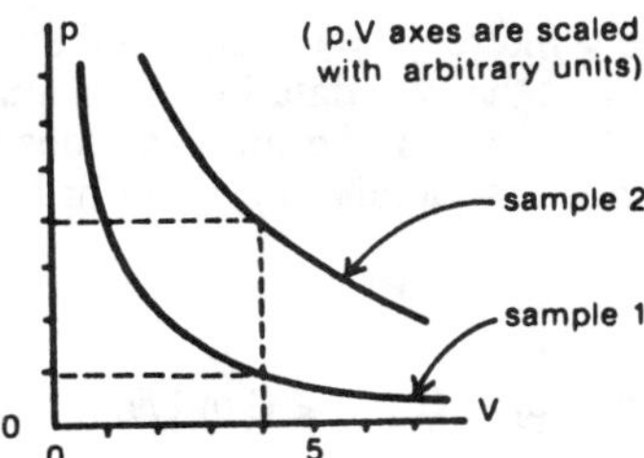

Problem 9.
The relation between two variables x and y, can be described by the equation

$$y = \frac{ax}{b + x^2}$$

where a,b = positive constants. Looking at only x ≥ 0, how does the slope of this curve vary? (Hint: to graph this equation and analyze how its slope varies, split the graph into three regions: x << b, x ≈ b, and x >> b. This is analogous to what was done for the graph of y = ax/(b+x) discussed above.)

Semi-Log and Log-Log Graphs and Functions:

The scales on the axes of the graphs discussed so far have all been linear. For some graphs, alternative scales—semi-log and log-log—are useful. A semi-log plot of a graph has a log scale on one axis (usually the ordinate) and a linear scale on the other axis (usually the abscissa). Semi-log paper looks like:

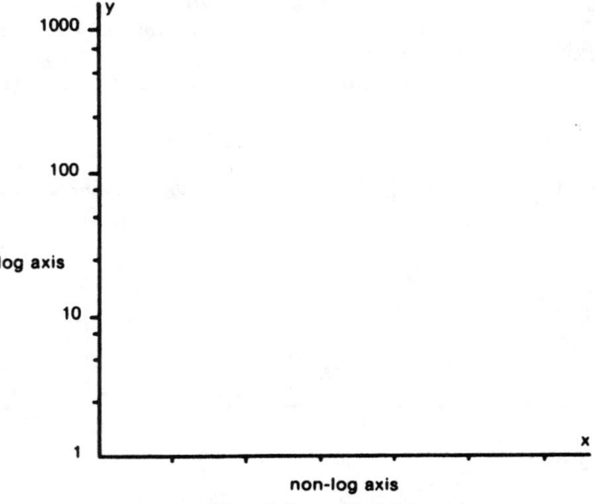

Fig. 4.6.g—Semi-log Axes

A semi-log scale is particularly useful for plotting exponential graphs because they become linear on semi-log graph paper. For example, consider:

$y = ae^{bx}$ where a,b = constants

Taking log of both sides,

$\log_{10} y = \log_{10} (ae^{bx}) = \log_{10} a + (b \log_{10} e)x$

$= \log_{10} a + (0.4343)bx$ $[\log_{10} e \cong 0.4343]$

This could be used to plot data to verify Newton's law of cooling (temperature difference versus time).

Observe that a plot of log y versus x is linear with the y-intercept = log a and the slope = 0.4343b. As another example, consider:

$s = s_0 10^{kt}$

$\log_{10} s = \log_{10} (s_0 10^{kt}) = \log_{10} s_0 + kt$

Observe that a plot of log s versus t is also linear with the y-intercept = log s_0 and the slope = k.
When plotting data on semi-log paper, one does **not** convert the raw data into logs and plot them on the paper; instead, one just plots the raw values on the paper since the scale on the log axis does the conversion. Semi-log plots of exponential graphs are valuable because it is easier to analyze a straight line than it is to analyze a curved line.

Example 1.
Graph $y = 500(10^{-1/2x})$ on both regular and semi-log graph paper (for $x \geq 0$ only).

regular graph : $y = 500(10^{-1/2x})$

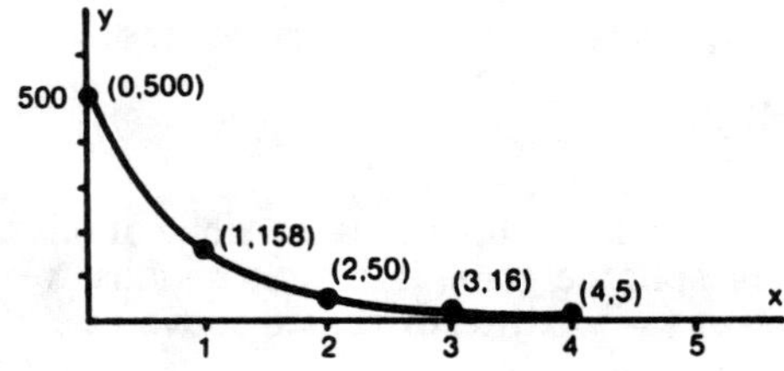

semi-log graph: $y = 500(10^{-1/2x})$ $\rightarrow$ $\log y = \log 500 - 1/2x$

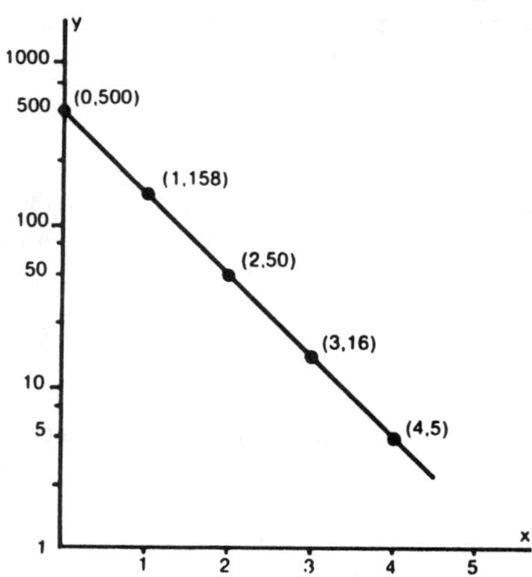

Observe:

(1) That the points on the log axis are not labelled by values of log y but by the corresponding values of y; that is, the point for log 10 = 1 is labelled by 10, not 1; the point for log 100 = 2 is labelled by 100, not 2, etc. This allows one to read the value of y for a particular value of x directly off the graph. But, **remember**, the slope of a semi-log graphical function, which here is -1/2, is

$$\frac{\Delta(\log y)}{\Delta x}, \text{ not } \frac{\Delta y}{\Delta x}.$$

(2) What if, instead, we had been given experimentally determined values of y for x = 1, 2, 3, 4, and had been told that x and y were related by the equation $y = a(10^{kx})$; it would have been much easier to determine a and k from the semi-log plot of these points than from their regular plot (these points are indicated on both graphs above). This is because k = the slope of, and a = the y-intercept extrapolated from, the line drawn through these points.

Problem 10.
The relation between two variables, x and y, is described by the equation $y = a(10^{bx})$ where a,b = constants. Using the data presented in the semi-log graph below, determine a and b (actual data points are marked with a dot).

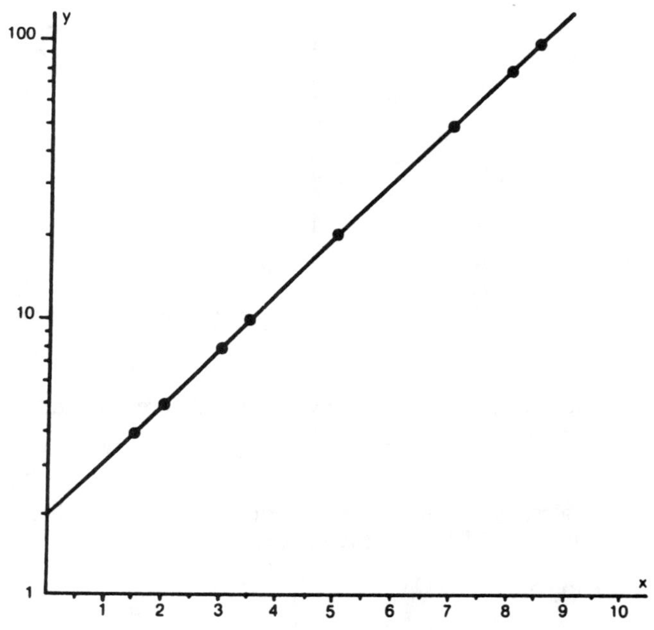

A log-log plot of a graph has log scales on both axes. Typically, it can be employed advantageously when two variables are directly or inversely proportional. When two variables, x and y, are directly proportional, a log-log plot is especially useful when their values range over several powers of 10. In this case, a log-log plot of x and y spreads out the data points while preserving the graph's linearity, i.e.:

if $y = kx$, $k > 0$,
then $\log y = \log x + \log k$.

Note that, in general, if $y = ax^n$ (a,n = constants), then y is directly proportional to x^n and so could be linearly plotted on log-log paper, i.e., $\log y = n\log x + \log a$. In this general case, a non-linear graph (for $n \neq 1$) is transformed into a linear graph of slope n and y-intercept = log a.

We have already observed that a linear function is easier to analyze than a non-linear function.

Example 2.

Graph $y = x$ on both linear and log-log paper for $1 \leq x \leq 1000$, identifying the points corresponding to x = 1, 10, 100, 1000.

linear graph: $y = x$
(linear scale, both axes)

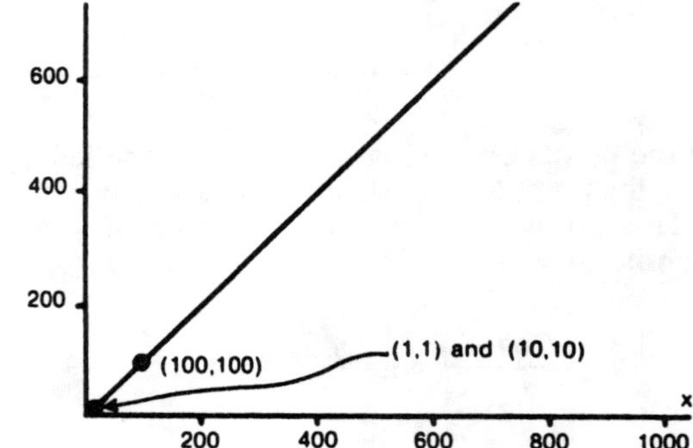

(Note, it is hard to show difference on a linear graph.)

log-log graph: $\log y = \log x$

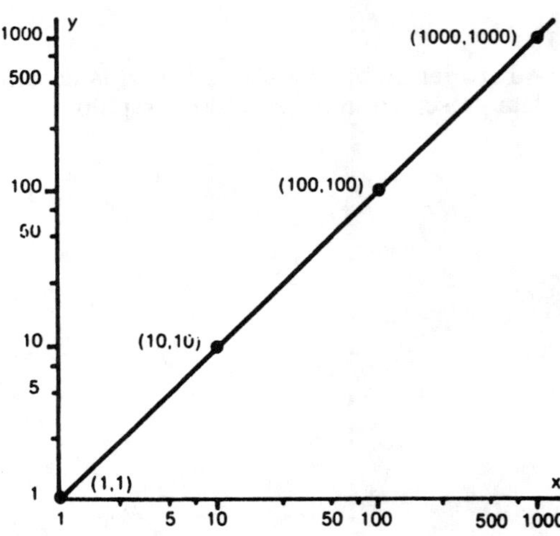

Note, in this example, how the plotted points in the log-log graph are "spread out," compared to the corresponding points in the linear graph, without losing linearity.

Example 3.

In the discussion of basic graphs, we already saw what the parabola $y = mx^2$ looks like when plotted as a graph with both linear axes. Plot $y = 5x^2$, for $1 \leq x \leq 10$, on log-log paper.

log-log graph is: $\log y = 2\log x + \log 5$

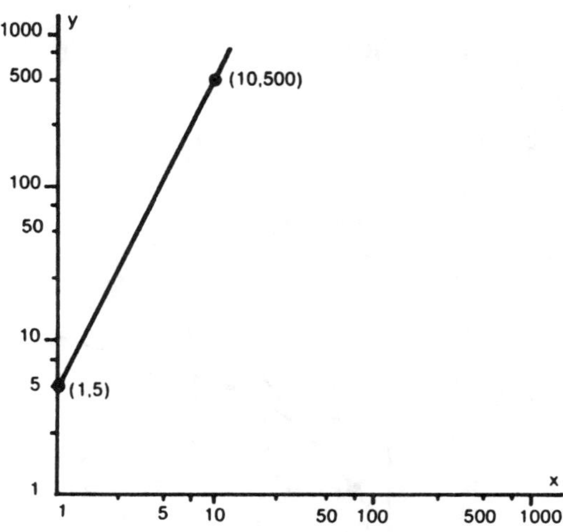

When two variables, x and y, are inversely proportional, a log-log plot converts their hyperbolic function into a linear function, i.e.,

if $y = \frac{k}{x}$, $k > 0$, (hyperbolic equation)
then $\log y = \log k - \log x$ (straight line transformation equation).

Actually, $y = k/x$ is just a special case of $y = kx^n$ (when $n = -1$), which we took note of above.

4.2.3.3 Solutions to the Analytic Geometry Problems

(1) $y = \frac{5x}{1+x}$; the ordered pairs requested are:

$(0,0)$, $(1,\frac{5}{2})$, $(4,4)$, $(9,4.5)$

Plotting these four points and drawing a curve through them for $x \geq 0$:

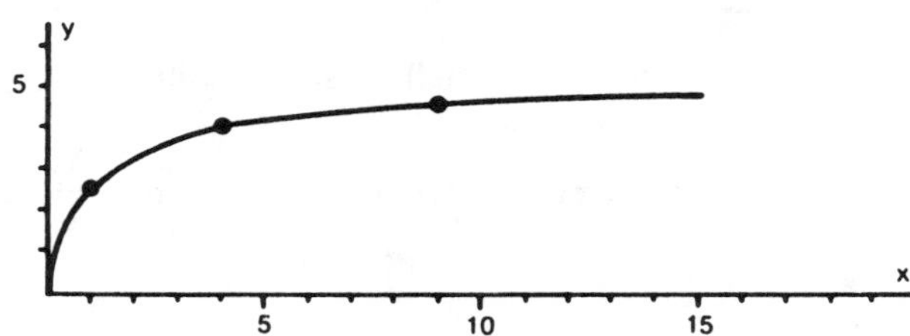

As x gets very large, $x >> 1$, so $y = \frac{5x}{1+x} \cong \frac{5x}{x} = 5$. Thus, the value of y approaches 5 as x gets very large.

(2) The two points indicated are (-4,4) and (6,-4). Let $(x_2,y_2) = (6,-4)$ and $(x_1,y_1) = (-4,4)$; then:

$$\text{slope} = \frac{y_2-y_1}{x_2-x_1} = \frac{-4-4}{6-(-4)} = \frac{-8}{10} = -\frac{4}{5}$$

(3) For line 1, let $(x_2,y_2) = (2,-1)$ and $(x_1,y_1) = (-7,6)$; then:

$$\text{slope of line 1} = \frac{y_2-y_1}{x_2-x_1} = \frac{-1-6}{2-(-7)} = -\frac{7}{9};$$

The magnitude of the slope of line 1 $= \frac{7}{9}$.

For line 2, let $(x_2,y_2) = (10,8)$ and $(x_1,y_1) = (2,1)$; then:

$$\text{slope of line 2} = \frac{y_2-y_1}{x_2-x_1} = \frac{8-1}{10-2} = \frac{7}{8};$$

The magnitude of the slope of line 2 $= \frac{7}{8}$;

Therefore, line 2 has the slope of greater magnitude $\left(\frac{7}{8} > \frac{7}{9}\right)$

(4) Draw the tangent at each of the three points:

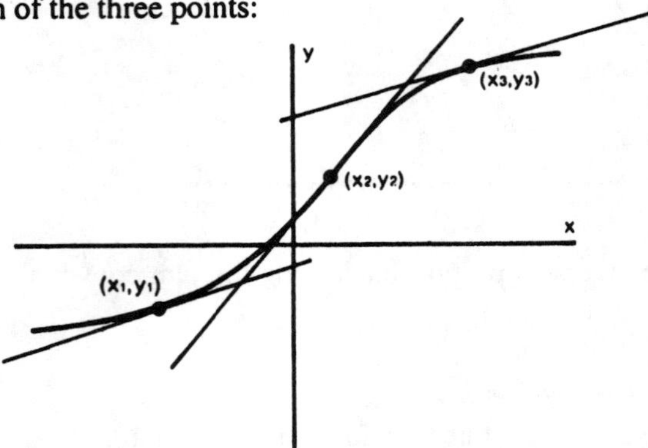

By inspection, the slope at (x_2,y_2) is the greatest. (See interpretation of sigmoid curve in the discussion of basic graphs.)

(5) The inflection point graph I is (with tangents drawn in at three points):

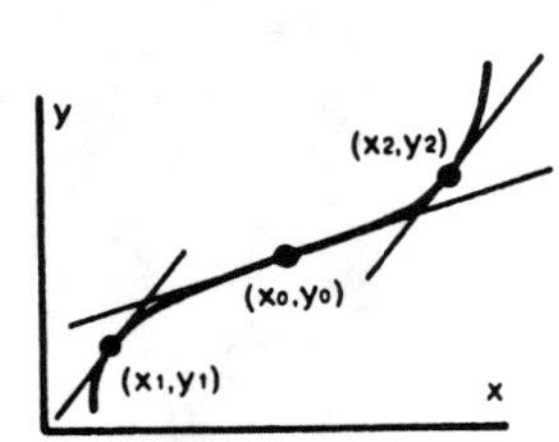

slope has minimum value at (x_0,y_0)

We observe that the slope, $\frac{\Delta y}{\Delta x}$, has a minimum (of small, positive value) at (x_0,y_0). As the points (x_1,y_1) and (x_2,y_2) move away from (x_0,y_0), $F(\Delta y,\Delta x)$ increases. Therefore, the graph of $\frac{\Delta y}{\Delta x}$ versus x looks like:

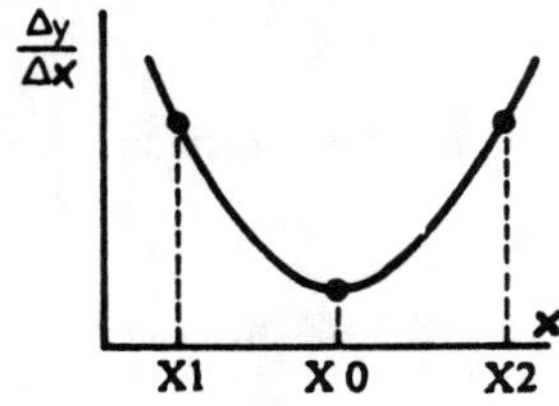

This curve is roughly parabolic.

(6) Based on the discussion of maximum, minimum, and inflection points:

B is a maximum point;
D is a minimum point;
C, E, G are inflection points.

(7) The slope-intercept form of $8x - 6y = 18$ is: $y = \frac{4}{3}x - 3$. Its graph is:

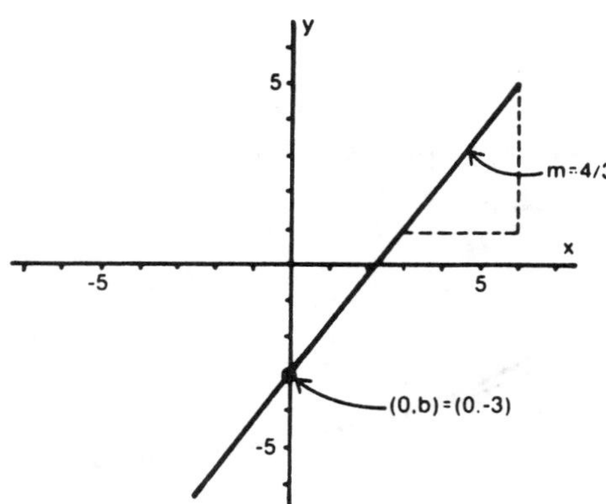

(8) Recall that the ideal gas law is $PV = nRT$. Note then that since n,T = constants for both samples, both P,V-graphs are hyperbolic (P and V being inversely proportional). To get the relative magnitudes of the constant temperatures T_1 and T_2, they have to be expressed in terms of common constant(s) so that their numerical ratio can be obtained.

For sample 1: $PV = RT_1$ $(n = 1)$

Since PV = constant, we can select any point on sample 1 graph to evaluate it numerically. Selecting point $(V,P) = (4,1)$: $(4)(1) = RT_1$ which implies that $T_1 = \frac{4}{R}$.

For sample 2: $PV = 2RT_2$ $(n = 2)$

Selecting point $(V,P) = (4,4)$: $(4)(4) = 2RT_2$ which implies that $T_2 = \frac{8}{R}$.

Taking the ratio $\frac{T_2}{T_1} = \frac{\frac{8}{R}}{\frac{4}{R}} = 2$; or, $T_2 = 2T_1$.

(9) $y = \frac{ax}{b+x^2}$; a,b = positive constants. Splitting the graph (for $x \geq 0$) into three regions corresponding to:

(A) $x \ll b,\ y = \frac{ax}{b+x^2} \cong \frac{a}{b}x$ (linear);

(B) $x \approx b,\ y = \frac{ax}{b+x^2}$ (no approximation);

(C) $x \gg b,\ y = \frac{ax}{b+x^2} \cong \frac{ax}{x^2} = \frac{a}{x}$ (hyperbolic).

To graph this equation, use the same three regions. For region A, the function looks linear; for region C, the function looks hyperbolic; and, for region B, these two partial graphs are connected by a smooth curve that must have a maximum point and an inflection point. The graph looks like:

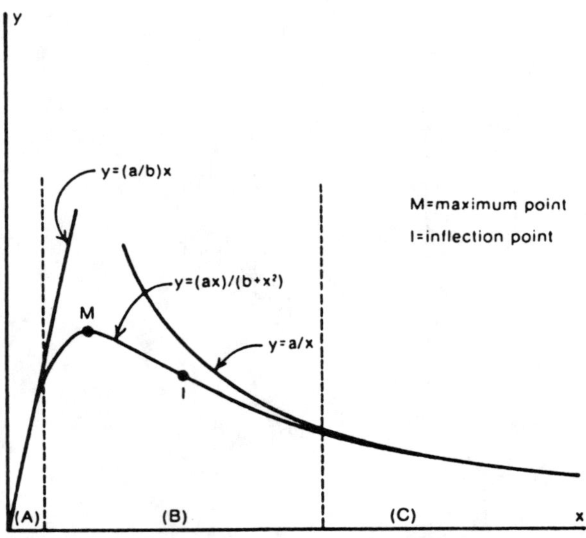

Segmental analysis for a compound curve (split into simpler curves)

The slope starts off at a finite, nearly constant value (region A). As x increases, it starts to decrease, being zero at the maximum point M and negative thereafter (region B). In the right-hand side of region B, the graph passes through an inflection point I where the slope reaches a minimum value and then begins to increase slightly. In region C, the slope approaches zero as the graph asymptotes to the x-axis.

(10) $y = 2(10^{x/5})$. For the y-intercept (x = 0), $y = a(10^{b \cdot 0}) = a$.

Reading directly from the graph,the y-intercept = a = 2. For determining b, consider:

$$y = a(10^{bx}) \quad \rightarrow \quad \log y = bx + \log a$$

the slope of this line = $b = \frac{\Delta(\log y)}{\Delta x}$. Selecting two points, $(x_1,y_1) = (3.5,10)$ and $(x_2,y_2) = (8.5,100)$, the slope equals:

$$b = \frac{\log y_2 - \log y_1}{x_2 - x_1} = \frac{\log 100 - \log 10}{8.5 - 3.5} = \frac{2 - 1}{5} = \frac{1}{5}$$

Thus, $y = 2(10^{x/5})$.

MCAT MATHEMATICS CONCEPT 13: Quadratic equations

The MCAT student encounters these equations in the physical sciences. For example, uniformly accelerated motion equations, projectiles, rate law and reaction order in chemical reactions. Problems in these physical sciences topics usually require solution of second order or quadratic equations in one variable. The general quadratic equation can be given by: $ax^2 + bx + c = 0$, where a,b,c are constant with $b^2 - 4ac > 0$. For these special values, the general form of solution is represented as:

$$x_1, x_2 = \frac{-b \pm \sqrt{b^2 - 4ac}}{2a}$$

where x_1 and x_2 are the two possible solutions.

As an example, consider a reversible biochemical reaction in which:

Reactant $\rightleftharpoons$ Product 1 + Product 2

The equilibrium constant, $K = \frac{[\text{Product 1}][\text{Product 2}]}{[\text{Reactant}]}$

Assume equimolar amount of product 1 and product 2 and let each be represented by m. Assume we started with a unimolar solution of the reactant.

	Reactant $\rightleftharpoons$	Product 1 +	Product 2
At start,	1	0	0
At equilibrium,	1-m	m	m

$$K = \frac{(m)(m)}{(1-m)}$$

$$K(1-m) = m^2$$

$$m^2 + mK - K = 0$$

Comparing this with the quadratic equation, $ax^2 + bx + c = 0$; $a = 1$, $b = K$, $c = -K$.

To obtain the solutions use the formula, $m_1, m_2 = \frac{-K \pm \sqrt{K^2 - 4(1)(-K)}}{2(1)}$

$$\text{Hence, } m_1 = \frac{-K + \sqrt{K^2 + 4K}}{2} \text{ and}$$

$$m_2 = \frac{-K - \sqrt{K^2 + 4K}}{2}$$

As you notice, both roots depend on the equilibrium constant. The negative root m_2 is usually hypothetical because equilibrium constants and concentrations cannot be negative. There is only one realistic root (m_1) as shown in the above solution. Another important observation! Students should memorize the fact that, for small numbers, the squares are smaller than the numbers. e.g., if $K = 10^{-8}$, then $K^2 = 10^{-16}$, which is negligible for all practical purposes. The interpretation of a quadratic equation will help you waste less precious time in solving it. Do not overdo the mathematical operations if they are not significant to arrive at the correct answers.

MCAT MATHEMATICS CONCEPT 14: Simultaneous equations

This section shows you how to solve two equations (linear equations) in two variables. A set of simultaneous equations may be represented as:

$$AX + BY = C \quad \text{(i)}$$
$$DX + EY = F \quad \text{(ii)}$$

The two equations shown have two variables X and Y and can be solved (i) either algebraically or (ii) graphically. A,B,C,D,E,F are real constants.

Algebraic Solution of Simultaneous Equations

Consider the equations, $3X + 2Y = 9$ .... (i)
$4X + 1Y = 11$ ....(ii)
Multiply equation (ii) by 2 (double both sides),
$8X + 2Y = 22$ ....(iii)

Subtract equation (iii) from equation (i) giving, $3X + 2Y - 8X - 2Y = 9-22$
$-5X = -13$
$X = 13/5 = 2.6$

Use X = 2.6 in either (i), (ii), or (iii) to obtain Y.

$4(2.6) + Y = 11$ gives $10.4 + Y = 11$ or $Y = 0.6 = 3/5$
$\therefore$ $X = 13/5$, $Y = 3/5$ is the solution set for these questions.

Graphical Solution of Simultaneous Equations

Use the graphic techniques discussed in MCAT Mathematics Concept 12 and graph both equations. You will get two straight lines intersecting at a point. The coordinates of that point will give you the <u>same</u> solution set as obtained earlier in the algebraic solution. On the MCAT, two experimental studies could be compared to see if they have a common point. Experiments in chemistry and biology can lead to simultaneous equations to arrive at one solution.

4.2.3.4 TRIGONOMETRY CONCEPTS

MCAT MATHEMATICS CONCEPT 15: Introduction to trigonometric functions

Trigonometry is concerned with the relationships between the angles and sides of triangles. Recall that for similar triangles, i.e., triangles that have the same angles but which are not necessarily the same size, the ratios of the corresponding sides are equal:

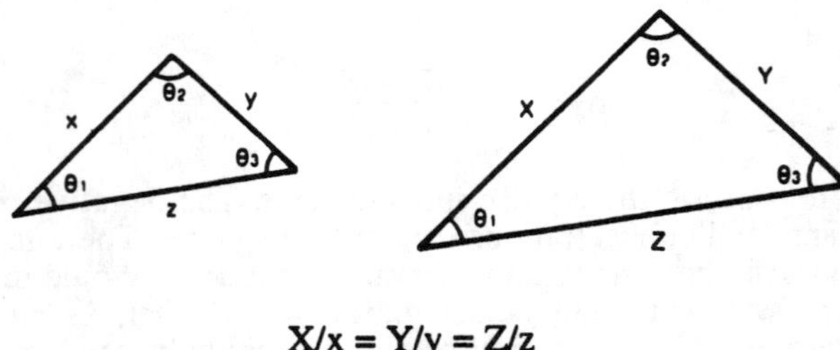

$$X/x = Y/y = Z/z$$
$$\theta_1, \theta_2, \theta_3 = \text{angles}$$

Fig. 4.7a—Similar Triangles

Focusing on right triangles, it can be directly deduced from this that the ratio of any two of the sides of a right triangle is the same for all similar right triangles. In other words, the possible ratios depend only on the angles of the right triangle. Thus, defining the sides and angles of a right triangle as:

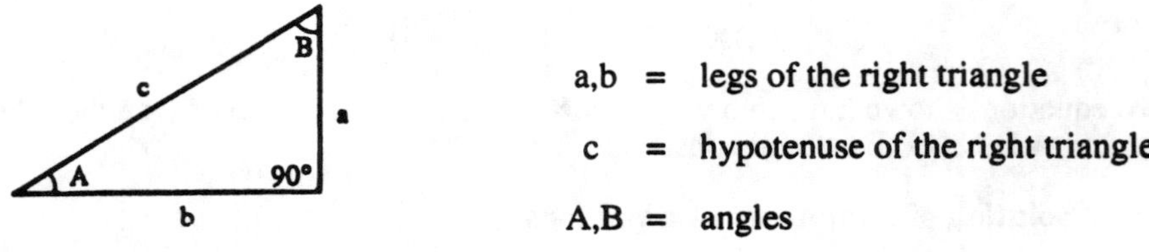

Fig. 4.7b—Right Triangles

The basic trigonometric functions are:

the sine of an angle $= \dfrac{\text{opposite side}}{\text{hypotenuse}}$, i.e., $\sin A = \dfrac{a}{c}$ and $\sin B = \dfrac{b}{c}$

the cosine of an angle $= \dfrac{\text{adjacent side}}{\text{hypotenuse}}$, i.e., $\cos A = \dfrac{b}{c}$ and $\cos B = \dfrac{a}{c}$

the tangent of an angle $= \dfrac{\text{opposite side}}{\text{adjacent side}}$, i.e., $\tan A = \dfrac{a}{b}$ and $\tan B = \dfrac{b}{a}$

Note that definitions are interrelated; for example, observe that $\sin A = \cos B$, $\sin B = \cos A$, and $\dfrac{\sin A}{\cos A} = \tan A$.

Problem 1.
Find sin A, cos A, and tan A.

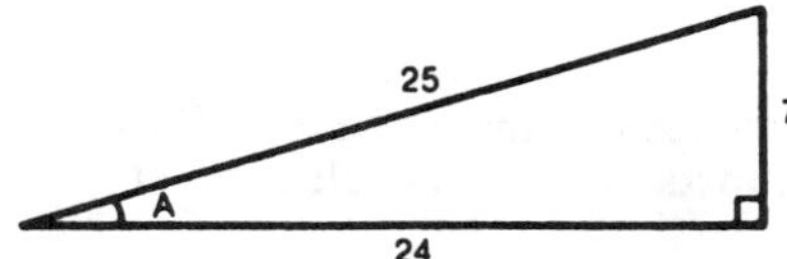

Problem 2.
Find sin B, cos B, and tan B.

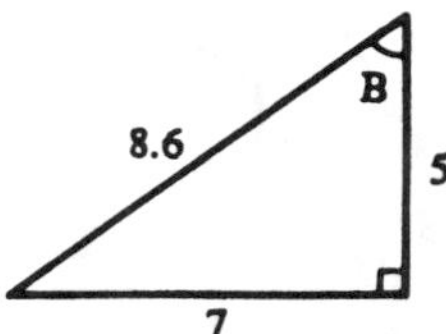

These right triangle definitions of the basic trigonometric functions are restricted to angles between 0° and 90°. However, the definitions of the trigonometric functions can be extended to include all angles. Without showing how this can be done (see textbook treatment of trigonometry), the trigonometric functions for angles between 0° and 360° are graphically represented by:

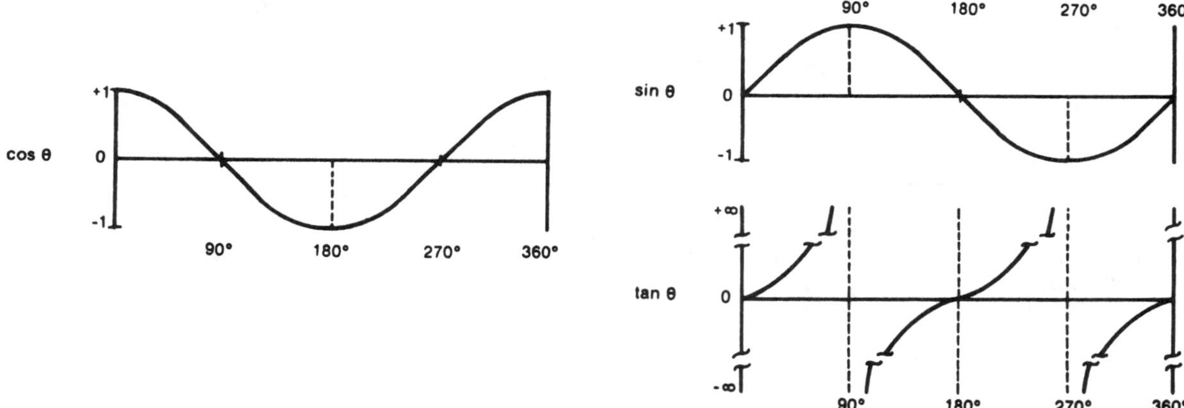

Fig. 4.7c—Graphical Representation of Trigonometric Functions

Problem 3.
Using the graphs above, find sin θ, cos θ, and tan θ for θ = 0°, 90°, 180°, and 270°.

The trigonometric functions are typically represented graphically for angles between 0° and 360° because they have repeating values, i.e., because they are periodic:

sin (x + 360°n) = sin x; where x = angle, n = integer

cos (x + 360°n) = cos x

tan (x + 180°n) = tan x

Based on the brief discussion above, two things should be observed and remembered:

(1) Trigonometric functions should logically turn up when considering quantities that are periodic in nature, e.g., wave phenomena in physics.

(2) Trigonometry should be useful when it is advantageous to represent a quantity as the hypotenuse or a leg of a right triangle, e.g., vectors—see below, MCAT Concept #18.

MCAT MATHEMATICS CONCEPT 16: Characteristics of 30⁰, 45⁰, 60⁰ right triangles

The characteristics of a few basic right triangles are shown below. They should be memorized for the MCAT along with the values of the trigonometric functions for the angles in them.

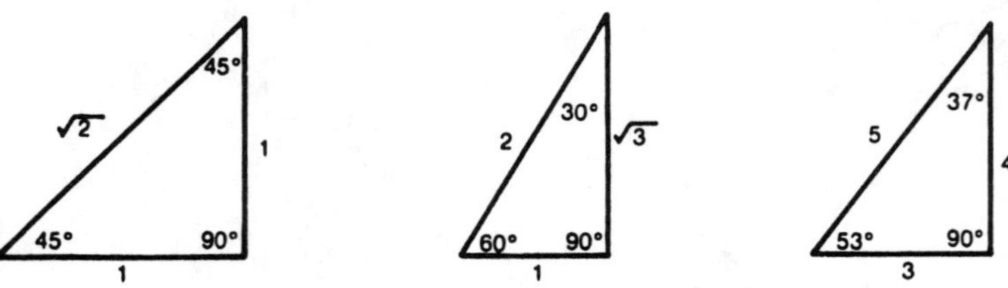

Fig. 4.8—Three Special Right Triangles

Problem 4.
Using the right triangles above, find sin θ , cos θ, and tan θ for θ = 30°, 45°, and 60° (these should be memorized).

$\sin(45^\circ) = \frac{1}{\sqrt{2}}$ $\cos(45^\circ) = \frac{1}{\sqrt{2}}$ $\tan(45^\circ) = 1$

$\sin(30^\circ) = \frac{1}{2}$ $\cos(30^\circ) = \frac{\sqrt{3}}{2}$ $\tan(30^\circ) = \frac{1}{\sqrt{3}}$

Problem 5.
Find x:

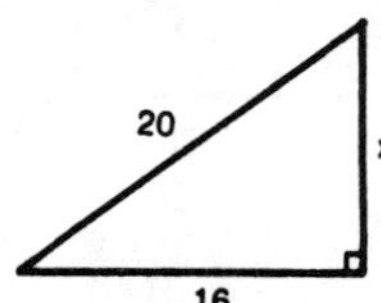

Problem 6.
Find x and y:

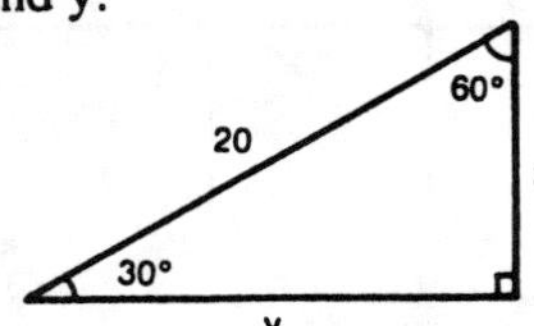

Up to this point, we have used degrees to measure angles; an alternative angular measure that you should be familiar with is the radian. A complete revolution about a point, it should be recalled, is 360°; the same revolution is alternatively represented by 2π radians (normally it is written as just 2π; the units of radians is assumed). The 2π to 360° equivalence determines the proportionality of the two angular measures, e.g., 180° = π, $90^\circ = \frac{\pi}{2}$, 720° = 4π; etc. (1 radian = 57.3°).

Problem 7.
What are 30°, 45°, and 60° in radian units?

The Pythagorean Theorem finds many applications in solving problems on the MCAT as well:

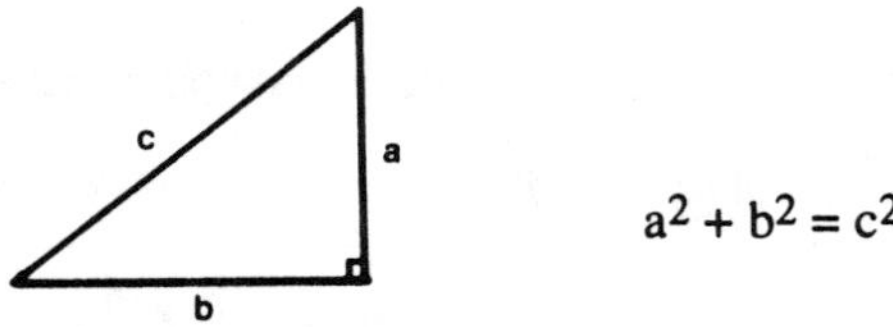

$$a^2 + b^2 = c^2$$

Problem 8.
Find b:

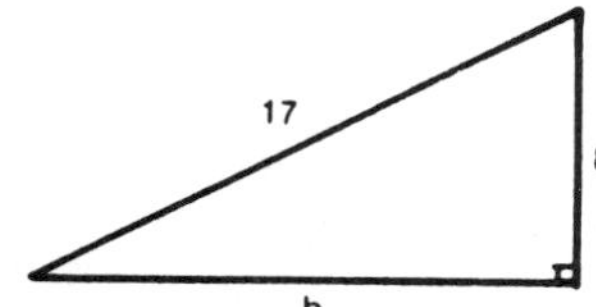

Problem 9.
Evaluate $\sin^2 \theta + \cos^2 \theta$, giving the answer in its simplest form.

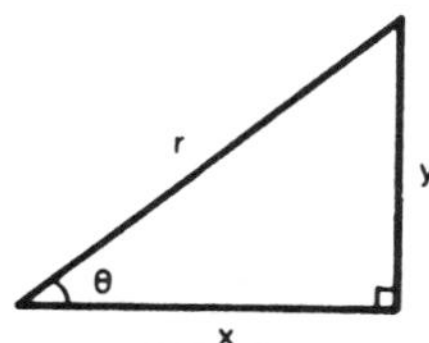

MCAT MATHEMATICS CONCEPT 17: Inverse trigonometric functions

Inverse trigonometric functions are used to determine the angle corresponding to a given value of any trigonometric function. e.g., Find the angle given sine angle = 0.5 or $\frac{1}{2}$. The backward operation of finding the angle from the function is also called inverting the function or finding the inverse of the given function. The angle for which the sine = $\frac{1}{2}$ is 30°.

Inverse trigonometric functions are represented as arcsin, arccos, arctan or $\sin^{-1}$, $\cos^{-1}$, and $\tan^{-1}$. <u>Important:</u> values of commonly used inverse trigonometric functions are shown below:

$\sin^{-1} 0$	=	0°	$\cos^{-1} 0$	=	90°
$\sin^{-1} \frac{1}{2}$	=	30°	$\cos^{-1} \frac{1}{2}$	=	60°
$\sin^{-1} \frac{1}{\sqrt{2}}$	=	45°	$\cos^{-1} \frac{1}{\sqrt{2}}$	=	45°
$\sin^{-1} \frac{\sqrt{3}}{2}$	=	60°	$\cos^{-1} \frac{\sqrt{3}}{2}$	=	30°
$\sin^{-1} 1$	=	90°	$\cos^{-1} 1$	=	0°

The inverse functions are used when the length of sides of triangles are given. In a right triangle, if the hypotenuse = 11 units and the altitude measures 9 units, then $\sin\frac{9}{11} = \sin^{-1}0.818$. The angle corresponding to $\sin^{-1} 0.818$ will be approximately between 45° and 60° ($\sin^{-1}\frac{1}{\sqrt{2}} = \sin^{-1} 0.707$ and $\sin^{-1} \frac{\sqrt{3}}{2} = \sin^{-1} 0.866$). These calculations can be used in physical sciences, to determine unknown angles from given lengths of various sides of a triangle.

Rules for Inverse Trigonometric Functions:

1. For any angle $0 < \theta < 90°$,
   (a) $\sin^{-1}(\sin\theta) = \theta$
   (b) $\cos^{-1}(\cos\theta) = \theta$
   (c) $\tan^{-1}(\tan\theta) = \theta$

2. For any $-1 \leq A \leq 1$,
   (a) $\sin(\sin^{-1} A) = A$
   (b) $\cos(\cos^{-1} A) = A$

3. For any A, $\tan(\tan^{-1} A) = A$

4. If $\theta = \sin^{-1}(y/r) = \cos^{-1}(x/r)$ with $x \neq 0$,
   then $\theta = \tan^{-1}(y/x)$.

Solutions to the Trigonometry Problems

(1) Using the right triangle definitions of the trigonometric functions:

$$\sin A = \frac{7}{25},\ \cos A = \frac{24}{25},\ \text{and } \tan A = \frac{7}{24}$$

(2) As in (1), using the right triangle definitions:

$$\sin B = \frac{7}{8.6},\ \cos B = \frac{5}{8.6},\ \text{and } B = \frac{7}{5}$$

(3) Reading values directly from the graph, the following table can be constructed:

θ

Function	0°	90°	180°	270°
sin θ	0	1	0	-1
cos θ	1	0	-1	0
tan θ	0	∞ (undefined)	0	∞ (undefined)

(4) Using the right triangles shown, the following table can be constructed:

θ

Function	30°	45°	60°
sin θ	$\frac{\sqrt{1}}{2}$	$\frac{\sqrt{2}}{2}$	$\frac{\sqrt{3}}{2}$
cos θ	$\frac{\sqrt{3}}{2}$	$\frac{\sqrt{2}}{2}$	$\frac{\sqrt{1}}{2}$
tan θ	$\frac{\sqrt{1}}{\sqrt{3}}$	1	$\frac{\sqrt{3}}{\sqrt{1}}$

Note: It is easier to memorize the table in the way it is presented.

(5) This should be recognized as a 3-4-5 right triangle. A 3-4-5 right triangle is recognized by noting some combination of two sides in ratio 3:4, 4:5, or 3:5 corresponding to the positions shown on the standard 3-4-5 triangle; the third is the missing side. The triangle in this problem corresponds to the known triangle:

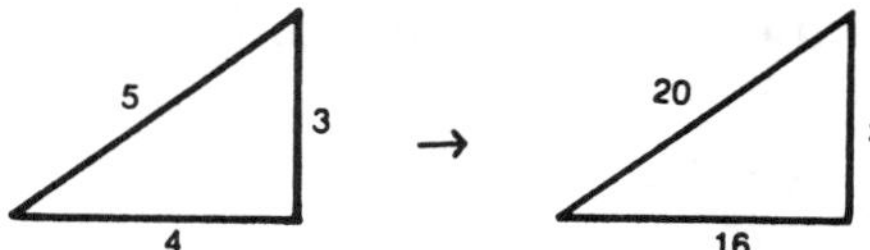

since these are similar triangles, the corresponding sides are proportional, i.e.,

$$\frac{x}{3} = \frac{20}{5} \quad \text{or} \quad \frac{x}{3} = \frac{16}{4}$$

In either case, x = 12

(6) $\sin 30° = \frac{x}{20}$; $x = 20\sin 30° = 20\left(\frac{1}{2}\right) = 10$

$\cos 30° = \frac{y}{20}$; $y = 20\cos 30° = 20\left(\frac{\sqrt{3}}{2}\right) = 10\sqrt{3}$

(7) Using the proportionality based on the equivalence of 360° and 2p:

$\frac{30°}{360°} = \frac{x}{2\pi}$ → $x = \frac{\pi}{6}$; 30° → $\frac{\pi}{6}$

$\frac{45°}{360°} = \frac{x}{2\pi}$ → $x = \frac{\pi}{4}$; 45° → $\frac{\pi}{4}$

$\frac{60°}{360°} = \frac{x}{2\pi}$ → $x = \frac{\pi}{3}$; 60° → $\frac{\pi}{3}$

(8) Using the Pythagorean Theorem:

$b^2 + 8^2 = 17^2$

$b^2 + 64 = 289$

$b^2 = 225$

$b = 15$

(9) $\sin \theta = \frac{y}{r}$ and $\cos \theta = \frac{x}{r}$

$$\sin^2 \theta + \cos^2 \theta = \frac{y^2}{r^2} + \frac{x^2}{r^2} = \frac{x^2 + y^2}{r^2} = \frac{r^2}{r^2} = 1$$

($x^2 + y^2 = r^2$ by the Pythagorean Theorem)

MCAT MATHEMATICS CONCEPT 18: Vector operations and rules

A **vector quantity** is one that is completely specified by a magnitude and a direction. A **scalar quantity** is one that is completely specified by its magnitude, there being no sense of direction. A vector is graphically symbolized by an arrow—the tail being the origin point, the head being the finish point, the length being proportional to its magnitude, and its angle (in relation to a reference) being indicative of its direction):

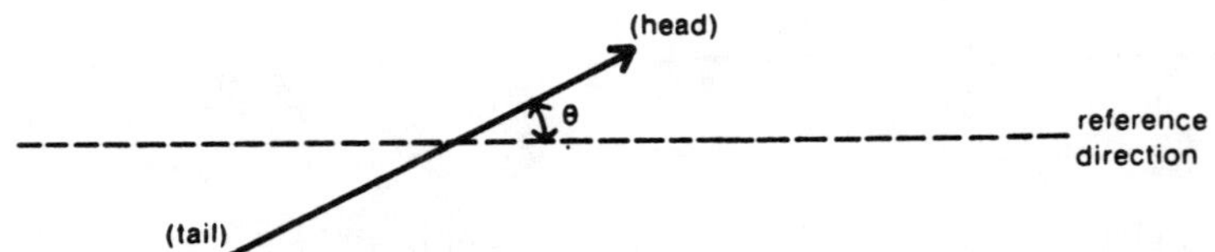

Fig. 4.9a—Definition Sketch for a Vector

Vectors are **added** graphically by placing the heads to tails in order and connecting the first tail with the last head:

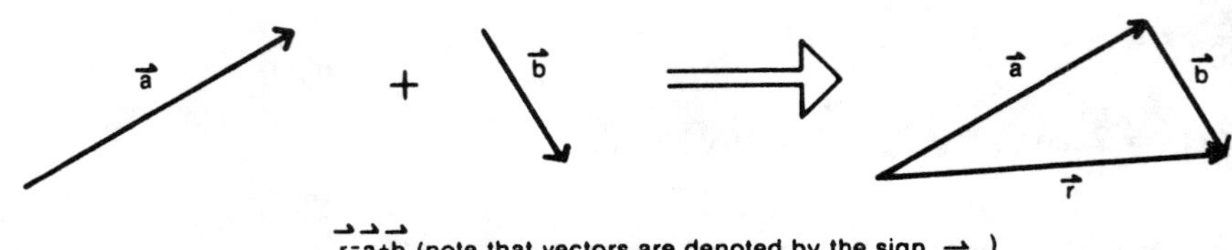

$\vec{r} = \vec{a} + \vec{b}$ (note that vectors are denoted by the sign ⇀)

Fig. 4.9b—Addition of Vectors

Vectors are **subtracted** by changing the direction(s) of the subtracted vector(s) and then adding as shown above:

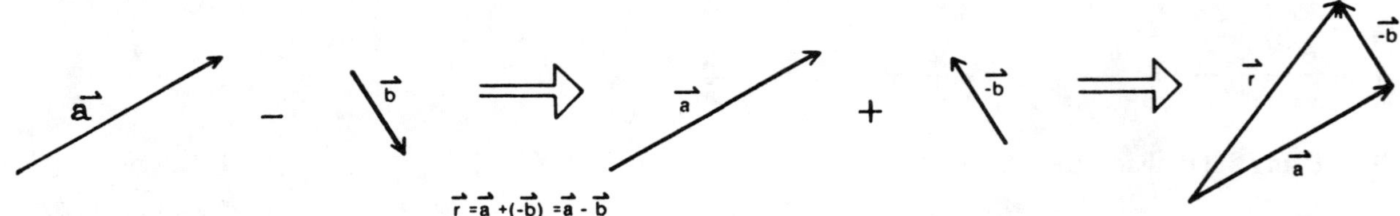

$\vec{r} = \vec{a} + (-\vec{b}) = \vec{a} - \vec{b}$

Fig. 4.9c—Subtraction of Vectors

In doing the vector subtraction above, the vector $\vec{b}$ is effectively multiplied by -1 to get $-\vec{b}$ which is equal in magnitude (length) to $\vec{b}$ but is in the opposite direction to it. Generalizing this, when a vector $\vec{r}$ is multiplied by a scalar c, the result is a new vector $\vec{R} = c\vec{r}$. The magnitude of $\vec{R}$ is c times the magnitude of $\vec{r}$. When c is positive, $\vec{R}$ has the same direction as $\vec{r}$; when c is negative, $\vec{R}$ has the opposite direction of $\vec{r}$. The MCAT explicitly does not require knowledge of any of the products of one vector with another vector, e.g., the dot and cross products.

Right-hand Rule for Vectors

The right-hand rule is used to determine the sense of the resultant vector which results from the cross product of two vectors. e.g. The torque or rotational moment resulting from the product of the moment arm and the force has a certain sense. Place the vectors (Moment arm $= \vec{r}$ and acting force on the object $= \vec{F}$) $\vec{r}$ and $\vec{F}$ in the same imaginary or fictitious plane. Imagine a line perpendicular to the plane of these two vectors. Call this the axis or line of action of the resulting moment of the force $\vec{F}$. Grasp this axis or action line with your right hand, but be sure to wrap your fingers around this line in a way that the fingers point as if moving from $\vec{r}$ to $\vec{F}$. The curling of the fingers should point in the same order as the product of $\vec{r}$ and $\vec{F}$. The direction of your thumb point will then point in the direction of the resulting moment. The figure drawn below shows how the sense of the resulting vector is determined. Note that $\vec{r}$ and $\vec{F}$ are in the plane of the paper.

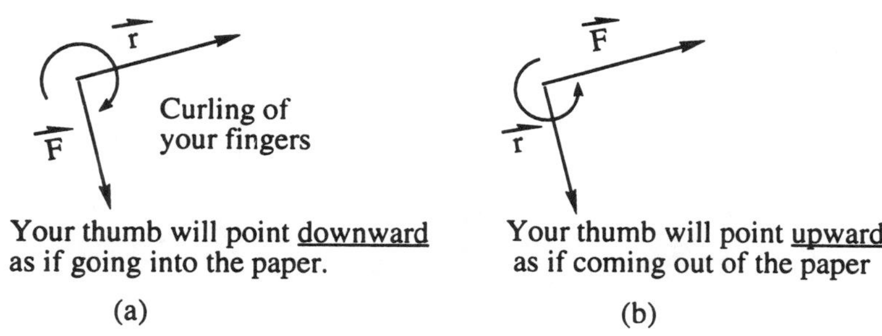

Fig. 4.9d—Demonstration of Right-hand Rule for Vectors

In problem solving, each vector is usually broken down into perpendicular components (here identified as x and y, which add together to give the original vector:

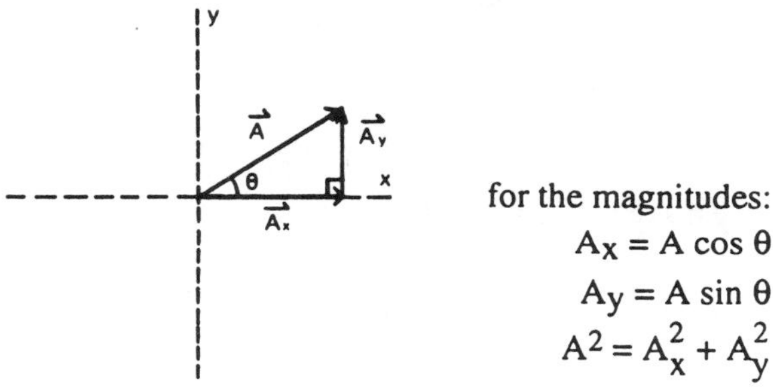

for the magnitudes:

$$A_x = A \cos \theta$$

$$A_y = A \sin \theta$$

$$A^2 = A_x^2 + A_y^2$$

(Note: when referring to the magnitude of $\vec{A}$, we write A)

Fig. 4.9e—Orthogonal Components of a Vector

In essence, the vector is represented as the hypotenuse of a right triangle where the legs (i.e., the components of the vector) are chosen to lie parallel to the axes of a convenient Cartesian coordinate system (as shown in the diagram above). To add (or subtract) two or more vectors, in each reference direction the component of the resulting vector is obtained by adding (subtracting) together all the components of these vectors in that direction; the resulting vector is constructed from its components thus obtained, e.g., for $\vec{A} + \vec{B} = \vec{C}$:

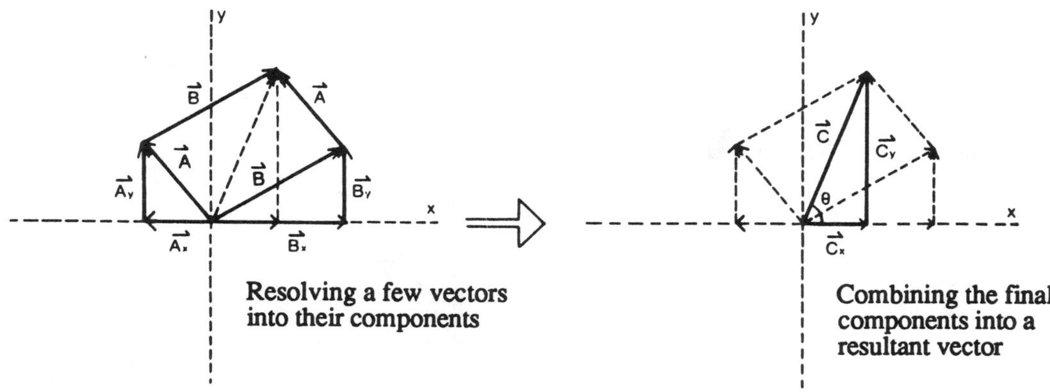

Fig. 4.9f—Orthogonal Components of Multiple Vectors

$\vec{C_x} = \vec{A_x} + \vec{B_x}$, $C_x = A_x + B_x$; $\vec{C_y} = \vec{A_y} + \vec{B_y}$, $C_y = A_y + B_y$

$\vec{C} = \vec{C_x} + \vec{C_y}$

$C^2 = C_x^2 + C_y^2$; $\tan\theta = \frac{C_y}{C_x}$

Example 1.

Given $\vec{A} + \vec{B} = \vec{C}$ find $\vec{C}$

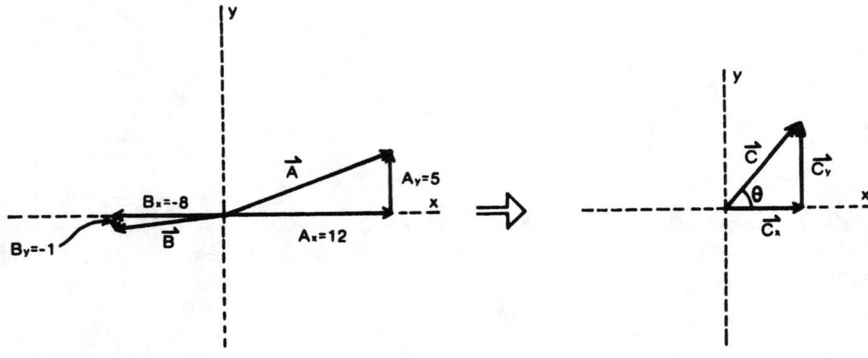

$C_x = A_x + B_x = 12 - 8 = 4$; $C_y = A_y + B_y = 5 - 1 = 4$

$C = \sqrt{C_x^2 + C_y^2} = \sqrt{4^2 + 4^2} = 4\sqrt{2}$

$\tan\theta = \frac{C_y}{C_x} = \frac{4}{4} = 1 \quad \rightarrow \quad \theta = 45°$

Problem 1.

What is the x-component of the vector $\vec{F}$?

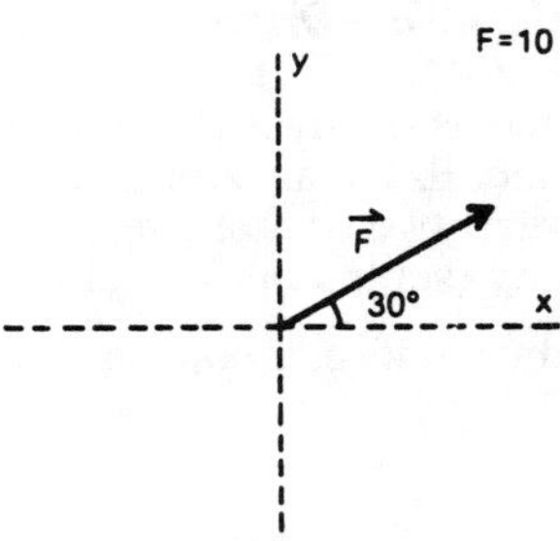

Problem 2.

What is the y-component of the vector $\vec{H}$?

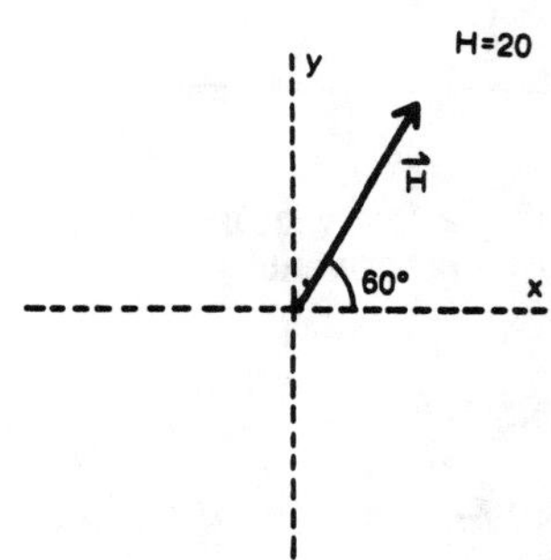

Problem 3.

What are the x- and y-components of $\vec{A} + \vec{B}$?

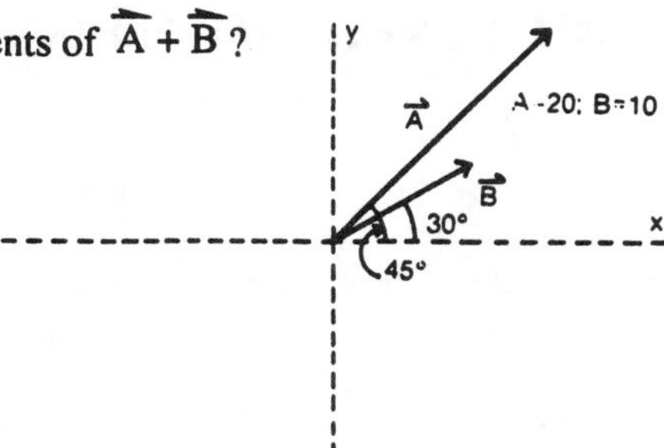

Solutions to Vector Problems

(1) Resolving the vector $\vec{F}$:

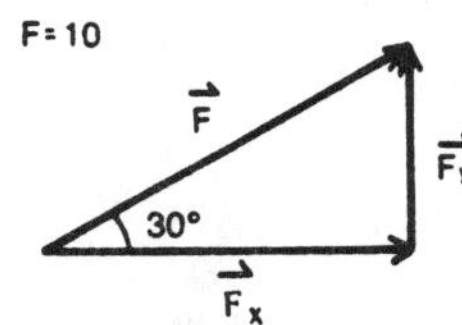

$$F_x = F \cos \theta = 10 \cos 30° = 10\left(\frac{\sqrt{3}}{2}\right) = 5\sqrt{3}$$

(2) Resolving the vector $\vec{H}$:

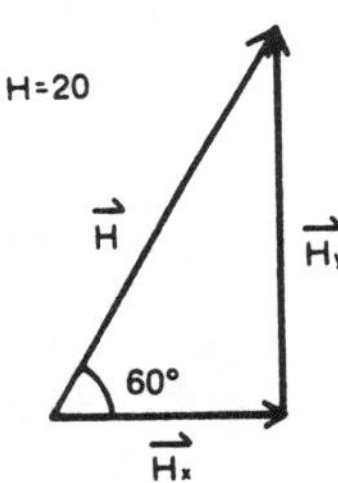

$$H_y = H \sin \theta = 20 \sin 60° = 20\left(\frac{\sqrt{3}}{2}\right) = 10\sqrt{3}$$

(3) Resolving the vectors $\vec{A} + \vec{B}$:

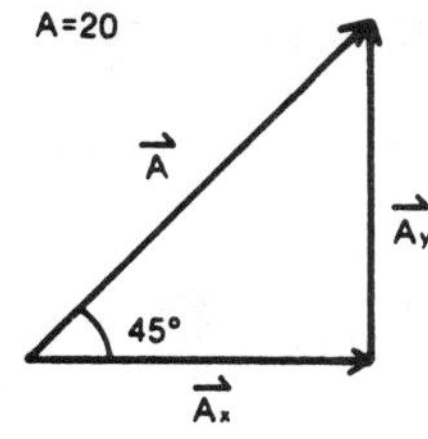

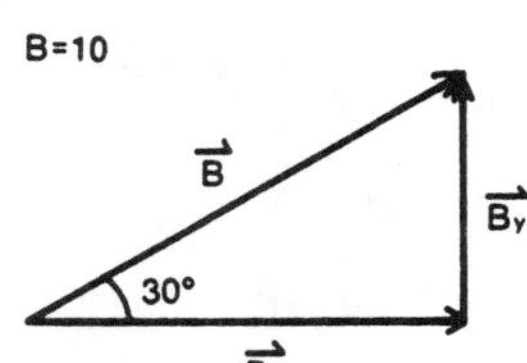

$$A_x + B_x = A \cos 45° + B \cos 30° = 20\left(\frac{1}{\sqrt{2}}\right) + 10\left(\frac{\sqrt{3}}{2}\right) = 10\sqrt{2} + 5\sqrt{3}$$

$$A_y + B_y = A \sin 45° + B \sin 30° = 20\left(\frac{1}{\sqrt{2}}\right) + 10\left(\frac{1}{2}\right) = 10\sqrt{2} + 5$$

MCAT MATHEMATICS CONCEPT 19: Using Metric and British Unit Systems

Basic Units and Conversions

The **metric system** is based on the decimal system. There are three basic units:

length: meter (m)

mass: gram (g)

volume: liter (l)

All other units of the metric system depend on using the following prefixes:

pico	-	(p) . . . . . 10^{-12}	deca . . . . 10^{1}
nano	-	(n) . . . . . 10^{-9}	kilo - (k) . . . . . .10^{3}
micro	-	(m) . . . . . 10^{-6}	mega - (M) . . . 10^{6}
milli	-	(m) . . . . . 10^{-3}	giga . . . . 10^{9}
centi	-	(c) . . . . . 10^{-2}	tera . . . . 10^{12}
deci	-	(d) . . . . . 10^{-1}	

Examples are:

kilometer = 1000 m

centimeter = $\frac{1}{100}$ meter

kilogram = 1000 g

milligram = $\frac{1}{1000}$ g

deciliter = $\frac{1}{10}$ liter

The English System has no rational basis. The basic units of it can be said to be:

length: foot (ft)

mass: pound (lb)

volume: gallon (gal)

But multiples of these are used just as often:

1 foot (ft)	=	12 in		
1 yard (yd)	=	3 ft	=	36 in
1 mile	=	1760 yds	=	5280 ft
1 pound (lb)	=	16 oz		

1 ton	=	2000 lbs
1 quart	=	2 pts
1 gallon (gal)	=	4 qts
1 pt	=	16 fluid ounces.

The key **conversions** between the metric and English systems are:

length:	2.54 cm	=	1 inch
mass:	454 g	=	1 pound
volume:	0.95 liters	=	1 quart.

Converting Units and Balancing Units in Equations

The MCAT requires: (1) the ability to convert units (conversion factors between metric and English systems being provided where needed), and (2) the ability to balance physical units in equations. To convert any unit in the metric to any corresponding unit in the English (or vice versa):

(1) Write all necessary conversions between units as equations, e.g.,

1 ton = 2000 lbs

(2) Each equation can be rewritten as either of two ratios, e.g.,

$$1 \text{ ton} = 2000 \text{ lbs} \rightarrow \frac{1 \text{ ton}}{2000 \text{ lbs}} \text{ or } \frac{2000 \text{ lbs}}{1 \text{ ton}}$$

(3) Convert between units by multiplying the correct sequence of these ratios together so that the desired units are obtained, the undesired units cancel out.

Example 1.
Convert 50 kg to ounces.

$$(50 \text{ kg})\left(\frac{1000 \text{ g}}{1\text{kg}}\right)\left(\frac{1 \text{ lb}}{454 \text{ g}}\right)\left(\frac{16 \text{ oz}}{1 \text{ lb}}\right) = \frac{(50)(1000)(16)}{454} \text{ oz} = 1762 \text{ oz}$$

Observe that kilograms are converted to grams, which are converted to pounds, which are converted to ounces. At each step, the ratio is so chosen as to cancel out the unwanted unit. In this example, all the units except ounces cancel out.

The physical units of the quantities in any equation have to balance. Consequently, in a formula, the units of one quantity can be determined from knowledge of the units of the other quantities. Also, examining to see if the units in a formula balance is a way of checking it for dimensional accuracy.

Example 2.

The kinetic energy E of a particle of mass m, moving at a speed v, is $E = \frac{1}{2} mv^2$. If E is in units of ergs $\left(\frac{\text{g-cm}^2}{\text{sec}^2}\right)$ and m is in units of grams, what are the units of speed?

$$E = \frac{1}{2} mv^2$$

$\text{g-cm}^2/\text{sec}^2 = (\text{g})\ (\text{units of speed})^2$

$(\text{units of speed})^2 = \text{cm}^2/\text{sec}^2$

units of speed = cm/sec

Problem 1.
Convert 20 kg to ounces.

Problem 2.
Convert 40 km to miles.

Problem 3.
Convert 10 liters to pints.

Problem 4.
Since the electric field $E = \frac{F}{q}$, where F = force = (mass x acceleration) and q = charge, what are the units of E in terms of mass (m), length (l), time (t), and charge (q)?

Problem 5.
The equation for the force F of gravity is:

$$F = k\frac{m_1 m_2}{r^2},$$

where m_1 and m_2 are masses and r is the distance between them.

What are the units in terms of mass (m), length (l), and time (t) of the constant k?

Solutions to Unit Conversion Problems

(1) $(20\ \text{kg})\left(\frac{1000\ \text{g}}{1\text{kg}}\right)\left(\frac{1\ \text{lb}}{454\ \text{g}}\right)\left(\frac{16\ \text{oz}}{1\ \text{lb}}\right) = \frac{(20)(1000)(16)}{454}\ \text{oz} = 705\ \text{oz}$

(2) $(40\ \text{km})\left(\frac{1000\ \text{m}}{1\ \text{km}}\right)\left(\frac{100\ \text{cm}}{1\text{m}}\right)\left(\frac{1\ \text{in}}{2.54\ \text{cm}}\right)\left(\frac{1\ \text{ft}}{12\ \text{in}}\right)\left(\frac{1\ \text{mi}}{5280\ \text{ft}}\right)$

$= \frac{(40)(1000)(100)}{(2.54)(12)(5280)}\ \text{mi} = 24.9\ \text{mi}$

(3) $(10\ \text{liters})\left(\frac{1\ \text{qt}}{0.95\ \text{liters}}\right)\left(\frac{2\ \text{pts}}{1\ \text{qt}}\right) = \frac{(10)(2)}{(0.95)}\ \text{pts} = 21\ \text{pints}$

(4) $E = \frac{F}{q} = \frac{ma}{q} = \frac{(m)\left(\frac{1}{t^2}\right)}{q} = \frac{m \cdot 1}{q \cdot t^2}$

(5) $F = \frac{k m_1 m_2}{r^2} \quad \rightarrow \quad k = \frac{r^2 F}{m_1 m_2} = \frac{r^2 (ma)}{m_1 m_2}$ for units calculations

$k = \frac{(1^2)(m)\left(\frac{1}{t^2}\right)}{(m)^2} = \frac{1^3}{m \cdot t^2}$

MCAT MATHEMATICS CONCEPT 20: Experimental Error: 1) Relative Magnitude 2) Propagation

Evaluating error: For the MCAT, it is important that one be able to identify the possible sources of error in a set of data. Determining the precision of a measurement is usually straightforward. The accuracy of a measurement is another matter. When comparing two equivalent groups of data, if it is safe to assume that there are no unique sources of error in one of the groups, it is probably true that the group whose measurements are more precise are also more accurate.

Example 1: (Physical sciences data) - Physics
We perform an experiment in which we measure the voltage drops across a set of complicated circuits; we anticipate results of the order of 0.10 volts. The voltmeter used to measure the voltage drops is precise to 0.0001 volts. However, there is a voltage noise in our apparatus separate from the voltmeter, of ± 0.01 volts. Therefore, the accuracy of our measurements is about ± 0.01 volts; the precision of the voltmeter readings has a negligible effect on the accuracy of our results. In this experiment, the data obtained is very precise but has a relatively low (about ± 10%) accuracy.

Example 2: (Physical sciences data) - Chemistry-related physics
We perform an experiment to determine the temperature dependence of the solubility of a particular organic salt in water. Our experimental apparatus is capable of maintaining a constant temperature of ± 1°C. Say we are particularly interested in measuring the salt's solubility at 37°C. Although we take it to be 37°C, each time we take a solubility measurement the true temperature is actually somewhere between 36°C and 38°C. Since the salt's solubility is temperature dependent, this variability in the true temperature results in a random error in the solubility measurements at 37°C. This random error, of course, directly affects the accuracy of these solubility measurements.

Types of Errors:

Errors can be classified under three headings: mistakes, systematic errors, and random errors. **Mistakes** are usually non-repetitive errors that might result from human errors such as misreading an instrument or occasions of performing a step wrong in an experimental procedure. The error that results from a mistake is largely unpredictable and unless caught will probably affect the data in some unknown way. An example of a mistake would be the miscounting of the pulses of one of the patients in a hospital.

A **systematic error** is a repetitive error caused by human error, instrument error, or experimental design error. It is repeated in every measurement, usually, to the same extent. If a systematic error is detected, there is a possibility that it can be corrected to some extent. An example of a systematic error would be a case where we are measuring a series of temperatures in an experiment and the thermometer being used to make these measurements is miscalibrated 2°C too high. In this case, the set of temperature measurements would have a systematic error of 2°C (too high).

We always attempt to do experiments under uniform conditions. Nevertheless, in practice, there is always some variability in these "uniform" conditions that cannot be removed. Thus, even if all human, instrument, and experimental design errors are corrected in an experiment, a variability which is called **random error** will still probably exist in its measurements. In other cases, for instance Example 1 above, the conditions under which the experiment is done have to be considered for sources of possible error (e.g., the ± 0.01 voltage noise in Example 1). As it turns out, it appears that accuracies are usually given when needed for comparison or for the calculation of other accuracies (see **propagation of error** below). Mistakes are difficult to identify. A measurement can be suspected of being mistaken only when it is out of line with a group of other identical measurements. To identify systematic error, we usually need direct evidence of a comparative nature. Basically, two groups of measurements are required where the **only** difference in obtaining them is the measurement of the quantity suspected of having a systematic error. For example, in the solubility experiment discussed above (Example 2), we might have monitored the temperature simultaneously with two thermometers in order to determine any specific error in one of them or, at least, any systematic difference in the temperatures simultaneously recorded by them. Random error is expected in all experiments as a contributor to the accuracy.

Error Propagation:

The MCAT requires that one be able to not only evaluate possible sources of error in a group of measurements, but also be able to calculate/estimate the possible error in quantities calculated from these measurements, i.e., **the propagation of error**. For the MCAT, simple calculations of error propagation should be sufficient. Specifically, when determining the value of y from a formula relating it to x and a measured value of x, one can calculate the high/low possible true values of y using the high/low possible true values of x (it is assumed that we are given the absolute or percentage accuracy of x). This can be illustrated by some examples:

Example 3.
We are given that $y = 2.303x$; x is measured to be $10 \pm 5\% = 10 \pm 0.5$. The possible true values of x range from 9.5 to 10.5; the possible true values of y range from $2.303\ (9.5) = 22$ to $2.303\ (10.5) = 24$.

Example 4.
We are given that $y = 75/x$; x is measured to be 0.250 ± 0.010. The possible true values of x range from 0.240 to 0.260; the possible true values of y range from

$$\frac{75}{0.260} = 288 \text{ to } \frac{75}{0.240} = 313 .$$

Problem
The relation between x and y is described by the equation $y = 20x - x^2$. If x is measured to be 5.0 ± 0.1, what are the possible true values of y?

Comparative Precision and Accuracy Analysis:

Data from sample experiments (called A, B and C) are presented below. These data will be used to compare the accuracy and precision in these experiments.

Experiment A:
A psychology experiment designed to test the difficulty of a particular maze for rats is done by having ten rats run the maze. The results for their solution times to the nearest 0.1 seconds are:

8.3, 7.1, 8.8, 11.1, 7.0, 13.7, 9.5, 10.3, 10.8, 9.9

Experiment B:
As a practice exercise, the students in a medical school class have to determine the pulse (number of heartbeats/minute) of 30 patients. One student's results (which have been frequency grouped instead of being recorded individually) to the nearest 5 are:

50: I (1)	65: V (5)	80: III (3)
55: II (2)	70: VII (7)	85: II (2)
50: III (3)	75: VI (6)	90: I (1)

Experiment C:
Two groups of 35-year-old subjects, one of men and one of women, have their blood cholesterol levels (mg/100 ml) measured. The data obtained (rounded to the nearest 1 mg/100 ml) are:

Group I: (men)	195, 198, 199, 196, 195, 196, 191, 194, 195, 196.
Group II: (women)	196, 193, 194, 201, 202, 205, 204, 202, 199, 204.

These data will be used in the examples to illustrate instrumentation used and how to analyze the relative degree of error.

In analyzing data, we are also interested in examining the nature of (e.g., the limitations of) the measurements that a set of data comprises. These considerations lead to the notion of error which stems from a desire to know the possible difference between the exact, true value of a quantity and our measured (or calculated) value of it.

Before embarking on a discussion of error, the **significant digits** of a number must be understood. A digit is significant when it has been measured exactly. Examples of determining the number of significant digits are:

(1) 7.000 4 significant digits; digits listed after a decimal point are assumed to be accurately measured.

(2) 7000 1 significant digit; no decimal point—see (3) below.

(3) 7000. 4 significant digits; the decimal point implies that all zeros are accurately measured.

(4) 7001 4 significant digits; all zeros between nonzero digits are significant.

When adding, multiplying, etc., the number of significant digits in the result cannot be such that it is any more precise than the least precise number involved in its calculation (see discussion of precision below). Consider as examples:

Experiment A.
Each piece of data in this experiment has 2 (e.g., 8.3) or 3 (e.g., 10.3) significant digits. When the mean for these data is calculated, it comes out initially as 9.65 but is rounded off to 9.7 because some of the numbers used to calculate this mean have only 2 significant digits. Likewise, the variance of these data is initially calculated as 3.643 but has to be rounded off to 3.6 (2 significant digits). See these calculations in examples above.

Experiment B.
The mean for these data is initially calculated as about 70.17 but is rounded off to 70 where the "0" is not significant. The data in this experiment have only one significant digit because they are rounded off to the nearest 5.

Errors occur in data because it is not possible to get exact numbers from experiments. In any experiment, there is a limit to how close we can get to knowing the true value of the quantity being measured. Consequently, there are several definitions/concepts with which you should be familiar that are used to describe and assess the error in a measurement or calculation.

The **precision** of a number or an experimental value is the smallest unit of measurement and is therefore closely related to the significant digits in a measured number. Consider as examples:

Experiment A.
The solution times for the rats running the maze are recorded to the nearest 0.1 seconds; therefore, the precision of these time measurements is 0.1 seconds. It is also called the "least count" of the measuring instrument.

Experiment B.
The pulse rates measured for this group of patients are recorded to the nearest 5; however, the precision of these measurements depends on how the student measured the pulse rate. If the student counts the pulses in a 30 second interval and then doubles this count to get the pulse rate in beats/minute, then the precision is 2 beats/minute as this is the smallest unit of measurement in terms of beats/minute. As another example, if the student counts the pulses in a 1-minute interval, then the precision is 1 beat/minute.

The **accuracy** of a number is how far the measured value of a variable may be from its true value. The true value is normally considered as an "average" obtained from a large set of data values. Consider as examples:

Experiment A.
The precision of the watch used to measure each maze solution time is 0.1 seconds. Neglecting any other possible sources of error, the accuracy of each time measurement is ± 0.05 seconds. Specifically, when a rat's measured solution time is 8.8 seconds, the true solution time is 8.8 ± 0.05 seconds, i.e., it is known to be between 8.75 and 8.85 seconds.

Experiment B:
Suppose the student measuring the pulse rates of the 30 patients took a pulse count in a 30-second interval and then doubled this count to get the pulse rate in beats/minute. We already observed above that in this case the precision is 2 beats/minute. Yet, this has little bearing on the accuracy of the data as presented. Neglecting the possibility of mistakes or systematic error (see below), the accuracy of the data as presented is ± 2.5 beats/minute, since the data has been rounded off to the nearest 5 beats/minute.

Experiment C.
The precision in the blood cholesterol level experiments is 1 mg/100 ml; therefore, their accuracy is ± 0.5 mg/100 ml. A measured value of 196 corresponds to a true value that is somewhere between 195.5 and 196.5.

However, when error results from sources other than the limitations of the measuring device, the accuracy and the precision are not usually so simply related. In many experiments, there may be factors other than the precision of the measurements involved which decrease the accuracy of their results. What you should understand from these experiments is that all sorts of factors can affect the accuracy of experimental results. With this in mind, we will next consider types of error more formally.

Solution to Problem

(1) For $x = 5.0$, $y = 20\,(5.0) - (5.0)^2 = 75$
For $x = 4.9$, $y = 20\,(4.9) - (4.9)^2 = 74$
For $x = 5.1$, $y = 20\,(5.1) - (5.1)^2 = 76$

The possible true values of y are 74, 75, and 76

MCAT MATHEMATICS CONCEPT 21: Approximation and Estimations

A useful skill that should be practiced by students is the art of reasonable estimation, which is used instead of exact answers. A large part of the MCAT pool of questions involves the ability to estimate an *approximate* answer quickly. The approximate answer is then compared to the actual answer choices provided. Do not spend too much time finding an exact answer when an approximated answer will give you the information you require.

Part of approximation and estimation is the ability to convert an arithmetic problem into one that can be done quickly in your head. To do this, learn to simplify the problem first. The generalization that multiplication and division may be done in any order is one means of doing this. You probably do this already without being aware of it.

Example 1.

$$40 \times 22 = (4 \times 10) \times 22 = (4 \times 22) \times 10 = 88 \times 10 = 880$$

By leaving the 10 until last, you have less to keep in mind for the multiplication.

A less obvious (but very useful) simplification can be made when you are required to multiply by 50 or 25 (or by the same numbers with the decimal moved, such as 5, 0.5, 2.5, 0.25, etc.) Remember that 50 is 100/2 and 25 is 100/4.

Example 2.

66 x 50

$$66 \times 50 = 66 \times \frac{100}{2} = \frac{66}{2} \times 100 = 33 \times 100 = 3300$$

Example 3.

66 x 2.5

$$66 \times 2.5 = 66 \times \frac{10}{4} = \frac{66}{4} \times 10 = \frac{660}{4} = 165$$

Example 4.

$\frac{320}{25}$

$$\frac{320}{25} = 320 / \frac{100}{4} = 320 \times \frac{4}{100} = \frac{320}{100} \times 4 = 3.2 \times 4 = 12.8$$

Problem 1.
Mentally multiply the following (simplify the operation as before, then multiply and add or subtract):

(a) 89 x 3 (b) \$1.05 x 9 (c) \$1.98 x 9
(d) \$3.95 x 8 (e) 72 x 30 (f) 44 x 60

Problem 2.
Mentally multiply or divide the following:

(a) 36 x 5.0 (b) $\frac{440}{50}$ (c) 28 x 25

(d) $\frac{120}{25}$ (e) 120 x 0.25 (f) 89 x 33.3

Answers to Problems 1 and 2

(1) (a) $89 \times 3 = (90 - 1)\,3$
$= 270 - 3 = 267$

(b) $1.05 \times 9 = 1.05\,(10 - 1)$
$= 10.50 - 1.05 = 9.45$

(c) $1.98 \times 9 = (2.00 - 0.02)\,9$
$= 18.0 - 0.18 = 17.82$

(d) $3.95 \times 8 = (4 - 0.05)\,8$
$= 32 - 0.40 = 31.60$

(e) $72 \times 30 = 72 \times 3 \times 10$
$= 216 \times 10 = 2160$

(f) $44 \times 60 = (40 + 4)\,60$
$= 2400 + 240 = 2640$

(2) (a) $36 \times 5.0 = 36 \times \frac{10}{2} = \frac{36}{2} \times 10 = 18 \times 10 = 180$

(b) $\frac{440}{50} = \frac{440}{1} \times \frac{2}{100} = \frac{88}{10} = 8.8$

(c) $28 \times 25 = 28 \times \frac{100}{4} = \frac{28}{4} \times 100 = 700$

(d) $\frac{120}{25} = \frac{120}{1} \times \frac{4}{100} = \frac{480}{100} = 4.8$

(e) $120 \times 0.25 = 120 \times \frac{1}{4} = 30$

(f) $89 \times 33.3 = 89 \times \frac{100}{3} = \frac{89}{3} \times 100 \approx \frac{90}{3} \times 100 = 3000$

Approximate Calculations and Percent Errors

Rapid mental calculation to find an approximate answer is a useful skill. This most often means rounding off to easily handled numbers. Sometimes, the most useful procedure is not obvious rounding. This is especially true in the type of calculation so often encountered in science, in which several numbers are to be multiplied and divided in one problem.

When simple rounding off can be used, it is, of course, a given easy method. Furthermore, it permits estimation of error type (is the result too large or too small?), and, if necessary, the size of error as a percentage of the answer.

Example 1.
What is the approximate price of three items that cost $7.98 each? Round off the price to $8. Then 3 x $8 = $24. The actual price is less than that used in the calculation. Therefore, the actual total is less than $24.

Sometimes it is desirable to know not only whether the approximate answer is too large or too small, but also by how much. Then it is useful to calculate the percent introduced by an approximation. (Usually, an approximate percent is sufficient or you might find yourself spending more time calculating the percent than you saved by making the rapid approximation.)

Percent error in any calculation is defined by the equation:

$$\%\ \text{error} = \frac{\text{error}}{\text{true value}} \times 100\%$$

Usually, the absolute value of error is used without any plus or minus signs.

Example 2.
Calculate the percent error: (a) 14 is rounded down to 10 and (b) 1004 is rounded down to 1000. For each, the error is 4.

(a) $\% \text{ error} = \frac{4}{14} \times 100\% = 28.6\%$

(b) $\% \text{ error} = \frac{4}{1004} \times 100\% = 0.4\%$

As the calculation above shows, the same size change can result in very different percent errors. This calculation should be used to understand "proportional reasoning."

Problem 1.
Calculate the approximate percent error introduced by the indicated rounding off for each example given below:

(a) Round 750 to 800
(b) Round 750 to 700
(c) Round 798 to 800
(d) Round 198 to 200
(e) Round 210 to 200

Answer to Problem 1

(a) Error = 800 - 750 = 50

$\% \text{ error} = \frac{50}{750} \times 100 = \frac{500}{75} = \frac{100}{15} = \frac{20}{3} = 6\frac{2}{3}\% \text{ (positive)}$

(b) Error = 750 - 700 = 50

$\% \text{ error} = \frac{50}{750} \times 100 = \frac{500}{75} = \frac{100}{15} = \frac{20}{3} = 6\frac{2}{3}\% \text{ (negative)}$

(c) Error = 800 - 798 = 2

$\% \text{ error} = \frac{2}{798} \times 100 = \frac{200}{798} = 0.25\% \text{ approx.}$

(d) Error = 200 - 198 = 2

$\% \text{ error} = \frac{2}{198} \times 100 = \frac{200}{198} = 1\% \text{ approx.}$

(e) Error = 210 - 200 = 2

$\% \text{ error} = \frac{10}{210} \times 100 = \frac{1000}{210} = \frac{100}{21} = 5\% \text{ approx. (negative)}$

Example 3.
How much solution should you mix to do measurements on eight samples if each requires 110 ml? You will make up somewhat more than the minimum required in case of waste, spills, etc., so you do not need to know the precise amount needed. But calculate it just to make sure you are making enough.

Rounding off, approximately 100 ml per sample is needed.

8 samples x 100 ml/sample = 800 ml

The number used in calculation, 100, was less than the amount actually needed (110), so the amount calculated is too small. The error is approximately 10 percent:

$$\frac{10 \text{ ml error}}{110 \text{ ml needed}} \times 100\% \approx 10\%$$

An additional 100 ml will more than make up for the 10 percent error and 100 ml more to allow for waste would indicate that you should make up at least 1000 ml of solution.

Rule 1.
In some problems it is possible to minimize errors caused by rounding off. When two numbers are to be multiplied and one is rounded down to a smaller number, try to round the other up to a larger number, as in the example below:

$$93 \times 69 \approx 90 \times 70$$

Example 4.
Multiply 2.7 x 38:

The usual way to round off would make both numbers larger and the resulting answer too large.

$$2.7 \times 38 \approx 3 \times 40 = 120$$

Rounding 2.7 all the way down to 2 would be such a large percentage change that again a large error would be introduced. However, 2.7 could be rounded down to 2.5, which in this calculation is a convenient number to use.

$$2.7 \times 38 \approx 2.5 \times 40 = 100$$

For comparison, the correct answer is 2.7 x 38 = 103. Therefore, the second method gave a more nearly correct answer.

Rule 2.
In a calculation involving division, it is desirable to round off in the same direction in both numerator and denominator. That is, if the numerator is rounded to a larger number, the denominator should also be rounded to a larger number. This is especially important if the rounding off introduces a large percentage change, e.g.,

$$\frac{68}{47} \approx \frac{70}{50}$$

Example 5.
Find the approximate quotients:

(a) $\frac{387}{750}$ (b) $\frac{419}{850}$

In each fraction, the denominator might be rounded up or down equally well. For (a) it would also be convenient to round the denominator up.

$$\frac{387}{750} \approx \frac{400}{800} = 0.5$$

If the denominator had been rounded down to 700, the result would have been 0.57. Since the correct answer is 0.52, the procedure of rounding numerator and denominator in the same direction gave a more nearly correct answer.

For (b) the numerator will be rounded down, from 419 to 400. There, the denominator should also be rounded down.

$\frac{419}{850} \cong \frac{400}{800} = 0.5$ the correct answer is 0.49.

Rule 3.
When one number is to be divided by another, rounding off can sometimes be done in such a way that one number is especially easy to divide by another.

Example 6.

$\frac{298}{2 \times 15} \approx \frac{300}{30} = 10$ means "is approximately equal to"

$\frac{685}{702} \approx \frac{700}{700} = 1$ the actual quotient should be less than 1, since the numerator is less than 700

Rule 4.
There are some combinations that cancel quite well. For example, 9 x 11 is very close to 10 x 10. Notice that where 9 is 1 less than 10, 11 is 1 more than 10. Similarly, 8 x 12 is also close to 10 x 10 and, of course, to 9 x 11.

Example 7.
Find the approximate answer.

$$\frac{8 \times 6 \times 93}{(7)^2}$$

Since 8 x 6 is close to 7 x 7, they can be cancelled.

$$\frac{8 \times 6 \times 93}{7 \times 7} \cong 93$$

Rule 5.
In some calculations there may be several numbers to be cancelled in order to reach a setup that allows a rapid mental calculation.

Example 8.
What is the approximate answer?

$$\frac{273 \times 775 \times 350}{298 \times 760}$$

You can make a very gross approximation and consider 273 ≅ 298 so that they cancel.

$\frac{273}{298} \cong 1$ This would make your answer too large, since you are pretending that 273 is actually a larger number, 298.

On the other hand, cancelling 775 with 760 causes far less error (about 2 percent rather than the 10 percent above). Here it would be suitable to cancel the numbers, but note that the true answer will be a bit larger than the calculation shows. (You cancel by assuming that 775 ≅ 760. Since, in fact, it is larger, the true answer should be larger.) Similarly, if 273 is cancelled with 298, you would have known that the true answer should be smaller. The two effects will not entirely counteract each other, since the percent error is not the same. You could write:

$$\frac{273}{298} \times \frac{773}{760} \times 350 \cong 350$$

Since this is too large, at a guess the answer might be near 330.

However, if you wish to be more accurate, you might notice that the numbers 273 and 298 are close to 270 and 300, and that these are divisible by 30.

$$\frac{273}{298} \approx \frac{270}{300} = \frac{9}{10} = 0.9 = 1 - 0.1$$

$$\frac{273}{298} \times \frac{775}{760} \times 350 \approx (1 - 0.1) \times 350 = 350 - 35 = 315$$

This is a little too small (error from 775/760), and you might guess the correct answer to be about 320.

Example 9.
Find the approximate answer:

$$\frac{2(450)}{(0.082)(298)}$$

There are several possible approaches to solving this problem, three of them are outlined below:

Method 1.

In rounding 298 to 300, notice that:

$$2 \times 450 = 900 \text{ thus } \frac{900}{0.082 \times 300} = \frac{3}{0.082}$$

To simplify the division, you might round 0.082 to 0.1, an increase of about 25 percent:

$$\frac{3}{0.1} = 30$$

If a more accurate answer is needed, consider that this is too small, since the denominator used was too big. Estimate that the result should be about 25 percent larger or about 37.

Method 2.

Round both 450 and 0.082:

$$\frac{2(450)}{0.082(298)} \approx \frac{2(500)}{0.1(300)} = \frac{10}{0.3} = \frac{100}{3} = 33$$

Method 3.

Rewrite in exponential notation with slight initial rounding off.

$$\begin{aligned} \frac{2(450)}{0.082(298)} &\approx \frac{2 \times 4.5 \times 10^2}{8 \times 10^{-2} \times 3 \times 10^2} \\ &= \frac{9}{8 \times 3} \times \frac{10^2}{10^{-2} \times 10^2} \\ &= \frac{3}{8} \times 10^2 \\ &= .37 \times 10^2 = 37 \end{aligned}$$

Problem

Make rapid approximate calculations for each.

(a) $\frac{27 \times 720}{59}$ (b) $\frac{760 \times 22.4 \times 330}{900 \times 273}$ (c) $\frac{9^2 \times 620}{99 \times 0.8}$

Answers to Problem

(a) $\frac{27 \times 720}{59} \approx \frac{30 \times 720}{60} = \frac{720}{2} = 360$ correct answer: 329.5

(b) $\frac{760 \times 22.4 \times 330}{900 \times 273} \approx \frac{760 \times 20 \times 330}{900 \times 270}$

$$= \frac{76 \times 2 \times 33}{9 \times 27} = \frac{152 \times 33}{9 \times 27}$$

$= \frac{150 \times 50}{10 \times 30} = 20$ correct answer: 22.9

(c) $\frac{9^2 \times 620}{99 \times 0.8} \approx \frac{81 \times 620}{100 \times 0.8}$

$= \frac{80 \times 620}{10 \times 8} = 620$ correct answer: 634

MCAT MATHEMATICS CONCEPT 22: Permutations, Combinations and Probability

This section includes the study of permutations, combinations, and probability. You will find it useful in determining the number of logical possibilities of some event without necessarily enumerating each case. Some formulas are included in the section and you should try to memorize them.

Fundamental Principles of Counting

If an event can occur in x different ways, and if, following this event, a second event can occur in y different ways, and, following this second event, a third event can occur in z different ways, then the number of ways the events can occur in the order indicated is $x \cdot y \cdot z$. This is called "multiplication rule of counting."

Formula: total number of ways in which event occurs = $x \cdot y \cdot z$

Example 1.
License plates of a certain state contain three letters followed by three digits, where the first digit cannot be zero. One calculates the number of possible different license plates as follows: Each letter can be selected in twenty-six different ways, the first digit in nine ways, and each of the other two digits in ten ways.

letters			digits		
26	26	26	9	10	10

$26 \cdot 26 \cdot 26 \cdot 9 \cdot 10 \cdot 10 = 15{,}818{,}400$. In other words, about 16 million distinct plates are possible. This principle is really useful in understanding genetic codes for the MCAT; see chapter 7, "Problem Solving in the Biological Sciences," below.

Factorial Symbol

The notation n! (read: "n factorial") denotes the product of the positive integers from 1 to n, inclusive:

$$n! = 1 \cdot 2 \cdot 3 \ldots (n-2)(n-1)n \text{ (in ascending order)}$$

Equivalently, n! is defined by

$$n! = n \cdot (n-1)!$$

It is also convenient to define $0! = 1$, $1! = 1$.

Example 2.

(a) $2! = 1 \cdot 2 = 2$ $\quad 3! = 1 \cdot 2 \cdot 3 = 6$
$4! = 1 \cdot 2 \cdot 3 \cdot 4 = 24$ $\quad 5! = 5 \cdot 4! = 5 \cdot 24 = 120$
$6! = 6 \cdot 5! = 6 \cdot 120 = 720$ $\quad 7! = 7 \cdot 6! = 7 \cdot (720) = 5040$

(b) $\frac{8!}{6!} = \frac{8 \cdot 7 \cdot 6!}{6!} = 8 \cdot 7 = 56$

(c) $\frac{9!}{7!3!} = \frac{9 \cdot 8 \cdot 7!}{7!\, 3 \cdot 2 \cdot 1} = 12$

Combination Factorial Symbol

The combination factorial symbol is defined as:

$$\binom{n}{r} = {}^{n}C_{r} = {}_{n}C_{r}$$

Read "en-see-are," where r and n are positive integers with r £ n, by

$$\binom{n}{r} = \frac{n(n-1)(n-2)\ldots(n-r+1)}{1 \cdot 2 \cdot 3 \ldots (r-1)r}$$

$$\binom{n}{r} = \frac{n!}{r!\,(n-r)!}$$

Example 3.

(a) $\binom{8}{3} = \frac{8!}{3!5!} = \frac{8 \cdot 7 \cdot 6 \cdot 5!}{3 \cdot 2 \cdot 1 \cdot 5!} = 56$

(b) $\binom{10}{4} = \frac{10!}{4!6!} = \frac{10 \cdot 9 \cdot 8 \cdot 7 \cdot 6!}{4 \cdot 3 \cdot 2 \cdot 1 \cdot 6!} = 210$

(c) $\binom{12}{1} = \frac{12!}{1!11!} = \frac{12\cdot 11!}{11!} = 12$

Permutations

Any arrangement of a set of *n* objects in a **given order** is called a permutation of the objects (taken all at a time). The arrangement has a **specific** possible order. Any arrangement of any $r \leq n$ of these objects in a given order is called a permutation of the *n* objects taken *r* at a time. Consider, for example, the set of P, Q, R, S.

(a) Permutations of four letters (taken all at a time):

P,Q,R,S	Q,P,R,S	R,P,Q,S	S,P,Q,R
P,Q,S,R	Q,P,S,R	R,P,S,Q	S,P,R,Q
P,S,Q,R	Q,R,S,P	R,S,P,Q	S,R,P,Q
P,S,R,Q	Q,R,P,S	R,S,Q,P	S,R,Q,P
P,R,S,Q	Q,S,P,R	R,Q,S,P	S,Q,P,R
P,R,Q,S	Q,S,R,P	R,Q,P,S	S,Q,R,P

There are 24 permutations in all.

(b) Permutations of four letters (taken three at a time):

P,Q,R	Q,P,S	R,P,S	S,P,Q
P,R,Q	Q,S,P	R,S,P	S,Q,P
P,Q,S	Q,S,R	R,Q,S	S,Q,R
P,S,Q	Q,R,S	R,S,Q	S,R,Q
P,R,S	Q,P,R	R,P,Q	S,P,R
P,S,R	Q,R,P	R,Q,P	S,R,P

There are 24 permutations in **all** for this case also. A formula to find possible permutations is given below, instead of writing each possible outcome.

(c) Permutations of four letters (taken two at a time):

P,Q	P,R	P,S
Q,P	R,P	S,P
Q,S	R,Q	S,Q
Q,R	R,S	S,R

There are 12 permutations in all.

The number of permutations of *n* objects taken *r* at a time is denoted by:

$P(n,r)$ or ${}_nP_r$

To find an expression for P(n,r) observe that the first element in an r-permutation of *n* objects can be chosen in n different ways; following this, the second element in the permutation can be chosen in n-1 ways; and, following this, the third element in the permutation can be chosen in n-2 ways. Continuing in this manner, the rth (last) element in the r-permutation can be chosen in $n - (r - 1) = n - r + 1$ ways. Thus, by the fundamental principle of counting,

$$P(n,r) = n(n-1)(n-2) \ldots (n-r+1)$$

Formula: $$P(n,r) = \frac{n!}{(n-r)!}$$

In the special case in which $r = n$,

$$P(n,n) = n(n-1)(n-2) \ldots 3\cdot 2\cdot 1 = n!$$

Solve the problem with sets of letters using P(4,4), P(4,3), P(4,2) and check your answers with arrangements shown in the above examples with letters P, Q, R, S. The above material should be carefully studied in conjunction with genetic codes, gene mapping and other pertinent topics as outlined in chapter 7.

Example 4.
In how many ways can five people sit in five chairs? In four chairs?

5 people, 5 chairs Assume all chairs are in a straight row.

n = 5 = people $P(5,5) = \frac{5!}{(5-5)!} = \frac{5!}{0!} = 5! = 120$ ways

r = 5 = chairs

5 people, 4 chairs

n = 5 = people $P(5,4) = \frac{5!}{(5-4)!} = \frac{5!}{1!} = 5! = 120$ ways

r = 4 = chairs

Solving the above cases shows that whether you provide 5 or 4 seats the number of arrangements does not change. It would be **hard** to guess at the possible answer without the formula given.

<u>5 chairs</u>	<u>4 chairs</u>
A B C D E	A B C D
A B C E D	A B D C
A B D C E	A B C E
A B E C D	A B E C
and so on.	and so on.

Compare these permutations with the "letter set" (P, Q, R, S) permutations.

Combinations

Suppose we have a collection of *n* objects. Remember combinations represent **groups**, not arrangements. A combination of these *n* objects taken *r* at a time is any selection of *r* of the objects **where order doesn't count.** In other words, an r-combination of a set of *n* objects is any subset containing *r* objects. For example, the combinations of the letters *a, b , c, d,* taken three at a time are:

(a,b,c), (a,b,d), (a,c,d), (b,c,d) or simply abc, abd, acd, bcd

Observe the following combinations are equal:

abc, acb, bca, cab, bac, cba

That is, each denotes the same set (a,b,c). The number of combinations of *n* objects taken *r* at a time is denoted by C(n,r). The symbols ${}_nC_r$, C_{nr} and C_r^n also appear in various texts. To find the general formula for C(n,r), we note that any combination of *n* objects taken *r* at a time determines r! permutations of the object in the combination. Consequently,

$$P(n,r) = r!\ C(n,r)$$

$$C(n,r) = \frac{P(n,r)}{r!} = \frac{n!}{r!\ (n-r)!} = \binom{n}{r}$$

Example 5.
In how many ways can three people sample the following drinks: iced tea, soft drink, mineral water, lemonade?

(a) If each person samples only one drink?
(b) If each person samples only two drinks?

Solutions to Example 5

(a) Each person must select 1 of the 4 drinks, so each has C (4,1) $= \binom{4}{1} = \frac{4!}{1!3!} = 4$ different possible choices.

$$\begin{pmatrix} n = 4 \text{ drinks} \\ r = 1 \text{ drink selected} \end{pmatrix}$$

Since each person makes the selection independently, there are

$4 \times 4 \times 4 = 64$ possible ways.

↑ ↑ ↑

(b) Each person must select 2 of the 4 drinks (in any order), so each has C (4,2) $= \binom{4}{2} = \frac{4!}{2!2!} = 6$ possible 2-drink combinations. Since each selects his/her 2 drinks independently, there are

$6 \times 6 \times 6 = 216$ possible ways.

↑ ↑ ↑

This illustrates the "multiplication principle" of counting.

Note: This question involves combinations rather than permutations (together with the "multiplication of choices" principle).

Example 6.
How many committees of three can be created from nine people? Each committee represents a combination of the nine people taken three at a time. Thus,

$$C(9,3) = \binom{9}{3} = \frac{9!}{3!\,(9-3)!} = \frac{9 \times 8 \times 7 \times 6!}{6 \cdot 6!} = 84 \text{ different committees can be formed.}$$

Example 7.
A farmer buys three cows, one pig, and four hens from a man who has seven cows, five pigs, and eight hens. How many choices does the farmer have?

The farmer can choose the cows in C(7,3) ways, the pigs in C(5,1) ways, and the hens in C(8,4) ways. Hence, he can choose the animals in

$$\binom{7}{3}\binom{5}{1}\binom{8}{4} = \frac{7 \cdot 6 \cdot 5}{3 \cdot 2 \cdot 1} \times \frac{5}{1} \times \frac{8 \cdot 7 \cdot 6 \cdot 5}{4 \cdot 3 \cdot 2 \cdot 1} = 12{,}250 \text{ ways}$$

Probability of an Event

The premedical student contemplating the MCAT should feel confident with the basic concept of probability as applied to genetics (Hardy-Weinberg principle) and physical chemistry (quantum numbers). Probability of something happening is a measure of "how likely" an event may occur. Probability lies between 0 (impossible) to 1 (certain).

Probability of an event = p(E)

(1) $p(E) = \frac{\text{Number of desired outcomes of E}}{\text{Number of possible outcomes of E}}$

(2) p(success) + p(failure) = 1

(3) $0 \leq p(E) \leq 1$. Note probability cannot be negative.

Example 8a.
A bag of candy-coated chocolates contains five greens and three yellows. What is the probability of selecting a green candy (a) in one try and (b) on the second try? (After the first try, put the candy back into the bag before you take the second one.)

(a) $p(g) = \frac{5}{5+3} = \frac{5}{8} = \frac{\text{Total no. of green candies}}{\text{Total no. of candies}}$

(b) During first try: $p(g) = \frac{5}{8}$ as shown in part (a) above.

During second try: $p(g) = \frac{5}{8}$ again, because nothing has changed.

It may be observed that under the same given conditions, the probability p(g) does not change for each try. Do not imagine that two trials will double the probability. This is the key to learning the definition of probability and its application. To answer the question "What is the probability of selecting a green candy after two tries when selection is done with replacement from a bag containing 5 greens and 3 yellows?" you must apply the principle of probabilistic independence (see statistically independent events):

$$
\begin{aligned}
p\binom{\text{green in}}{\text{2 tries}} &= 1 - p\binom{\text{no green in}}{\text{2 tries}} \\
&= 1 - p\binom{\text{no green on}}{\text{1st try}} \cdot p\binom{\text{no green on}}{\text{2nd try}} \\
&= 1 - \frac{3}{8} \cdot \frac{3}{8} \\
&= 1 - 9/64 = 55/64
\end{aligned}
$$

Note: If an identical experiment is repeated under identical conditions in numerous independent trials, the probability for success will remain the same for each individual trial.

Visual solution: A more graphical solution is illustrated for students who are using genetics (Punnett squares).

Probability Matrix:

Probability of green on 1st try = 5/8
Probability of no green on 1st try = 3/8
Probability of green on 2nd try = 5/8
Probability of no green on 2nd try = 3/8

Sample Space: This is a map showing <u>all</u> possible outcomes.

yellow	green	green
yellow	green	green
yellow	green	

<u>Note</u>: There are eight possible outcomes.

		2nd try		
		green	**yellow**	
1st try	**green**	green, green	green, yellow	Possible outcomes for 1st and 2nd tries
	yellow	yellow, green	yellow, yellow	

(i) Probability of 1st candy being green and 2nd candy being green

$$= \left(\frac{5}{8}\right)\left(\frac{5}{8}\right) = \frac{25}{64}$$

(ii) Probability of 1st candy being green and second candy being yellow

$$= \left(\frac{5}{8}\right)\left(\frac{3}{8}\right) = \frac{15}{64}$$

(iii) Probability of 1st candy being yellow and second candy being green

$$= \left(\frac{3}{8}\right)\left(\frac{5}{8}\right) = \frac{15}{64}$$

Probability of 1st candy being yellow and second candy being yellow

$$= \left(\frac{3}{8}\right)\left(\frac{3}{8}\right) = \frac{9}{64}$$

Adding (i), (ii) and (iii) gives you the probability of getting a piece of green candy in either of two tries.

$$\frac{25}{64} + \frac{15}{64} + \frac{15}{64} = \frac{55}{64}$$

Mutually Exclusive Events:

Certain events cannot occur simultaneously, e.g., you cannot attend anthropology class and biology lab at the same time. If in Scholastic College there are 12 classes offered at 2:30 p.m., the probability that a certain student, known to be in class at that time, will be in Anthropology or Biology is:

p(A or B) = p(A) + p(B)

p(Anthropology or Biology) = $\frac{1}{12} + \frac{1}{12} = \frac{2}{12} = \frac{1}{6}$

Statistically Independent Events:

Events that **can** occur simultaneously, but the first event does not affect the second event, e.g., there is a probability that it rains in Miami, Florida, at 4 p.m. **and** a football game is played at 4 p.m. in Tampa, Florida, on the same day.

p(A) = p(rains in Miami) = $\frac{1}{100}$ (assume)

p(B) = p(game played in Tampa) = $\frac{2}{29}$ (assume)

p(A and B) = p(A)•p(B) = $\frac{1}{100} \cdot \frac{2}{29} = \frac{1}{1450}$

MEMORIZE:

p(A **or** B) = p(A) + p(B)	Mutually exclusive
p(A **and** B) = p(A) • p(B)	Statistically independent

Remember, the probability of the union of mutually exclusive events is **higher** than the probability of either event. On the other hand, the probability of the simultaneous occurrence of statistically independent events is **lower** than the probability of either event.

Example 9.
In a bag are five peaches and four plums. Michelle selects one, replaces it and selects another. What is the probability that both selections are peaches?

These are **independent events.**

p(A) = p(peach) in first selection = $\frac{5}{5+4} = \frac{5}{9}$

p(B) = p(peach) in second selection = $\frac{5}{5+4} = \frac{5}{9}$

p(A and B) = $\frac{5}{9} \cdot \frac{5}{9} = \frac{25}{81}$ is less than $\frac{5}{9}$

Example 10.
Andrew has four nickels, seven pennies, and three dimes in his pocket. He selects one. What is the probability it is a penny or a dime?

These are **mutually exclusive** events because there is no coin which is both a penny and a dime.

p(penny **or** dime) = p(penny) + p(dime) = $\frac{7}{14} + \frac{3}{14} = \frac{5}{7}$

is more than $\frac{7}{14}$.

4.2.4 MATHEMATICS CONCEPTS TEST

(1) Solve for x: $x^3 = 216a^6b^9$

(2) Solve for y: $\frac{1}{y-1} + \frac{1}{y+2} = \frac{1}{5(y-1)}$

(3) Solve for b: 6-2(3-2(5-3(b-2)-4)-2)-1 = 50b

(4) The potential of an electric dipole

$$V = \frac{p\cos\theta}{r^2},$$

where p = the strength of the electric dipole, r = the distance from the electric dipole to the point of observation, and θ = the angle between the line to the point of observation and the direction of the dipole. If p is tripled, r is halved, and θ is changed from 0° to 60°, how are the original and final dipole potentials related?

(5) The dose of a drug is 5 mg per kilogram of body weight. If a person weighs 70 kg, what amount of drug should be given?

(6) The dose of a drug is 5 mg per 40 kg of body weight. If a person weighs 60 kg, what amount of drug should be given?

(7) The cost of item A in 1986 was $64. Its cost in 1987 was $89.60. What was the percent increase in the price of item A between 1986 and 1987?

(8) Evaluate: $4 \times 10^{-4} + 17 \times 10^{-6}$

(9) Evaluate: $(2 \times 10^4)(5 \times 10^{-5})$

(10) Solve for x: $x = \left(\frac{5 \times 10^3}{25 \times 10^{-5}}\right)^3$

(11) Evaluate: $7.15 \times 10^3 + 0.025 \times 10^1$

(12) The ideal-gas law is PV = nRT. If the absolute temperature T is doubled, the pressure P is decreased by 1/4 of its original value, and the number of moles n is left unchanged, what is the new volume in relation to the original volume?

(13) Find the value of: $\left(\frac{2}{3}\right)^{-6}\left(\frac{16}{27}\right)^2$

(14) Solve for x: log(4x) = 2

(15) What is the slope of the line segment connecting the points (17,-16) and (2,24)?

(16) The specific heat c (per unit volume) of a metal is described by the formula $c = aT + bT^3$, where T = absolute temperature and a,b = constants. If T is doubled, is the new specific heat less than eight times, exactly eight times, or more than eight times greater than the original specific heat?

(17) Calculate the slope of the line graphed below (use two points indicated):

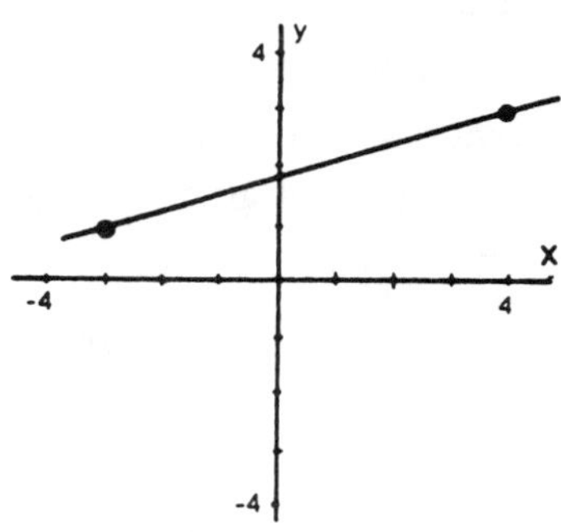

(18) Which of the following slopes has the largest magnitude (neglecting signs)?

(a) 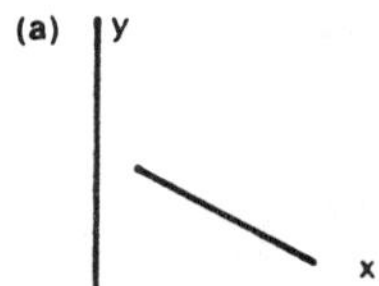

(b) 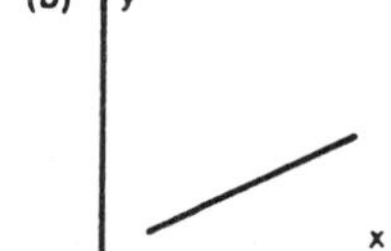

(c) 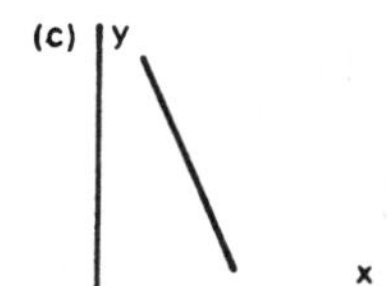

(d) 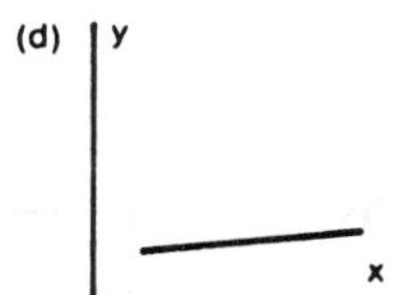

(19) Which points, if any, are: maximum points? minimum points? inflection points?

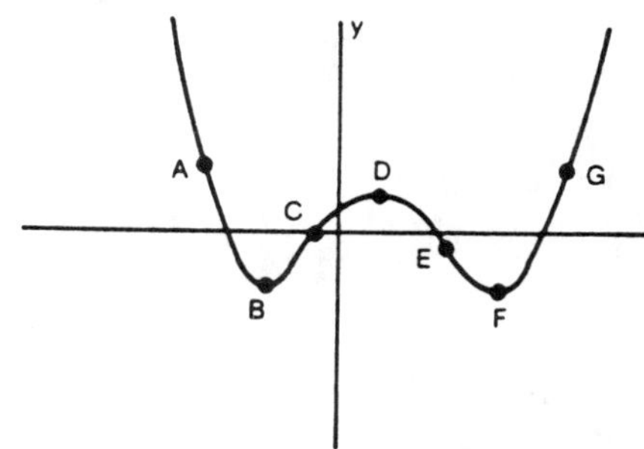

(20) A linear graph can be algebraically described by the equation $2 + 9y = 15x$. What are the slope and y-intercept of this line?

(21) The ideal-gas law for one mole of an ideal gas is $PV = RT$. For a constant temperature T, the P,V-graph looks like:

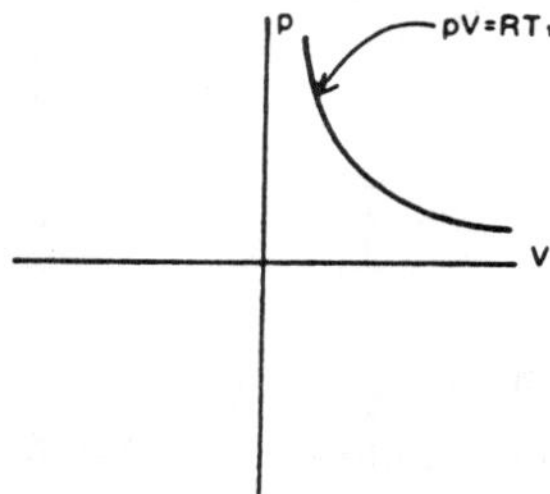

On the basis of this graph, for constant temperatures T_2 and T_3 such that $T_2 < T_1$ and $T_3 > T_1$, draw possible P,V-graphs.

(22) The relation between two variables, C and t, can be described by the equation:

$$C = C_o(1 - e^{-kt})$$

where C_o,k = positive constants. Looking at $t \geq 0$ only, how does the slope of this curve vary? (Hint: to graph this equation and analyze how its slope varies, split the graph into three regions: $kt << 1$ — in this region $e^{-kt} \approx 1 - kt$, $kt \approx 1$, and $kt >> 1$). Plot a segmental graph and explain the connection between various segments.

(23) A semi-log plot of $y = a(10)^{bx}$ has a y-intercept = 64 and a slope = 3. What are a and b?

(24) Find b:

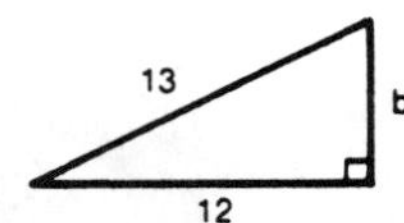

(25) Evaluate: sin 30° cos 60° - tan 45° sin 90°

(26) Find $\frac{\tan A}{\tan(A+B)}$:

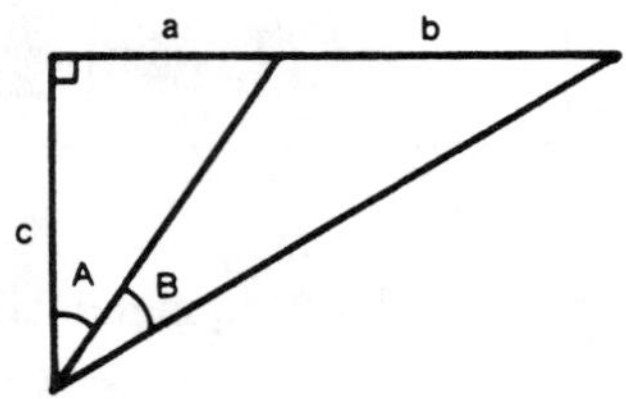

(27) What are the x- and y-components of A + B?

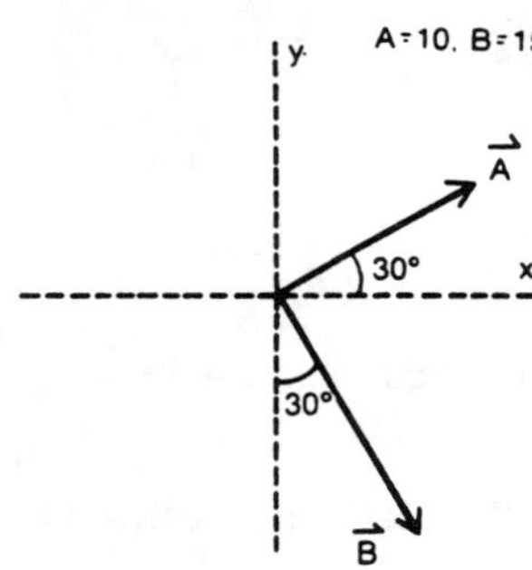

(28) Convert 2 tons to grams.

(29) Convert 100 ft. to centimeters.

(30) Convert 128 fluid ounces to milliliters.

(31) The electric potential V between two points is given by the formula V = Er, where E = electric field and r is the distance between the two points. The electric field is given by $E = \frac{F}{q}$, where F = the electrical force and q = charge. The unit of V is the volt. What is the volt equal to in terms of mass (m), length (l), time (t), and charge (q)?

(32) Solve for R: $\frac{1}{R} = \frac{1}{R_1} + \frac{1}{R_2}$. Having a formula for R, rewrite the formula explicitly in terms of R_1 and $\left(\frac{R_1}{R_2}\right)$.

As the value of $\left(\frac{R_1}{R_2}\right)$ goes to infinity, what value does R approach?

Solutions to the Mathematics Concepts Test

(1) $x = 6a^2b^3 \quad x^3 = 216a^6b^9$

$$\sqrt[3]{x^3} = \sqrt[3]{216a^6b^9} = \sqrt[3]{216}\ a^{6/3}b^{9/3}$$

$$x = 6a^2b^3$$

(2) $y = -\frac{1}{3} \qquad \frac{1}{y-1} + \frac{1}{y+2} = \frac{1}{5(y-1)}$

$$5(y+2) + 5(y-1) = y + 2$$

$$10y + 5 = y + 2$$

$$9y = -3\ ;\ y = -\frac{1}{3}$$

(3) $b = \frac{1}{2} \qquad 6 - 2(3-2(5-3(b-2)-4)-2) - 1 = 50b$

$$5 - 2(3-2(1-3b+6)-2) = 50b$$

$$5 - 2(1-14+6b) = 50b$$

$$5 + 26 - 12b = 50b$$

$$31 = 62b\ ;\ b = \frac{31}{62} = \frac{1}{2}$$

(4) $V_2 = 6V_1 \qquad$ Let $V_1 = \frac{p_1\cos\theta_1}{r_1^2}$, $V_2 = \frac{p_2\cos\theta_2}{r_2^2}$,

$$\text{then } \frac{V_2}{V_1} = \frac{\frac{p_2\cos\theta_2}{r_2^2}}{\frac{p_1\cos\theta_1}{r_1^2}} = \frac{p_2}{p_1}\cdot\frac{\cos\theta_2}{\cos\theta_1}\cdot\frac{r_1^2}{r_2^2}$$

$$\cos\theta_1 = \cos 0° = 1,\ \cos\theta_2 = \cos 60° = \frac{1}{2}$$

$$p_2 = 3p_1 \text{ and } r_2 = \frac{1}{2}r_1$$

$$\frac{V_2}{V_1} = \frac{3p_1}{p_1}\cdot\frac{\frac{1}{2}}{1}\cdot\frac{r_1^2}{\left(\frac{1}{2}r_1\right)^2} = 3\cdot\left(\frac{1}{2}\right)\cdot 4 = 6\text{, or } V_2 = 6V_1$$

(5) $x = 350$ mg The dose of the drug is directly proportional to body weight.The ratio of drug dose to body weight is $\frac{5 \text{ mg}}{1 \text{ kg}}$; therefore,

if x = the amount of the drug for a person weighing 70 kg, then:

$$\frac{5 \text{ mg}}{1 \text{ kg}} = \frac{x}{70 \text{ kg}} \rightarrow \quad x = 350 \text{ mg}$$

(6) $x = 7.5$ mg The dose of the drug is directly proportional to body weight.

The ratio of drug dose to body weight is $\frac{5 \text{ mg}}{40 \text{ kg}}$; therefore,

if x = the amount of the drug for a person weighing 60 kg, then:

$$\frac{5 \text{ mg}}{40 \text{ kg}} = \frac{x}{60 \text{ kg}} \rightarrow \quad x = 7.5 \text{ mg}$$

(7) $p = 40\%$ increase The price of A in 1986 = \$64; its price in 1987 = \$89.60.
If p = % increase, then: \$89.60 =

$$\$64\left(1 + \frac{p}{100}\right). \; 1.4 = 1 + \frac{p}{100} \rightarrow p = 40\% \text{ increase}$$

(8) 4.17×10^{-4} $4 \times 10^{-4} + 17 \times 10^{-6}$

$$= 4 \times 10^{-4} + .17 \times 10^{-4} = 4.17 \times 10^{-4}$$

(9) 1 $(2 \times 10^{4})(5 \times 10^{-5})$

$$= 10 \times 10^{4-5} = 10^{1} \times 10^{-1} = 10^{1-1} = 10^{0} = 1$$

(10) $x = 8 \times 10^{21}$ $x = \left(\frac{5 \times 10^{3}}{25 \times 10^{-5}}\right)^{3} = \left(\frac{5}{25} \times 10^{3-(-5)}\right)^{3}$

$$= (.2 \times 10^{8})^{3} = (2 \times 10^{7})^{3} = 8 \times 10^{21}$$

(11) 7.15025×10^{3} $7.15 \times 10^{3} + 0.025 \times 10^{1}$

$$= 7.15 \times 10^{3} + 0.00025 \times 10^{3}$$

$$= 7.15025 \times 10^{3}$$

(12) $V_2 = \frac{8}{3} V_1$ Let $V_1 = \frac{n_1 R T_1}{P_1}$ and $V_2 = \frac{n_2 R T_2}{P_2}$, then

$$\frac{V_2}{V_1} = \frac{\frac{n_2 R T_2}{P_2}}{\frac{n_1 R T_1}{P_1}} = \frac{n_2}{n_1} \bullet \frac{T_2}{T_1} \bullet \frac{P_1}{P_2}$$

$$n_2 = n_1. P_2 = \frac{3}{4} P_1 \, . \, T_2 = 2T_1$$

$$\frac{V_2}{V_1} = \frac{n_2}{n_2} \bullet \frac{2T_1}{T_1} \bullet \frac{P_1}{\frac{3}{4} P_1} = 1 \bullet 2 \bullet \left(\frac{4}{3}\right) = \frac{8}{3}, \text{ or } V_2 = \frac{8}{3} V_1$$

(13) 4 $\left(\frac{2}{3}\right)^{-6} \left(\frac{16}{27}\right)^{2} = \left(\frac{2}{3}\right)^{-6} \left(\frac{2^4}{3^3}\right)^{2} = \frac{2^{-6} \bullet 2^{8}}{3^{-6} \bullet 3^{6}} = \frac{2^2}{3^0} = 4$

(14) $x = 25$ $\qquad \log(4x) = 2$

$4x = 10^2 = 100 \qquad \rightarrow \qquad x = 25$

(15) $m = \frac{-8}{3}$ $\quad$ Let $(x_1,y_1) = (17,-16)$ and $(x_2,y_2) = (2,24)$;

$$m = \frac{y_2-y_1}{x_2-x_1} = \frac{24-(-16)}{2-17} = \frac{40}{-15} = \frac{-8}{3}.$$

(16) Less than 8x. $\qquad$ Let $c_1 = aT_1 + bT_1^3$ and $c_2 = aT_2 + bT_2^3$; $T_2 = 2T_1$.

$$\frac{c_2}{c_1} = \frac{aT_2 + bT_2^3}{aT_1 + bT_1^3} = \frac{2aT_1 + 8bT_1^3}{aT_1 + bT_1^3} < \frac{8aT_1 + 8bT_1^3}{aT_1 + bT_1^3} = 8$$

Thus, $c_2 < 8c_1$.

(17) $m = \frac{2}{7}$ $\qquad$ The two points on the graph are $(x_1,y_1) = (-3,1)$ and $(x_2,y_2) = (4,3)$:

$$m = \frac{y_2 - y_1}{x_2 - x_1} = \frac{3-1}{4-(-3)} = \frac{2}{7}$$

(18) $\quad$ c $\qquad$ By inspection, graph (c) has the slope of the largest magnitude.

(19) Based on the discussion of maximum, minimum, and inflection points in section 4.2.3.3:

D is a maximum point;

B, F are minimum points;

C, E are inflection points.

(20) $m = \frac{5}{3}, b = -\frac{2}{9}$

$2 + 9y = 15x$; putting this in slope-intercept form:

$y = \frac{5}{3}x - \frac{2}{9}$. The slope, $m = \frac{5}{3}$ and the y-intercept $b = -\frac{2}{9}$.

(21) $pV = RT$ is a hyperbolic graph when T = constant. If $T_2 < T_1$ and $T_3 > T_1$, possible graphs for $pV = RT_2$ and $pV = RT_3$ are:

(See discussion of hyperbolic graphs)

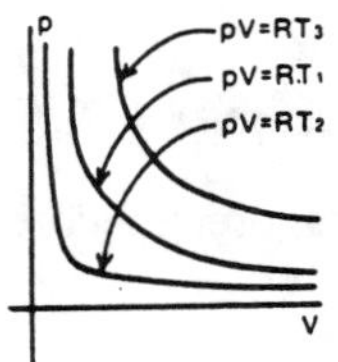

(22) $C = C_o(1 - e^{-kt})$; C_o,k = positive constants. Splitting the graph (for $t \geq 0$) into three regions corresponding to:

(A) $\quad kt \ll 1, C = C_o(1 - e^{-kt}) \cong C_o(1-(1-kt)) = C_okt$ $\qquad$ (linear);
(note that we used the approximation $e^{-kt} \approx 1-kt$ for $kt \ll 1$)

(B) $\quad kt \approx 1, C = C_o(1 - e^{-kt})$ $\qquad$ (no approximation);

(C) $kt >> 1, C = C_o(1 - e^{-kt}) \cong C_o$ (zero slope).
(note that $e^{-kt} \cong 0$ for $kt >> 1$)

To graph this equation, use the three regions above. For region A, the graph looks linear; for region C, the graph looks flat (zero slope); and, for region B, these two partial graphs are connected by a smooth curve. The graph looks (not to scale) like this:

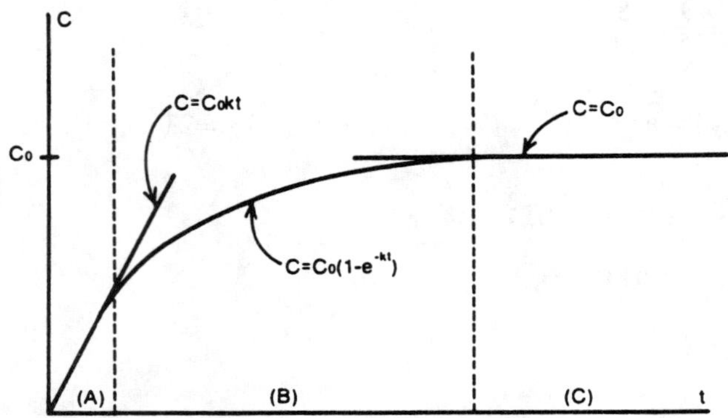

(Assign different values to 'kt' from 0 to +5 and see if you can get segments I, II, and III, and then join them with a smooth curve.)

The slope starts off at a finite ($= C_ok$), nearly constant value (region A). As t increases, the slope decreases (region B) until it becomes zero (region C).

$kt << 1$ $C = C_okt$ (segment I)

For region A $0 \leq kt \leq 0.5$

$kt \approx 1$ $C = C_o(1 - e^{-kt})$ (segment II)

For region B $0.5 < kt < 3$

$kt >> 1$ $C = C_o$ (segment III)

For region C $3 \leq kt \leq \infty$

(23) $y = 64(10)^{3x}$ For the y-intercept ($x = 0$), $y = a(10)^{b \cdot 0} = a = 64$. The slope of the semi-log plot $= b = 3$.

(24) $b = 5$ Using the Pythagorean theorem:

$12^2 + b^2 = 13^2$

$b^2 = 13^2 - 12^2 = 169 - 144 = 25$

$b = 5$

(25) $-\frac{3}{4}$ $\sin 30° \cos 60° - \tan 45° \sin 90°$

$= \left(\frac{1}{2}\right)\left(\frac{1}{2}\right) - (1)(1) = \frac{1}{4} - 1 = -\frac{3}{4}$

(26) $\frac{\tan A}{\tan(A+B)} = \frac{a}{a+b}$ $\qquad \frac{\tan A}{\tan(A+B)} = \frac{\frac{a}{c}}{\frac{a+b}{c}} = \frac{a}{a+b}$

(27) Recomposing the vectors $\vec{A}$ and $\vec{B}$:

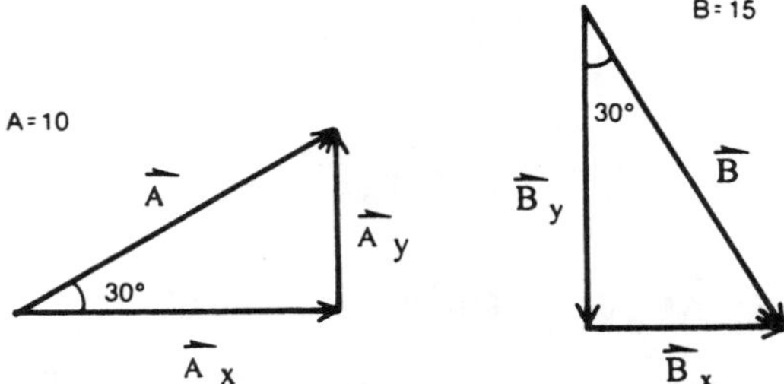

$$A_x + B_x = A \cos 30° + B \sin 30° = 10\left(\frac{\sqrt{3}}{2}\right) + 15\left(\frac{1}{2}\right) = 5\sqrt{3} + 7.5$$

$$A_y + B_y = A \sin 30° - B \cos 30° = 10\left(\frac{1}{2}\right) - 15\left(\frac{\sqrt{3}}{2}\right) = 5 - \frac{15\sqrt{3}}{2}$$

(28) $1.816\text{x}10^6$ g $\qquad (2 \text{ tons})\left(\frac{2000 \text{ lb}}{1 \text{ ton}}\right)\left(\frac{454 \text{ g}}{1 \text{ lb}}\right) = \frac{(2)(2000)(454)}{1} \text{ g}$

$= 1{,}816{,}000 \text{ g} = 1.816\text{x}10^6 \text{ g}$

(29) 3048 cm $\qquad (100 \text{ ft})\left(\frac{12 \text{ in}}{1 \text{ ft}}\right)\left(\frac{2.54 \text{ cm}}{1 \text{ in}}\right) = \frac{(100)(12)(2.54)}{1} \text{ cm}$

$= 3048 \text{ cm}$

(30) 3800 ml $\qquad (128 \text{ oz})\left(\frac{1 \text{ pt}}{16 \text{ oz}}\right)\left(\frac{1 \text{ qt}}{2 \text{ pt}}\right)\left(\frac{0.95 \text{ liters}}{1 \text{ qt}}\right)\left(\frac{1000 \text{ ml}}{1 \text{ liter}}\right)$

$= \frac{(128)(0.95)(1000)}{(16)(2)} \text{ ml} = 3800 \text{ ml}$

(31) $\frac{m \bullet l^2}{q \bullet t^2}$ volts $= V = Er = \frac{Fr}{q} = \frac{(ma)r}{q}$ for units analysis

$$= \frac{(m)\left(\frac{1}{t^2}\right)(l)}{q} = \frac{m \bullet l^2}{q \bullet t^2}$$

(32) $\frac{1}{R} = \frac{1}{R_1} + \frac{1}{R_2}$ $\quad\rightarrow\quad$ $R_1R_2 = R(R_1 + R_2)$

$R = \frac{R_1R_2}{R_1+R_2}$. Alternatively, $R = \frac{R_1}{\left(\frac{R_1}{R_2}\right)+1}$ (as requested).

As $\left(\frac{R_1}{R_2}\right) \rightarrow \infty$, $R = \frac{R_1}{\left(\frac{R_1}{R_2}\right)+1} \rightarrow \frac{R_1}{\frac{R_1}{R_2}} = R_2$.

4.3 DATA ANALYSIS IN PHYSICAL/BIOLOGICAL SCIENCES

This part of chapter 4 contains two different kinds of information. Concepts 23-26 indicate how to think about the three basic formats of data presentation. They should be read carefully, and right now, as they may change the way you work with data. Concepts 27 through 32 is a brief encyclopedia of data analysis techniques. It should be reviewed quickly and then used for reference whenever you need it. Most of the material in this section should already be familiar to you.

The new MCAT, as mentioned earlier does not include a separate Quantitative Skills subtest. The data analysis tasks, according to the MCAT Student Manual and the AAMC practice tests boil down to the following list of questions:

- Are you able to interpret information presented in graphic or tabular format?
- Are you familiar with various types of data, such as graphs, tables or figures that are presented in passage-based problems?
- What are the basic principles and methods used in the presentation of data?
- Can you explain, identify or compare the components of graphs, tables, figures, diagrams and charts?
- Are you capable of identifying trends and relationships inherent in data?
- Do you always try to understand and determine the background knowledge relevant to a particular interpretation of data?
- Do you know how to select the most appropriate format for representing numerical information?
- Can you perform calculations on a set of numerical data for statistical analysis?

    (i) Do you know how to determine the arithmetic average, range, and standard deviation?
    (ii) Do you understand statistical association and correlation as applied to multiple data sets (from various instruments or different experimental investigations)?

The practice MCAT items have aimed at testing the student's skills on one or more of the above topics. The student should focus on the above skills and keep a closer eye on graphs obtained from plotting complex functions. Science rules and laws lead to quadratic or exponential functions which should be thoroughly reviewed. Histograms and bar charts are not very common in scientific analysis. In both physical and biological sciences the data collected is normally arranged in multiple columns and plotted as line graphs or functional plots in most laboratory research.

The test items following each passage may cover topics ranging from biological to physical sciences; the data displays will be in many different forms. In this section we will focus on data displays: how to interpret them and how to relate information they contain to other sources of information that may be in the test item or problem. Questions that ask you to relate and synthesize information coming from several different sources are a part of what is new on the MCAT and you may have had very little previous experience with these complex passage-based items.

MCAT MATHEMATICS CONCEPT 23: Reading Data Tables

The purpose of a data table is to show how two or more variables are related by giving several specific instances. In some cases you will need to do nothing more than read some numbers off the tables; we assume you know how to do that. But other questions may expect you to do much more. To understand a table you should look for a pattern or relationship between the variables. For example, one variable may always be larger than the other; there is usually a quantitative relationship such as variable x is three times variable y. To find this relation read from left to right across the columns, not down along one column. Look for relationships by trying to derive the elements of one column from the other. On multiple column tables compare two columns at a time. Occasionally one column will depend on the values in two or more other columns but this level of complexity is less likely to appear on a timed test and should only be examined after the first possibility has been examined.

TV Viewers	TV Soap Operas No.Programs/Day	Pre-Exam Hours Studied	Exam Score by Percent
Peter	2	80	60
Susan	3	90	60
Howard	0	95	95
Beth	1	85	75
Paul	0	45	45
Henry	2	60	40
Carol	1	90	80

Fig. 4.10a—Data Table Showing Four Variables

First notice that there is no pattern to the numbers in the vertical columns. There is also no clear pattern between the TV viewed and the hours studied. There is a weak pattern between the hours studied and the exam scores. The three highest scores were from people who watched one or fewer programs per day so TV viewing may be lowering exam performance. See if you can determine a numerical relation between the hours studied, soap operas viewed and the exam score.

Spreadsheets

Spreadsheets look like data tables but they are quite different. In a data table all the rows are of the same character; each is a specific example of values the variables can hold. In the example above, each row represents a person. On a spreadsheet each row may contain a very different kind of information from that in the other rows. The first row might be the number of days spent on a trip; the second row the cost of hotel rooms; and the third various nondeductible expenses. While it is usually best to begin by looking for relationships that exist across columns, it may also be useful to search for relationships within a column (the longer the trip the more paid for hotels).

Data tables and spreadsheets are sometimes represented in pictorial form. The two most common examples are the histogram and the pie chart. The histogram below illustrates the first column of the "TV Soap Operas" data table above in Concept #23. Pie charts are used to illustrate how a total is divided among its component parts; it is often marked in percentages of the whole. The pie chart below also displays the first column of the "TV Soap Operas" data table.

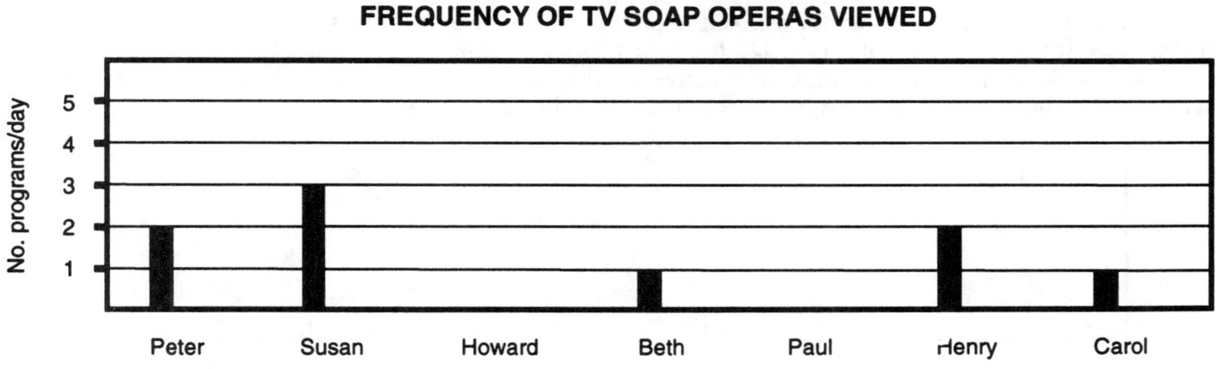

Fig. 4.10b—Histogram Showing Frequency Analysis

DISTRIBUTION OF TOTAL TV SOAP OPERAS VIEWED

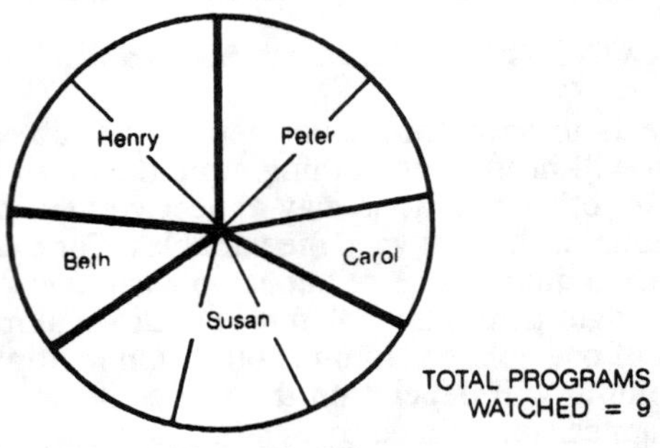

Fig. 4.10c—Pie Chart

MCAT MATHEMATICS CONCEPT 24: Graphs and Data Tables

Graphs and data tables are closely related. A data table is a list of specific points that could be plotted on a graph. Graphs usually contain more information than tables because they show how the points are connected, i.e., what intermediate values exist. But graphs can be deceptive, if the lines connecting the points were simply drawn in by hand there is no guarantee that the real data will choose to follow the line. The graph may suggest that values are known in regions where no data has been measured.

Before drawing a line through a collection of plotted points it is important to know how precisely each point has been located. This is usually indicated by error bars. The line may go through any part of the error bar and still fit the point. Graphs 1 and 2 show how the same points may suggest different graphs as the size of the error bars changes. The components of a graph are: Horizontal and vertical axes, origin, scales, the graphical line connecting various data points.

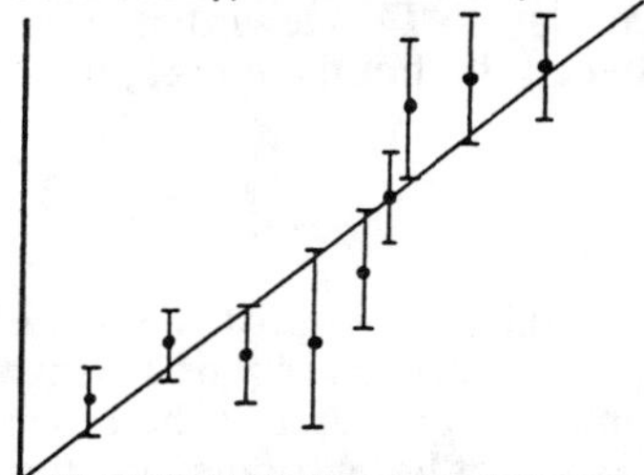

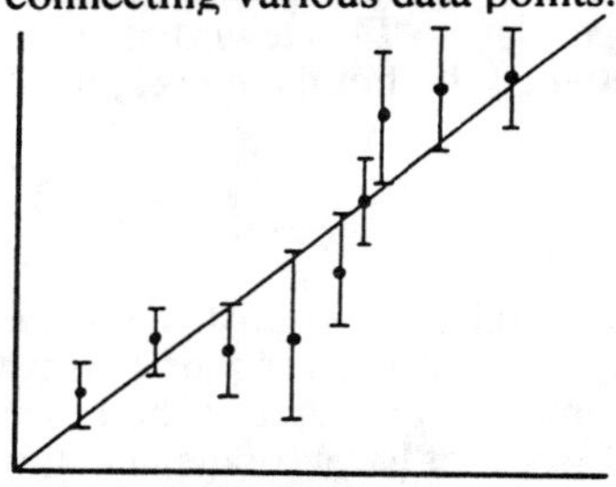

Fig. 4.11a—Graph 1

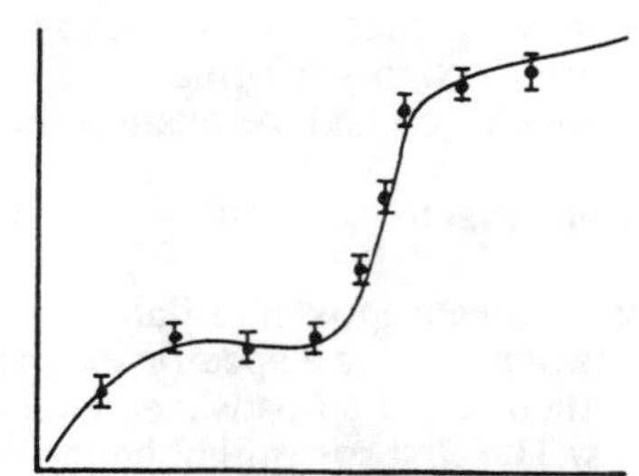

Fig. 4.11b—Graph 2

The simplest type of graph is a straight line. It is obtained from data that satisfies the familiar equation $y = mx + b$. You should be very comfortable with this sort of graph, but if you are not, review the math concepts in this book or in any college algebra text. The most important characteristic of a linear function is its slope. It will tell you what factor to multiply x by in order to obtain y. It may then be necessary to add a correcting constant b, but the fundamental essence of the relationship is contained in the slope.

Because straight line graphs are the easiest to draw and understand, data is often plotted so as to make the graph appear to be linear. Graphs 3 and 4 represent the same data, but graph 4 has an x-axis made up of values for t^2 rather than t. Another common transformation is to plot log x rather than x. This is particularly useful in biology where many functions are logarithmic. Do not forget to check how the graph axes are labeled. Avoid the common mistake of reading the graph as y versus x, when in fact it is y versus x^2. In the first case y will increase at roughly the same rate as x, in the second case it will increase much faster.

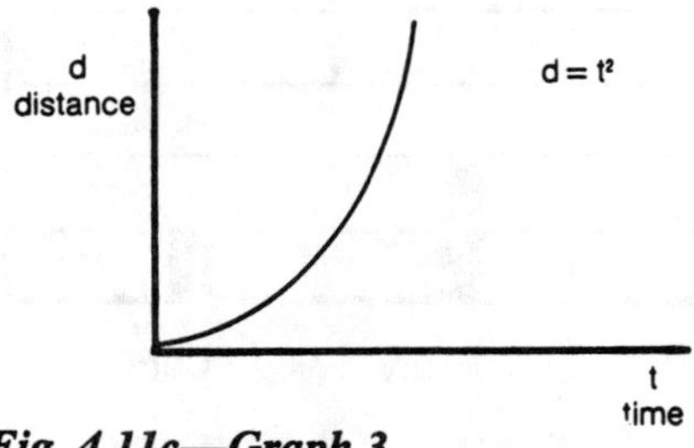

Fig. 4.11c—Graph 3

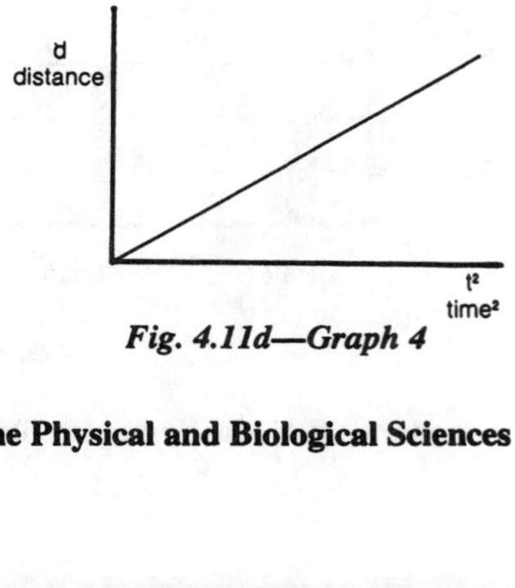

d
distance

t²
time²

Fig. 4.11d—Graph 4

You should be familiar with a number of curves representing mathematical functions, including y vs. x^2 (quadratic), x^3 (cubic), ln x (logarithmic), e^x (exponential), and the trig functions. In each case you should be able to compare these non-linear functions with a linear function; the y values in y vs. x^2 increase faster than in y vs. x; on the other hand y vs. ln x increases less rapidly than the linear case. You should also understand how the slope changes, it keeps getting steeper in y vs. x^2, it increases then decreases and then increases again in y vs. x^3

Complicated graphs can be broken up and viewed as a composite of several linear pieces or a mixture of basic forms: quadratic, cubic, etc. The common "s" curve for population growth starts out as an exponential and then switches to logarithmic as predators and a limited food supply restrict growth.

MCAT MATHEMATICS CONCEPT 25: Interpretation of Equations

Equations can be very complicated, but as with graphs, they can be broken down into simple parts. Unlike graphs, where the parts are visually separate, the sections of an equation are often all mixed up. There are three basic forms to consider; y may depend on: x plus something, x times something and something divided by x. In the first case x and y increase at the same rate; in the second, one variable increases faster than the other; in the third case one variable increases as the other decreases.

The most important thing to remember about interpreting equations is that they are rules for *calculating* numbers. They tell you what to *do* to some numbers to generate a new number. The equation: y = 8x tells you to take a value for x and to multiply it by 8 to generate the value for y. Although glancing at the equation may make you think that the x is bigger than the y the reverse is in fact the case. This is a very common mistake so take extra care to avoid it.

The following two samples will test whether you understand how to read equations.

1. Six out of ten doctors recommend brand A. Write an equation relating the number of doctors recommending brand A to the number of doctors recommending other brands.

2. In a certain large hospital, the number of patients with smallpox (P_{sp}) is related to the number of patients with AIDS (P_a) by the equation:

$$1{,}000\ P_a = P_{sp}$$

What is unusual about this situation? (Answers at the end of the section.)

Complicated equations can be understood by holding everything constant except for one pair of variables. For example, if

$$z = [a(u + v) - s^2]/t\,(w - b),$$

then z depends linearly on u (or v) and inversely on t (or w). To see this, lump everything together that is not the variable of interest.

$$\begin{aligned} z &= [a(u + v) - s^2]/t(w - b) \\ &= [au/t(w - b)] + (av - s^2)/t(w - b) \\ &= ku + c \\ \text{where } k &= a/t(w - b) \text{ and } c = [av - s^2]/t(w - b) \end{aligned}$$

With practice you will learn to make these transformations very quickly in your head so that you can just look at a complicated expression and see how the different variables affect the value of the total expression.

Functions are often written in the form y = f(x) = x + 2, instead of y = x + 2. For complex expressions this notation can be very useful and you should know what it means and how to use it. The term f(u,v,w) means that the function f depends on the variables u, v and w and not on others. In the expression above for z, it would mean that you should consider u, v and w to be variables and the other letters to be constants. On the other hand, if we had written f(s,t), it would mean that u, v, w were constants and that only s and t would be considered variables.

Tables, graphs, and equations all tell the same type of story but each has its own particular format. You should know how to relate these three notation systems. Practice taking information from one system and expressing it in the other. Exercises to practice this skill can be found in *Beyond Problem Solving and Comprehension* by Whimbey and Lochhead (see Section 4.6).

Answers to Interpretation of Equations Problems

1. Correct answers are: $4D_A = 6D_X$ or, $D_A/D_X = 6/4$.

   Common incorrect answers include:
   $6D_A = 4D_X$, $6D_A + 4D_X = 10$, $6D_A = 10D_X$, $D_A/D_X = 6/10$.

2. This equation indicates that there are many more cases of smallpox than of AIDS: 1,000 people with smallpox for every one who has AIDS. Since smallpox has been eradicated world-wide, cases of it are very rare. AIDS on the other hand is increasingly common. The expected ratio would be the reverse of that indicated by the equation.

MCAT MATHEMATICS CONCEPT 26: Other modes for displaying data

We have already considered the principle designs and methods for displaying data, but there are many variations on these. In the following sections we review those variations most likely to appear on the MCAT. Try to view these not as a collection of different devices but rather as extensions of the basic techniques described above. Do not dwell unnecessarily on sections you already understand; look for topics where you feel you may be weak and spend time there. Solving problems will teach you far more than reading text; so get to the problems quickly and come back to the text as you find you need it.

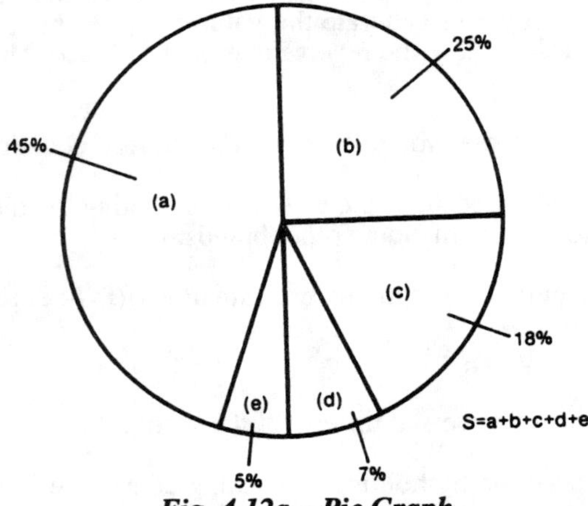

Fig. 4.12a—Pie Graph

4.3.1 Data Presentation

Percentage or Pie Graphs

Percentage graphs in the form of circles (also called pie graphs) are used to represent the breakdown of a quantity into its component parts. A total quantity S is represented by the whole area of a circle; the percentage that each of its components—say a, b, c, d, and e—is of S is represented by a corresponding fraction of the area of the circle (in the form of a sector):

Pie graphs provide a visual reinforcement of numerical percentages.

Bar Graphs and Histograms

Bar graphs or histograms are very common and may be constructed in several alternate forms. In general, they are used to show relations between distinct groups by virtue of the length or height of a rectangle. In other words, one coordinate represents the groups being compared while the other coordinate represents the quantity of interest. The various forms that histograms can take include:

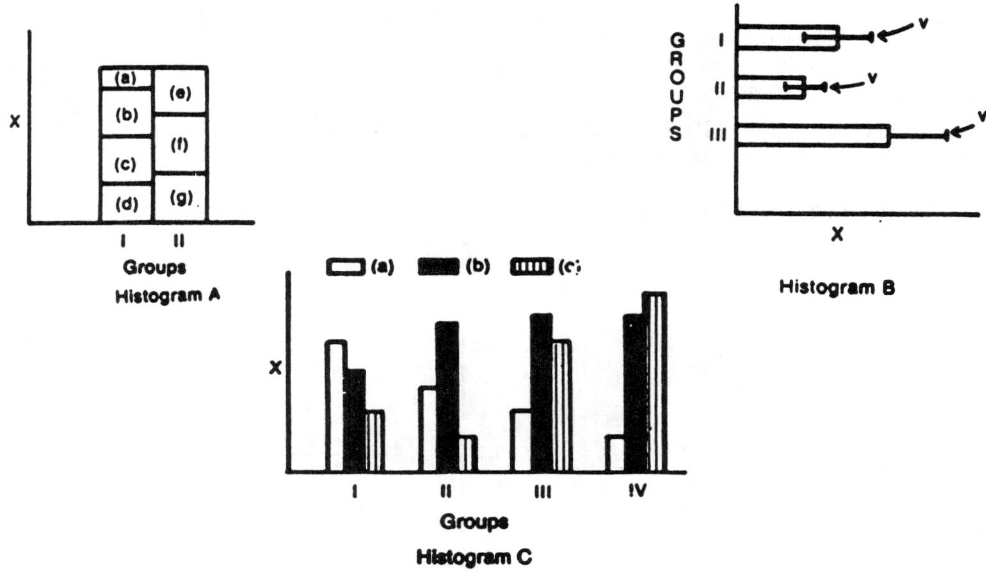

Fig. 4.12b—Histogram Types

In all three histograms, X is the variable of interest. In histogram A, two groups are being compared. Since the totals, a + b + c + d and e + f + g respectively, for both groups are identical, this bar graph is actually a type of percentage graph. That is, the data in this bar graph could be alternatively presented as two pie graphs, one for each group. Histogram B is straightforward: three groups are compared to each other with respect to the variable X. In histogram C, each "bar" represents the specification of the value of three variables: X, group number, and a third variable that can be specified as a, b, or c. This type of bar graph format could represent two different situations: (1) it might represent the comparison of four groups where each group as a totality is separated into components a, b, and c; or (2) it might represent the comparison of twelve groups that are specified by a group number and by a third variable that can be specified as a, b, or c. Remember that the group number is a variable that might specify a group of subjects in an experiment, an age group, etc. Sometimes a logical order exists for the groups, e.g., sex or ethnic background. As an added point, the lines marked "v" on histogram B represent the margin of error in X for each group. Margins of error are sometimes included on graphs—see Concept #20 for a discussion of error.

Presentation of Data Points by Graphs

In a histogram such as B above, the value of X for each group might be some sort of "average" value of X for the members in that group. We might instead wish to graph the data such that the value of X for each member of a group was represented. This graph would take the form:

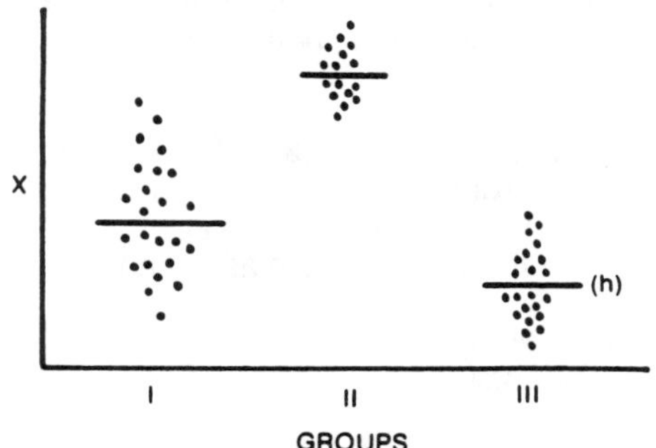

Fig. 4.12c—Grouped Data Graph

Each dot (circle) represents one member of the group and its value for the variable X. The horizontal spread of the points is just to prevent crowding and is meaningless, i.e., only the points themselves have meaning. The horizontal line (h) usually gives the average value or some similar measure of central tendency (see Concept #29) for that group. An important value of this data presentation is that it gives a sense of overlap (or separation) between the different groups, and this is often crucial in medicine.

Example 1. (Biological Sciences Data: Biology)
Two groups of 35-year-old subjects, one of men and one of women, have their blood cholesterol levels (mg/100 ml) measured. The data is:

Group I (men): 195, 198, 199, 196, 195, 196, 191, 194, 195, 196.
Group II (women): 196, 193, 194, 201, 202, 205, 204, 202, 199, 204.

Represent these data as data points by group:

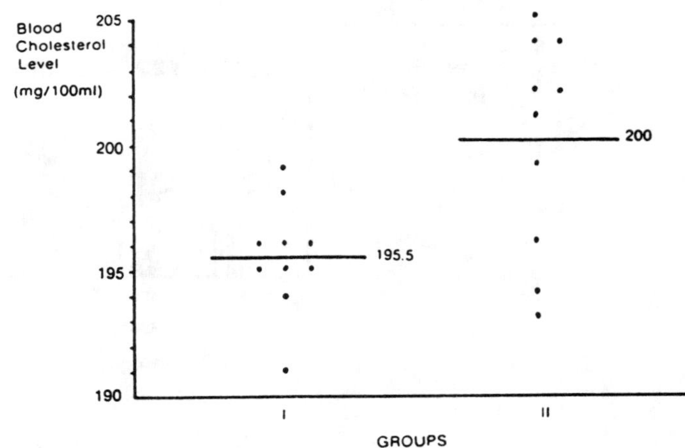

The horizontal line for each group represents the average blood cholesterol level for that group.

Graphs Involving "Before and After" Groups

Another graph often found in medical literature is used to show the change of a variable with a "before and after" set of conditions:

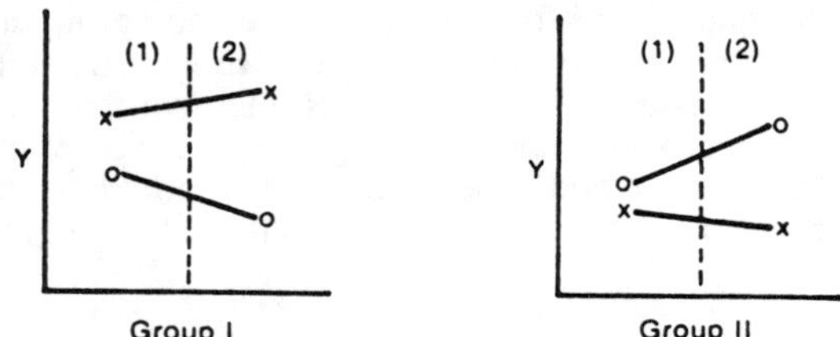

Fig. 4.12d—Before and After Graphs

In these two graphs, two groups are being looked at, Y being the variable of interest. Region (1) is the "before" condition and region (2) is the "after" condition; o and x represent subgroups or values of other variables being assessed for each group. The only information in these graphs is at the points, e.g., x and o. The horizontal axis has no meaning as the dotted lines separate condition (1) points from condition (2) points.

Example 2. (Social Sciences Data: Psychology)
Two groups of subjects, one of boys and one of girls, are timed in solving a puzzle. Each group is divided into two age (5-year-olds and 10-year-olds) subgroups. On Day 1, the time it takes each subject to solve a standard puzzle is recorded. The next day, Day 2, they are given a similar puzzle and the time it takes each of them to solve it is again recorded. The average solution time for each age/gender group is shown below:

	Average Solution Time (minutes)	
Group I	Day 1	Day 2
Boys (5-years old)	12	10
Boys (10-years old)	3	1
Group II		
Girls (5-years old)	13	11
Girls (10-years old)	4	1

Construct "before and after" graphs from this data.

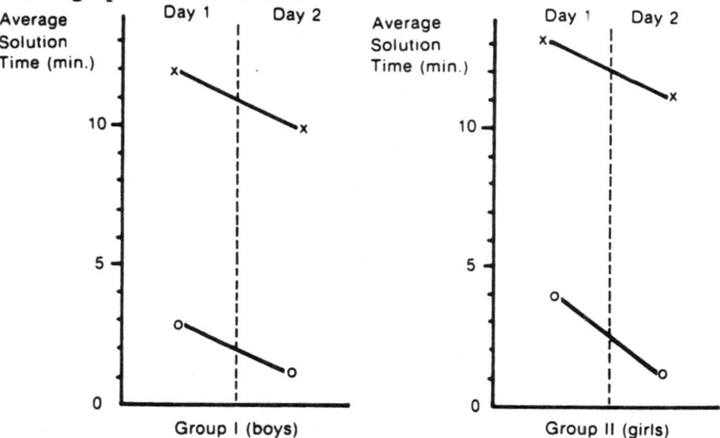

(In these graphs, x represents 5-year olds and o represents 10-year olds.)

MCAT MATHEMATICS CONCEPT 27: Determining Inherent Trends and Relationships in Data

This section returns to graphs based on the Cartesian coordinate system. Usually, when presented with a set of data involving two variables, say x and y, one plots the data as points in an xy-coordinate system in an effort to identify the relation between x and y. Unfortunately, all data so plotted do not always indicate a clear relation between x and y. The result of such a plot might be just a scatter of points or a graph with no apparent regularity:

I)

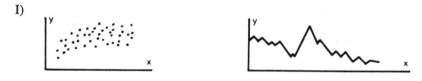

Figure 4.13a—I) Scatter Plots for Data II) Continuous Line Graph

In these cases, it is important not to over-read the graphs. It may be necessary to restrict the analysis of the data to specific regions of the graph or just to make a general observation (such as "no relationship between x and y obvious"). Some graphs of data points may allow curves to be fitted or approximately drawn through them. When eyeballing a curve through points, in general, if there are as many points at (approximately) equal distances above and below the eyeballed curve, then it should be a reasonably accurate approximation; for example:

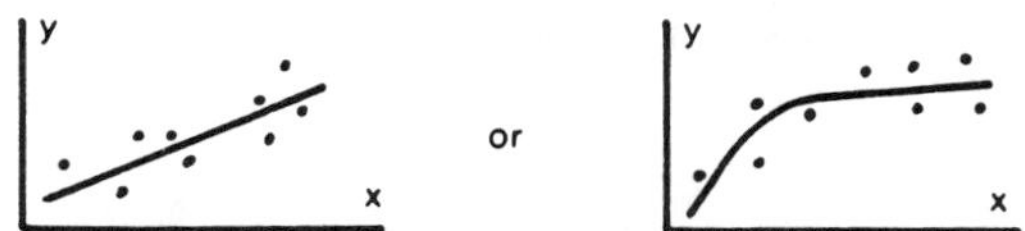

Figure 4.13b—Approximate Curve Fitting for a Scatter Plot

It should be remembered that these curve fits are tentative assignments that are best when one already has an idea of the relation (linear, hyperbolic, etc.) between x and y. Curve fitting is an art and comes with practice and experience. It involves fitting a simple equation to a set of data points.

Although it is not really related to curve fitting in its normal sense, this is a good place to observe the following: one should be aware of the graphical presentation of data in the form of a smooth curve when the curve that has been "fit" to discrete data points has no purpose other than for aesthetics. Typically, this occurs when one of the two variables, usually the independent variable, is discrete—for example, it represents years, ages, etc.—and, therefore, only the discrete data points in the graph have meaning. That is, the points on any line drawn between them do not have meaning. This is best illustrated by an example. Consider a set of data that plots the variation in a quantity y over the years between 1970 and 1979 inclusive:

The graph could also be drawn as:

or as:

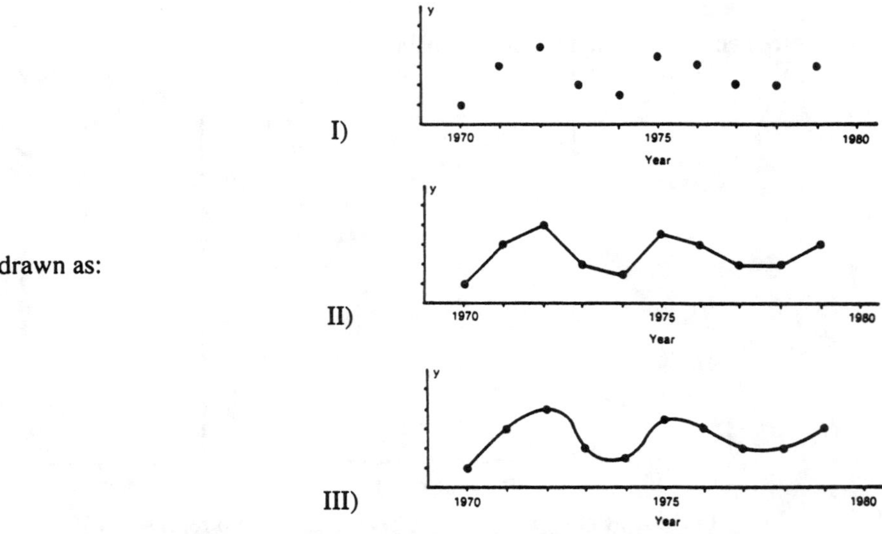

Fig. 4.13c—I) Raw Data Plot II) Broken Line Graph III) Smooth Curve

As explicitly shown in the first graph above, in the latter two graphs only the data points corresponding to each of the years have meaning; the points on the straight line segments or smooth curves drawn between them have no meaning. The smooth curve drawn through the points in the last graph drawn above only decorates (perhaps obscures?) the presentation of the real data in it.

MCAT MATHEMATICS CONCEPT 28: Statistical Data Analysis

Having discussed data presentation above in Concept #27, we turn next to the quantitative interpretation of a set of data, i.e., statistics. Before looking at how data can be analyzed, the data from three sample experiments (called A, B, and C) are presented below. In the discussion that follows, these data will be used for examples and practice problems.

Experiment A:
A psychology experiment designed to test the difficulty of a particular maze for rats is done by having ten rats run the maze. The results for their solution times to the nearest 0.1 second are:

8.3, 7.1, 8.8, 11.1, 7.0, 13.7, 9.5, 10.3, 10.8, 9.9.

Experiment B:
As a physiology experiment, the students in a medical school class have to determine the pulse (number of heartbeats/minute) of 30 patients. One student's results (which have been frequency grouped instead of being recorded individually) to the nearest 5 are:

50:	I	(1)	65:	V	(5)	80:	III	(3)
55:	II	(2)	70:	VII	(7)	85:	II	(2)
60:	III	(3)	75:	VI	(6)	90:	I	(1)

Experiment C:
In a physiological study, two groups of 35-year old subjects, one of men and one of women, have their blood cholesterol levels (mg/100 ml) measured. The data obtained (rounded to the nearest 1 mg/100 ml) are:

Group I (men):	195, 198, 199, 196, 195, 196, 191, 194, 195, 196.
Group II (women):	196, 193, 194, 201, 202, 205, 204, 202, 199, 204.

Having this data, the problem now becomes one of how to organize and analyze them so that they can be interpreted/presented to someone else clearly and meaningfully. The information above reflects two types of data that are commonly encountered in raw form (as taken during an experiment and not manipulated into graphs, means, ranges, etc.). In Experiment A, the data are of a **continuous** nature because all decimal values of time are possible (e.g., 8.003, 9.1083, etc.) even though they are not recorded. In Experiment B, the data are of a discrete, or **count** nature, because only integer values of pulse rate are possible. That is, as measured, a pulse can be 6 or 7; it cannot be 7.1 or 6.983. The fact that they are count data is particularly evident for categories such as age or sex where the number in each group is recorded. The distinction between discrete and continuous data can be important.

Problem 1.
Are the data in Experiment C count data or continuous data?

Sorting the Data:

Often it is a good idea, when presented a set of data, to make some simple observations. The easiest way to do this is to organize the data in ascending or descending order (or groups). Experiment B's data are already in ascending order; Experiment A's data will also be organized into an ascending order:

7.0, 7.1, 8.3, 8.8, 9.5, 9.9, 10.3, 10.8, 11.1, 13.7

Next, get a feeling for the data in Experiments A and B by using the simple steps below:

Experiment A.

(1) smallest value = 7.0
(2) largest value = 13.7
(3) range is 7.0 to 13.7: 13.7 - 7.0 = 6.7
(4) average might be about 10: $\frac{13.7 + 7.0}{2} \cong 10$

Experiment B.

(1) smallest value = 50
(2) largest value = 90
(3) range is 90 - 50 = 40
(4) most values are around 70, so the average is probably about 70
(5) there are few values at the ends of the range (50 and 90), but many at the middle (65 to 75)

These simple observations, which can be made rapidly, gives one some idea about the limits of the data, the average value of the data, the variability of the data, and the distribution of the data over its possible values.

Problem 2.
Do the same type of simple analysis on the data for Groups I and II in Experiment C as was done for Experiments A and B above.

Structuring the Data

If it has not already been done, the next steps in the analysis will probably be to construct graphs and/or tables from the data; our concern now is mostly with tables. When interpreting **tables**, like interpreting graphs, it is essential to read the headings at the tops and sides of the tables to determine what is being presented. Then, survey the whole table to get a feel for the data and any noticeable general trends there. Next, look for more specific points or regions of data that may be of interest. Whether or not in conjunction with a table, another simple way to structure a set of data is to determine what **percentages** (or proportions) of it meet specified classifications. This is best illustrated by examples:

Experiment A.

For some reason, you are interested in the percentage of rats with times less than 9.0 seconds:

% with times less than 9.0 seconds = $\frac{4}{10} \times 100 = 40\%$

Experiment B.

An arbitrary definition of bradycardia (slow pulse) is rates less than or equal to 60. What proportion of the patients in the sample have bradycardia?

proportion with bradycardia = $\frac{6}{30} = 0.20$

Observe that it is arbitrary whether one uses percentages or proportions. In some cases, a percentage or proportion can be used to calculate a desired result; for example:

Experiment B.

Suppose that you do not know the total number of patients in this experiment. You are told that there are 12 people with pulses 75 or greater and that this constitutes 40% of the total number of patients. How many people, N, are there in total?

$12 = \frac{40}{100} N \quad ; \quad N = 30$ patients

Experiment A.

You are told that 40% of the rats ran the maze in times greater than 10.0 seconds. How many rats, T, ran the maze in times greater than 10.0 seconds?

$$T = \frac{40}{100} \times 10 = 4$$

Problem 3.
What are the respective percentages of subjects in Groups I and II of Experiment C who had blood cholesterol levels of 196 or lower?

Once a set of data is structured in a desired format and preliminary analysis has been done, more formal statistical calculations can be made to describe it. Statistically, the two key features of a set of data are its central tendency and its variation.

Central Tendency

The central tendency of a set of data is the value it seems to approach. It is also called the "expected value." It is the one value that is taken to be representative of the whole set of data. The common measures of central tendency are the mode, the median, and the average (or mean). Only the computation of averages is required for the MCAT. The mode and the median are not required; however, their definitions will be given if they are needed on the MCAT. For this reason, you should be familiar with them beforehand.

MCAT MATHEMATICS CONCEPT 29: Calculating Expected Value or Average

The **average** takes into account directly the value of each piece of data. It is calculated by adding together each piece of data and then dividing the sum by the total number of pieces of data:

$$\text{The average} = x = \frac{x_1 + x_2 + \ldots + x_n}{n},$$

where $x_1, x_2, \ldots, x_n$ = the individual pieces of data and n = the total number of pieces of data. For example:

Experiment A.

$$\text{The average} = \frac{7.0+7.1+8.3+8.8+9.5+9.9+10.3+10.8+11.1+13.7}{10}$$

$$= (9.65) \approx 9.7$$

(remember that the eyeballed average was about 10)

Experiment B.

$$\text{The average} = \frac{1(50)+2(55)+3(60)+5(65)+7(70)+6(75)+3(80)+2(85)+1(90)}{30}$$

$$= (70.17) \approx 70$$

The **median** is the value in a set of data that is positionally halfway between the lowest and highest values in the set. It is determined by listing all the values in the set of data in ascending order and then identifying the one that is positionally in the middle. In general, when there is an even number of values in a set of data, the median is calculated by taking the average of the middle two numbers. Examples of medians are:

Experiment A.

The values in ascending order are:

7.0, 7.1, 8.3, 8.8, 9.5, 9.9, 10.3, 10.8, 11.1, 13.7

Since there is an even number of values (10), the two middle values are 9.5 and 9.9.
The median =

$$\frac{9.5 + 9.9}{2} = 9.7$$

Experiment B.

The data for this experiment are presented in ascending order in its initial presentation above. Again, since there is an even number of pieces of data, the median is the average of the two middle values (the 15th and 16th values counting from either end).

The median =

$$\frac{70 + 70}{2} = 70$$

The **mode** is the most frequent value that appears in a set of data. It exists only if one value occurs more often than any of the other values. Examples are:

Experiment A.

None exists—each value occurs only once.

Experiment B.

Mode = 70; it appears seven times, which is more often than any of the other values.

The question naturally arises as to which measure of central tendency is the best; the answer is that it depends on the distribution of the data. Consider three sets of data, which are presented graphically in histograms, where N = the frequency of a particular value of the variable x:

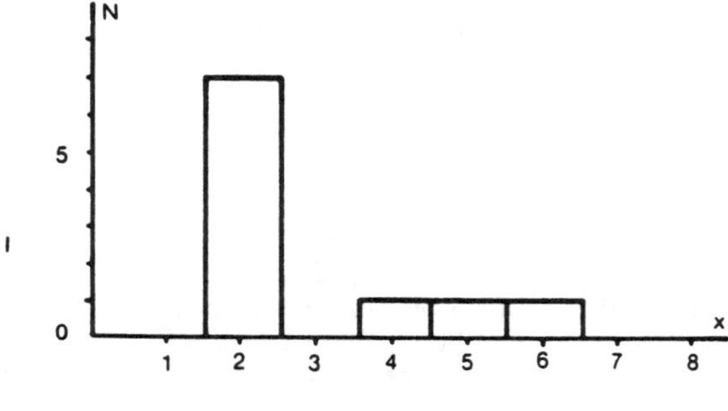

$$\text{mean} = 2.9 = \frac{7(2)+1(4)+1(5)+1(6)}{7+1+1+1} \approx 3$$

median = 2

mode = 2

data = 2,2,2,2,2,2,2,4,5,6

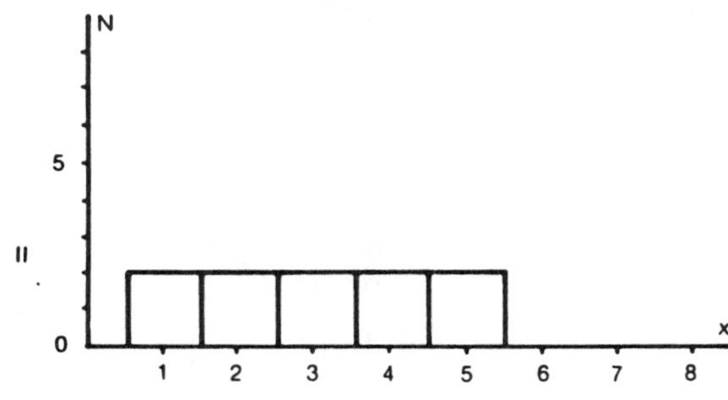

$$\text{mean} = 3 = \frac{2(1)+2(2)+2(3)+2(4)+2(5)}{2+2+2+2+2}$$

median = 3

one mode does not exist

data = 1,1,2,2,3,3,4,4,5,5

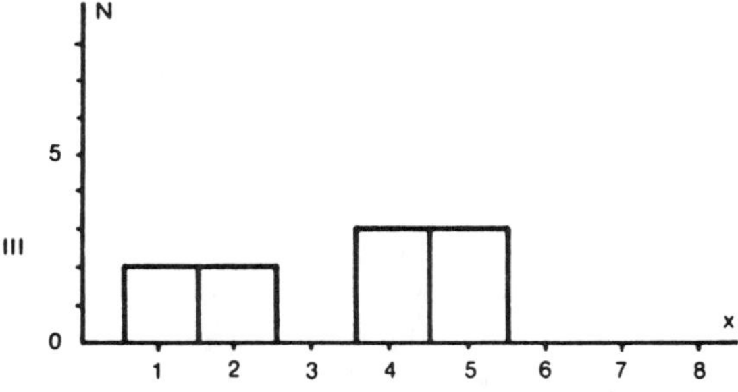

$$\text{mean} = 3.3 \cong 3 = \frac{2(1)+2(2)+3(4)+3(5)}{2+2+3+3}$$

median = 4

two modes = 4,5 (bi-modal)

data = 1,1,2,2,4,4,4,5,5,5

Fig. 4.14—Histograms Showing Mean, Median, and Mode

For the data in histogram I, both the mode and the median are good measures of central tendency; the average (mean) is probably not. Whenever the frequency of one value predominates in a set of data, the mode is usually a good measure of central tendency. Unique modes do not exist for the data in histograms II and III. For the data in histogram II, both the average and the median are good measures of central tendency. When the values of a set of data are distributed fairly evenly over the range of the data (as in this case) the average is sometimes considered better because it takes into account directly the value of each piece of data. The median is probably a better measure of central tendency than the average for the data in histogram III. Typically, the median is preferable to the average in cases where the values in a set of data are clustered toward one end of the range, but not in a way where the mode would become a good measure of central tendency as in histogram I.

Problem 4.
Calculate the mode, the median, and the average for each group in Experiment C. Identify, if possible, which of the three measures of central tendency is probably best for each group.

MCAT MATHEMATICS CONCEPT 30: Variation or Dispersion Around Average

The measures of central tendency discussed above each give one value to describe a whole set of data. This one value is inadequate to "completely" describe the data because it gives no sense of the variation (or the dispersion) of the data about this value. In other words, we need a knowledge of the variation in a set of data to complement our knowledge of its central tendency. The common measures of variation are the range, the variance, and the standard deviation. Only the computation of the range is required for the MCAT. The variance and the standard deviation are not required; however, their definitions will be given if they are needed on the MCAT. For this reason, you should be familiar with them beforehand.

The **range** is simply the difference between the highest and lowest values in a set of data. For example:

Experiment A.
Range = 13.7 - 7.0 = 6.7

Experiment B.
Range = 90 - 50 = 40

Because the range takes into account only the highest and lowest values in a set of data, it is a rough measure of variation. In some cases, it is really not a reasonable measure of variation. When either or both of the extreme values in a set of data are far out of line with the rest of the data, the range is a questionable measure of variation. For example, consider the data presented in the histograms below (N = the frequency of a particular value of the variable x):

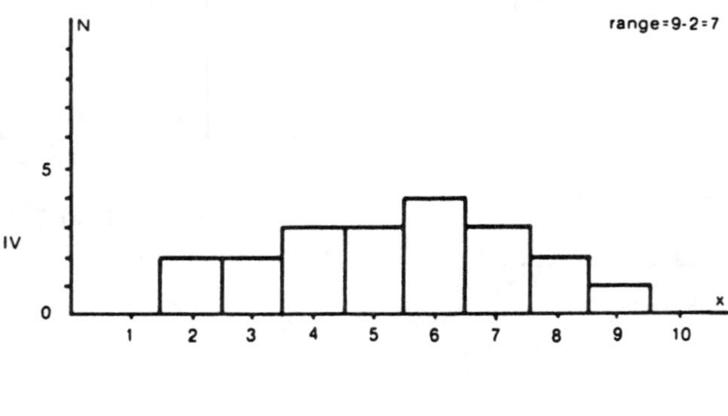

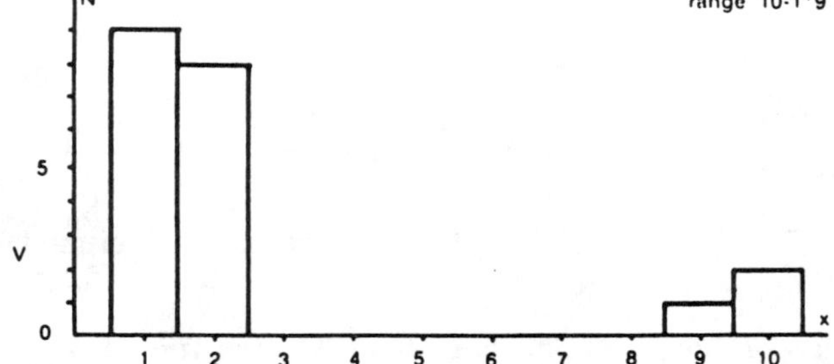

Fig. 4.15—Histograms Showing Dispersion of Data Around the Mean

The range of the data in histogram IV gives a good idea of that data's variability. On the other hand, the range of the data in histogram V does not really give a good idea of that data's variability.

The **variance** (V) and the **standard deviations** (S.D.) are intimately related:

$$\text{S.D.} = \sqrt{V}$$

The MCAT requires that you understand the concepts, but you will not have to make calculations. The following should be reviewed and understood but need not be memorized.

The variance, like the mean, takes into account each value in a set of data. It is calculated by taking the average value of the squares of the deviation for each data point from the mean:

$$\text{variance} = \frac{(x_1 - \bar{x})^2 + (x_2 - \bar{x})^2 + ... + (x_n - \bar{x})^2}{n},$$

where $x_1, x_2, \ldots, x_n$ = values of individual pieces of data, x = the mean, and n = the total number of pieces of data. The standard deviation is simply calculated by taking the square root of the variance so calculated:

$$\text{standard deviation} = \left(\frac{(x_1 - \bar{x})^2 + (x_2 - \bar{x})^2 + ... + (x_n - \bar{x})^2}{n}\right)^{1/2}.$$

Examples of calculation of the standard deviation and the variance are:

Experiment A.

$$V = \frac{(7.0\text{-}9.7)^2 + (7.1\text{-}9.7)^2 + ... + (11.1\text{-}9.7)^2 + (13.7\text{-}9.7)^2}{10}$$

$$= (3.643) \cong 3.6$$

$$\text{S.D.} = \sqrt{V} = \sqrt{3.6} = 1.9 .$$

Experiment B.

$$V = \frac{(50\text{-}70)^2 + 2(55\text{-}70)^2 + ... + 2(85\text{-}70)^2 + (90\text{-}70)^2}{30}$$

$$= (85.833) \cong 86$$

$$\text{S.D.} = \sqrt{V} = \sqrt{85} = (9.22) \approx 9$$

(Recall that this data was rounded off to the nearest 5.)

A rough way to estimate the standard deviation of a set of data is to take its range and divide by 4:

$$\text{S.D.} \cong \frac{\text{Range}}{4}.$$

Experiment A.

$$\text{S.D.} \cong \frac{13.7\text{-}7.0}{4} = (1.675) \cong 1.7$$

Experiment B.

$$\text{S.D.} \cong \frac{90\text{-}50}{4} = (10) .$$

Comparing these estimates of the standard deviation to the exact calculations above, we can observe that, when the range is a good indicator of the variation in a set of data, this S.D. approximation using it is also good.

Problem 5.
Calculate the range, the variance, and the standard deviation for each group in Experiment C.

MCAT MATHEMATICS CONCEPT 31: Graphical Interpolation

The final topic of data analysis to be considered is **interpolation**. Consider a set of data which relates two variables, x and y. Linear interpolation is a way of approximating the value of one of the variables, e.g., y, for a value of the other variable, e.g., x, which we do not have as a measurement in our set of data. Specifically, if we know that y either always increases or always decreases when x increases in our set of data, we can linearly approximate the relation between x and y between any two adjacent data points and thereby be able to calculate an approximate value of y for any value of x between these two points. An example of this can be shown with the following data:

x	y
0	10
10	40
20	60
30	75
40	85
50	90

graphically →

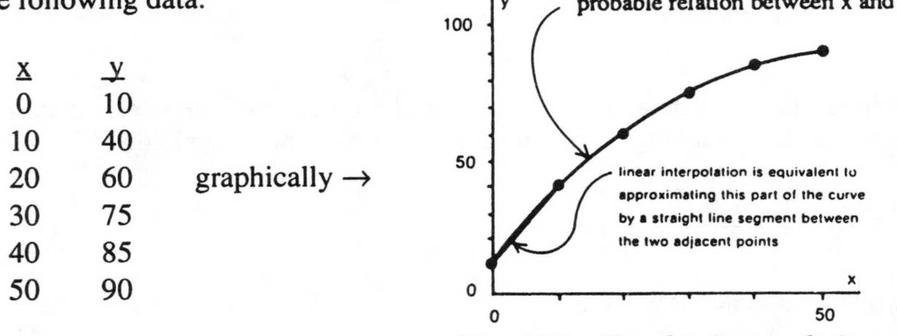

Fig. 4.16—Graphic Interpolation

We are interested in knowing the value of y when x = 7. We observe (or know for a fact) that as x increases, y increases; thus, linear interpolation is possible. We interpolate the value of y at x = 7 by approximating the relation between x and y as linear between x = 0 and x = 10 (see graph above). Since y increases by 30 in this interval while x increases by 10, y is taken as increasing by 3 when x increases by 1. Therefore, the interpolated value of y at x = 7 is y = 10 + (7)(3) = 31. Note that when considering the use of interpolation, it is important to verify (or at least be very confident) that an increasing/increasing or increasing/decreasing relation exists between the two variables, x and y.

Problem 6.
Using the data above, interpolate the values of y for x = 16, 32, and 48.

MCAT MATHEMATICS CONCEPT 32: Problem Solving Using Data Analysis Techniques

(1) Take enough time to understand what each number, axis, line, etc., means before trying to answer the questions in a problem. In other words, quickly assess the nature of the information being presented. This is also called "conquer the given".

(2) Read statements/questions carefully, i.e., make sure that you are answering the questions being asked. This is also called "What is the question?" Especially look out for qualifiers because their presence or absence can determine whether a statement is true/supported or false/contradicted. Examples are:

- (a) "exactly" versus "approximately"
- (b) "never" versus "sometimes" (or usually) versus "always" (or "consistently")
- (c) "are greater" versus "tend to be greater"
- (d) "on the average"

(3) Select relevant data or information pertinent to the question only:

- (a) Sometimes all this involves is the extraction of a particular piece of information from a table or graph.
- (b) However, in other instances, this can involve having to decide which data are pertinent and which are irrelevant or inconclusive. This is especially true when analyzing a set of data for a possible correlation between two variables.

Say we are given data relating three variables (A,B, and C). If we wish to detect a correlation between the values of A and the values of B (if one exists), we have to look at subsets of these data in which C is a constant in order to isolate this correlation. Any subset of the data in which C is not constant in value cannot be used to determine a possible correlation between A and B; the only exception is if we already know that there is no correlation between the values of C and the values of A or B. Simply put, it is the "rule of comparison"—you can compare only two things at a time.

(4) Do **not** overextend stated facts or assumptions. Consider as an example a composite group C, which consists of two subgroups A and B (C = A + B). If we are told that 40% of C falls into a certain category, it is not reasonable to assume that it is true that approximately 40% of A and 40% of B each separately fall into this category. In other words, do not ask questions that are more detailed than the question itself. Your task is to answer the question the test-maker asked, not one that you feel should have been asked.

(5) If the data in a problem are not presented in a good format for answering its questions, reorganize the data into a more appropriate format. Typically, this is useful in situations in which one is presented raw data. For example, consider Experiment B at the beginning of Concept #20. Suppose that its data had been originally presented in a raw format consisting of a list of 30 patients, numbered 1 through 30, with a pulse rate recorded for each. If then asked questions about the distribution of pulse rate values in this set of data, it would have been advantageous to reorganize it into the frequency format in which it is actually presented in Concept #29.

(6) Be careful to distinguish between "**what**" data and "**why**" data. Consider, as an example, a set of data, say in the form of a graph, which shows the annual birth rate in the U.S. for the years between 1935 and 1955. The information that can be derived from this graph is only how the annual birth rate varied during this period. These data do not address any explanations for why it varied the way it did. That is, the information is insufficient for answering any questions concerning possible explanations for the birth rate's behavior during this period.

(7) Be very cautious in making value judgments. For instance, a set of data might show that the smoking of tobacco products predisposes smokers to mouth and lung diseases. However, it cannot be concluded from these data that the sale of tobacco products should be restricted or banned because they are health hazards. This is because this conclusion is a value judgment; to say that it is true or false would be to do so using one's own opinions concerning the regulation of products that are health hazards, not the data presented. You could conclude that doctors ought to warn their patients of the danger.

(8) In general, **do not make assumptions about missing information** unless explicitly told to do so. For example, suppose we are given data which show that 4% of the men who get diabetes subsequently suffer blindness as a result, while only 3% of the women who get it subsequently suffer blindness. We are then presented with the statement: "More men suffer blindness as a result of being diabetic than do women." It might seem attractive to make the assumption that about as many men get diabetes as do women and thereby judge this statement as true/supported. However, this assumption is not justified because we are not told to assume this (or anything else). The correct answer here is that the information is insufficient to decide the truth or falsity of this statement.

(9) In general, all the information needed to answer questions is given in the problem. Nevertheless, general knowledge is to be used to interpret the information presented in a problem, e.g., in situations where there are known relationships between the variables involved. On the other hand, do not use general knowledge to supply missing data or to answer a question on which the problem's data have no bearing.

(10) When data is presented in a graphical format, be aware of the fact that sometimes we will be more interested in the slope of the graph than in the graph itself. That is, for two variables x and y, there will be cases where our interest is in how the slope varies with x, not in how y varies with x (see discussion of slope in MCAT Mathematics Concept #11). For example, consider a reaction A + B= C. We might be given a graph that plots the amount of C formed versus time. If we are interested in the kinetics of the reaction, we are more interested in the rate of change of concentration (which is the slope of the graph) at a time t than in the total amount of C formed at the time t..

(11) Interpolate values of a variable only when both of the following conditions are met (let the two variables be x and y; we wish to interpolate a value of y for a given value of x for which there is not a measured value of y):

(a) There is a known increasing/increasing or increasing/decreasing relationship between x and y.

(b) We are interpolating the value of y for a given value of x which is between two measured data points. In other words, interpolation cannot be done outside the range of the data. (See discussion of interpolation in MCAT Mathematics Concept #31).

(12) Be aware of possibly different information-gathering procedures when comparing two groups of similar data. For example, suppose that in Experiment B at the beginning of MCAT Mathematics Concept #20 that a second student had measured the pulse rates of another group of 30 patients, rounding the beats off to the nearest 1 beat/minute. The pulse rates of the group whose data are actually given is rounded off to the nearest 5 beats/minute. Consequently, when comparing the data for these two groups of patients, this difference in how their respective pulse rates were recorded would have to be considered.

(13) Be careful, when using the range as a measure of variability (see discussion of the range in Concept #30). Often the best way to make simple comparisons of the distributions and relative variabilities of equivalent groups of data is to use frequency representations of them such as the one for the data in Experiment B at the beginning of Concept #20.

Solutions to Data Analysis Problems

(1) The data in Experiment C is continuous data.

(2) Group I: Put the data in ascending order:191, 194, 195, 195, 195, 196, 196, 196, 198, 199; then:

(1) smallest value = 191
(2) largest value = 199
(3) range is 199 - 191 = 8
(4) most values are around 195 or 196, so the average is probably about 195 or 196
(5) there are few values at the ends of the range (191 and 199), but many at the middle (195 to 196)

Group II: Put the data in ascending order: 193, 194, 196, 199, 201, 202, 202, 204, 204, 205; then:

(1) smallest value = 193
(2) largest value = 205
(3) range is 205 - 193 = 12
(4) average might be about 199 : $\frac{193+205}{2} = 199$
(5) the values cluster toward the higher end of the range

(3) Group I: Percentage with blood cholesterol levels of 196 or lower = $\frac{8}{10} \times 100 = 80\%$

Group II: Percentage with blood cholesterol levels of 196 or lower = $\frac{3}{10} \times 100 = 30\%$

(4) Group I: A unique mode does not exist, as 195 and 196 both appear three times.

The median $= \frac{195+196}{2} = 196\ (195.5)$

The average $= \frac{191+194+3(195)+3(196)+198+199}{10} = 196\ (195.5)$

Both the average and the median are good measures of the central tendency of Groups I's data.

Group II: A unique mode does not exist, as 202 and 204 both appear twice.

The median $= \frac{201 + 202}{2} = 202\ (201.5)$

The average $= \frac{193+194+196+199+201+2(202)+2(204)+205}{10}$

$= 200$

It is a toss-up as to which measure of central tendency, the median or the average, is probably better. Qualitatively, the average tends to reflect the spread of data at the lower end of the range more than the median does, while the median tends to reflect the cluster of data at the high end of the range more than the average does.

(5) Group I:
The range = 199 - 191 = 8

$$V = \frac{(191\text{-}196)^2 + (194\text{-}196)^2 + ... + (198\text{-}196)^2 + (199\text{-}196)^2}{10}$$

$$= (4.5) \cong 5$$

$$S.D. = \sqrt{V} = \sqrt{5} = (2.236) \cong 2$$

Group II:
The range = 205 - 193 = 12

$$V = \frac{(193\text{-}200)^2 + (194\text{-}200)^2 + ... + 2(204\text{-}200)^2 + (205\text{-}200)^2}{10}$$

$$= (16.8) \cong 17$$

$$S.D. = \sqrt{V} = \sqrt{17} = (4.123) \cong 4$$

(6) For x = 16: Slope of line segment between x = 10 is x = 20 is
$\frac{60 - 40}{20 - 10} = 2$, i.e., y increases by 2 when x increases by 1.
Thus, at x = 16, y = 40 + 6(2) = 52.

For x = 32: Slope of line segment between x = 30 and x = 40 is
$\frac{85 - 75}{40 - 30} = 1$, i.e., y increases by 1 when x increases by 1.
Thus, at x = 32, y = 75 + 2(1) = 77.

For x = 48: Slope of line segment between x = 40 and x = 50 is
$\frac{90 - 85}{50 - 40} = \frac{1}{2}$, i.e., y increases by 1 when x increases by 2.
Thus, at x = 48, y = 85 + 8(1/2) = 89.

4.4 PRACTICE PROBLEMS IN DATA ANALYSIS AND REASONING

The problems in the remainder of this chapter are designed to give you practice in data analysis and reasoning to prepare you for the new, passage-based MCAT. The problems in this section present you with passages in several different forms, primarily written text and graphs or tables. You will need to extract information from all of these sources, which were introduced with exercises in earlier sections.

These problems are not intended to be exactly like those you will find in the MCAT; some are a little harder, others may be a bit more fun. There are serious reasons for the sometimes wacky nature of the text that adjoins a few of the problems. Humor is a very effective memory aid; it also eases the tedium of study.

Biological and physical sciences problems have so far been multiple choice, but in this section several formats are used, including true/false and short answer. The purpose is partly to make sure you are prepared in case there is a shift in the MCAT format (the SAT has already announced such a change), but more important it is to give you the best possible preparation in areas where multiple choice may not provide a suitable test of your skill. Short answer questions help you practice evaluation skills such as judging the soundness of an argument or the credibility of a source (see pages 12, 30, 31 of *The MCAT Student Manual* for a full list of such skills).

Little in the way of science content is included in this section. This is so that you can practice essential skills without having the facts (or lack of facts) get in your way. Once you have mastered the problem-solving techniques, you will need to combine them with knowledge of science, which is the province of chapters 5 and 7 to follow. Practicing the different components separately is the surest way to make certain you have all the pieces working before you enter the examination room.

A wise strategy when doing problems is to read the questions quickly before reading the text and graphs. You will then be looking for specific information. In some cases you will only be trying to confirm your first guess or to make sure there is nothing in the data that contradicts your expectations. In other cases you will be searching for specific data that you need just to start work on a question. It is always easier to find things when you know what you are looking for. But be careful; it is also easy to miss things you do not expect. After you have decided on an answer, you should search for evidence that might contradict your choice.

It may also be possible to guess the answer to some questions before you read the information provided. Some test-takers can do quite well without reading through a test passage. We do not recommend you use this strategy on the exam, but as a practice exercise you may want to try it now with these data analysis problems for the following reason: the MCAT does not penalize for guessing; your final score may benefit from fast educated guesses as time runs out and some questions remain unanswered.

Each set of problems has been selected from physical sciences, biological sciences or social sciences to give a good variety. These problems are only intended to be "skill-testers". Do not be surprised if the actual MCAT passages and problems are harder.

Passage I (Questions 1 - 11) - Social sciences data

A lumber company ran a four-man crew during the first ten working days of August. On Wednesday, August 15, three lumberjacks fell ill and the fourth quit. Production figures for the month of August are given in the table.

Trees Cut Down on Ten Consecutive Days (all work is on approximately the same size trees):

Day	Man A	Man B	Man C	Man D
1	12	12	12	8
2	11	17	13	9
3	13	5	12	7
4	9	16	11	7
5	10	10	12	8
6	11	8	10	8
7	12	7	13	9
8	14	18	14	20
9	9	6	15	9
10	10	12	12	7

Keyed choice
Based on the given information, choose:

(A) If the statement is true or probably true.
(B) If the information in the table is not sufficient to indicate whether there is any degree of truth or falsity in the statement.
(C) If the statement is false or probably false.

1. Man A's average trees per day is greater than man B's.
2. Man A's average trees per day is greater than man C's.
3. It is easier to predict how many trees man A will cut on any given day than it is to do the same for man B.
4. It is easier to predict how many trees man A will cut on any given day than it is to do the same for man C.
5. A total of 8 is a better prediction of how many trees man D will cut in a day than is 20.
6. The variability of man B's daily totals is greater than the variability of man C's.
7. The range of man D's daily totals is less than the range of man A's.
8. Except for day 8, man D had duties other than cutting down trees for days 1 through 10.

Multiple choice

9. How many trees were cut on Fridays?

   A. 78
   B. 84
   C. 103
   D. 101

10. On what date in August were the lumberjacks most productive?

   A. August 1
   B. August 2
   C. August 10
   D. August 14

11. Which of the following best describes the average production for the month of August?

   A. 19 trees/working day
   B. 39 trees/working day
   C. 4.9 trees/working day
   D. 10 trees/working day

Passage II (Questions 12 - 19) - Social sciences data

Although 50% of fatal automobile accidents involve drivers who are or who have been alcoholics, less than 1% of the drivers in such accidents belong to Alcoholics Anonymous. A study was conducted in New York to determine whether AA drivers were significantly more cautious than the general public.

Alcoholism Cure Rates in New York State:	
Members of Alcoholics Anonymous	20,000
% regarded as cured	65%
% who have successfully resumed social drinking	3%
Estimated number of alcoholics and ex-alcoholics	750,000
Estimated % regarded as cured	20%
Estimated % who could resume social drinking successfully	12%

Keyed choice

Based on the given information, choose:

(A) If the statement is true or probably true.
(B) If the information in the table is not sufficient to indicate whether there is any degree of truth or falsity in the statement.
(C) If the statement is false or probably false.

12. Members of AA comprise less than 1/10 of the estimated alcoholics in New York.

13. The cure rate in AA is higher than in New York as a whole.

14. The cure rate in AA is higher than in New York as a whole because those who join AA are more highly motivated than those who don't.

15. AA discourages its members from attempting to resume social drinking.

16. Something in the methods used by AA makes it more difficult for the people it cures to resume social drinking than it is for the average alcoholic.

17. There is a strong reason not to draw conclusions from the relative size of the 3% and 12% entries in this table.

Multiple choice

18. Is the percentage of AA drivers involved in fatal accidents unexpectedly high or low?

19. In order to determine how much more likely it is for an alcoholic to be involved in a fatal accident, you would need to:

A. factor out the percent cured
B. know the total population of New York State
C. calculate the ratio of drinkers to alcoholics
D. know the number of drivers in the population from which the number 750,000 was obtained.

Passage III (Questions 20 - 33) - Social sciences data

An environmental psychologist performed five experiments with rats to investigate the effect of room color on the rate of problem-solving.

Experiment 1—Group I rats were run in a red-colored maze. In the first experiment they were deprived of food for 30 hours prior to the experiment but were otherwise in very good health.
Experiment 2—Group II rats were also run in a red maze. They were well-fed and healthy.
Experiment 3—Group III rats were the same as those used in experiment 1. Feeding conditions were identical, but the maze walls were painted blue. The experiment was conducted two weeks after the conclusion of the first experiment.
Experiment 4—Group IV rats were the same as those used in experiment 2. They were well-fed and healthy. The maze walls were painted blue. The experiment was carried out 2 weeks after the conclusion of experiment 2.
Experiment 5—using Group V rats, this experiment was conducted two months after the others. Several rats had died and a new group was formed by combining the healthiest members of the two groups. The rats used in this study were all well-fed. The maze walls were painted red, but the floor was blue.

Rates at Which Rats Solve a Maze:

	Average time to solve (sec.)	No. solving in less than 12 sec.	Median time (sec.)	Range of times (sec.)
Group I (50 rats)	15.3	15	15.1	10.5
Group II (50 rats)	12.9	20	12.7	8.4
Group III (50 rats)	18.5	10	17.8	17.0
Group IV (50 rats)	21.0	7	21.3	30.1
Group V (80 rats)	15.7	13	15.6	12.1

Multiple choice

20. Support for the hypothesis that color affects maze solving times can be found by comparing:

A. Groups I and III with II and IV
B. Groups I and II with III and IV
C. Groups I and V
D. Groups V and IV with II

21. The hypothesis that hungry rats are less adept at problem solving than well-fed rats might be partially supported by comparing:

A. Groups I and III with II and IV
B. Groups I and II with III and IV
C. Groups I and V
D. Groups V and IV with II

22. The experiments taken as a whole prove that the color red makes rats better at problem solving than does the color blue. True or false?

23. A reasonable hypothesis to propose from the data in the experiments is that the color blue makes rats slow. True or false?

Keyed choice
Based on the information given, select:

(A) If the statement is supported by the information given.
(B) If the statement is contradicted by the information given.
(C) If the statement is neither supported nor contradicted by the information given.

24. On the average, the rats in Group III were quicker at solving the maze than the rats in Group II.

25. The slowest rat in Group IV finished the maze in less than 43 seconds.

26. The number of rats in Group II that finished the maze in less than 12 seconds is less than the number of rats in Group I that finished the maze in less than 16 seconds.

27. The percentage of rats in Group IV that finished the maze in less than 12 seconds is less than the percentage of rats in Group V that finished the maze in less than 12 seconds.

28. The slowest rat in Group V was faster than the slowest rat in Group III.

29. If no rat finished faster than in 5 seconds, then the slowest rat in Group II was faster than the slowest rat in Group III.

30. The time of the slowest rat in Group III is farther from the average time for Group III than is the time of the fastest rat in that group.

31. Calculate the average time for the rats in the first four groups.

32. Calculate the average time for all the rats in the study.

33. It makes sense to say that the measurements in columns 1, 3, and 4 are less accurate than the measurements in column 2.

Passage IV (Questions 34 - 43) - Physical sciences data

A group of introductory physics students were given the task of drawing a variety of graphs for five different situations. The first situation was a coconut on top of a palm tree and the second was a coconut falling from the top of the tree to the ground. The third situation involved a skateboarder, who was actually the professor in the course, coasting across the parking lot; the fourth involved his return hopping with his feet tied together in a bag. The final situation involved the launching of a Sprint missile during the power build-up phase when the missile continues to gain acceleration. Unfortunately, when the coconut was dropped it landed on the head of the student who was keeping track of which graphs referred to which situations and the other students were left with the task of sorting out what had been done.

Distance, Velocity, Acceleration and Time:

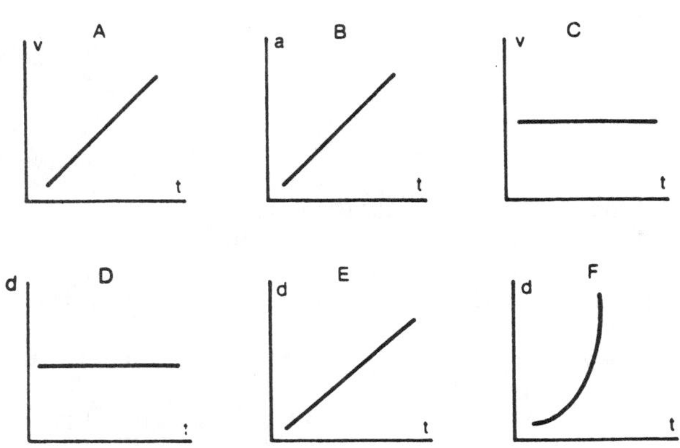

34. Do the students have at least one graph for each of the five kinds of motion? If not, which kinds of motion have been left out?

35. Which graph represents an object at rest?

36. Which graph represents uniform acceleration?

37. Which graphs represent the same kind of motion?

38. For which of these graphs is a graph of a versus t **not** a straight line?

39. Over a long time period, which of these motions will have the largest average velocity? (Assume in graph F that d goes as t^2.)

As additional exercises, construct the four graphs asked for in questions 40 - 43 below.

40. Draw an a versus t graph that represents the same motion as graph A.

41. Draw an a versus t graph that represents the same motion as graph C.

42. Draw a v versus t graph that represents the same motion as graph E.

43. Draw a v versus t graph that represents the same motion as graph F. (Assume d goes as t^2 in graph F.)

Passage V (Questions 44 - 54) - Biological sciences data

Each patient represented in the graph below received only one type of treatment, and percentages are of total number of patients receiving that treatment. The only dosages that were actually used are those explicitly indicated on the horizontal axis, i.e., all integral doses from 1 to 22.

Percentage of Lung Cancer Patients Surviving Longer than Five Years After Receiving Six Weeks of Radiation Therapy in Indicated Dosage Along with Indicated Chemotherapeutic Agent:

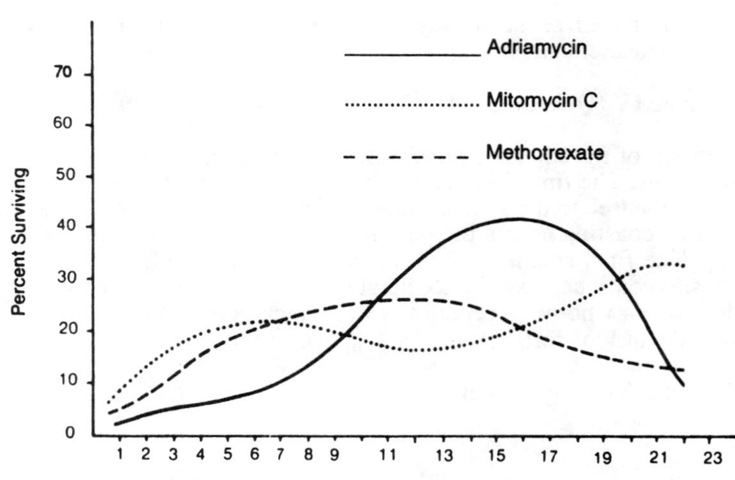

Based on the information given, select:

(A) If the first item is larger than the second.
(B) If the second item is larger than the first.
(C) If they are equal.
(D) If the difference cannot be evaluated on the basis of the information given.

44. 1. Actual dosage which is less than 14 units that is closest to the intersection of Mitomycin C and Adriamycin lines.
2. Actual dosage which is less than 14 units that is closest to the intersection of Methotrexate and Adriamycin lines.

45. 1. Number of dosages for which Mitomycin C has a higher 5-year survival percentage than Methotrexate.
    2. Number of dosages for which Methotrexate has a higher 5-year survival percentage than Mitomycin C.

46. 1. Highest dosage for which Mitomycin C has a higher 5-year survival percentage than does Methotrexate.
    2. Highest dosage for which Methotrexate has a lower 5-year survival percentage than does Adriamycin.

47. 1. Lowest dosage for which Mitomycin C is more effective than both Methotrexate and Adriamycin.
    2. Highest dosage for which Mitomycin C is less effective than both Methotrexate and Adriamycin.

48. 1. Dosage for which Adriamycin has a higher 5-year survival percentage than does Mitomycin C and a lower 5-year survival percentage than does Methotrexate.
    2. Half of lowest dosage for which Adriamycin has a higher 5-year survival percentage than does Methotrexate and a lower 5-year survival percentage than does Mitomycin C.

49. 1. Range of 5-year survival percentages experienced by groups receiving Mitomycin C.
    2. Range of 5-year survival percentages experienced by those receiving Adriamycin.

50. Can one tell what the average 5-year survival percentage of those receiving Adriamycin was?
If so, what was it?
If not, why not?

51. If one is told that each dosage of radiation was received by the same number of patients, can one tell what the average 5-year survival percentage of those receiving Mitomycin C was?
If so, what was it?
If not, why not?

52. Can one tell what the average 5-year survival percentage of those receiving 12 units of radiation was?
If so, what was it?
If not, why not?

53. If one is given the further information that the total number of people who received Mitomycin C was the same as the respective total numbers of people who received Methotrexate and Adriamycin, can one tell what the average 5-year survival percentage of those receiving 12 units of radiation was?
If so, what was it?
If not, why not?

54. If one is given the further information that of those receiving 12 units of radiation the number who received Mitomycin C was the same as the respective numbers who received Methotrexate and Adriamycin, can one tell what the average 5-year survival percentage of those receiving 12 units of radiation was?
If so, what was it?
If not, why not?

Passage VI (Questions 55 - 59) - Biological sciences data

Cumulative Percentage of U.S. Population that has had 14-Day Measles by Age Group and Gender:

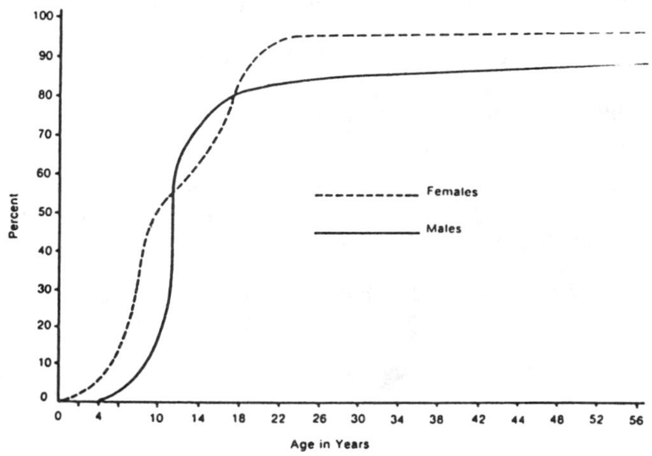

55. Explain why at first glance it seems wrong for these graphs to have a negative slope anywhere.

56. Explain how it actually is possible for them to have a negative slope.

57. Show where these graphs have a negative slope.

58. Which is more closely tied to a high percentage of people catching measles at a particular age, a high percentage on this graph or a high positive change in percentage with respect to a change in age on this graph?

59. What quantity from these graphs indicates change in percent with respect to change in age?

Passage VII (Questions 60 - 65) - Biological sciences data

Epidemics in Country X Between 1950 and 1963

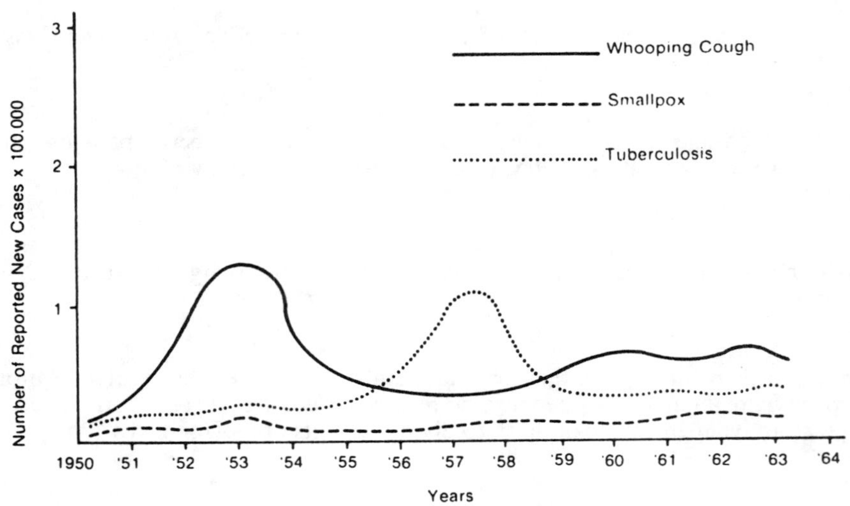

Based only on the information given, select:

(A) If the statement is true or probably true.
(B) If the information in the graph is not sufficient to indicate whether there is any degree of truth or falsity in the statement.
(C) If the statement is false or probably false.

60. There were more reported cases of whooping cough in country X in 1953 than in any other year studied.

61. In 1954 there were more people living in country X who had had whooping cough than in any other year.

62. In country X a higher percentage of the population was reported to have fallen ill with smallpox in 1963 than in 1961.

63. If 10% of those reported to have contracted smallpox in 1957 died of it that year and 3% of those reported to have contracted whooping cough in 1953 died of it in that year, then these figures represent more smallpox deaths than whooping cough deaths.

64. If 2% of the reported new cases of smallpox and .1% of the reported new cases of tuberculosis in 1957 died in that same year, then more people in country X died of tuberculosis in 1957 than died of smallpox.

65. On the average, of the three diseases, whooping cough was the greatest threat to public health in the period between 1950 and 1963.

4.4.1 Solutions to Practice Problems

Answer Key

1.	**C**	**23.**	**True**	**44.**	**B**
2.	**C**	**24.**	**B**	**45.**	**A**
3.	**A**	**25.**	**A**	**46.**	**A**
4.	**C**	**26.**	**A**	**47.**	**B**
5.	**A**	**27.**	**A**	**48.**	**C**
6.	**A**	**28.**	**C**	**49.**	**B**
7.	**C**	**29.**	**A**	**50.**	**No**
8.	**B**	**30.**	**C**	**51.**	**No**
9.	**C**	**31.**	**16.9 sec.**	**52.**	**No**
10.	**C**	**32.**	**16.6 sec.**	**53.**	**No**
11.	**A**	**33.**	**C**	**54.**	**Yes, about 25%**
12.	**A**	**34.**	**No, does not include the hopping motion**	**55.**	**(See explanations)**
13.	**A**			**56.**	**(See explanations)**
14.	**B**	**35.**	**D**	**57.**	**Nowhere**
15.	**B**	**36.**	**A**	**58.**	**(See explanations)**
16.	**B**	**37.**	**C and E**	**59.**	**Slope**
17.	**A**	**38.**	**A,B,or F**	**60.**	**A**
18.	**Indeterminate**	**39.**	**B**	**61.**	**B**
19.	**D**	**40.**	**(See explanations)**	**62.**	**B**
20.	**B**	**41.**	**(See explanations)**	**63.**	**C**
21.	**A**	**42.**	**(See explanations)**	**64.**	**B**
22.	**False**	**43.**	**(See explanations)**	**65.**	**B**

4.4.2 Explanatory Solutions for Practice Problems

Passage I

1. C. False. Average trees per day for man A = 11.1; average trees per day for man B = 11.1. Thus the average of man A equals the average of man B.

2. C. False. Average trees per day for man A = 11.1; average trees per day for man C = 12.4. Thus the average of man A is less than the average of man C.

For answering questions 3-7, it may be helpful to make a table such as the one below.

Frequency of Occurrence in Ten-Day Period

No. of trees cut down per day	Man A	Man B	Man C	Man D
5		1		
6		1		
7		1		3
8		1		3
9	2			3
10	2	1	1	
11	2		1	
12	2	2	4	
13	1		2	
14	1		1	
15			1	
16		1		
17		1		
18		1		
19				
20				1

3. A. Probably true. It should be easier to predict the number of trees cut down on any given day for the man whose data have a smaller relative variation. Thus, this statement is probably true because man A's data do cluster substantially closer about their average value than do man B's data. Since man A and man B have the same average, this is very easy to see in the table above.

4. C. Probably false. Although the data for man A and those for man C have the same range (both have ranges equal to 5), the data for man C are more tightly distributed about their average value than those for man A and therefore should be easier to predict.

5. A. Probably true. Excluding the single occurrence of 20, the average for man D is 8 with the data (for the nine days) being distributed evenly and tightly about 8.

6. A. True. Since the lowest and highest values of the data for both man B and man C are not out of line with the rest of the respective data for both men, the ranges in the data for both men are reasonable measures of the variabilities in their respective data. The range for man B = 13, while the range for man C = 5; thus, the variability for man B is greater than for man C.

7. C. False. Range for man D = 20 - 7 = 13; range for man A = 14 - 9 = 5. Thus, the range for man D is greater than the range for man A.

8. B. Information insufficient. Although this statement is a plausible explanation for the distribution of man D's data, there is no information in this problem that pertains to evaluating explanations to account for the distributions of the respective data for the four men.

9. C. We know from the written text that on Wednesday, August 15, all work stopped. Make a calendar for August where August 15 falls on a Wednesday:

S	M	T	W	T	F	S
			1	2	3	4
5	6	7	8	9	10	11
12	13	14	15	16	17	18
19	20	21	22	23	24	25
26	27	28	29	30	31	

Fridays are the third and eighth working days. The trees cut are13+5+12+7+14+18+14+20 = 103.

10. C. The most productive day was the eighth working day (66 trees cut), which was August 10.

11. A. The number of working days in August is 23 (see calendar). Add up all the trees cut and divide by 23.

Passage II

12. A. True. In order to answer the questions in this problem, we have to make sense of the information on the table because it is not altogether clear as it stands. It is reasonable to presume that Alcoholics Anonymous (AA) has both alcoholics and ex-alcoholics as members with an ex-alcoholic being a person who has been cured of his/her alcoholism. Thus, based on the data given in the table, 35% of the members of AA in New York and 80% of the estimated alcoholics and ex-alcoholics in New York as a whole are alcoholics. Consequently, the number of alcoholics who are members of AA which = (.35)(20,000) = 7,000 is less than 1/10 of the estimated alcoholics in New York which = (.1)(.8)(750,000) = 60,000.

13. A. True. Reading directly from the data in the table, the cure rate in AA (= 65%) is higher than that in New York as a whole (= 20%).

14. B. Information insufficient. Although this is a possible explanation for the higher cure rate in AA than in New York as a whole, there is no information in this problem which supports it over another explanation(s) for the higher cure rate in AA.

15. B. Information insufficient. While the table tells us that only 3% of AA's members have successfully resumed social drinking, it does not tell us anything about why—for example, AA's policy on advising its members with regard to resuming social drinking. Consequently, we cannot deduce much from this percentage. Anyway, in most cases, the existence of a policy cannot be determined

from a set of numerical data, except in the rare situation where only one policy could have led to the given outcome.

16. B. Information insufficient. As was the case in (15) above, this statement is too complicated to be judged as true or false on the basis of the information in the table. We have been told nothing about the different methods that are used to cure alcoholism, especially any special methods used by AA. (Issues such as whether or not members of AA are typical of alcoholics and ex-alcoholics in New York as a whole, the importance of abstinence as a cure for alcoholism, and the higher cure rate in AA than in New York would have to be considered in judging this statement as true or false.)

17. A. True. We cannot draw conclusions from comparisons of these two percentages because they do not represent the same quantity, i.e., do not confuse "could" with "have."

18. Indeterminate. The text states that 1% of AA drivers are involved in accidents. They are part of the 50% who are or were alcoholics. The ratio of these groups is 1/50 = .02.

But in terms of the total pool of such drivers, the ratio is 20,000/750,000 = .026. The fraction of AA drivers involved in accidents is a little less than that of this group as a whole. No precise comparison to the general public is possible, since we have no data on the number of people in that group; however, the driving population of New York State is certainly much larger than 750,000, so we could conclude that both components of the alcoholic population are more likely to be in an accident than is a member of the general public. In most cases it is best to stick with the data given; in this case we would conclude that the answer is "indeterminate." But some problems will expect you to make a judgement using general knowledge. You may have to guess what the test graders are after; the various multiple-choice answers may help you decide.

19. D. We know that alcoholics, who number 750,000, account for 50% of the accidents. We also know that nonalcoholics account for the other 50%, but we do not know how many there are. Both B and D give us a population number, but B includes many people who are not drivers, such as young children. Therefore, D is probably the best answer.

Note: this problem includes a mixture of realistic and nonrealistic data. This often happens on tests. The number of fatal automobile accidents involving alcohol is about 50%, but it is not true that all of these people are or were alcoholics, at least not under a definition of alcoholic that produces only 750,000 of them in the State of New York. Part of the art of being a good test-taker is to know how to mix your real world knowledge with the imaginary world of the test questions. Here practice is the best teacher.

Passage III

20. B. Color information is given in the written text: answer A confounds color; answer B makes a reasonable comparison of two red conditions with two blue conditions; C compares red with red and blue, it also does not control other factors; in answer D, experiments 2 and 4 could be compared, but the inclusion of 5 introduces uncontrolled factors.

21. A. Answer A compares well-fed vs. hungry and controls for color; answer B confounds fed and hungry; in answer C, populations differ and color is poorly controlled; in answer D, all groups are well-fed and no comparison is possible.

22. False. Rats in the red mazes did solve the fastest. They may have been better at problem solving, but many other explanations are also possible.

23. True. Rats in the blue mazes solved the slowest.

24. B. Contradicted. The average time it took group III rats to solve the maze (= 18.5 sec.) was longer than that for group II rats (= 12.9 sec.); so group III rats were slower.

25. A. Supported. We need to find the maximum time it could have taken a group IV rat to solve the maze. Since the table tells us that 7 group IV rats solved the maze in less than 12 sec., the fastest solution time for a group IV rat was less than 12 sec. The range of solution times for group IV was 30.1 sec.; consequently, the slowest solution time for a group IV rat was less than 12 + 30.1 = 42.1 sec. which is less than 43 sec.

26. A. Supported. The number of group II rats that solved the maze in less than 12 sec. = 20. Since the median solution time for group I rats = 15.1 sec., at least half of group I, which = 25 rats, solved the maze in less than 16 sec.

27. A. Supported. The percentage of group IV rats that solved the maze in less than 12 sec. = (7/50) x 100 = 14%; the percentage of group V rats that solved the maze in less than 12 sec. = (13/80) x 100 = 16.25%.

28. C. Neither supported nor contradicted. We have not been told the slowest or fastest times in either group. Yet, we can observe that both groups had rats who solved the maze in less than 12 sec.; so, we know that the fastest time in each group was between 0 sec. and 12 sec. Using the range in solution times for each group, we can determine minimum and maximum possible values for the slowest time in each group. That is, for group V, the slowest time was between 0 + 12.1 = 12.1 and 12 + 12.1 = 24.1; for group III, the slowest time was between 0 + 17 = 17 sec. and 12 + 17 = 29 sec. However, before comparing the possible values of the slowest times in groups V and III respectively, we should examine the data to see if their ranges can be reduced further in size. Thus, these two ranges become 15.7-24.1 sec. (group V) and 18.5-29 sec. (group III) because the slowest time in each group cannot be less than that group's average time (or median time). Since the ranges for the slowest time in groups III and V overlap, we cannot tell which group's slowest rate was faster than the other's.

29. A. Supported. We can approach this question the same way as we did (28) above. However, in this case, the fastest time in each group was between 5 sec. and 12 sec. Using the range in solution times of each group, the slowest time for group II was between 5 + 8.4 = 13.4 sec. and 12 + 8.4 = 20.4 sec., while the slowest time in group III was between 5 + 17 = 22 sec. and 12 + 17 = 29 sec. Since these two ranges do not overlap, we can conclude that the slowest rat in group II (13.4-20.4 sec.) was faster than the slowest rat in group III (22-29 sec.).

30. C. Neither supported nor contradicted. As we reasoned in (28) above, the time of the slowest group III rat was between 18.5 sec. and 29 sec. Since the average for group III was 18.5 sec., the range in possible time differences between the slowest group III rat and the "average" group III rat = 0-10.5 sec. Since the time of the fastest group III rat was between 0 sec. and 12 sec., the range in possible time differences between the fastest group III rat and the "average" group III rat = 6.5-18.5 sec. Thus, as the ranges overlap, we cannot determine which solution time, the slowest or the fastest, is farther from the average solution time of group III. In general, it should be remembered that when given just an average and a range for a set of values, where the average falls in the range cannot be determined.

31. 16.9 seconds (use standard definition of the average). Average of first four groups =

$$\frac{50(15.3 + 12.9 + 18.5 + 21.0)}{50(4)} = 16.9 \text{ sec.}$$

32. 16.6 seconds. Average of all five groups =

$$\frac{50(15.3 + 12.9 + 18.5 + 21.0) + 80(15.7)}{50(4) + 80} = 16.6 \text{ sec.}$$

33. C. Neither supported nor contradicted. We do not know the respective percentage accuracies of the two groups of measurements. We have to talk about their percentage, not absolute, accuracies because the two groups of measurements involve two different quantities. This question is complicated by the fact that the accuracy of the number of rats which solve the maze in less than 12 sec. is dependent on the accuracy of the time measurements when a rat's solution time is near 12 sec. For example, if three of the solution times for one of the groups happened to be 11.9, 12.0, and 12.1 sec., the accuracy of the number of rats solving the maze in less than 12 sec. in this group would be critically dependent on the accuracy of these three times. This relationship between the two accuracies cannot be extracted from the data in the table; so, we cannot tell which group of measurements is more accurate.

Passage IV

34. No. Graphs A and F both refer to constant acceleration. Graphs C and E both refer to constant velocity. Thus there are only four different kinds of motion represented. The hopping motion would involve a velocity that cycled up and down and an acceleration that also stepped up and down. The distance vs. time graph would look like a staircase.

35. D. In graph D, d = constant; so object is at rest.

36. A. Uniform acceleration = constant acceleration which means constant change in velocity per unit time. In graph A, v is constantly increasing; so a is constant.

37. C,E. In graph C, v = constant; so $a = 0$ (no graph for this) and d = (constant) x t, as in E.

38. A, B or F Graph of d versus t is a line in D and E. It is also a line if v = constant, as in C. In A, v goes as t, so d goes as t^2. In B, a goes as t, so v goes as t^2 and d goes as t^3. In F, d versus t is obviously not a line.

39. B. Eventually the motion in which d goes as t^3 will have the largest d and hence the largest average velocity. That d goes as t^3 in B was identified in (38) above.

40. Velocity changing constant amount per unit time, as in graph A, is equivalent to a constant acceleration.

41. Constant velocity, as in graph C, is equivalent to $a = 0$.

42. Position changing constant amount per unit time, as in graph E, is equivalent to a constant velocity.

43. If d goes as t^2, then v goes as t; so v is constantly increasing.

Passage V

Remember that the real data in the graph for this problem are represented by the distinct points for each of the three chemotherapeutic agents at each of the integral radiation dosages from 1 to 22. The lines that have been drawn through the points of each drug over the range of radiation dosages tend to obscure this fact. These lines serve to clarify the presentation of the data by distinctly separating the data for the three drugs; however, the line segments between any two data points do not themselves represent data to be used in answering the questions for this problem.

44. B. (1) Actual dosage which is less than 14 units that is closest to the intersection of Mitomycin C and Adriamycin lines = 9 units
(2) Actual dosage which is less than 14 units that is closest to the intersection of Methotrexate and Adriamycin lines = 10 units

45. A. (1) Number of dosages for which Mitomycin C has a higher 5-year survival percentage than Methotrexate = (22-15) + (6-0) = 13
(2) Number of dosages for which Methotrexate has a higher 5-year survival percentage than Mitomycin C = 15 - 6 = 9

46. A. (1) Highest dosage for which Mitomycin C has a higher 5-year survival percentage than does Methotrexate = 22 units
(2) Highest dosage for which Methotrexate has a lower 5-year survival percentage than does Adriamycin = 21 units

47. B. (1) Lowest dosage for which Mitomycin C is more effective than both Methotrexate and Adriamycin = 1 unit
(2) Highest dosage for which Mitomycin C is less effective than both Methotrexate and Adriamycin = 15 units

48. C. (1) Dosage for which Adriamycin has a higher 5-year survival percentage than does Mitomycin C and a lower 5-year survival percentage than does Methotrexate = 10 units
(2) Half of lowest dosage for which Adriamycin has a higher 5-year survival percentage than does Methotrexate and a lower 5-year survival percentage than does Mitomycin C = (1/2)(20) = 10 units

49. B. (1) Range of 5-year survival percentages experienced by groups receiving Mitomycin C = about (30 - 8) = about 22%
(2) Range of 5-year survival percentages experienced by those receiving Adriamycin = about (43-1) = about 42%

Keep in mind when answering questions 50 - 54 that each experimentally unique group of patients is characterized both by the receipt of one of the three chemotherapeutic agents and by the receipt of a specific dosage of radiation therapy.

50. No. In addition to the 5-year survival percentage data for Adriamycin shown in the graph, we would also have to be told how the total number of patients receiving Adriamycin was distributed over the range of radiation dosages in order to be able to calculate the average 5-year survival percentage of those receiving Adriamycin. It is not reasonable to assume that the total number of patients receiving Adriamycin was distributed evenly over the range of radiation dosages.

51. No. In order to calculate the average 5-year survival percentage of those receiving Mitomycin C, it is not sufficient to know that each dosage of radiation was received by the same number of patients. This is because we have not also been told how this same number of patients is split between the three chemotherapeutic agents for each dosage of radiation. Like (50) above, it is not reasonable to assume that this same number of patients was split between the three chemotherapeutic agents in the same manner for each of the dosages of the radiation.

52. No. To calculate the average 5-year survival percentage of those receiving 12 units of radiation, we would also have to be told how the total number of patients who received a radiation dosage of 12 units was split between the three groups of patients who received 12 units of radiation and one of the chemotherapeutic agents.

53. No. The information that the total number of patients who received a particular chemotherapeutic agent was the same for all three drugs does not necessarily mean that the number of patients who received 12 units of radiation and a particular chemotherapeutic agent was the same for all three drugs. Thus, like the case in (52) above, a lack of information about how the total number of patients who received 12 units of radiation was split between the three groups of patients who each received 12 units of radiation and one of the three drugs makes the requested calculation impossible.

54. Yes, about 25%. The information given in this question allows us simply to average the survival percentages at 12 units of radiation for the three chemotherapeutic agents shown in the graph to get the average 5-year survival percentage of those who received 12 units of radiation. Observing that the averages are about 33% for Adriamycin, 26% for Methotrexate, and 16% for Mitomycin C, the average = about (33 + 26 + 16)/3 = 25%.

Passage VI

55. In general, one would expect the cumulative percentage of people who have had 14-day measles always to increase as occurrences of it in older people became included in this percentage. If this percentage does only increase, then the slope can only be positive in this graph. See (56) below.

56. If the relative number of those who have had 14-day measles to those who have not had 14-day measles decreased from one age to the next, then a negative slope would occur in this graph. This decrease in the relative number would occur if: (a) those people who have had 14-day measles were removed from the population, or (b) new individuals who have not had 14-day measles were added to the population, e.g., through immigration.

57. Nowhere. All slopes are positive in this graph.

58. High positive change in percentage with respect to a change in age. The ages at which the change from one age to the next in the cumulative percentage who have had 14-day measles are high can be expected to be those ages at which the chance of catching measles is high. Thus, the slope, the change in cumulative percentage with respect to a change in age, is more closely tied to the chance of catching measles of a particular age than is the cumulative percentage. The cumulative percentage at a particular age is tied to the cumulative chance of catching measles up to that age.

59. Slope. In this graph, the slope indicates the change in cumulative percentage with respect to change in age.

Passage VII

60. A. True. A straightforward graph reading shows that there were about 130,000 reported new cases of whooping cough in country X in 1953, more than in any other year between 1950 and 1963.

61. B. Information insufficient. The number of people in country X in a particular year who have had whooping cough cannot be calculated from data on the incidence of newly reported cases of it. Factors such as whooping cough's percentage death rate over the years before the year in question would also have to be known before this number could be determined.

62. B. Information insufficient. In order to compute and then compare the percentage of country X's population that contracted smallpox in 1963 to the percentage that contracted it in 1961, we would also have to be told the size of country X's population in 1963 relative to that in 1961. It is not reasonable to make any assumptions with respect to the size of country X's population in 1963 relative to that in 1961.

63. C. False. From the graph, approximately 10,000 people contracted smallpox in 1957 and approximately 130,000 people contracted whooping cough in 1953. Then:

number of smallpox deaths = (.10)(10,000) = 1,000 deaths
number of whooping cough deaths = (.03)(130,000) = 3,900 deaths
Thus, these figures represent fewer smallpox deaths than whooping cough deaths.

64. B. Information insufficient. Between the information in this statement and that in the graph, the respective numbers of reported new cases of tuberculosis and smallpox in 1957 that died in that same year can be calculated—about 200 for smallpox and just over 100 for tuberculosis. However, reading the statement carefully, it asks for a comparison of the total number of deaths (including those occurring in cases reported prior to 1957) caused by tuberculosis in 1957 to the total number caused by smallpox in 1957. The respective numbers of deaths caused by tuberculosis and smallpox in 1957 for cases of these diseases reported prior to 1957 cannot be determined; so this comparison cannot be accomplished.

65. B. Information insufficient. Value judgements such as this one cannot be made on the basis of the simple incidence data such as those presented in the graph for this problem.

4.5 MATHEMATICS DEFINITIONS

With Illustrations [*]

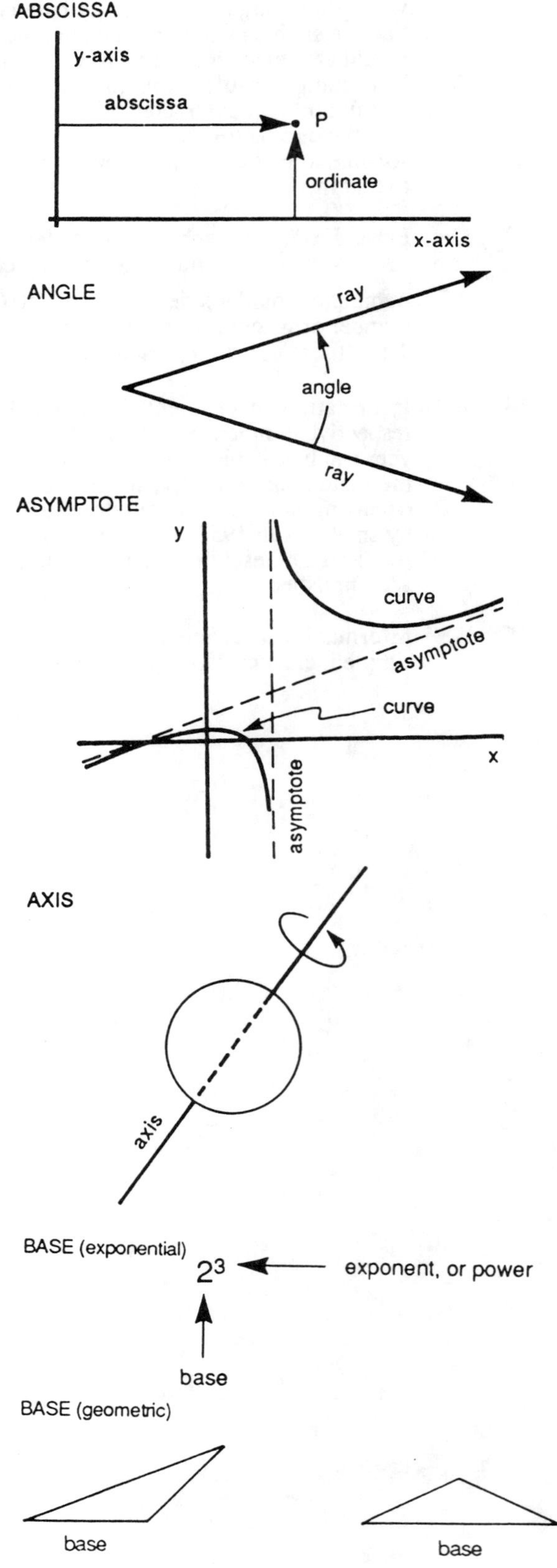

Abscissa*
Within a system of coordinates, the distance of a point from the vertical (or *y*) axis measured along a line parallel to the horizontal (or *x*) axis. (See *ordinate.)*

Absolute value
The size of a number without regard to its sign; the distance from zero of a number on a number line.

Analysis (noun), **analyze** (verb)
To separate any complex whole into simpler parts in order to perceive its nature or function. Analysis is a powerful tool when used to make a complex problem simpler and more easily understood, e.g., to analyze water quality in a lab, to analyze trends graphs in the MCAT quantitative subtest, or to analyze a reading text. (See also *synthesis, quantitative analysis.)*

Angle*
An angle is formed at the point two rays or plane surfaces converge. (See *ray.*)

Asymptote*
A straight line associated with a curve in a way that, as a point moves along an extremity of the curve, the distance from the point to the line approaches zero and the direction of the curve at the point approaches the direction of the line.

Average
The numerical result obtained by dividing the sum of two or more quantities by the number of those quantities.

Axis*
A real or imaginary straight line on which an object can be thought of as translating or rotating, e.g., the axis around which the earth rotates, the spin axis of a top or phonograph disc. In a graph, an axis is a straight line for reference or measure. The vertical axis is the y-axis; the horizontal axis is the x-axis. (See *abscissa.)*

Base (exponential)*
The number that is raised to various powers to produce the main counting units of a number system.

Base (geometric)*
The length of a side of a figure which has been oriented so that the side in question is "horizontal" or parallel to the bottom edge of the page. Any side can be the base but as the base changes so will the height.

Characteristic
The integer part of a common (base-10) log. (See *mantissa.)*

Cone (*see next page)
A solid with a circle for its base and a curved surface tapering evenly to a point, e.g., cone for ice cream.

Concave
Having a surface or boundary that curves like the inner surface of a sphere.

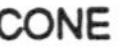

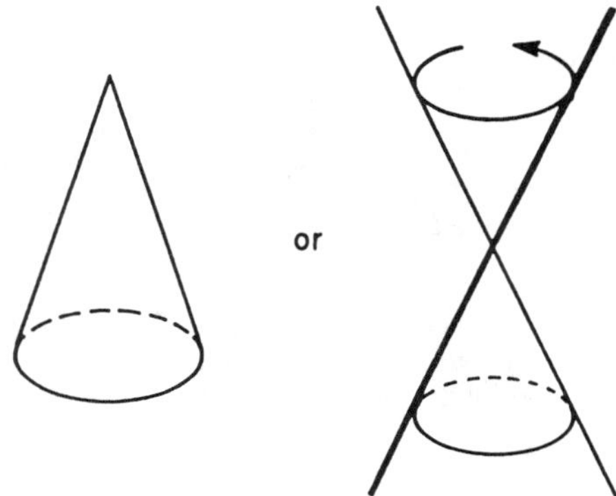

Constant (noun)

A symbol or number that has a fixed value under certain given conditions. (A physics problem may state, usually in parentheses, "assume the wind velocity is a constant"; in chemistry note the constant used in each of the ideal-gas laws.)

Convex

Having a surface or boundary that curves like the outer surface of a sphere.

Coordinates

A system of one or more numbers used to define the position of a point. (See *abscissa.)*

Critical point*

(Math) A point on the graph of a function where the line tangent to the curve is vertical or horizontal. The function may have a local maximum or minimum at a critical point.

(Chem) A combination of temperature and pressure above which it is not possible to liquify a gas, e.g., for CO_2 gas the critical point is 31.1° C. at 73 atm.

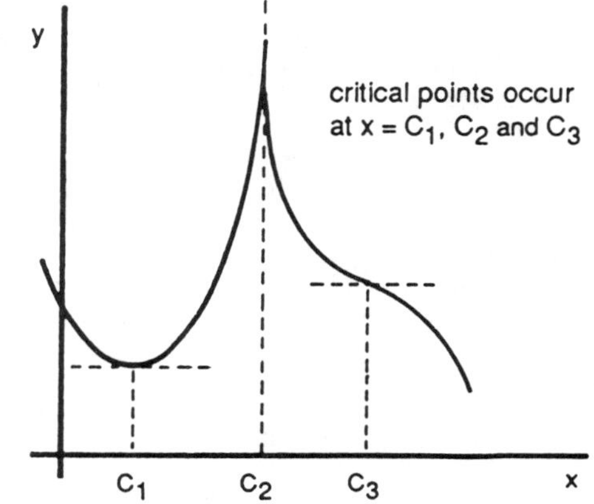

Deci-

Prefix representing the number 10.

Decimal

A set of numerals that represent a fraction (after the decimal point). A decimal indicates a multiple of a positive or negative power of 10. (See *decimal point.)*

Decimal point

A dot that separates the integer part of a number from the decimal fraction part of the number.

Degree

A unit of measure for angles or arcs.

Distance

The length of a line segment between two points.

Equation

A mathematical assertion that two expressions are equal.

Exponent

A superscript above a number that indicates repeated multiplication and shows the number of times the base is to be multiplied by itself. (see *base*.)

Expression

A mathematical phrase. (An equation is a mathematical sentence.) An expression indicates a finite number of mathematical operations, such as addition or multiplication, to be performed on the variables.

Fraction

A part of a whole expressed as numerator over denominator. (If you are given 1/5 of an apple pie, what percentage of the pie do you receive? Review converting fractions to percentages and vice versa. Practice estimating the conversions; for example, approximately what fraction of the whole pie is 47%.)

Function

A rule that relates two quantities in such a way that for every first coordinate there is exactly one corresponding second coordinate. A function may be specified by a list of ordered pairs, a graph or a formula.

Graph*

A visual representation of mathematical information. The word "graph" comes from Greek and it means "to write or draw."

The most common types of graphs on the MCAT are bar graphs, pie graphs, and line graphs. Bar graphs are used to make comparisons, i.e., between categories. Pie or circle graphs are often used to show some kind of distribution of a whole, for example, the distribution of wealth, of population, etc. Multiple line graphs are often used to show change in one or more variables.

Learning to read graphs is a little like learning to read a language in which virtually everything that is said is both quantitative and comparative. (In any given election year, graphs can tell you how many Democrats voted Republican and vice versa, but it will not show you why.)

GRAPH

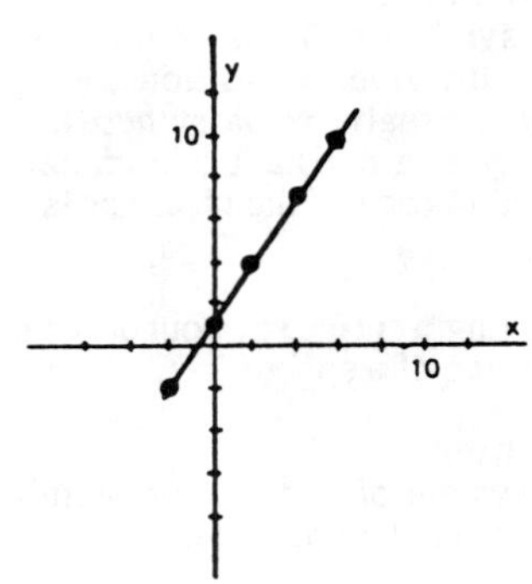

Note that this graph can also be algebraically represented by

$$y = \frac{3}{2}x + 1.$$

Height*

The height of a geometric figure is usually not one of its sides. It is the distance from the base to a line parallel to the base that goes through the point on the figure which is farthest above the base.

HEIGHT

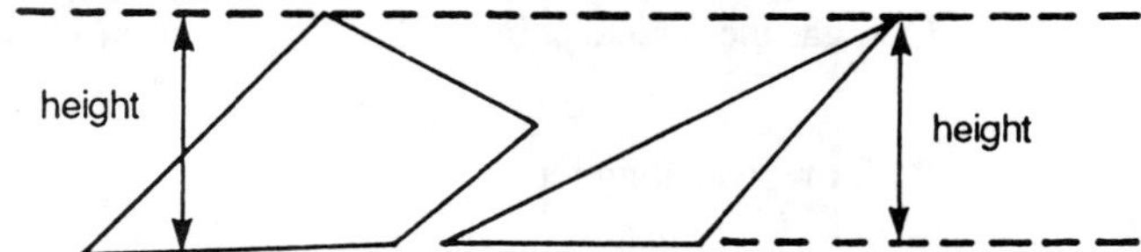

Hyperbola*

A plane curve formed by the intersection of a cone with an oblique plane cut at an angle steeper than the angle of the side of the cone.

HYPERBOLA

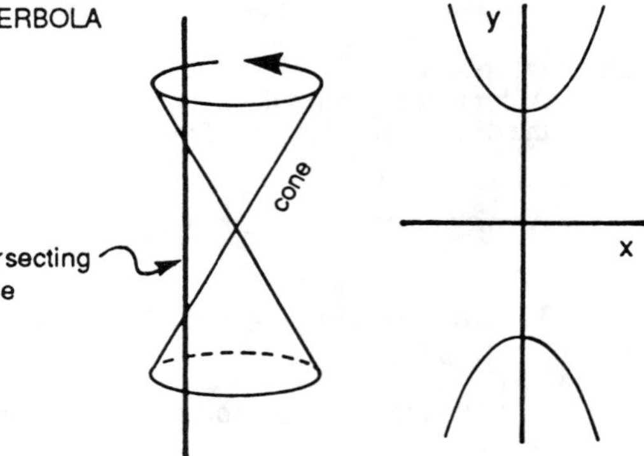

Inflection

The act or result of curving or bending.

Inflection point*

A point on a curve that separates an arc that is concave upward from one that is concave downward and vice versa.

INFLECTION POINT

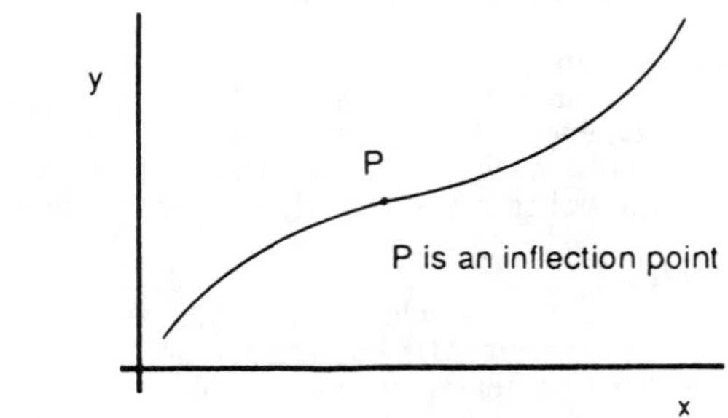

Logarithm

Another name for an exponent, an alternative form for exponential notation. For example, if $2^3 = 8$, then $\log_2 8 = 3$, read "the base-2 log of 8 is 3." (Ten is the base for the common log system, and e = 2.718... is the base for the natural log system.)

Mantissa

The decimal part of a common (base-10) logarithm. (See *characteristic*.)

Median

The middle number in a series arranged in order of size, or, if there is no middle value, the average of the two middle numbers.

Mode

The value, number, etc., used most frequently in a given distribution.

Ordinate*

Within a system of coordinates, the distance of a point from the horizontal (or x) axis measured along a line parallel to the vertical (or y) axis. (See illustration for *abscissa.*)

Origin

The intersection of coordinate axes.

Parabola*

A curve formed when a plane cuts a cone in a direction parallel to the side of the cone. The graph of a quadratic equation is a parabola. A parabola is also the set of points that are equidistant from a fixed line and a fixed point.

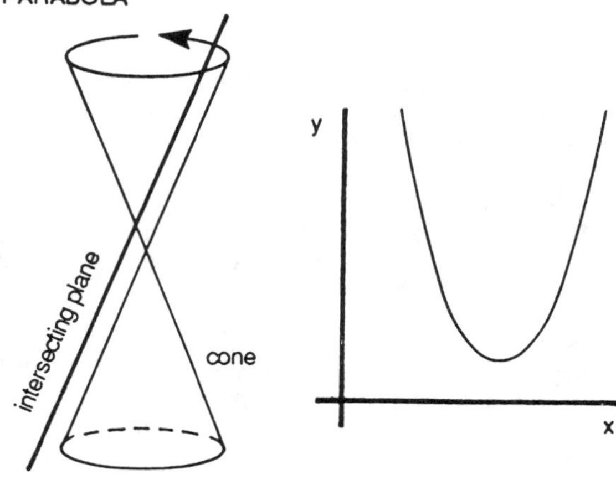

Percent, percentage

A fraction with a denominator of 100 (1/100); a given part or amount in every hundred.

Parallel lines/planes*

A term that describes two or more lines (or two or more planes) that extend in the same direction at a constant distance apart so that they never meet. (In gymnastics, exercise is done on parallel bars. An MCAT biology question might ask about parallel evolution; if you know what parallel bars in a gym are, can you say what parallel evolution is?)

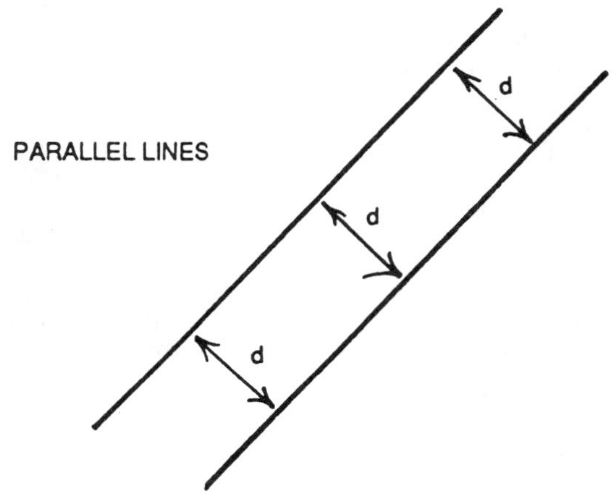

Proportion

Having the same ratio; a quantity in a mathematical proportion.

Quadratic

An equation of the form $y = ax^2 + bx + c$, where a, b and c are constants. The graph of a quadratic is a parabola.

Quantitative analysis

Analysis by the amount or quantity of a variable.

Rate

The ratio of one variable to another representing how a change in one relates to a change in the other, e.g., slope.

Ratio

The quotient of one quantity divided by another, e.g., probability is a ratio or fraction.

Ray*

Any one of several lines coming out from a point, as in the spokes of a wheel; one of the lines of light that appear to radiate from a light source. (See *angle*.)

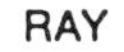

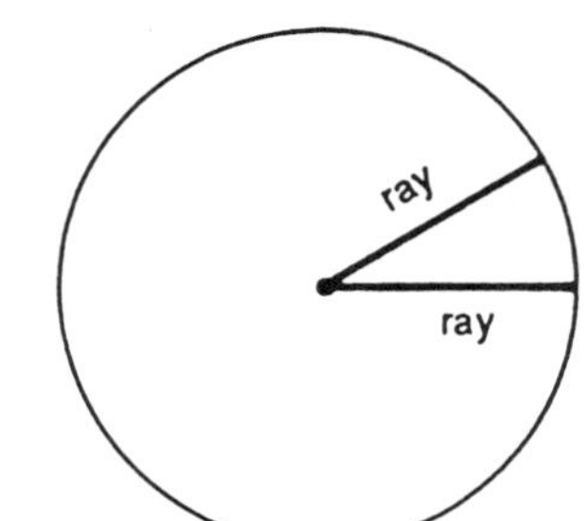

Root

A quantity which, when multiplied by itself a specified number of times, produces a given quantity.

Scalar quantity

A quantity that has magnitude described by a real number, but no direction in space, e.g., temperature, time, or mass.

Slope*

A number that describes the direction of a straight line; a ratio that measures the rate at which a line rises or falls with respect to a horizontal change.

SLOPE

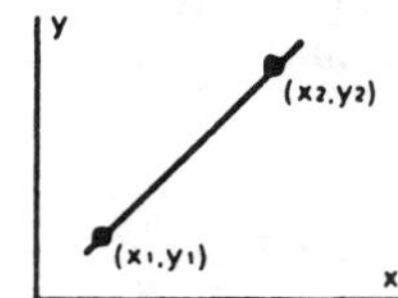

The slope of the straight line graphed here is:

$$\text{slope} = m = \frac{y_2-y_1}{x_2-x_1} = \frac{\Delta y}{\Delta x} = \text{constant}$$

Synthesis (noun), **synthesize** (verb)

Synthesis is to put parts together to form a whole. (Analysis is to break up the whole into its parts in order to understand it better.)

When studying, analysis is only half of what is required for understanding; synthesis is the other half. In quantitative analysis, graphs or charts are first analyzed, then the information is synthesized in order to combine concepts to answer the questions. Analysis and synthesis are complements of each other. (See *analysis.*)

Tangent*

A line or plane that touches, but does not intersect, a curved line or surface at <u>one</u> point only.

TANGENT

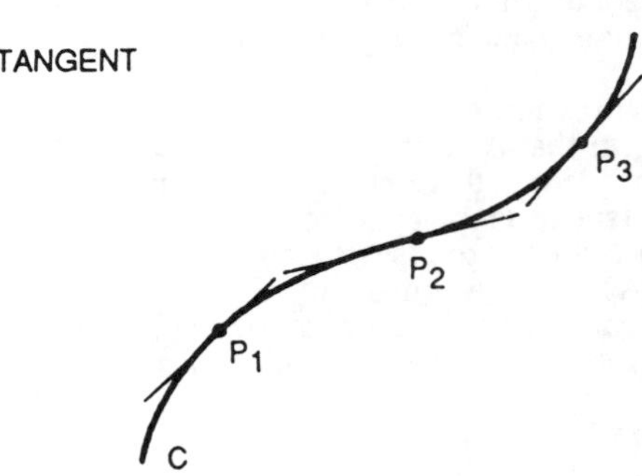

Lines are drawn tangent to the curve C at the points P_1, P_2 and P_3

Vacuum

The absence of matter.

Variable (mathematical)

A quantity, usually represented by a letter such as x, that can take on a range of different values. Two variables are often linked through a function (represented by an equation or graph) that gives a rule for determining the value of one variable from the other.

Vector*

A quantity with both magnitude and direction, such as a force or velocity.

VECTOR

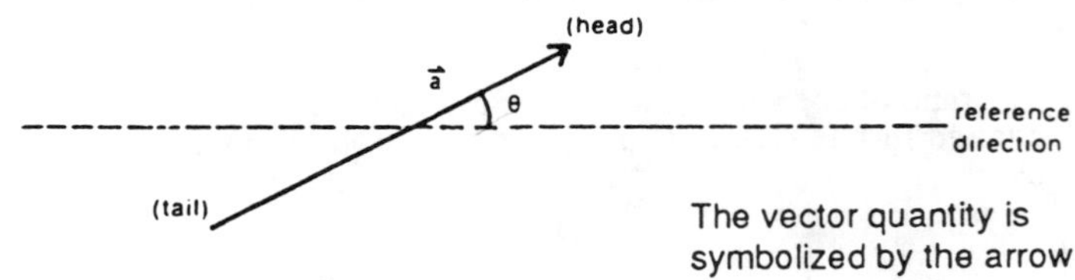

The vector quantity is symbolized by the arrow

4.6 REFERENCES

Beyond Problem Solving and Comprehension, 1984. Arthur Whimbey and Jack Lochhead. Hillsdale, N.J.: Lawrence Erlbaum Associates.

Drawing on the Right Side of Your Brain, 1979. Betty Edwards. Los Angeles: Jeremy P. Tarcher, Inc.

How to Study in College, 4th or later ed. Walter Pauk. Boston: Houghton Mifflin Co.

Knowledge as Design, 1986. Ed. by D. N. Perkins. Hillsdale, N.J.: Lawrence Erlbaum Associates.

Learning to Learn, 2nd or later ed. J. D. Novak and D. B. Gowin. New York: Cambridge University Press.

Problem Solving and Comprehension, 5th or later ed. Arthur Whimbey and Jack Lochhead. Hillsdale, N.J.: Lawrence Erlbaum Associates.

The Complete Problem Solver, 2nd or later ed. John R. Hayes. Hillsdale, NJ: Lawrence Erlbaum Associates.

Unicorns are Real: A Right-Brained Approach to Learning, 1986. Barbara M. Vitale. New York: Warner Books.

Using Both Sides of Your Brain, 1983. Tony Buzan. New York: E. P. Dutton, Inc.

With Good Reason: An Introduction to Informal Fallacies, 3rd or later ed. S. Morris Engel. New York: St. Martin's Press.

PASSAGE TYPES IN PHYSICAL AND BIOLOGICAL SCIENCES

These passage types were developed in accordance with the passage formats shown on page 30 of the MCAT Student Manual and Appendix A in this book. MCAT-type passages in physical and biological sciences usually belong to one of the following categories:

- Descriptive information passages
- Descriptive information passages with diagrams
- Instrument information passages
- Descriptive problem-solving passages
- Descriptive problem-solving passages with diagrams
- Instrument problem-solving passages
- Problem-solving passages using laboratory devices
- Experimental problem-solving passages
- Experimental problem-solving passages with diagrams
- Problem-solving passages with diagrams only
- Research study passages with diagrams
- Instrumental research study passages
- Research study passages using laboratory devices
- Experimental research study passages
- Research study passages with persuasive arguments
- Descriptive persuasive argument passages
- Persuasive argument passages with diagrams
- Experimental persuasive argument passages
- Persuasive argument passages using medical instruments

Interactive Learning Tutorial for the MCAT

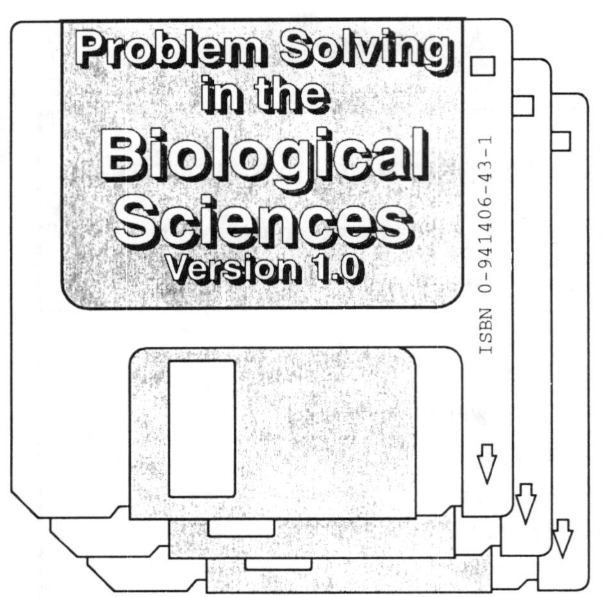

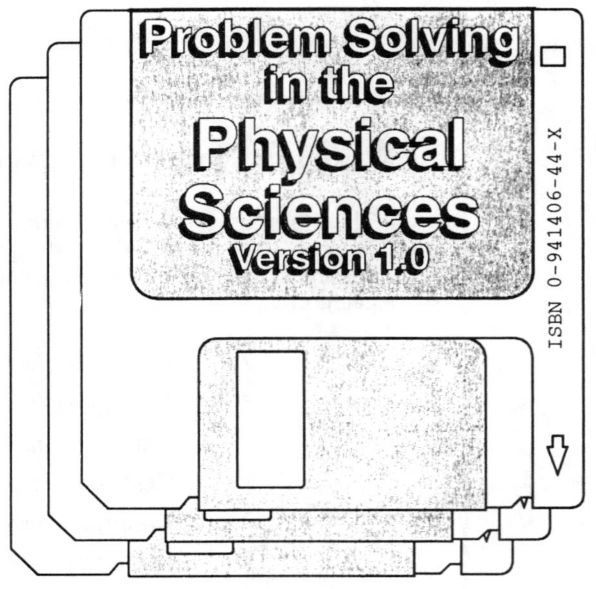

YOUR BEST COMBINATION FOR MCAT SUCCESS

This easy-to-use software from Betz Publishing Company is a tutorial for self-managed learning. You learn the important skills essential for problem solving in the MCAT. It is the only software of its kind, designed to help you become highly efficient and productive in MCAT preparation. It is an interactive resource to link advanced premedical concepts in Physical and Biological Sciences with related chapters from *A Complete Preparation for the MCAT*, based on the outline according to the *MCAT Student Manual* (AAMC).

The **Biological Sciences** software intentionally focuses on anatomy and physiology fundamentals. This shows you how to interpret diagrams, figures, and medical terms, and how to apply concepts learned in physics, mathematics, chemistry, and biology courses. Special verbal reasoning and test-taking skills in bioorganic chemistry are used in this software to show you how indirect recall of information plays a major role in learning organic chemistry.

The **Physical Sciences** software takes experimental physics and general chemistry laboratory experiences and blends them with typical MCAT passages. Users are required to perform mathematical operations, apply various reasoning patterns, and decipher physical principles as required in actual MCAT problems.

NO FORMAL REVIEW OF ORGANIC CHEMISTRY, PHYSICS, OR BIOLOGY IS DUPLICATED IN THESE SOFTWARE PACKAGES. A complete science review is provided in chapters 5 and 7 of *A Complete Preparation for the MCAT.* Software packages are fully integrated for "passage-linked science review," and they reflect the way passage types are incorporated in the Physical and Biological Sciences of the MCAT. The arguments and types of reasoning required to make scientific decisions are a special highlight of this software. Use it regularly as you read journal articles and newspapers, watch science videos, and above all, as you are learning to work MCAT passages and problems. **CALL 1 (800) 634-4365 TO PLACE YOUR ORDER.**

Chapter 5

Problem Solving in the Physical Sciences

EXPANDED TABLE OF CONTENTS FOR PHYSICAL SCIENCES

Introduction to Problem Solving in the Physical Sciences 5–4
General Chemistry 5–8
Sec. 5.1 Electronic Structure of the Atom 5–8
5.1.1 Review of Electronic Structure of the Atom 5–8
5.1.2 Questions to Review Electronic Structure of the Atom 5–11
5.1.3 Answers to Questions in Section 5.1.2 5–13
5.1.4 Discussion of Answers to Questions in Section 5.1.2 5–13
5.1.5 Checklist for Electronic Structure of the Atom 5–14
5.2 The Periodic Table 5–14
5.2.1 Review of the Periodic Table 5–14
5.2.2 Questions to Review the Periodic Table 5–16
5.2.3 Answers to Questions in Section 5.2.2 5–19
5.2.4 Discussion of Answers to Questions in Section 5.2.2 5–20
5.2.5 Checklist for the Periodic Table 5–20
5.3 Chemical Bonding 5–21
5.3.1 Review of Chemical Bonding 5–21
5.3.1.1 Ionic Bonding 5–21
5.3.1.2 Covalent Bonding 5–21
5.3.1.3 Intermolecular Forces in Liquids and Solids 5–24
5.3.2 Questions to Review Chemical Bonding 5–25
5.3.3 Answers to Questions in Section 5.3.2 5–28
5.3.4 Discussion of Answers to Questions in Section 5.3.2 5–28
5.3.5 Checklist for Chemical Bonding 5–29
5.4 Stoichiometry 5–29
5.4.1 Review of Stoichiometry 5–29
5.4.2 Questions to Review Stoichiometry 5–30
5.4.3 Answers to Questions in Section 5.4.2 5–31
5.4.4 Discussion of Answers to Questions in Section 5.4.2 5–31
5.4.5 Checklist for Stoichiometry 5–33
5.5 Electrochemistry 5–33
5.5.1 Review of Electrochemistry 5–33
5.5.2 Questions to Review Electrochemistry 5–36
5.5.3 Answers to Questions in Section 5.5.2 5–41
5.5.4 Discussion of Answers to Questions in Section 5.5.2 5–42
5.5.5 Checklist for Electrochemistry 5–46
5.6 Quantitative Chemistry: Compounds and Chemical Reactions 5–46
5.6.1 Review of Quantitative Chemistry 5–46
5.6.2 Questions to Review Quantitative Chemistry 5–49
5.6.3 Answers to Questions in Section 5.6.2 5–53
5.6.4 Discussion of Answers to Questions in Section 5.6.2 5–53
5.6.5 Checklist for Quantitative Chemistry 5–58
5.7 Solution Chemistry 5–58
5.7.1 Review of Solution Chemistry 5–58
5.7.1.1 Concentration Units 5–58
5.7.1.2 Ions in Solution, Solubility, Chemical Separations 5–60
5.7.2 Questions to Review Solution Chemistry 5–61
5.7.3 Answers to Questions in Section 5.7.2 5–63
5.7.4 Discussion of Answers to Questions in Section 5.7.2 5–63
5.7.5 Checklist for Solution Chemistry 5–65

5.8 Acids and Bases 5–65
5.8.1 Review of Acids and Bases 5–65
5.8.1.1 Neutralization Reactions and Acid/Base Titrations 5–67
5.8.1.2 Buffers 5–68
5.8.2 Questions to Review Acids and Bases 5–69
5.8.3 Answers to Questions in Section 5.8.2 5–73
5.8.4 Discussion of Answers to Questions in Section 5.8.2 5–73
5.8.5 Checklist for Acids and Bases 5–76
5.9 Phases and Phase Equilibria 5–76
5.9.1 Review of Phases and Phase Equilibria 5–76
5.9.1.1 Colligative Properties (Freezing and Boiling Points) 5–77
5.9.2 Questions to Review Phases and Phase Equilibria 5–79
5.9.3 Answers to Questions in Section 5.9.2 5–81
5.9.4 Discussion of Answers to Questions in Section 5.9.2 5–81
5.9.5 Checklist for Phases and Phase Equilibria 5–82
Chemistry-Related Physics 5–83
5.10 Gas Properties 5–83
5.10.1 Review of the Gas Properties 5–83
5.10.1.1 Applications of Gas Properties to the Human Body 5–86
5.10.2 Questions to Review Gas Properties 5–86
5.10.3 Answers to Questions in Section 5.10.2 5–89
5.10.4 Discussion of Answers to Questions in Section 5.10.2 5–89
5.10.5 Checklist for Gas Properties 5–91
5.11 Solid and Fluid Properties 5–91
5.11.1 Review of Solid and Fluid Properties 5–91
5.11.1.1 Elastic Properties of Solids 5–91
5.11.1.2 Density and Its Physical Meaning 5–92
5.11.1.3 Static and Dynamic Properties of Fluids 5–93
5.11.1.4 Applications of Solid and Fluid Properties to the Human Body 5–96
5.11.2 Questions to Review Solid and Fluid Properties 5–97
5.11.3 Answers to Questions in Section 5.11.2 5–100
5.11.4 Discussion of Answers to Questions in Section 5.11.2 5–100
5.11.5 Checklist for Solid and Fluid Properties 5–101
5.12 Thermodynamics and Thermochemistry 5–101
5.12.1 Review of Thermodynamics and Thermochemistry 5–101
5.12.1.1 Thermodynamics 5–101
5.12.1.2 Thermochemistry 5–106
5.12.1.3 Applications of Thermodynamics and Thermochemistry to the Human Body 5–107
5.12.2 Questions to Review Thermodynamics and Thermochemistry 5–107
5.12.3 Answers to Questions in Section 5.12.2 5–114
5.12.4 Discussion of Answers to Questions in Section 5.12.2 5–114
5.12.5 Checklist for Thermodynamics and Thermochemistry 5–117
5.13 Rate Processes in Chemical Reactions—Kinetics and Equillibrium 5–118
5.13.1 Review of Rate Processes in Chemical Reactions 5–118
5.13.1.1 Kinetics 5–118
5.13.1.2 Equilibrium 5–120
5.13.1.3 Applications of Rate Processes in Chemical Reactions to the Human Body 5–122
5.13.2 Questions to Review Kinetics and Equilibrium 5–123
5.13.3 Answers to Questions in Section 5.13.2 5–125
5.13.4 Discussion of Answers to Questions in Section 5.13.2 5–125
5.13.5 Checklist for Kinetics and Equilibrium 5–126
Physics 5–127
5.14 Force and Motion, Gravitation 5–127
5.14.1 Review of Force and Motion, Gravitation 5–127
5.14.2 Questions to Review Force and Motion, Gravitation 5–129
5.14.3 Answers to Questions in Section 5.14.2 5–132
5.14.4 Discussion of Answers to Questions in Section 5.14.2 5–132
5.14.5 Checklist for Force and Motion, Gravitation 5–133
5.15 Work and Energy 5–133
5.15.1 Review of Work and Energy 5–133
5.15.2 Questions to Review Work and Energy 5–135
5.15.3 Answers to Questions in Section 5.15.2 5–137

5.15.4 Discussion of Answers to Questions in Section 5.15.2 5–137
5.15.5 Checklist for Work and Energy 5–138
5.16 Translational Motion 5–138
5.16.1 Review of Translational Motion 5–138
5.16.2 Questions to Review Translational Motion 5–141
5.16.3 Answers to Questions in Section 5.16.2 5–143
5.16.4 Discussion of Answers to Questions in Section 5.16.2 5–143
5.16.5 Checklist for Translational Motion 5–145
5.17 Equilibrium and Momentum 5–146
5.17.1 Review of Equilibrium and Momentum 5–146
5.17.1.1 Equilibrium 5–146
5.17.1.2 Momentum 5–147
5.17.2 Questions to Review Equilibrium and Momentum 5–147
5.17.3 Answers to Questions in Section 5.17.2 5–149
5.17.4 Discussion of Answers to Questions in Section 5.17.2 5–149
5.17.5 Checklist for Equilibrium and Momentum 5–151
5.18 Electrostatics and Electromagnetism 5–151
5.18.1 Review of Electrostatics and Electromagnetism 5–151
5.18.1.1 Electrostatics 5–151
5.18.1.2 Electromagnetism 5–153
5.18.2 Questions to Review Electrostatics and Electromagnetism 5–155
5.18.3 Answers to Questions in Section 5.18.2 5–159
5.18.4 Discussion of Answers to Questions in Section 5.18.2 5–159
5.18.5 Checklist for Electrostatics and Electromagnetism 5–161
5.19 Electric Circuits 5–161
5.19.1 Review of Electric Circuits 5–161
5.19.1.1 Electric Circuits 5–161
5.19.1.2 Alternating Electric Circuits 5–164
5.19.2 Questions to Review Electric Circuits 5–166
5.19.3 Answers to Questions in Section 5.19.2 5–172
5.19.4 Discussion of Answers to Questions in Section 5.19.2 5–172
5.19.5 Checklist for Electric Circuits 5–174
5.20 Wave Characteristics and Periodic Motion 5–174
5.20.1 Review of Wave Characteristics and Periodic Motion 5–174
5.20.2 Questions to Review Wave Characteristics and Periodic Motion 5–177
5.20.3 Answers to Questions in Section 5.20.2 5–180
5.20.4 Discussion of Answers to Questions in Section 5.20.2 5–180
5.20.5 Checklist for Wave Characteristics and Periodic Motion 5–183
5.21 Sound 5–184
5.21.1 Review of Sound 5–184
5.21.1.1 The Human Ear 5–184
5.21.2 Questions to Review Sound 5–186
5.21.3 Answers to Questions in Section 5.21.2 5–189
5.21.4 Discussion of Answers to Questions in Section 5.21.2 5–189
5.21.5 Checklist for Sound 5–191
5.22 Light and Geometrical Optics 5–191
5.22.1 Review of Light and Geometrical Optics 5–191
5.22.1.1 The Human Eye 5–191
5.22.1.2 Reflection 5–193
5.22.1.3 Refraction 5–195
5.22.2 Questions to Review Light and Geometrical Optics 5–197
5.22.3 Answers to Questions in Section 5.22.2 5–203
5.22.4 Discussion of Answers to Questions in Section 5.22.2 5–204
5.22.5 Checklist for Light and Geometrical Optics 5–206
5.23 Nuclear and Atomic Structure 5–206
5.23.1 Review of Nuclear and Atomic Structure 5–206
5.23.1.1 Review of Nuclear Structure 5–206
5.23.1.2 Review of Atomic Structure 5–208
5.23.2 Questions to Review Nuclear and Atomic Structure 5–210
5.23.3 Answers to Questions in Section 5.23.2 5–213
5.23.4 Discussion of Answers to Questions in Section 5.23.2 5–213
5.23.5 Checklist for Nuclear and Atomic Structure 5–214
5.24 References 5–214

INTRODUCTION TO PROBLEM SOLVING IN THE PHYSICAL SCIENCES

Merely memorizing scientific facts and solving physics and chemistry problems with mathematical calculations are not adequate for the new MCAT. In order to work the new scientific passages and accommodate the various types of reasoning they present beyond rote memory, Chapter 5 has been divided into 3 parts: General Chemistry, Chemistry-related Physics and Physics. Each section should be reviewed to develop a *conceptual understanding* of scientific facts and their application to medically or health-related situations.

Reading a conceptual section such as 5.3.1.1 (Ionic Bonding) involves the use of critical verbal reasoning skills to extract information and precise scientific reasoning, which includes definitions, perception, and association with previous knowledge. Reading this section will help you to read longer passages filled with text, formulas and equations in association with various sketches and schematic drawings. Apply the concepts you have learned to the "Questions for Review . . ." at the end of each section.

Chemistry-related Physics should be reviewed with an intent to link concepts in physics and chemistry. This part is also written to demonstrate common areas in physical sciences which may be classified either as chemistry or physics. Medical problem-solving always aims at solving scientific problems which include a mix of physiology, anatomy, pharmacology and biochemistry. Each section ends with a list of interrelated medical topics which should be included in your physical sciences review.

Finally, we suggest that you refer to introductory textbooks in anatomy, physiology and biochemistry to answer the following questions:

(i) How will you relate to information presented in the book?
(ii) How will you extract basic concepts from the information?
(iii) How will this information relate to passages in the new MCAT?
(iv) What forms of reasoning will you use to master new information?
(v) How will you use this new information to construct questions in the review style of *A Complete Preparation for the MCAT?*
(vi) Why is it more difficult for you to extract basic concepts from a new book?

Chapters 2, 3, and 4 in this book are designed to provide intellectual tools to help you become a good problem solver. These intellectual tools consist of reasoning, critical reading, interpretation of graphical information and acquiring scientific knowledge. The new MCAT emphasizes the use and application of these intellectual tools. Look at the following physical science passage and apply your own intellectual skills to it.

> "As a scientist, I boil water in a pot and observe the chaotic mixture of water, steam and bubbles. As I become more curious, but bored with boiling plain water, I choose to boil an egg. I take an egg and carefully lower it with a spoon into the boiling pot. I know that adding sodium chloride or table salt will make it much easier to peel the egg."

To answer specific questions relating to the above situation, employ the following intellectual tools or skills:

- Reading for scientific information—see Chapters 2, 4 and Appendix A
- Developing scientific vocabulary—refer to a thesaurus or dictionary
- Deriving any conclusion (based on supported or unsupported claims)—see Chapter 3
- Constructing science problems—see Chapters 4 and 8
- Looking for missing information (including unstated assumptions)—see Chapter 3

- *Reading for cause and effect.* The passage explains that boiling water (implied word is "heating" water to a certain temperature) increases its temperature. The heat causes the bubbles of dissolved air to expand and escape at the surface of the water. The heating of the liquid yolk and white inside the porous egg shell causes it to solidify. Why? Remember, heating a cube of ice changes it from a solid to a liquid, which is a physical change. Hence, boiling an egg is a chemical reaction. Studying the chemical compo-sition of egg yolk and egg white would explain that. Salt in the water provides salt molecules which travel through the egg shell making it easier to peel. Is that a valid conclusion? Does the salt lower or raise the boiling point? All these questions can be connected to biology, physics, or chemistry concepts.

- *Reading for scientific information.* This builds your knowledge of physics, chemistry, biology and mathematics. Knowing the definitions of scientific words makes comparative and analogical reasoning much easier. Important scientific words in this passage would be: water, boiling, steam, bubbles (air), egg, sodium chloride, temperature. Try to define these words and their usage in physics, chemistry and biology—learn to integrate definitions and develop concepts, e.g., would sodium chloride create an acidic medium or a basic medium?

- *Deriving any conclusions.*

  The following conclusions are *obvious (direct)*;

  (1) Heat is required to boil water.
  (2) Eggs solidify after a certain time if put in boiling water.
  (3) Peeling an egg shell is easier if salt is added to the water.

  The following conclusions are *implied (indirect)*:

  (1) The scientist is trying to explain a very simple everyday situation in a highly sophisticated scientific and logical way.
  (2) Egg shells can be hard to peel.
  (3) Water should be boiling at a certain temperature before eggs are lowered into it.
  (4) The specific heat of an egg and the specific heat of water are different.
  (5) Thermodynamic equilibrium is achieved when water boils.
  (6) Elevation of boiling point by adding salt can be measured by using a thermometer.
  (7) The egg used in the experiment could be fresh, stale or rotten.

- *Constructing science problems.* These are multiple-choice or mixed-choice questions based on the scientific situation explained. In this exercise, ask yourself the following questions:

  (1) What is egg yolk made of?
  (2) What is the egg shell made of?
  (3) What is egg white made of?
  (4) At what temperature does water boil? Why?
  (5) Are egg molecules biological molecules?
  (6) How long does it take to boil an egg? Why?
  (7) How much water should you boil?
  (8) How much salt should you add to the water? Why?
  (9) When should you peel the egg?
  (10) How should you lower the egg into the water (with what size spoon)?
  (11) Who is a scientist?
  (12) Does this experiment represent a scientific situation?
  (13) Do egg molecules arrange themselves differently when salt is added? If so, why?

Be sure to add "why?" after each question as shown and double check your answers. Feel free to open a chemistry or physics book for basic help.

The last two steps, "Solving science problems" and "Looking for missing information," are well covered in chapter 4. In this instance, an unstated assumption or missing information would be as follows, "A raw egg should be lowered very carefully to prevent it from breaking or cracking." Review diagramming and reasoning skills carefully before moving ahead in this chapter. Take note of how the above situation reflects integration of physics, chemistry, reading, reasoning and some mathematics. The new MCAT focuses on the integration of various subject areas. In physical sciences, the focus is on integration of physics concepts and chemistry concepts with reading and reasoning to improve your overall performance. As a reminder, the short passage above is extremely simple compared to MCAT science problems. Review and integrate various sections or subsections of chapters as you progress in your overall MCAT review, e.g., electronic structure of an atom should be linked with atomic and nuclear structure in physics.

The introduction in chapter 1 emphasizes that the arrangement of various topics in a subsection or section is *not* in the same sequence as in the MCAT Student Manual outline. It should be realized that logical continuity, conceptual building blocks and coherent subject matter were important objectives in developing the sequence of this book. See the charts that follow for direction in studying general chemistry and physics. The coverage of topics and the amount of detail in the background knowledge for these topics has been kept to bare essentials to let you grasp *all* related concepts. The reordering of sections is actually beneficial because on the actual MCAT test items are arranged rather randomly.

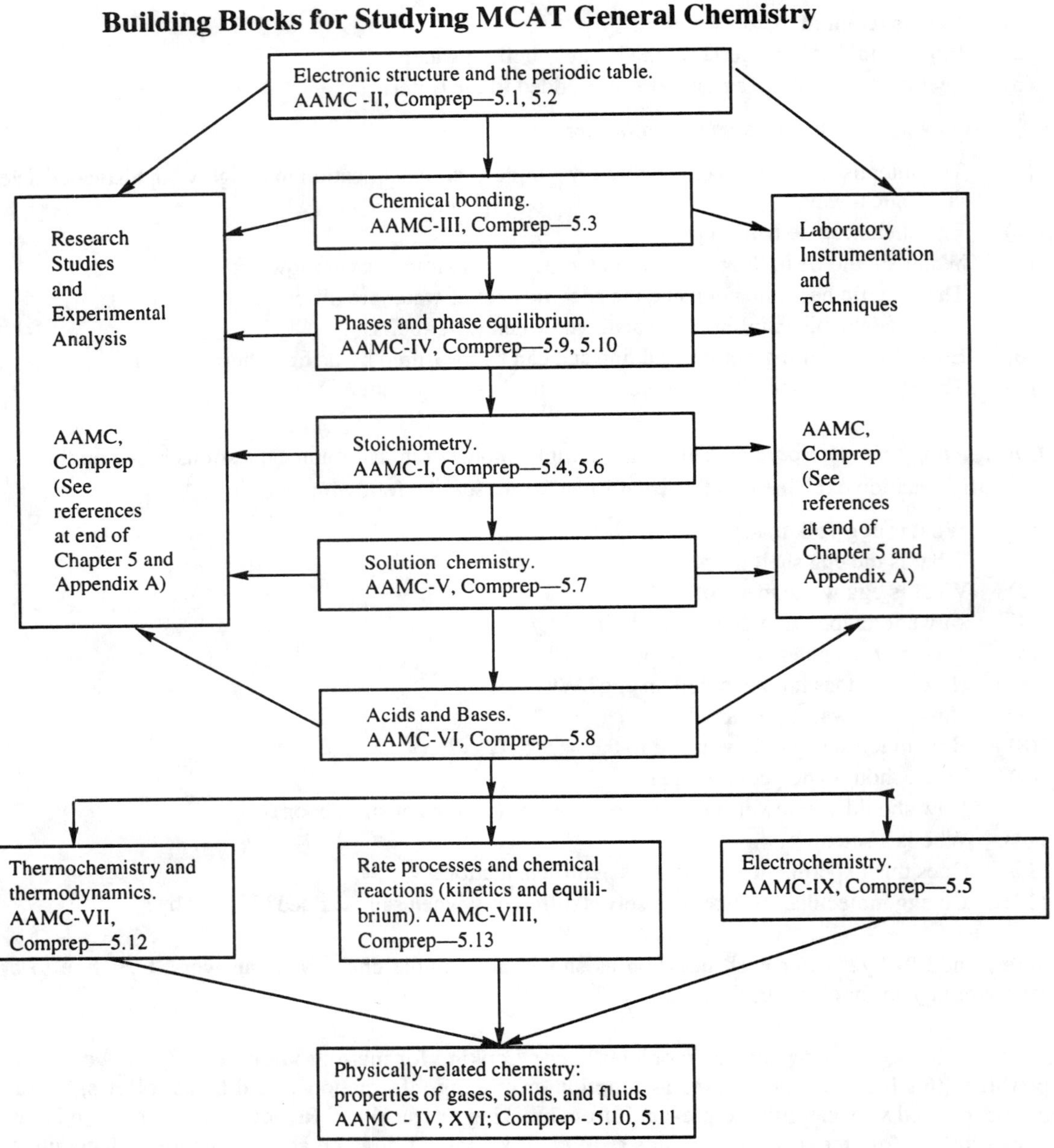

Building Blocks for Studying MCAT Physics

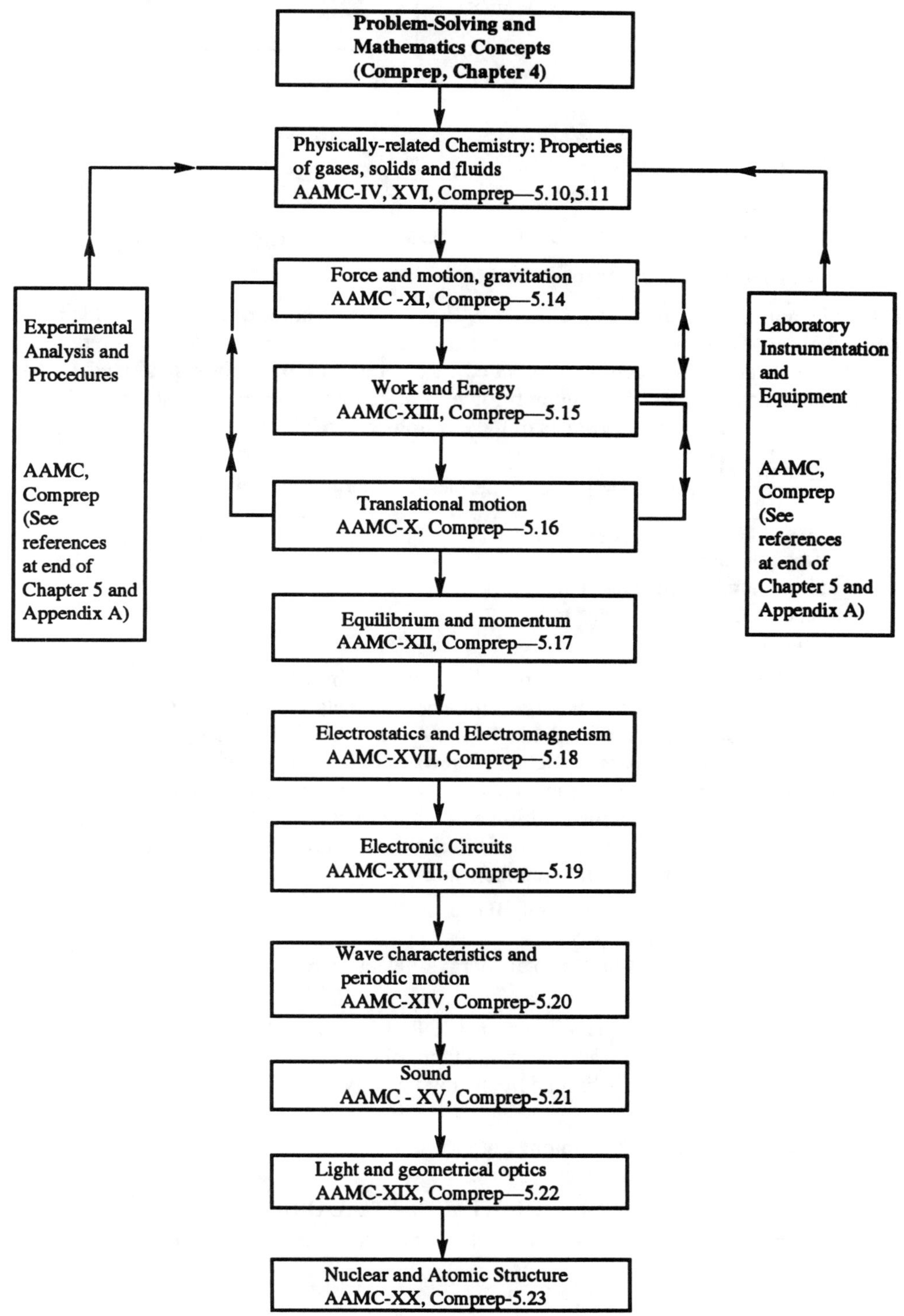

GENERAL CHEMISTRY

5.1 ELECTRONIC STRUCTURE OF THE ATOM

5.1.1 Review of Electronic Structure of the Atom

Bohr used the theories and experimental data of Planck, Einstein and Rutherford to develop his theory of the atom. He thought the angular momentum of the electron was in multiples of $h/2\pi$ (or $mvr = nh/2\pi$) (see "momentum" in Physics), and that electrons circulated in discrete circular orbits stabilized by having the centrifugal force on the electron equal the Coulomb force of attraction between the nucleus and the electron. From these inferences he derived the energy states of the electrons given by:

$$E = -\frac{2\pi^2 m Z^2 e^4}{n^2 h^2}$$, where n = 1,2,3, . . . defines the energy states or levels

m = mass of electron
e = charge on electron
Z = atomic number (nuclear charge)
h = Planck's Constant
ν,f = frequency

Energy transitions occur between states with energy change equal to $h\nu$ which could be calculated from above ($h = |E_f - E_i|$). Note that $E \propto 1/n^2$ and as n gets larger, the energy levels get closer together. Bohr was able to explain some of the hydrogen spectrum lines with his theory. Another key to his theory was that electrons in any one of the energy states do not radiate energy. The major flaws in Bohr's theory were the discrete orbits and the determination of exact momentum of the electron concurrently. *Heisenberg's uncertainty principle* stated that it is impossible to determine simultaneously the position and momentum of an electron as in Bohr's theory. This led to the probabilistic theory of electronic structure as derived by Schroedinger. The quantum theory and its natural quantum numbers resulted. The quantum numbers are:

(1) n = principle quantum number (ORBITAL SIZE)
takes values n = 1,2,3,4,5 . . . .
higher n means that higher total energy of electron represents higher energy levels
1 = K, 2 = L, 3 = M, 4 = N, etc.

(2) l = angular momentum quantum number (ORBITAL SHAPE)
higher l means higher angular momentum of electron
angular momentum is limited by the total energy (n)
$l = 0,1,2 \ldots n-1$
defines orbitals of atom (along with n)
0 = s, 1 = p, 2 = d, 3 = f, etc.

(3) m_l = magnetic quantum number (ORBITAL SPATIAL ORIENTATION)
orientation of the electron's magnetic field in an external field—limited by the angular momentum (l)
$m_l = l, l-1, \ldots 0, \ldots, -l+1, -l$
(i.e., takes all values between $+l$ and $-l$) determines spatial orientation of orbitals and, consequently, the *number* of orbitals of type l

(4) m_s = spin quantum number (ORBITAL SPIN ORIENTATION)
does not arise from solution of the Schroedinger equation
the spin of an electron in its axis also generates a magnetic field which can orient two ways with an external field
values have been chosen as + 1/2, – 1/2 for the direction of spin (refer to section 5.18.1.2 on electromagnetism).

Each electron in an atom has a set (n, l, m_l, m_s) of quantum numbers that uniquely defines it. *Pauli's Exclusion Principle* states that no two electrons in the same atom may have the same set of quantum numbers. Only a certain number of electrons is allowed for each quantum number:

n: a maximum of $2n^2$ electrons
for n = 1, get 2 electrons
for n = 2, get 8 electrons
for n = 3, get 18 electrons

l: a maximum of $4l + 2$ electrons
for $l = 0$ (s orbital), get 2 electrons
for $l = 1$ (p orbital), get 6 electrons
for $l = 2$ (d orbital), get 10 electrons
for $l = 3$ (f orbital), get 14 electrons

m_l: a maximum of two electrons for each m_l

An example of how one gets these numbers is shown for n = 3 (maximum numbers of electrons are in parentheses) in Fig. 5.1.

n	l	m_l	m_s
3 (18)	0 (2)	0 (2)	+1/2, –1/2
	1 (6)	+1 (2)	+1/2, –1/2
		0 (2)	+1/2, –1/2
		–1 (2)	+1/2, –1/2
	2 (10)	+2 (2)	+1/2, –1/2
		+1 (2)	+1/2, –1/2
		0 (2)	+1/2, –1/2
		–1 (2)	+1/2, –1/2
		–2 (2)	+1/2, –1/2

Fig. 5.1—Example of the Quantum Number Relationships

Each orbital is symbolized by using the n and l quantum numbers as follows: ls, 3p, 5f (n ↗ ↖ l)

where n = 1, 3, 5 . . . . . represents principal quantum numbers and l = s, p, f . . . . represents angular momentum quantum numbers.

The *orbitals are filled* in sequence, from the lowest energy to the highest energy. The pattern of orbitals filled is called the *electron configuration*. The sequence is not that expected because some orbitals, especially those with $s(l = 0)$, penetrate (get closer to the nucleus than others) and are consequently lowered in energy more and are filled first. A useful way to remember the sequence is to add the n and l numerical values. The lowest sum is filled first. In the case of a tie, the lowest n value is filled first (remember s = 0, p = 1, d = 2, f = 3). For example: 1s 2s 2p 3s 3p 3d 4s vs. 1s 2s 2p 3s 3p 4s 3d. In the first configuration 3d is written before 4s. Using the rule for 3d, n(= 3) + d(= 2) = 5, whereas for 4s, n(= 4) + s(= 0) = 4; therefore second configuration should be used.

The orbitals are filled by knowing the number of electrons in the atom (if neutral, this is the atomic number AN), and then filling each orbital sequentially up to its maximum number of electrons. For example:

Al = 13: $1s^2\ 2s^2\ 2p^6\ 3s^2\ 3p^1$
Ca = 20: $1s^2\ 2s^2\ 2p^6\ 3s^2\ 3p^6\ 4s^2$

If the atom is charged, the extra electrons (if negative) are added or the lost electrons (if positive) are removed. For example:

Al^{+3} (AN = 13): $1s^2\ 2s^2\ 2p^6$
O^{-2} (AN = 8): $1s^2\ 2s^2\ 2p^6$

Fig. 5.2 shows another way to remember the sequence of filling:

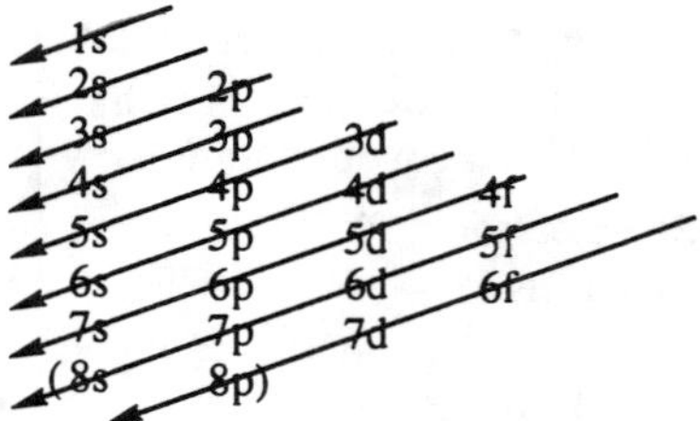

The sequence: 1s 2s 2p 3s 3p 4s 3d 4p 5s, etc.

Fig. 5.2—A Way of Remembering the Sequence of Filling of Orbitals

Hund's rule describes the way electrons are to be put into each orbital (n, l). Electrons go into each orbital of same energy (m_l) with parallel spins (same m_s) until each orbital is half filled (i.e., all electrons unpaired), then they are paired (put in the same orbital with opposite m_s's) (Fig. 5.3).

correct way:	$2p^4$	↑↓	↑	↑	incorrect way:	↑↓	↑↓	(empty)
	m	+1	0	−1				
	m_s	+1/2, −1/2	+1/2	+1/2				

Fig. 5.3—Hund's Rule

Orbitals (Fig. 5.4) are determined by the n, l, and m_l numbers. The n and l are important for determining the energy and shape of the orbital. The m_l determines the orientation (direction in space) of the orbitals. Remember that an orbital describes the probability of an electron being in a region of space; it is not the electron spread out.

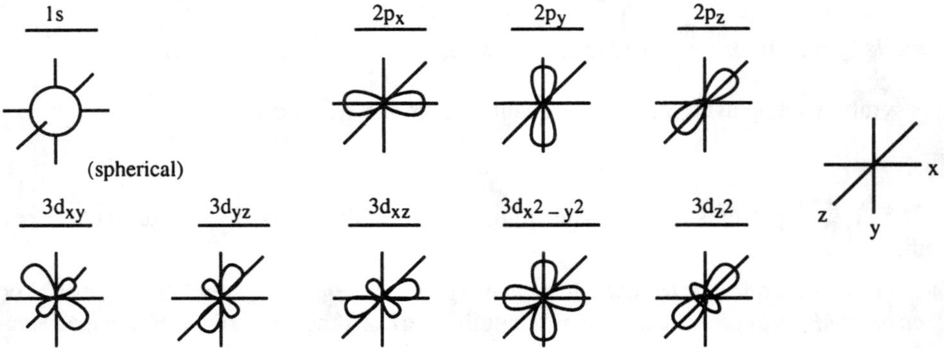

Fig. 5.4—Orbitals

The *ground state* of the electrons of an atom is when the electrons are in the lowest energy states available to the electrons. For example, the ground state of the aluminum was

$1s^2\ 2s^2\ 2p^6\ 3s^2\ 3p^1$

An *excited state* of the atom occurs when one or more electrons occupy orbitals (energy levels) other than the lowest available to the atom. This occurs by "exciting" the electron (by input of some type of energy) to the higher state. For example, for the aluminum:

$$1s^2\ 2s^2\ 2p^6\ 3s^2\ 3p^1 \xrightarrow{\text{energy}} 1s^2\ 2s^2\ 2p^6\ 3s^0\ 3p^3$$

both 3s electrons are now in the higher energy level 3p.

For the electrons, the higher the n or l quantum numbers, the higher the energies. When electrons shift between the different orbitals, energy is absorbed or emitted as a frequency of light. When energy is emitted (the electron moves from higher orbitals to lower orbitals, i.e., closer to the nucleus in general), a bright band appears at that frequency (or wavelength) in a spectrum (the continuum of all frequencies or wavelengths)—this results in *emission spectra*. When energy is absorbed by the electron (as must occur in the example above), a dark band appears at that frequency because energy is removed from the spectrum. This results in *absorption spectra*. Look at the spectrum as a source of light containing all the frequencies (wavelengths) representing different energies. As this passes through a substance, energy may be added (by emission from atoms) and certain frequencies become more intense (brighter) or energy may be removed (by absorption by atoms) and certain frequencies become less intense (less bright).

5.1.2 Questions to Review Electronic Structure of the Atom

1. All of the following were theorized by Bohr in his description of the atom except:

A. angular momentum of electrons in multiples of $h/2\pi$.
B. electrons circulate in discrete circular orbits.
C. energy of each electron is inversely proportional to n^2.
D. electrons radiate energy continuously in a given orbit.

2. The statement, "it is impossible to determine simultaneously the position and momentum of an electron," is attributable to:

A. Heisenberg.
B. Einstein.
C. Planck.
D. Schroedinger.

3. The following shape represents what type of orbital?

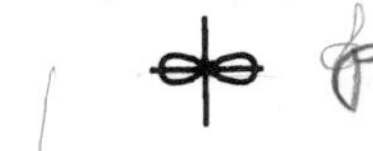

A. p
B. s
C. d
D. f

4. The letters s,p,d and f are used to represent which quantum numbers?

A. angular momentum (l)
B. principal (n)
C. magnetic (m_l)
D. spin (m_s)

5. The magnetic quantum number (QN) has its values limited *directly* by the value of:

A. principal QN.
B. angular momentum QN.
C. spin QN.
D. none of the above.

6. Hund's Rule states:

A. Electrons fill orbitals with parallel spins until all the orbitals of the same energy are half filled, then they go into suborbitals with anti-parallel (opposite) spins.
B. Two electrons in the same atom cannot have the same four quantum numbers.
C. There is a maximum of two electrons in any orbital.
D. None of the above.

7. Pauli's Exclusion Principle states:
   A. The position and momentum of an electron cannot be simultaneously determined.
   B. Electrons with the same spin cannot go into the same orbital.
   C. No two electrons in an atom may have the same set of the four quantum numbers.
   D. None of the above.
8. When an atom emits energy as light, bands in the spectrum will appear which are:
   A. brighter.
   B. darker.
   C. colorless.
   D. hard to locate.
9. The maximum number of electrons in an orbital with m_l (magnetic quantum number) = 3 is:
   A. 6
   B. 4
   C. 3
   D. 2
10. The maximum number of electrons in a shell with n (principal quantum number) = 3 is:
   A. 6
   B. 8
   C. 18
   D. 32
11. The maximum number of electrons in an orbital with l (angular momentum quantum number) = 3 is
   A. 6
   B. 10
   C. 14
   D. 18
12. An element with atomic number = 22 has how many electrons in the 2p orbital?
   A. 6
   B. 4
   C. 3
   D. 1
13. The electron configuration of magnesium (Mg) with atomic number 12 is:
   A. $1s^2\ 2s^2\ 2p^6\ 3s^2$
   B. $1s^2\ 2s^2\ 3s^2\ 3p^6$
   C. $1s^2\ 2s^2\ 2p^2\ 3s^2\ 3p^2\ 3d^2$
   D. None of the above
14. Sodium has an atomic number = 11. The electron configuration of the sodium ion (NA^{+1}) is:
   A. $1s^2\ 2s^2\ 2p^6\ 3s^2$
   B. $1s^2\ 2s^2\ 2p^5\ 3s^2$
   C. $1s^2\ 2s^2\ 2p^6\ 3s^1$
   D. $1s^2\ 2s^2\ 2p^6$

Use the following information for Questions #15-#17

The atomic number of manganese (Mn) is 25.

15. The electron configuration of the ground state is:
   A. $1s^2\ 2s^2\ 2p^6\ 3s^2\ 3p^6\ 3d^7$
   B. $1s^2\ 2s^2\ 2p^6\ 3s^2\ 3p^6\ 4s^2\ 4p^5$
   C. $1s^2\ 2s^2\ 2p^6\ 3s^2\ 2d^{10}\ 3p^3$
   D. None of the above

16. An excited state of the atom may be:

A. $1s^2\ 2s^2\ 2p^6\ 3s^2\ 3p^6\ 4s^1\ 3d^6$
B. $1s^2\ 2s^2\ 2p^6\ 3s^2\ 3p^6\ 4s^2\ 3d^5$
C. $1s^2\ 2s^2\ 2p^6\ 2d^{10}\ 3s^2\ 3p^3$
D. None of the above

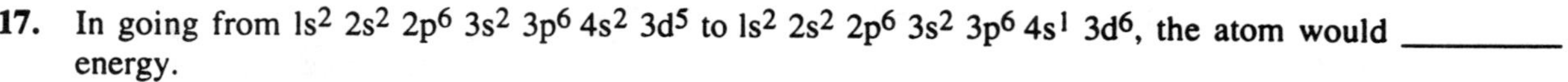

17. In going from $1s^2\ 2s^2\ 2p^6\ 3s^2\ 3p^6\ 4s^2\ 3d^5$ to $1s^2\ 2s^2\ 2p^6\ 3s^2\ 3p^6\ 4s^1\ 3d^6$, the atom would ________ energy.

A. absorb
B. emit
C. not change energy states

5.1.3 Answers to Questions in Section 5.1.2

(1) D (2) A (3) A (4) A (5) B (6) A (7) C (8) A (9) D (10) C (11) C (12) A (13) A (14) D (15) D (16) A (17) A

5.1.4 Discussion of Answers to Questions in Section 5.1.2

Questions #1 to #8: Adequately discussed in Section.

Question #9 (Answer: D) All orbitals contain a maximum of two electrons.

Question #10 (Answer: C) Using the formula given in Section, $2n^2 = 2(3)^2 = 2(9) = 18$. See example in Section for alternative method to determine it.

Question #11 (Answer: C) Using the formula given in the Section, $4l + 2 = 4(3) + 2 = 12 + 2 = 14$.

Question #12 (Answer: A) There are 22 electrons (from AN = 22). The electron configuration is:

$$1s^2\ 2s^2\ 2p^6\ 3s^2\ 3p^6\ 4s^2\ 3d^2$$

It might have been clear that the 2p orbital would have been filled. So, the answer would be a filled p orbital which has *six* electrons.

Question #13 (Answer: A) There are 12 electrons because AN = 12. The sequence of filling is:

1s 2s 2p 3s 3p 4s 3d

The *s* orbital has a maximum of 2 electrons, and the *p* orbital has a maximum of 6 electrons. The electron configuration is:

$$1s^2\ 2s^2\ 2p^6\ 3s^2$$

Question #14 (Answer: D) There are 10 electrons in the sodium ion whereas in the neutral atom there are 11 (from atomic number = 11). Since the ion is a positive one, there must be one less electron available. The electron configuration is then:

$$1s^2\ 2s^2\ 2p^6$$

Question #15 (Answer: D) The ground state is when the electrons are in the lowest energy levels available. The sequence of filling for 25 electrons is:

$$1s^2\ 2s^2\ 2p^6\ 3s^2\ 3p^6\ 4s^2\ 3d^5$$

So, none of the answers given is correct.

Question #16 (Answer: A) An excited state occurs when electrons in the ground state orbitals are "excited" to higher energy orbitals. In (A), a 4s electron is excited to a 3d electron.

Question #17 (Answer: A) Here the 4s electron is being excited to become a 3d electron. Since 3d electrons are of higher energy than 4s (due to the penetrance of this orbital and consequent lowering of its energy), it would require energy to move 4s to 3d levels. Therefore, the atom must absorb this energy.

5.1.5 Checklist for Electronic Structure of the Atom

______	Heisenberg's Uncertainty Principle	______	emission spectra
______	angular momentum of electron	______	n
______	Pauli's Exclusion Principle	______	l
______	orbital	______	m_l
______	shell	______	m_s
______	Hund's rule	______	Bohr theory of atomic structure
______	ground states	______	quantum numbers and filling of electron orbitals (electronic structure)
______	absorption spectra		
______	excited states	______	relation of spectra to atomic structure

5.2 THE PERIODIC TABLE

5.2.1 Review of the Periodic Table

The periodic table is an orderly arrangement of elements by their atomic numbers based on the quantum theory of the atom. Mendeleev was the first to arrange elements by their atomic numbers. Features of the organization of the chart are (see also Fig. 5.5):

(1) Rows or *periods* represent the principal quantum number (n) and have values from n = 1 to n = 7. Each period is the sequential filling of the orbitals within a shell.

(2) Columns or *groups* represent elements with the same electron configuration in the *outermost shell.* There is the A set of elements called *representative*, and these have the *s* and *p* orbitals as the outermost. The *nonrepresentative*, or B set, elements have the *d* or *f* orbitals as the outermost. The Roman Numerals (I, II, etc.) give the number of electrons in the outermost orbitals. From this, the electron configuration and valance can be determined. For the VI A group, for example, there are six electrons in s and p orbitals. This gives an $s^2\ p^4$. Remember that the second period atoms prefer the *octet state* and that they will gain or lose electrons to reach it, whichever is easier. The common valence in VI A is – 2 because it is easier to gain 2 electrons to go to $s^2\ p^6$ (octet) than to lose 6 electrons and go to $s^0\ p^0$ (which would be the next lower octet) and have a + 6 valence. Elements in the same group tend to have similar chemical properties. Remember the mnemonic, "**Asp body fang**" for group A-s-p and group b-d-f orbitals.

(3) The different *blocks* represent the angular momentum quantum number (l). The number of spaces from left to right in each block is the maximum number of electrons for each quantum number: *s* has a maximum of 2, *p* has a maximum of 6, *d* has a maximum of 10, and *f* has a maximum of 14.

(4) The magnetic quantum number (m_l) and spin quantum number (m_s) are not represented on the chart.

(5) Representative elements, transition elements, inner transition elements (actinides, lanthanides), inert gases and other special groups are labeled on the chart (Fig. 5.5).

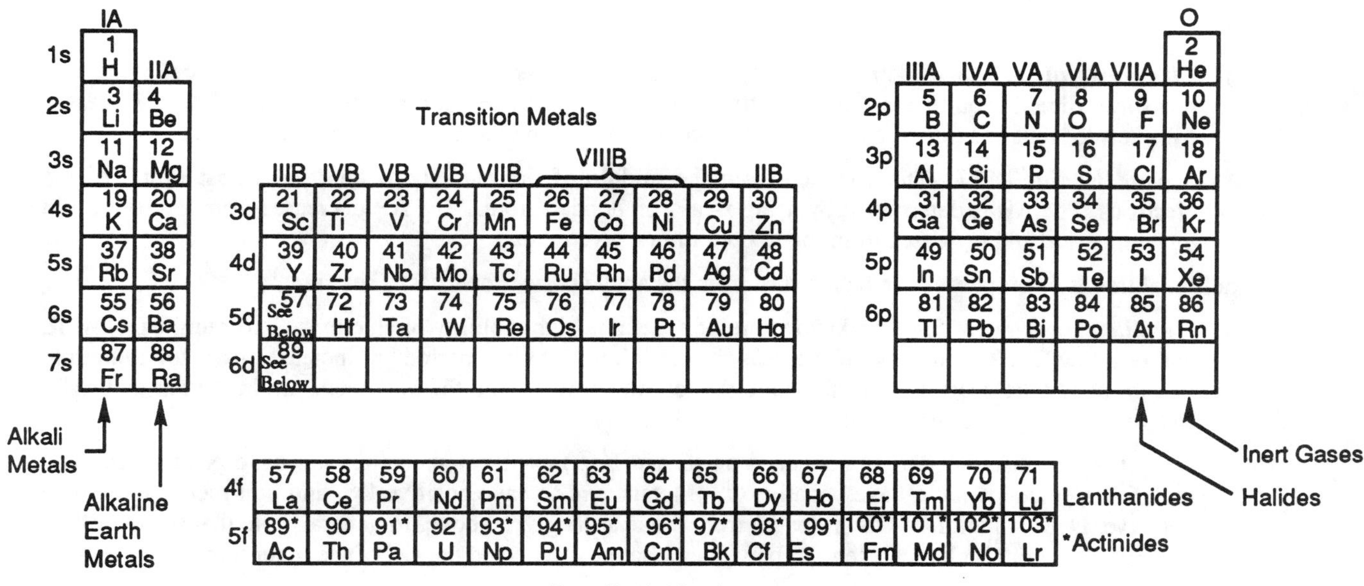

Fig. 5.5—The Periodic Chart/Table

The *periodic properties* are properties of the elements which vary in a more or less regular pattern as a function of the atomic numbers, and, hence, electron configuration. The horizontal and vertical structure of the periodic table can be understood as follows:

(1) As one reads from left to right in a given period, the nuclear pull on the outermost electrons increases. This causes the electrons to be bound tighter and to be closer to the nucleus.

(2) As one reads down a given column, the outermost electrons are bound less tightly because more electrons are between the nucleus and the outermost electrons, and because a shell has been completed and this effectively shields the outer electrons.

Based upon the above discussion, the gross atomic trends of the periodic properties are shown below:

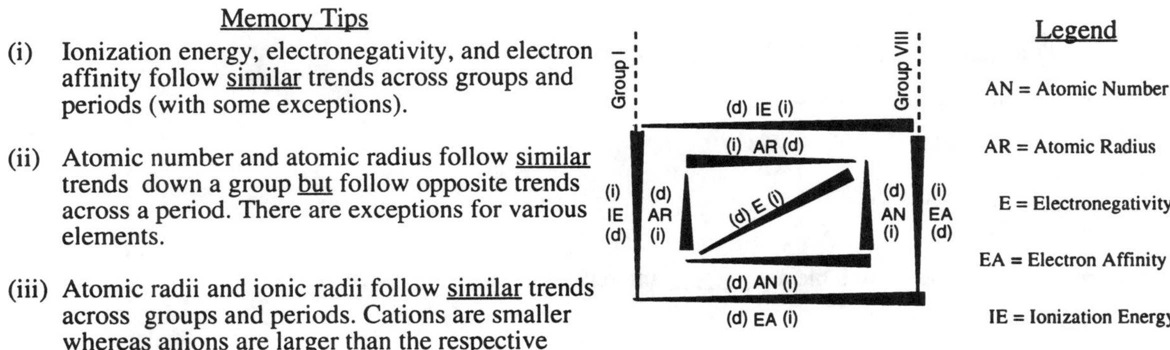

Sketch Showing Conceptual Model to Study Increase (i) or Decrease (d) in Various Periodic Properties

(1) *Ionization energy (IE)*—The energy (or voltage) measured in kJ/mol. required to ionize a gaseous atom, i.e., take the outermost electron away from the atom. The higher the IE, the more difficult it is to remove an electron, and this means the nucleus is holding on tighter. IE increases, generally, from left to right in a period, and it decreases from top to bottom in a group. Ionization energy is always positive and the process of ionization is always endothermic.

(2) *Electron Affinity (EA)*—The energy released when an electron is moved from infinity into the lowest energy vacant orbital in the gaseous atom. The stronger the nuclear attraction for electrons, the higher the EA (absolute value). The EA is subject to configuration variations (Be $2s^2$ < Li $2s^1$ but C>B) and repulsion of electrons in the same energy level (F<Cl but Br<Cl). No overall trend is observed. It may be endothermic or exothermic.

(3) *Electronegativity (E)*—The relative attraction of the nucleus for the electrons in a chemical bond. Not measured directly, but it can be indirectly obtained from EA, IE and/or bond energies. The E increases from left to right in a period and decreases from top to bottom in a group—this is similar to IE.

(4) *Atomic Radius (AR)*—The distance from the middle of the nucleus to the "outermost limit" of the electrons. The AR is determined by using x-rays on bonded atoms. The AR decreases from left to right in a given period and increases from top to bottom in a given group.

Additional trends of properties can be inferred from the above basic properties. These are:

(1) *Metallic character (MC)*—The key feature of a metal is high mobility of electrons. This requires a low IE and/or a low EA. This means MC decreases from left to right in a period but increases from top to bottom in a group. In the chart, the metals are to the left and bottom, and the nonmetals are in the top and right. Between is a region of transition called the semi-metals.

(2) *Oxidation State (OS)*—The OS depends on IE and EA. Low IE elements tend to have positive OS, and high EA elements tend to have negative OS. Metals tend to have positive OS, and non-metals tend to be negative. Determination of OS (valence) from the chart is given above. In general, note that the OS of the transition (d orbital) elements tend to be variable but positive. And the OS of the inner transition elements (f-orbitals) tend to be + 3.

(3) *Chemical Activity (CA)*—This depends on the ease of removing an electron (low IE) or the ease of adding an electron (high EA). Either situation leads to high CA. Hence, CA trends are not usually discussed across a period (because the balance of IE and EA changes), but trends are meaningful for groups. On the left side of the chart, CA increases as you go down the chart in a given group (because IE decreases). On the right side of the chart, CA increases as you go up the chart in a given group (because EA generally increases).

(4) *Acidity Trends*—See Section 5.8.1.

(5) *Hydrogen Bonding (HB)*—HB exists for F, O, N and Cl but would theoretically increase as one ascended a given group.

(6) Substances may be paramagnetic, ferromagnetic or dimagnetic depending on m_s. Review section 5.18.1.2 (Electromagnetism).

5.2.2 Questions to Review the Periodic Table

1. The periodic table is based upon:

A. atomic weights.
B. mass number.
C. neutron number.
D. atomic number.

2. The periods of the periodic table are ______ and represent the ______ quantum number.

A. horizontal; principal
B. horizontal; angular momentum
C. vertical; principal
D. vertical; angular momentum

3. Groups of the periodic table:

A. represent the magnetic quantum number.
B. represent elements with the same outer electron configuration.
C. are horizontal.
D. all of the above are correct.

4. Which of the following quantum numbers is not represented on the periodic chart?

   A. principal
   B. angular momentum
   C. magnetic
   D. all are

5. The transition elements have the _____ -orbital as the outermost.

   A. s
   B. p
   C. d
   D. f

6. Inert gases:

   A. have incomplete shells.
   B. are found in the same period.
   C. are found at the beginning of a period.
   D. are found in the same group.

7. All of the following are correct except:

   A. the nuclear attraction for the outermost electrons decreases from right to left in a given period.
   B. in moving down a given column, the outermost electrons are bound less tightly.
   C. half-filled or completely filled orbitals have more stability than other incompletely filled orbitals.
   D. all of the above are correct.

8. The energy required to ionize a gaseous atom is called the:

   A. ionization energy.
   B. electron affinity.
   C. electronegativity.
   D. none of the above.

9. The relative attraction of the nucleus for the electrons in a chemical bond is called the:

   A. ionization energy.
   B. electron affinity.
   C. electronegativity.
   D. none of the above.

10. The energy released when an electron is moved from infinity into the vacant orbital (with the lowest energy) is termed as:

    A. electron affinity.
    B. electronegativity.
    C. ionization energy.
    D. none of the above.

11. The ionization energy:

    A. generally increases from left to right in a period.
    B. does not change in a period.
    C. increases from top to bottom in a group.
    D. does not change in a group.

12. The electron affinity:

    A. decreases from left to right in a period.
    B. measures the attraction of the atom for electrons.
    C. increases from top to bottom in a group.
    D. variations follow no overall trend.

13. The electronegativity:

    A. is measured directly from physical characteristics.
    B. does not vary in a group.
    C. decreases from left to right in a period.
    D. decreases from top to bottom in a group.

14. The atomic radius:

    A. is calculated from bond energies.
    B. decreases from left to right in a period.
    C. decreases from top to bottom in a group.
    D. all of the above.

15. Metallic character:

    A. depends upon the mass number.
    B. decreases from bottom to top in a group.
    C. requires a high ionization energy and a high electron affinity.
    D. decreases from top to bottom in a group.

16. Which of the following statements is true concerning oxidation states (OS)?

    A. High ionization energy elements have positive OS.
    B. Metals tend to have negative OS.
    C. Low electron affinity elements tend to have positive OS.
    D. Non-metals tend to have negative OS.

17. Chemical activity in groups:

    A. increases as ionization energy increases.
    B. decreases as electron affinity decreases.
    C. increases as you read down the left side of the periodic chart.
    D. increases as electron affinity decreases.

18. Phosphorus (P) is in group VA; the electron configuration of its outermost shell is:

    A. $s^2 p^3$
    B. p^5
    C. d^5
    D. cannot be determined

19. Bromine (Br) is in group VII A; its most common oxidation state (OS) is probably:

    A. + 1
    B. − 1
    C. − 2
    D. cannot be determined

20. The electron configuration of selenium is:
    $1s^2 2s^2 2p^6 3s^2 3p^6 4s^2 3d^{10} 4p^4$. It is probably in what group?

    A. VI A
    B. IV A
    C. VI B
    D. need more information

21. The atomic number of chlorine is 17. It is in what group?

    A. VII A
    B. IV A
    C. I A
    D. cannot be determined by trends

22. Fluorine (F) has an atomic number (AN) = 9 and chlorine (Cl) has an AN = 17. Which one has the higher electron affinity?

A. both are equal
B. Cl
C. F
D. cannot be determined

23. Sodium (Na) has an atomic number (AN) = 11 and aluminum (Al) has an AN = 13. Which one has the higher ionization energy?

A. both are equal
B. Na
C. Al
D. cannot be determined

24. Oxygen (O) has an atomic number (AN) = 8 and sulfur (S) has an AN = 16. Which one has the greater electronegativity?

A. S
B. O
C. both are equal
D. cannot be determined

25. The atomic number (AN) of magnesium (Mg) is 12, and the AN of sulfur (S) is 16. Which one has the larger atomic radius?

A. Mg
B. S
C. both are equal
D. cannot be determined

26. Lithium (Li) has an atomic number (AN) = 3 and potassium (K) has an AN = 19. Which one has the greater metallic character?

A. both are equal
B. Li
C. K
D. cannot be determined

27. Berylium (Be) has an atomic number (AN) = 4, and strontium (Sr) has an AN = 38. Which one has the greater chemical activity?

A. both are equal
B. Sr
C. Be
D. cannot be determined

28. Magnesium (Mg) has an atomic number (AN) = 12 and Bromine (Br) has an AN = 35. Which one has the greater chemical activity?

A. both are equal
B. Mg
C. Br
D. cannot be determined

5.2.3 Answers to Questions in Section 5.2.2

(1) D (2) A (3) B (4) C (5) C (6) D (7) D (8) A (9) C (10) A (11) A
(12) D (13) D (14) B (15) B (16) D (17) C (18) A (19) B (20) A (21) A (22) D
(23) C (24) B (25) A (26) C (27) B (28) D

5.2.4 Discussion of Answers to Questions in Section 5.2.2

Questions #1 to #17: Adequately discussed in Section.

Question #18 (Answer: A) The A means that P is a representative element in the group and that its outer-most shell contains s and p orbitals. The V means that P is a fifth group element with 5 outer electrons, and these give the following electron configuration, s^2 p^3.

Question #19 (Answer: B) Since Br is in group VII A the electron configuration of its outermost shell is s^2 p^5. The closets octet is s^2 p^6, and this requires an extra electron to give it an OS of – 1.

Question #20 (Answer: A) Since the outermost incomplete orbitals are *s* and *p* (the d orbital is complete), the selenium is an *A* element. The *s* and *p* contain 2 + 4 = 6 electrons. This means selenium is in group VI A.

Question #21 (Answer: A) The electron configuration of chlorine is ls^2 $2s^2$ $2p^6$ $3s^2$ $3p^5$. The outermost incomplete orbitals are *s* and *p*—this makes it *A* (representative). There are 2 + 5 = 7 electrons in the *s* and *p* orbitals—this makes it a group VII element.

Question #22 (Answer: D) EA has no overall trend useful for predictions.

Question #23 (Answer: C) The electron configuration of Na is ls^2 $2s^2$ $2p^2$ $3s^1$ and Al is ls^2 $2s^2$ $2p^6$ $3s^2$ $3p^1$. This places them in the same period—highest *n* number is 3 in each. Ionization energy (IE) increases from left to right on the table. Then Al has a higher IE than Na.

Question #24 (Answer: B) O has an electron configuration of ls^2 $2s^2$ $2p^4$, and sulfur has an electron configuration of ls^2 $2s^2$ $2p^6$ $3s^2$ $3p^4$. This places both in group VI A. In a group, the electronegativity decreases from top to bottom. Then O has the greater electronegativity.

Question #25 (Answer: A) The electron configurations are: Mg = ls^2 $2s^2$ $2p^6$ $3s^2$; S = ls^2 $2s^2$ $2p^6$ $3s^2$ $3p^4$. They are, therefore, in the same period. The atomic radius decreases from left to right in a period. Then Mg is larger than S.

Question #26 (Answer: C) The electron configurations are: Li = ls^2 $2s^2$; K = ls^2 $2s^2$ $2p^6$ $3s^2$ $4s^1$. Therefore, both are in group IA. In a group the metallic character increases from top to bottom. Then K has more metallic character than Li.

Questions #27 (Answer: B) The electron configurations are: Be = ls^2 $2s^2$; Sr = ls^2 $2s^2$ $2p^6$ $3s^2$ $3p^6$ $4s^2$ $3d^{10}$ $4p^6$ $5s^2$. Therefore, they are both in group II A. In a group on the left side, the chemical activity increases from top to bottom. Then Sr is more reactive than Be.

Question #28 (Answer: D) The electron configurations are: Mg = ls^2 $2s^2$ $2p^6$ $3s^2$; Br = ls^2 $2s^2$ $2p^6$ $3s^2$ $3p^6$ $4s^2$ $3d^{10}$ $4p^5$. This means they are neither in the same group nor period and cannot be compared by general periodic trends.

5.2.5 Checklist for the Periodic Table

______ periods
______ groups
______ representative elements
______ octet state
______ periodic properties
______ oxidation state
______ ionization energy
______ electron affinity
______ electronegativity
______ atomic radius
______ metallic character
______ chemical activity
______ basis for the periodic table
______ organization of the table, especially in relation to the quantum numbers
______ general basis for the variation of the periodic properties
______ paramagnetism
______ ferromagnetism
______ dimagnetism

5.3 CHEMICAL BONDING

5.3.1 Review of Chemical Bonding

5.3.1.1 IONIC BONDING

When metal (e.g., Na) and nonmetal (e.g., Cl_2) elements are mixed together, oppositely charged ions are quickly formed. This readily occurs when the atoms involved differ greatly in their attraction for electrons (e.g., a metal of low ionization energy and a nonmetal with a high ionization energy). The resulting ionic compound is more stable (lower in energy) than its elements and owes this stability to the packing of the oppositely charged ions into a lattice.

5.3.1.2 COVALENT BONDING

A chemical bond formed by sharing a pair of electrons is called a covalent bond. Covalent bonds are more prevalent in nonmetallic compounds. Gases such as hydrogen (H_2) or chlorine (Cl_2) are the simplest examples of covalent bonding. Each of these gas molecules shares one pair of electrons:

$$H\cdot + \cdot H \rightarrow H:H \qquad :\ddot{\underset{..}{Cl}}\cdot + \cdot\ddot{\underset{..}{Cl}}: \rightarrow :\ddot{\underset{..}{Cl}}:\ddot{\underset{..}{Cl}}:$$

Organic compounds, many of them being of prime interest in medicine, can have multiple covalent bonds per molecule. The major elements involved in organic compounds are carbon (C), hydrogen (H), oxygen (O), nitrogen (N) and halides (fluorine-F, chlorine-Cl, bromine-Br, iodine-I). Sulfur (S) and phosphorus (P) are also in many organic compounds. Carbon forms 4 bonds, N forms 3 and has one unshared pair of electrons, O forms 2 and has 2 unshared pairs of electrons. H forms one bond and each halogen forms one bond and has 3 unshared pairs of electrons—all of the above are assumed to be neutral. The possible bonds are *single bonds* (SB, one shared pair of electrons), *double bonds* (DB, two shared pairs of electrons) and *triple bonds* (TB, three shared pairs of electrons). C and N form all three types, O forms DB and SB and H and the halides (in organic compounds) form SB's only.

The C atom has one s orbital and three p orbitals in its outer bonding electron shells. (See Section 5.1.1). In organic molecules, these original atomic orbitals are recombined into *hybrid orbitals* made of part *s* and part *p*. If one *s* and three *p's* are mixed, there result four hybrid sp^3 *orbitals* (each consisting of one part *s* and three parts *p*) on the carbon atom. If one s orbital and two p orbitals mix, there result three sp^2 orbitals and one original p orbital on each carbon atom. If one *s* and one *p* mix, there result two *sp orbitals* and two original p orbitals on each carbon. The electron pair geometry of the orbitals and the valence-shell electron pair repulsion models (VSEPR) are sp^3-tetrahedral, sp^2-trigonal and sp-linear (Fig. 5.6).

The VSEPR theory or the **V**alency **S**hell **E**lectron **P**air **R**epulsion theory explains the different shapes of molecules. The word 'valency' or 'valence' dictates strength of an atomic bond. Valence electrons are the electrons in the outermost shell or orbit of the atom.

The VSEPR theory states:

(1) The geometrical or structural arrangement of bonds around an atom (in a molecule) depends on the *total number* of electron pairs in the valence shell of the atom. This includes *both* bonding (shared) pairs *and* nonbonding (unshared) pairs.

(2) *Two* pairs of electrons have a *linear* arrangement, *three* pairs of electrons have an *equilateral triangle* arrangement, and *four* pairs of electrons have a *tetrahedral* arrangement.

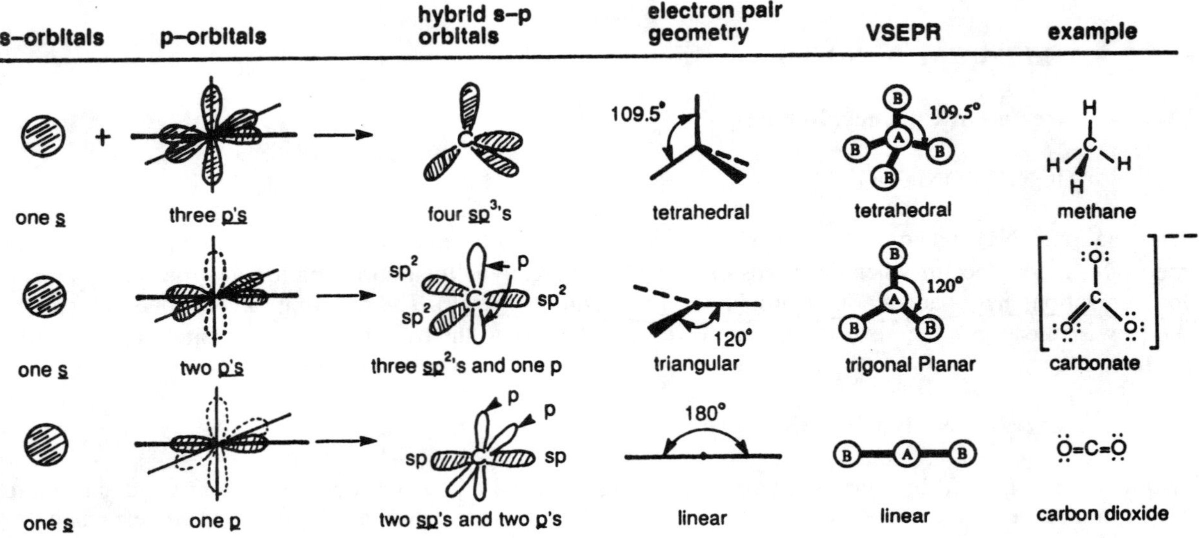

Fig. 5.6—Hybrid Bonding Orbitals

Sigma (σ) bonds have electron density between the nuclei. Sigma bonds are formed when hybrid orbitals (sp, sp^2, sp^3) overlap directly. *Pi (π) bonds* have electron density (overlap) above and below the axis (and plane) of the atoms. They are formed by "sideways" overlap of the p orbitals. *Single bonds* are σ bonds. *Double bonds* are made of one σ bond and one π bond, *triple bonds* include one σ and two π bonds. Note that σ bonds are symmetric about the axis and can rotate freely. *Multiple bonds* (DB, TB), with π components, are not symmetric about the axis and are not free to rotate about it (Fig. 5.7).

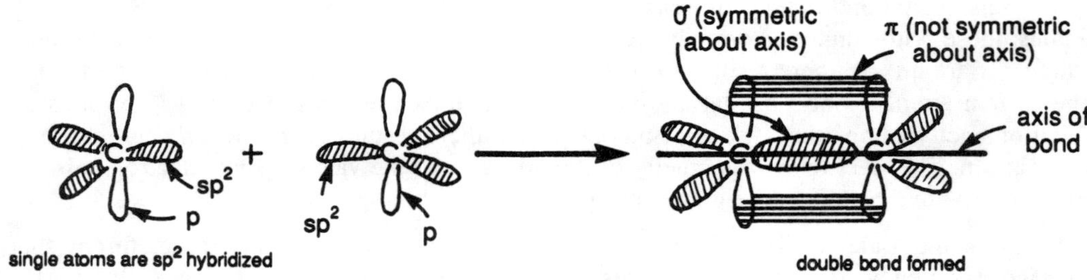

Note that the sp^2's overlap between the nuclei to form the σ bond; the p's overlap above and below the axis between the C's to form a π bond.)

Fig. 5.7—Sigma and Pi Bonds

When adjacent atoms are sp^2 or sp hybridized, there is the possibility of side to side overlap of the leftover p orbitals over all of these atoms. This is called delocalization of the electrons in the π bonds of the molecule. Two ways of depicting these molecules are by the molecular orbital (MO) or the valence bond (resonance) approach. The MO approach takes a linear combination of atomic orbitals (LCAO) to form molecular orbitals which electrons go into to form bonds. These molecular orbitals cover the whole molecule, and, hence, the delocalization of electrons is depicted. In the *valence bond (resonance) approach,* there is a linear combination of different structures with localized π bonds (and unpaired electrons), which together depict the true molecule (the resonance hybrid). There is no one structure that is representative of the molecule (Fig. 5.8).

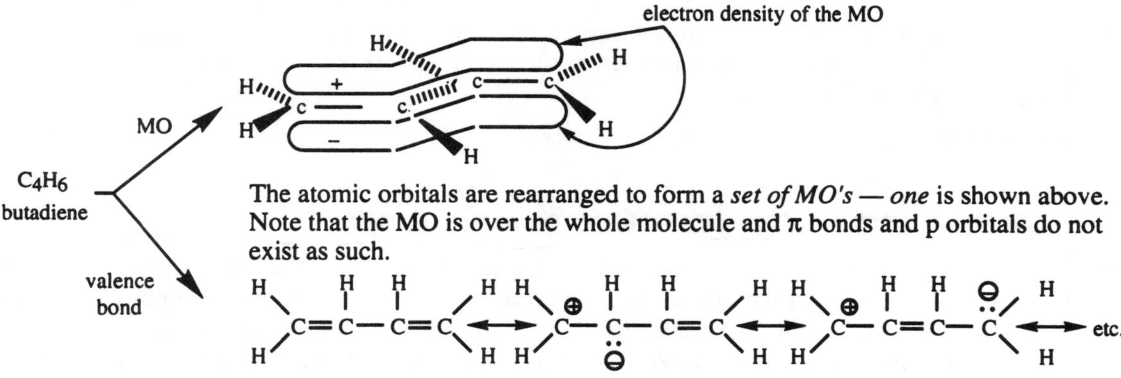

electron density of the MO
MO
C_4H_6
butadiene
valence
bond
The atomic orbitals are rearranged to form a *set of MO's — one* is shown above. Note that the MO is over the whole molecule and π bonds and p orbitals do not exist as such.
etc.
Note that no one structure represents the molecule which is a composite of all of them. The π bonds and p orbitals do exist in each structure above.

Fig. 5.8—Comparison of MO and Valence Bond Approaches

It is the *valence electrons* (outer shell electrons) that enter into the formation of chemical bonds. (See sections 5.1.1 and 5.2.1). *Electron dot structures* are a means of illustrating the valence electrons and how they enter into bond formation. They are used in conjunction with the octet rule stating that a maximum of eight electrons is possible in the outermost shell of atoms. This rule holds only for the second row elements (C, N, O, F). Third row elements (Si, P, S, Cl) can use d orbitals and, hence, can have more. Examples of the use of the electron dot formulas:

(1) CO_2 C-4 valence electrons
O-6 valence electrons
combine single electrons (may have to make double or triple bonds)

(2) CO_3^{-2} (an example of resonance)
C-4 valence electrons
O-6 valence electrons
-2 means two extra electrons to place on the atoms

Each element, in the final structure, counts one half the electrons in a bond as its own and counts all unpaired electrons as its own. The sum of these two numbers should equal the number of valence electrons the element began with.

When atoms of differing electronegativity form the chemical bond, a situation of charge separation exists. For example,

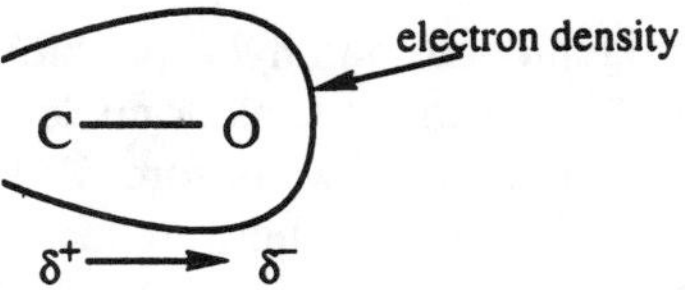

There is a slight pulling of electron density by the oxygen (the more electronegative) from the carbon (the less electronegative) as shown. This results in the C-O bond having *partial ionic character*. The separation of charge also causes an electrical dipole to be set up in the direction of the arrow as shown. A dipole has a positive end (the C above) and a negative end (the O above). A dipole will line up in an electric field (see Section 5.18.1). The most electronegative elements are: fluorine (4.0) > oxygen (3.5) > nitrogen (3.0) = chlorine (3.0). These are often combined with hydrogen (2.1) and carbon (2.5) and, hence result in bonds with partial ionic character. The numbers in parentheses show electronegativity of various elements. The *dipole moment* is a measure of the charge separation and, hence, the electronegativities of the elements that make up the bond. The larger the dipole moment, the larger the charge separation.

See Section 5.8.1.1 for a discussion of Lewis acids and bases.

5.3.1.3 INTERMOLECULAR FORCES IN LIQUIDS AND SOLIDS

The *intermolecular forces* are forces that exist between the molecules of the liquid or solid. These forces depend upon the chemical characteristics of the molecules and play a large part in determining the physical behavior (e.g., phase changes, solubility) of the liquid or solid. The types of forces that exist between molecules are van der Waals, hydrogen bonds, and hydrophobic. *Van der Waals* forces are very weak attractive forces due to the net attraction between the nucleus of one atom and the electrons in another. These forces are effective only over short distances and increase as the molecular weights increase, i.e., as the number of atoms or electrons in a molecule increase. This type of van der Waals force merges with the slightly stronger forces (may also be considered van der Waals) that exist between polar molecules or between molecules that are inductible (i.e., a separation of charge in a molecule can be induced by the presence of a second). *Polar molecules* are those made up of elements differing in electronegativity, e.g.,

$\overset{\delta+}{C}$—$\overset{\delta-}{O}$, $\overset{\delta+}{C}$—$\overset{\delta-}{Cl}$, and are asymmetric in geometry.

Hydrogen bonds are weak attractive bonds, but stronger than van der Waals, between the hydrogens on chlorine, fluorine, nitrogen or oxygen and the nonbonding electrons on these same elements. These are the only elements for which hydrogen bonding exists. Bonding becomes stronger when the electronegativity of the atoms increases and when the hydrogen bond can have a 180° orientation. (Fig. 5.9.)

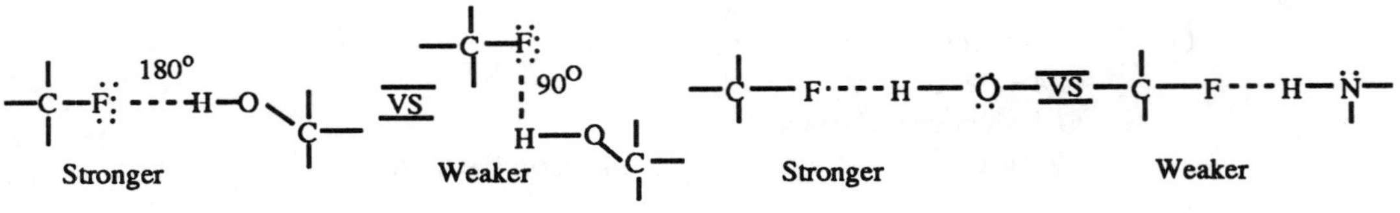

180°
—C—F: - - - H—O—C—   VS   —C—F: 90° H—O—C—
Stronger   Weaker

—C—F····H—O—   VS   —C—F···H—N—
Stronger   Weaker

Fig. 5.9—Hydrogen Bonding

Hydrophobic bonds are weak attractive bonds between molecules that are nonpolar (no net separation of charges in molecules). These bonds exist because nonpolar molecules (e.g. hydrocarbons, fats, aromatics) decrease the entropy (see Section 5.12.1) of water when the molecules are apart. When these nonpolar molecules come together and form hydrophobic bonds, the entropy increases and the free energy is lowered and the bonds become stable. *Ionic forces* exist between ions, i.e., positive and negative ions. These can be very strong forces and are exemplified in ionic solids (e.g. NaCl, table salt). Ionic forces are due to Coulomb forces (see Section 5.18.1)

The weak forces (van der Waals, hydrogen bonds and hydrophobic), although very weak individually, are very strong when many exist between molecules as in proteins or nucleic acids. A large part of the stability of these and other polymers is due to the multitude of these weak forces. When solids melt or liquids evaporate, these are the forces that must be overcome. The greater the number of these intermolecular bonds, or the more different types of these bonds present, the greater the stability of the substance and the more difficult it is to melt or evaporate. Temperature increases tend to disrupt these weak inter-molecular forces easily, especially when they are few in number.

Also, molecules of similar types (e.g. hydrophobic or polar or with hydrogen bonding) tend to be soluble in each other because the forces are similar. Similarly, molecules of different types, especially polar versus nonpolar, tend to be insoluble.

The basic organization of *ionic crystals* is based on the assumption that maximum stability of the crystal is achieved by maximizing the attractive forces between cations (positive) and anions (negative) and minimizing the repulsive forces between ions of the same charge. Hence, anions and cations try to be as close together as possible while minimizing anion-anion repulsion.

5.3.2 Questions to Review Chemical Bonding

1. Which type of bond has electron density directly between the nuclei?

A. pi (π)
B. sigma (σ)
C. both
D. neither

2. Which type of bond is formed by overlap of p orbitals perpendicular to the 2 nuclei?

A. pi (π)
B. sigma (σ)
C. both
D. neither

3. Single bonds are composed of _________ bonds.

A. pi (π)
B. sigma (σ)
C. both
D. neither

4. Double bonds are composed of _________ bonds.

A. pi (π)
B. sigma (σ)
C. both
D. neither

5. Rotation about the bonding axis can occur with:

A. pi (π) bonds.
B. double bonds.
C. both.
D. neither pi nor double bonds.

6. Delocalization of electrons (i.e., resonance) occurs over:

A. sigma bonds between separated atoms.
B. sigma bonds on adjacent atoms.
C. pi bonds on adjacent atoms.
D. pi bonds between separated atoms.

7. The resonance approach implies that:

A. one structure cannot be drawn which accurately depicts the electrons in the true molecule.
B. one structure can be drawn which accurately depicts the electrons in the true molecule.
C. two structures can be drawn which accurately depict electrons in the true molecule.
D. none of the above.

8. The octet rule does not have to hold for which of the following elements?

A. C
B. O
C. F
D. P

9. An acceptable resonance form of the following ion is:

H H H H
H–C5–C4–C3=C2–C1(⊕)(H)(H)
H H

A. H–C5–C4–C3=C2=C1(H)(H)

B. H–C5–C4–C3=C2–C1(H)(H) ⊕H

C. H–C5–C4=C3–C2=C1(H)(H)

D. H–C5–C4–C3(⊕)–C2=C1(H)(H)

10. All of the following are acceptable resonance forms of the following ion except:

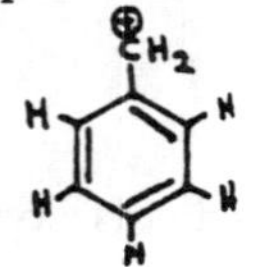

A.

B.

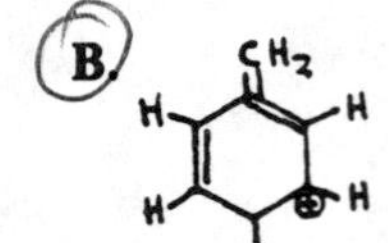

C.

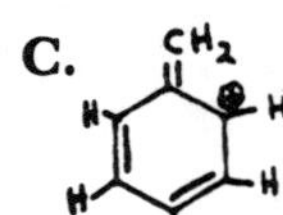

D.

11. What is the electron dot formula of H_2O?
(Atomic numbers: H = 1, O = 8)

A. H:H:Ö: B. H:Ö:H C. ·H:Ö:H· D. Ḧ:Ḧ:Ö:

12. What is the electron dot formula for SO_4^{-2}?
(Atomic numbers: O = 8, S = 16)

A. :S̈:Ö:Ö:Ö:Ö:$^{-2}$ B. Ö::S::Ö$^{-2}$ (with :O: above and :Ö: below) C. $^{-}$:Ö:Ö::S::Ö:Ö:$^{-}$ D. Ö::S::Ö (with :Ö:$^{-}$ above and :Ö:$^{-}$ below)

For the following questions use the electronegativities given in the section.

13. In which compound does the starred carbon have the largest partial positive charge?

A. $H_3C{-}C^{*}H_2{-}F$

B. $H{-}C^{*}H_2{-}Cl$

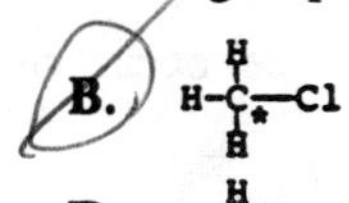

C.

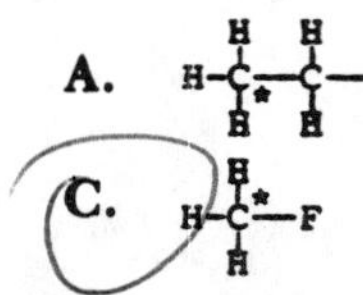

D. $H{-}C^{*}H_2{-}O{-}H$

14. Select the following compound with the largest dipole moment:

A. CH_3-CH_2-CH_3
B. CH_3-CH_2-Cl
C. CH_3-CH_2-OH
D. CH_3-CH_2-H

15. Select the compound with the largest dipole moment:

A. CCl_4

B. Cl–C₆H₄–Cl (para-dichlorobenzene)

C. H(Cl)C=C(Cl)H

D. Cl(H)C=C(Cl)H

16. Which of the following is not considered as an intermolecular force between molecules?

  A. covalent bonds
  B. hydrogen bonds
  C. hydrophobic bonds
  D. van der Waals forces

17. van der Waals forces depend upon:

  A. repulsion of the molecules from water.
  B. Coulomb attractions between ions.
  C. attraction between the nucleus of one atom and the electrons of another.
  D. none of the above.

18. All of the following factors increase the strength of van der Waals forces between molecules except an:

  A. increase in the molecular weight of the molecules.
  B. increase in the number of atoms in the molecule.
  C. increase in the number of electrons in the molecule.
  D. increase in the ionic strength of the molecule.

19. The weakest (in strength) of the following intermolecular forces is:

  A. hydrogen bonding.
  B. the typical van der Waals.
  C. forces between polar molecules.
  D. ionic.

20. Hydrogen bonds are possible between all the following elements except:

  A. carbon.
  B. nitrogen.
  C. oxygen.
  D. fluorine.

21. Hydrophobic bonds:

  A. are interactions between polar molecules.
  B. do not occur for hydrocarbons.
  C. are due to an increase in entropy of the system.
  D. all of the above.

22. The strongest of the forces between molecules is:

  A. van der Waals.
  B. hydrogen bonding.
  C. hydrophobic.
  D. polar.

23. For the three atoms involved in the hydrogen bond (e.g., $-\ddot{\underset{\cdot\cdot}{A}}:$ and $H-\ddot{\underset{\cdot\cdot}{B}}-$), the angle that allows the greatest strength (using H as the vertex) is:

  A. less than 90°
  B. 90°
  C. 90° to 180°
  D. 180°

24. The stability of some polymers may be due to:

  A. many of the weak intermolecular forces (bonds).
  B. a few of the weak intermolecular bonds.
  C. cannot be due to the weak intermolecular bonds.
  D. none of the above.

5.3.3 Answers to Questions in Section 5.3.2

(1) B (2) A (3) B (4) C (5) D (6) C (7) A (8) D (9) D (10) B (11) B (12) D
(13) C (14) C (15) D (16) A (17) C (18) D (19) B (20) A (21) C (22) D (23) D (24) A

5.3.4 Discussion of Answers to Question in Section 5.3.2

Questions #1 to #8 Adequately discussed in the Section.

Question #9 (Answer: D) Pi (π) electrons can be delocalized over charges (+ or –) and over radicals. So, view the plus charge as if it were an adjacent p orbital ready to overlap. Option (A) is not acceptable because an atom is displaced (the H)—resonance forms are of the same molecule, so no atoms can move. This is also true of option (C). Option (C) also places a p orbital on C where none existed. Hydrogen has no p orbitals and can form only one bond so option (B) is incorrect. Option (D) is correct which shows a simple 'shift' of the bond from C_3-C_2 to C_2-C_1.

Question #10 (Answer: B) Options (A), (C) and (D) are arrived at by simple 'shifts' of the π bonds around the ring. There is no way to get the structure in option (B)—also, one carbon has five bonds.

Question #11 (Answer: B) Oxygen has an electron configuration of $ls^2\ 2s^2\ 2p^4$, so there are 6 valence electrons (see sections 5.1.1 and 5.2.1). The hydrogen's is ls^1, and it has one valence electron. These are symbolized and combined as:

H• + •Ö• + •H ⟶ H:Ö:H.

Note: (1) that the single element is usually the central element, (2) single electrons are paired up, (3) the octet rule is followed for oxygen, and (4) the number of electrons that belong to each element is the same as the number of valence electrons it started with (see section discussion).

Question #12 (Answer: D) If you thought that none of the structures accurately depicts the true SO_4^{-2} ion, you are correct because resonance is possible with this structure. The electron configurations are:

$$O = ls^2\ 2s^2\ 2p^4\ S = 1s^2\ 2s^2\ 2p^6\ 3s^2\ 3p^4.$$

The valence electrons (in the outer shell only) are:

O = 6 and S = 6 plus two electrons for charge (– 2).

The electron dot formula is:

(2) (1) (3) (4) +2e⁻ (2) (4)

Note: (1) The electron "pairs" on S (I → II) are broken up to accommodate the free electron pairs of O (esp. #1 and #3). Hence, sulfur does not follow the octet rule (II, III). (2) The O's in II (i.e., #2 and #4) have one unpaired electron each; these are paired with the two extra electrons (II → III) to make the O's follow the octet rule. (3) An equivalent structure is,

(4) In counting up the valence electrons for each atom, remember the two extra electrons are spread out among the O's (actually the O's and S). See Question #11 for other points.

Question #13 (Answer: C) The element with the highest electronegativity is F, so this pulls the most electron density away from the C making it slightly positive. The F is more effective when attached directly to the C as in (C) than when another atom (the other C) intervenes as in (A).

Question #14 (Answer: C) The reasoning is the same as in #13. The O is the most electronegative and causes the largest charge separation,

$$\underset{\longrightarrow}{\overset{\text{C—O}}{\delta^{+}\ \ \delta^{-}}}$$

and, hence, the largest dipole moment.

Question #15 (Answer: D) This is to point out that dipole moments are vectors (directions and magnitude) and are additive as such. The molecules in (A), (B) and (C) are all symmetric and the dipoles are opposite and equal and, hence, cancel. This is not true for (D):

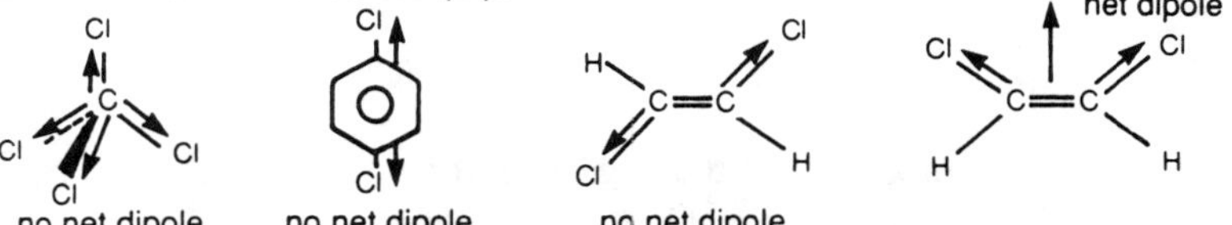

Questions #16 to #24: Adequately explained in Section.

5.3.5 Checklist for Chemical Bonding

- ______ ionic bonding
- ______ sigma bonds
- ______ pi bonds
- ______ resonance
- ______ intermolecular forces
- ______ van der Waals forces
- ______ polar molecules
- ______ weak intermolecular forces
- ______ general idea of ionic forces in crystals
- ______ nonpolar molecules
- ______ role of weak forces in stability of molecules
- ______ role of weak forces in phase changes and solubility
- ______ dipole moment
- ______ electron dot structures
- ______ partial ionic character
- ______ hydrogen bonds
- ______ hydrophobic bonds
- ______ ionic forces
- ______ VSEPR theory

5.4 STOICHIOMETRY

5.4.1 Review of Stoichiometry

Stoichiometry refers to the use of atomic theory to make quantitative assessments related to atoms, compounds and chemical reactions.

Chemical equations should be balanced prior to doing stoichiometric calculations. Balancing is by trial and error (for non-redox), and the check is to see if there are equal numbers of each element on each side of the equation. A hint to aid in balancing equations is:

> balance the element(s) which appear in only one compound on each side of the equation, save elements which appear in more than one compound until last.

Practice is the key to balancing equations. An example of a balanced equation is:

$$N_2(g) + 3H_2(g) \rightarrow 2NH_3(g).$$

The numbers in front of the molecules give the smallest ratios of these molecules that will react with each other. That is, they are the number of moles of each that must be present to get a complete reaction. See also Section 5.5.1 for oxidation-reduction reactions.

5.4.2 Questions to Review Stoichiometry

1. Balance the following equation, and determine the coefficient in front of $KClO_3$:

$$KClO_3 \rightarrow KCl + KClO_4$$

A. 1
B. 2
C. 3
D. 4

2. The coefficient in front of Zn in the following equation is:

$$Zn + HCl \rightarrow ZnCl_2 + H_2$$

A. 1
B. 2
C. 3
D. 4

3. Which of the following reactants or products has the largest coefficient in the balanced equation?

$$C_{12}H_{22}O_{11} + O_2 \rightarrow CO_2 + H_2O$$

A. O_2
B. CO_2
C. H_2O
D. O_2 and CO_2

4. What is the coefficient in front of $Ca(OH)_2$ in the following equation when balanced?

$$(NH_4)_2SO_4 + Ca(OH)_2 \rightarrow NH_3 + H_2O + CaSO_4$$

A. 1
B. 2
C. 3
D. 4

5. What is the sum of coefficients in the following equation when balanced?

$$CuO + H_3PO_4 \rightarrow Cu_3(PO_4)_2 + H_2O$$

A. 6
B. 7
C. 8
D. 9

6. What is the sum of coefficients in the following equation when balanced?

$$Na_2O_2 + H_2O \rightarrow NaOH + O_2$$

A. 5
B. 7
C. 9
D. 11

Use the following unbalanced equation for question #7.

$$N_2H_4(l) + N_2O_4(l) \rightarrow N_2(g) + H_2O(l) \qquad (H = 1, N = 14, O = 16)$$

7. The sum of coefficients in the balanced equation is:

A. 4
B. 6
C. 8
D. 10

8. In the equation below, the sum of the balanced coefficients is:

$FeS(s) + O_2(g) + H_2O(l) \rightarrow Fe_2O_3(s) + H_2SO_4(l)$ (H = 1, O = 16, S = 32, Fe = 56)

A. 8
B. 13
C. 18
D. 23

5.4.3 Answers to Questions in Section 5.4.2

(1) D (2) A (3) D (4) A (5) D (6) C (7) D (8) D

5.4.4 Discussion of Answers to Questions in Section 5.4.2

Question #1 (Answer: D) The O's appear in only one compound on each side of the equation, so balance it first. In this type of situation, simply multiply each compound by the number of atoms of the element (i.e., O in this case) in the other compound:

unbalanced: $KClO_3 \rightarrow KCl + KClO_4$

balanced O: $4KClO_3 \rightarrow KCl + 3KClO_4$

There is no apparent clear choice between K or Cl so just pick one to balance. Luckily both K and Cl are already balanced. Check by counting total number of each element on each side of the equation:

check:	$4KClO_3$	$KCl + 3KClO_4$
K:	4	4
Cl:	4	4
O:	12	12

Question #2 (Answer: A) Can select Zn, H or Cl because all appear in only one compound on each side. In this case, select the one that appears most complicated which is H or Cl in this case:

unbalanced: $Zn + HCl \rightarrow ZnCl_2 + H_2$

balanced H: $Zn + 2HCl \rightarrow ZnCl_2 + H_2$

Zn and Cl: both are balanced also

check:	$Zn + 2HCl$	$ZnCl_2 + H_2$
Zn:	1	1
Cl:	2	2
H:	2	2

Question #3 (Answer: D)

unbalanced: $C_{12}H_{22}O_{11} + O_2 \rightarrow CO_2 + H_2O$

balance C: $C_{12}H_{22}O_{11} + O_2 \rightarrow 12CO_2 + H_2O$

balance H: $C_{12}H_{22}O_{11} + O_2 \rightarrow 12CO_2 + 11H_2O$

balance O: $C_{12}H_{22}O_{11} + 12O_2 \rightarrow 12CO_2 + 11H_2O$

check:	$C_{12}H_{22}O_{11} + 12O_2$	$12CO_2 + 11H_2O$
C:	12	12
H:	22	22
O:	11 + 24 = 35	24 + 11 = 35.

Question #4 (Answer: A)

unbalanced: $(NH_4)_2SO_4 + Ca(OH)_2 \rightarrow NH_3 + H_2O + CaSO_4$

Note: Treat SO_4^{-2} as a group in this case.

SO_4^{-2} and Ca are already balanced

balance N: $(NH_4)_2SO_4 + Ca(OH)_2 \rightarrow 2NH_3 + H_2O + CaSO_4$

balance O: $(NH_4)_2SO_4 + Ca(OH)_2 \rightarrow 2NH_3 + 2H_2O + CaSO_4$

(note that the O's in the SO_4^{-2}'s balance themselves and do not have to be accounted for in this balancing of the O's)

balance H: already balanced.

check:	$(NH_4)_2SO_4 + Ca(OH)_2$	$\rightarrow$	$2NH_3 + 2H_2O + CaSO_4$
N:	2	|	2
H:	8 + 2 = 10	|	6 + 4 = 10
S:	1	|	1
O:	4 + 2 = 6	|	2 + 4 = 6.

Question #5 (Answer: D)

unbalanced: $CuO + H_3PO_4 \rightarrow Cu_3(PO_4)_2 + H_2O$

Note: the PO_4^{-3} can be treated as a group since it is not changed in the reaction.

Can select Cu, PO_4^{-3} or H to balance first, the H's appear the most complicated so do them first.

balance H: $CuO + 2H_3PO_4 \rightarrow Cu_3(PO_4)_2 + 3\ H_2O$

balance PO_4: already balanced

balance Cu's: $3CuO + 2H_3PO_4 \rightarrow Cu_3(PO_4)_2 + 3\ H_2O$

balance O: already balanced (note again that the O's on the PO_4^{-3}'s were balanced by balancing the PO_4^{-3}'s)

check:	$3CuO + 2H_3PO_4$	$\rightarrow$	$Cu_3(PO_4)_2 + 3\ H_2O$
Cu:	3	|	2
O:	3 + 8 = 11	|	8 + 3 = 11
H:	6	|	6
P:	2	|	2

Question #6 (Answer: C)

unbalanced: $Na_2O_2 + H_2O \rightarrow NaOH + O_2$

balance Na: $Na_2O_2 + H_2O \rightarrow 2NaOH + O_2$

balance H: already balanced

balance O: $Na_2O_2 + H_2O \rightarrow 2NaOH + {}^1/2O_2$

remove fractions by multiplying through by 2:

check:	$2Na_2O_2 + 2H_2O$	$\rightarrow$	$4NaOH + O_2$
Na:	4	|	4
O:	4 + 2 = 6	|	4 + 2 = 6
H:	4	|	4

Question #7 (Answer: D)

unbalanced: $N_2H_4 + N_2O_4 \rightarrow N_2 + H_2O$

balance O: $N_2H_4 + N_2O_4 \rightarrow N_2 + 4H_2O$

balance H: $2N_2H_4 + N_2O_4 \rightarrow N_2 + 4H_2O$

balance N: $2N_2H_4 + N_2O_4 \rightarrow 3N_2 + 4H_2O$

check:	$2N_2H_4 + N_2O_4$	$\rightarrow$	$3N_2 + 4H_2O$
N:	4 + 2 = 6	|	6
H:	8	|	8
O:	4	|	4

Question #8 (Answer: D)

unbalanced:	$FeS + O_2 + H_2O \rightarrow Fe_2O_3 + H_2SO_4$
balance H, S:	already balanced
balance Fe:	$2FeS + O_2 + H_2O \rightarrow Fe_2O_3 + H_2SO_4$
rebalance S:	$2FeS + O_2 + H_2O \rightarrow Fe_2O_3 + 2H_2SO_4$
rebalance H:	$2FeS + O_2 + 2H_2O \rightarrow Fe_2O_3 + 2H_2SO_4$
balance O:	$2FeS + 9/2\ O_2 + 2H_2O \rightarrow Fe_2O_3 + 2H_2SO_4$
multiply by 2:	$4FeS + 9O_2 + 4H_2O \rightarrow 2Fe_2O_3 + 4H_2SO_4$

check:	$4FeS + 9O_2 + 4H_2O \rightarrow 2Fe_2O_3 + 4H_2SO_4$	
Fe:	4	4
S:	4	4
O:	18 + 4 = 22	6 + 16 = 22
H:	8	8

5.4.5 Checklist for Stoichiometry

______ symbolism of chemical equations
______ balancing of chemical equations
______ use of chemical equations in solving problems

5.5 ELECTROCHEMISTRY

5.5.1 Review of Electrochemistry

Electrochemistry is the study of chemical reactions in which the reactants undergo a change in oxidation state (i.e., there is a transfer of electrons between atoms). The *oxidation state* (OS) of an atom is a convenient bookkeeping device for keeping track of the electrons in a reaction. The atoms do not actually possess the charge (when in a molecule) designated by the OS. The following rules (general with exceptions) are useful for determining the OS:

(1) all elements have an OS = 0 in the elemental form, e.g., O_2, Fe, Na (these can exist as ions but then they are not in the elemental form);

(2) hydrogen is + 1 except when combined with metals as hydrides (− 1);

(3) oxygen is − 2 except when combined with fluorine, then it is + 2, or in peroxides (−1), or in superoxides (− 1/2);

(4) fluorine is always = − 1;

(5) Group I metals (Li, Na, K, etc.) are + 1;

(6) Group II metals (Mg, Ca, Sr, Ba) are + 2;

(7) Halogens (Cl, Br, I) are − 1 unless combined with F or O;

(8) Al = + 3;

(9) charges (not OS) of some common complex ions:

SO_4^{-2}	sulfate	CO_3^{-2}	carbonate
NO_3^{-1}	nitrate	$CH_3CO_2^-$	acetate
PO_4^{-3}	phosphate	ClO_4^-	perchlorate
OH^-	hydroxide		

In an oxidation-reduction reaction, one (or more) atom(s) is always oxidized, and one (or more atoms is always reduced. *Oxidation* is the loss of electrons (or equivalently the loss of hydrogen in organic chemistry), and *reduction* is the gain of electrons (or equivalently the gain of hydrogen in organic chemistry). Remember the mnemonic "OIL RIG" meaning oxidation is loss and reduction is gain of electrons. An *oxidizing agent* is a substance that can take electrons from other atoms and is reduced. A *reducing agent* is a substance that can give electrons to other atoms and is oxidized. The overall reaction can be divided into the *oxidation half-reaction* and the *reduction half-reaction*, for example:

overall reaction:	$Zn + Cu^{+2} \rightleftharpoons Zn^{+2} + Cu$
oxidation half-reaction:	$Zn \rightleftharpoons Zn^{+2} + 2e^-$
reduction half-reaction:	$Cu^{+2} + 2e^- \rightleftharpoons Cu$

Note: (1) the e^- (electrons) in the oxidation (loss) half-reaction are on the right side (of the arrow), and for the reduction (gain) half-reaction they are on the left; (2) the sum of the electrons in the balanced half-reactions must cancel out when added (algebraically) to get the overall reaction.

These half-reactions may occur at electrodes (substances made of metal or carbon at which electrons may be exchanged). Electrodes are of two types: cathode and anode. A cathode is an electrode that attracts cations (positively charged ions such as H^+, Ca^{++} and NH_4^+) and it is where reduction of electrode occurs. In electrochemical cells (voltaic, galvanic) the reaction is spontaneous, whereas in electrolytic cells the reaction is nonspontaneous. The cathode is positive in electrochemical cells and is negative in electrolytic cells. An anode is the electrode that attacts anions (negatively charged ions such as Cl^-, OH^-, SO_4^{--}) and it is where oxidation of electrode occurs. The anode is negative in electrochemical cells and positive in electrolytic cells. Electrons enter the anode by oxidation of a substance and move to the cathode where they exit by reduction of some substance. A conducting connector, e.g., a wire or a salt bridge, acts as a link between the anode and the cathode.

	CONTRAST				**COMPARE**
Electrochemical cells	voltaic & galvanic	cathode +	anode -	spontaneous	• oxidation occurs at anode • reduction occurs at cathode • cathode attracts cations in solution • anode attracts anions in solution
Electrolytic cells	N/A	cathode -	anode +	nonspontaneous	

The capacity of one substance to give or take electrons from another substance is complex. Suffice it to say that electron affinities, ionization potentials, concentrations, pressures and temperature are all important. Fortunately, the relative ability of a substance to give or take electrons can be quantified in one number symbolized by E. E is the potential difference (or voltage, Section 5.18) that is generated when two substances are connected. This potential, when standardized, is called the *standard half-cell potential* (E°) as follows:

(1) a *reference half-reaction* is established and its E° = 0,
$2H^+ (1M) + 2e^- \rightarrow H_2(1\ atm)$
atm = atmosphere and M = molar
(2) all other half-reactions are compared to this and the E° for each of them is determined,
(3) to be E°, these standard conditions must hold;
concentration of all solutes is 1M (one molar),
pressure of all gases is 1 atm,
temperature is 25°C (298°K).

The *standard half-cell potential* (E°) can be written as an oxidation half-reaction,

$A \rightarrow A^{+n} + ne^-$, or, as a reduction half-reaction $A^{+n} + ne^- \rightarrow A$.

The first is called an *oxidation cell potential*; the second is called a *reduction cell potential*. Usually the reduction cell potentials are used. Regardless of which one is used, the *interpretation* of E° is the same. The more positive the E°, the more likely the reaction to proceed to the right as written. Please note:

(1) if the direction of the equation is reversed, the sign of E° changes to the opposite ($+ \rightarrow -$) or ($- \rightarrow +$),
(2) the value of E° *is not* affected by the stoichiometry of the reaction.

To determine the *potential for a reaction*, call it $\Delta E°$, the appropriate $E°$ for the half-cell reactions must be looked up, given the correct sign, and then added up. For example, given the reaction,

$$2A + B^{+2} \rightarrow 2A^{+1} + B$$

the oxidation half-reaction (O) is,

$$(O): 2A \rightarrow 2A^{+1} + 2e^-$$

the reduction half-reaction (R) is,

$$(R): B^{+2} + 2e^- \rightarrow B.$$

Then if a table of reduction potentials is available, one will find these (in the table)

$$A^{+1} + e^- \rightarrow A \qquad E° = -1.10V$$
$$B^{+2} + 2e^- \rightarrow B. \qquad E° = +0.50V$$

These half-reactions from the reduction potential table are rewritten as they occur (the direction) in the given reaction:

$$(O): 2A \rightarrow 2A^{+1} + 2e^- \qquad E° = +1.10V$$
$$(R): 2e^- + B^{+2} \rightarrow B \qquad E° = +0.50V$$

overall: $2A + B^{+2} \rightarrow 2A^{+1} + B \qquad \Delta E° = +1.60V$

Note:
(1) when balancing the half-reaction, the $E°$ is not affected as for the (O) above,
(2) when reversing the equation as found in the table, the sign of $E°$ (from the table) is reversed as for the (O),
(3) if the overall $\Delta E°$ is positive, then the reaction proceeds from left to right as written,
(4) if the overall $\Delta E°$ is negative, then the reaction proceeds in the reverse direction and it should be rewritten as such.

The value of $\Delta E°$ determines the maximal amount of work the reaction can perform. The relation is:

$$\text{work (joules)} = (\Delta E)(q) = (\Delta E)(I)(\Delta t)$$

ΔE = volts q = charge in coulombs
I = current in amperes (coulombs/sec)
t = time in seconds

The equation is valid for electrolysis (below).

Galvanic cells produce a current and voltage internally by a chemical reaction. For example, a lead storage battery. The size of the potential, $\Delta E°$, is as calculated by the methods above.

Concentration cells can produce a current and voltage by differences in concentrations of the same substance. The larger the concentration difference, the larger the potential produced by the cell.

Electrolysis is the process whereby electrons are pushed into a system by an external voltage, and a reaction can be forced to go in a direction it could not go spontaneously. This is one way metals may be recovered from their salts. Also, gold or silver electroplating is done this way. The key relations are:

1F (faraday) = 96,500 coulombs = 1 mole of electrons (Faraday's Relation)

1 ampere of current = 1 coulomb/sec.

These relations are used to determine how much of a metal can be plated out by a given current acting over a certain time, or they can be used to calculate the reverse.

The suggested sequence of steps to *balance oxidation-reduction equations is:*

(1) identify which substance(s) is(are) oxidized and reduced in the net ionic equation,

(2) write half-reactions for each substance oxidized and reduced,

(3) balance each half-reaction,

(4) add half-reactions and the electrons should cancel out (multiply each half-reaction by a small whole number as necessary),

(5) check by counting elements on each side,

(6) Note: for each half-reaction and the overall reaction, the charges should be equal on each side of the equation as should the mass (number of each element on each side); often H^+, OH^-, or H_2O can be added as needed depending on the pH of the solution.

5.5.2 Questions to Review Electrochemistry

1. The oxidation state of an element in its elemental form is:

A. + 1
B. 0
C. − 1
D. need electron configuration

2. All of the following elements generally have an oxidation state of + 1 except:

A. F
B. Na
C. H
D. K

3. All of the following elements generally have an oxidation state of + 2 except:

A. Al
B. Ca
C. Ba
D. Mg

4. Which complex ion below has a charge of − 2?

A. $NO_3{}^{-?}$
B. $PO_4{}^{-?}$
C. $ClO_4{}^{-?}$
D. $SO_4{}^{-?}$

5. Oxidation of a molecule:

A. results in a gain of electrons.
B. results in a more negative oxidation state.
C. may be viewed as the loss of hydrogen in some cases.
D. all of the above.

6. An oxidizing agent is a species that:

A. goes to a more negative oxidation state.
B. gains electrons.
C. is reduced.
D. all of the above.

7. In the reduction half-reaction, the electrons appear on the ____________ of the equation.

A. right side
B. left side
C. either side
D. cannot be determined

8. When the oxidation and reduction half-reactions are added, the sum of the electrons is:

A. positive.
B. negative.
C. zero.
D. any of the above.

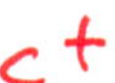

9. Oxidation of the solution (or solute) occurs at the:

   A. anode.
   B. cathode.
   C. neither.
   D. anode and cathode.

10. "Positive" substances are attracted to the:

   A. anode.
   B. cathode.
   C. neither.
   D. anode and cathode.

11. The direction of electron flow is:

   A. from anode to cathode.
   B. from cathode to anode.
   C. either way.
   D. not determinable.

12. All of the half-cell potentials (ΔE) use the ____________ as the reference.

   A. hydrogen (H_2) half-cell
   B. oxygen (O_2) half-cell
   C. carbon (C) half-cell
   D. arbitrarily set zero point

13. The ΔE° depends on all the following variables except:

   A. temperature.
   B. concentrations.
   C. pressures of gases.
   D. all of the above.

14. Half-cell potentials are usually written as:

   A. oxidation half-reactions.
   B. reduction half-reactions.
   C. reactant half-reactions.
   D. product half-reactions.

15. The more negative the value of ΔE°:

   A. the more likely the reaction is to proceed left to right.
   B. the more likely the reaction is to proceed right to left.
   C. the less likely the reaction is to proceed left to right.
   D. the less likely the reaction is to proceed right to left.

16. If the coefficients in a half-reaction are doubled, the ΔE° is:

   A. doubled.
   B. halved.
   C. not affected.
   D. tripled.

17. If ΔE = electrical potential, I = current and Δ*t* = time the current is flowing, then the work (or energy) = W generated is:

   A. $W = \frac{(\Delta E)(I)}{\Delta t}$
   B. $W = \frac{(\Delta E)}{(I)(\Delta t)}$
   C. $W = (\Delta E)(I)(\Delta t)$
   D. none of the above

18. If the potential created by a chemical reaction is used to move a current, the cell created is called a:

A. concentration cell.
B. galvanic cell.
C. electrolytic cell.
D. mixed cell.

19. One faraday corresponds to:

A. one volt of cell potential.
B. 96,487 amperes.
C. one mole of electrons.
D. all of the above.

20. What is the oxidation state of Pt in $PtCl_4^{-2}$?

A. + 2
B. − 2
C. + 4
D. − 4

21. The oxidation state of Co in $Co_3(PO_4)_2$ is:

A. + 2
B. + 3
C. − 2
D. − 3

22. The oxidation state of Cr in $K_2Cr_2O_7$ is:

A. + 3
B. + 6
C. + 12
D. − 12

23. The oxidation state of Fe in $FeCl_2$ is:

A. − 4
B. − 2
C. + 4
D. + 2

24. Which of the following would be considered a reduction half-reaction?

A. $A^{+2} + 2e^- \rightarrow A$
B. $A \rightarrow A^{+2} + 2e^-$
C. both
D. neither

25. The reduction half-reaction of $A^{+2} + 2B \rightarrow A + 2B^{+1}$ is:

A. $2B \rightarrow 2B^{+1} + 2e^-$
B. $A \rightarrow A^{+2} + 2e^-$
C. $A^{+2} + 2e^- \rightarrow A$
D. $2B^{+1} + 2e^- \rightarrow 2B$

26. Suppose A and B^{+2} are placed in the same solution. Will there be a spontaneous reaction? If so, what is the balanced equation? Below are the pertinent reduction potentials:

$A^{+1} + e^- \rightarrow A$ $E° = -1.50V$
$B^{+2} + 2e^- \rightarrow B$ $E° = -1.00V$

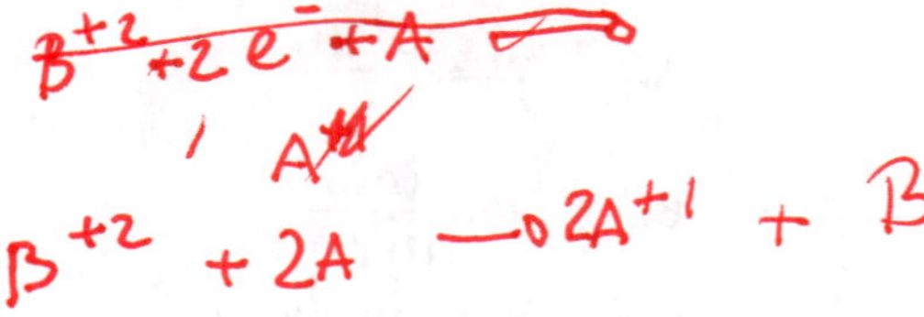

A. no, because the $\Delta E°$ of the reaction is negative
B. yes, $A + B^{+2} \rightarrow A^{+1} + B$
C. yes, $2A + B^{+2} \rightarrow 2A^{+1} + B$
D. yes, $2A + B \rightarrow 2A^{+1} + B^{+2}$

Use the following data for the remainder of the problems.

Standard Reduction Potentials at 25° C in Aqueous Solutions

Half-Reaction	**E° (volts)**	
$Ca^{+2} + 2e^- \rightarrow Ca$	-2.9	
$Na^+ + e^- \rightarrow Na$	-2.7	
$Al^{+3} + 3e^- \rightarrow Al$	-1.7	
$Mn^{+2} + 2e^- \rightarrow Mn$	-1.2	
$Zn^{+2} + 2e^- \rightarrow Zn$	-0.8	
$Cu^{+2} + 2e^- \rightarrow Cu$	$+0.3$	
$I_2(s) + 2e^- \rightarrow 2I^-$	$+0.5$	
$PtCl_4^{-2} + 2e^- \rightarrow Pt + 4Cl^-$	$+0.7$	(See Question #20)
$Ag^+ + e^- \rightarrow Ag$	$+0.8$	
$O_2 + 4H^+ + 4e^- \rightarrow 2H_2O(l)$	$+1.23$	
$Cr_2O_7^{-2} + 6e^- \rightarrow Cr^{+3}$	$+1.33$	
$Cl_2 + 2e^- \rightarrow 2Cl^-$	$+1.36$	
$MnO_4^- + 5e^- \rightarrow Mn^{+2}$	$+1.51$	

Equations:

$$\Delta E = \Delta E^\circ - \frac{0.059}{n} \log \frac{[C]^c[D]^d}{[A]^a[B]^b} = \Delta E^\circ - \frac{0.059}{n} \log K \text{ at } 25^\circ C = \Delta E^\circ - \frac{RT}{nF} \log K$$

(the Nernst Equation) $\Delta E = 0$

for $aA + bB \rightarrow cC + dD$

ΔE° = standard cell potential

ΔE = cell potential at new set of concentrations

n = number of electrons exchanged in the reaction as written

K = equilibrium constant

$$\Delta G^\circ = -nF\Delta E^\circ \quad \text{or} \quad \Delta G = -nF\Delta E$$

F = faraday = 23,000 cals/volts (= 96,500 coulombs)

n = number of electrons exchanged in reaction as written

ΔE = cell potential

ΔG = free energy of reaction = cals

RT = (8.3145)(298) M-K-S units

27. The sum of all the coefficients in the following equation when balanced (the solution is *acidic* and *aqueous*) is: $Ag + NO_3^- \rightarrow Ag^+ + NO$

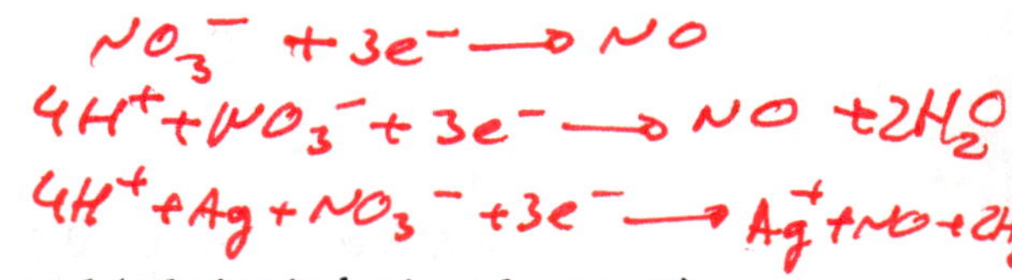

A. 9
B. 14
C. 15
D. 18

28. The sum of all the coefficients in the following equation when balanced (solution is *basic* and *aqueous*) is: $N_2H_4 + Cu(OH)_2 \rightarrow N_2 + Cu$

A. 8
B. 10
C. 12
D. 14

29. The sum of all the coefficients in the following equation when balanced (solution is *basic* and *aqueous*) is: $ClO_2 + OH^- \rightarrow ClO_2^- + ClO_3^-$

A. 5
B. 7
C. 9
D. 10

Use the following information for Questions #30 to #39.

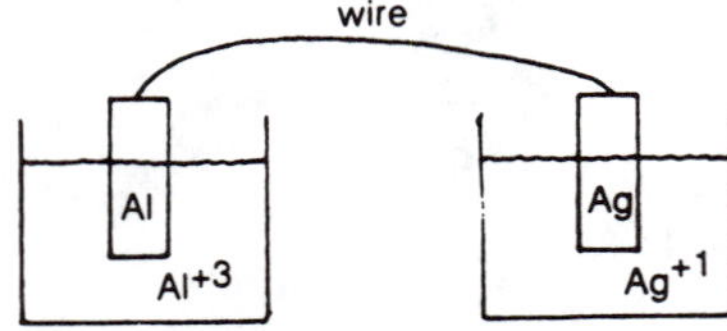

30. Which substances are the reactants in the above cell assuming concentrations are all standard (1M)?

A. $Al + Ag$
B. $Al^{+3} + Ag^{+}$
C. $Al + Ag^{+}$
D. $Ag + Al^{+3}$

31. Write the balanced oxidation half-reaction of the above cell:

A. $Ag^{+} + e^{-} \rightarrow Ag$
B. $Al^{+3} + 3e^{-} \rightarrow Al$
C. $Ag \rightarrow Ag^{+} + e^{-}$
D. $Al \rightarrow Al^{+3} + 3e^{-}$

32. Reduction of the solution is occurring at the ____________electrode.

A. Al
B. Ag
C. neither
D. both

33. The Al electrode is ___________ and is called the ____________.

A. positive, anode
B. positive, cathode
C. negative, anode
D. negative, cathode

34. The flow of electrons is from the ___________ electrode to the ___________ electrode.

A. Al, Ag
B. Ag, Al

35. The sum of coefficients in the balanced equation for the reaction is:

A. 4
B. 6
C. 8
D. 10

36. The *standard* cell potential ($\Delta E°$) for the reaction is __________ volts.

A. – 0.9
B. 0.9
C. 2.5
D. 4.1

37. Using the Nernst equation, what is the cell potential (ΔE), in volts, of the above reaction? Note: At 25°C the electrolyte concentrations are $[Al^{+3}] = 0.1M$ and $[Ag^{+}] = 0.1M$).

A. – 1.14
B. 1.14
C. 2.46
D. 2.10

38. The free energy (ΔG) of the reaction for the conditions, given in calories, is:

A. + 169,740
B. − 169,740
C. + 56,580
D. − 56,580

39. This type of cell may be *best* considered a(n):

A. concentration cell
B. galvanic cell
C. electrolytic cell
D. none of these

40. Which of the following substances will oxidize Mn?

A. Al^{+3}
B. Na
C. Zn^{+2}
D. Ca^{+2}

41. Which of the following substances will reduce $I_2(s)$?

A. Pt
B. Ag^+
C. Cl^-
D. Zn

42. Which of the following is a stronger oxidizing agent than $Cr_2O_7^{-2}$?

A. Cl^-
B. MnO_4^-
C. O_2
D. Ag^+

43. Which of the following is a stronger reducing agent than Zn?

A. Cu^{+2}
B. Na^+
C. Al
D. Pt

44. A current of 10 amps is passed through a solution of Ag^+ for one hour. What weight of Ag (GAW = 108) will be plated out?

A. 40.3g
B. 22.4g
C. 5.6g
D. 1.2g

5.5.3 Answers to Questions in Section 5.5.2

(1) B (2) A (3) A (4) D (5) C (6) D (7) B (8) C (9) A (10) B (11) A (12) A
(13) D (14) B (15) B (16) C (17) C (18) B (19) C (20) A (21) A (22) B (23) D (24) A
(25) C (26) C (27) B (28) B (29) B (30) C (31) D (32) B (33) C (34) A (35) C (36) C
(37) C (38) B (39) B (40) C (41) D (42) B (43) C (44) A

5.5.4 Discussion of Answers to Questions in Section 5.5.2

Questions #1 to #19: Adequately explained in Section.

Question #20 (Answer: A) An equation is:

$Pt + 4Cl = -2$ (Cl = − 1 from rules in Section)
$Pt + 4(-1) = -2$
$Pt - 4 = -2$
$Pt = +2.$

Question #21 (Answer: A) An equation is:

$3Co + 2\ PO_4 = 0$ ($PO_4 = -3$ from Section)
$3Co + 2(-3) = 0$
$3Co - 6 = 0$
$3Co = +6$
$Co = +2$

Question #22 (Answer: B) An equation is:

$2K + 2Cr + 7O = 0$
$2(+1) + 2Cr + 7(-2) = 0$
$2Cr - 12 = 0$
$2Cr = +12$
$C = +6$

Question #23 (Answer: D) The equation is:

$Fe + 2Cl = 0$
$Fe + 2(-1) = 0$
$Fe - 2 = 0$
$Fe = +2.$

Question #24 (Answer: A) A reduction half-reaction has the electrons on the left side (so that there is a gain) as in (A).

Question #25 (Answer: C) In the reaction as written, the A^{+2} is being reduced to A: i.e., $A^{+2} \rightarrow A$ is a change to a more negative (less positive) oxidation state which is reduction.

Question #26 (Answer: C) The half-reactions would be:

$A \rightarrow A^{+1} + e^-$ $E° = +1.50V$ (because reversed)
$B^{+2} + 2e^- \rightarrow B$ $E° = -1.00V$

This is because A and B^{+2} are the reactants given. Then balance electrons by multiplying half-reactions as necessary) so they sum to zero:

$2A \rightarrow 2A^{+1} + 2e^-$ $E° = +1.50V$ (note E° does not change)
$B^{+2} + 2e^- \rightarrow B$ $E° = -1.0V$

Sum: $2A + B^{+2} \rightarrow 2A^{+1} + B$ $\Delta E° = +0.50V$

Since the ΔE° is positive, the reaction will occur spontaneously as written.

Question #27 (Answer: B) Follow the scheme given in the Section:

(1) Ag is oxidized; the N in NO_3^- is reduced

$Ag + NO_3^- \rightarrow Ag^+ + NO$
oxidation states: 0 +5, −2 +1 +2, −2

(2) (a) oxidation half-reaction

$Ag \rightarrow Ag^+ + e^-$

(b) reduction half-reaction

$3e^- + NO_3^- \rightarrow NO$

(3) (a) $Ag \rightarrow Ag^+ + e^-$ already balanced

(b) $NO_3^- + 3e^- \rightarrow NO$ N's are balanced

$4H^+ + NO_3^- + 3e^- \rightarrow NO$ Add H^+ to left to balance charge on *both* sides

$4H^+ + NO_3^- + 3e^- \rightarrow NO + 2H_2O$ Add H_2O to right to balance H's and O's

(4) $3\,Ag \rightarrow 3\,Ag^+ + 3e^-$

$$\frac{4H^+ + NO_3^- + 3e^- \rightarrow NO + 2H_2O}{4H^+ + 3Ag + NO_3^- \rightarrow 3Ag^+ + NO + 2H_2O}$$

sum of coefficients = 4 + 3 + 1 + 3 + 1 + 2 = 14

(5) everything checks

Note that for acidic or basic solutions the H^+ or OH^-, respectively, are usually on the left side of the equation. Also, the balancing of charge does not have to make the overall charge neutral but must make the net charge on one side equal to the net charge on the other.

Question #28 (Answer: B) As in #27 above,

(1) N is oxidized, Cu is reduced

$N_2H_4 + Cu(OH)_2 \rightarrow N_2 + Cu$

oxidation states: – 2, + 1 + 2, – 2, + 1 0 0

(2) (a) oxidation half-reaction

$N_2H_4 \rightarrow N_2 + 4e^-$ (each N loses two electrons)

(b) reduction half-reaction

$2e^- + Cu\,(OH)_2 \rightarrow Cu$

(3) balance each half-reaction

(a) $N_2H_4 \rightarrow N_2 + 4e^-$ N's are already balanced

$4\,OH^- + N_2H_4 \rightarrow N_2 + 4e^-$ Add OH^- to left to balance charge

$4\,OH^- + N_2H_4 \rightarrow N_2 + 4e^- + 4\,H_2O$ Add H_2O to right to balance the O's (and H's)

(b) $2e^- + Cu\,(OH)_2 \rightarrow Cu$ Cu's are balanced

$2e^- + Cu\,(OH)_2 \rightarrow Cu + 2OH^-$ balance charge by adding OH^- to the right side, H's and O's are then balanced

(4) $4\,OH^- + N_2H_4 \rightarrow N_2 + 4H_2O + 4e^-$

$$\frac{4e^- + 2Cu\,(OH)_2 \rightarrow 2Cu + 4OH^-}{N_2H_4 + 2Cu(OH)_2 \rightarrow N_2 + 2Cu + 4H_2O}$$ (multiply by 2)

sum of coefficients = 1 + 2 + 1 + 2 + 4 = 10

(5) everything checks out

Question #29 (Answer: B) Follow steps as in #27:

(1) Cl is oxidized, Cl is reduced

$ClO_2 + OH^- \rightarrow ClO_2^- + ClO_3^-$

oxidation states: + 4, – 2 – 2, + 1 + 3, – 2 + 5, – 2

(2) (a) oxidation half-reaction

$ClO_2 \rightarrow ClO_3^- + e^-$

(b) reduction half-reaction

$e^- + ClO_2 \rightarrow ClO_2^-$

(3) balance each half-reaction

(a) $ClO_2 \rightarrow ClO_3^- + e^-$ Cls already balanced, add OH^- to left to balance charge

$2\,OH^- + ClO_2 \rightarrow ClO_3^- + e^-$

$2\,OH^- + ClO_2 \rightarrow ClO_3^- + H_2O + e^-$ Add H_2O to right to balance O and H

(b) $e^- + ClO_2 \rightarrow ClO_2^-$ Cl's, O and charge are already balanced

(4) $$\begin{array}{l} 2\,OH^- + ClO_2 \rightarrow ClO_3^- + H_2O + e^- \\ \quad e^- + ClO_2 \rightarrow ClO_2^- \\ \hline 2OH^- + 2ClO_2 \rightarrow ClO_2^- + ClO_3^- + H_2O \end{array}$$
sum of coefficients = 2 + 2 + 1 + 1 + 1 = 7

Question #30 (Answer: C) There are four possible substances for reactants Al, Al^{+3}, Ag and Ag^+ ; only two can be reactants. One will be oxidized and one will be reduced. The candidates for oxidation are Al and Ag; the candidates for reduction are Al^{+3} and Ag^{+1}. Since the ΔE° for $Al \rightarrow Al^{+3} + 3e^-$ (+ 1.7) is larger than the ΔE° for $Ag^+ + e^- \rightarrow Ag$ (+ 0.8) which is larger than the ΔE° for $Al^{+3} + 3e^- \rightarrow Al$ (– 1.7), the Al must be oxidized and the Ag^+ reduced.

Question #31 (Answer: D) From #30, the Al is oxidized to get: $Al \rightarrow Al^{+3} + 3e^-$.

Question #32 (Answer: B) From #30, the Ag^+ is being reduced causing reduction at the Ag electrode.

Question #33 (Answer: C) Oxidation occurs at the Al electrode from #32. Oxidation occurs at the anode which is negative.

Question #34 (Answer: A) The Al electrode is losing electrons ($Al \rightarrow Al^{+3} + 3e^-$) which travel through the wire to the Ag electrode where they are used ($Ag^+ + e^- \rightarrow Ag$).

Question #35 (Answer: C) Following the steps in the Section for balancing equations:

(1) Al is oxidized, Ag^+ is reduced

$$Al + Ag^+ \rightarrow Al^{+3} + Ag$$

oxidation states: 0 +1 +3 0

(2) (a) oxidation half-reaction

$$Al \rightarrow Al^{+3} + 3e^-$$

(b) reduction half-reaction

$$e^- + Ag^+ \rightarrow Ag$$

(3) both are already balanced

(4) $$\begin{array}{l} Al \rightarrow Al^{+3} + 3e^- \\ \quad 3e^- + 3Ag^+ \rightarrow 3Ag \\ \hline Al + 3Ag^+ \rightarrow Al^{+3} + 3Ag \end{array}$$ (multiplied by 3)

sum of coefficients = 1 + 3 + 1 + 3 = 8

(5) everything checks

Question #36 (Answer: C) Using the balanced half-reactions from #35 and the E° from the table:

$$\begin{array}{lll} & Al \rightarrow Al^{+3} + 3e^- & E° = +1.7 \text{ (sign reversed)} \\ & 3e^- + 3Ag^+ \rightarrow 3Ag & E° = +0.8 \\ \hline \text{Sum:} & Al + 3Ag^+ \rightarrow Al^{+3} + Ag & \Delta E° = +2.5 \text{ volts} \end{array}$$

Question #37 (Answer: C) The Nernst equation for the balanced reaction is:

$$\Delta E = \Delta E° - \frac{0.059}{n} \log \frac{[Al^{+3}]}{[Ag^+]^3} \approx 2.5 - \frac{0.06}{3} \log \frac{0.1}{(0.1)^3} \approx 2.5 - 0.02 \log \frac{10^{-1}}{(10^{-1})^3}$$

$$\approx 2.5 - 0.02 \log \frac{10^{-1}}{10^{-3}} \approx 2.5 - 0.02 \log 10^2$$

$$\approx 2.5 - 0.02(2) \approx 2.5 - 0.04 \approx 2.46 \text{ volts.}$$

Question #38 (Answer: B) The equation for ΔG is,

$$\Delta G = nF\Delta E = -(3)(23{,}000)(2.46) \approx (-3)(2.5)(23{,}000) \approx -(7.5)(23{,}000)$$
$$\approx -(7)(23{,}000) - (1/2)(23{,}000) \approx -161{,}000 - 11{,}500 = -172{,}500 \text{ cals}$$
$$= -172.5 \text{ kcals}$$

Exact answer by calculator = – 169,740 cals.

Question #39 (Answer: B) The voltage in this cell is generated by a chemical reaction. The difference in concentrations reflect that the conditions are not standard. The classic concentration cell would have either Al^{+3}/Al or Ag^{+}/Ag in both beakers but in different concentrations in each.

Question #40 (Answer: C) If a substance (X) oxidizes Mn, it must take electrons from it and be reduced. The half-reactions are

oxidation:	$Mn \rightarrow Mn^{+2} + 2e^-$	$E° = +1.2$
reduction:	$X^{+n} + ne^- \rightarrow X.$	

Therefore any substance will oxidize Mn if its reduction potential is greater than – 1.2 volts (more positive than). Since the reduction potentials for Ca^{+2} (– 2.9) and Al^{+3} (– 1.7) are too negative and Na cannot be reduced normally, Zn^{+2} (– 0.8) is the best answer. Or any substance on the left side of the arrows below Mn will oxidize Mn.

Question #41 (Answer: D) If a substance (X) reduces $I_2(s)$, it must be oxidized in the process. The half-reactions are:

reduction:	$I_2(s) + 2e^- \rightarrow 2I$	$E° = +0.5$
oxidation:	$X \rightarrow X^{+n} + ne^-.$	

Therefore, any substance will reduce $I_2(s)$ if its oxidation potential (reverse of that found in table) is more positive than – 0.5 volts. This makes Zn, with an oxidation potential = + 0.8 volts, the only possibility given.

Question #42 (Answer: B) Since oxidizing agents are reduced, another way of asking the problem is which substance has a more positive reduction potential. Referring to the table, MnO_4^- is the only possibility.

Question #43 (Answer: C) This question can be rephrased to ask which substance has a more positive oxidation potential than Zn. This is because reducing agents are oxidized. Remembering that the signs of the ΔE° and the directions of the equations are reversed to get oxidation potentials, the table shows that Al is the only possibility.

Question #44 (Answer: A) This is an electrolysis problem. First, moles of electrons are determined.

$$\text{moles of electrons} = \frac{\text{charge passed}}{96{,}500 \text{ coulombs/mole of elec.}} = \frac{36{,}000}{96{,}500} = \frac{360}{965}$$

charge passed = (current)(time in secs) = coulombs

Since $Ag^{+} + e^- \rightarrow Ag$, the moles of electrons correspond to the moles of Ag plated out. (If, e.g., one had $Ni^{+2} + 2e^- \rightarrow Ni$, then each mole of electrons would plate out only 1/2 mole of Ni). Then,

moles of electrons = moles of AG = weight of AG/GAW of Ag

and,

weight of Ag = (moles of Ag)(GAW of Ag)

= (360/965)(108) ≈ (360/970)(110) ≈ (3/8)(110)

≈ (3/4)(55) ≈ 165/4 ≈ 41.25.

Exact answer by calculator = 40.29.

5.5.5 Checklist for Electrochemistry

______ Reduction half-cell potential
______ oxidation
______ reduction
______ oxidizing agent
______ reducing agent
______ half-reactions
______ anode
______ cathode
______ reference half-reaction
______ oxidation state
______ Galvanic cells/voltaic cells
______ concentration cells
______ electrolysis
______ Nernst equation
______ Faraday
______ Coulomb
______ amperes
______ current
______ standard half-cell
______ potential
______ terminology of electrochemistry
______ writing and balancing half-reactions and electrochemical equations
______ determination of cell potentials
______ reactions at electrodes
______ Faraday's relation and its application
______ electrolytic cells

5.6 QUANTITATIVE CHEMISTRY: COMPOUNDS AND CHEMICAL REACTIONS

5.6.1 Review of Quantitative Chemistry

Compounds are made of discrete individual atoms (which, however, can be divided into neutrons, protons and electrons). These atoms then combine in specific ratios with each other, depending upon their chemical characteristics, to form compounds. The elements (a set of atoms with the same atomic number) have a constant weight, and these weights are maintained when combined into chemical compounds (a combination of two or more elements).

A *mole* of any substance contains 6.02×10^{23} particles *(Avogadro's Number)*. A mole of an element contains this many atoms. A mole of a compound contains this many molecules. For an element, the number of moles present is,

$$\text{moles} = \frac{\text{weight of sample in grams}}{\text{atomic weight of element in grams (GAW)}}$$

GAW = *gram-atomic weight.*

For a compound, the *gram-molecular weight* (GMW) is found by adding the (GAWs) of all the elements that make it up (need the molecular formula). Then, the moles of a compound is found as follows:

$$\text{moles} = \frac{\text{weight of sample in grams}}{\text{GMW}}$$

Moles can be calculated in many other ways (see below) and all of these are interconvertible via moles. *Mole is important* because it gives the number of molecules (or atoms) in a given weight of a substance, whereas the weight itself does not. Mole is the key to solving most quantitative mass problems in chemistry. In general, think about how to calculate the number of moles, and, usually the rest of the problem will be easier to complete.

Different substances have differing combining powers with each other. That is, one molecule may be two or more times more reactive than another for a specific purpose. A familiar example should be H_2SO_4 (a diprotic acid) and HCl (a monoprotic acid) in terms of donation of hydrogen ions (H^+). A mole would contain the same number of molecules of H_2SO_4 and HCl, but this does not give us their relative strength in giving H^+. What is needed is a measure, like mole, which would give us the relative or equivalent effectiveness of given weights of substances for specific characteristics. For this reason, the measure called *equivalents* was established. When weights are converted to equivalents, one can be sure, for example, that one equivalent of an acid will react completely and equally with one equivalent of a base. It cannot be stated, without additional information, that one mole of an acid will react exactly with one mole of a base for the reasons above. Note that in one equivalent of a substance there are 6.02×10^{23} particles of interest (e.g. H+ or OH− for acids and bases). The formula for calculating equivalents is:

$$\text{equivalents} = \frac{\text{weight of sample in grams}}{\text{gram equivalent weight (GEW)}}$$

The GEW is calculated as follows:

$$\text{GEW} = \frac{\text{gram molecular weight}}{n}$$

The value of n depends on the chemical nature of the compound. For acids, it is the number of hydrogens used in the reaction per molecule. For bases, it is the number of exchangeable OH^-s used in the reaction per molecule. For oxidation-reduction reactions, it depends on the number of electrons transferred by a given compound in a given reaction. For examples and further explanation of n, refer to 5.5.1, 5.7.1 and 5.8.1.

The percentage composition of compounds is the percent of the total weight of a given element in that compound:

$$\%\ \text{composition of element A} = \frac{\text{total weight in grams of A}}{\text{GMW of the compound}} \times 100.$$

An example is: % of oxygen (O) in $KClO_3$ (K = 39, Cl = 36, O = 16)

$$\%\ \text{of O} = \frac{(3)(16)}{39 + 36 + 3(16)} \times 100 = 39\%.$$

Of course, the percentages of all components should sum to 100%. An *empirical formula* is the formula with the smallest ratio of atoms to each other. The *molecular formula* is the actual formula of the molecule of the substance. For example, for benzene:

structural formula (benzene ring with H on each C) **molecular formula = C_6H_6**
empirical formula = C_1H_1

Of course, it is possible for the empirical formula to be the same as the molecular formula. It is possible to determine empirical formulas if the percentage composition of the compound is known. This is done as follows:

(1) Assume the given percent of each element as the number of grams of that element (i.e., assume you are given 100 grams = 100% of the compound);
(2) Divide the given percentage of each element by its atomic weight to give the moles of each in the compound;
(3) Divide each of these numbers by the smallest of the numbers obtained from step #2;
(4) Determine what small number (to multiply the result of #3), usually 2-5, if any, is needed to convert the numbers from #3 into (approximately) whole numbers. These whole numbers are the ratio of the elements to each other.

What has been done is to convert weights (from percent) into moles by step #2. These moles are, themselves, the ratios of elements to each other. Steps #3 and #4 are just simple techniques to get whole numbers because elements are made of atoms and not fractions of atoms. To *determine the molecular formula* from the empirical formula, the gram-molecular weight (GMW) must be known from some other source, usually the given. (You can find GMW if weight of compound and number of moles is known—see below). Then determine the gram-empirical formula weight (i.e., add up the elements in the empirical formula) and then divide the GMW by the gram-empirical formula weight. The resulting number is how many times each element in the empirical formula is to be multiplied to get the molecular formula. An example is:

> A compound of 2.04% H, 32.65% S, and 65.31% O has a GMW = 98 (from other experiments). What is the empirical formula and molecular formula?
>
> (H = 1, S = 32, O = 16)

By the steps above:

(1) $H = 2.04g$ $S = 32.5g$ $O = 65.31g$

(2) H: 2.04/1 = 2.04

S: 32.65/32 = 1.02

O: 65.31/16 = 4.08

(3) H: 2.04/1.02 = 2

S: 1.02/1.02 = 1

O: 4.08/1.02 = 4

(4) Not needed because step #3 results in whole numbers. Therefore the empirical formula is H_2SO_4.

Gram-empirical formula weight is calculated as follows:

$2(1) + (32) + 4(16) = 98.$

Then, divide gram-molecular weight by the gram-empirical formula weight:

98/98 = 1

Then multiply each element in the empirical formula by the 1 to get the molecular formula which is the same as the empirical formula in this case.

In the following balanced equation, $N_2(g) + 3H_2(g) \rightarrow 2NH_3(g)$ the numbers in front of the molecules give the smallest ratios of these molecules that will react with each other. That is, they are the number of moles of each that must be present to get a complete reaction. If there is too much (or too little) of a reactant present, then that reactant is in excess (or is deficient), and the reaction when finished will have some reactants left over. The amount and which reactant is left over is calculated from the balanced equation using the *ratio of moles*. Note again that moles are the intermediary between weights, volumes, etc. and that the numbers in the equations reflect ratios of moles and nothing else. See also Section 5.5.1 for oxidation-reduction reaction.

Various means of determining the mole of substances are discussed in other Sections. The methods are:

(1) mole = weight in grams/GMW;

(2) MV = mole; M = molarity; V = liters (Section 5.7.1);

(3) NV = equivalents; N = normality, V = liters (Section 5.7.1);

(4) mV = mole; m = molality, V = kg's of solvent (Section 5.7.1);

(5) freezing point depression (or boiling point elevation) calculations (Section 5.9.1.1)
T = km. First determine m, then use m to determine mole as in #4 above;

(6) one mole of any gas at STP occupies 22.4 liters (Section 5.10.1);

(7) at the same temperature and pressure, equal volumes of ideal gases contain equal numbers of moles (Avogadro's Principle) (Section 5.10.1);

(8) PV = nRT (Section 5.10.1)
Ideal Gas Equation;

(9) $P_1 = X_1 P_T$ (Section 5.10.1)
P_1 = partial pressure of gas #1
P_T = total pressure
X_1 = mole fraction of gas #1;

(10) one mole of electrons is one faraday, a faraday is 96,500 coulombs; an ampere (measure of current) is 1 coulomb/sec (Section 5.5.1);

(11) Law of Dulong and Petit:
6.3 = (SH)(GAW)
SH = specific heat in cals/gram
GAW = gram-atomic weight of element.

Note that from the moles, the gram-molecular weight can be calculated, and that moles provide a means of conversion between the diverse situations above.

5.6.2 Questions to Review Quantitative Chemistry

1. A chemical compound:

A. is made of discrete individual atoms.
B. is made of atoms (of different elements) combined with each other in specific ratios.
C. has the weight equal to sum of the weights of the elements that make it up.
D. all of the above.

2. Avogadro's number is based upon:

A. the number of liters that make up one mole of gas.
B. 6.023×10^{23} particles per mole.
C. the number of molecules in a chemical compound.
D. none of the above.

3. Given that mole = m and the weight = w of a compound with a gram-molecular weight = GMW, which is the correct relationship between these?

A. m = (w) (GMW)
B. m = w/GMW
C. m = GMW/w
D. m = l/(w)(GMW)

4. Equivalents:

A. are the same as the mole of a substance.
B. contain $\frac{6.023 \times 10^{23}}{n}$ particles, n = number of atoms under concern.
C. depend on the specific number of groups, e.g., H^+ or electrons transferred, by a molecule.
D. are not determinable for monovalent elements.

5. If equivalents = E, weight of sample = W and the gram equivalent weight = GEW, the correct relation between these is

A. E = 1/(W)(GEW)
B. E = GEW/W
C. E = W/GEW
D. E = (W)(GEW)

6. If gram-molecular weight = GMW, gram equivalent weight = GEW and the number of groups of interest per molecule = n, the correct relationship between these is:

A. GEW = (n)(GMW)
B. GEW = 1/(n)(GMW)
C. GEW = n/GMW
D. GEW = GMW/n

7. If the percent composition of element B in a compound = P, the number of atoms of element B in the compound = n_1, the gram atomic weight of element B = GAW, and the gram molecular weight of the compound = GMW, then the correct relationship between these is:

A. P = (n)(GAW)/(GMW) × 100
B. P = (n)(GAW)/(GMW)
C. P = (n)(GAW)(GMW)
D. P = GMW/(n)(GAW) × 100

8. All of the following formulas give moles except:

   A. (normality)(volume) = moles.
   B. (molality) (kilograms of solvent) = moles.
   C. liters of gas at STP/22.4 = moles.
   D. (Pressure)(Volume)/(Ideal gas constant)(Temperature) = moles.

9. Moles may be calculated from all of the following types of data except:

   A. freezing point depressions.
   B. partial pressures.
   C. electrochemistry (Faradays of charge consumed).
   D. valency number of elements.

The following information is provided for the remainder of the questions. Atomic weights: H = 1, C = 12, N = 14, O = 16, F = 19, Na = 23, Al = 27, P = 31, S = 32, Cl = 35, K = 39, Ca = 40, Cr = 52, Fe = 56, Cu = 63, Br = 80, Ag = 108, and Pb = 207.

10. What is the gram-molecular weight of NH_4Cl?

    A. 53
    B. 50
    C. 49
    D. none of the above

11. What is the gram-molecular weight of $C_6H_{12}O_6$?

    A. 180
    B. 130
    C. 29
    D. none of the above

12. How many moles are 34 g of $AgNO_3$?

    A. 0.20
    B. 0.30
    C. 0.40
    D. none of the above

13. How many grams are there in 0.5 mole of NaOH?

    A. 5g
    B. 20 g
    C. 30 g
    D. none of the above

14. It is known that 5g of a compound is 0.1 mole of that substance. What is its gram-molecular weight (GMW)?

    A. 25
    B. 100
    C. 150
    D. none of the above

15. The gram-equivalent weight (GEW) of HNO_3 when it acts as an acid (donation of H^+) is approximately.

    A. 21
    B. 63
    C. 126
    D. none of the above

16. The gram-equivalent weight of H_3PO_4 when it acts as an acid (donation of H^+) is approximately:

    A. 33
    B. 49
    C. 98
    D. all of the above

17. In a reaction where HNO_3 is used, the nitrogen of the HNO_3 gains 5 electrons. The equivalent weight of HNO_3 in terms of its ability to exchange electrons is approximately:

A. 3
B. 13
C. 63
D. none of the above

18. In a reaction where KNO_3 is used, the nitrogen gains 2 electrons. The equivalent weight of KNO_3 in terms of its ability to gain electrons is approximately:

A. 21
B. 32
C. 63
D. none of the above

19. In a reaction, the Cr of $K_2Cr_2O_7$ gains 6 electrons. The equivalent weight of $K_2Cr_2O_7$ in this reaction in terms of its ability to exchange electrons is approximately:

A. 147
B. 49
C. 25
D. none of the above

20. How many equivalents of base (OH^-) are there in 5g of Al $(OH)_3$ if all OHs react?

A. 0.10
B. 0.20
C. 0.75
D. none of the above

21. Two equivalents of H^+ would require what weight of H_2SO_4?

A. 196
B. 98
C. 49
D. none of the above

22. Approximately what percentage of $CuSO_4$ is sulfur?

A. 20
B. 30
C. 40
D. none of the above

23. The approximate percentage of H in $(NH_4)_2\ SO_4$ is:

A. 6
B. 7
C. 4
D. none of the above

24. What is the empirical formula of the following compound?

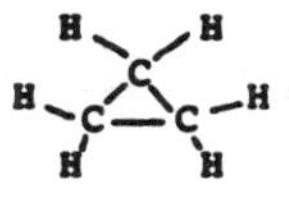

A. C_3H_6
B. C_2H_2
C. C_1H_2
D. none of these

25. A compound contains 39.8% Cu, 20.1% S and 40.1% O. Its empirical formula is:

A. $CuSO_2$
B. Cu_2SO_3
C. $CuSO_4$
D. none of these

26. A compound contains 39.9% C, 6.7% H and 53.4% O. The empirical formula is:

A. CH_2O
B. C_2H_2O
C. CHO
D. none of the above

27. A compound contains 2.6 gms of N, 0.8 gms of H, and 6.6 gms of Cl. The empirical formula is:

A. N_2H_2Cl
B. $N(HCl)_2$
C. NH_4Cl
D. none of the above

28. A compound of carbon and hydrogen contains 92.3% C. The molecular weight (from other experiments) is known to be 52. What is the molecular formula?

A. C_2H_2
B. C_4H_4
C. C_3H_6
D. none of these

29. The specific heat of an element is 0.03, its gram atomic weight is:

A. 18.9
B. 210
C. 189
D. need more information

Use the following unbalanced equation for questions #30 through #32.

$$N_2H_4(l) + N_2O_4(l) \rightarrow N_2(g) + H_2O(l)$$

$$(H = 1, N = 14, O = 16)$$

30. How many moles of N_2 will be produced if 3 moles of N_2H_4 are used up in the reaction?

A. 2
B. 3
C. 4 1/2
D. 9

31. There are 8 gms of N_2H_4 and 92 gms of N_2O_4 available. What weight of water in grams can be made from this?

A. 4 1/2
B. 9
C. 18
D. 36

32. If 36g of H_2O is produced in the above reaction, what volume of nitrogen is also produced assuming the reaction is at STP?

A. 1.5 liters
B. 10 liters
C. 33.6 liters
D. 44.8 liters

Use the following information for questions #33 through #35.

$$FeS(s) + O_2(g) + H_2O(l) \rightarrow Fe_2O_3(s) + H_2SO_4(l)$$
$$(H = 1, O = 16, S = 32, Fe = 56)$$

33. If 22.4 liters of O are allowed to react with 44g of FeS, approximately what weight of H_2SO_4 is produced (assume reaction run at STP)?

   A. 98g
   B. 49g
   C. 44g
   D. 2g

34. If 5 moles of FeS are used in the reaction, what is the maximum number of moles of Fe_2O_3 that can be produced?

   A. 1.0
   B. 2.5
   C. 5.0
   D. 7.5

35. If 98g of H_2SO_4 is desired, what volume of O_2 must be used in the reaction (assume STP)?

   A. 50.4 liters
   B. 22.4 liters
   C. 11.2 liters
   D. 1 liter

5.6.3 Answers to Questions in Section 5.6.2

(1) D	(2) B	(3) B	(4) C	(5) C	(6) D	(7) A	(8) A	(9) D	(10) A
(11) A	(12) A	(13) B	(14) D	(15) B	(16) D	(17) B	(18) D	(19) C	(20) B
(21) B	(22) A	(23) A	(24) C	(25) C	(26) A	(27) C	(28) B	(29) B	(30) C
(31) B	(32) C	(33) C	(34) B	(35) A					

5.6.4 Discussion of Answers to Questions in Section 5.6.2

Questions #1 to #9: Adequately discussed in this Section.

Question #10 (Answer: A) GMW $= N + 4(H) + Cl = 14 + 4(1) + 35 = 53$

Question #11 (Answer: A) GMW $= 6C + 12H + 6O = 6(12) + 12(1) + 6(16)$
$= 72 + 12 + 96 = 180$

Question #12 (Answer: A) Moles $= \frac{\text{weight}}{\text{GMW}} = 34/169 = 0.20$

GMW $= Ag + N + 3(O) = 107 + 14 + 3(16)$
$= 21 + 48 = 169$

Question #13 (Answer: B) weight $=$ (moles(GMW) $= (0.5)(40) = 20$ g
GMW $= Na + O + H = 23 + 16 + 1 = 40$

Question #14 (Answer: D) GMW $=$ weight/moles $= 5/0.1 = 50.$

Question #15 (Answer: B) GEW $=$ GMW/n $= 63/1 = 63$
GMW $= H + N + 3(O) = 1 + 14 + 3(16)$
$= 15 + 48 = 63$
n $=$ # of exchangeable H's per molecule $= 1$

Question #16 (Answer: D) H_3PO_4 can give 1, 2, or 3 protons in a reaction; therefore the reaction must be specified. $3(1) + 31 + 4(16) = 98 =$ GMW. Then $98/1 = 98$, $98/2 = 49$, $98/3 \approx 33$.

Question #17 (Answer: B) GEW $= \frac{GMW}{n} = 63/5 \approx 13$

GMW $= H + N + 3(O) = 1 + 14 + 3(16)$
$= 15 + 48 = 63$
n = # of exchangeable electrons per molecule = 5

Question #18 (Answer: D) GEW $= \frac{GMW}{n} = 101/2 \approx 50$

GMW $= K + N + 3(O) = 39 + 14 + 3(16)$
$= 53 + 48 = 101$
n = # of exchangeable electrons per molecule = 2

Question #19 (Answer: C) GEW $= \frac{GMW}{n} = 294/12 \approx 25$

GMW $= 2(K) + 2(Cr) + 7(O) = 2(39) + 2(52) + 7(16)$
$= 78 + 104 + 112 = 294$
n = # of exchangeable electrons per molecule
= (2)(6) = 12 because there are two Cr's per molecule

Question #20 (Answer: B) Equivalents $= \frac{weight}{GEW} \approx 5/26 \approx 0.20$

GEW $= \frac{GMW}{n} = 78/3 = 26$
GMW $= Al + 3(O) + 3(H) = 27 + 3(16) + 3(1)$
$= 27 + 48 + 3 = 78$
n = # of exchangeable OH's per molecule = 3

Question #21 (Answer: B) Weight = (GEW)(Equivalents) = (49)(2) = 98

GEW = GMW/n = 98/2 = 49
GMW $= 2(H) + S + 4(O) = 2(1) + 32 + 4(16)$
$= 2 + 32 + 64 = 98$
n = # of exchangeable H's per molecule = 2

Question #22 (Answer: A) % S = (weight of S/GMW)(100) = (32/159)(100) ≈ 20

weight of S = (1)(S) = (1) (32) = 32
GMW = Cu + S + 4(O) = 63 + 32 + 4(16) = 95 + 64 = 159

Question #23 (Answer: A) % H = (weight of H/GMW)(100) = (8/132)(100) ≈ 6

weight of H = 8(H) = 8(1) = 8
GMW $= 2(N) + 8(H) + S + 4(O) = 2(14) + 8(1) + 32 + 4(16)$
$= 28 + 8 + 32 + 64 = 132$

Question #24 (Answer: C) The molecular formula is C_3H_6 (by counting all the atoms). The smallest ratio of this is C_1H_2.

Question #25 (Answer: C) By these steps enumerated in the Section,

(1) Cu 39.8 g S = 20.1g O = 40.1g
(2) moles Cu = 39.8/63 = 0.63
moles S = 20.1/32 = 0.63
moles O = 40.1/16 = 2.51
this gives $Cu_{0.63}\,S_{0.63}\,O_{2.51}$
(3) dividing each number by 0.63:
$Cu_{\frac{0.63}{0.63}}\;S_{\frac{0.63}{0.63}}\;O_{\frac{2.51}{0.63}} = Cu_1S_1O_{3.98}$
(4) not needed since 3.98 ≈ 4, and this yields $CuSO_4$

Question #26 (Answer: A) Follow the same steps as in #25,

(1) C = 39.9g H = 6.7g O = 53.4g
(2) moles C = 39.9/12 = 3.33
moles H = 6.7/1 = 6.7
moles O = 53.4/16 = 3.34
this gives $C_{3.33}\,H_{6.7}\,O_{3.34}$

(3) dividing each number by 3.33:

$$C_{\frac{3.33}{3.33}} H_{\frac{6.7}{3.33}} O_{\frac{3.34}{3.33}} = C_1H_2O_1 = CH_2O$$

(4) not needed

Question #27 (Answer: C)

(1) just use the grams as given
N = 2.6g H = 0.8g Cl = 6.6g

(2) moles N = 2.6/14 = 0.19 (≈ 0.20!)
moles H = 0.8/1 = 0.80
moles Cl = 6.6/35 = 0.19 (≈ 0.20!)
$N_{0.2}\,H_{0.8}\,Cl_{0.2}$

(3) Divide all by 0.2

$$N_{\frac{0.2}{0.2}} H_{\frac{0.8}{0.2}} Cl_{\frac{0.2}{0.2}} = N_1H_4Cl_1 = NH_4Cl$$

(4) not needed

Question #28 (Answer: B) The correct answer can be obtained just by determining the molecular weights of the options. The procedure outlined in the Section is first to determine the empirical formula and then the molecular formula from it.

(1) C = 92.3g H = 100 - 92.3 = 7.7g

(2) moles C = 92.3/12 = 7.7
moles H = 7.7/1 = 7.7
$C_{7.7}\,H_{7.7}$

(3) Divide both by 7.7

$$C_{\frac{7.7}{7.7}} H_{\frac{7.7}{7.7}} = C_1H_1 = CH$$

(4) not needed

The gram-empirical formula weight is C + H = 12 + 1 = 13. This goes into the gram-molecular weight 52/13 = 4 times. This means the ratios of elements in the empirical formula must be multiplied by 4 and this gives C_4H_4.

Question #29 (Answer: B) This is a direct application of the Law of Dulong and Petit (see Section)

$$6.3 = (SH)(GAW)$$
$$GAW = 6.3/SH = \frac{6.3}{0.03} = 210$$

Question #30 (Answer: C) These types of problems are solved by using the known ratios of the moles of the compounds from the balanced equation.

Known ratios from equation:

$$\frac{x \text{ moles } N_2}{3 \text{ moles } N_2H_4} = \frac{3 \text{ moles } N_2}{2 \text{ moles } N_2H_4}$$

x = (3/2)(3) = 9/2 = 4 1/2.

Question #31 (Answer: B) First convert weights to moles:

GMWs (gram-molecular weight):
N_2H_4 = 2(14) + 4(1) = 28 + 4 = 32
N_2O_4 = 2(14) + 4(16) = 28 + 64 = 92
H_2O = 2(1) + 16 = 2 + 16 = 18

$$\text{moles} = \frac{\text{weight}}{\text{GMW}}$$

$$\text{moles of } N_2H_4 = \frac{8}{32} = \frac{1}{4}$$

$$\text{moles of } N_2O_4 = \frac{92}{92} = 1$$

Then determine if one of these is in limiting amount by using the ratios of the compounds in the balanced equation:

if all of the N_2H_4 were used up, then:

$$\frac{x \text{ moles } N_2O_4}{1/4 \text{ mole } N_2H_4} = \frac{1 \text{ mole } N_2O_4}{2 \text{ moles } N_2H_4}$$

$$\frac{x}{1/4} = \frac{1}{2}$$

$$x = (1/2)(1/4) = \frac{1}{8} \text{ moles of } N_2O_4 \text{ would be required.}$$

if all of the N_2O_4 were used up, then:

$$\frac{x \text{ moles } N_2H_4}{1 \text{ mole } N_2O_4} = \frac{2 \text{ moles } N_2H_4}{1 \text{ mole } N_2O_4}$$

$$\frac{x}{1} = \frac{2}{1}$$

$$x = \left(\frac{2}{1}\right)(1) = 2 \text{ moles of } N_2H_4 \text{ would be required.}$$

Since only 1/4 mole of N_2H_4 is available, and not 2 moles as would be required to use up all of the N_2O_4, the N_2H_4 is the limiting reagent. Then, using the moles of the limiting reagent, calculate the expected moles of the desired product.

$$\frac{x \text{ moles } H_2O}{1/4 \text{ mole } N_2H_4} = \frac{4 \text{ moles } H_2O}{2 \text{ moles } N_2H_4}$$

$$\frac{x}{1/4} = \frac{4}{2}$$

$$x = \left(\frac{4}{2}\right)(1/4) = 1/2 \text{ mole } H_2O.$$

Now calculate the grams of H_2O:

$$\text{moles} = \frac{\text{weight}}{\text{GMW}}$$

$$\text{weight} = (\text{moles})(\text{GMW}) = (1/2)(18) = 9 \text{ gms.}$$

Question #32 (Answer: C) Use moles in the intermediate step, after determining GMWs wherever possible:

GMWs:

$H_2O = 2(1) + 16 = 18$

$N_2 = 2(14) = 28$

$$\text{moles} = \frac{\text{weight}}{\text{GMW}}$$

$$\text{moles of } H_2O = \frac{36}{18} = 2$$

Then use equation to find moles of N_2:

$$\frac{x \text{ moles } N_2}{2 \text{ moles of } H_2O} = \frac{3 \text{ moles } N_2}{4 \text{ moles } H_2O}$$

$$\frac{x}{2} = \frac{3}{4}$$

$$x = (3/4)(2) = 1\,1/2 \text{ mole } N_2.$$

Then since at STP and 22.4 liters = 1 mole of gas:

$$\frac{\text{x liters of } N_2}{\text{3/2 moles of } N_2} = \frac{\text{22.4 liters of } N_2}{\text{1 mole of } N_2}$$

$$\frac{x}{3/2} = \frac{22.4}{1}$$

x = (22.4)(3/2) = 33.6 liters.

Question #33 (Answer: C) Again convert to moles:

moles of O_2: $\frac{\text{x moles } O_2}{\text{22.4 liters } O_2} = \frac{\text{1 mole } O_2}{\text{22.4 liters } O_2}$

$$\frac{x}{22.4} = \frac{1}{22.4}$$

$$x = \left(\frac{1}{22.4}\right)(22.4) = 1 \text{ mole}$$

moles of FeS: GMW of FeS = 56 + 32 = 88

$$\text{moles of Fe} = \frac{\text{weight}}{\text{GMW}} = \frac{44}{88} = \frac{1}{2}$$

Then determine if either reagent is in limiting amounts;

if all the O_2 is used up

$$\frac{\text{x moles FeS}}{\text{1 mole } O_2} = \frac{\text{4 moles FeS}}{\text{9 moles } O_2}$$

$$\frac{x}{1} = \frac{4}{9}$$

x = 4/9 mole of FeS would be required

if all the FeS is used up

$$\frac{\text{x moles } O_2}{\text{1/2 mole FeS}} = \frac{\text{9 moles } O_2}{\text{4 moles FeS}}$$

$$\frac{x}{1/2} = \frac{9}{4}$$

$x = \left(\frac{9}{4}\right)\left(\frac{1}{2}\right) = \frac{9}{8}$ moles of O_2 would be required

So, the O_2 is in limiting amounts because less than 9/8 mole is available. Note that more than 4/9 mole of FeS is available to react with the O_2. Then use moles of O_2 to determine how much of H_2SO_4 will be produced:

$$\frac{\text{x moles } H_2SO_4}{\text{1 mole } O_2} = \frac{\text{4 moles } H_2SO_4}{\text{9 moles } O_2}$$

$$\frac{x}{1} = \frac{4}{9}$$

x = 4/9 moles of H_2SO_4 will be produced

since moles = $\frac{\text{weight}}{\text{GMW}}$ and

GMW of H_2SO_4 = 2(1) + 32 + 4(16) = 2 + 32 + 64 = 98

then,

weight of H_2SO_4 = (moles)(GMW) = $\left(\frac{4}{9}\right)$ (98) ≈ (4)(11) = 44 gms.

Question #34 (Answer: B)

$$\frac{x \text{ moles } Fe_2O_3}{5 \text{ moles FeS}} = \frac{2 \text{ moles } Fe_2O_3}{4 \text{ moles FeS}}$$

$$\frac{x}{5} = \frac{2}{4}$$

$$x = \left(\frac{2}{4}\right)(5) = \frac{5}{2} = 2^1/2 \text{ moles of } Fe_2O_3$$

Question #35 (Answer: A)

GMWs: $H_2SO_4 = 2(1) + 32 + 4(16) = 2 + 32 + 64 = 98$

$O_2 = 2(16) = 32$

moles: moles $H_2SO_4 = \frac{98}{98} = 1$ mole

moles of O_2 required:

$$\frac{x \text{ moles } O_2}{1 \text{ mole } H_2SO_4} = \frac{9 \text{ moles } O_2}{4 \text{ moles } H_2SO_4}$$

$$\frac{x}{1} = \frac{9}{4}$$

$$x = \left(\frac{9}{4}\right)(1) = \frac{9}{4} = 2^1/4 \text{ moles of } O_2$$

Volume of O:

$$\frac{x \text{ liters of } O_2}{9/4 \text{ moles of } O_2} = \frac{22.4 \text{ liters of } O_2}{1 \text{ mole of } O_2}$$

$$\frac{x}{9/4} = \frac{22.4}{1}$$

$$x = \left(\frac{22.4}{1}\right)\left(\frac{9}{4}\right) = 50.4 \text{ liters}$$

5.6.5 Checklist for Quantitative Chemistry

_____ mole concept and related calculations
_____ Avogadro's Number
_____ equivalent
_____ gram-molecular weight
_____ gram atomic weight
_____ gram-equivalent weight
_____ percent composition
_____ concept of equivalents and related calculations using equivalents
_____ empirical versus molecular formulas
_____ alternative methods of determining mole
_____ use of chemical formulas to solve problems
_____ limiting reagent reactions

5.7 SOLUTION CHEMISTRY

5.7.1 Review of Solution Chemistry

5.7.1.1 CONCENTRATION UNITS

A *liquid solution* is a homogenous, liquid mixture of variable composition over a limited range consisting of two or more components. Note that a solution may also be gaseous or solid. Given a two component solution, the *solvent* is the component in greater amount (herein, usually a pure liquid), and the *solute* is the component in lesser amount (herein, usually a solid or second liquid). Note that solids, gases or other liquids can be dissolved in a given pure liquid to make a solution.

There are many possible ways of *measuring the composition of solutions.* The common ones are:

(1) *Percent composition* can be weight/volume, weight/weight, volume/volume, etc. It must be designated as to the type and the units of mass and volume used.

$$\% = \frac{\text{amt. of solute}}{\text{total amt. of solution}} \times 100 \text{ (usual form).}$$

(2) *Density* (ρ)

$$\rho = \frac{\text{mass of solution}}{\text{total volume of solution}}$$

(3) *Mole Fraction (X)*

$$x_1 = \frac{\text{moles of one component}}{\text{total moles of one component}} = \frac{n_i}{\sum_{i=1}^{m} n_i}$$

n_1 = moles of component #1, for i = 1

i = 1, 2, 3 . . . . . , m = component number

Σn_i = sum over moles of all m components.

For component #1, if m = 3,

$$X_i = \frac{n_i}{\sum_{i=1}^{3} n_i} \quad \frac{n_1}{n_1 + n_2 + n_3}$$

This is useful when emphasizing the relation between concentration-dependent properties of solutions and the relative amounts of the components (see below).

(4) *Molarity (M)*

$$M = \frac{\text{moles of solute}}{\text{liter of solution}}$$

Varies with the temperature. (The term "formality" rather than "molarity" may be used in some older textbooks.)

(5) *Molality (m)*

$$m = \frac{\text{moles of solute}}{\text{kilogram of solvent}}$$

Does not vary with temperature. Note that the molality and molarity of a given solution *cannot* be the same. (However, for dilute solutions molality and molarity are *almost* the same.)

(6) *Normality (N)*

$$N = \frac{\text{equivalents of solute}}{\text{liter of solution}}$$

N = nM relates normality and molarity. The formula is used to calculate the gram-formula weight (e.g., NaCl is the formula for table salt with an equivalent or formula weight of 58.5). n = number of protons (H^+) or (OH^-) ions.

The following concept is important for solving problems dealing with solutions and concentrations. Most problems can be solved by realizing there is usually a *conservation of mass.* This means:

$$\text{given: } C = \text{concentration unit} = \frac{\text{amt. of solute}}{\text{volume of solution}}$$

(all of the above are like this except for molality; just substitute kilograms for volume and solvent for solution)

V = volume of solution

then: $(C)(V)$ = amount of solute
amount = gms, moles, equivalents, etc., depending on the concentration unit (C) used

then: this amount of solute is conserved

(1) as solutions are diluted,
$C_1V_1 = C_2 V_2$ = amount
e.g., $M_1 V_1 = M_2 V_2$ = moles
$(\%_1)(V_1) = (\%_2)(V_2)$ = grams if % is (W/V).

(2) as solutions are made from solid and liquids,
CV = amount of solute used to make the solution, e.g.,

$$(M)(V) = \text{moles} = \frac{\text{weight}}{\text{gram-molecular weight}}$$

$$(\%)(V) = \text{grams } (\% \text{ is W/V here}).$$

Then the correct combination of formulas is chosen depending upon the problem.

5.7.1.2 IONS IN SOLUTION, SOLUBILITY, CHEMICAL SEPARATIONS

Electrolytes are substances that dissociate into positive and negative ions when dissolved in a solvent. The ions are positive (cations) and negative (anions) and are surrounded by solvent molecules in solution (a process called solvation; when the solvent is H_2O, this is hydration). Our discussion will refer to water as a solvent.

Some substances are only partially soluble in water. The *ion product* is a means of quantifying the solubility:

$$M_mA_a + H_2O \rightarrow mM^{+a}(aq) + aA^{-m}(aq)$$

(aq) = dissolved in water

$$\text{ion product} = [M^{+a}]^m[A^{-m}]^a$$

[ ] = concentration in moles/liter, i.e. molarity.

e.g. For $Ca_3(PO_4)_2$, m = 3, a = 2
Ion product = $(Ca^{+2})^3(PO_4^{-3})^2$

The ion product can be calculated for any solution. The *solubility product* (K_{sp}) is the ion product for a *saturated solution* (as much as possible of the solute has been dissolved at a given temperature):

$$K_{sp} = [M^{+a}]^m[A^{-m}]^a$$

for a saturated solution. The smaller the K_{sp}, the less soluble is a solid. The K_{sp} is larger than the ion product except at saturation where they are equal. As long as the ion product is less than the K_{sp}, more solute can be dissolved.

The *common ion effect* on solubility can be understood in terms of Le Chatelier's Principle (Section 5.13.1.2). Explanation of the effect is based on analysis of the following equation:

$$M_mA_a + H_2O \rightleftharpoons mM^{+a}(aq) + aA^{-m}(aq)$$

The common ions would be M^{+a} or A^{-m}. These are increased by adding compounds that dissociate into them and add them to solution, and they are decreased by adding species that react with them and remove them from solution. If M^{+a} or A^{-m} are increased, the reaction shifts to the left and less of M_mA_a dissolves. If M^{+a} or A^{-m} are decreased, the reaction shifts to the right and more of the M_mA_a dissolves. Note that K_{sp} is not affected—the ion not changed compensates (by increasing or decreasing) for the ion changed (the common ion). For example:

for $CaSO_4$ $\quad K_{sp} = 2.4 \times 10^{-5}$

$$CaSO_4(s) + H_2O \rightarrow Ca^{+2}(aq) + SO_4^{-2}(aq)$$

On adding Na_2SO_4 which gives SO_4^{-2}, the reaction shifts to the left and more solid $CaSO_4$ forms, this leaves less $Ca^{+2}(aq)$ in solution.

However, on adding Na_3PO_4, the PO_4^{-3} reacts with $Ca^{+2}(aq)$ to form $Ca_3(PO_4)_2$ which has a $K_{sp} = 1.3 \times 10^{-32}$ and is very insoluble, this removes $Ca^{+2}(aq)$ from the solution which causes the reaction to shift to the right, this causes more of the $CaSO_4(s)$ to dissolve and this results in more $SO_4^{-2}(aq)$ in solution.

5.7.2 Questions to Review Solution Chemistry

1. Fifty grams of sugar are dissolved in enough water (approximately 168 ml) to make 200 ml of solution. The percent composition of sugar in solution in terms of gms/ml is:

   A. 40%
   B. 0.25%
   C. 2.5%
   D. 25%

2. The density of the sugar solution in question #1 in gms/ml (assume water weighs 1 gm/ml) is:

   A. 0.8
   B. 1.00
   C. 1.05
   D. 1.09

3. What weight of salt is in 50 mls of solution with a density of 1.05 gms/ml? Assume the volume is due mostly to water and water weighs 1 gm/ml.

   A. 1.05
   B. 2.5
   C. 3.25
   D. 5.0

4. A gas mixture contains 84g of N_2 (N = 14), 64g of O_2 (O = 16), and 10g of H_2 (H = 1). What is the mole fraction of O_2 in this mixture?

   A. 0.4
   B. 0.3
   C. 0.2
   D. need more information

5. A solution is made by dissolving 23g of ethyl alcohol (C_2H_5OH; C = 12, O = 16, H = 1) in 500 mls of water. Water has a density of 1 gm/ml. What is the molality of ethyl alcohol?

   A. 0.25
   B. 0.5
   C. 1.0
   D. none of the above

6. Seventy-five grams of Na_2CO_3 (Na = 23, C = 12, O = 16) are dissolved in enough water to make 1 liter of solution. What is the molarity of the solution?

   A. 1.1
   B. 1.0
   C. 0.71
   D. none of the above

7. One-hundred milliliters of a 2M solution of H_2SO_4 contains how many moles of H_2SO_4?

   A. 0.2
   B. 2
   C. 200
   D. none of the above

8. A 3M solution of H_3PO_4 (all H's react) contain how many equivalents of H_3PO_4 in 500 mls?

A. 1
B. 2
C. 6
D. none of the above

9. What weight of NaCl (Na = 23, Cl = 35) would be required to make 2 liters of a 1.5F solution?

A. 174
B. 116
C. 58
D. none of the above

10. How many mls will need to be added to 500 mls of a 1.5M solution in order to make a 1.0M solution?

A. 100 mls
B. 250 mls
C. 5000 mls
D. none of the above

11. Given the following data:

Ion	*Radius (A)*	*Charge*
Li	0.68	+ 1
K	1.33	+ 1
Cs	1.67	+ 1

Which ion would *most likely* have the largest hydration shell in solution?

A. Li^+
B. K^+
C. Cs^+
D. cannot be predicted

Use the following information for Questions #12 through #15. (The numbers are K_{sp}'s)

$BaSO_4$	1×10^{-10}	BaF_2	2×10^{-6}
PbS	7×10^{-29}	$PbSO_4$	1×10^{-8}
$PbCO_3$	2×10^{-13}	AgCl	3×10^{-10}
Ag_2S	1×10^{-51}	FeS	1×10^{-19}
HgS	3×10^{-53}		

12. If a saturated solution of $Cu(OH)_2$ contains $[Cu^{+2}] = 3.4 \times 10^{-7}$ and $[OH^-] = 6.8 \times 10^{-7}$ the K_{sp} is:

A. 8.2×10^{-21}
B. 1.6×10^{-19}
C. 4.6×10^{-13}
D. none of the above

13. A saturated solution of $Cu(IO_3)_2$ is 3.0×10^{-3} moles/liter (M). The K_{sp} is:

A. 6×10^{-6}
B. 2.7×10^{-8}
C. 9×10^{-9}
D. none of the above

14. A saturated solution of $BaSO_4$ contains what concentration of Ba^{+2}?

A. 2×10^{-10}
B. 1×10^{-5}
C. 0.5×10^{-10}
D. none of the above

15. If enough Na_2SO_4 is added to a saturated solution of $PbSO_4$ to make the total $[SO_4^{-2}] = 2 \times 10^{-2}$M, how much $[Pb^{+2}]$ is in solution?

- **A.** 2×10^{-16}
- **B.** 1×10^{-4}
- **C.** 5×10^{-7}
- **D.** none of the above

5.7.3 Answers to Questions in Section 5.7.2

(1) D (2) D (3) B (4) C (5) C (6) C (7) A (8) D (9) A (10) B
(11) A (12) B (13) D (14) B (15) C

5.7.4 Discussion of Answers to Questions in Section 5.7.2

Question #1 (Answer: D)

$$\% = \frac{\text{weight of solute}}{\text{volume of solution}} \times 100 = \frac{50}{200} \times 100 = \frac{50}{2} = 25\%$$

Question #2 (Answer: D)

$$\text{density} = \frac{\text{total weight of solution}}{\text{total volume of solution}} = \frac{\text{weight of sugar + weight of water}}{\text{total volume of solution}}$$

$$= \frac{50 + 168}{200} = \frac{218}{200} = \frac{22}{20} = \frac{5}{4} = 1.10 \text{ gms./ml. (exact answer = 1.09)}$$

Question #3 (Answer: B)

$$\text{density } (\rho) = \frac{\text{total weight (w)}}{\text{total volume (v)}}$$

$$\rho = \frac{w}{v}$$

$w =$ (v)(ρ) = (50 mls)(1.05 gm/ml) = 52.5 gms total

$w =$ total weight = weight of salt + weight of water

weight of water = (1 gm/ml)(50 mls) = 50 gms

52.5 = weight of salt + 50

weight of salt = 2.5 gms.

Question #4 (Answer: C)

$$^{n}O_2 = \frac{\text{weight}}{\text{GMW}} = \frac{64}{32} = 2; = {}^{n}H_2\ \frac{10}{2} = 5;\ {}^{n}N_2 = \frac{84}{28} = 3$$

$$X_{O_2} = \frac{^{n}O_2}{^{n}O_2 + {}^{n}N_2 + {}^{n}H_2} = \frac{2}{2+3+5} = \frac{2}{10} = 0.2$$

Question #5 (Answer: C)

$$\text{GMW} = C_2H_5OH = 2(12) + 5(1) + 16 + 1 = 24 + 5 + 17 = 46$$

$$\text{moles of } C_2H_5OH = \frac{\text{weight}}{\text{GMW}} = \frac{23}{46} = \frac{1}{2}$$

$$\text{kgs of water} = (500 \text{ mls}) \left(\frac{1 \text{ gm}}{1 \text{ ml}}\right) \left(\frac{1 \text{ kg}}{1000 \text{ gm}}\right) = \frac{500}{1000} \text{kg} = \frac{1}{2} \text{kg}$$

$$m = \frac{\text{moles of solute}}{\text{kg's of solvent}} = \frac{1/2}{1/2} = 1.0$$

Question #6 (Answer: C)

GMW of $CaCO_3 = 2(23) + 12 + 3(16) = 58 + 48 = 106$

$\text{moles of } Na_2CO_3 = \frac{\text{weight}}{\text{GMW}} = \frac{75}{106} = .71$

$M = \frac{\text{moles of solvent}}{\text{liters of solution}} = \frac{.71}{1} = 0.71$

Question #7 (Answer: A)

$V = (100\text{mls})\left(\frac{1l}{1000\text{ mls}}\right) = \frac{100}{1000} = \frac{1}{10} = 0.1$

moles = (M)(V) = (2)(0.1) = 0.2

Question #8 (Answer: D)

For H_3PO_4 there are three hydrogen protons, therefore n = 3.

N = nM = (3)(3) = 9

$V = (500\text{ mL})\left(\frac{1L}{1000\text{ mL}}\right) = 1/2\text{ L}$

No. of equivalents = (N)(V) = (9)($^1/2$) = 4.5

Question #9 (Answer: A) First find the number of moles that are required, then find the weight from this:

moles = (F) (V) = (1.5)(2) = 3

since moles $= \frac{\text{weight}}{\text{GMW}}$

weight = (GMW)(moles) = (58)(3) = 174

GMW of NaCl = 23 + 35 = 58

Question #10 (Answer: B)

$M_2V_2 = M_1 V_1$

$V_2 = \frac{M_1 V_1}{M_2} = \frac{(1.5)(500)}{1.0} = 750$ mls is the total volume.

Then 750 – 500 = 250 mls for the added volume (pure water, e.g.).

Question #11 (Answer: A) In general, the ion with the highest charge to volume (or radius) ratio will be the most hydrated. Since all the charges are the same, the ion with the smallest radius will be the most densely charged and have the greatest hydration—this is Lithium.

Question #12 (Answer: B)

$Cu(OH)_2 \rightleftharpoons Cu^{+2} + 2OH^-$

$Ksp = [Cu^{+2}][OH^-]^2 = (3.4 \times 10^{-7})(6.8 \times 10^{-7})^2$

$\approx (3 \times 10^{-7})(7 \times 10^{-7})^2 \approx (3 \times 10^{-7})(49 \times 10^{-14})$

$\approx (3 \times 10^{-7})(50 \times 10^{-14}) \approx 150 \times 10^{-21} \approx 1.5 \times 10^{-19}$

Note that estimation works well here.

Question #13 (Answer: D)

$Cu(IO_3)_2 \rightleftharpoons Cu^{+2}\ 2IO_3^-$

$K_{sp} = [Cu^{+2}][IO_3^-]^2$

$[Cu^{+2}]$ = amt dissolved = 3×10^{-3}

$[IO_3^-]$ = twice the amount dissolved = $2(3 \times 10^{-3}) = 6 \times 10^{-3}$

$K_{sp} = (3 \times 10^{-3})(6 \times 10^{-3})^2 = (3 \times 10^{-3})(36 \times 10^{-6}) = 108 \times 10^{-9}$

$= 1.08 \times 10^{-7}$

Note that when the options are very nearly equal then estimation should not be used.

Question #14 (Answer: B)

$$BaSO_4 \rightleftharpoons Ba^{+2} + SO_4^{-2}$$

$$K_{sp} = [Ba^{+2}][SO_4^{-2}]$$

$$[Ba^{+2}] = [SO_4^{-2}]$$

$$K_{sp} = 1 \times 10^{-10} = [Ba^{+2}][Ba^{+2}] = [Ba^{+2}]^2$$

$$[Ba^{+2}] = (1 \times 10^{-10})^{1/2} = 1 \times 10^{-5}$$

Question #15 (Answer: C)

$$PbSO_4 \rightleftharpoons Pb^{+2} + SO_4^{-2}$$

$$K_{sp} = [Pb^{+2}][SO_4^{-2}] = 1 \times 10^{-8}$$

$$[Pb^{+2}][2 \times 10^{-2}] = 1 \times 10^{-8}$$

$$[Pb^{+2}] = \frac{1 \times 10^{-8}}{2 \times 10^{-2}} = 0.5 \times 10^{-6} = 5 \times 10^{-7}$$

Note that since each $PbSO_4$ gives only one Pb^{+2} per molecule, the $[Pb^{+2}]$ in solution is the same as the amount of $PbSO_4$ that dissolves in the solution. The above is an example of the common ion effect.

5.7.5 Checklist for Solution Chemistry

______ solvent
______ solute
______ solubility product
______ density
______ mole fraction
______ molality
______ molarity
______ normality

______ ion product
______ percent composition
______ common ion effect
______ concentration units and their use in solving problems
______ ions in solution
______ common ion effect

5.8 ACIDS AND BASES

5.8.1 Review of Acids and Bases

There are three common definitions of acids and bases:

(1) **Arrhenius**
Substances that can dissociate into H^+ are acids. Substances that can dissociate into OH^- are bases.

(2) **Brønsted-Lowry**
An acid is a substance that can donate H^+. A base is a substance that can accept H^+.

(3) **Lewis**
An acid is an electron pair acceptor, so it must have a vacant orbital. A base is an electron pair donator, so it should have a free pair of electrons.

Certain acids or bases fall under one classification; others may fall under more than one. The Brønsted-Lowry concept is stressed herein.

The *strength* of an acid (protic, esp.) is determined by its ability to donate protons (H^+). The strength of a base is determined by its ability to accept protons. This strength is measured by the acid (or base) dissociation constant:

Acid

$$HA \rightleftharpoons H^+ + A^-$$ (neglecting solvent, $H^+(H_2O)$ or H_3O^+ is more realistic)

$$K_A = \frac{[H^+][A^-]}{[HA]}$$ at equilibrium

Base

$$MOH \rightleftharpoons M^+ + OH^-$$ (for hydroxy bases)

$$K_B = \frac{[M^+][OH^-]}{[MOH]}$$ at equilibrium

The larger the $K_A(K_B)$, the stronger the acid (base). The smaller the pK_A (pK_B), the stronger the acid (base)—see below for pH. If an acid is strong its *conjugate base* is weak and vice versa. The same is true for bases and their *conjugate acids*. This terminology is:

HA	+	B	$\rightleftharpoons$	A^-	+	HB^+
$acid_1$		$base_2$		conjugate $base_1$		conjugate $acid_2$

A strong acid is one that dissociates completely. A weak acid is one that dissociates incompletely. The conjugate base (acid) of a weak acid (base) is strong.

Strong acids react with strong bases to produce neutral solutions. Strong acids and weak bases produce acidic salts, whereas strong bases and weak acids produce basic salts. Salts of weak acids or bases are basic and acidic, respectively. This is because they hydrolyze in water; the process in hydrolysis:

a salt of a weak acid is basic

CH_3CO_2H (acetic acid) is a weak acid

$CH_3CO_2^-Na^+$ (sodium acetate) is the salt

$CH_3CO_2^-Na^+ + HOH \rightleftharpoons [CH_3CO_2H + Na^+ + OH^-$ solution is basic

a salt of a weak base is acidic

NH_4OH is a weak base

NH_4Cl is the salt

$NH_4Cl + HOH \rightleftharpoons NH_4OH + H^+ + Cl^-$ solution is acidic

Examples of strong acids are H_2SO_4, HCl, HNO_3, HI, HBr, $HClO_4$. Examples of weak acids are H_2CO_3, H_3PO_4 and CH_3CO_2H. Examples of strong bases are NaOH, KOH, LiOH and $Ca(OH)_2$. The important weak base is NH_3 (ammonia) or NH_4OH. Organic acids and some phenols may be strong or weak acids. The organic bases are amines and are weak.

The *pH* is defined as follows:

$$pH = -\log[H^+] = \log(1/[H^+])$$

$[H^+]$ = hydrogen ion concentration in moles/liter as molarity or normality (both are the same in this case).

The pK_A and pOH are similarly defined. The pH of water solutions at 25°C range from pH = 1 to pH = 14. A pH = 7 is neutral, a pH <7 is acid and a pH >7 is basic. The dissociation of water is:

$$H_2O \rightleftharpoons H^+ + OH^-$$

$$K_W = [H^+][OH^-] = 10^{-14}$$

Note that K_W is *not the equilibrium constant*. This results in this relationship:

$$pH + pOH = 14.$$

The *H^+ of a strong acid* or the OH^- of a strong base can be calculated from the normality (discussed in Section 5.7.1) of the acid or base. The *$H^+(OH^-)$ from a weak acid (base)* cannot be calculated from the normality of the acid (base) because they are only partially dissociated. These problems are rigorously solved by using the equations below:

$$(1)\ K_A = \frac{[H^+][A^-]}{[HA]}$$

$$(2)\ K_W = [H^+][OH^-]$$

Equation (1) can be simplified if $K_A \ll [HA_0]$(original concentration of acid), then,

$$[H^+] \approx \sqrt{K_A[HA_0]}$$

The $[H^+]$ can also be arrived at as follows:

	HA	$\rightleftharpoons$	H^+	+	A^-	
original:	$[HA_0]$		0		0	
at equilibrium:	$[HA_0]-x$		x		x	(assume negligible H^+ from H_2O)

$$\text{then } K_A = \frac{[H^+][A^-]}{[HA]} = \frac{(x)(x)}{[HA_0]-x}$$

x = amount of HA that dissociates in moles/liter = $[H^+]$

The equation can be solved using the quadratic formula, or if the x is small relative to $[HA_0]$, then neglect x in the expression $[HA_0]-x$, and solve to get $[H^+] \approx \sqrt{K_A[HA_0]}$ as before.

5.8.1.1 NEUTRALIZATION REACTIONS AND ACID/BASE TITRATIONS

Neutralization reactions are solved using the following equation:

$N_AV_A = N_BV_B$

N = normality

V = volume in liters

A = acid

B = base

A neutralization reaction is one in which the number of equivalents of acid is exactly neutralized by an equal number of equivalents of base.

A *titration* is a neutralization reaction in which a given amount of acid (base) is neutralized by a base (acid) which is added gradually (usually in the form of falling drops from a burette). A titration may be done as follows:

f = fraction of acid neutralized = equivalents of base added/n_o

n_o = original equivalents of acid

V = original volume of acid

v = volume of base added

$[H^+]$ (from acid and water) = $[OH^-]$ at the equivalence point

then,

$[H^+]$ = $(n_o)(1-f)/(V+v)$ + contribution from the H_2O (usually negligible)

= acid concentration at any given point during the titration up to neutralization by base (f = 1.0)

note that $(n_o)(1-f)/(V+v)$ = amount of acid not neutralized by added base.

Titrations can be used to calculate the normality of unknown acid (base) solutions, the equivalent weight of an unknown base or acid or the pK_A's (pK_B's). The point in a titration at which the acid has been exactly neutralized by addition of a base is the equivalence point. Examples of titration curves are in Fig. 5.10.

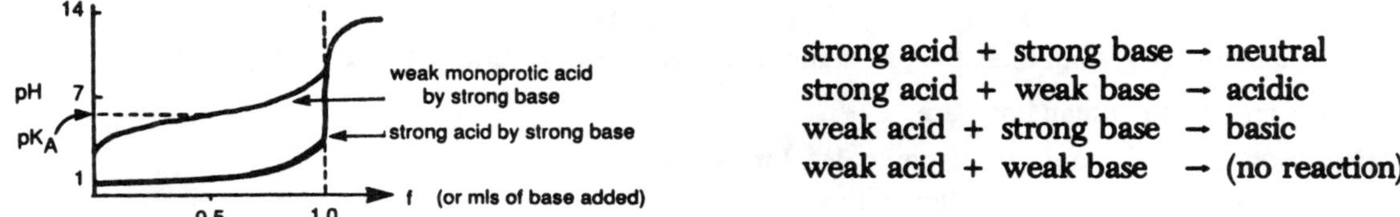

Fig. 5.10—Titration Curves

Note that the curve differs for strong and weak acids, and that the pK_A = pH where the acid is half neutralized.

5.8.1.2 BUFFERS

A *buffer solution* resists changes in pH. For biological substances buffers make the pH values rather stable. The pH of blood is around 7.4. Carbonate, bicarbonate and phosphate ions act as buffers for blood. The multiple acid-base groups in biological molecules such as proteins and lipids act as buffers in the human body. This means a buffer solution is able to hold the pH of a solution relatively constant when an acid or base is added to that solution. *Buffers* are mixtures of weak acids or bases and their salts. For example:

(1)	acetic acid CH_3CO_2H	sodium acetate $CH_3CO_2^-Na^+$
(2)	carbonic acid H_2CO_3	sodium bicarbonate $NaHCO_3$
(3)	ammonium hydroxide NH_4OH	ammonium chloride NH_4Cl

Most strong acids or bases and their salts do not make good buffers because they cannot hold the pH constant (see below).

A buffer works by having an acid component to neutralize added bases and a basic component to neutralize added acids. This can be accomplished by using weak acids or bases and their salts. For example:

for acetic acid-acetate buffer

CH_3CO_2H combines with added base

$$CH_3CO_2H + OH^- \rightleftharpoons CH_3CO_2^- + H_2O$$

$CH_3CO_2^-$ combines with added acid

$$CH_3CO_2^- + H^+ \rightleftharpoons CH_3CO_2H$$

Hence the pH which depends on free H^+ or OH^- is held nearly constant. It may be obvious that it is the ratio of salt and weak acid or base that is important.

The *Henderson-Hasselbalch* relation points out the importance of the ratio:

$$HA + H_2O \xrightarrow{K_A} H_3O^+ + A^-$$

$$K_A = \frac{[H_3O^+][A^-]}{[HA]}, \text{ for } H_2O$$

(HA = acid and A^- = salt of the acid)

solving for $[H_3O^+]$

$$(1)\ [H_3O^+] = \left(\frac{[HA]}{[A^-]}\right)(K_A) \text{ or,}$$

$$(2)\ pH = pK_A + \log\frac{[A^-]}{[HA]}$$

(1) and (2) are equivalent expressions of the Henderson-Hasselbalch relation.

The *effectiveness of a buffer* can be understood in terms of this relation. The key points are:

(1) buffers are most effective when the desired pH (of the solution) is near the pK_A,

(2) ratios ($[A^-]/[HA]$) in the range of 0.1 to 10 are where buffers are effective. Note that this is because the ratio changes slowly and, thus, the pH changes slowly when the ratio = 1 (i.e., $[A^-] = [HA]$).

Important buffers in the human body are:

(1) phosphates—inorganic and organic (least important)
(2) carbonic acid—bicarbonate (most important)
(3) proteins—moderate importance.

Example: Calculate the ratio of $[HCO_3^-]$ to $[H_2CO_3]$ required to maintain a pH of 7.2 in the bloodstream of a mammal. The value of $K_A = 8 \times 10^{-7}$ for H_2CO_3 in blood. The reaction equation is:

$$HCO_3^- + H^+ \rightarrow H_2CO_3$$

Solution:

$$\text{pH} = -\log [H^+]$$
$$7.2 = -\log [H^+]$$
$$\log[H^+] = -8.0 + 0.8 \text{ (Refer to Math Concept \#1)}$$

From definition of log, (Refer to Math Concept #8)

$$[H^+] = 10^{-8.0+0.8} = 10^{-8}\ 10^{0.8} \text{ (Refer to Math Concept \#6)}$$
$$[H^+] = (10^{-8})\,(6.31)$$
$$8 \times 10^{-7} = K_A = \frac{[H^+][HCO_3^-]}{[H_2CO_3]} = (6.31)(10^{-8})\,\frac{[HCO_3^-]}{[H_2CO_3]}$$
$$\frac{[HCO_3^-]}{[H_2CO_3]} = \frac{8(10^{-7})}{(6.31)(10^{-8})} = 12.7 \approx 13$$

Hence the required ratio is 13.

5.8.2 Questions to Review Acids and Bases

1. An acid is a substance that can donate hydrogen ion (H^+); this is a definition of acids given by:
   - **A.** Lewis.
   - **B.** Arrhenius.
   - **C.** Brønsted-Lowry.
   - **D.** none of the above.

2. A base is an electron pair donor; this is a definition of bases given by:
   - **A.** Arrhenius.
   - **B.** Brønsted-Lowry.
   - **C.** Lewis.
   - **D.** none of the above.

3. The conjugate base of a weak acid (one that dissociates incompletely) is:
   - **A.** weak.
   - **B.** strong.
   - **C.** highly alkaline.
   - **D.** highly acidic.

4. Given the reaction of acid (HA) and base (B) below: $HA + B \rightleftharpoons A^- + HB^+$
   - **A.** A^- is the conjugate of acid of HA
   - **B.** A^- is the conjugate base of B
   - **C.** HB^+ is the conjugate acid of B
   - **D.** HB^+ is the conjugate base of HA

5. The salt of a strong acid is:
   - **A.** basic.
   - **B.** neutral.
   - **C.** acidic.
   - **D.** none of the above.

6. The salt of a weak acid is:
   - **A.** basic.
   - **B.** neutral.
   - **C.** acidic.
   - **D.** none of the above.

7. The salt of a weak base is:

A. basic.
B. neutral.
C. acidic.
D. none of the above.

8. Select the weakest acid:

A. HCl
B. HNO_3
C. H_2SO_4
D. CH_3CO_2H

9. Select the strongest acid:

A. CH_3CO_2H
B. H_3PO_4
C. H_2CO_3
D. H_2SO_4

10. Select the weakest base:

A. NaOH
B. KOH
C. NH_3
D. $Ca(OH)_2$

11. All of the following are important buffer systems of the body except:

A. carbonic acid-bicarbonate.
B. phosphates.
C. proteins.
D. nucleic acids.

12. A buffer solution is most effective when:

A. a strong acid or base and its salt are used.
B. the desired pH is near the pK of the acid or base.
C. the ratio of salt to acid (base) is less than 1/10 or greater than 10.
D. a strong acid is mixed with a weak acid.

13. A buffer solution:

A. is made of strong acids and their salts.
B. is made of strong bases and their salts.
C. resists changes in pH when acids or bases are added.
D. is made of strong bases, salts and strong acids.

14. Borane, H–B(–H)–H

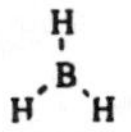

with boron having an atomic number of five and B-H bonds being relatively strong covalent bonds, is a(n):

A. acid according to Brønsted-Lowry.
B. acid according to Lewis.
C. acid according to Arrhenius.
D. base according to Lewis.

15. Ammonia, H–N̈(–H)–H is a(n):

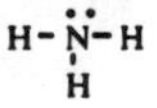

A. acid according to Brønsted-Lowry.
B. base according to Brønsted-Lowry.
C. base according to Lewis.
D. both (**B**) and (**C**).

16. Pyruvic acid is a weak acid. Sodium hydroxide is a strong base. These are combined to form water and sodium pyruvate (a salt). If this salt is placed in water, the solution will be:

- **A.** basic.
- **B.** neutral.
- **C.** acidic.
- **D.** slightly basic.

17. Given the acid HA that dissociates into H^+ and A^-, the acid dissociation constant (K_A) is:

- **A.** $K_A = \frac{[HA^+][A^-]}{[HA]}$
- **B.** $K_A = \frac{[HA]}{[HA^+][A^-]}$
- **C.** $K_A = [HA][HA^+][A^-]$
- **D.** $K_A = \frac{[HA][HA^+]}{[A^-]}$

18. Acid #1 has an acid dissociation constant (K_{A1}) of 5×10^{-5}. Acid #2 has a $K_{A2} = 9 \times 10^{-7}$:

- **A.** Acid #1 is a weaker acid than acid #2
- **B.** The conjugate base of acid #1 is a weaker base than the conjugate base of acid #2
- **C.** Both (A) and (B)
- **D.** Neither (A) nor (B)

19. Fifty mls of a 2M solution of HCl contains how many milliequivalents of acid?

- **A.** 100
- **B.** 10
- **C.** 1
- **D.** 0.1

20. What volume of a 0.1M acid would be required to neutralize 50 mls of a 0.3M base?

- **A.** about 17 mls
- **B.** about 150 mls
- **C.** about 300 mls
- **D.** about 450 mls

21. If 100 mls of a 2M solution of acid neutralizes 25 mls of a solution of base, the molarity of the base is:

- **A.** 0.5M
- **B.** 2M
- **C.** 4M
- **D.** 8M

22. Select the incorrect expression for pH, where ($[H^+]$ = hydrogen ion concentration):

- **A.** $pH = -\log [H^+]$
- **B.** $pH = \log[H^+]^{-1}$
- **C.** $pH = 1/\log[H^+]$
- **D.** $pH = \log(1/[H^+])$

23. A solution has a hydroxide ion concentration of 10^{-8}, the pH is:

- **A.** 0
- **B.** 1
- **C.** 6
- **D.** 8

24. A solution has a hydrogen ion concentration $[H^+]$ of 2×10^{-6}. If log 2 = 0.30 the pH is :

- **A.** 4.3
- **B.** 5.7
- **C.** 6.3
- **D.** 12.3

25. A solution has a pH = 9.3. The hydrogen ion concentration is (antilog 0.30 = 2, antilog 0.70 = 5):
   A. 5×10^{-9}
   B. 2×10^{-9}
   C. 5×10^{-10}
   D. 2×10^{-10}

26. A solution has a pOH = 9, the hydrogen ion concentration is:
   A. 10^{-9}
   B. 10^{9}
   C. 10^{5}
   D. 10^{-5}

27. The pH of a 0.01M solution of HCl (strong acid) is:
   A. 1
   B. 2
   C. − 1
   D. cannot be determined

28. Calculate the pH of a 0.001M solution of NaOH (strong base):
   A. 11
   B. 4
   C. 1
   D. 3

29. A 0.10M solution of monoprotic weak acid is 10% ionized, the pH is:
   A. 0.01
   B. 0.1
   C. 1
   D. 2

30. If the K_A is much less than the original concentration HA_o of a *weak* acid in solution, and H^+ = hydrogen ion concentration, then:
   A. $K_A \approx [H^+] + [HA_o]$
   B. $[H^+] \approx \sqrt{K_A[HA_o]}$
   C. $K_A \approx [H^+]/[HA_o]$
   D. $[H^+] \approx \sqrt{K_A/[HA_o]}$

31. The acid dissociation constant (K_A) of a weak monoprotic acid is 4×10^{-5}. The $[H^+]$ of a 0.1M solution is:
   A. 4×10^{-6}
   B. 4×10^{-5}
   C. 2×10^{-4}
   D. 2×10^{-3}

32. Which point (or line) on the graph below showing the titration of a weak monoprotic acid by a base represents the pK_A of the acid?

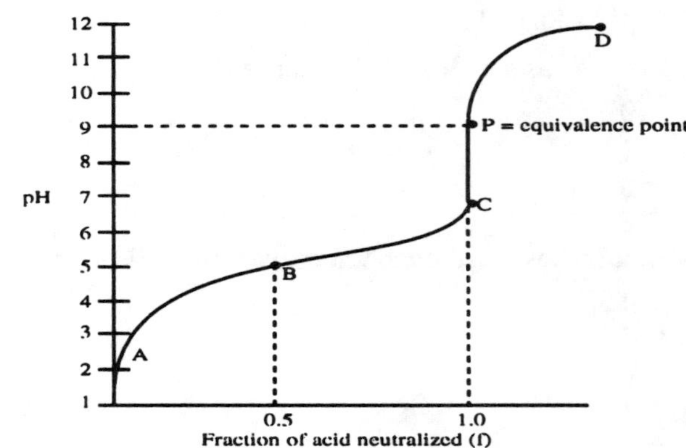

   A. A
   B. B
   C. C
   D. D

33. All of the following may be used to make a buffer solution except:

A. H_2CO_3
B. H_2SO_4
C. NH_4OH
D. CH_3CO_2H

34. A buffer solution made up of 0.1M acid (with a $pK_A = 5$) and its salt which is 1.0M would have a pH of:

A. 5.1
B. 6
C. 6.1
D. 7

35. A buffer solution with a pH = 3.3 is desired. An acid (with a $pK_A = 4.3$) and its salt are available. What ratio of salt to acid is required?

A. 10
B. 1
C. 1/10
D. 1/100

5.8.3 Answers to Questions in Section 5.8.2

(1) C (2) C (3) B (4) C (5) B (6) A (7) C (8) D (9) D (10) C (11) D (12) B
(13) C (14) B (15) D (16) A (17) A (18) B (19) A (20) B (21) D (22) C (23) C (24) B
(25) C (26) D (27) B (28) A (29) D (30) B (31) D (32) B (33) B (34) B (35) C

5.8.4 Discussion of Answers to Questions in Section 5.8.2

Questions #1 to #13: Adequately discussed in Section.

Question #14 (Answer: B) Since the atomic number is five, the electron configuration is $1s^2\ 2s^2\ 2p^1$. Then there are only 3 bonding electrons ($2s^2\ 2p^1$) to fill the four possible bonding orbitals (2s, $2p_x$, $2p_y$, $2p_z$). This means there is one vacant orbital that can accept an electron pair. Lewis' definition of an acid is an electron pair acceptor. The information about the covalent bond is to suggest that the H's do not dissociate, and, therefore, the Arrhenius and Brønsted-Lowry definitions do not hold.

Question #15 (Answer: D) Ammonia is a base by Brønsted-Lowry because it is a proton acceptor. It is also a base by Lewis because it is an electron pair donor.

Question #16 (Answer: A) The reaction is,

$$\text{pyruvic acid} + NaOH \rightarrow H_2O + \text{Na pyruvate}$$
$$\text{Na pyruvate} + HOH \rightleftharpoons \text{pyruvic acid} + Na^+ OH^-$$

It is the free OH^- in solution that makes the solution basic. Undissociated acid (e.g., pyruvic acid) has no effect on the acidity or basicity of the solution.

Question #17 (Answer: A) The K_A is defined as the equilibrium constant of this reaction:

$$HA \rightleftharpoons H^+ + A^- \text{ at equilibrium}$$

This is given as:

$$K_A = \frac{[H^+][A^-]}{[HA]}$$

Question #18 (Answer: B) The larger the K_A, the stronger the acid. Also, stronger acids have weaker conjugate bases (see Section for terminology). Note that $10^{-5} > 10^{-7}$, this means acid #1 is stronger than acid #2 and its conjugate base is weaker.

Question #19 (Answer: A)

$MV = \text{moles}$ if $V = \text{liters}$, $M = \text{moles/liter}$

$MV = \text{millimoles (mm)}$ if $V = \text{mls}$, $M = \text{mm/ml}$

$(2\text{mm/ml})(50 \text{ mls}) = 100 \text{ mm}.$

Question #20 (Answer: B)

$$M_A V_A = M_B V_B$$

$$V_A = \frac{M_B V_B}{M_A} = \frac{(0.3)(50)}{(0.1)} = (3)(50) = 150 \text{ mls.}$$

Question #21 (Answer: D)

$$M_A V_A = M_B V_B$$

$$M_B = \frac{M_A V_A}{V_B} = \frac{(2)(100)}{(25)} = (2)(4) = 8 \text{ M}$$

Question #22 (Answer: C) Recall that,

$$-\log x = \log x^{-1} = \log\left(\frac{1}{x}\right).$$

Question #23 (Answer: C) Since,

$$K_w = [H^+][OH^-] = 10^{-14}$$

$$[H^+] = \frac{10^{-14}}{[OH^-]} = \frac{10^{-14}}{10^{-8}} = 10^{-6}$$

then:

$$pH = -\log [H^+] = -\log 10^{-6} = -(-6) = +6$$

($\log 10^{-6} = -6$, the log of any power of 10 is the exponent).

Or:

$$pOH = -\log [OH^-] = -\log 10^{-8} = -(-8) = 8$$

$$pH + pOH = 14$$

$$pH = 14 - pOH = 14 - 8 = 6$$

Question #24 (Answer: B)

$$pH = -\log [H^+] = -\log 2 \times 10^{-6} = -(\log 2 + \log 10^{-6})$$

$$= -(0.30 - 6) = -(-5.7) = 5.7$$

Question #25 (Answer: C)

$$pH = -\log [H^+]$$

$$9.3 = -\log [H^+] = \log [H^+]^{-1}$$

$$10^{9.3} = 10^{\log [H^+]^{-1}} = [H^+]^{-1} = 1/[H^+]$$

$$[H^+] = 1/10^{9.3} = 10^{-9.3} = 10^{-10+0.7} = 10^{0.7} \times 10^{-10} = 5 \times 10^{-10}$$

(antilog of 0.7 = 5 or $10^{0.7} = 5$).

Study the steps carefully. Several important log relationships are shown as discussed in Chapter 4.

Question #26 (Answer: D) First method:

Step (a): $pH + pOH = 14$

$$pH = 14 - pOH = 14 - 9 = 5$$

Step (b):

$$pH = -\log [H^+]$$

$$5 = -\log [H^+]$$

$$-5 = \log [H^+]$$

$$10^{-5} = [H^+]$$

Second method:

Step (a):
$$\begin{aligned} pOH &= -\log [OH^-] \\ 9 &= -\log [OH^-] \\ -9 &= \log [OH^-] \\ 10^{-9} &= [OH^-] \end{aligned}$$

Step (b): $[H^+][OH^-] = 10^{-14}$

$[H^+] = 10^{-14}/[OH^-] = 10^{-14}/10^{-9} = 10^{-5}$

Question #27 (Answer: B) The $[H^+]$ of a strong acid is the normality of the acid. For HCl (a monoprotic acid), the molarity and normality are equal.

(a) $[H^+] = 0.01 = 1 \times 10^{-2}$

(b) $pH = -\log [H^+] = -\log (10^{-2}) = -(-2) = 2$

Question #28 (Answer: A) The hydroxide concentration of a strong base is its normality. The molarity (M) is the same as normality (N) for NaOH. Then:

(a) $[OH^-] = 0.001 = 1 \times 10^{-3} = 10^{-3}$

(b) $[H^+][OH^-] = 10^{-14}$

$[H^+] = 10^{-14}\ [OH^-] = 10^{-14}/10^{-3} = 10^{-11}$

(c) $pH = -\log [H^+] = -\log 10^{-11} = -(-11) = 11.$

Or, the problem may be solved by:

(a) $pOH = -\log [OH^-] = -\log (10^{-3}) = -(-3) = 3$

(b) $pH + pOH = 14$

$pH = 14 - pOH = 14 - 3 = 11.$

Question #29 (Answer: D) For the reaction given:

	HA	**H^+**	**A^-**
original:	HA_0	0	0
equilibrium:	$0.9HA_0$	$0.1HA_0$	$0.1HA_0$

Then:

$[H^+] = (0.1)(0.1) = 0.01 = 10^{-2}$

Then:

$pH = -\log [H^+]$

$= -\log(10^{-2}) = -(-2) = 2.$

Question #30 (Answer: B) This serves to point out a formula to determine K_A for weak acids.

Question #31 (Answer: D) The $[H^+]$ of a weak acid must be calculated from K_A. Since $0.1 \gg 4 \times 10^{-5}$, use the formula:

$$[H^+] = \sqrt{K_A[HA_0]} = \sqrt{(4 \times 10^{-5})(10^{-1})} = \sqrt{4 \times 10^{-6}}$$
$$= \sqrt{4} \times \sqrt{10^{-6}} = \sqrt{2 \times 10^{-3}}$$

and:

$2 \times 10^{-3} \ll 10^{-1} (0.002 \ll 0.1)$ so the assumption is correct. An alternative method to solve the problem is:

	HA ⇌	**H^+**	**A^-**
start:	0.1	0	0
equilibrium:	0.1-x	x	x

$$K_A = \frac{[H^+][A^-]}{[HA]} = \frac{[x][x]}{[0.1 - x]} = \frac{x^2}{0.1 - x} = \frac{x^2}{0.1} \text{ (assume } x \ll 0.1)$$

$4 \times 10^{-5} = x^2/10^{-1}$

$x^2 = (10^{-1})(4 \times 10^{-5}) = 4 \times 10^{-6}$

$x = \sqrt{4 \times 10^{-6}} = \sqrt{4} \times \sqrt{10^{-6}} = 2 \times 10^{-3}$

Question #32 (Answer: B) This is shown in the review of titration curves. The pK_A of an acid is the pH at which it can be half neutralized or f = 0.5.

Question #33 (Answer: B) H_2SO_4 is a strong acid. Strong acids or bases do not make good buffers.

Question #34 (Answer: B) Use Henderson-Hasselbalch relation.

$$pH = pK_A + \log\frac{[A^-]}{[HA]} = 5 + \log\frac{1.0}{0.1} = 5 + \log 10 = 5 + 1 = 6$$

Question #35 (Answer: C) Use the Henderson-Hasselbalch relation.

$$pH = pK_A + \log\frac{[A^-]}{[HA]}$$

$$3.3 = 4.3 + \log\frac{[A^-]}{[HA]}$$

$$-1 = \log\frac{[A^-]}{[HA]}$$

$$10^{-1} = [A^-]/[HA]$$

$$\frac{1}{10} = \frac{[A^-]}{[HA]}$$

5.8.5 Checklist for Acids and Bases

_____	Arrhenius	_____	biological buffers
_____	Brønsted-Lowry	_____	pH, pK_a
_____	Lewis	_____	definitions of acids and bases
_____	conjugate base	_____	strengths of acids/bases and their salts
_____	conjugate acid	_____	definition and calculations using pH, pK_a
_____	titration curves	_____	titrations
_____	buffers	_____	neutralizations
_____	Henderson-Hasselbalch	_____	buffer solutions and calculations

5.9 PHASES AND PHASE EQUILIBRIA

5.9.1 Review of Phases and Phase Equilibria

The *three phases* are gases, liquids and solids. Following are the conversions between the three states (or phases):

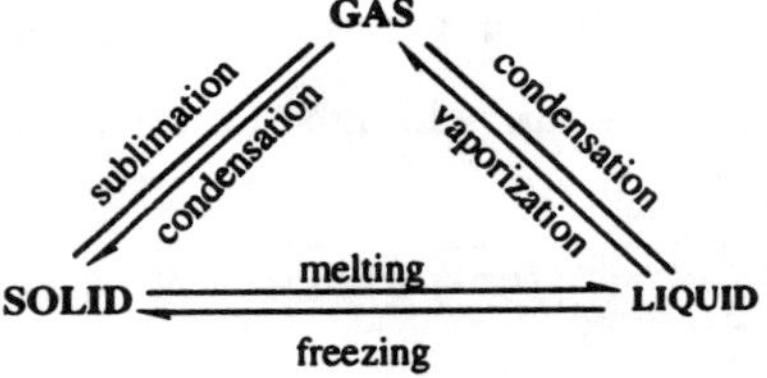

As a *substance moves from solid to liquid to gas*, several changes occur: (1) the molecules become more disordered, (2) the kinetic energy of the molecules increases, (3) the intermolecular forces become weaker, and (4) the molecules become farther separated (density decreases).

The relative magnitudes of the heats of phase changes ($\Delta H_v > \Delta H_f$) imply that the liquid state is more like the solid state than the gaseous state. When going in the forward direction, heat must be put into the system and the surroundings become cooler (e.g. vaporization of sweat cools the body). When going in the reverse direction, heat is given off from the system and the surroundings become warmer (e.g., condensation of water vapor from the air warms the body). *Brownian motion* (e.g. the random motion of a pollen grain due to collision with the liquid molecules) is evidence for the motion and kinetic energies of liquid molecules. Molecules have a range of kinetic energies. The number in a given energy range (ΔE) is proportional to $e^{-\Delta E/kT}$ (from the Boltzmann distribution). Molecules above a certain kinetic energy level can escape into the vapor phase (i.e., evaporate). To evaporate, the molecules must have enough energy to overcome the intermolecular forces (the stronger the attractive forces, the more energy required—see Section 5.3.1.3 for intermolecular forces). The molecules that evaporate become gases and exert a pressure called the *vapor pressure*. Solids also have a vapor pressure based on a similar argument. Generally, substances with stronger intermolecular attractive forces have lower vapor pressures. Substances with weak intermolecular forces tend to have high vapor pressures. Note: as the temperature increases, the average kinetic energy per molecule increases, and the liquid (or solid) evaporates faster (Fig. 5.11).

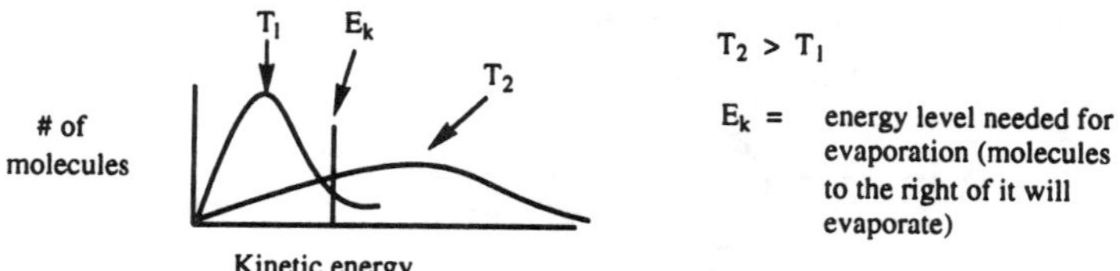

Note: as Temperature (T) increases (T_1 Æ T_2) more molecules have E_k's high enough to evaporate.

Fig. 5.11—Kinetic Energy of Molecules

The *boiling point* (BP) of a liquid is the temperature at which the vapor pressure of the liquid equals the atmospheric (opposing) pressure. For the standard BP, this pressure is taken to be one atmosphere. Note, as the atmospheric pressure decreases, the liquid can boil at lower temperatures. Boiling points have great dependence upon intermolecular forces. Remember that nonpolar molecules have weaker forces. Note that symmetric molecules tend to have smaller intermolecular attractive forces also. The *freezing point* (FP) of the liquid (or melting point, MP, of the solid) is that temperature at which the vapor pressure of the solid equals the vapor pressure of the liquid.

Another way of describing the relationships above is the *phase diagram* (Fig. 5.12).

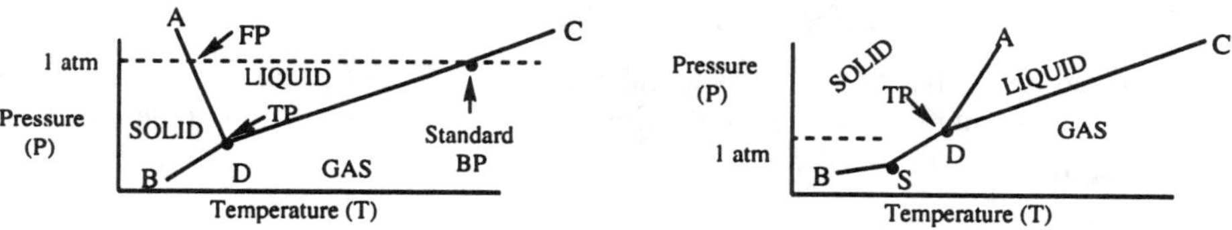

Fig. 5.12—Phase Diagrams: Water (a) and Carbon Dioxide (b)

(1) this is a plot of *pressure (P) versus temperature (T)*,
(2) TP = *Triple point* which is the value of P and T where solid, liquid and gas all coexist in equilibrium,
(3) *regions* marked solid, liquid and gas signify the existence of only that phase,
(4) the *lines* represent the coexistence of two phases in equilibrium and the vapor pressures (below)
    - AD = solid and liquid in equilibrium, transition is melting (freezing)
    - BD = solid and gas in equilibrium, transition from solid to gas is called sublimation (reverse is condensation)
    - CD = liquid and gas in equilibrium, transition is vaporization (condensation),
    - CD = vapor pressure of the liquid at different temperatures
    - BD = vapor pressure of the solid at different temperatures
(5) Note that all the lines except AD for H_2O have *positive slopes*. This means that as the pressure is increased on solid H_2O (ice), its melting point decreases and ice can melt at a lower temperature. This is the basis for ice skating.
(6) *The location of the 1 atmosphere of pressure relative to the TP* determines if a solid melts at atmospheric pressure or sublimes. If 1 atm is above the TP, get solid → liquid as for water. If the 1 atm is below the TP get solid → gas (sublimation) as for CO_2.

5.9.1.1 COLLIGATIVE PROPERTIES (FREEZING AND BOILING POINTS)

A solute added to a pure liquid changes some properties of that liquid. The effect of a solute on a pure liquid depends, primarily, on the relative number of particles present and not their identity. Properties that are affected by the number of particles present and not by the characteristics of the particles are called *colligative properties* (boiling point elevation, freezing point depression, vapor pressure and osmotic pressure). The effect of the number of solute particles (usually non-volatile, so there is no contribution to the overall vapor pressure) on the boiling point (BP) and freezing point (FP) can be understood by considering their effect on vapor pressure (VP) and using the phase diagram. When a solute is dissolved in a pure liquid, the solute molecules are bound by liquid molecules. This represents an increase in potential energy which must be overcome by kinetic energy if the molecules are to escape. This causes fewer to have enough kinetic energy to escape into the vapor phase, resulting in a lowering of the VP (Fig. 5.13).

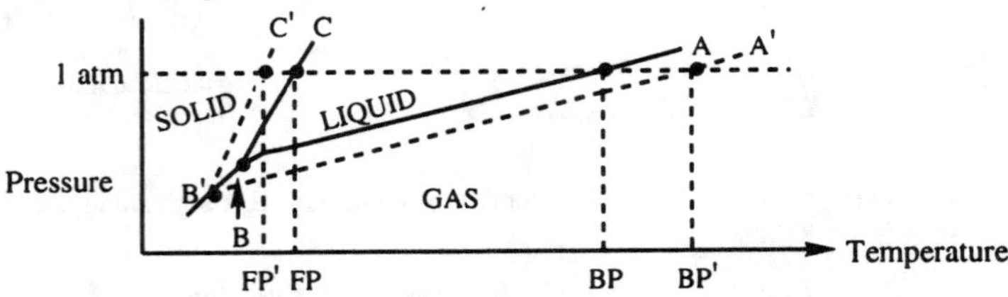

Fig. 5.13—Effect of Solutes on BP and FP

AB	= original VP line of the liquid
CB	= original FP line of the solid
A′B′	= lowering of the VP of the liquid by added solute
C′B′	= lowering the FP of the solid by the solute
ΔBP	= BP′ - BP = boiling point elevation
FP	= original freezing point
FP′	= new FP caused by solute
ΔFP	= FP′ - FP = freezing point depression

Equations can be derived using thermodynamics to calculate the effect of a solute on the FP or BP of a liquid. Following are the simplified equations for freezing point depression and boiling point elevation:

$$\Delta T = +k_b m$$

$$\Delta T = -k_f m$$

ΔT = elevation (for BP) or depression (for FP) of BP or FP respectively

$$m = \text{molality} = \frac{\text{moles of solute particles}}{\text{kilogram of solvent}}$$

Note that the equation calls for moles of solute particles. This means that if a solute dissociates (e.g. NaCl), the moles of particles are greater than the moles of solute. If the solute dimerizes, the moles of particles are less. An alternative way to write the formula to take this into account is:

$\Delta T = -i\, k_f\, m$

i = # of particles the solute dissociates into

$m = \frac{\text{moles of solute}}{\text{kilogram of solvent}}$

k_b = boiling point elevation constant depends on the pure liquid being used

k_b = 0.51 for H_2O

k_f = freezing point depression constant depends on the pure liquid being used

k_f = 1.86 for H_2O

The above equations can be used for a variety of purposes:

(1) k's can be calculated, $k = \frac{\Delta T}{m}$

(2) The number of actual particles can be inferred—make a known *m* for a liquid with a known k and calculate the expected ΔT. If ΔT (by experiment) is greater than that calculated, then more particles than expected were present and the solute must have dissociated. If ΔT (by experiment) is less than that calculated, then fewer particles than expected were present, and the solute must have aggregated (e.g. dimerized). The actual molality of the particles can then be calculated because ΔT (from experiment) and k are known.

(3) Most often, the equations are used to estimate molecular weights = MW (given that corrections are made for dissociation or aggregation)

take a liquid with a known k
dissolve x grams of solute (MW unknown) in y kg's of the liquid (solvent)
then determine the ΔT experimentally
the MW is found by going through these calculations

(a) $m = \frac{\Delta T}{k}$ $\quad\quad$ ΔT, k are known

(b) $m = \frac{\text{moles of solute}}{\text{kg of solvent}} = \Delta T/k$

(c) $m = (\text{g solute/MW solute})/\text{kg of solvent} = \Delta T/k$

(d) $\text{MW solute} = (\text{g solute})(k)/(\text{kg solvent})(\Delta T)$

(4) Definitions:

(a) *Suspension*—a heterogeneous mixture of solute suspended in solvent, e.g., clay particles suspended in water.

(b) *Colloids*—solutes that, when mixed with water, do not pass through parchment membranes, e.g., starch, glue (substances in solution that do pass through parchment membranes are called *crystalloids*, e.g., sugar, salt.)

(c) *Emulsion*—a colloidal suspension of two liquids that are not soluble in each other, e.g., oil and vinegar in a salad dressing.

(d) *Foam*—a mixture of a gas in a liquid, e.g., aerosol shaving cream.

(e) *Gel*—colloids that flow at a very slow rate and behave more like solids, e.g., jelly, stick antiperspirant.

5.9.2 Question to Review Phases and Phase Equilibria

1. The conversion of a gas to a liquid is called:

A. melting.
B. vaporization.
C. freezing.
D. condensation.

2. As a solid changes to a liquid, all of the following occur except

A. molecules become more disordered
B. kinetic energy of the molecules decreases
C. intermolecular forces become weaker
D. molecules become farther separated

3. The liquid state is more like the ________ state than the ________ state.

A. gaseous; solid
B. solid; gaseous
C. equally similar to both
D. plasma; ionic

4. Vaporization of a liquid from the skin will cause the skin to become:

A. cooler.
B. warmer.
C. extremely hot.
D. extremely cold.

5. Which of the following forces in liquids have the highest vapor pressure?

A. strong intermolecular forces
B. weak intermolecular forces
C. tangential viscous forces
D. intermolecular forces have no effect on vapor pressure

6. As the temperature of a substance increases, the average kinetic energy per molecule:

A. decreases.
B. increases.
C. is not affected.
D. cannot be determined.

7. As the atmospheric pressure decreases, the boiling point of a liquid:

A. cannot be determined.
B. is not affected.
C. increases.
D. decreases.

Use the following data for questions #8 to #12.

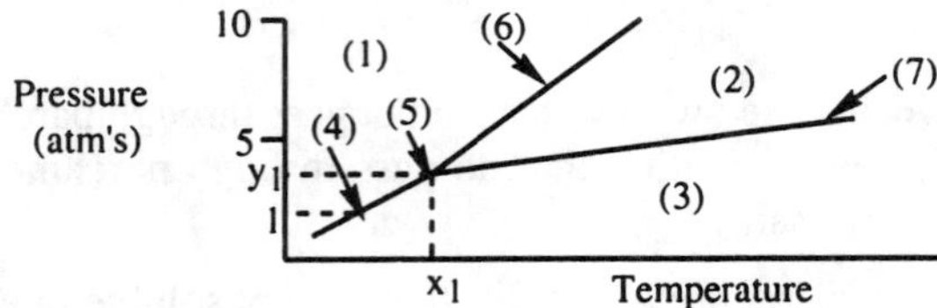

8. Gaseous state is represented by:

A. 1
B. 3
C. 4
D. 7

9. The vapor pressure of the liquid is represented by:

A. 3
B. 4
C. 6
D. 7

10. The triple point is:

A. 1
B. 4
C. 5
D. 7

11. Liquid state can exist only in region ________________________.

A. 1
B. 2
C. 3
D. 5

12. At atmospheric pressure the solid phase of this substance will only:

A. remain a solid.
B. melt.
C. freeze.
D. vaporize.

13. Colligative properties depend upon:

A. the chemical properties of the solute.
B. the physical properties of the solute.
C. the chemical properties of the solvent.
D. the number of solute particles present in solution.

14. Examples of colligative properties include all except:

- **A.** boiling point elevation.
- **B.** solubility.
- **C.** vapor pressure.
- **D.** osmotic pressure.

15. The effect of a solute on the vapor pressure of a liquid is to:

- **A.** have no effect.
- **B.** increase it.
- **C.** decrease it.
- **D.** increase it and then decrease it.

16. The equation relating the freezing point depression (ΔT) with the freezing point constant (k_f) and the molality (m) of the solution is (excluding the minus sign and i):

- **A.** $\Delta T = k_f/m$
- **B.** $\Delta T = m/k_f$
- **C.** $\Delta T = 1/k_f m$
- **D.** $\Delta T = k_f m$

Use the following for Questions #17 to #19:

Five grams of a compound with a molecular weight of 80 is placed in 500g of a liquid which has a normal freezing point of 58.5°C. The freezing point of the solution is now 57°C. Next, 2g of an unknown compound is placed in 250g of the same liquid, and the freezing point is now 58°C.

17. What is the freezing point depression constant (k_f) of the liquid?

- **A.** 12
- **B.** 6
- **C.** 3
- **D.** 1.5

18. What is the expected molecular weight of the unknown compound by freezing point analysis?

- **A.** 192
- **B.** 96
- **C.** 48
- **D.** 72

19. A mass spectograph analysis shows the true molecular weight of the compound to be 384. What inference can be made about the compound's behavior in the liquid?

- **A.** it dissociates
- **B.** it forms dimers
- **C.** it forms tetramers
- **D.** no inference can be made

5.9.3 Answers to Questions in Section 5.9.2

(1) D (2) B (3) B (4) A (5) B (6) B (7) D (8) B (9) D (10) C (11) B (12) D
(13) D (14) B (15) C (16) D (17) A (18) A (19) A

5.9.4 Discussion of Answers to Questions in Section 5.9.2

Questions #1 to #16: Adequately discussed in Section.

Question #17 (Answer: A) The complete formula is:

$k = \Delta T / - im$

where i = the number of particles the substance dissociates into and the negative in the denominator offsets the negative temperature drop. If the absolute value of ΔT is taken the minus sign may be ignored, and if the molecule does not dissociate, then i = 1 and may be ignored.

m = moles/kg of solvent = (1/16)/(1/2) = (1/16)(2/1)
= 2/16 = 1/8

(moles = weight/molecular weight = 5/80 = 1/16, and kg = grams of substance/1000 grams = 500/1000 = 1/2).

$\Delta T = 58.5°C - 57°C = 1.5°C = 1\frac{1}{2} = 3/2$

(Note, if the formula,

$k = \Delta T / - im$

is used, the ΔT must be determined as follows,

$\Delta T = T_f - T_i = 57 - 58.5 = -1.5°C$

f = final, i = initial).

Finally,

k = (3/2)/(1/8) = (3/2)(8/1) = 24/2 = 12

Question #18 (Answer: A) Use the results from #17 and the procedure outlined in the Section:

(a) $m = \Delta T/k = {}^{1}/_{2}/12 = {}^{1}/_{2} \cdot 1/12 = 1/24$
$\Delta T = 58.5 - 58 = 0.5 = {}^{1}/_{2}$

(b) moles of solute = (m)(y) = (1/24)($^{1}/_{4}$) = 1/96
y = kg of solute = 250/1000 = $^{1}/_{4}$

(c) MW = x/moles of solute = 2/(1/96) = (2)(96/1) = 192
x = weight of solute = 2g

Question #19 (Answer: A) The expected freezing point depression using the molecular weight given is

ΔT = km = (12)(1/48) = 12/48 = 1/4 = 0.25°C
m = moles/kg solvent = (2/384)/(1/4) = (2/384)(4/1)
= (2)(4)/384 = 1/48

So, the expected ΔT is 0.25°C. Since the actual is 0.5°C, this means there must have been more particles present than expected, and that the compound must have dissociated, or,

$i = \Delta T / - km = -(1/2)/-(12)(1/48) = (1/2)(48/12) = 48/24 = 2.$

This means 2 particles per original molecule.

5.9.5 Checklist for Phases and Phase Equilibria

______ vaporization
______ condensation
______ heat of fusion
______ heat of vaporization
______ Brownian motion
______ vapor pressure
______ interpretation of phase diagrams
______ triple point
______ colligative properties
______ sublimation
______ molality
______ boiling point elevation
______ freezing point depression
______ suspension
______ colloid
______ emulsion
______ foam
______ gel

CHEMISTRY-RELATED PHYSICS

This part of chapter 5 presents concepts learned both in Physics and Chemistry. The MCAT Student Manual states that problem-solving in the physical sciences will be tested in an integrated form. Chemistry-related physics presents an integrated approach to learning the interconnected concepts of the physical sciences on topics such as gases and liquids and their relationship to medical situations.

5.10 GAS PROPERTIES

The chart below summarizes the physical characteristics of solids, liquids, and gases.

Solids	Liquids	Gases
1. Solids are rigid.	1. Liquids are fluid.	1. Gases are extremely fluid.
2. Solids have a definite shape.	2. Liquids have no definite shape, but have a well-defined surface.	2. Gases are shapeless; they occupy the entire container.
3. Solids have a definite volume.	3. Liquids have a definite volume.	3. Gases have no definite volume.
4. Solids have a higher density because their molecules are closely packed together.	4. Liquids are lighter than solids because molecules are farther apart.	4. Gases are extremely light because their molecules are far apart.
5. Solids are extremely cohesive.	5. Liquids, except for mercury, are less cohesive.	5. Gases have almost no cohesion at all. There is almost no interaction between their molecules.
6. Solids diffuse at an extremely slow rate, e.g., lead and gold diffuse into each other when left for six months or more.	6. Liquids exhibit various types of diffusion such as confective, turbulent, and molecular, e.g., preparing coffee or tea in boiling water.	6. Gases diffuse at high speeds, e.g., air freshener in a room.
7. Well-known theories and laws have been established to study solid behavior.	7. As of today, there is a large gap in the study of liquid behavior. No good model exists to represent a liquid.	7. Well-known theories have been established to study behavior of gases.
8. Solids are almost incompressible.	8. Liquids are slightly compressible (do not confuse the slipping of liquid molecules under pressure with compression).	8. Gases are highly compressible, which gives them the property of resiliency.

5.10.1 Review of the Gas Properties

This section discusses gas laws and theories used in both chemistry and physics. Gases have relatively high translational kinetic energies per molecule as compared with liquids. Gases take the shape of the container they are in, like liquids; but, unlike liquids, they completely fill any container. The *key characteristics* of gases are the pressure (P), the volume (V), the temperature (T), and the quantity (moles = n). Gases are broadly considered as ideal or non-ideal. An *ideal gas* has no intermolecular forces, and the gas molecules occupy no volume (they are points in space). This means the gases should have low density. In general, at high temperatures and low pressures, most gases can be considered to be ideal. A *non-ideal* gas has intermolecular forces, and the molecules do have a finite volume. Laws covering the behavior of ideal gases will be covered first. The metric *pressure* units are mmHg = torr. The English system uses atmospheres (atm). The conversion is 760 torrs = 1 atm. See Section 5.12.1.2 for temperature scales.

Boyle's law states that pressure and volume are inversely related ($P \propto 1/V$), i.e., as the pressure increases, the volume decreases and vice versa. *Charles' law* states that the temperature and volume are directly related, i.e., as the temperature increases, the volume increases and vice versa. These laws are combined to give the *Ideal gas law* which is:

$$PV = n\,RT$$

P = pressure, V = volume, n = moles, T = absolute temperature
R = Ideal gas constant = 0.0821 *l* -atm/°K-mole

Another useful way of writing the Ideal gas law is,

$$\frac{PV}{T} = \text{constant or,}$$

$$\frac{P_1V_1}{T_1} = \frac{P_2V_2}{T_2}$$

Also, note that *22.414 liters of an ideal gas at S.T.P. (Standard Temperature and Pressure—273° K and 1atmosphere pressure) represent 1 mole of that gas. Avogadro's principle* is also important for solving problems and states that equal volumes of ideal gases at the same temperature and pressure contain the same number of moles (or molecules). *Dalton's law* states that the total pressure (P_t) of a mixture of gases is equal to the sum partial pressures (P_i) of the gases:

$$P_t = P_1 + P_2 + P_3 + \ldots$$

The *partial pressure* (P_i) of a gas in a mixture of gases is determined as follows:

$$P_i = X_i\,P_t$$

P_t = total pressure
X_i = mole fraction of gas in the mixture

$$X_i = \frac{n_i}{n_1 + n_2 + n_3 + \ldots} = \frac{n_i}{\Sigma n_i}$$

n_i = moles of a gas
Σn_i = sum of the moles of all gases.

The Kinetic theory of gases attempts to describe the energy characteristics of gases as a whole by analyzing the motion and mass characteristics (e.g. forces, momentum) of individual molecules. The theory is based on basic postulates mentioned below:

(1) *All* gases consist of small, spherical particles called molecules, which are similar to mini-tennis balls bouncing in a box.

(2) These molecules are in constant or perpetual motion. They move at high velocities. The size of these molecules is around 2Å-5Å and they travel in random directions with speeds of about 1000 meters/sec (almost 0.5 miles/second)

(3) The distance between individual molecules is great as compared to their diameter, may be up to 70Å or more apart.

(4) Collisions between molecules are perfectly elastic, of the order of 5 billion collisions per second.

The kinetic theory for gases can also be applied to liquids and solids. The kinetic theory illustrates the concept of solubility as shown in the sketch below.

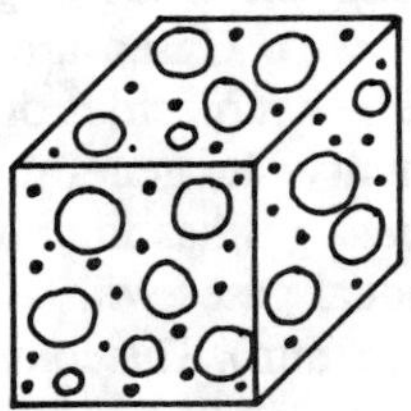

Model illustrating "Kinetic Molecular Theory" and "Solubility of Molecules"

Stirring grains of salt or sugar in water results in a homogenous solution. The salt or sugar molecules do not disappear but occupy the intermolecular spaces in H_2O. The result of this mixing, according to the kinetic molecular theory of liquids and solids, is a solution.

Motion of molecules relates to kinetic energy of molecules. The temperature of the medium is a measure of the average kinetic energy of the molecules. The sketch at right shows the energy of molecules as related to internuclear distance between atoms. Looking in greater detail at the sketch, the curve first goes down, then turns up, forming a "potential well."

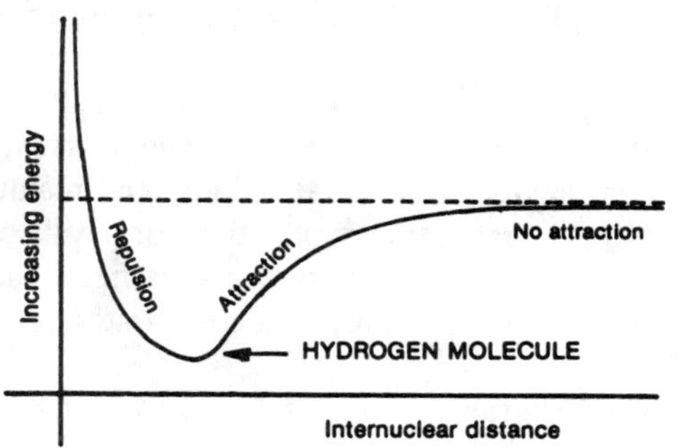

An atom residing in the bottom of a potential well carries out small thermal oscillations about its equilibrium position. Movements from left to right in the diagram represent phase changes from solids to liquids to gases. This illustrates "cohesion" and "adhesion" between molecules which results in internuclear or van der Waals forces for real gases.

The kinetic theory of gases has its limitations but important results of it are:

(1) Boyle's law, Charles' law, and the Ideal gas law are derivable from it;

(2) P and V can be related to the kinetic energy of molecules,

$PV = 2/3\ NE_k$ (on a molecular scale)
N = # of molecules, E_k = translational energy/molecule
or, $E_k = (3/2)\ RT$ (on a mole scale)
also at a given temperature, all molecules have the same average E_k;

(3) *Graham's law of diffusion* can be determined from E_k as follows:

$E_{k_1} = E_{k_2}$ i.e., the average E_ks are equal (kinetic energies of molecules)
1, 2 = molecules
also $1/2 m_1 v_1^2 = 1/2\ m_2 v_2^2$
$v_1/v_2 = \sqrt{m_2} / \sqrt{m_1} = \sqrt{m_2/m_1}$
v = velocities of diffusion (e.g., mls/min)
m = molecular weights or densities.

(4) Values for heat capacities of monoatomic gases:

C_v = specific heat at constant volume
C_p = specific heat at constant pressure
$C_v = \frac{3}{2}\ R$
$C_p = C_v + R$
$C_p/C_v = 1.67$
R = 1.99 cals/mole- °K = gas constant

One of the simpler equations for nonideal gases is the *van der Waals equation* which applies corrections to account for the false assumptions of ideal gases:

$$\left(P + \frac{n^2a}{V^2}\right)(V\text{-}nb) = nRT$$

a, b are constants
n^2a/V^2 corrects for intermolecular forces = pressure correction
nb corrects for the volume occupied by gas molecules = volume correction.

Note that if the density is very low, then V»nb and $n^2a/V^2 \rightarrow 0$, and the ideal gas law results. The effect of the intermolecular forces is to decrease the pressure of the gas. The effect of the volume of molecules is to increase the volume occupied by the gas. The terms above bring the pressure and volume back to ideal levels.

5.10.1.1 Applications of Gas Properties to the Human Body

The premedical student should also review applications of the gas theories and laws to the human respiratory system (inhalation and exhalation). The working of a spirometer should be understood in order to solve problems as they relate to tidal volume and residual volume in the human lungs. Passages in biological and physical sciences reflecting applications of gas theories may appear on the MCAT. The student should relate the human respiratory system to concepts learned in section 5.10.1 (Review of Gas Properties). Following are the gas laws related to physiology of the respiratory system:

Definition of Dalton's Law: Each gas in a mixture of gases in a closed space exerts its own characteristic pressure as if no other gases were present. This is also called partial pressure, or P. Atmospheric pressure = the sum of the partial pressures of all the different gases in the closed space.

Application: Partial pressures are important to study the movement of gases in the lungs, blood and tissues. A gas will diffuse from a region where its partial pressure is higher to a region where its partial pressure is lower. For example, PO_2 is 105 mm Hg in the alveoli and 40 mm Hg in deoxygenated blood, thus the oxygen will diffuse into the blood to oxygenate it.

Definition of Henry's Law: The volume of a gas that will dissolve in a liquid depends on its partial pressure and its solubility coefficient.

Application: Air gases dissolve in different amounts in the blood. For example, the solubility coefficient of O_2 is 0.024 and of CO is 0.57. Some traumas such as near-drowning or carbon monoxide poisoning cause the body to need more O_2 in the blood. By increasing the partial pressure of O_2 in the patient's environment, more O_2 can get in to the blood. This occurs in a hyperbaric chamber, where the PO_2 becomes around 3000 mm Hg, thus raising the solubility of O_2 in the blood.

5.10.2 Questions to Review Gas Properties

1. The variables used to describe gases include all except:

A. pressure.
B. volume.
C. moles.
D. all of the above.

2. All of the following are characteristics of ideal gases except:

A. absence of intermolecular forces.
B. nonideal gases may exhibit ideal behavior at high pressure and low temperature.
C. the molecules occupy no space.
D. all of the above are correct.

3. Boyle's law states that:

A. volume varies inversely as temperature at constant pressure.
B. volume varies directly as temperature at constant pressure.
C. pressure varies inversely as volume at constant temperature.
D. pressure varies directly as volume at constant temperature.

4. Charles' law states that:

A. volume varies inversely as temperature at constant pressure.
B. volume varies directly as temperature at constant pressure.
C. pressure varies inversely as volume at constant temperature.
D. pressure varies directly as volume at constant temperature.

5. All are expressions for the ideal gas law except:

A. $PV = nRT$

B. $\frac{PV}{T} = \text{constant}$

C. $\frac{P_1V_1}{T_1} = \frac{P_2V_2}{T_2}$

D. $\left(P + \frac{n^2a}{V^2}\right)(V\text{-}nb) = nRT$

6. One mole of an ideal gas at STP has all of the following characteristics except:

A. volume = 1 liter.
B. temperature = 273°K.
C. pressure = 1 atmosphere.
D. all of the above are correct.

7. Each gas in a mixture exerts a pressure. The total pressure of all the gases in the container is:

A. less than the sum of the separate pressures of each gas.
B. more than the sum of the separate pressures of each gas.
C. equal to the sum of the separate pressures of each gas.
D. the sum is variable.

8. The correct expression for the partial pressure (P_A) of n_A moles of a gas in a mixture of gases with a *total* of n_T moles and a total pressure = P_T is:

A. $P_A = (n_A + n_T)\, P_T$
B. $P_A = (n_T - n_A)\, P_T$
C. $P_A = n_A P_T$
D. $P_A = (n_A/n_T)P_T$

9. All of the following are conclusions of the Kinetic theory of gases except:

A. derivation of the van der Waals equation.
B. derivation of Boyle's and Charles' law.
C. relation of average kinetic energy of gases to temperature.
D. Graham's law of diffusion.

10. In the van der Waals equation for nonideal gases,
$\left(P + \frac{n^2a}{V^2}\right)(V\text{-}nb) = nRT$, it is *not true* that:

A. $\frac{n^2a}{V^2}$ corrects for intermolecular forces.

B. nb corrects for the volume occupied by gas molecules.
C. at high densities the equation reduces to the ideal gas law.
D. all of the above are correct.

11. The pressure on a sample of gas is tripled, the new volume is:

A. 9 times the original volume.
B. 3 times the original volume.
C. 1/3 of the original volume.
D. 1/9 of the original volume.

12. If the temperature of a gas is increased four times, the volume is:

A. increased 16 times.
B. increased 4 times.
C. increased 2 times.
D. decreased 4 times.

13. One mole of an ideal gas occupies 3 liters at 37°C. Approximately what pressure, in atmospheres, does the gas exert?

A. 1.1 atm
B. 4.2 atm
C. 8.5 atm
D. 12.3 atm

14. What volume will 2 liters of a gas at 27°C and 2 atm occupy at S.T.P.?

A. 3.6 liters
B. 5.1 liters
C. 1.1 liters
D. cannot be determined

15. Two moles of an ideal gas occupy what volume at S.T.P.?

A. 22.4 liters
B. 44.8 liters
C. 67.2 liters
D. cannot be determined

16. If is found that 2 grams of a vaporized liquid occupy 0.82 liters at S.T.P. What is the molecular weight of the gas?

A. 13.5 grams
B. 27 grams
C. 54 grams
D. cannot be determined

17. A container of pure oxygen has a pool of water at its bottom. The atmospheric pressure is 760 torrs and equals the total pressure of the container. If the temperature is 37°C and the vapor pressure of water is 47 torrs at this temperature, what is the pressure of the dry oxygen?

A. 700 mm Hg
B. 684 mm Hg
C. 807 mm Hg
D. 713 mm Hg

18. A mixture of 2 moles of O_2, 3 moles of N_2, and 5 moles of H_2 exerts a pressure of 700 torrs. The partial pressure of N_2 is:

A. 700 torrs
B. 210 torrs
C. 490 torrs
D. 760 torrs

19. A mixture of 5 moles of O_2, 4 moles of N_2, and 1 mole of CO is collected above water at a temperature of 27°C. The total pressure is 760 torrs and the vapor pressure of water at 27°C is 27 torrs. What is the partial pressure exerted by O_2?

A. 76 torrs
B. 100 torrs
C. 367 torrs
D. 380 torrs

20. Oxygen (molecular weight = 32) diffuses at a rate of 10 mls/min. Under the same conditions of temperature and pressure, how fast will hydrogen (molecular weight = 2) diffuse?

A. 20 mls/min
B. 40 mls/min
C. 160 mls/min
D. need more information

5.10.3 Answers to Questions in Section 5.10.2

(1) D (2) B (3) C (4) B (5) D (6) A (7) C (8) D (9) A (10) C (11) C (12) B (13) C (14) A (15) B (16) C (17) D (18) B (19) C (20) B

5.10.4 Discussion of Answers to Questions in Section 5.10.2

Questions #1 to #10: Adequately discussed in Section.

Question #11 (Answer: C) This is a direct application of Boyle's law. Volume varies inversely as pressure. So, if pressure is increased by a factor of 3, the volume is decreased by a factor of 3. That is, the volume is $1/3$ of the original.

Question #12 (Answer: B) A direct application of Charles' law. Volume varies directly as temperature. Since temperature is increased by a factor of 4, the volume is increased by a factor of 4.

Question #13 (Answer: C) This problem deals with one gas under one set of n-P-V-T; this suggests that the equation to use is PV = nRT. Solving for pressure, one gets,

$$P = nRT/V$$

The value of R is required. By knowing the units used, this can be determined as follows:

$$R = \frac{PV}{nT} = \frac{(1 \text{ atm})(22.4 \text{ liters})}{(1 \text{ mole})(273^{o}K)} = 0.082 \ \frac{\text{atm-liters}}{\text{mole-}^{o}K}$$

(Because 1 mole of an ideal gas at STP—273°K, 1 atm—occupies 22.4 liters.)

Also, remember, that the temperature is the absolute temperature: $T = 37^{o} + 273^{o} = 310^{o}K$
Then,

$$P = \frac{(1)(0.082)(310)}{(3)} \approx 8.2 \text{ atms}$$

$$\text{note } \frac{310}{3} \approx 100 \text{ and then } (100)(0.082) \approx 8.2$$

Note the approximations made. The 8.2 is closes to 8.5 atms.

Question #14 (Answer: A) Note that this problem requires the gas be compared at two different conditions of P-V-T; the best equation to use in this instance is,

$$\frac{P_2V_2}{T_2} = \frac{P_1V_1}{T_1}$$

(STP) (Original)

Solving for V_2,

$$V_2 = V_1\left(\frac{T_2}{T_1}\right)\left(\frac{P_1}{P_2}\right) = (2)\left(\frac{273}{300}\right)\left(\frac{2}{1}\right) \approx 3.6$$

$$T_1 = 27 + 273 = 300$$

the approximation is made as follows

$$\frac{273}{300} \approx \frac{270}{300} \approx \frac{27}{30} \approx \frac{9}{10}$$

$$\text{then, } (2)\left(\frac{9}{10}\right)(2) = \left(\frac{36}{10}\right) = 3.6$$

Question #15 (Answer: B) Since one mole of an ideal gas occupies 22.4 liters at STP, two moles would occupy twice as much or 2 × 22.4 = 44.8 liters.

Question #16 (Answer: C) First the number of moles is determined. Since the substance is a gas and there is one set of PV-T conditions use:

$$PV = nRT.$$

Solving for n,

$$n = \frac{PV}{RT} = \frac{(1)(0.82)}{(0.082)(273)} \approx \frac{1}{27}$$

the approximation for n is as follow

$$\frac{0.82}{0.082} = 10, \text{ then } \frac{10}{273} \approx \frac{10}{270} \approx \frac{1}{27}$$

The definition of moles (n) in (Section 5.6.1):

$$\text{moles} = \frac{\text{weight}}{\text{molecular weight}} \text{ or,}$$

$$\text{molecular weight} = \frac{\text{weight}}{\text{moles}} \approx \frac{2}{1/27} \approx (2)\left(\frac{27}{1}\right) \approx 54 \text{ gms.}$$

alternate: Since n = wt/mw, PV = (wt/mw)RT; mw = wt(RT/PV).

Question #17 (Answer: D) The only point of this problem is to stress that when gases are collected over a liquid (e.g. water), the vapor pressure of that liquid must be subtracted from the total pressure to get the pressure of the gases without the added effect of the liquid's vapor pressure. The vapor pressure varies with temperature. Note that the total pressure of the gases is still the sum of the partial pressures (Dalton's Law),

$$P_{tot} = P_{O_2} + P_{H_2O} \text{ vapor}$$

$$P_{O_2} = P_{tot} - P_{H_2O} \text{ vapor} = 760 - 47 = 713.$$

Question #18 (Answer: B) This is a direct application of Dalton's Law of partial pressures. The partial pressure of $N_2(P_{N_2})$ is,

$$P_{N_2} = X_{N_2}P_T$$

$$P_T = 700 \text{ torrs}$$

$$X_{N_2} = \frac{n_{N_2}}{n_{N_2} + n_{O_2} + n_{H_2}} = \frac{3}{3+5+2} = \frac{3}{10}$$

$$P_{N_2} = \frac{3}{10}(700) = 210 \text{ torrs.}$$

Question #19 (Answer: C) This is just a combination of the principles of questions #17 and #18. First, the effect of the water vapor on the total pressure is taken into account:

P_T(Total pressure of gases) = total pressure – water vapor pressure

$$P_T = 760 - 27 = 733 \text{ torrs.}$$

Then Dalton's Law is applied using this 733 torrs:

$$P_{O_2} = X_2P_T$$

$$X_2 = \frac{n_{O_2}}{n_{O_2} + n_{N_2} + n_{CO_2}} = \frac{5}{5+4+1} = \frac{5}{10} = \frac{1}{2}$$

$$P_{O_2} = (1/2)(733) = 367 \text{ torrs.}$$

Question #20 (Answer: B) In general, the lighter gas will diffuse faster. Using the formulation of Graham's law of diffusion,

$$\frac{V_{H_2}}{V_{O_2}} = \sqrt{\frac{MW_{O_2}}{MW_{H_2}}}$$

$$\frac{V_{H_2}}{10} = \sqrt{\frac{32}{2}} = \sqrt{16} = 4$$

$$V_{H_2} = (10)(4) = 40 \text{ mls/min.}$$

5.10.5 Checklist for Gas Properties

______ pressure
______ ideal gas
______ nonideal gas
______ Boyle's law
______ Charles' law
______ Avogadro's principle
______ Dalton's law
______ partial pressure
______ mole fraction
______ spirometer
______ Graham's law of diffusion
______ van der Waals equation
______ characteristics of ideal gases
______ concept of partial pressures
______ ideal gas law
______ kinetic theory of gases
______ volume-mole relationship of ideal gas at STP
______ characteristics of nonideal gases
______ tidal volume
______ residual volume

5.11 SOLID AND FLUID PROPERTIES

5.11.1 Review of Solid and Fluid Properties

5.11.1.1 ELASTIC PROPERTIES OF SOLIDS

When a force acts on a solid, the solid is deformed. If the solid returns to its original shape, it is called *elastic*. The effect of a force depends on the area over which it acts. Stress is defined as the ratio of the force to the area over which it acts. Strain is defined as the relative change in dimensions or shape of the object caused by the stress. This is embodied in the definition of the modulus of elasticity (ME) as:

$$ME = \text{stress/strain}.$$

An important reminder for the MCAT student is to understand elastic solids. As an example, steel is more elastic than rubber. Rubber is more stretchable, but not more elastic, than steel. Do not confuse the words "elastic" and "stretchable."

Some different types of stresses are *tensile stress* (equal and opposite forces directed away from each other), *compressive stress* (equal and opposite forces directed toward each other), and *shearing stress* (equal and opposite forces which do not have the same line of action). There are two commonly useful moduli of elasticity:

(1) Young's Modulus (Y) for compressive or tensile stress:
Y = longitudinal stress/longitudinal strain = $(F/A)/(\Delta l/l)$ = $Fl/A\Delta l$
l = original length
Δl = change in length

The A is the area normal (perpendicular) to the force

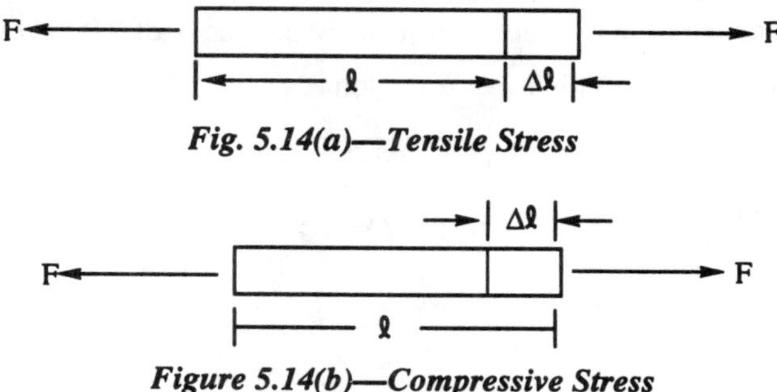

Fig. 5.14(a)—Tensile Stress

Figure 5.14(b)—Compressive Stress

(2) Shear modulus (S) or the modulus of rigidity is:
S = shearing stress/shearing strain = (F/A)/ ϕ = (F/A)/tan ϕ = (F/A)/(d/l) = Fl/dA. See Fig. 5.14(c)

The A is the area tangential to the force $\phi = \tan \phi$ for small angles.

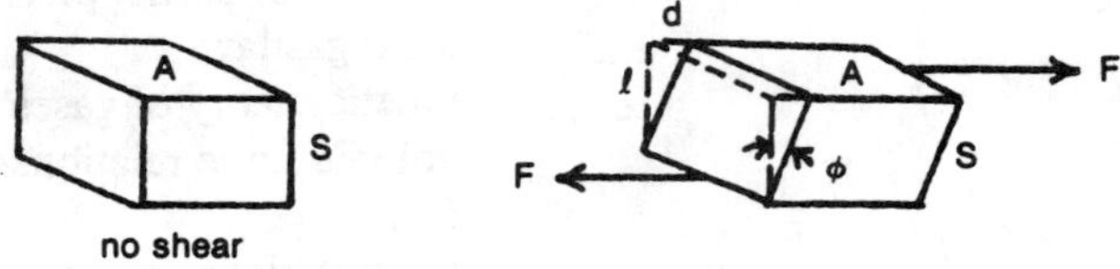

Fig. 5.14(c)—Shear Stress

5.11.1.2 DENSITY AND ITS PHYSICAL MEANING

What is meant by "heavy as lead" and "light as a feather?" Clearly, a grain of lead is light, while a mountain of feathers has considerable weight. Use of such comparisons are based not on a body's mass, but on the density of the material from which it is made.

The mass of a unit volume of a body is called its *density*. A grain of lead and a massive block of lead have the same density. Density is an *intensive* property.

In denoting density, usually shown is the number of grams (g) a cubic centimeter $(cm)^3$ of the body weighs—the symbol g/cm^3 is placed after this number. In order to determine the density, the number of grams is divided by the number of cubic centimeters (the fractional line in the symbol is a reminder).

Certain metals are among the heaviest materials—osmium, whose density is equal to 22.5 g/cm^3, iridium (22.4), platinum (21.5), tungsten and gold (19.3). The density of iron is 7.88, that of copper is 8.93. Lighter substances include air with density .0013 g/cm^3.

It should be stipulated that this discussion assumes continuous bodies. If there are pores in a solid, it will be lighter. Porous bodies—cork, sponge, steel wool—are frequently used in technology. The density of sponge may be less than 0.5, although the solid matter from which it is made has a higher density. As all other bodies whose density is less than one, sponge floats superbly on water unless soaked.

The lightest liquid is liquid hydrogen; it can only be obtained at extremely low temperatures. One cubic centimeter of liquid hydrogen has a mass of 0.07 g. Organic liquids—alcohol, benzene, kerosene—do not differ significantly from water in density. Mercury is very heavy—it has a density of 13.6 g/cm^3.

Gases occupy whatever volumes contain them. Even though emptied into vessels of different volumes, gas-bags with the same mass of gas will always fill the volumes uniformly.

The density of gases is defined under so-called normal conditions or at STP (temperature of 0°C and pressure of one atmosphere). The density of air under normal conditions is equal to 0.00129 g/cm^3; chloride is 0.00322 g/cm^3. Gaseous hydrogen, like the liquid, is the lightest gas with density of 0.00009 g/cm^3.

Density represents the packing of material in a certain volume.

Mass density $\rho = \dfrac{\text{mass}}{\text{volume}}$

Weight density $\gamma = \dfrac{\text{weight}}{\text{volume}}$

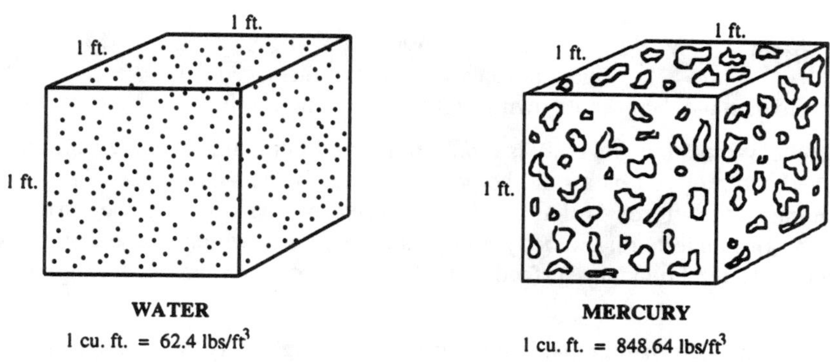

Fig. 5.15—Illustration of the Concept of Density

As an example, an average human being weighing 150 lbs. with 90% water is like a container of water about the same weight:
150 x 0.90 = 135 lbs. The weight density of water = 62.4 lbs./ft^3.
Using, weight density = weight/volume:

$$62.4 = \frac{135}{\text{volume}}$$

This results in the average volume of the human body at 2.16 ft^3. The above example shows the fundamental use of the density equation.

Generally, solids are more dense than liquids, which are more dense than gases. The *specific gravity* (SG) is defined as:

$$SG = \left(\frac{\text{density of a substance}}{\text{density of water}}\right) \text{ at a given temperature.}$$

The density of water is about 1 gm/ml over most common temperatures. So in most instances the specific gravity of a substance is the same as its density. Note that the units of density are mass/volume, whereas SG has no units.

5.11.1.3 STATIC AND DYNAMIC PROPERTIES OF FLUIDS

Density is one of the key properties of fluids (liquids or gases) and the other is pressure. Pressure (P) is defined as force (F) per unit area (A):

$$P = F/A.$$

F is the normal (perpendicular) force. Fluids can only exert P at an enclosed surface or body. Otherwise, fluids will flow under a shearing stress instead of being deformed elastically as solids would (see above). Pressure is also formulated as potential energy per unit volume as follows:

$$P = F/A = mg/A = (mg/A)(h/h) = mgh/V = \rho gh$$

$$\rho = \text{density} \qquad h = \text{depth below surface.}$$

Characteristics of force and pressure of fluids are:

(1) Forces exerted by fluids are always perpendicular to the container.
(2) The fluid pressure (hydrostatic) is directly proportional to the depth of the fluid and to its density:

$$P \propto \rho h$$

(3) At any particular depth, the fluid pressure is the same in all directions.
(4) Fluid pressure is independent of the shape or area of its container.
(5) An external pressure applied to an enclosed fluid is transmitted uniformly throughout the volume of the liquid (Pascal's law).
(6) An object which is completely or partially submerged in a fluid experiences an upward force equal to the weight of the fluid displaced (Archimedes' principle). This *buoyant force* (F_B) is:

$$F = V\rho g = mg$$

buoyant force = weight of displaced fluid

An object that floats must displace its own weight (not volume) in fluid.

Looking at Fig. 5.16 below, assume the body is totally immersed in the liquid. Now suppose the fluid inside the surface to be removed and replaced by a solid body having exactly the same shape. The pressure at every point will be exactly the same as before, so that the force exerted on the body by the surrounding fluid will be unaltered. That is, the fluid exerts on the body an upward force, F_y, which is equal to the weight, mg, of the fluid originally occupying the boundary surface and whose line of action passes through the original center of gravity.

The submerged body, in general, will not be in equilibrium. Its weight may be greater or less than F_y, and if it is not homogeneous, its center of gravity may not be on the line of F_y.

The weight of a dirigible floating in air, or of a submarine floating at some depth below the surface of the water, is just equal to the weight of a volume of air, or water, that is equal to the volume of the dirigible or submarine. That is, the average density of the dirigible equals that of the air, and the average density of the submarine equals the density of the water.

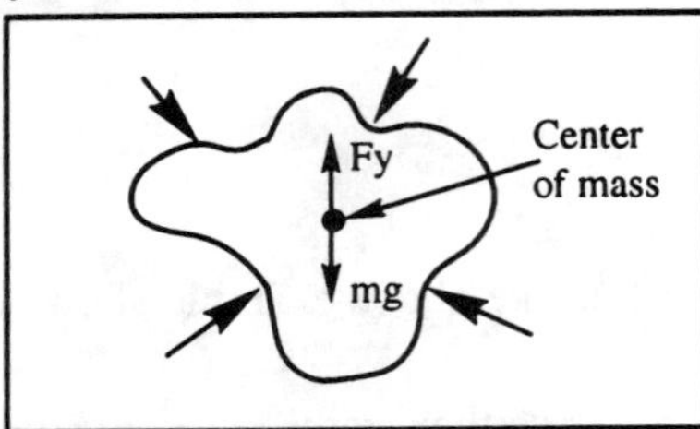

Fig. 5.16—Buoyancy

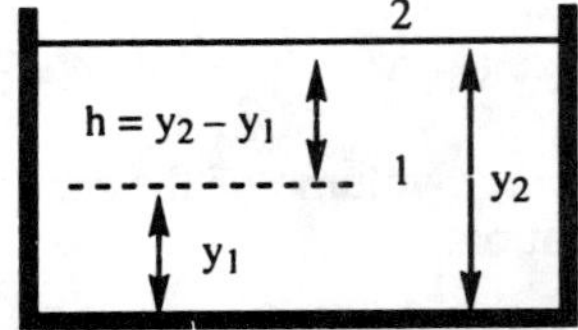

Fig. 5.17—Hydrostatic Pressure

If p_1 and p_2 are the pressures at elevations y_1 and y_2 above some reference level and when ρ and g are constant,

$$p_2 - p_1 = -\rho g\,(y_2 - y_1).$$

Apply this equation to a liquid in an open vessel, as in Fig. 5.17 above. Take point 1 at any level and let p represent that pressure at this point. Take point 2 at the top where the pressure is atmospheric pressure, p_a. Then:

$$p - p_a = \rho g\,(y_2 - y_1),$$

$$p = p_a + \rho gh.$$

Note that the shape of the containing vessel does not affect the pressure, and that the pressure is the same at all points at the same depth.

Concept of Mass Flux

Mass flux can be defined as the rate of change of mass of a fluid. It represents mass flow per unit time. It is an extremely important parameter to measure flow of blood from the heart, flow of substances into the kidneys, and also the flow of air into the lungs. Remember, mass flux is proportional to the rate of flow R mentioned below.

Fluids in motion are described by two equations, the continuity equation and Bernoulli's Equation. Fluids are assumed to have streamlined flow which means that the motion of every particle in the fluid follows the same path as the particle that preceded it. Turbulent flow occurs when one path is not followed, molecules collide, energy is dissipated and frictional drag is increased. Rate of flow (R) is:

$$R = \text{volume past a point/time} = Avt/t = Av$$

$$\text{volume} = (\text{cross-sectional area})(\text{length}) = (A)(vt) = Avt$$

$$\text{length} = \text{distance} = (\text{velocity})(\text{time}) = vt$$

The equation can also be written as (the continuity equation):

$$A_1v_1 = A_2v_2 = \text{constant (see Fig. 5.18)}$$

where subscripts 1 and 2 refer to different points in the line of flow. Note that the velocity of the fluid is faster where the cross-sectional area is smaller and vice versa. Also, where the velocity is faster, the pressure (P) exerted is smaller and vice versa.

Bernoulli's Equation is an application of the Law of Conservation of Energy and is:

$$P + \rho gh + {}^1/_2\rho v^2 = \text{constant}$$

pressure energy + potential energy + kinetic energy = constant

This can be equivalently written as:

$$P_1 + \rho gh_1 + {}^1/_2\rho v_1{}^2 = P_2 + \rho gh_2 + {}^1/_2\rho v_2{}^2 \text{ (See Fig. 5.18)}$$

where the subscripts 1 and 2 refer to different points in the flow. All symbols are as defined previously.

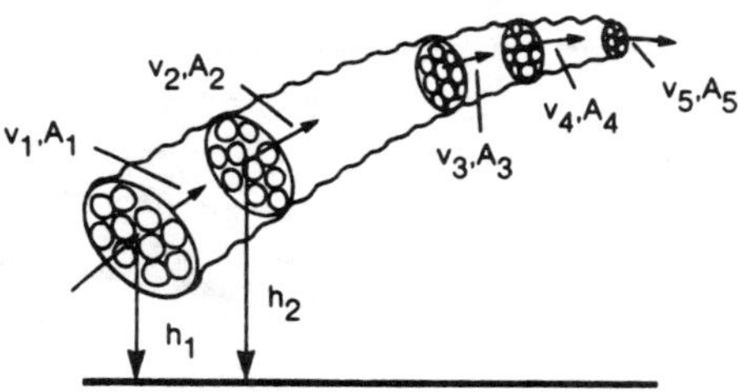

Fig. 5.18—Concept of Mass Flux/Bernoulli's Equation

Another important property of fluids is viscosity. Viscosity is analogous to friction between moving solids. It may, therefore, be viewed as the resistance to flow between layers of fluid (as in streamline or laminar flow) sliding relative to each other. This also means that viscosity, as friction, results in dissipation of mechanical energy. As one layer slides over another, its motion is transmitted to the second layer and causes this layer to be set in motion. Since a mass (m) of the second layer is set in motion (v) and some of the energy of the first layer is lost, there is a transfer of momentum (mv) between the layers. The greater the transfer of this momentum from one layer to another, the more kinetic energy (αv^2) that is lost and the slower the layers move. The viscosity coefficient (η) is a measure of the efficiency of transfer of this loss of mechanical energy and, consequently, greater loss of velocity. The reverse situation holds of low viscosity coefficients. Then a high viscosity (coefficient) substance flows slowly (e.g., molasses), and a low viscosity (coefficient) substance flows relatively fast (e.g., water or, especially, helium). Note that the transfer of momentum to adjacent layers is, in essence, the exertion of a force upon these layers to set them in motion (Newton's 1st Law—see Section 5.17.1). Whether flow is streamlined (laminar) or turbulent (chaotic loss of layers flowing past each other and their replacement with eddies and whirlpool, etc., with the resultant dissipation of more mechanical energy) depends on a combination of factors already discussed. A convenient measure is Reynolds Number (R):

$$R = vd\rho/\eta$$

v = velocity of flow; d = diameter of tube; ρ = density of fluid; η = viscosity coefficient. In general, if $R<2000$ the flow is streamlined; if $R>2000$ the flow is turbulent. Note that as $v\uparrow$, $d\uparrow$, $\rho\uparrow$ or $\eta\downarrow$, the flow becomes more turbulent.

Flow of Blood in Small Arterioles, Venuoles

The Hagen-Poiseuille law for laminar viscous flow of blood through small size tubes can be calculated by:

$$\text{Flow rate } = Q = \frac{\pi R^2 F_v}{8\eta L} = v\pi R^2 \text{ (from continuity equation)}$$

- Q = Flow rate = m^3/sec
- R = Radius of flow tube or blood vessel (m)
- F_v = Viscous force causing flow (nt)
- η = Viscosity of blood $\frac{nt\cdot s}{m^2}$
- L = Length of tube or blood vessel (m)
- v = Average velocity of blood flow (m/s)

Use proportional reasoning to remember that flow rate is directly proportional to $(\text{Radius})^2$, pressure difference is inversely proportional to $(\text{Radius})^2$. In order to determine vicous force per unit area, divide Fv by the cross sectional area, which is represented by Δp or pd.

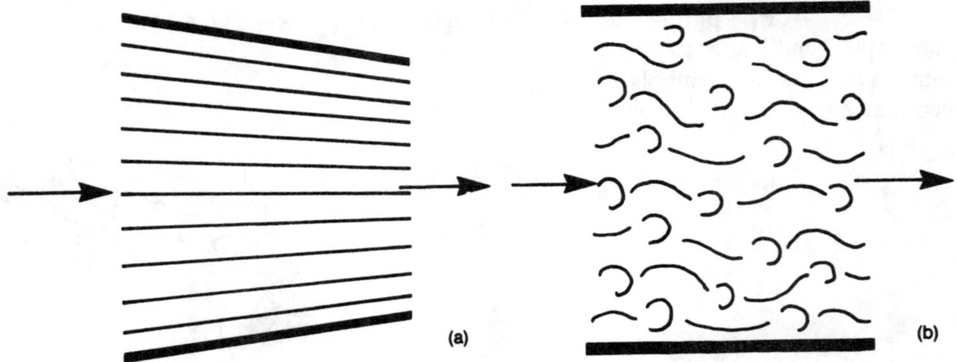

Fig. 5.19—Illustrations of Laminar Flow and Turbulent Flow

Surface Tension

Molecules of a liquid exert attractive forces toward each other (*cohesive forces*), and exert attractive forces toward surfaces they touch (*adhesive forces*). If a liquid is in a gravity-free space without a surface, it will form a sphere (smallest area relative to volume). If the liquid is lining an object, the liquid surface will contract (due to cohesive forces) to the lowest possible surface area. The forces between the molecules on this surface will create a membrane-like effect. Due to the contraction, a potential energy (PE) will be present in the surface. This PE is directly proportional to the surface area (A). An exact relation is formed as follows:

$$PE = s_t A$$

$$s_t = \text{surface tension} = PE/A = \text{joules/m}^2$$

An alternative formulation for surface tension (s_t) is:

$$s_t = F/l$$

F = force of contraction (of surface)
l = length along surface.

Because of the contraction, small objects which would ordinarily sink in the liquid may "float" on the surface membrane.

The liquid will rise or fall on a wall or in a capillary tube if the adhesive forces are greater than cohesive or cohesive are greater than adhesive forces, respectively:

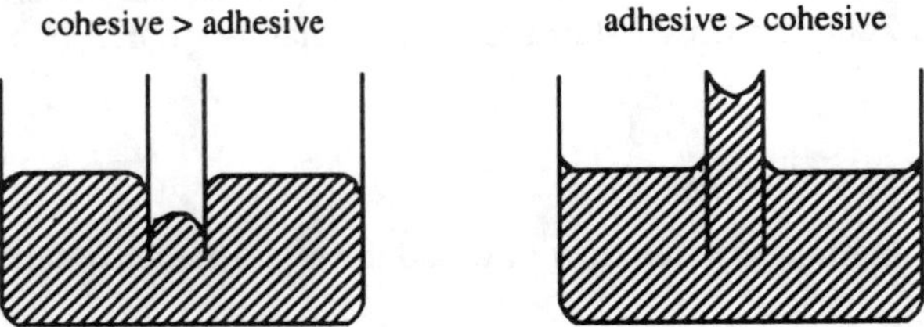

The distance the liquid rises or falls in the tube is directly proportional to the s_t and inversely proportional to the liquid density and radius of the tube.

5.11.1.4 APPLICATIONS OF SOLID AND FLUID PROPERTIES TO THE HUMAN BODY

Solids and fluids have numerous applications in human physiology. The following basic concepts and applications should be learned as an extension of your knowledge base during your review:

(a) External and internal homeostatic balance related to optimal quantities of ions, water and cellular fluids at optimal pressure and temperature.

(b) Structural differences: (i) between short, long, flat and irregular bones (ii) between compact and spongy bone; mechanical stress and the piezoelectric effect in bones; bone fracture.

(c) Various types of joints, ligaments and tendons, as related to movement, which includes gliding, rotating, hinged, pivotal, ball and socket, etc.

(d) Types of contractions in muscles: isotonic, isometric and treppe.

(e) Relationships of heart beats to atrial pressure, arterial pressure, atrial systole, ventricular systole and diastole, cardiac output and stroke volume.

(f) Working of an artificial heart as a fluid pump.

(g) Hydrostatic and osmotic pressure related to filtration through capillaries.

(h) Glomerular filtration rate, renal clearance.

(i) Operation of an artificial kidney or a hemodialysis machine.

(j) Physical characteristics of urine and blood such as volume, color, pH, specific gravity, temperature and pressure.

The above applications to pre-medical physiology are based on fundamental properties of solids and fluids. Students should understand how these applications can be related directly to physics of solids and fluids by learning definitions, formulas and various types of modern instruments used in the laboratory.

5.11.2 Questions to Review Solid and Fluid Properties

1. Mechanical stress, as used in physics, is defined as:

A. the maximum weight an object can support.
B. the force per unit length.
C. the ratio of the force to the area over which it acts.
D. the relative change in dimensions of an object caused by a force.

2. When an object is deformed by forces acting away from the object along the same line of action but in the opposite direction, the resulting stress is called:

A. tensile stress.
B. traction stress.
C. compressive stress.
D. shearing stress.

3. If D = density, m = mass and V = volume occupied by that mass, then density is:

A. D = (m)(V)
B. D = l/(m)(V)
C. D = m/V
D. D = V/m

4. Pressure is defined as:

A. force per unit volume.
B. force per unit area.
C. mass per unit volume.
D. work times volume.

5. Pressure may be conceptualized as:

A. force per unit volume.
B. work times volume.
C. potential energy per unit volume.
D. weight per unit volume.

6. All are characteristics of forces and pressures exerted by fluids except:

   A. forces are always perpendicular to the container walls.
   B. pressure is directly proportional to the product of depth and fluid density.
   C. pressure depends on the shape and size of the container.
   D. buoyant force of submerged object equals the weight of the displaced fluid.

7. Pascal's Law (of fluids) states that:

   A. an external pressure applied to an enclosed fluid is transmitted uniformly through the volume of the fluid.
   B. at any depth, the fluid pressure is the same in all directions.
   C. fluid pressure is dependent on the shape or area of its container.
   D. an object completely or partly submerged in a fluid experiences an upward force equal to the weight of the fluid displaced.

8. Bernoulli's Equation is an application of:

   A. the 2nd Law of Thermodynamics.
   B. the Law of Conservation of Momentum.
   C. the Law of Conservation of Mass.
   D. the Law of Conservation of Energy.

9. All are true of viscosity except:

   A. it is analogous to friction.
   B. there is no dissipation of mechanical energy.
   C. there is transfer of momentum between adjacent layers.
   D. as viscosity increases, rate of flow decreases.

10. A certain metal has a mass (m) = 36 gm and occupies a volume (V) = 4 mls. The density (d) of it is:

   A. 144 gm-mls
   B. 9 gms/ml
   C. $^1/_9$ mls/gm
   D. $^1/_{444}$ gms^{-1} mls^{-1}

11. A substance has a density (d) of 7 gms/ml. If 42 gms are required, what volume (V) of the substance is this?

   A. $^1/_6$ mls
   B. 6 mls
   C. 294 mls
   D. need more information

12. A fluid has a density (d) of 5 gms/ml and fills a container up to a height (h) of 10 cm's. The pressure (P) on the floor of the container is:

   A. 49,000 $dynes/cm^2$.
   B. 50 nts/m^2.
   C. 50 V $dynes/cm^2$ where V = volume in mls.
   D. not determinable with the data provided.

13. If an object is moved from a depth of 4 meters to a depth of 8 meters beneath the surface of a large tank of water, the pressure on it will:

   A. remain the same.
   B. quadruple.
   C. halve.
   D. double.

14. At a depth of 10 meters in a large container of water, 3 sheets of glass are placed parallel to the surface. Sheet A is 3m × 5m, sheet B is 4 × 4 and sheet C is 2 × 9. Which sheet has the greatest fluid pressure on its surface?

A. A
B. B
C. C
D. all are equal

15. The buoyant force (F_B) on an object that has a mass of 10 gms, a volume of 10 mls and displaces 2 mls of a liquid with a density of 5 gms/ml is:

A. 10 dynes
B. 9800 dynes
C. 1000 dynes
D. 40 dynes

16. In order for an object to float in a fluid, it must:

A. be made of a substance more dense than the fluid.
B. be made of a substance less dense than the fluid.
C. displace its own weight in the fluid.
D. displace its own volume in the fluid.

17. The key feature of an object that sinks when placed in a fluid is that:

A. it displaces its weight in the fluid.
B. it displaces less than its weight in the volume it displaces.
C. it displaces its weight before it displaces its volume.
D. it displaces its volume in the fluid.

18. A pipe has a section A of diameter = 10 meters and a section B of 5 meters. A given quantity of fluid flowing through it would:

A. move at the same speed at A and B.
B. move faster at A.
C. move faster at B.
D. would need volume of fluid to evaluate.

19. Fluid is flowing as shown in the pipe below. At what point is the pressure exerted by the fluid the highest (pipe is filled with fluid at all points)? Points A, B, C and D are at the same elevation.

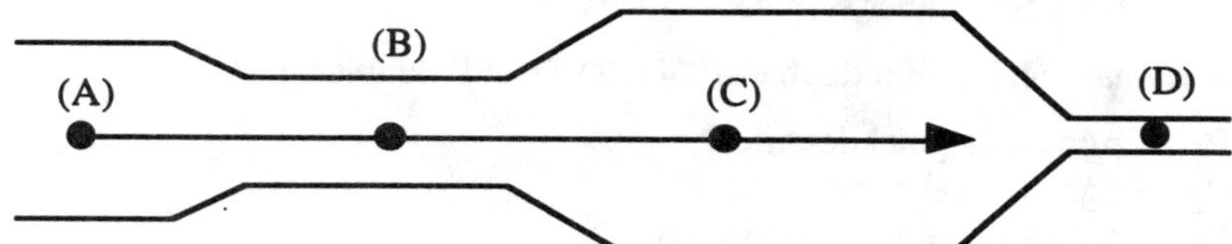

A. A
B. B
C. C
D. D

20. At which point is the pressure exerted by the fluid the *least* in the constant diameter pipe below? Assume all pipes are of constant diameter and points A, B, C and D are not at the same elevation.

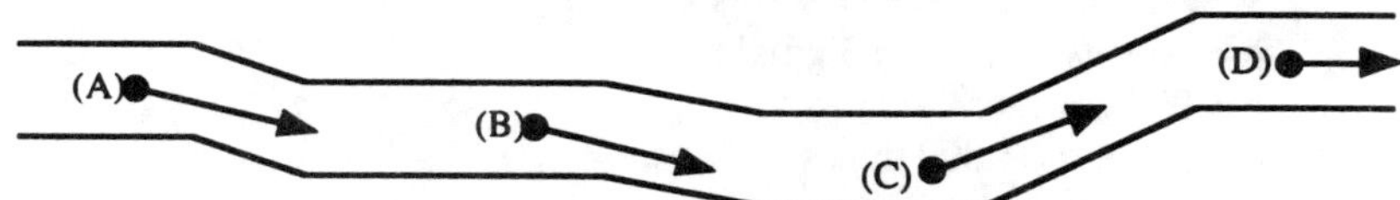

A. A
B. B
C. C
D. D

21. The relative diameters of the blood vessels of the body and the relative flows are:

arteries > arterioles > capillaries.

In which of the above is turbulent flow most likely?

A. artery
B. arteriole
C. capillary
D. all equal

5.11.3 Answers to Questions in Section 5.11.2

(1) C (2) A (3) C (4) B (5) C (6) C (7) A (8) D (9) B (10) B (11) B (12) A
(13) D (14) D (15) B (16) C (17) B (18) C (19) C (20) D (21) A

5.11.4 Discussion of Answers to Questions in Section 5.11.2

Questions #1 to #9: Adequately discussed in the text.

Question #10 (Answer: B)

$$d = m/V = 36 \text{ gms}/4 \text{ mls} = 9 \text{ gms/ml}$$

Question #11 (Answer: B)

$$d = m/V$$
$$V = m/d = 42 \text{ gms}/7 \text{ gms per ml} = 6 \text{ mls}$$

Question #12 (Answer: A)

$$P = F/A = \rho gh$$
$$P = (5 \text{ gms/cm}^3)(980 \text{ cms/sec}^2)(10 \text{ cms}) = 49{,}000 \text{ (gm-cm/sec}^2\text{)/cm}^2$$
$$P = 49{,}000 \text{ dynes/cm}^2$$
$$\text{dyne} = \text{(gm-cm)/sec}^2.$$

Question #13 (Answer: D) The pressure (P) exerted by the fluid is:

$$P = \rho gh \text{ or } P \propto h$$
$$h = \text{depth under surface.}$$

So, P is directly proportional to h and if h doubles (8/4 = 2) Then P doubles. *OR*

$$P_1 = \rho gh_1 = \text{original depth}$$
$$P_2 = \rho gh_2 = \text{final depth}$$
$$P_2/P_1 = \rho gh_2/\rho gh_1 = h_2/h_1 = 8\text{m}/4\text{m} = 2$$
$$P_2 = 2P_1.$$

Question #14 (Answer: D) Fluid pressure (P) is independent of the area or shape of its container or objects. The $P \propto \rho h$ where ρ = density and h = depth. So at any particular depth the pressure is equal in all directions.

Question #15 (Answer: B) From Archimedes' Principle:

$$F = V\rho g$$
$$V = \text{volume displaced} = 2 \text{ mls}$$
$$\rho = \text{density of fluid} = 5 \text{ gms/ml}$$
$$g = 980 \text{ cms/sec}^2$$
$$F = (2)(5)(980) = 9800 \text{ dynes.}$$

Question #16 (Answer: C) Two factors determine floating of an object: i) the overall density of the object, not the substance it is made of, and ii) the buoyant force vs. the weight of the object. According to i) B is incorrect, and according to ii) C is correct.

Question #17(Answer: B) According to Archimedes' Principle an object must displace its weight to float. The maximum volume of fluid that an object can displace is its (the object's) own volume. If a weight of fluid displaced in that maximum volume is not greater than the weight of the object, then it will sink.

Question #18 (Answer: C) The continuity equation is:

$$A_1v_1 = A_2v_2.$$

Note that the larger the cross section, the smaller the fluid velocity and vice versa.

Question #19 (Answer: C) The velocity (v) is slowest where the cross-sectional area (A) is greatest from the continuity equation ($A_1v_1 = A_2v_2$). At faster velocities, the pressure is lower, and at slower velocities the pressure (P) is higher from Bernoulli's Equation:

$$P + \rho gh + {}^1/_2\, \rho v^2 = \text{constant}$$

ρgh does not change if h = constant

then ${}^1/_2\, \rho v^2$ increases as v increases, and P must decrease because the whole expression is constant.

As the fluid moves faster, pressure energy (P) is converted to kinetic energy (${}^1/_2\, \rho v^2$) and the pressure drops.

Question #20 (Answer: D) Since the diameter is constant, the velocity of fluid flow is constant by the continuity equation ($A_1v_1 = A_2v_2$). From Bernoulli's Equation:

$$P + \rho gh + {}^1/_2\, \rho v^2 = \text{constant}$$

${}^1/_2\, \rho v^2$ does not change

ρ = density   v = velocity

ρgh changes because h (height above some arbitrary reference point) is changing, the larger h means the larger this term; the larger ρgh means the smaller the P term becomes; then, the higher the pipe (due to h), the smaller the pressure (P).

Question #21 (Answer: A) Turbulence is best estimated using Reynolds number (R) or by remembering the relations from R. The viscosity and density of the fluid (i.e., the blood) is constant. Since diameter (d) and velocity (v) are greatest in the arteries and

$$\text{turbulence} \propto (v)(d)$$

they have the highest turbulence. The velocity is greater in the arteries because the sum total of all cross-sectional areas of the arteries in the human body is less than the total cross-sectional areas of all the capillaries.

5.11.5 Checklist for Solid and Fluid Properties

______ density
______ elastic properties
______ specific gravity
______ buoyancy
______ hydrostatic pressure
______ fluid statics
______ Pascal's Law
______ viscosity
______ Bernoulli's Equation
______ tensile forces
______ compressive forces
______ fluid dynamics

5.12 THERMODYNAMICS AND THERMOCHEMISTRY

5.12.1 Review of Thermodynamics and Thermochemistry

Thermodynamics deals with the physical laws that determine transfer and flow of heat whereas thermo-chemistry deals with the heat absorbed or given out during chemical reactions.

5.12.1.1 THERMODYNAMICS

Heat is a form of energy. Bodies *do not contain* heat; they either emit or absorb energy as heat. When a body absorbs or emits energy, all of the energy need not be in the form of heat. For example, a body emitting energy may emit some as heat and some as light energy. A body contains *thermal energy* (or internal energy) which is the *sum* of the potential and kinetic energies associated with the position or motion, respectively, of the molecules, as mentioned earlier in the kinetic theory of gases.

Thermal equilibrium results when the average kinetic energies per molecule of two bodies are equal. This is also when the heat flow between the bodies is zero, and when the temperatures of the two bodies are equal. *Temperature* is taken to be a measure of the average thermal energy of a body; it is also a measure of the amount of energy absorbed or emitted as heat by a body. Thus when temperature rises, the average kinetic energy per molecule rises, and the object absorbs more energy as heat, and vice versa.

Temperature of molecules = Constant x mv^2 (average)

Measurement of temperature is by thermometers. A *thermometer* has (1) a thermometric property (e.g., pressure, density, linear expansion, resistance) which varies directly as temperature; (2) a lower fixed point (e.g., freezing point (FP) of water); (3) a higher fixed point (e.g., boiling point (BP) of water); and (4) a scale calibrated between these two points and extrapolated beyond them. Relative temperature scales are the *Celsius* or *Centigrade* (FP of water = 0°C, BP of water = 100°C) and the *Fahrenheit* (FP of water = 32°F, BP of water = 212°F). Absolute scales (the zero point of the scale is the true absolute zero) are the *Rankine* (°R) calibrated in °F units and the *Kelvin* (°K) calibrated in °C units. Interconversions of the scales are:

°C = 5/9 (°F-32) or °F = (9/5) °C + 32 and 5 units Celsius = 9 units Fahrenheit

°K = °C + 273 °R = °F + 460

The Celsius and Fahrenheit scales are equal at -40°.

Heat capacity is a measure of the amount of heat a body can gain (or lose) per change in temperature (Δt),

heat capacity = heat gained/temperature change = $Q/\Delta t$.

Specific heat capacity (C) is the heat capacity per unit mass of substance:

$C = (Q/\Delta t)/m = Q/m\Delta t$.

This can be rearranged to give the amount of heat exchanged (gained or lost) by a substance:

$Q = (C)(m)(\Delta t)$.

The units of heat most commonly used are calories. A calorie is the amount of heat required to raise the temperature of 1 gram of water one degree Celsius.

A kilocalorie is 1000 calories. Since heat is a form of energy, its units must be equivalent to the unit of other energies (kinetic or potential) or work which is the Joule (or other similar units). *The interconversion of calories and joules is:*

(Memorize for the MCAT!)

4.184 joules = 1 calorie
4.2 joules ≈ 1 calorie

The *specific heat of water is then:*

1 (calorie/gm - °C).

It is in the understanding of *phase transitions* that specific heat, heat of fusion and heat of vaporization have particular value. Below are the important features of phase transitions (See Sections 5.3.1.3 and 5.9.1):

Phase Transition	Conditions	Heat Associated
(1) solid ⇌ liquid (melt →, ← freeze)	Solid and liquid vapor pressure in equilibrium. Temperature called melting (or freezing) point (MP or FP).	heat of fusion (H_f) H_f = Q/m at MP or Q = m H_f Q = heat transferred m = mass
liquid ⇌ gas (evaporate (boil) →, ← condense)	Gas and liquid vapor pressure in equilibrium. Temperature called the boiling point (BP)	Heat of evaporation (H_v) H_v = Q/m at BP or Q = H_v m

Note that $H_V > H_f$ because usually more kinetic energy per molecule is required to separate liquid molecules to become gaseous than to separate solid molecules to become liquid. As a substance gains or loses energy as heat, it passes through the various phases. A scheme for substances gaining heat is:

Phases & Temps	Solid Below MP (1) →	Solid at MP (2) →	Liquid at MP (3) →	Liquid at BP (4) →	Gas at BP (5) →	Gas above BP

	(1)	(2)	(3)	(4)	(5)
Heat changes	Heat is absorbed to raise the temperature as the specific heat of the solid: $Q = C\,m\Delta t$	Heat is absorbed as heat of fusion to cause solid to melt to the liquid. Note that the temperature does not change: $Q = H_f\,m$	Heat is absorbed as the specific heat of the liquid to raise its temperature: $Q = C\,m\Delta t$	Heat is absorbed as heat of vaporization to cause the liquid to be converted to gas. The temperature does not change. $Q = H_v\,m$	Heat is absorbed as the specific heat of the gas to raise its temperature: $Q = C\,m\Delta t$

Note: C represents specific heat constant for a solid, liquid, or gas.

The reverse steps would hold if the substance was losing energy as heat. To summarize, heat is used to change the phase or the temperature of a substance. When two objects are in contact and at different temperatures, heat flows from the one with the higher temperature to the one with the lower temperature until the temperatures are equal. The above equations can be used to calculate heat flows and temperatures by using:

Heat flow law: heat loss = heat gain (Memorize this equation and how to use it on the MCAT.)

As an illustration, study the following example and how it relates to the heat flow law.

> You are preparing a small pot of chicken soup in the kitchen. The pot is made of a special alloy with a specific heat of 0.10. The specific heat of chicken soup is 0.83. Suddenly you drop a large gold bracelet in the soup. The bracelet has a mass of 75 grams. There are about 1000 grams of chicken soup in the pot and the pot has a mass of 500 grams. The bracelet you were wearing had a temperature of 50°F. The specific heat of the bracelet is 0.032. The temperature of the pot and the soup inside it is 88°C. Find the final temperature of the bracelet.

Solution: Heat lost by hot substances = heat gained by cold substances.

The problem shows that chicken soup and the pot are *hot*, whereas the bracelet is *cold*. Convert the temperature of the bracelet to °C, using,

$$\frac{F-32}{9} = \frac{C}{5}, \quad \frac{50-32}{9} = \frac{C}{5}$$

which gives temperature of bracelet to be 10°C.

Heat lost by pot + heat lost by chicken soup = Heat gained by gold bracelet.

Subscripts used are as follows:
s = chicken soup
b = gold bracelet
p = cooking pot

$$C_p\,(m_p)(t_p - t_f) + C_s\,(m_s)(t_s - t_f) = C_b\,(m_b)(t_f - t_b)$$

t_f = Final temperature of bracelet and resulting mixture.

$$0.1\,(500)(88 - t_f) + 0.83\,(1000)(88 - t_f) = 0.032\,(75)(t_f - 10)$$

Solving for t_f one obtains 87.8°C. In other words, the bracelet's temperature is *almost* the same as the chicken soup, but it rose rapidly from 10°C to 87.8°C. On the MCAT you *could* have approximated the answer to this problem by looking at the relative *masses* of various objects. This illustrates the use of the heat flow equation.

When substances gain (or lose) heat they usually undergo *expansion (or contraction)*. Expansion (contraction) can be by linear dimensions, by area, or by volume. These are:

Type	Final	Original	Change caused by heat
(1) Linear	L	L_o	$\alpha \Delta t L_o$

$L = L_o + \alpha \Delta t L_o = L_o(1 + \alpha \Delta t)$

α = coefficient of linear thermal expansion, Δt = change in temp

Type	Final	Original	Change caused by heat
(2) Area	A	A_o	$\beta \Delta t A_o$

$A = A_o + \beta \Delta t A_o = A_o(1 + \beta \Delta t)$

β = coefficient of area thermal expansion = 2α

Type	Final	Original	Change caused by heat
(3) Volume	V	V_o	$\gamma \Delta t V_o$

$V = V_o + \gamma \Delta t V_o = V_o(1 + \gamma \Delta t)$

γ = coefficient of volume thermal expansion = 3α

Heat flows between substances by three mechanisms: conduction, convection and radiation. *Conduction* is a process in which heat energy is transferred by adjacent molecular collisions throughout a material medium—the medium does not move. The heat energy is carried off by the motion of the electrons. Good electrical conductors, therefore, are usually good heat conductors. The rate of heat transfer (H) by conduction is:

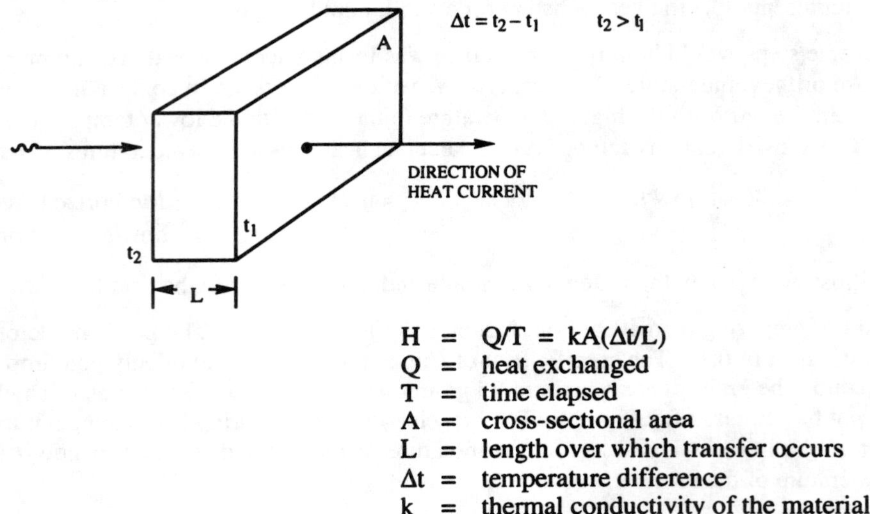

$H = Q/T = kA(\Delta t/L)$
Q = heat exchanged
T = time elapsed
A = cross-sectional area
L = length over which transfer occurs
Δt = temperature difference
k = thermal conductivity of the material

Fig. 5.20—Heat Conduction

Note that the rate (H) is directly proportional to A and Δt and inversely proportional to L. The thermal conductivity, k is a property of the substance.

Convection is a process in which heat energy is transferred by the actual mass motion of a fluid (gas or liquid). Convection currents are set up which may be natural (caused by density differences, e.g., wind) or forced (as in a house ventilation system). The rate of energy transfer (H) is:

$H = Q/T = hA\Delta t$ (note the relations shown).

The convection coefficient h is not a property of the substance.

Radiation is a process in which heat energy is transferred by electromagnetic waves absorbed or emitted at the atomic level. All substances radiate heat regardless of the temperature. In general, as the absolute temperature (T) increases, the wavelength of the emitted heat decreases. The rate of radiation (heat) emitted per unit area (R) is:

$R = e\delta T^4$ (Stefan-Boltzmann Law)
T = absolute temperature
e = emissivity = the ability to absorb or emit thermal radiation
δ = Stefan-Boltzmann's constant.

The *key relation* is that R is proportional to the fourth power of the absolute temperature. A body at the same temperature as its surroundings will radiate and absorb heat at the same rate. If not at the same temperature, the net rate of radiation is:

net rate of radiation = rate of energy emission – rate of energy absorption

$R = e\delta\, T_1^4 - e\delta\, T_2^4 = e\delta(T_1^4 - T_2^4)$

T_1 = temperature of body

T_2 = temperature of surroundings.

Thermodynamics is concerned with physical laws governing the energy states of molecules and chemical reactions. A system is comprised of a large number of molecules, the so-called "object" under study. It is the reference point. When the system gains energy, the (energy) change is positive. The environment is everything outside the system. Systems exchange energy by the processes of work or heat exchange. Systems do not contain work or heat. Work or heat exchange depends upon the path from the initial to the final state. This is in contrast to state functions which are independent of the path taken but depend upon the initial and final states only. The state functions to be discussed are pressure (P), volume (V), temperature (T), internal energy (E) and entropy (S). See section 5.12.1.2 for the discussion of other state functions, enthalpy (H) and free energy (G).

Energy is a property of a system and not a process (like heat or work). Specifically, the internal energy change (ΔE), of a system depends on the work done and heat exchanged as follows:

$\Delta E = q - W$ *First Law of Thermodynamics*

$q = +$ if heat is added to the system

$q = -$ if heat is lost from the system

$W = + p\Delta V$ if work is done by the system

p = external pressure

$\Delta V = V_f - V_i$ change in volume of the system

Note: this gives the sign to the work done by the system.

The internal energy depends on the kinetic energies of the molecules, on the potential energies of forces between molecules, and the kinetic and potential energies of the electrons and nuclei. The First Law of Thermodynamics is a restatement of the law of Conservation of Energy. The ΔE of a reaction is determined by running the reaction at constant volume and measuring the amount of heat exchanged:

$\Delta E = q - W = q - p\Delta V = q_v$

$\Delta V = 0$

q_v = heat at constant volume.

A reversible process is one that occurs in such small increments that it can be reversed at any point. An irreversible process is one that cannot be easily reversed. As a concrete example, if you walked down a flight of stairs one step at a time, it would be fairly easy to reverse your direction at any step—this would be a reversible process. But if you jumped out of a window, equivalent to going down a flight of stairs, you could not reverse yourself—this would be an irreversible process. For reversible (rev) and irreversible (irrev) processes, the following are true:

$W_{rev} > W_{irrev}$

$q_{rev} > q_{irrev}$

These concepts lead into entropy (S) and the Second Law of Thermodynamics, which is

$\Delta S = (q_{rev}/T)$ for a reversible path = change in entropy

Note: (1) ΔS is still independent of a particular reversible path,

(2) $\Delta S = \Delta S$ system $+ \Delta S$ environment $= 0$,

(3) ΔS exists for an irreversible path but it is not equal to (q_{rev}/T)

(4) ΔS is increasing for an irreversible path.

Entropy is further discussed in Section 5.12.1.2.

5.12.1.2 THERMOCHEMISTRY

Enthalpy (ΔH) is the energy change (in terms of heat content) in a chemical reaction that occurs at constant pressure. The natural tendency of systems is toward minimum energy—the lower the energy of the system, the more stable the system. This means that a reaction that occurs with loss of energy (or negative energy) is a favorable reaction. The *standard enthalpy of formation* (ΔH_f°) is the enthalpy change when one mole of a compound is formed from its elements at 298°k. An example is:

$$C + 1/2\ O_2\ (g) \rightarrow CO(g) \quad \Delta H_f^\circ\ (CO) = -26.4\ \text{kcal.}$$

The *standard enthalpy change of a reaction* (ΔH°) is:

$$\Delta H_f^\circ = \Sigma\Delta H_f^\circ\ (\text{products}) - \Sigma\Delta H_f^\circ\ (\text{reactants})$$

That is, the ΔH_f° of all the products are added together and the ΔH_f° of all the reactants are subtracted from them. Note: the enthalpy of elements as they exist at 298°K is zero. *Hess's Law of Constant Heat Summation* states that ΔH°'s of the reactions can be added algebraically to get the overall ΔH° for the overall reaction. Note that when the direction of a reaction is reversed, the sign of the ΔH° is changed (from + → –, or from – → +). Also, if the reaction as written is multiplied (or divided) by a number, the ΔH° must also be multiplied (or divided) by the same number. An example:

Q: Find the enthalpy of formation (ΔH_f°) of $Ca(OH)_2(s)$ given the following:

$$2H_2(g) + O_2(g) \rightarrow 2H_2O(l) \qquad \Delta H = -136.6\ \text{kcal}$$
$$CaO(s) + H_2O(l) \rightarrow Ca(OH)_2(s) \qquad \Delta H = -15.3\ \text{kcal}$$
$$2CaO(s) \rightarrow 2Ca(s) + O_2(g) \qquad \Delta H = +303.6\ \text{kcal}$$

A: ΔH_f° of $Ca(OH)_2$ means its formation from $Ca(s)$, $H_2(g)$ and $O_2(g)$. The answer by using the principles above is:

$$1/2\ [2H_2(g) + O_2(g) \rightarrow 2H_2O(l)] \qquad \Delta H = 1/2\ (-136.6\ \text{kcal})$$
$$CaO(s) + H_2O(l) \rightarrow Ca(OH)_2(s) \qquad \Delta H = -15.3\ \text{kcal}$$
$$1/2\ [2Ca(s) + O_2(g) \rightarrow 2CaO(s)] \qquad \Delta H = 1/2\ (-303.6\ \text{kcal})$$

rewriting the above,

$$H_2(g) + 1/2\ O_2(g) \rightarrow H_2O(l) \qquad \Delta H = -68.3\ \text{kcal}$$
$$CaO(s) + H_2O(l) \rightarrow Ca(OH)_2(s) \qquad \Delta H = -15.3\ \text{kcal}$$
$$Ca(s) + 1/2\ O_2(g) \rightarrow CaO(s) \qquad \Delta H = -151.8\ \text{kcal}$$

---

net:

$$Ca(s) + H_2(g) + O_2(g) \rightarrow Ca(OH)_2(s) \qquad \Delta H = -235.4\ \text{kcal}$$

Note: the $CaO(s)$ and $H_2O(l)$ cancel because they are on opposite sides of the equation.)

Entropy (ΔS) is another measure of the stability of a system. It represents that part of the total energy not available for useful work. Entropy can be viewed as a measure of the number of microscopic states associated with a given macroscopic state. The more microscopic states a given macroscopic state has, the higher its entropy. This is also the same as saying the more probable (in the sense of probability) a state is, the higher its entropy. This is also the same as saying the more random a state, the higher its entropy. Systems tend toward maximum entropy for the greatest stability.

ΔH and ΔS represent two tendencies of systems. These may oppose each other or be in the same direction. *Free energy* (ΔG) is a measure of the tendency of a system which takes into account ΔH and ΔS. It gives the net tendency of the system. The formulation of ΔG is

$$\Delta G = \Delta H - T\Delta S$$

T = absolute temperature.

For chemical reactions, the following conditions hold:

if $\Delta G = 0$, then the reaction is at equilibrium
$\Delta G < 0$, then a spontaneous reaction (no energy input) is possible
$\Delta G > 0$, then no reaction spontaneously

The system tends toward a minimal value of ΔG which is the maximal stability.

The more negative ΔG, the more probable the reaction will go as written. In summary, the ΔG represents the useful energy the system has to do work. As before, with ΔH

$$\Delta G^\circ = \Sigma\Delta G_f^\circ \text{ (products)} - \Sigma\Delta G_f^\circ \text{ (reactants)}$$

Bonded molecules have lower energy than separate atoms; therefore, when atoms combine to form molecules, they lose energy (when spontaneous). The *bond dissociation energy* (D) is the enthalpy change of the reaction in which a specific bond in a gaseous molecule is broken. The D is positive (i.e., it requires input of energy to break a bond). The *average bond energy (E)* is the approximate energy required to break a bond of a particular type (e.g., C-H) in any compound it may occur in. Note that each C-H in CH_4 has a different D, but the E would be the average of all four of these. The larger the numerical value (all are positive by definition) of the bond energy, the stronger the bond.

Exothermic reactions proceed with a negative ΔH, and *endothermic* reactions proceed with a positive ΔH.

That is:

exothermic: reactants → products + heat
endothermic: heat + reactants → products.

5.12.1.3 APPLICATIONS OF THERMODYNAMICS AND THERMOCHEMISTRY TO THE HUMAN BODY

Thermodynamics and thermochemistry have numerous applications to the physiology and biochemical processes in the human body. The following basic concepts and applications will help you learn how to expand your knowledge base during your review:

(a) Thermal regulation and internal/external homeostasis leading to optimal temperature in the average human. Concepts relating input and output of heat energy changes in the body, e.g., hot temperatures lead to sweating to regulate body temperature.

(b) Heat productivity by skeletal muscles.

(c) Basal metabolic rate; loss of heat from the body by conduction, convection and radiation; control of body temperature by the hypothalamus.

(d) Sunstroke, fever and hypothermia analysis.

(e) Biochemical reactions.

The above mentioned applications should be linked with your study of thermodynamics and thermochemistry to make your review more medically oriented. Pay special attention to modern lab instruments used to measure some of the terms discussed in thermodynamics and thermochemistry.

5.12.2 Questions to Review Thermodynamics and Thermochemistry

1. A measure of the heat of a chemical reaction is:

A. entropy.
B. enthalpy.
C. free energy.
D. none of these.

2. The more stable systems with regard to H are systems that have:

A. zero ΔH.
B. maximum ΔH.
C. minimum ΔH.
D. none of the above.

3. A measure of the total energy not available for useful work is the:

   A. entropy.
   B. enthalpy.
   C. free energy.
   D. none of the above.

4. The more stable systems with regard to entropy are systems that have:

   A. minimum ΔS.
   B. maximum ΔS.
   C. zero ΔS.
   D. none of these.

5. High values of entropy are associated with all of the following except:

   A. a large number of microscopic states for a given macroscopic state.
   B. high probability of a state.
   C. high randomness of a state.
   D. all of the above are correct.

6. The net energy available to a system is given by the:

   A. entropy.
   B. enthalpy.
   C. free energy.
   D. none of the above.

7. The relationship between free energy (ΔG), enthalpy (ΔH), entropy (ΔS) and absolute temperature (T) is:

   A. $\Delta G = \Delta H + \Delta S$
   B. $\Delta G = \Delta H + T\Delta S$
   C. $\Delta G = \Delta H - T\Delta S$
   D. $\Delta G = T\Delta H - \Delta S$

8. If $\Delta G<0$, then:

   A. the reaction is at equilibrium.
   B. a spontaneous reaction is possible.
   C. no reaction is possible.
   D. none of the above are possible.

9. With regard to ΔG a system is most stable when:

   A. ΔG is a maximum.
   B. ΔG is a minimum.
   C. ΔG is zero.
   D. ΔG is infinite.

10. The larger the numerical value of chemical bond energy, the:

    A. stronger the bond.
    B. weaker the bond.
    C. more complex is the bond.
    D. longer the bond.

11. The following reaction is:

    reactants $\rightarrow$ products, ΔH = negative

    A. exothermic.
    B. endothermic.
    C. hydrostatic.
    D. electromagnetic.

Use the following information for the remainder of the Questions.

Enthalpies of Formation, ΔH_f° (kcals/mole) at 298°K

$H_2O(g)$	–58	$NO_2(g)$	8	$Ca(OH)_2$	–236	$CH_3CH_2OH(l)$	–66
$H_2O(l)$	–68	$NH_3(g)$	–11	$CaCO_3(s)$	–288	$C_2H_4(g)$	13
$SO_3(g)$	–94	$CO_2(g)$	–94	$C_2H_6(g)$	–20	$C_4H_{10}(g)$	–30
$NO(g)$	19	$CaO(s)$	–152	$CH_3OH(l)$	–57		

Bond Energies (ΔH in kcals/mole)

H-H	104	O-H	111	N = N	226	C-Cl	79	H-Cl	103
O= O	118	C-C	83	C-N	70	C = O	170	C-H	99
Cl-Cl	58	C-O	84	C = C	147				

12. Calculate the ΔH_f° of $H_2SO_4(l)$ given the following equation:

$$H_2O(l) + SO_3(g) \rightarrow H_2SO_4(l) \quad \Delta H^\circ = -32 \text{ kcals}$$

A. – 6
B. – 58
C. – 162
D. – 194

13. Calculate the heat (ΔH°) of reaction for the following reaction:

$$CaO(s) + CO_2(g) \rightarrow CaCO_3(s)$$

A. – 534
B. + 534
C. + 42
D. – 42

14. Calculate the heat (ΔH°) of reaction for the following reaction:

$$C_2H_4(g) + H_2O(l) \rightarrow CH_3CH_2OH(l)$$

A. – 121
B. + 15
C. – 15
D. – 11

15. Calculate the heat (ΔH°) of a reaction for the combustion of n-butane (C_4H_{10})

$$C_4H_{10}(g) + O_2(g) \rightarrow CO_2(g) + H_2O(l)$$
(unbalanced)

A. – 132
B. – 192
C. – 310
D. – 686

16. Which of the following steps requires the most energy?

$$\text{(I) } C=O \rightarrow C-O$$
$$\text{(II) } C=C \rightarrow C-C$$

(neglect other bonds that might be formed)

A. I
B. II
C. both equal
D. not enough information to solve problem

17. Which of the following steps releases the most energy?

(I) H_2 + $H_2C{=}CH_2 \rightarrow H_3C{-}CH_3$

(II) H_2 + $H_2C{=}O \rightarrow H_3C{-}OH$

A. I
B. II
C. neither releases energy
D. both release same amount of energy

18. Heat:

A. is contained by an object.
B. is absorbed or emitted by an object.
C. is defined by statements (A) and (B).
D. is defined by neither statement (A) nor statement (B).

19. Temperature:

A. is a measure of the average thermal energy of a body.
B. is a measure of the amount of heat a body absorbs or emits.
C. increases when the average kinetic energy per molecule increases.
D. all of the above.

20. Thermal equilibrium occurs when:

A. the average kinetic energy per molecule of two bodies is equal.
B. the heat flow between two bodies is zero.
C. the temperature between two bodies is equal.
D. all are correct.

21. Heat capacity is:

A. the amount of heat a body contains per degree of temperature.
B. the amount of heat a body can gain or lose per degree change in temperature.
C. represented as: temperature/heat.
D. both (A) and (C).

22. Specific heat capacity is:

A. the amount of heat contained by a substance.
B. the amount of heat contained per unit change of temperature by a substance.
C. the heat capacity per unit change in temperature.
D. the heat capacity per unit mass.

23. If C = specific heat capacity, Δt = change in temperature and m = mass, then the amount of heat (Q) exchanged is:

A. $Q = C/m\Delta t$
B. $Q = C\, m\Delta t$
C. $Q = Cm/\Delta t$
D. $Q = C\Delta t/m$

24. Heat of fusion refers to the phase change between:

A. gas and solid.
B. liquid and gas.
C. liquid and solid.
D. all phases.

25. When a solid is converted to a liquid:

A. heat is released.
B. heat is required.
C. temperature increases.
D. heat is neither released nor required.

26. A net release of heat to the environment occurs during:

A. condensation.
B. sublimation.
C. evaporation.
D. melting.

27. Heat flows between substances by all the following processes except:

A. conjugation.
B. conduction.
C. convection.
D. radiation.

28. The process whereby heat is transferred by adjacent molecular collisions throughout a medium is:

A. convection.
B. conduction.
C. radiation.
D. momentum.

29. In heat transfer in a substance (e.g., a heat-conducting rod), the rate of heat transfer is:

A. directly proportional to the length of the conductor.
B. indirectly proportional to the temperature difference.
C. directly proportional to the cross-sectional area of the conductor.
D. independent of the nature of the substance.

30. The process of transferring heat energy in a moving fluid mass is called:

A. bulk flow.
B. radiation.
C. conduction.
D. convection.

31. Heat loss or gain by the process of radiation:

A. occurs in all substances regardless of temperature.
B. occurs only if the temperature is above the critical temperature of a substance.
C. is independent of the nature of a substance.
D. occurs only if the temperature is below the critical temperature of a substance.

32. As the absolute temperature increases, the wavelength of radiation emitted by a substance tends to:

A. increase.
B. decrease.
C. remain the same.
D. change periodically.

33. The reference point in thermodynamics is called the:

A. surroundings.
B. environment.
C. state.
D. system.

34. Which of the following is independent of the path taken?

A. internal energy
B. work
C. heat
D. none of these

35. A statement of the First Law of Thermodynamics is:

A. $\Delta S = q_{rev}/T$
B. $\Delta G = \Delta H - T\Delta S$
C. $\Delta E = q - W$
D. none of these

36. The internal energy (ΔE) depends upon:

A. kinetic energy of molecules.
B. potential energy of forces between molecules.
C. kinetic and potential energies of electrons and nuclei.
D. all of these.

37. The Second Law of Thermodynamics involves the term:

A. internal energy.
B. enthalpy.
C. entropy.
D. free energy.

38. During the conversion of a liquid to a gas, the heat is:

A. used to overcome intermolecular forces between liquid molecules and convert them to gaseous molecules.
B. used to raise the temperature of the gas.
C. used to raise the temperature of the liquid.
D. all of the above.

39. The conversion of 10 grams of a solid to 10 grams of its liquid at the freezing point (25°C) requires 100 cals of heat. The heat of fusion of this substance is:

A. 0.40 cals/gm·°C
B. 40 cals·gm/°C
C. 10 cals/gm
D. 250 cals· °C/gm

40. An object weighing 10 gms has a specific heat of 2 cals/gm/°C. To raise its temperature from 10°C to 60°C would require how many calories?

A. 10 cals
B. 100 cals
C. 1000 cals
D. 5000 cals

41. A substance weighing 5 gms has its temperature raised from 25° to 75°C without a phase change while absorbing 45 calories of heat. Its specific heat capacity is:

A. 11,250 cals/gm·°C
B. 450 cals/gm· °C
C. 0.18 cals/gm· °C
D. 4.50 cals/gm·°C

42. The amount of heat required to convert 10 gms of water (solid) at 0°C to water (liquid) at 50°C (specific heat of solid water is 0.5 cals/gm·°C; specific heat of liquid water is 1.0 cals/gm·°C; heat of fusion of water is 80 cals/gm) is:

A. 1300 kilocalories
B. 350 cals
C. 1300 cals
D. 1500 cals

43. If a heating coil is supplying 50 cals/min to a tank containing water (ice) at 0°C, the amount of water (as a liquid) that can be formed in 10 min. (use specific heat and heat of fusion from question #42) is:

A. 3.5 gms
B. 6.25 gms
C. 420 gms
D. 500 gms

44. A temperature of 50°C (Celsius) corresponds to what temperature Fahrenheit (F)?

A. 122°F
B. 90°F
C. 82°F
D. 27.8°F

45. At what temperature are the Celsius (°C) andf Fahrenheit (°F) scales equal?

A. 100
B. 37
C. –40
D. 0

46. The coefficient of linear expansion (α) of a substance is 2×10^{-5}°C^{-1} . The coefficient of volume expansion (γ) would be:

A. 6×10^{-5} °C^{-1}
B. 8×10^{-5} °C^{-1}
C. 2×10^{-15} °C^{-3}
D. 9×10^{-5} °C^{-1}

47. An object with a linear expansion coefficient (α) of 2×10^{-4o} °C^{-1} has the volume of 10.000 liters. If the temperature increases 100°C, the new volume will be:

A. 10.020 liters
B. 10.008 liters
C. 10.600 liters
D. 10.060 liters

48. Heat is being conducted through a square-faced metal block 4 meters long with sides 2 meters in length. If another block of the same metal is constructed but with a square face of 4 meters on a side and 8 meters long, what is the rate of heat conduction through it, compared with the first block, for a given temperature difference? *Note:* the heat is passing through the square faces along the complete length.

A. The second rate is four times the first rate.
B. The second rate is twice the first rate.
C. The second rate is one-half the first rate.
D. The second rate is one-fourth the first rate.

49. If the temperature of an object is changed from 20°C to 10°C, the rate of heat loss due to radiation is how much of the original?

A. slightly more than the original
B. slightly less than the original
C. 1/2 as much
D. 1/16 as much

5.12.3 Answers to Questions in Section 5.12.2

(1) B (2) C (3) A (4) B (5) D (6) C (7) C (8) B (9) B (10) A (11) A (12) D (13) D (14) D (15) D (16) A (17) A (18) B (19) D (20) D (21) B (22) D (23) B (24) C (25) B (26) A (27) A (28) B (29) C (30) D (31) A (32) B (33) D (34) A (35) C (36) D (37) C (38) A (39) C (40) C (41) C (42) C (43) B (44) A (45) C (46) A (47) C (48) B (49) B

5.12.4 Discussion of Answers to Questions in Section 5.12.2

Questions #1 to #11: Adequately discussed in Section.

Question #12 (Answer: D) The ΔH_f° is the formation of one mole of the $H_2SO_4(l)$ from its elements:

$$H_2(g) + S(s) + 2O_2(g) \rightarrow H_2SO_4(l) \qquad \Delta H_f^\circ = ?$$

Now using the information given, a set of equations must be put together that adds up to this net equation. This is done as follows:

$$(1)\ H_2(g) + 1/2O_2(g) \rightarrow H_2O(l) \qquad \Delta H_f^\circ = -68$$

$$(2)\ S(s) + \frac{3}{2}O_2(g) \rightarrow SO_3(g) \qquad \Delta H_f^\circ = -94$$

Rearrange these to show how they add up to the equation wanted:

$$H_2(g) + 1/2O_2(g) \rightarrow H_2O(l) \qquad \Delta H_f^\circ = -68 \text{ kcals}$$

$$S(s) + \frac{3}{2}O_2(g) \rightarrow SO_3(g) \qquad \Delta H_f^\circ = -94 \text{ kcals}$$

$$H_2O(l) + SO_3(g) \rightarrow H_2SO_4(l) \qquad \Delta H_f^\circ = -32 \text{ kcals}$$

$$\text{sum: } H_2(g) + 2O_2(g) + S(s) \rightarrow H_2SO_4(l) \qquad \Delta H_f^\circ = -194 \text{ kcals}$$

Or, an alternative method:

$$\Delta H^\circ \text{ (product)} - \Delta H^\circ \text{ (reactant)} = \Delta H^\circ \text{ reaction}$$

$$\Delta H_f^\circ\ H_2SO_4 - \{\Delta H_f^\circ\ H_2O(l) + \Delta H_f^\circ\ SO_3(g)\} = -32 \text{ kcal}$$

$$\Delta H_f^\circ\ H_2SO_4 - (-68 \text{ kcal} - 94 \text{ kcal}) = -32 \text{ kcal}$$

$$\Delta H_f^\circ\ H_2SO_4 = -194 \text{ kcal}$$

Question #13: (Answer: D) This is a direct application of Hess' Law.

$$\Sigma\Delta H_f^\circ \text{ (products)} = -288$$

$$\Sigma\Delta H_f^\circ \text{ (reactants)} = -94 - 152 = -246$$

then,

$$\Delta H^\circ = \Sigma\Delta H_f^\circ \text{ (products)} — \Sigma\Delta H_f^\circ \text{ (reactants)}$$

$$\Delta H^\circ = -288 - (-246) = -288 + 246 = -42.$$

Question #14: (Answer: D) This is also a direct application of Hess' Law.

$$\Sigma\Delta H_f^\circ \text{ (products)} = -66$$

$$\Sigma\Delta H_f^\circ \text{ (reactants)} = -68 + 13 = -55$$

and,

$$\Delta H^\circ = \Sigma\Delta H_f^\circ \text{ (products)} — \Sigma\Delta H_f^\circ \text{ (reactants)}$$

$$= -66 - (-55) = -66 + 55 = -11.$$

Question #15 (Answer: D) First balance the equation (Section 5.4):

$$\begin{array}{rlcl} \text{unbalanced:} & C_4H_{10} + O_2 & \rightarrow & CO_2 + H_2O \\ \text{balance H:} & C_4H_{10} + O_2 & \rightarrow & CO_2 + 5H_2O \\ \text{balance C:} & C_4H_{10} + O_2 & \rightarrow & 4CO_2 + 5H_2O \\ \text{balance O:} & C_4H_{10} + \frac{13}{2}O_2 & \rightarrow & 4CO_2 + 5H_2O \end{array}$$

(leave as 1 mole C_4H_{10} because ΔH° based on one mole of the substance)

$$\begin{array}{rl|c} \text{check: C:} & 4 & 4 \\ \text{H:} & 10 & 10 \\ \text{O:} & 13/2(2) = 13 & 13 \end{array}$$

Now apply Hess' Law:

$$\Sigma\Delta H_f^\circ \text{ (products)} = 4\ \Delta H_f^\circ \text{ of } CO_2(g) + 5\Delta H_f^\circ \text{ of } H_2O(l)$$

$$= 4(-94) + 5(-68) = -376 - 340 = -716$$

$$\Sigma\Delta H_f^\circ \text{ (reactants)} = \Delta H_f^\circ \text{ of } C_4H_{10} + 13/2\Delta H_f^\circ \text{ of } O_2(g)$$

$$= -30 + 13/2(0) = -30$$

and,

$$\Sigma\Delta H^\circ = \Delta H_f^\circ \text{ (products)} = \Delta H_f^\circ \text{ (reactants)}$$

$$= -716 - (-30) = -716 + 30 = -686 \text{ kcals.}$$

Question #16 (Answer: A) This is an application of Hess' Law using bond energies:

	ΔH
C = O → C + O	170
C + O → C – O	– 84
C = O → C – O	86
C = C → 2C	147
2C → C – C	– 83
C = C → C – C	64

Question #17 (Answer: A) Again apply Hess' Law to each by adding all bond energies in products and reactants:

		ΔH
I	$H_2 + C_2H_4 \rightarrow 6H + 2C$	
	104 + 4(99) + 147	
	H-H 4C-H C=C	647 kcal
	$6H + 2C \rightarrow C_2H_6$	
	83 + 6(99)	– 677 kcal
	C-C + 6CH	
net	$H_2 + C_2H_4 \rightarrow C_2H_6$	– 30 kcal
II	$H_2 + CH_2O \rightarrow 4H + C + O$	
	104 + 2(99) + 170	472 kcal
	H-H CH C = O	
	$4H + C + O \rightarrow CH_3OH$	
	3(99) + 84 + 111	– 492 kcal
	3C-H + C-O + OH	
net	$H_2 + CH_2O \rightarrow CH_3OH$	– 20 kcal

Questions #18 to #37: Adequately discussed in the Section.

Question #38 (Answer: A) During a phase conversion step, energy is used to break intermolecular bonds and is not used to increase the average kinetic energy of the molecules (raise the temperature).

Question #39 (Answer: C)

heat of fusion = calories required for phase change/mass undergoing phase change
= 100 cals/10 gms = 10 cals/gm

Question #40 (Answer: C)

$Q = C\,m\Delta t = (2\text{ cals/gm}\cdot{}^\circ C)(10\text{ gms})(60 - 10^\circ C) = (2)(10)(50)\text{ cals}$
$Q = 1000\text{ cals}$

Question #41 (Answer: C)

$C = Q/m\Delta t = 45\text{ cals}/(5\text{ gms})(75 - 25^\circ C) = 9/50 = 0.18\ (\text{cals/gm}\cdot{}^\circ C)$

Question #42 (Answer: C) The scheme is:

water (solid) at 0°C →(1) water (liquid) at 0°C →(2) water (liquid) at 50°C

(1) heat of fusion (H_f) of water for phase change
cals = (H_f)(mass) = (80 cals/gm)(10 gms) = 800 cals

(2) SH of water (liq) to raise temperature
cals = (SH)(mass)(temp change) = $C\,m\Delta t$
= (1.0)(10)(50 – 0) = (10)(50) = 500 cals

Total: (1) + (2) = 800 + 500 = 1300 cals.

Question #43 (Answer: B) The total heat delivered in 10 mins. is:

cals = (50 cals/min)(10 mins) = 500 cals.

The scheme for water changes is:

water (solid) at 0°C →(1) water (liquid) at 0°C

(1) heat of fusion (H_f) of water for phase change
H_f = heat change/mass = Q/m
m = Q/H_f = 500 cals/(80 cals/gm) = 6.25 gms.

Question #44 (Answer: A) Use ratio and proportion and known facts about temperature scales:

$$\begin{aligned}(50-0)/(100-0) &= (F-32)/(212-32) = (F-32)/180\\ (50)(180)/100 &= F-32\\ 90 &= F-32\\ 122 &= F\end{aligned}$$

°C		°F
100	BP	212
50		?°F
0	FP	32

BP = boiling point
FP = freezing point

(The key to understanding this is noting that the distances on the scales are equal even though the calibrations differ.)

Question #45 (Answer: C) This is similar to Question #27:

°C		°F
100	BP	212
?°C		?°F
0	FP	32

$$\begin{aligned}C-0/100-0 &= F-32/212-32\\ C/100 &= F-32/180\\ \text{now } C &= F \text{ for problem}\\ F/100 &= F-32/180\\ 180F/100 &= F-32\\ 9F/5 &= F-32\\ 9F &= 5F-160\\ 4F &= -160\\ F &= -40^\circ = C\end{aligned}$$

Question #46 (Answer: A) The following relationship holds:

$$\gamma = 3\alpha = (3)(2 \times 10^{-5}{}^\circ C^{-1}) = 6 \times 10^{-5}{}^\circ C^{-1}.$$

Question #47 (Answer: C) The coefficient of volume expansion (γ) is:

$$\gamma = 3\alpha = (3)(2 \times 10^{-4}{}^\circ C^{-1}) = 6 \times 10^{-4}{}^\circ C^{-1}.$$

The formula for volume expansion is:

$$\begin{aligned} V &= V_o(1 + \gamma\Delta t) \\ &= (10.000)[1 + (6 \times 10^{-4})(100)] = 10.000\,[1 + (6 \times 10^{-4})(10^2)] \\ &= (10.000)(1 + 6 \times 10^{-2}) = (10.000)(1 + 0.06) \\ &= (10.000)(1.06) = 10.600 \text{ liters.} \end{aligned}$$

Question #48 (Answer: B) The formula for heat rate in conduction is:

$$H = k(A/L)\Delta t$$

$$H \propto A \text{ and } H \propto 1/L \text{ or,}$$
$$H \propto A/L.$$

Then k and Δt are constants. And,

$$\begin{aligned} A_1 &= (2)(2) = 4\ m^2 \quad \text{(area of a square)} \\ L_1 &= 4\ m \\ A_2 &= (4)(4) = 16\ m^2 \\ L_2 &= 8\ m \end{aligned}$$

Putting these in either of the formulas above

$$\frac{H_2}{H_1} = \frac{k\frac{A_2}{L_2}\Delta t}{k\frac{A_1}{L_1}\Delta t} = \frac{\frac{A_2}{L_2}}{\frac{A_1}{L_1}} = \frac{A_2}{L_2} \cdot \frac{L_1}{A_1} = \frac{(16)}{(8)} \cdot \frac{(4)}{(4)} = 2$$

$$H_2 = 2H_1$$

Question #49 (Answer: B) Using the Stefan-Boltzmann Law:

$$R = e\delta T^4$$

1 = original 2 = final

$$T_1 = 20^\circ + 273^\circ = 293^\circ, \qquad T_2 = 10^\circ + 273^\circ = 283^\circ$$

$$\frac{R_2}{R_1} = \frac{e\delta T_2^4}{e\delta T_1^4} = \frac{T_2^4}{T_1^4} = (283/293)^4 = 0.87$$

$$R_2 = 0.87R_1$$

5.12.5 Checklist for Thermodynamics and Thermochemistry

______ enthalpy
______ standard enthalpy of formation
______ standard enthalpy of a reaction
______ Hess' Law
______ entropy
______ free energy
______ exothermic
______ endothermic
______ relation between ΔH, ΔS and ΔG and meaning of each
______ use of Hess' Law
______ use of meaning of bond energies
______ First Law of Thermodynamics
______ Second Law of Thermodynamics
______ equivalence of joules and calories

______ celsius (centigrade)
______ Fahrenheit
______ Rankine
______ Kelvin
______ interconversions of temperature scales
______ coefficients of thermal expansion
______ conduction
______ convection
______ radiation (of heat)
______ specific heat
______ heat capacity
______ heat of fusion
______ heat of vaporization
______ internal energy

5.13 RATE PROCESSES IN CHEMICAL REACTIONS—KINETICS AND EQUILIBRIUM

5.13.1 Review of Rate Processes in Chemical Reactions

5.13.1.1 KINETICS

Kinetics deals with the rates (how fast) of chemical reactions. This means it relates to the activation energy (see below) rather than the ΔH (enthalpy change) of a reaction as in thermodynamics (Section 5.12.1).

For a chemical reaction to occur, several conditions must be met. They are:

(1) the molecules must *collide* (make contact). The more they collide, the greater the chance of a reaction.

(2) The molecules must have enough energy to react once they have collided. Remember that molecules have a distribution of kinetic energies (Boltzmann distribution), and only some of the molecules will have enough energy to react. Note: Kinetic energy is proportional to the average temperature of the molecules.

(3) Given a collision and sufficient energy, a molecule may not react unless the *orientation* is correct. The energy requirements and orientation are related in that some orientations require less energy for reaction to occur.

The three factors above help determine the *activation energy* (E_A). The E_A is the energy barrier which must be overcome for a reaction to occur. The higher the E_A, the slower the reaction. A *catalyst* (a substance not used up or changed in a reaction) speeds up reactions by lowering the E_A. This is how *enzymes* work.

Most reactions proceed as a series of steps which are exemplified by chain reactions. *Chain reactions* are exemplified by radical reactions such as halogenation. The steps are as follows:

(1) *Initiation* — the production of radicals

$$Cl_2 \rightarrow 2Cl^-$$

(2) *Propagation* — the production of radicals by reaction with radicals, this keeps the reaction going:

$$Cl^- + R_3CH \rightarrow R_3C^{\bullet} + HCl$$
$$R_3C^{\bullet} + Cl_2 \rightarrow R_3CCl + Cl^-$$

(3) *Termination* — the destruction of radicals by the reactions of two radicals with each other or by the reactions of radicals with the walls of the container:

$$Cl^- + R_3C^{\bullet} \rightarrow R_3CCl$$
$$R_3C^{\bullet} + R_3C^{\bullet} \rightarrow R_3C - CR_3$$

There are many possible overall paths (reaction coordinates) which may be taken by reactants being converted to products. The path taken will be the one with the lowest E_A. Each step, i.e., each E_A in an overall path, is called an *elementary process.* The elementary process with the highest E_A is the *slowest step (rate determining* step) and determines the overall rate of the reaction. If one molecule is involved in an elementary process, it is said to be *unimolecular.* If two molecules, it is said to be bimolecular, if three, then *trimolecular*, etc. Given an overall path (with its composite elementary processes), the *principle of microscopic reversibility* states that the elementary processes of the reverse reaction are the same as the forward reaction (Fig. 5.21).

$$\text{reactants} \rightleftharpoons I_1 \rightleftharpoons I_2 \rightleftharpoons I_3 \rightleftharpoons \text{products}$$

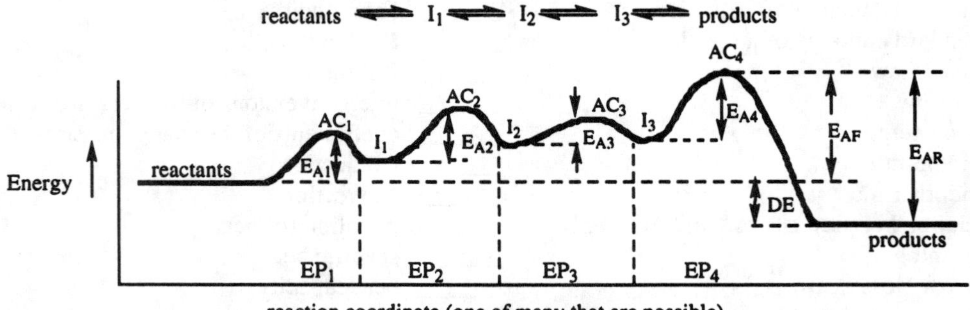

Fig. 5.21—A Reaction Coordinate

EP = elementary process

AC = activated complex, a transient species that may be converted to products or reactants, cannot be isolated; also called the *transition state complex*

I = intermediates, transient species that may be isolated in some instances; note they are like "rest points" between the EP's

E_A = activation energies

E_{A_F} = overall E_A for forward reaction

E_{A_R} = overall E_A for reverse reaction

ΔE = energy of the reaction = $E_{A_R} - E_{A_F}$

The *rates of reactions* are quantified in terms of *rate expressions* which relate the change in concentration of one reactant (or product) with time to the concentration of other reactants (or products):

for,

$$aA + bB \rightarrow cC + dD \text{ (overall reaction)}$$

the rate expression might be,

$$\text{rate} = \frac{\Delta[A]}{\Delta t} = -k\,[A]^m\,[B]^n$$

the minus sign (–) is because [A] is decreasing with time,

k = rate constant for the reaction

[ ] = concentration in moles/liter (molarity).

Note that the exponents of $A^{(m)}$ and $B^{(n)}$ do not, in general, equal the coefficients of A(a) and B(b). This points out that rate expressions cannot be determined from the stoichiometric equations; they must be determined by experiment. The rate of reaction, and hence, the rate expression, varies during the course of the reaction. This is because the net reaction rate is,

net rate = forward rate – reverse rate,

forward rate = $k_f\,[A]^m[B]^n$

reverse rate = $k_r\,[C]^x[D]^y$.

The *forward rate* depends on the concentration of the reactants, and the *reverse rate* depends on the concentration of the products. Early (initially) in the reaction, there are more reactants and the forward rate dominates. As reactants are converted to products, there accumulates more products and the reverse rate increases until it equals the forward rate. This point is equilibrium (Fig. 5.22).

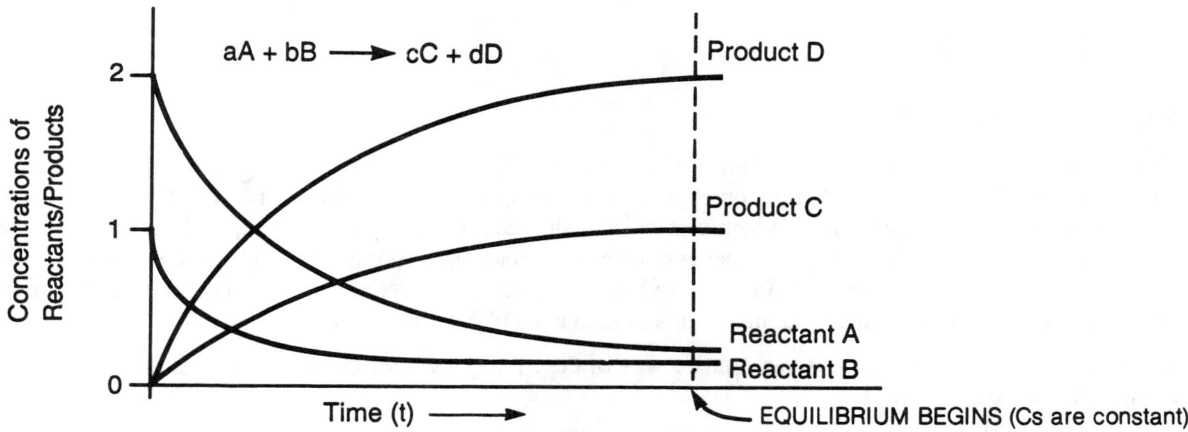

The rate is Δc/Δt = slope, and this changes going from t=0 to equilibrium.

Fig. 5.22—Course of a Reaction

For the reason above, most rate expressions are for *initial rates* (reactants present but no products) and, hence, are forward rates and take the form:

$$\text{rate} = k[A]^m[B]^n$$

The problem then is to determine the values of m and n. This is done by varying the concentration of one reactant while holding other reactants constant and determining how the rate is affected by this. The *order* of the reaction (contrasted with molecularity) is the sum of the exponents in the experimentally derived rate expression. For example:

given: $\text{rate} = k[A]^2[B]^{1/2}$

then: order of reaction = $2 + {}^1/2 = 2{}^1/2$
order of reactant in $\underline{A} = 2$
order of reactant in $\underline{B} = {}^1/2$

First order kinetics means the order is one, second order is two, etc. The rate constant can be calculated once the orders in each reactant is known:

$$k = \frac{\text{rate}}{[A]^2[B]^{1/2}}$$

From the collision theory of gaseous reactions, the following equation is derived:

$k = Ae^{-E_A/RT}$
k = rate constant
A = a constant which includes collision, orientation, and molecular factors
e = base of natural logs
E_A = activation energy
R = 1.99 cal/mole – °K
T = absolute temperature

The E_A can be calculated by determining the rate constant at a number of different temperatures and making this plot:

$$\ln k = \ln A - \frac{E_A}{R} \cdot \frac{1}{T}$$

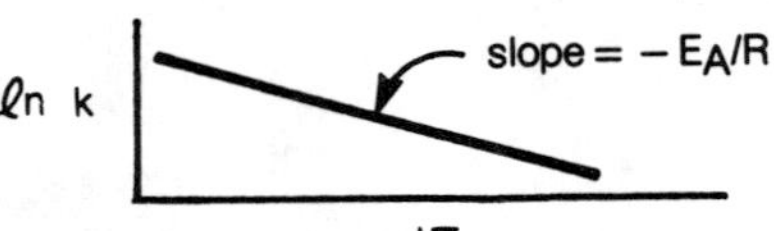

Comparing with the slope-intercept form of a straight line equation (y = b + mx), Intercept, b = lnA

Slope, m = $-E_A/R$
y = ln k
x = 1/T

5.13.1.2 EQUILIBRIUM

All chemical reactions proceed toward an equilibrium state. The *equilibrium state* exists when the forward rate equals the reverse rate: hence, there is no change in the components of the reaction (see 5.13.1.1). This points out that the equilibrium state is a dynamic state; i.e., the reactions have not ceased, and reactants are being converted to products and products are being converted to reactants. At equilibrium, ΔG (free energy) is zero, ΔH (enthalpy) is a minimum, and ΔS (entropy) is maximum (see Section 5.12.1). This means that there is *minimum energy* and *maximum randomness* in a system at equilibrium.

The *equilibrium constant* (K) is a quantitative way of describing the interrelationships of the concentrations of components at equilibrium. It is:

given the reaction: $aA + bB \underset{K_2}{\overset{K_1}{\rightleftharpoons}} cC + dD$

forward rate = $K_1\,[A]^a[B]^b$

backward rate = $K_2\,[C]^c[D]^d$

then the equilibrium constant is:

forward rate = backward rate

$K_1 [A]^a[B]^b = K_2 [C]^c[D]^d$

$K = \frac{K_1}{K_2} = \frac{[C]^c[D]^d}{[A]^a[B]^b}$ depends only on temperature

[ ] = concentration in moles/liter (molarity)
[gases] = atmospheres
[pure solids] = constant

The constant K is a measure of the capacity of reactants to be converted to products. The larger the K, the more reactants will be converted to products. The expression:

$$\frac{[C]^c[D]^d}{[A]^a[B]^b}$$

can be determined *at points other than equilibrium. The direction the reaction must proceed to get to equilibrium* can be determined by comparing the values of the expression with the K:

$$\text{if } \frac{[C]c[D]^d}{[A]^a[B]^b} < K$$

then the reaction proceeds to equilibrium from left to right as written (the numerator, products, must increase and/or the denominator, reactants, must decrease for the expression to equal K);

$$\text{if } \frac{[C]^c[D]^d}{[A]^a[B]^b} > K$$

then the reaction proceeds to equilibrium from right to left as written (the reverse of the above).

Note that the equilibrium constant for the reverse (K_R) of a given reaction (K) is:

$$K_R = 1/K.$$

The overall equilibrium constant (K) for a series of reactions is the product of the individual equilibrium constants:

$K = K_1K_2K_3 \ldots\ldots$ (Memorize for the MCAT)

When a reaction is *exothermic* (ΔH is negative), K actually decreases as the temperature increases. The reverse is true for an endothermic reaction (see 5.12.1).

Le Chatelier's Principle is a good way to determine what the effect of a change in condition (e.g., concentration) will do to the relative concentrations of reactants/products and other factors (e.g., heat, volume) in a reaction. The Principle is:

> Any perturbation (change) to a system initially at equilibrium will cause that system (if left alone) to adjust in such a way as to offset that perturbation.

This means the system will go toward a new equilibrium but with concentrations and other factors appropriately adjusted. A practical way of using Le Chatelier's Principle is:

(1) Write all the components and conditions of the reaction on the appropriate side of the equation. This includes all the reactants, products, heat and volume. The heat is the heat of the reaction. If positive, it is a reactant; if negative, it is a product (see 5.12.1). Remember that an increase in temperature is like increasing the energy (heat) and vice versa. The volume can be related to the moles (in the balanced equation) of gases in the reaction. Put the volume on the side with the fewer moles of gas ("balances" out the volume). Remember that as pressure increases, the volume decreases and vice versa.

(2) Apply these rules (from Le Chatelier's) to determine how the equilibrium will shift:

(a) if a component or condition increases, the reaction is shifted to the opposite side; i.e., components/conditions on the other side will increase and those on the same side will decrease;

(b) if a component/condition decreases, the reaction is shifted to its side, the other components/conditions on that side increase and the components/conditions on the opposite decrease.

An example is:

given the reaction,

$$M_2(g) + 3E_2(g) \rightleftharpoons 2ME_3(g) \qquad \Delta H = +\ 10\ \text{kcals}$$

Rewrite using the rules above.

$$\text{heat} + M_2(g) + 3E_2(g) \rightleftharpoons 2ME_3(g) + \text{volume}$$

Examples of effects of perturbations are:

if $\uparrow M_2$,
reaction shifts to right

If $\downarrow E_2$,
reaction shifts to left

if $\uparrow$ pressure,
this causes volume to decrease
reaction shifts to right

if $\downarrow$ temperature,
same as decreasing heat and decreasing volume
reaction shift is indeterminate

if add a catalyst
no shift in equilibrium by a catalyst,
catalyst *only affects rate of reaction.*

5.13.1.3 APPLICATIONS OF RATE PROCESSES IN CHEMICAL REACTIONS TO THE HUMAN BODY

Biochemical reactions in the human body are dependent on rate processes in chemical reactions—both kinetics and equilibrium. The study of biochemistry requires a fairly good background in activation energy and metabolic processes applied to the average human body. The following basic concepts and terms should be thoroughly reviewed and understood as you finish your review in general chemistry.

(a) Maximum catalytic rates of enzymes; fundamentals of enzyme kinetics in relation to Michaelis-Menten equations and graphs, analysis of kinetic tabular data and enzyme inhibitors.

(b) The relation of pH to rate of enzymatic reactions.

(c) Metabolic pathways—catabolism and anabolism including experimental techniques to study metabolic inhibitors; use of isotopes and autoradiography.

(d) Glycogen metabolism related to blood glucose levels—graphing enzyme activity versus glucose concentration.

(e) Kinetics of mediated transport.

(f) Physiology of protein, carbohydrate, lipid metabolism in the human body.

The physical and chemical concepts related to biochemical reactions should be reviewed before studying sections 7.1 and 7.2 in the Biological Sciences (chapter 7). Kinetics and equilibrium concepts should be directly linked to more advanced biological concepts, which are essential for the study of medicine.

5.13.2 Questions to Review Kinetics and Equilibrium

1. All of the following conditions must be met in order for a chemical reaction to occur except:

   A. collisions.
   B. sufficient energy per molecule to react.
   C. appropriate orientation of colliding molecules.
   D. homeostasis.

2. The energy that must be overcome for a chemical reaction to occur is called the:

   A. enthalpy.
   B. activation energy.
   C. entropy.
   D. free energy.

3. The steps in a chain reaction include all except:

   A. initiation.
   B. propagation.
   C. acceleration.
   D. termination.

4. The step in which radicals already present are used to generate new radicals is called:

   A. initiation.
   B. propagation.
   C. acceleration.
   D. extermination.

Use the following diagram to answer Questions #5 through #7.

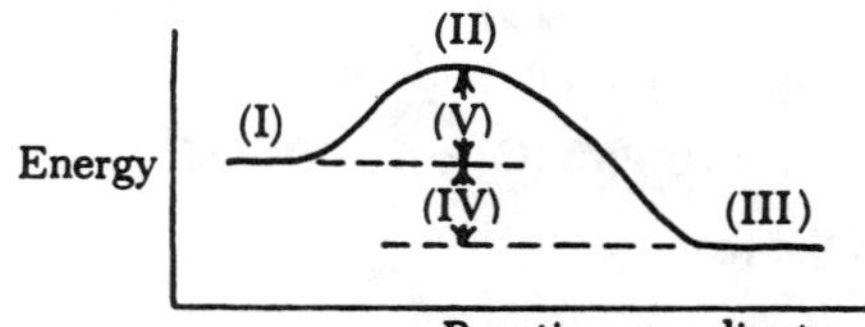

5. The activation energy of the forward reaction is given by:

   A. II
   B. III
   C. IV
   D. V

6. The heat of the reaction is given by:

   A. II
   B. III
   C. IV
   D. V

7. The activated complex would be located at:

   A. I
   B. II
   C. III
   D. none of the above

8. The rate determining step of a reaction with a series of steps is characterized by:

   A. the lowest energy of activation.
   B. the highest energy of activation.
   C. the highest enthalpy.
   D. none of the above.

9. The role of a catalyst is to:

A. shift the equilibrium of the reaction in favor of the products.
B. speed up the reaction by raising the activation energy.
C. speed up the reaction by lowering the activation energy.
D. shift the equilibrium of the reaction in favor of the reactants.

10. At equilibrium:

A. the forward reaction continues.
B. the reverse reaction continues.
C. there is minimum energy and maximum randomness.
D. all of the above statements are true.

11. As the value of K (the equilibrium constant) becomes larger:

A. more products will be present at equilibrium.
B. less products will be present at equilibrium.
C. the faster the reaction will proceed.
D. the slower the reaction will proceed.

12. Given the reaction symbolized as: $A \overset{K}{\rightleftharpoons} B$,
if $[B]/[A] = 2 \times 10^{-5}$ and it is known that $K = 5 \times 10^{-4}$ from other experiments, in what direction must the reaction proceed to reach equilibrium?

A. [B] must increase and/or [A] decrease
B. [B] must decrease and/or [A] decrease
C. [B] and [A] should be equal to start the reaction
D. cannot be determined from the information given

13. For the reaction: $A + 2B \overset{K}{\rightleftharpoons} 2C$, the concentration, in moles/liter, of the components at equilibrium are:

$$[A] = 1 \times 10^{-2}M,\ [B] = 2 \times 10^{-3}M,\ [C] = 5 \times 10^{-6}\ M.$$

What is the equilibrium constant (K) of the reaction?

A. 6.25×10^{-4}
B. 0.225
C. 25
D. none of the above

Use the following information for Questions #14 through #17.

$$C_2H_5OH(l) + 3O_2(g) \rightleftharpoons 2CO_2(g) + 3H_2O(l) \quad \Delta H° = -327 \text{ kcals}$$

14. If the temperature is increased, the equilibrium:

A. shifts to the left.
B. shifts to the right.
C. is unchanged.
D. can never be achieved.

15. If the pressure is increased, the equilibrium:

A. shifts to the left.
B. shifts to the right.
C. is unchanged.
D. depends on volume.

16. If $O_2(g)$ is added, the equilibrium:

A. shifts to the left.
B. shifts to the right.
C. is unchanged.
D. can never be achieved.

17. A chemical is added which absorbs $CO_2(g)$. This will cause the equilibrium to be:

A. shifted to the left.
B. shifted to the right.
C. unchanged.
D. independent of any catalysts.

Use the following information for Questions #18 through #21.

$$CH_4(g) + H_2O(l) \rightleftharpoons CH_3OH(l) + H_2(g) \quad \Delta H = +29 \text{ kcal}$$

18. If the $H_2(g)$ formed is allowed to escape from the reaction, the equilibrium will be:

A. shifted to the left.
B. shifted to the right.
C. unchanged.
D. unattainable in thirty seconds or less.

19. If the pressure is doubled, the equilibrium:

A. shifts to the left.
B. shifts to the right.
C. is unchanged.
D. is acquired within two minutes.

20. Suppose CO_2 catalyzes this reaction. If it is added, the equilibrium:

A. shifts to the left.
B. shifts to the right.
C. is unchanged.
D. cannot be achieved.

21. If the temperature is decreased, the equilibrium:

A. shifts to the left.
B. shifts to the right.
C. is unchanged.
D. is unchanged forever.

5.13.3 Answers to Questions in Section 5.13.2

(1) D (2) B (3) C (4) B (5) D (6) C (7) B (8) B (9) C (10) D (11) A (12) A

(13) A (14) A (15) B (16) B (17) B (18) B (19) C (20) C (21) A

5.13.4 Discussion of Answers to Questions in Section 5.13.2

Questions #1 to #11: Adequately discussed in the text.

Question #12 (Answer: A) In this case [B] / [A] <K because $2 \times 10^{-5} < 5 \times 10^{-4}$. Then for [B] / [A] to become equal to K, the [B] must increase and the [A] must decrease.

Question #13 (Answer: A) The equilibrium constant (K) is,

$$K = \frac{[\,C\,]^2}{[\,A\,][\,B\,]^2} = \frac{[5 \times 10^{-6}]^2}{[1 \times 10^{-2}][2 \times 10^{-3}]^2} = \frac{25 \times 10^{-12}}{(10^{-2})(4 \times 10^{-6})}$$

$$K = \frac{25 \times 10^{-12}}{4 \times 10^{-8}} = \frac{25}{4} \times 10^{-12+8} = 6.25 \times 10^{-4}$$

Question #14 (Answer: A) The complete equation is

$$C_2H_5OH(l) + 3O_2(g) \rightleftharpoons 2CO_2(g) + 3H_2O(l) + \text{vol.} + \text{heat.}$$

Volume goes on the right side because there are fewer moles of gas on that side. Heat goes on the right because the reaction is exothermic, i.e., heat is a product. hen an increase in temperature causes an increase in heat which shifts the reaction to the opposite side (the left).

Question #15 (Answer: B) See #14. An increase in pressure causes a decrease in volume. A decrease in volume pulls a reaction to its side (the right).

Question #16 (Answer: B) The added O_2 shifts the reaction to the opposite side (the right). Increased temperature also increases the volume (Charles' law). This also shifts the reaction to the left.

Question #17 (Answer: B) The $CO_2(g)$ decreases and this pulls the reaction to its side (the right).

Question #18 (Answer: B) The overall equation is:

$$\text{heat} + CH_4(g) + H_2O(l) \rightleftharpoons CH_3OH(l) + H_2(g).$$

The heat is on the left because the reaction is endothermic which means heat is used as a reactant. There is no volume factor because there is an equal number of moles of gases on both sides. Since the H_2 is being removed, the reaction is pulled to its side (the right).

Question #19 (Answer: C) See #18. There is no volume factor so the pressure has no effect.

Question #20 (Answer: C) Catalysts do not affect the equilibrium of a reaction.

Question #21 (Answer: A) A decrease in temperature is like decreasing the heat which shifts the reaction to that side (the left).

5.13.5 Checklist for Kinetics and Equilibrium

______ kinetics
______ Le Chatelier's Principle
______ activation energy
______ equilibrium constant
______ propagation
______ intermediates
______ transition states
______ catalyst
______ chain reactions
______ initiation
______ termination
______ requirements for a chemical reaction to occur
______ steps in chain reactions
______ meaning of equilibrium and the equilibrium constant
______ use of Le Chatelier's Principle

5.14 FORCE AND MOTION, GRAVITATION

5.14.1 Review of Force and Motion, Gravitation

"Body" and "object" are used interchangeably in Physics. A body generally refers to a rigid body. A body consists of a large number of particles.

The *center of mass* (COM) of a body is that point whose motion can be described like a particle (e.g., as linear, circular, parabolic) even if the motion of the object cannot be so described. In collisions, the COM velocity (of the system) is not changed. The *center of gravity* (COG) is the COM but is conceptualized as that point where the sum of gravitational forces acting on an object can be represented by a summation force (acting at the COM). An object suspended from the COG is in rotational equilibrium (Section 5.17.1). The COG can be determined experimentally by suspending an object by a string at different points and noting that the direction of the string passes through the COG. The intersections of the projected lines in the different suspensions is the COG. The COG of a regular geometric object is the geometric center. The COG of an irregular object may be inside or outside the object. An object is in *stable equilibrium* if the COG is as low as possible, and any change in orientation will lead to an elevation of the COG. *Unstable equilibrium* is when the COG is high (relative to a surface supporting it, e.g.), and any change in orientation would lead to a lowering of the COG. *Neutral equilibrium* is an intermediate location of the COG and a change in orientation would not change the level of the COG. A force acting through the COG causes translational motion. A force acting off the COG causes rotational motion. *Mass* is a dimension that cannot be broken down into simpler units. This is to be contrasted with *weight* which is a force. Units of mass are slugs (weight in pounds divided by g = 32 ft/sec^2), kilograms, grams, etc. Units of weight are pounds (defined differently from the pounds of mass), dynes (gms·cm/sec^2) and newtons (kg·m/sec^2).

Newton's Second Law relates an unbalanced force acting upon an object, producing an acceleration in the direction of the force that is directly proportional to the force and inversely proportional to the mass of the body:

$$a = F/m$$

$$\text{or, } F = ma$$

For every action, there is an equal and opposite reaction. This is *Newton's Third Law*. If one object exerts a force, F, on a second object, the second object exerts a force, –F, on the first. These forces cannot neutralize each other because they act on different objects. Every force relates to three basic forces. These are gravitational (below), electromagnetic (Section 5.18), and nuclear (Section 5.23).

Newton's Second Law of Motion is considered to be the *most* important one for the MCAT student. Applications and uses of the *Second Law* include driving a nail into the wall, putting your foot on the accelerator of your car while driving, freely falling objects, inclined plane motion with friction, running compared to jogging, the movement of blood and drugs in your arteries and veins. Make sure that you draw a "*free–body*" diagram to solve problems which involve the second and third laws of motion.

As shown earlier, Force = mass × acceleration.
Momentum = mass × velocity.

$$\text{Hence, } \frac{\text{Force}}{\text{Momentum}} = \frac{\text{acceleration}}{\text{velocity}}$$

$$F = ma = \frac{m(v_f - v_i)}{(t_f - t_i)} \text{ (definition of acceleration)}$$

$$F(t_f - t_i) = m(v_f - v_i) \quad = \text{Impulse–Momentum Principle}$$

Newton also formulated the *Law of Gravitation* as:

$F = K_G(m_1 m_2/r^2)$, $K_G = G$ = Gravitational constant (do not confuse with Gibbs Free energy, ΔG)

This states that there is a gravitational force existing between any two bodies of masses m_1 and m_2. The force is proportional to the product of the masses:

$$F \propto m_1 m_2$$

and inversely proportional to the square of the distance between them:

$$F \propto 1/r^2$$

K_G is the universal constant of gravitation, and its value depends upon the units being used.

Frictional forces are illustrated in Fig. 5.23.

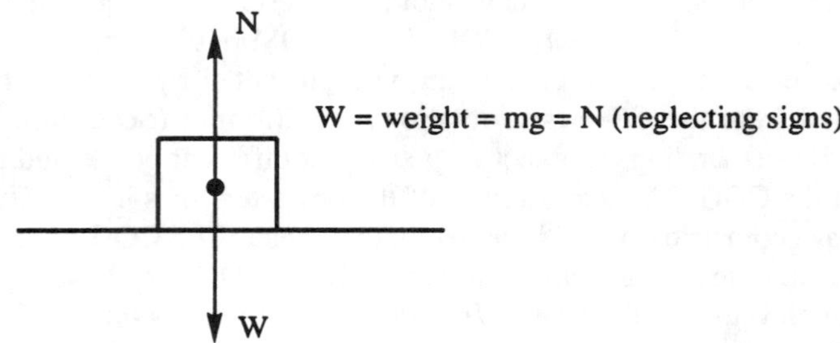

Fig. 5.23—Frictional Forces related to Normal Forces

F = μN, this is the maximal frictional force
μ = coefficient of friction
N = normal (perpendicular) force to the surface the object rests on.

Friction is the resistance offered to the motion of a body and is mostly caused by the roughness (ups and downs or indentations) between two rough bodies. Friction depends on the texture of the contact surface of two bodies.

Frictional forces are nonconservative (mechanical energy is not conserved) and are caused by molecular adhesions between tangential surfaces but are independent of the area of contact of the surfaces. Frictional forces always oppose motion. Static friction exists when the object is not moving, and it must be overcome for motion to begin. The coefficient of static friction, μ_s, is given as:

$$\mu_s = \tan\theta,$$

where Ø is the angle at which the object first begins to move. On an inclined plane as the angle is increased from 0° → Ø°, the object slips initially and later slides down the plane.

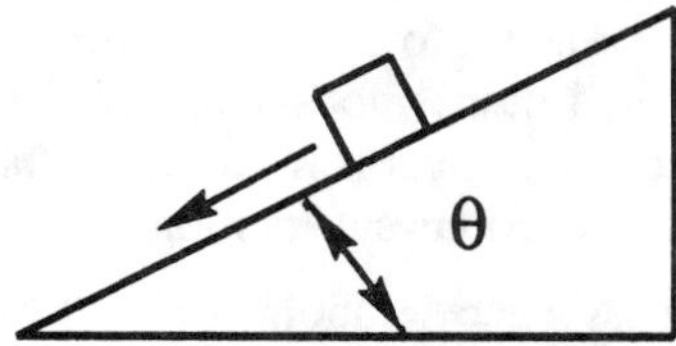

Fig. 5.24—Inclined Plane

There is also a coefficient of kinetic friction, μ_k, which exists when surfaces are in motion. Note that $\mu_s > \mu_k$ always, meaning that the static coefficient is always greater than the kinetic coefficient.

The analysis of *motion on an incline* is shown in Fig. 5.25.

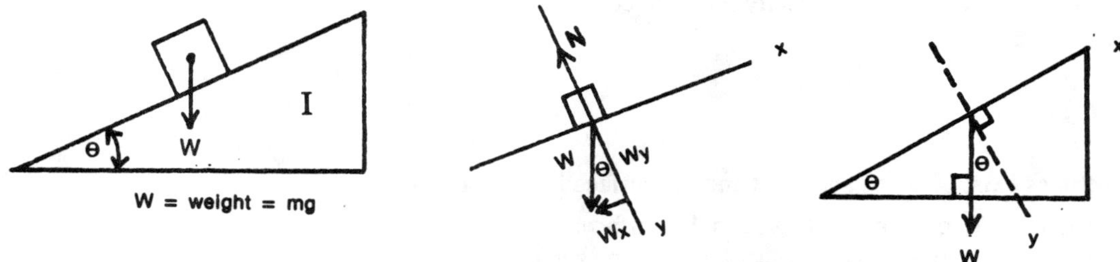

components of forces:

N = normal (perpendicular) force to the surface the object rests on.

$W_y = W\cos\Theta,\ W_x = W\sin\Theta$

Fig. 5.25—Motion on an Incline I (Neglecting Friction)

The weight (W) due to gravity (g) may be sufficient to cause motion if friction is overcome. The reference axes are usually chosen as shown such that one (the x) is along the surface of the incline. Additional forces such as tension (T) on the object added to the basic set above is shown in Fig. 5.26. Note that $m_2 > m_1$ and the free body diagram in Fig. 5.26 is for mass m_2.

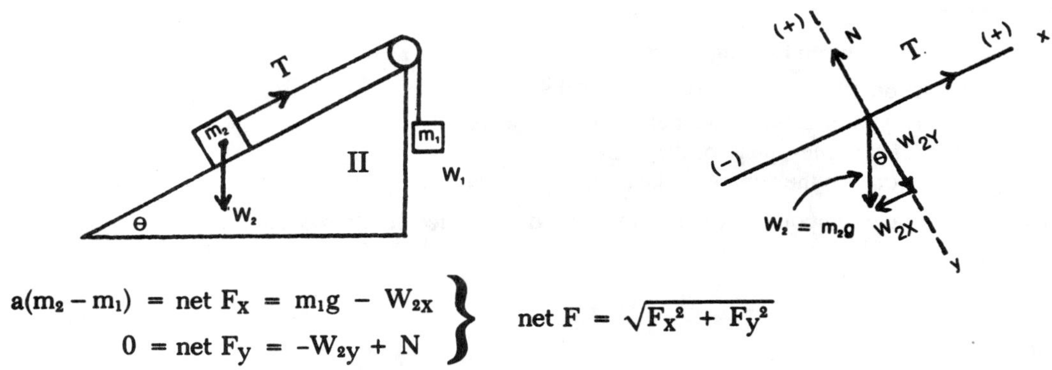

$$\left.\begin{aligned} a(m_2 - m_1) &= \text{net } F_x = m_1 g - W_{2x} \\ 0 &= \text{net } F_y = -W_{2y} + N \end{aligned}\right\} \quad \text{net } F = \sqrt{F_x^2 + F_y^2}$$

Fig. 5.26—Motion on an Incline II

Note that N is the reactive force to W_{2y}, the axes are assigned (+) and (−) as one desires.

5.14.2 Questions to Review Force and Motion, Gravitation

1. One of Newton's laws of motion states that:

- **A.** an unbalanced force acting upon an object produces an acceleration of that object.
- **B.** objects moving in circles at constant tangential velocity have no force acting upon them.
- **C.** the square of the period of revolution is proportional to the cube of the radius of revolution.
- **D.** objects falling to earth describe a hyperbolic projectory.

2. In order for any object to undergo an acceleration, it must:

- **A.** lose energy.
- **B.** gain energy.
- **C.** be acted upon by balanced (net zero) forces.
- **D.** be acted upon by unbalanced forces.

3. Newton's Second Law is mathematically represented by:

   A. $E = {}^1/2\ mv^2$
   B. $F = -kx$
   C. $U = mgh$
   D. $F = ma$

4. Frictional forces exist between an object and the surface it is on, and they:

   A. are proportional to the normal force to the surface.
   B. are dependent on the area of contact between the surfaces.
   C. always augment the motion of the object.
   D. are conservative forces.

5. For μ_S (coefficient of static friction) and μ_k (coefficient of kinetic friction):

   A. $\mu_S > \mu_k$
   B. $\mu_S = \mu_k$
   C. $\mu_S < \mu_k$
   D. $\mu_S \bullet \mu_k = 1$

6. The motion of the center of mass is like:

   A. the motion of a particle.
   B. the motion of an extended object.
   C. the motion of a rigid body.
   D. none of the above.

7. The force of gravitation between two objects is:

   A. inversely proportional to the products of the masses.
   B. inversely proportional to the distance between the objects.
   C. directly proportional to the square of the radius.
   D. inversely proportional to the square of the distance between the objects.

8. A force of 15 newtons acting upon a 5 kg object will produce an acceleration equal to:

   A. $^1/3$ m/sec^2
   B. $^1/75$ m/sec^2
   C. 3 m/sec^2
   D. 75 m/sec^2

9. An object has an acceleration of 2 m/sec^2 and a mass of a 5 kg. The force necessary to impart this acceleration is:

   A. 0.4 newtons
   B. 2.5 newtons
   C. 5 newtons
   D. 10 newtons

10. If F = force, ΔU = potential energy change, Δx = displacement over which ΔU occurs, then:

   A. $F = \Delta U \Delta x$
   B. $F = 1/\Delta U \Delta x$
   C. $F = -\Delta x/\Delta U$
   D. $F = -\Delta U/\Delta x$

11. An object first begins to slip down an inclined plane when the angle with the horizontal is 45°. The coefficient of static friction (μ_S) of the object–surface is:

   A. 0.5
   B. 1.0
   C. $\sqrt{2/2}$
   D. need more information

Use the following speed–time graph for Questions #12 through #16.

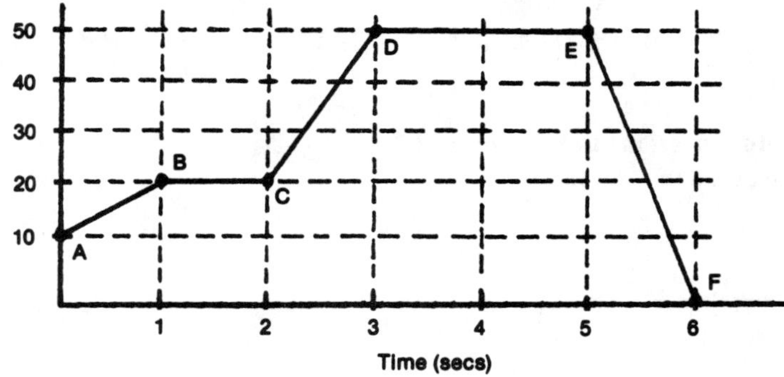

The above is a graph for a 2 kg object moving along a straight line to the right.

12. The area under the graph represents:

A. distance.
B. acceleration.
C. force.
D. velocity.

13. The greatest force is acting at:

A. AB
B. BC
C. CD
D. EF

14. No net force is acting along:

A. AB
B. BC
C. CD
D. EF

15. The distance traveled from A to B is:

A. 5 m
B. 10 m
C. 15 m
D. 20 m

16. At point F, the object is:

A. motionless.
B. moving backward.
C. moving forward.
D. at the origin.

17. What value of weight (W_1) is required such that the object (A) does not move down the incline (assume no friction):

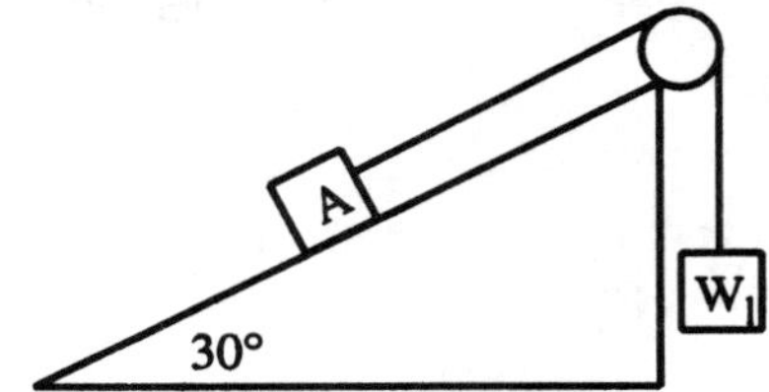

mass of A is 10 kg

A. 5 newtons
B. 10 newtons
C. 49 newtons
D. none of the above

5.14.3 Answers to Questions in Section 5.14.2

(1) A (2) D (3) D (4) A (5) A (6) A (7) D (8) C (9) D (10) D (11) B (12) A
(13) D (14) B (15) C (16) A (17) C

5.14.4 Discussion of Answers to Questions in Section 5.14.2

Questions #1 to #7: Adequately discussed in the Section.

Question #8 (Answer: C)

$$F = ma$$
$$a = F/m = 15 \text{ newtons}/5 \text{ kgs} = 3(\text{nts/kg})$$
$$= 3[\text{kg–m/sec}^2)/\text{kg}] = 3 \text{ m/sec}^2$$

Question #9 (Answer: D)

$$F = ma = (5 \text{ kg})(2 \text{ m/sec}^2) = 10 \text{ kg–m/sec}^2 = 10 \text{ newtons.}$$

Question #10 (Answer: D) If the relationship is not already known to you, it may be determined (in this case) by knowing unit interrelations (i.e., by doing dimensional analysis as shown):

energy = work = Fd (Section 5.15.1)
Force = energy/displacement, which is the *form* of answer (D).

Force = newtons and energy = joules = *newtons–meters* and d = meters, the only way to combine the units of energy and displacement to yield the units of force is:

$$\text{newtons (force)} \propto \frac{\text{newtons–meters (energy)}}{\text{meters (displacement)}} = \text{newtons}$$

or

$$\text{Force} \propto \frac{\text{energy}}{\text{displacement}}$$

Force is proportional to energy/displacement.

Question #11 (Answer: B) μ_s is found by:

$$\mu_s = \tan\theta$$
$$\mu_s = \tan 45°$$
$$\mu_s = 1/1 = 1$$

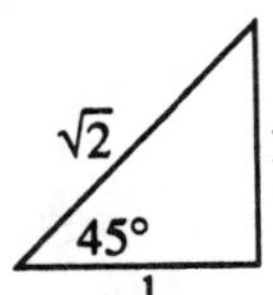

$\tan\theta$ = opposite/adjacent.

Question #12 (Answer: A) The area under any curve is proportional to the product of the quantities represented by the axes:

y–axis is speed (v)
x–axis is time (t)
product = (v)(t) = distance.

Question #13 (Answer: D) The greatest force acts where the greatest acceleration (positive or negative) acts. This is because:

$$F = ma \text{ and } F \propto a.$$

The greatest acceleration is where the slope $\Delta v/\Delta t$ is the greatest in absolute value (neglecting signs). For each of the above line segments, the slope, and acceleration, is:

	a	=	$\Delta v/\Delta t = (v_f - v_i)/(t_f - t_i)$				
AB:	a	=	(20 – 10)/(1 – 0)	=	10/1	=	10
BC:	a	=	(20 – 20)/(2 – 1)	=	0/1	=	0
CD:	a	=	(50 – 20)/(3 – 2)	=	30/1	=	30
EF:	a	=	(0 – 50)/(6 – 5)	=	–50/1	=	–50.

Hence, EF has the greatest acceleration and the greatest force.

Question #14 (Answer: B) Again, since F = ma and $F \propto a$, a zero acceleration gives a zero force. A zero acceleration occurs where the slope is zero. See the discussion in Question #13 for the slopes of the segments. BC is the only one with a zero slope and, therefore, a zero acceleration and a zero force.

Question #15 (Answer: C)

(I) By geometry:

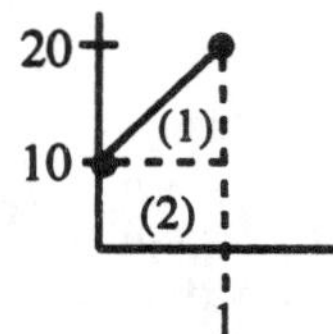

Area (1) = $(^1/_2)(10)(1) = 5$m
Area (2) = (10)(1) = 10m
total = 5 + 10 = 15 m

(II) By formulas:

$d = d_o + v_o t + {}^1/_2 at^2$ (Section 5.16.1)

$d_o = 0 \quad v_o = 10$ m/sec

$a = \Delta v/\Delta t = (20 - 10)/(1 - 0) = 10/1 = 10$ m/sec^2

$t = 1$ sec

$d = 0 + (10)(1) + (^1/_2)(10)(1)^2 = 10 + 5 = 15$ m.

Question #16 (Answer: A) The speed is zero at point F, so the object must not be moving. Also, note that at no point is the speed negative, so the object could not have returned to the origin.

Question #17 (Answer: C) The schematic showing the forces is:

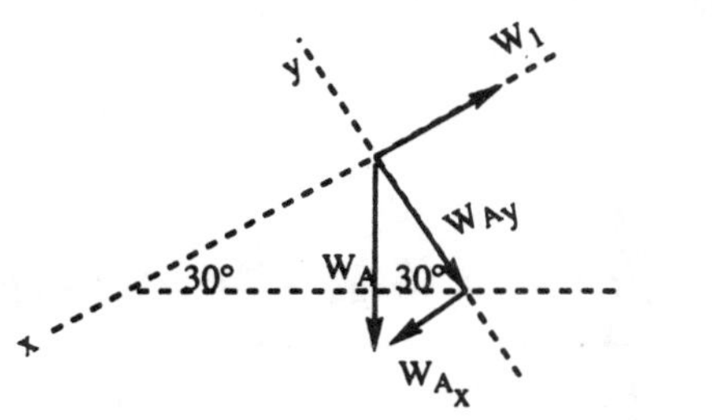

$W_A = mg = (10)(9.8) = 98$ nts

$W_{A_x} = W_A \sin 30° = (98)(1/2) = 49$nts

Remember:

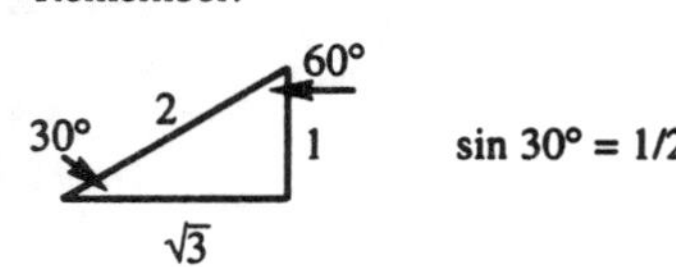

In order for the object not to move, W_1 should balance W_{Ax}. W_{Ay} has no effect on motion along x (the incline). Therefore, W_1 of 49 nts is required. The mass would be:

$$m = W_1/g = 49/9.8 = 5 \text{ kgs.}$$

5.14.5 Checklist for Force and Motion, Gravitation

______ center of mass
______ center of gravity
______ Newton's second law
______ motion on an incline
______ Newton's third law
______ Law of gravitation
______ friction
______ mass
______ weight

5.15 WORK AND ENERGY

5.15.1 Review of Work and Energy

Energy is a scalar and is generally conceptualized as the ability to do work. Note that objects exert forces upon other objects, and if a displacement results, work (see below) is performed which is not contained within the object. Energy, by contrast, is contained by the object (or system), and if work is performed, this energy either increases or decreases (for negative or positive work respectively).

$$\text{Work} = \text{Force times distance} = F \times d$$

Mechanical energy is divided into kinetic energy (K) and potential energy (U). *Kinetic energy* is the energy associated with the motion of objects. *Potential energy* is the energy that results by position or configuration (of a system); there is no motion. When motion begins, potential energy is converted into kinetic energy. The formulation of potential energy depends upon the system.

U = mgh = gravitational potential energy
m = mass
h = height above earth's surface.
k = $(1/2)mv^2$ = kinetic energy
v = speed of object

Additional features of potential energy are: (1) potential energy *cannot* be defined for frictional forces, and (2) the potential energy of a system is independent (in contrast to work) of the path to reach that system.

Potential energy can be of many types such as: magnetic, electric, chemical. Always remember potential energy as a *field* that exists around molecules.

The *Law of Conservation of Mechanical Energy* is:

Total Energy (TE) = kinetic energy (K) + potential energy (U) + energy due to dissipative forces (e.g., friction).

In the absence of dissipative forces, this can be taken as:

TE = K + U

On the actual MCAT the questions normally reflect applications of energy conservation. Remember that potential and kinetic energies at *any* two points, along the path of movement of the particle, can be easily found by the following formula: $K_1 + U_1 = K_2 + U_2$ (without considering friction).

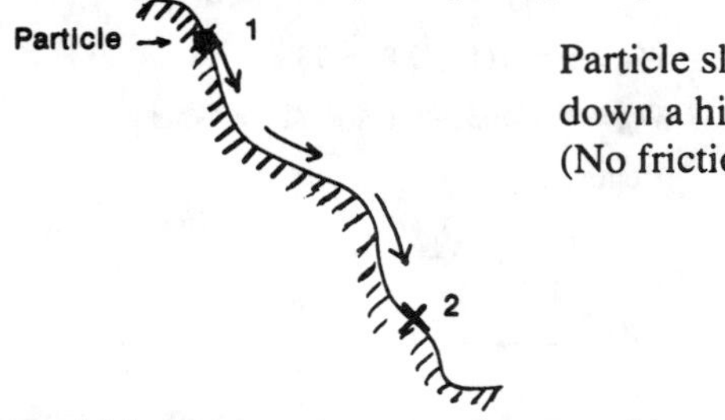

Particle sliding down a hill (No friction)

$$(1/2)mv_1^2 + mgh_1 = (1/2)mv_2^2 + mgh_2$$

$$\boxed{\frac{v_1^2}{2} + gh_1 = \frac{v_2^2}{2} + gh_2}$$

Potential and kinetic energy are scalar quantities.

Work (W) is a scalar. Work results when a force (F) causes displacement (d):

$$W = Fd\cos\theta$$

Note that F cos θ is the component of F along the displacement (d). When θ = 0°, then cos 0° = 1, and W = Fd which is the result for forces in the same direction as the displacement. When θ = 90°, then cos 90° = 0 and W = 0. That is, forces perpendicular to the displacement do no work. Remember, walking a dog illustrates the concept of work.

Work can also be defined in terms of the change in mechanical energy of an object. Remember that the potential energy between two points (or positions) is the amount of work that would be required to move an object between those two points. The change in kinetic energy of an object is the work performed by the object assuming all the energy goes into work. To summarize:

W = $E_f - E_i = \Delta E$
E = K + U = mechanical energy
f = final i = initial Δ = change.

This means work and energy have the same units:

W + (force)(distance) = newtons· meters = joules
= dynes· cms = ergs.

Joules and ergs are units of work or energy.
Pressure (P) times volume (V) also yields work (W), W = (P)(V).
This is used to study heat engines.

Power (P) is a scalar and is the rate at which work is done:

$$P = \text{work(W)/time(t)} = W/t$$

The units of power are:

$$P = \text{work/time} = \text{joules/secs} \equiv \text{watts}.$$

5.15.2 Questions to Review Work and Energy

1. When a system does work or work is done on a system:

A. the force of the system changes.
B. the momentum of the system changes.
C. the torque of the system changes.
D. the energy of the system changes.

2. All of the following statements are correct concerning potential energy (PE) except:

A. PE depends on the configuration rather than the motion of a system.
B. PE may be converted to kinetic energy.
C. PE cannot be defined for frictional forces.
D. PE depends upon the path taken to reach a certain state.

3. The law of conservation of energy takes into account all of the following except:

A. conversion of mass into energy.
B. potential energy.
C. kinetic energy.
D. energy loss due to dissipative forces.

4. If W = work and t = time, then power (P) is:

A. $P = W/t$
B. $P = t/W$
C. $P = Wt$
D. $P = 1/Wt$

5. At what angle to the direction of the displacement would a force perform no work?

A. 0°
B. 45°
C. 90°
D. 180°

6. All are expressions of work except:

A. changes in mechanical energy.
B. momentum times mass.
C. force times distance.
D. pressure times volume.

7. A 5kg object is moving in a straight line at a velocity of 4 meters/sec. The kinetic energy (K) is:

A. 40 joules
B. 20 joules
C. 10 joules
D. 80 joules

8. An object weighing 10 kg is at a distance of 10 m above the earth's surface. The potential energy (U) of this object is:

A. 980 joules
B. 100 joules
C. 9.8 joules
D. 1000 joules

9. If a 5 kg object is 20 meters above the earth's surface and it falls to 10 meters above the surface, what is the change in potential energy (U)?

A. gains 490 joules
B. loses 490 joules
C. loses 50 joules
D. The potential energy does not change, only the kinetic energy changes.

10. The shaded area under the graph represents:

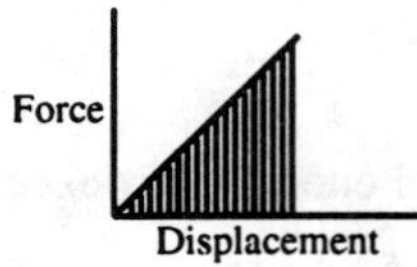

A. momentum
B. force field
C. work
D. pressure

11. A person does 20 joules of work in 10 seconds; the power (P) generated is:

A. 2000 watts
B. 200 watts
C. 2 watts
D. 0.5 watts

12. A force of 20 newtons is used to move an object 20 meters in 10 seconds; the power (P) used is:

A. 40,000 watts
B. 4,000 watts
C. 400 watts
D. 40 watts

13. A force of 10 newtons pushes a 5 kg object 20 meters. The work performed is:

A. 200 joules
B. 40 joules
C. 10 joules
D. 2.5 joules

14. How much work is performed in the diagram below?

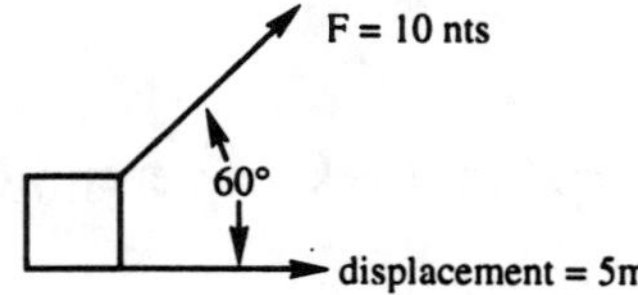

A. 50 joules
B. 50 cos 30° joules
C. 25 joules
D. 50 sin 60° joules

15. A 5 kg object moving at 4 m/sec strikes a second object. After the collision, the first object is moving at 2 m/sec. Assuming all the energy (E) was used to perform work (W) on the second object, the work performed is:

A. 30 joules
B. 60 joules
C. 90 joules
D. 120 joules

5.15.3 Answers to Questions in Section 5.15.2

(1) D (2) D (3) A (4) A (5) C (6) B (7) A (8) A (9) B (10) C (11) C (12) D
(13) A (14) C (15) A

5.15.4 Discussion of Answers to Questions in Section 5.15.2

Questions #1 to #6: Adequately discussed in the Section.

Question #7 (Answer: A)

$$K = \frac{1}{2}mv^2 = (\frac{1}{2})(5)(4)^2 = (5/2)(16) = 40 \text{ joules.}$$

Question #8 (Answer: A)

$$U = mgh = (10 \text{ kg})(9.8 \text{ m/sec}^2)(10\text{m}) = 980 \text{ joules.}$$

Question #9 (Answer: B)

$$U = U_2 - U_1 = mgh_2 = mgh_1 = mg(h_2 - h_1)$$
$$= (5)(9.8)(10 - 20) = (5)(9.8)(-10) = -490 \text{ joules.}$$

The minus sign means U is lost.

Question #10 (Answer: C) The area under the graph is given by the product of the quantities on the axes. This is (force)(displacement), which is work (or energy).

Question #11 (Answer: C)

P = work/time = 20 joules/10 secs = 2 joules/sec = 2 watts.

Question #12 (Answer: D)

P = work/time = 400 joules/10 secs = 40 joules/sec = 40 watts.
work = (force)(distance) = (20)(20) = 400 joules.

Question #13 (Answer: A)

$$W = Fd \cos \theta$$
$$\text{For } \theta = 0°, \cos \theta = 1$$
$$W = Fd = (10)(20) = 200 \text{ joules.}$$

Question #14 (Answer: C) According to the 30°–60°–90° triangle rules, the side lengths are shown:

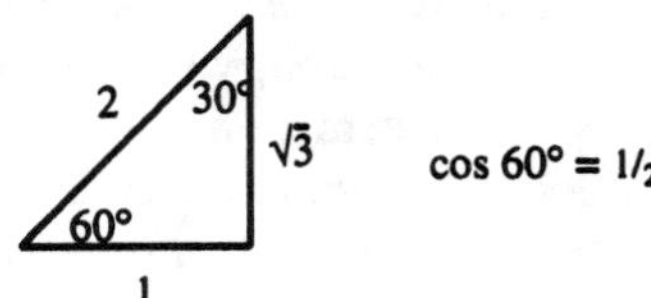

Then: $W = Fd \cos \theta = (10)(5) \cos 60° = 50(\frac{1}{2}) = 25$ joules.

Question #15 (Answer: A)

$$\Delta E = W = E_f - E_i$$
$$E = \frac{1}{2} mv^2$$
$$W = \frac{1}{2} mv_f^2 - \frac{1}{2} mv_i^2 = \frac{1}{2} m(v_f^2 - v_i^2)$$
$$W = \frac{1}{2}(5)(4^2 - 2^2) = (5/2)(16 - 4) = (5/2)(12) = 30 \text{ joules.}$$

5.15.5 Checklist for Work and Energy

______	work	______	power
______	kinetic energy	______	joules
______	gravitational potential energy	______	watts
______	Law of Conservation of Energy		

5.16 TRANSLATIONAL MOTION

5.16.1 Review of Translational Motion

Distance depends upon the path taken, has no fixed direction, and has magnitude only. *Speed* is the distance traveled divided by the change in time. Both speed and distance are scalar quantities—have magnitude but no fixed direction. They have positive values only. *Displacement* is independent of the path taken (i.e., depends only on initial and final positions of the object) and has a constant direction and magnitude. *Velocity* is the displacement divided by the change in time. Both velocity and displacement are vector quantities (i.e., have direction and magnitude). *Acceleration* is the change in velocity divided by the change in time, and it is a vector. (Fig. 5.27.)

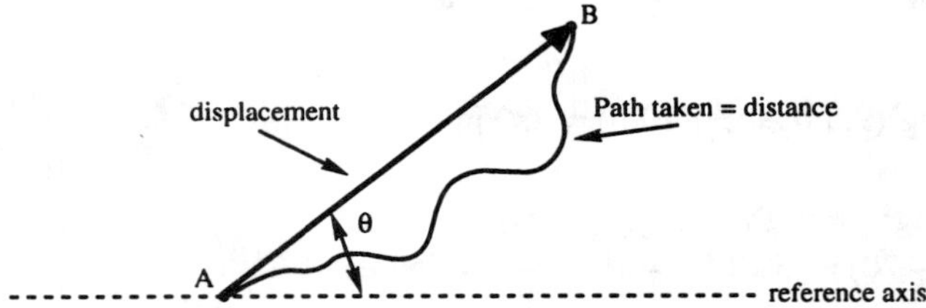

Note that displacement has a direction and magnitude and is independent of the path taken (there are many paths from A to B but the displacement is the same regardless of the path taken)

$$\text{speed} = \frac{\Delta\text{distance}}{\Delta\text{time}} = \frac{d_f - d_i}{t_f - t_i}$$

$$\text{velocity} = \frac{\text{displacement}}{\Delta\text{time}}$$

$$\text{acceleration} = \frac{\Delta\text{velocity}}{\Delta\text{time}} = \frac{v_f - v_i}{t_f - t_i}$$

Δ(delta) = change
f = final
i = initial

Fig. 5.27—Translational Motion Parameters

Displacement is the "net" area under the velocity–time graph, where area above the t–axis is counted as positive and area below this axis is counted as negative. However, in order to compute the total distance traveled, compute the "total" area between the velocity–time graph, where areas above and below the t–axis are both counted as positive. The *units* of distance and displacement are length such as feet (ft), meters (m), miles and kilometers (km). The units of speed and velocity are length divided by time such as feet/sec., miles/hour or meters/sec. Acceleration has the units of length/time/time (length/time^2) and examples are feet/sec^2, meters/sec^2 and miles/hour^2.

Note the *sign* (+ or –) of displacement, velocity or acceleration depends on the system under study and the specific values of the final (f) and initial (i) values. A displacement is negative if it is opposite to the direction designated as positive. The velocity is negative if the displacement is negative. The acceleration is negative if the velocity is decreasing. *Instantaneous* velocity or acceleration represent a given point in time. For instantaneous velocity, it is the slope of the graph of distance vs. time at the given time. The *average* velocity is defined for a period of time, and is expressed as:

$v = \frac{v_f + v_i}{2}$ if acceleration is constant.

Force is defined as the *action* of one particle on another, e.g., pushing a book with your hand.

Forces (Section 5.14.1) act upon objects to cause an acceleration. If a constant force is acting there is a constant (unchanging) acceleration. The motion produced in this case is called *uniform accelerated motion.* The acceleration (a) causes a change in velocity (v) over time (t):

If $a = -10$ m/sec^2, 5 secs elapse and the final velocity = 0,

then, $v_f = v_i + at$ gives $0 = v_i - (10)(5)$, hence $v_i = +50$ m/s

The acceleration and velocity are both causing a change in displacement (d)—the directions of acceleration, velocity and displacement are all the same:

d_{vo} = $v_o t$ displacement due to the initial velocity (v_o) at time = t;
d_a = $\frac{1}{2}at^2$ displacement due to the acceleration at time = t
d_o = initial displacement (if any) from a reference.

The total displacement (d) in a time (t) for uniform accelerated motion (equation for uniform accelerated motion) is:

$d = d_o + v_o t + \frac{1}{2}at^2$ [*uniform accelerated motion* equation: memorize]

or, final displacement (d) = initial displacement from a reference point (d_o) + change in displacement due to initial velocity ($v_o t$) + change in displacement due to acceleration ($\frac{1}{2}at^2$) = $d_o + d_{vo} + d_a$.

Translational motion is the movement of an object in a straight line. The above equations illustrate uniform accelerated motion along a straight line.

Displacement, velocity and acceleration are added (or subtracted) by methods of *vectors*.

It may be noted that speed, time and distance are *scalars*, whereas velocity, acceleration and displacement are *vectors.* In order to review vectors, study the section on vectors under mathematics in this book. Make sure that you really understand how to break or resolve a vector into the sine and cosine components. On the actual MCAT, if a problem is asked about finding the resultant of 3 or 4 vectors, use the "quick graphical method" illustrated below:

Quick graphical method:

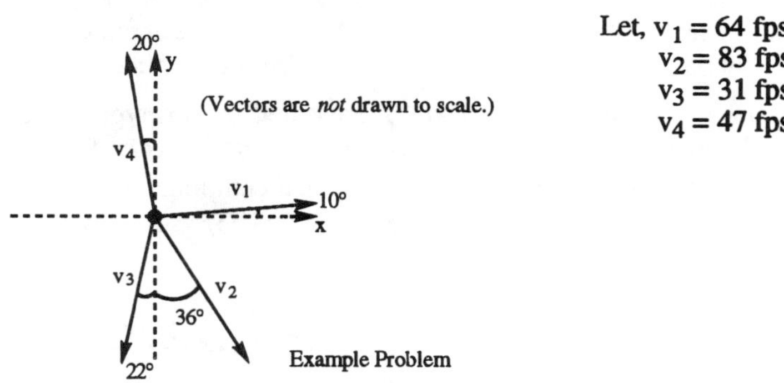

Let, $v_1 = 64$ fps
$v_2 = 83$ fps
$v_3 = 31$ fps
$v_4 = 47$ fps

In order to find the resultant of the four vectors v_1, v_2, v_3, v_4, you can use the long method, which involves breaking down each vector into two components.

Use of "quick graphical method"

Select any vector to start with. For this example problem, select v_3 as the starting vector. Remember each vector has a *tip* (the arrowhead) and a *tail* (where it is attached to the particle). Start by drawing the vector v_3, making sure *your* measurements of *direction* and *length of vector* are fairly accurate. Now select *any other* vector such as v_1, and draw it so that the tail of v_1 coincides with the tip of v_3. Proceed to vector v_2 and draw it so that the tail of v_2 coincides with the tip of v_1. You are now left with vector v_4. Using the sequential procedure outlined above, draw v_4 attached to v_2 so that the tail of v_4 coincides with the tip of v_2. The vector diagram is now complete. To determine the answer as to the *direction* and *length of the resultant*, join the tip of v_4 to the tail of v_3.

$AB = v_R$ = Resultant velocity vector for the problem.

This method is also called the "Tip–Tail method" and takes about one to two minutes. The question that might arise in your mind: "Can I use a protractor or ruler on the MCAT?" The answer is "NO." Use your answer sheet or the test booklet and your pencil to *measure* as you would with a ruler and a protractor. Your sense of direction and orientation will guide you. Draw the X–axis and Y–axis to improve your "angle sense" so that you have a better grip on finding the angles. PRACTICE THIS METHOD AT LEAST FIVE TIMES, before using it on the actual MCAT. Students who know this method have more confidence in solving such problems.

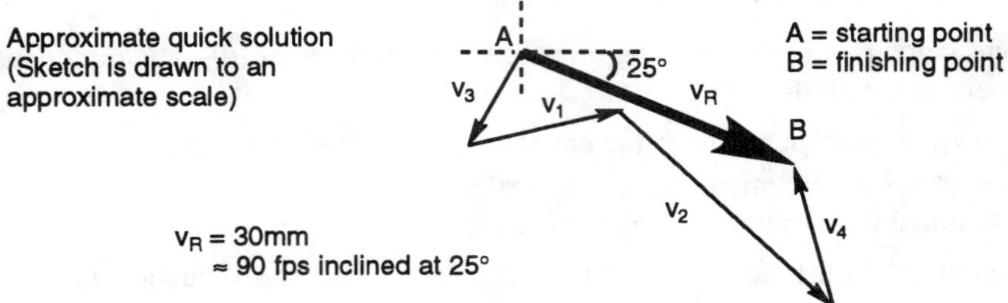

Free fall motion. This is vertical motion (in reference to the earth), that is, upward or downward in a straight line. It is always uniformly accelerated motion with the acceleration equal to g. Values of g are:

$$32 \text{ ft/sec}^2 \text{ or } 980 \text{ cms/sec}^2 \text{ or } 9.8 \text{ m/sec}^2.$$

The equations for uniform linear motion are applicable when *g* is substituted for *a*:

$$d = d_o + v_o t + 1/2\, gt^2$$
$$v = gt.$$

The reference point (origin) and positive and negative directions must be defined. As an example, in g = 32 ft/sec^2, what the *g* means is that for every second an object is falling under the influence of gravity (neglecting air resistance), the velocity is increasing by 32 ft/sec. For an object thrown straight up, its speed is decreasing by 32 ft/sec for every second.

In the free fall of actual objects, the value of g is modified by buoyancy of air and resistance of air. What results is drag force and depends on the location on earth, weight, shape and size of the object, and the velocity of the object (as free fall velocity increases, the drag force increases). When the drag force reaches the force of gravity, the object reaches a final velocity called the terminal velocity and continues to fall at that velocity.

Projectile motion is mathematically represented by two types of translational motion: vertical (affected by g) and horizontal (independent of g). The vertical motion (free fall) and the horizontal translational motion (with a=o) are represented as vertical and horizontal components. The projectile is generally fired at some angle (Ø) to the horizontal, and the motion is parabolic (see Fig. 5.28).

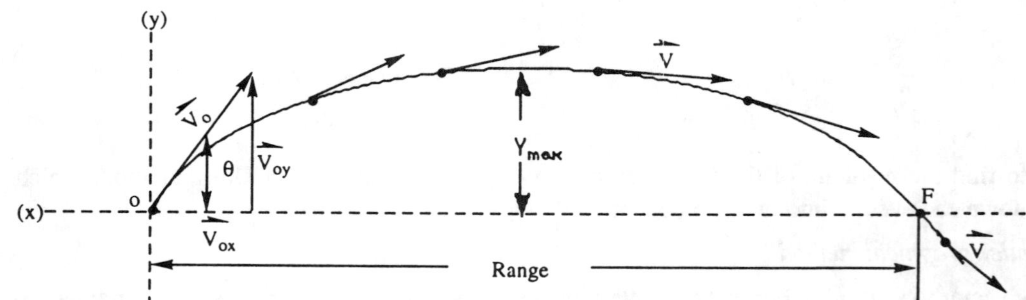

Fig. 5.28—Projectile Motion

Vertical component (free fall)

initial speed	$v_{oy} = v_o \sin\theta$
distance at time = t	$y = v_{oy}t + 1/2\, gt^2$
speed at any time = t	$v_y = v_{oy} + gt$

(note that g is negative if it is opposite to the original displacement)

Horizontal component (linear with constant speed)

initial speed	$v_{ox} = v_o \cos\theta$
distance at any time = t	$x = v_{ox}t$
speed at any time = t	$v_x = v_{ox}$ (speed is constant)

Initial velocity vector $\vec{v_o}$ *at any time = t*

magnitude	$v_o^2 = (v_{ox})^2 + (v_{oy})^2$ (Pythagorean Theorem)
direction (θ)	$\tan(\theta) = v_{oy}/v_{ox}$

(1) v_{ox} is constant
(2) v_y is zero at y_{max}, then $v_y = 0 = v_{oy} + gt$, $-v_{oy} = gt$ (and can solve for t)
(3) at O and F, the v's are equal
(4) the maximum range is attained when $\theta = 45°$

5.16.2 Questions to Review Translational Motion

1. Which of the following does not depend on direction?

A. distance
B. displacement
C. acceleration
D. all of the above

2. Which of the following is a vector?

A. distance
B. speed
C. velocity
D. all of the above

3. The variable with the dimension of length/time^2 is:

A. displacement.
B. velocity.
C. acceleration.
D. force.

4. A constant acceleration is caused by a:

A. constant force.
B. changing force.
C. constant displacement.
D. combination of (A) and (B).

5. A force was applied for 10 sec to an object moving at 10m/sec. The final velocity was 60m/sec. The acceleration was:

A. 3 m/sec^2.
B. 5 m/sec^2.
C. 7 m/sec^2.
D. none of the above.

6. An object initially moving at 15m/sec is accelerated at the rate of 5m/sec^2 for 5 sec. The final velocity of the object is:

A. 15 m/sec.
B. 25 m/sec.
C. 40 m/sec.
D. 100 m/sec.

7. An object starts 5m from a reference point with an initial velocity of 10 m/sec and an acceleration of 5 m/sec^2. How far is the object from the reference point after 5 secs?

A. 75m
B. 80m
C. 117.5m
D. 180.5m

Use the following velocity–time graph for Questions #8 through #12. The motion is in a straight line.

8. The slope of the graph at any point represents:

A. acceleration.
B. displacement.
C. force.
D. kinetic energy.

9. The instantaneous velocity at point B is:
A. 20 m/sec
B. 25 m/sec
C. 10 m/sec
D. 35 m/sec

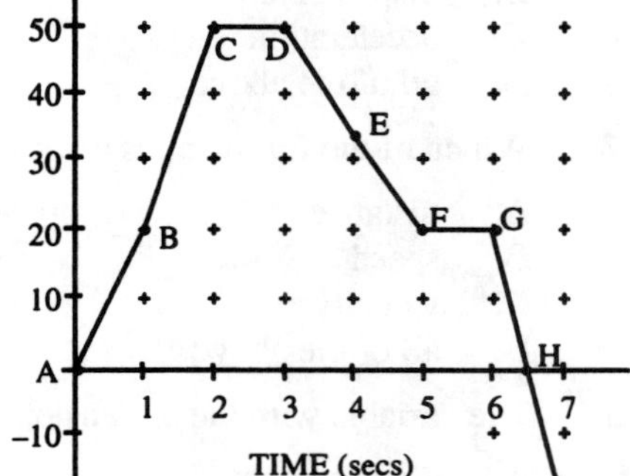

10. The instantaneous acceleration at point E is:

A. 15 m/sec^2
B. – 15 m/sec^2
C. 30 m/sec^2
D. – 30 m/sec^2

11. The total displacement of the particle between t = 0 to t = 7 secs is approximately:

A. – 145 m
B. 125 m
C. 185 m
D. 350 m

12. The average speed from 0 to 2 secs is:

A. 12.5 m/sec
B. 20 m/sec
C. 22.5 m/sec
D. 25 m/sec

13. The analysis of projectile motion is greatly simplified by which of the following statements:

I. Using the formula for describing the motion as a parabola
II. Realizing that the time of ascent is one-half the time of descent
III. Neglecting the effect of gravity if the object is considered a point mass
IV. Separating the motion into vertical (free fall) and horizontal (uniform accelerated motion) components

A. I and II only
B. II, III and IV
C. I and III only
D. I, III and IV

14. The maximum horizontal distance an object can attain is when the object is thrown at an angle to the horizontal. What is the value of that angle?

A. 15°
B. 30°
C. 45°
D. 60°

15. An unbalanced force acting upon an object causes:

A. a change in the mass of the object.
B. an acceleration of the object.
C. the object to maintain a constant velocity.
D. none of the above.

16. An object is thrown vertically upward at an initial velocity of 49 m/sec. It will rise to what height?

A. 122.5 m
B. 245 m
C. 490 m
D. the time must be given

17. An object dropped from the edge of a cliff will fall how far in 10 seconds?

A. cannot be determined without the mass of the object
B. 98 m
C. 980 m
D. 490 m

Use the following information for Questions #18 and #19.

An object is thrown with an initial speed of 19.6 m/sec at an angle of 30° with the horizontal.

18. The maximum height the object reaches is:

A. 2.45 m
B. 4.9 m
C. 9.8 m
D. 98 m

19. The range (horizontal distance) of the object is:

A. 19.6 m
B. $19.6\sqrt{3}$ m
C. 9.8 m
D. $9.8\sqrt{3}$ m

5.16.3 Answers to Questions in Section 5.16.2

(1) A (2) C (3) C (4) A (5) B (6) C (7) C (8) A (9) A (10) B (11) C (12) C
(13) D (14) C (15) B (16) A (17) D (18) B (19) B

5.16.4 Discussion of Answers to Questions in Section 5.16.2

Questions #1 to #4: Adequately discussed in the Section.

Question #5 (Answer: B) Use the formula for acceleration (a),

$$a = \Delta v/\Delta t = (v_f - v_i)/(t_f - t_i) = (60 - 10)/(10 - 0) = 50/10 = 5 \text{ m/sec}^2$$

Question #6 (Answer: C) The final velocity (v_f) is:

v_f = initial velocity + velocity change due to acceleration =
15 m/sec + at = 15 + (5 m/sec^2) (5 sec) = 15 + 25 = 40 m/sec

Question #7 (Answer: C) Use the formula for distance:

$$d = d_o + v_o t + {}^1\!/_2\, at^2 \quad = 5 + (10)(5) + {}^1\!/_2\,(5)(5)^2$$
$$= 5 + 50 + ({}^1\!/_2)(5)(25) = 55 + {}^1\!/_2\,(125)$$
$$= 55 + 62.5 = 117.5$$

Question #8 (Answer: A) The slope of the curve of any graph is the ratio of the change in the y-axis (Δy) to the corresponding change in the x-axis (Δx). In this case,

Δy = change in speed = Δv
Δx = change in time = Δt

then:

slope = $\Delta y/\Delta x = \Delta v/\Delta t$ = acceleration.

Question #9 (Answer: A) The answer is 20 m/sec as read from the graph. Instantaneous velocity is the velocity at a given point in time.

Question #10 (Answer: B) Since E is on the line DF, the instantaneous acceleration (i.e., the slope at a given point) at E is the same as the slope of line DF:

acceleration at E = $(20 - 50)/(5 - 3) = -30/2 = -15$ m/sec^2

Question #11 (Answer: C) The area of the graph for each time interval will be the displacement. Review equations for area of a triangle and a trapezoid to calculate values.

Triangle	AB	0–1 secs	$20 \times 1/2 = 10$ m
Trapezoid	BC	1–2 secs	$(20 + 50) \times 1/2 = 35$ m
Rectangle	CD	2–3 secs	$50 \times 1 = 50$ m
Trapezoid	DE	3–4 secs	$(50 + 34) \times 1/2 = 42$ m
Trapezoid	EF	4–5 secs	$(34 + 20) \times 1/2 = 27$ m
Rectangle	FG	5–6 secs	$20 \times 1 = 20$ m
Triangle	G-H-I	6–7 secs	$20 \times (1/2) - 20 \times (1/2) = 0$ m

Total of all displacements covered from t = 0 to t = 7 = 10 + 35 + 50 + 42 + 27 + 20 = 184m ≅ 185m.

Question #12 (Answer: C) The average speed is,

average speed = total distance/total time.

The total distance is the area under the graph from A to C.

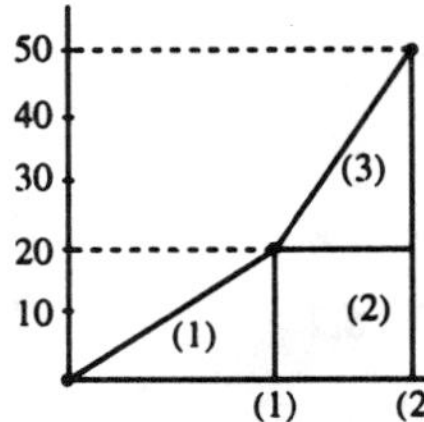

Total area = distance = Area #1 + Area #2 + Area #3
= (1/2)(20)(1) + (20)(1) + (1/2)(30)(1)
= 10 + 20 + 15 = 45m

Then: avg. speed = 45m/2 sec. = 22.5 m/sec. The formula $v = \frac{v_f + v_i}{2}$ cannot be used because the acceleration is not constant over this interval.

Questions #13 to #15: Adequately discussed in the Section.

Question #16 (Answer: A) The object will rise for as long as it takes the downward acceleration (due to gravity-g) to overcome the initial upward velocity, i.e.:

$v_o = gt$

$$t = \frac{v_o}{g} = \frac{49 \text{ m/sec}}{9.8 \text{ m/sec}^2} = 5 \text{ secs.}$$

Then using the formula for uniform accelerated motion:

$d = d_o + v_o t + 1/2\, gt^2 = 0 + 49\,(5) + 1/2\,(-9.8)(5)^2 = 245 - 122.5$
$d = 122.5$ m.

Note that g is negative because it is downward acceleration.

Question #17 (Answer: D) Using the equations for accelerated motion (Section 5.16.1) and the fact that gravity is the acceleration:

$$d = d_o + v_o t + {}^{1}\!/_{2}\, gt^2$$
$$= 0 + (0)(10) + ({}^{1}\!/_{2})(9.8)(10)^2 = (4.9)(100) = 490 \text{ m.}$$

This is an example of free fall motion.

Question #18 (Answer: B) The maximum height would correspond to the height reached if the object was thrown vertically upward with the vertical component of the initial velocity (v_o)

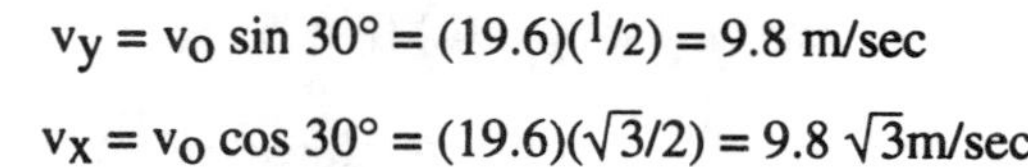

$v_y = v_o \sin 30° = (19.6)({}^{1}\!/_{2}) = 9.8$ m/sec

$v_x = v_o \cos 30° = (19.6)(\sqrt{3}/2) = 9.8\sqrt{3}$m/sec

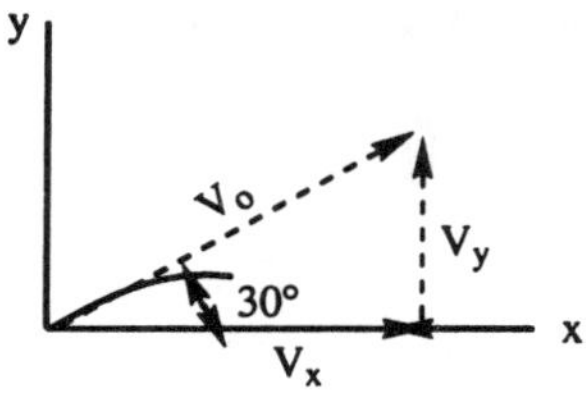

Remember: sin θ = opposite/hypotenuse
cos θ = adjacent/hypotenuse

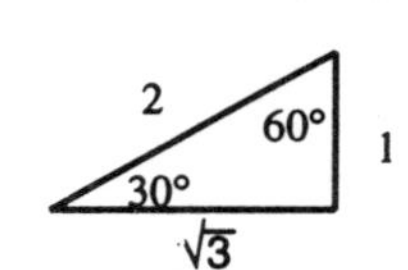

The height can be calculated using the formula for accelerated motion: $h = h_o + v_y t + {}^{1}\!/_{2}\, gt^2$.

Time is found, by reasoning that the object continues to rise until its upward motion is offset by the downward acceleration of gravity (g): $v_y = gt$

$$t = \frac{v_y}{g} = \frac{9.8 \text{ m/sec}}{9.8 \text{ m/sec}^2} = 1 \text{ sec.}$$

Note that 1 sec is the time required for half the trajectory. Using the above:

$$h = h_o + v_y t + {}^{1}\!/_{2}\, gt^2$$
$$d = 0 + (9.8)(1) + ({}^{1}\!/_{2})(-9.8)(1)^2 = 9.8 - 4.9 = 4.9\text{m.}$$

Question #19 (Answer: B) From question #18, the time for half the trajectory was 1 sec, so the total time is two secs. To find the range, use the horizontal component of the initial velocity (v_x) as calculated in question #18. There is no force in the horizontal direction so the acceleration is zero in this direction. Then using the equation for accelerated motion applied in the horizontal direction:

$$d = d_x + v_x t + {}^{1}\!/_{2}\, a_x t^2$$
$$d = 0 + (9.8\sqrt{3})(2) + ({}^{1}\!/_{2})(0)(2)^2$$
$$d = 19.6\sqrt{3} \text{ m.}$$

5.16.5 Checklist for Translational Motion

______ equation for uniform accelerated motion
______ speed
______ distance
______ displacement
______ velocity
______ acceleration
______ translational motion
______ projectile motion
______ free fall motion
______ Tip-Tail method

5.17 EQUILIBRIUM AND MOMENTUM

5.17.1 Review of Equilibrium and Momentum

5.17.1.1 EQUILIBRIUM

When a force (Section 5.14.1) acts upon an object, the object will undergo translational motion or rotational motion. Translational motion is the motion of the object through space when the force is acting along an axis and/or the center of mass (that point whose motion can be described like a particle, Section 5.14.1). Rotational motion is the rotation of an object about an axis caused by a force not directed along that axis. The effective force causing rotation about an axis is the *torque* (L) (Fig. 5.29).

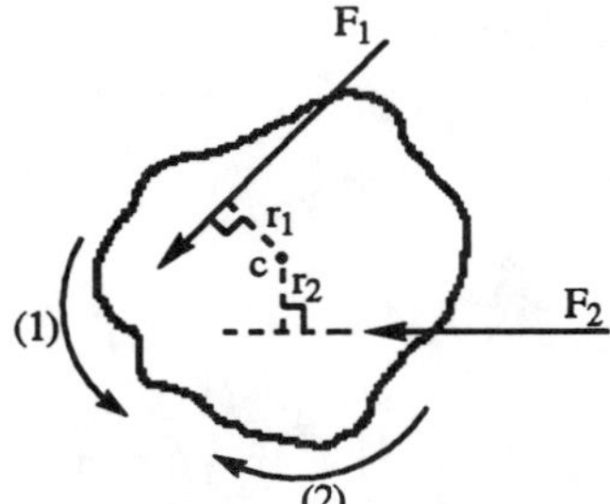

L = (force) × (moment arm),
moment arm is the perpendicular distance from the force to the axis
F = force
r = moment arm
c = center of mass or an axis
L_1 = $(F_1)(r_1)$ = counterclockwise (1) = positive
L_2 = $(F_2)(r_2)$ = clockwise (2) = negative

Fig 5.29—Torque (Rotational Moment)

To determine the direction of rotation caused by the torque, imagine the direction the object would rotate if the force is pushing against its moment arm (at right angles). The net forces acting on an object is best determined by resolving them into the x and y components. The net torques acting on an object is obtained by summing the counterclockwise (+) and clockwise (–) torques. An object is at equilibrium when the net forces and torques acting on it are zero. Note that this means there is no acceleration but does not mean there is no velocity; it means either the object is motionless or moving with a constant velocity. The conditions of equilibrium are:

for translational equilibrium

$\Sigma F_x = 0$ (Σ= sum over all)

$\Sigma F_y = 0$

for rotational equilibrium

$\Sigma L = 0$ (in a given geometric plane, must hold for three mutually perpendicular planes).

If the torques sum to zero about one point in an object, they will sum to zero about any point in the object. If the point chosen as reference includes the line of action of one of the forces, that force need not be included in calculating the torques.

Newton's First Law states that objects at rest or in motion tend to remain as such unless acted upon by an outside force. That is, objects have inertia (resistance to motion). For translational motion, the mass (m) is a measure of inertia. For rotational motion, a quantity derived from mass called the moment of inertia (I) is the measure of inertia. Thus, $I = \Sigma\ mr^2$ in general, but its exact formulation depends on the structure of the object. See Section 5.11.1 for compressive and tensile forces.

5.17.1.2 MOMENTUM

Momentum (M) is a vector quantity . Its formulation for magnitude is:

M = mv
m = mass
v = velocity

Linear momentum is a measure of the tendency of an object to maintain motion in a straight line. Notice that M is directly proportional to the mass of the object and its velocity (not acceleration). The larger the M, the greater the tendency of the object to remain moving along a straight line (in the same direction). Momentum is also a measure of the force needed to stop or change direction of the object The *impulse* (I) is given by:

$I = F\,\Delta t = M = mv$
F = force acting
Δt = elapsed time

Impulse is a measure of the force required to impart or change momentum of an object. Impulse is also a vector. Just like energy, *momentum is also conserved.* The total linear momentum of a system is constant when the resultant external force acting on the system is zero.

Remember, there are three conservation laws for ALL states of matter:

1. Law of Conservation of Mass
2. Law of Conservation of Momentum
3. Law of Conservation of Energy

Collisions are a form of interaction of matter during which momentum (remember, it is a vector) is conserved. During an elastic collision (objects do not stick), there is conservation of momentum and conservation of kinetic energy. During an inelastic collision (objects stick together), there is conservation of momentum but not of kinetic energy (the remainder of the energy is lost as heat or sound, so total energy is conserved).

Two special collisions will be mentioned. In the explosion of an object at rest, the total momentum of all the fragments must sum to zero (original momentum was zero). If one object collides elastically with a second identical object that is at rest, the first object comes to rest and the second moves off with the momentum of the first. Newton's Second Law and Third Law of Motion are discussed in Section 5.14.1.

5.17.2 Questions to Review Equilibrium and Momentum

1. Rotational motion represents:

A. movement of an object along a curved line.
B. movement of an object through space.
C. motion of an object about a fixed point.
D. motion of an object about an axis.

2. "An object at rest tends to remain at rest while objects in motion tend to remain in motion . . . ;" this is Newton's First Law and it reflects the property of:

A. velocity.
B. weight.
C. potential energy.
D. inertia.

3. If a force is acting on an object, but off an axis, what type of motion results?

A. rotational
B. translational
C. frictional
D. projectile

4. The product of force times the perpendicular moment arm is the:

A. energy.
B. work.
C. torque.
D. force.

5. The net force (in newtons) on the following object (answers in nts) is:

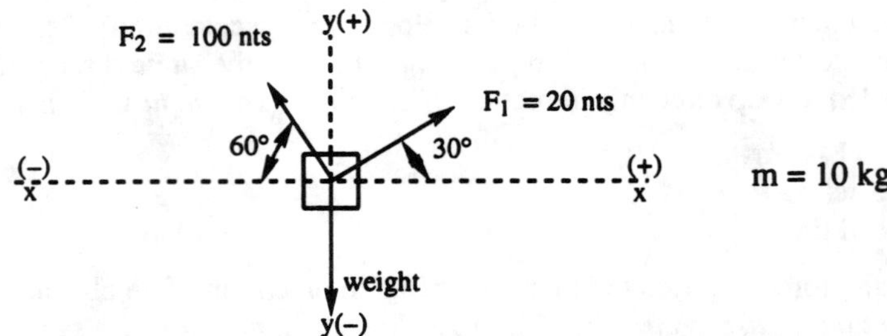

A. zero
B. 32.7 nts
C. 99.5 nts
D. 127.9 nts

6. What is the net force on the following object?

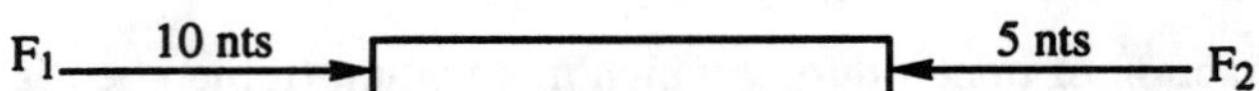

A. 15 nts
B. 5 nts to the right
C. 5 nts compressive force
D. none of the above

7. What is the net torque acting about the axis through the center A (perpendicular to the paper) of the square with sides equal to 4m?

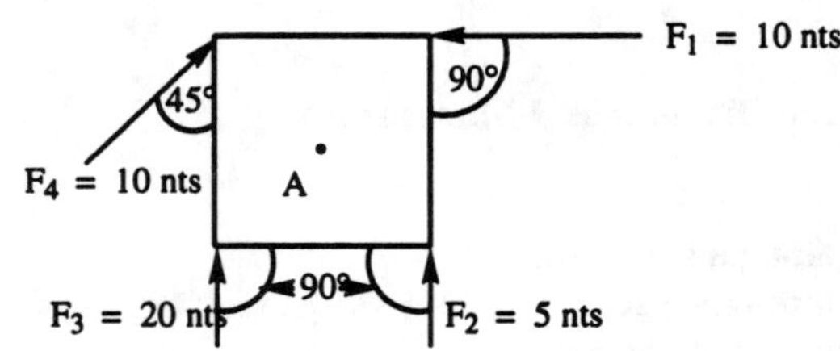

A. 38.2 nt – m counterclockwise
B. 76.4 nt – m clockwise
C. 38.2 nt – m clockwise
D. none of the above

8. The object below is in static and rotational equilibrium. What are the components of the force, F_1?

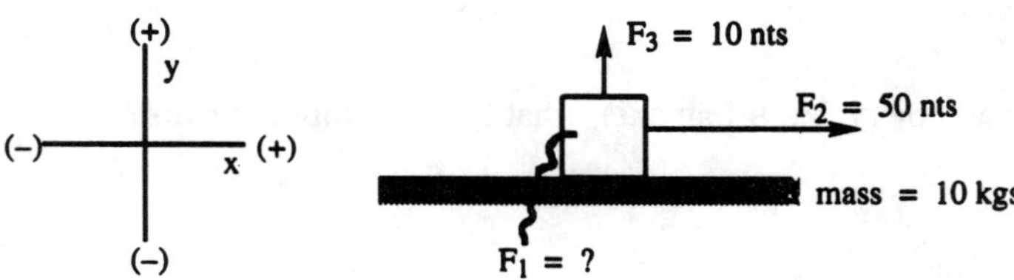

A. $F_x = -50$ nts; $F_y = -10$ nts
B. $F_x = -50$ nts; $F_y = +88$ nts
C. $F_x = +50$ nts; $F_y = -108$ nts
D. none of the above

9. The object below is in rotational equilibrium. What force, F_1, is required for this equilibrium (neglect the weight)?

A. counterclockwise, 17.5 nts
B. clockwise, 5 nts
C. clockwise, 35 nts
D. none of the above

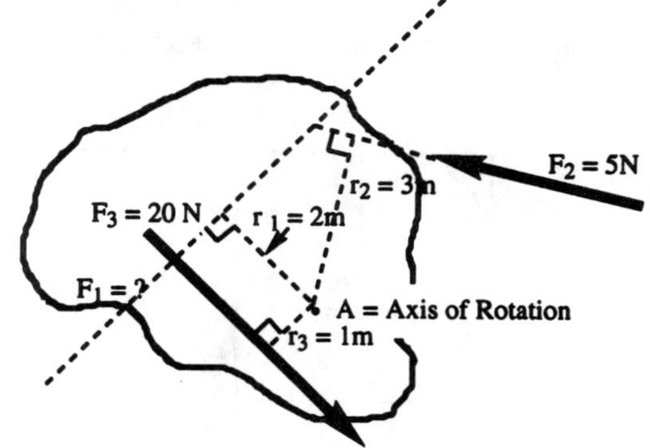

5.17.3 Answers to Questions in Section 5.17.2

(1) D (2) D (3) A (4) C (5) B (6) B (7) C (8) B (9) D

5.17.4 Discussion of Answers to Questions in Section 5.17.2

Questions #1 to #4: Adequately discussed in the text.

Question #5 (Answer: B) The forces may be rediagrammed as:

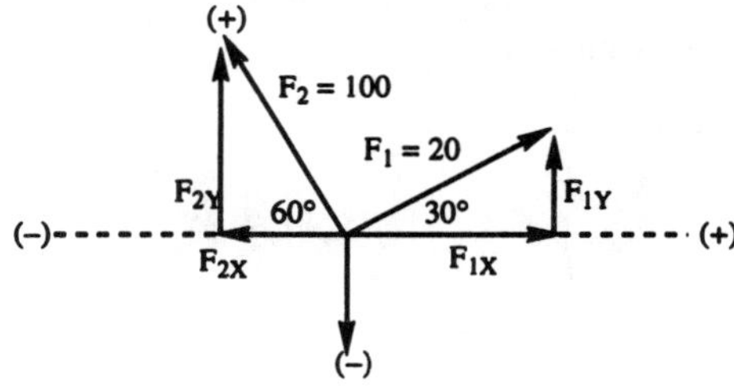

$W_y = mg = (10)(9.8) = 98$ nts
(Weight has no x-component in this case.)

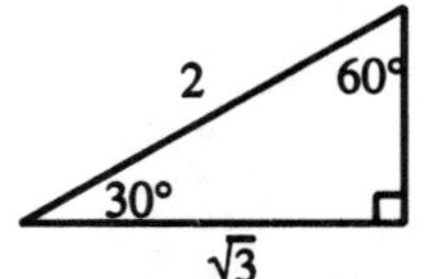

Then: for F_1: $F_{1y} = + (1/2)(20) = +10$ $F_1x = + (\sqrt{3}/2)20 = + 10\sqrt{3}$
for F_2: $F_{2y} = + (\sqrt{3}/2)(100) = +50\sqrt{3}$ $F_{2x} = - (1/2)(100) = -50$

Then $\Sigma F_x = F_{1x} + F_{2x} + W_x = 10\sqrt{3} - 50 + 0 = 17.3 - 50 = -32.7$ nts

REMEMBER: ($\sqrt{3} \sim 1.73$)

$\Sigma Fy = F_{1y} + F_{2y} + W_y = + 10 + 50\sqrt{3} - 98 = +50(1.73) - 88$
$= 86.5 - 88 = -1.5$ nts.

The net force (F) would be:

$F^2 = F_x^2 + F_y^2$

$F = \sqrt{F_x^2 + F_y^2} = \sqrt{(-32.7)^2 + (-1.5)^2} = 32.7$ nts

Question #6 (Answer: B). These are opposing forces acting along the same line of action. The net force is the algebraic sum (assume positive is to the right):

net force = + 10 nts – 5 nts = + 5 nts.

Question #7 (Answer: C), The forces, their moment arms (r) and directions of rotation (R) are:

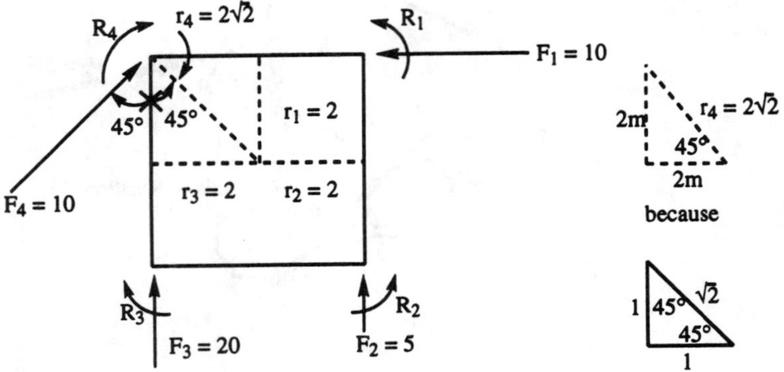

The torques are:

Counterclockwise (+)
$L_1 = F_1 \times r_1 = (10)(2) = +20$ nt · m
$L_2 = F_2 \times r_2 = (5)(2) = +10$ nt · m

Clockwise (–)
$L_3 = F_3 \times r_3 = -(20)(2) = -40$ nt · m
$L_4 = F_4 \times r_4 = -(10)(2\sqrt{2}) = -20\sqrt{2} = -28.2$ nt · m

The net torque (L) is:

$L = L_1 + L_2 + L_3 + L_4 = +20 + 10 - 40 - 28.2 = +30 - 68.2$
$L = -38.2$ nt · m (which is clockwise).

Question #8 (Answer: B). The force diagram is:

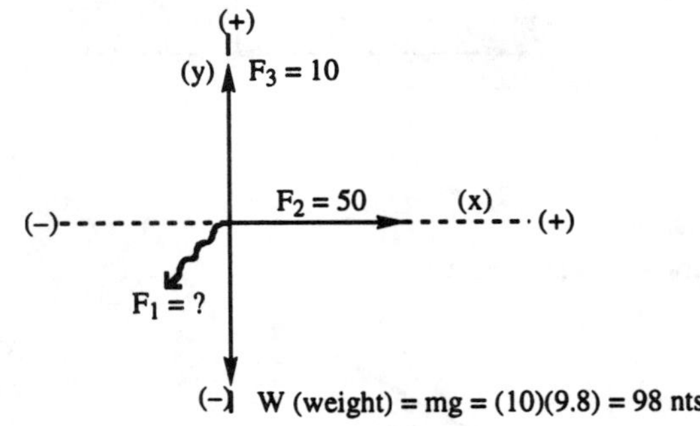

Components of forces:

$F_1 : F_{1x} = ?$	$F_{1y} = ?$
$F_2 : F_{2x} = +50$	$F_{2y} = 0$
$F_3 : F_{3x} = 0$	$F_{3y} = +10$
$W : W_x = 0$	$W_y = -98$

Net force (F):

$\Sigma F_x = 0 = F_{1x} + F_{2x} + F_{3x} + W_x = F_{1x} + 50 + 0 + 0 = F_{1x} + 50$
then, $F_{1x} + 50 = 0$
$F_{1x} = -50$ nts.

$\Sigma F_y = 0 = F_{1y} + F_{2y} + F_{3y} + W_y = F_{1y} + 0 + 10 - 98 = F_{1y} - 88$
then, $F_{1y} - 88 = 0$
$F_{1y} = 88$ nts.

Also, practice using quick graphical method as shown in Section 5.16.1.

Question #9 (Answer: D) The directions of rotations are:

F_2 causes counterclockwise (+) motion
F_3 causes counterclockwise (+) motion

The individual torques are:

$L_1 = F_1 \times r_1 = (F_1)(2) = 2F_1$ (sign unknown)
$L_2 = + F_2 \times r_2 = + (5)(3) = + 15$ nt • m
$L_3 = + F_3 \times r_3 = + (20)(1) = + 20$ nt • m.

Since rotational equilibrium exists the torques sum to zero:

$$\Sigma L = L_1 + L_2 + L_3 = 0$$
$$2F_1 + 15 + 20 = 0$$
$$2F_1 + 35 = 0$$
$$2F_1 = -35$$

$F_1 = -17.5$ nts and motion is clockwise.

5.17.5 Checklist for Equilibrium and Momentum

______	conditions for translational equilibrium	______	torque
______	conditions for rotational equilibrium	______	Law of Conservation of Mass
______	resolution of forces into their components	______	Law of Conservation of Momentum
______	Newton's First Law	______	Law of Conservation of Energy

5.18 ELECTROSTATICS AND ELECTROMAGNETISM

5.18.1 Review of Electrostatics and Electromagnetism

5.18.1.1 ELECTROSTATICS

The elementary charges are called positive (+) or negative (–). Each has a charge of 1.6×10^{-19} coulombs but differ in sign. The electron is the negative charge carrier, and the proton is the positive charge carrier. Substances with an excess of electrons have a net negative charge. Substances with a deficiency of electrons have a net positive charge. One way of charging substances is by rubbing them (i.e., by contact). For example, glass rubbed on fur becomes positive and rubber rubbed on fur becomes negative. Objects can also be charged by induction which occurs when one charged object brought near another causes a charge redistribution in the latter to give net charge regions. *Conductors* transmit charge readily. *Insulators* resist the flow of charge.

Charges exert *forces* upon each other Like charges repel each other and unlike charges attract. For two charges the force is given by *Coulomb's Law*:

$$F = k(q_1q_2/r^2) = (1/4\pi\varepsilon_0)(q_1q_2/r^2)$$

+ r –
q_1 q_2

Fig. 5.30—Illustration of Coulomb's Law

$q_1, q_2 =$ charges $k =$ constant $= 9.0 \times 10^9$ nt–m^2/coul^2
$\varepsilon_0 =$ permittivity of air to the forces $= 8.85 \times 10^{-12}$ coul^2/nt–m^2
$r =$ distance between the charges.

A charge generates an *electric field* (E) in the space around it. Fields (force fields) are vectors (have direction and magnitude). A field is generated by an object and is that region of space around an object that will exert a force on a second object when it is brought into the field. The field exists independently of the second object and is not altered by its presence The force exerted on the second object depends upon that object and the field. The electric field (E) is:

$E = F/q = kQ/r^2$ (i.e., $F = kQq/r^2$)
E and F are vectors
Q = charge generating the field
q = charge placed in it.

Charges exert forces upon each other through fields. The direction of a field is the direction a positive charge would move if placed in it. *Electric field* lines are imaginary lines which are in the same direction as E at that point. The direction is away from positive charges and toward negative charges.

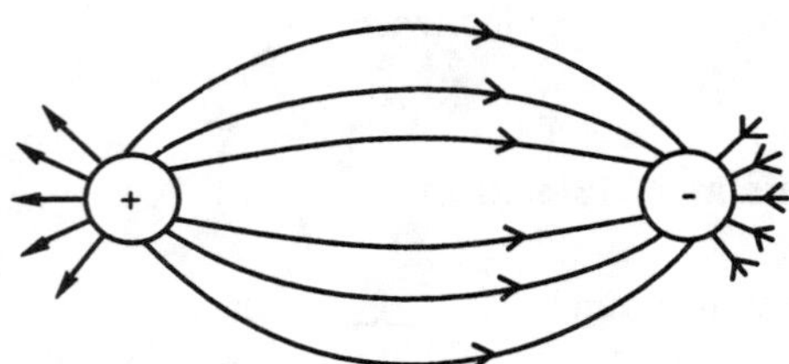

Fig. 5.31—Electric Field Lines

The *potential energy (PE)* of a charged object in a field would equal the work done on that object to bring it from infinity to a distance (r) from the charge setting up the electric field or,

PE = work = $Fr = (qE)r = kQq/r$
Q = charge setting up field
q = charge brought in to a distance r.

When a + q moves against E, its PE increases When a – q moves against E, its PE decreases. Realize that if you brought two positive charges together, work would have to be done to the system (and PE would increase), and vice versa for a + q and a – q.

The *electric potential (V)* is a scalar, and it is defined at each distance (r) from a charge (Q) generating an electric field It represents the negative of the work per unit charge in bringing a + q from infinity to r:

$V = PE/q = kQ/r$ = volts = joules/coulomb
$V = Ed$ for a parallel plate capacitor (Section 5.19.1).

Lines (and surfaces) of equal V are perpendicular to electric field lines. Work can only be done when moving between surfaces of electric potentials and is, therefore, independent of the path taken. No work is done when a charge (q) is moved along an equal potential (equipotential) surface (or line), because the component of force is zero along it. Potential (V) is defined in terms of positive charges such that V is positive when due to a + Q and negative when due to a – Q Potential (V) is added algebraically at a point (because it is a scalar).

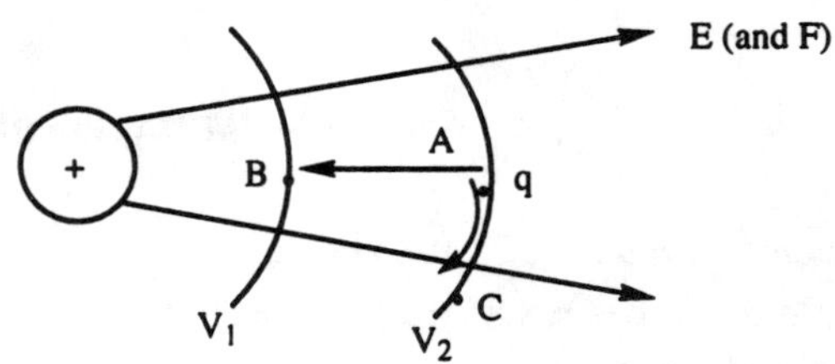

Fig. 5.32—Electrical Potential

(1) V_1, V_2 are two potential surfaces perpendicular to E and F; the values of V_1 or V_2 cannot be measured, only the difference between them can be measured.
(2) $V_2 - V_1$ (or $V_1 - V_2$) is the potential difference (PD, see below);
(3) charge (q) moved from A to B has work (W) done on it

$$W = q\,(V_1 - V_2) = q\,(PD) \text{ see below;}$$

(4) charge (q) moved from A to C has no work done because this is along an equipotential surface and the component of force (F) is perpendicular to it;
(5) the lines of F are along the lines of E.

The *potential difference (PD)* is the difference in V between two points, or it is the work per unit positive charge done by electric forces moving a small test charge from the point of higher potential to the point of lower potential (Fig. 5.32):

$$PD = V_A - V_B = \text{volts} = \text{work/charge or joules/coulomb}$$
$$\text{Work} = q\,(V_A - V_B) = q\,(PD).$$

An *electric dipole* consists of two charges separated by some finite distance (d). Usually the charges are equal and opposite. The laws of forces, fields etc., above, apply to dipoles. A dipole is characterized by its *dipole moment (D.M.)* which is the product of the charge (q) and d. Dipoles tend to line up with the electric field. Motion of dipoles against an electric field requires energy as discussed above.

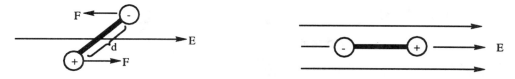

Dipole with equal and opposite charges

Alignment of dipole with E

E = electric field
F = forces exerted by E on the dipole

dipole moment = (distance)(charge) = qd.

Fig. 5.33—Dipoles

5.18.1.2 ELECTROMAGNETISM

This section will enable the student to link magnetism and its numerous applications to: electronic structure and the periodic properties of elements; interaction of mechanical, electrical and magnetic fields; and finally electromagnetic wave spectrum related to accelerating electric charges. Concepts related to electromagnetism are divided into the following categories:

(a) Definition of magnetism and its applications
(b) Types of magnetic materials
(c) Dimensions of common electromagnetic properties
(d) Fundamental rules and laws in electromagnetism
(e) Electromagnetic wave spectrum

A brief discussion of each category is given below:

(a) *Definition of magnetism and its applications:*

A magnet has two poles, similar to an electric dipole. Unlike an isolated resting electron that can exist as a monopole, the simplest magnetic structure that can exist is the magnetic dipole. Magnetism is caused by the arrangement of individual atoms in a substance. The applications of magnetism range from stick-on refrigerator magnets to the design of highly sophisticated particle accelerators. Some other applications include mechanisms inside galvanometers, voltmeters, ammeters; running of supermagnetic levitation trains, brain wave analysis related to hearing, storing data on floppy computer diskettes, walkman radios/tape recorders, credit card strips and cabinet door locks. As Blackmore discovered, bacteria are guided by the north-end of the magnetic compass, which allows the bacteria to orient themselves in chaotic waters. These *magnetotactic* bacteria have led to advanced research in microbiology The above applications make magnetism an important topic for premedical students to understand.

(b) *Types of magnetic materials:* Common household magnets are made of Fe_3O_4 molecules (composed of 2 FeO and Fe_2O_3 molecules) Fe_3O_4 molecules appear as reddish-brown rust when iron objects are exposed to both air and water for long time periods Magnetic materials are of three types:

(i) *Diamagnetic:* These are the weakest magnetic materials. The atoms of these materials *do not* have inherent magnetic dipoles. Magnetic polarities or moments can be induced in them by external fields e.g. bismuth, copper.

(ii) *Paramagnetic:* These substances are relatively stronger than diamagnetic materials. Paramagnetism is the tendency of individual atoms (each with a magnetic dipole) to align along the magnetic field. Atoms of these materials have inherent magnetic dipoles. The stronger the magnetic field the higher the magnetic tendency towards atomic alignment within the substance.

(iii) *Ferromagnetic:* These substances are highly magnetic even without an external magnetic field. These substances have strong inherent magnetic dipoles. Each surrounding or neighboring atom has a strong interaction with the strong dipoles. The arrangement is more permanent in ferromagnetic materials, e.g., lodestone.

(c) *Dimensions of common electromagnetic properties:* Electromagnetic properties are represented by a combination of electrical and magnetic variables and constants.

Magnetic field (B) $1B = \frac{1N}{1C \cdot 1m/s}$

As 1 ampere = 1C/s

$\therefore 1B = \frac{1N}{m \cdot A}$

$1T = 1 \text{ Tesla} = 1B = \frac{1N}{m\text{–}A} = 10^4 \text{ gauss}$

Permeability Constant $[\mu_0]$ $\mu_0 = 4\pi \times 10^{-7} T \cdot m/A$

Magnetic Flux (Wb)
1Wb = 1 Weber = 1 Tesla·m^2

Bohr Magneton $[\mu_B]$ $1\mu_B = \frac{he}{4\pi m}$

where, m = mass of electron
h = Planck constant = 6.63×10^{-34}J·s
e = unit charge on one electron (–)

(d) *Fundamental rules and laws in Electromagnetism:*

(i) Opposite magnetic poles attract each other and like magnetic poles repel each other.

(ii) A moving electric charge or current rearranges the atoms/molecules in a substance. This leads to magnetic fields and a conceptual development of a magnetic charge.

Magnetic fields (B) are generated by moving electrical fields (E). The force of the magnetic field F_B is related to the velocity (v) of the charge (q) as follows: $F_B = qv \cdot B$. The magnetic force acts at right angles to the velocity vector. This means that it cannot speed up or slow down a moving charged particle but it can deflect it. The magnitude of the magnetic deflecting force is:

$$F_B = qvB \sin\phi.$$

The maximal value for the deflecting force occurs when the test charge is moving at right angles to the magnetic field ($\phi = 90°$) and is 0 when ϕ corresponds to either 0° or 180°.

(iii) If a test charge q is moving at right angles to the magnetic field with $\phi = 90°$, for no deflection, electric force = magnetic force

$$qE = qvB \sin 90°$$

$$v = \frac{E}{B} \text{ speed of particles in an electron tube}$$

This principle is used in television, the cathode ray tube and computer terminal design.

On the other hand, if electrons go around in a circular path, then, centrifugal force = magnetic force.

$$F = ma = \frac{mv^2}{r} = qvB\sin\phi$$

For $\phi = 90°$, $\sin 90° = 1$

$$r = \frac{mv}{qB} = \text{radius of the electron path} \ldots\ldots(i)$$

Angular velocity, $\omega = \frac{v}{r}$, becomes

$\omega = \frac{qB}{m}$, using (i), which shows that angular velocity is <u>independent</u> of particle velocity.

(iv) *Biot and Savart law:* states that in a long straight wire conducting current I, the magnetic field is proportional to the current and inversely proportional to the perpendicular distance r.

Mathematically, $B = \frac{\mu_0 I}{2\pi r}$ gives the magnitude of the magnetic field for the simple case of a straight wire.

(v) *Right-Hand Rule:* This rule helps you determine the direction of the magnetic field set up due to electric current in a wire.

Grasp a wire in your right hand with your thumb laid out in the direction of the current. Your four fingers will curl around naturally indicating the direction of the lines of the magnetic field.

(vi) *Faraday's law of electromagnetic induction:* The induced electromotive force in an electric circuit is equal in magnitude to the time rate of change of magnetic flux Faraday's law was followed by Lenz's law to determine the direction of an induced current. Consult a physics reference book to understand Lenz's law.

(vii) *Gauss' law for magnetism* states that isolated magnetic poles (monopoles) do *not* exist.

(e) *Electromagnetic Wave Spectrum:* Review section 5.20.1 to understand the electromagnetic spectrum. It is important to realize that electric fields and magnetic fields are further interrelated. If a magnetic field changes, an electrical field is produced From the principle of symmetry the reverse is true. An electrical field produced by a changing magnetic field is expressed by Faraday's Law, and, a magnetic field produced by a changing electrical field (or by a current or both) is expressed by the Ampere-Maxwell Law Gauss' law, Faraday's law and the Ampere-Maxwell law can be combined to give the so-called "Maxwell's equations." With S = distance, μ = magnetic dipole and I = current, electromagnetic waves can be generated with widely varying wavelengths. See Figs. 5.46(a) and 5.46(b). Notice that x-rays are at the lower end of the electromagnetic spectrum, visible light toward the middle and radio bands toward the upper end of the spectrum:

5.18.2 Questions to Review Electrostatics and Electromagnetism

1. Concerning fields, which is *incorrect*?

A. They exist in space and are generated by objects (e.g., mass).
B. Gravitational and electrical fields are examples.
C. They are scalars.
D. They exist independently of other objects.

2. Coulomb's Law of electrical forces (q = charge, r = distance between charges, k = constant, F = force) is:

A. $F = k(q_1q_2/r^2)$
B. $F = k(q/r^2)$
C. $F = k(q_1q_2/r)$
D. $F = K(q_2/r)$

3. If F = force = kq_1q_o/r^2 and q_o = an electric charge, then F/q_o is:

A. the electric field generated by q_1.
B. the force acting on q_o.
C. the electric potential set up by q_o.
D. the work done by the force on q_1.

4. Electric field lines are:

   A. directed away from negative charges.
   B. directed away from positive charges.
   C. directed toward positive charges.
   D. none of the above.

5. An electric potential:

   A. represents the negative of the work per unit charge in bringing a positive charge from one point to another in an electric field.
   B. is a vector.
   C. has the units of henries.
   D. represents all of the above.

6. Following are formulations for electric potential (V) except: (q = charge, r = distance, E = electric field, F = force, ε_0 = permittivity)

   A. $V = (^1/4\pi\varepsilon_0)(q/r)$
   B. V = potential energy/charge
   C. V = Er
   D. V = Fq

7. A volt is:

   A. newton/coulomb.
   B. joule/coulomb.
   C. coulomb/newton.
   D. coulomb/joule.

8. Electrical work is:

   A. dependent on the path taken by a charge between equipotential surfaces.
   B. zero when a charge is moved along an equipotential (electric potential) line.
   C. zero when a charge moves between surfaces of different electric potential.
   D. both (A) and (C).

9. The potential difference as used in electrostatics is:

   A. the difference in potential energy between two points.
   B. the difference in electric potential between two points.
   C. the difference in work between two points.
   D. both (A) and (C).

10. Which of the following is a correct formulation of electrical work (W) done on moving a charge (q) in an electric field (E)? (V = electric potential, PD = potential difference, F = electrical force, r = distance between charges)

    A. W = q(PD)
    B. W = Fq
    C. W = Vr
    D. W = Eq

11. All are true about electric dipoles except:

    A. they consist of two charges separated by a finite distance.
    B. the dipole moment is a product of the charge and the distance between them.
    C. the motion of dipoles against an electric field requires no energy.
    D. the positive end of the dipole points in the direction of the electric field.

12. If the distance between two electrical charges is doubled, the force between them is:

    A. decreased by $^3/4$.
    B. decreased by $^1/2$.
    C. doubled.
    D. quadrupled.

13. The charge (q) on each of two objects is doubled and they are moved twice as far apart (r); the force between them is:

   A. multiplied by a factor of 8.
   B. quadrupled.
   C. doubled.
   D. unchanged.

14. As two electrical charges move further apart, the force between them:

   A. increases proportionally to the inverse square of the distance between them.
   B. increases proportionally to the distance between them.
   C. decreases proportionally to the inverse square of the distance between them.
   D. decreases proportionally to the distance between them.

15. If charge #1 (q_1) is doubled, charge #2 (q_2) is tripled and the distance (r) between them is not changed, the force (F) between them:

   A. divides by a factor of 36.
   B. multiplies by a factor of 36.
   C. multiplies by a factor of 6.
   D. does not change.

16. What is the force between charge #1 (q_1) and charge #2 (q_2) in the diagram below?

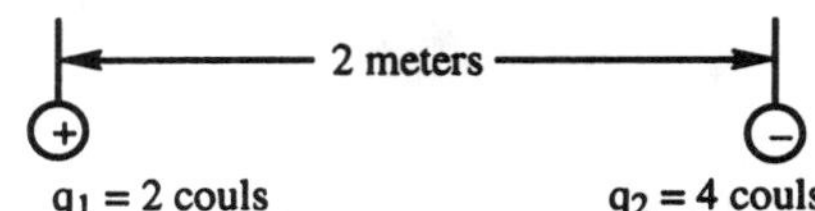

   A. repulsive, 2 nts
   B. attractive, 2 nts
   C. repulsive, 2k nts
   D. attractive, 2k nts

17. The net force on charge C (q_c) is:

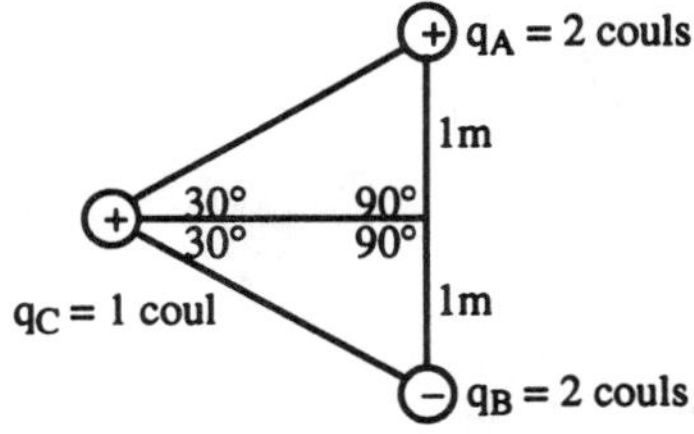

Assume, k = dielectric constant

   A. zero.
   B. horizontal and to the right, 0.5kN
   C. horizontal and to the left, 0.5kN
   D. vertical and down, 0.5kN

18. The electric field (E) generated by a charge:

   A. is constant at all distances from the charge.
   B. decreases directly as distance from the charge increases.
   C. decreases proportional to the inverse square of the distance from the charge.
   D. decreases proportional to the inverse distance from the charged.

19. All of the following are correct formulas for the potential energy (PE) of a charged object (q) in an electric field except:

   A. PE = Vq
   B. PE = Fr
   C. PE = Eq
   D. PE = qEr

F = force on charge
V = electric potential
E = electric field
r = distance of charge from object setting up the electric field

20. A positive charge is moved against (in the opposite direction of) an electric field. The potential energy of this positive charge:

A. remains the same.
B. decreases.
C. increases.
D. cannot be evaluated from the information given.

21. A negative charge is moved against (in the opposite direction of) an electric field. The potential energy of this negative charge:

A. stays the same.
B. increases.
C. decreases.
D. cannot be evaluated from the information given.

22. What is the electrical potential (V) at point A?

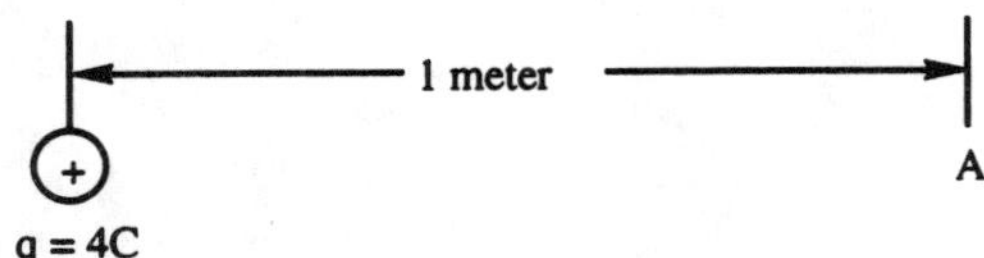

A. +4 volts
B. – 4 volts
C. +4k volts
D. – 4k volts

23. Determine the electric potential at point A.

$q_1 = +4C$ ⊕ —— 1m ——→ • A ←—— 2m ——→ ⊖ $q_2 = -16C$

A. – 28 volts
B. +28 volts
C. +4k volts
D. – 4k volts

24. What is the work done in moving a charge q_1 from A to B?

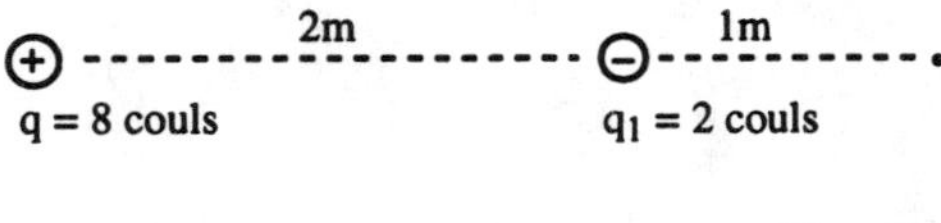

(A) ——→ (B)

A. – 10π joules
B. + 10π joules
C. + (8k/3) joules
D. – (8k/3) joules

25. Using Gauss' Law of Magnetism, which of the following statements is true:

A. The simplest magnetic structure is a dipole.
B. Magnetic flux varies with the charge.
C. Magnetic flux is not related to change in surface area of the magnetic field.
D. Magnetic flux varies with the velocity of the charge.

26. Some of the shortest electromagnetic waves are:

A. microwaves.
B. x-rays.
C. AM-radio waves.
D. FM-radio waves.

5.18.3 Answers to Questions in Section 5.18.2

(1) C (2) A (3) A (4) B (5) A (6) D (7) B (8) B (9) B (10) A (11) C (12) A (13) D (14) C (15) C (16) D (17) D (18) C (19) C (20) C (21) C (22) C (23) D (24) C (25) C (26) B

5.18.4 Discussion of Answers to Questions in Section 5.18.2

Questions #1 to #11 Adequately discussed in the Section.

Question #12 (Answer: A) From Coulomb's Law:

f = final   o = original

$$\frac{F_f}{F_o} = \frac{k\frac{q_1q_2}{r_f^2}}{k\frac{q_1q_2}{r_o^2}} = \frac{\frac{1}{r_f^2}}{\frac{1}{r_o^2}} = \frac{1}{r_f^2}\cdot\frac{r_o^2}{1} = \frac{r_o^2}{r_f^2} = \frac{r_o^2}{(2r_o)^2} = \frac{r_o^2}{4r_o^2} = \frac{1}{4}$$

$(r_f = 2r_o)$

$$\frac{F_f}{F_o} = \frac{1}{4}$$

$$F_f = 1/4F_o$$

Or reason from Coulomb's Law that force is proportional to the inverse square of distance ($1/r^2$); this is $(1/2)^2 =$ 1/4 for this case. Hence the force difference, $F_o - F_f = F_o - \frac{1}{4}F_o = \frac{3}{4}\ F_o$.

Question #13 (Answer: D) From Coulomb's Law:

f = final   o = original

$q_{1f} = 2q_{1o}$ $q_{2f} = 2q_{2o}$ $r_f = 2r_o$

$$\frac{F_f}{F_o} = \frac{k\frac{q_{1f}q_{2f}}{r_f^2}}{k\frac{q_{1o}q_{2o}}{r_o^2}} = \frac{q_{1f}q_{2f}}{r_f^2}\cdot\frac{r_o^2}{q_{1o}q_{2o}} = \frac{2q_{1o}2q_{2o}}{(2r_o)^2}\cdot\frac{r_o^2}{q_{1o}q_{2o}} = \frac{2\cdot 2\cdot q_{1o}\cdot q_{2o}\cdot r_o^2}{4\cdot r_o^2\cdot q_{1o}\cdot q_{2o}} = \frac{4}{4} = 1$$

$$\frac{F_f}{F_o} = 1 \text{ or } F_f = F_o$$

Reasoning from Coulomb's Law shows that force is directly proportional to the product of the charges; the doubling of each charge would increase the force by a factor of (2)(2) = 4. Since force is proportional to the inverse square of the separation, the increase in separation decreases the force by $(1/2)^2 = 1/4$. Multiplying these factors together to get the net change as (4)(1/4) = 1 or no change.

Question #14 (Answer: C) From Coulomb's Law:

$F \propto 1/r^2$, hence the force decreases proportionally to the square of the distance.

Question #15 (Answer: C) From Coulomb's Law:

f = final   o = original

$q_{1f} = 2q_{1o}$ $q_{2f} = 3q_{2o}$

$$\frac{F_f}{F_o} = \frac{k\frac{q_{1f}q_{2f}}{r^2}}{k\frac{q_{1o}q_{2o}}{r^2}} = \frac{q_{1f}q_{2f}}{q_{1o}q_{2o}} = \frac{(2q_{1o})(3q_{2o})}{(q_{1o})(q_{2o})} = \frac{2-3}{1} = 6$$

$$F_f = 6F_o$$

Reasoning from Coulomb's Law shows force is direcıly proportional to the product of the charges, since this product is increased (2)(3) = 6 times so the force must also be multiplied with 6.

Question #16 (Answer: D) From Coulomb's Law:

$F = k(q_1q_2/r^2) = k(+2)(-4)/(2)^2 = -2$ k nts. Since the sign is negative, the force is attractive.

Question #17 (Answer: D). This problem may be solved by the symmetry of the system, Coulomb's Law and geometry The forces (vectors) and their components exerted by $q_A(F_A)$ and $q_B(F_B)$ on qc are:

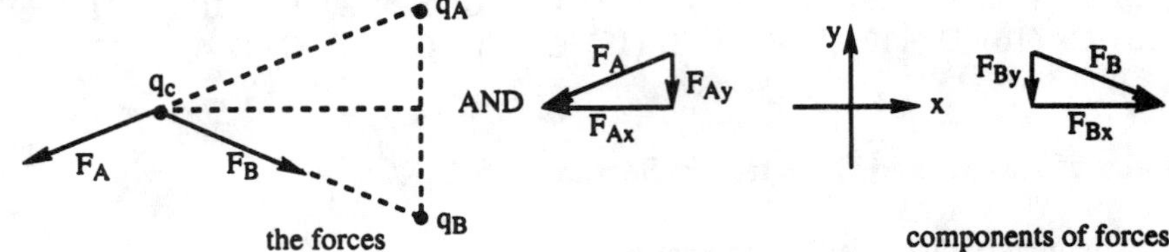

The x-components (F_{A_x} and F_{B_x}) cancel (because they are equal and opposite by the symmetry of the system) and the y-components sum to a vertically downward force. So, by elimination the answer is (D) ***OR***, first by applying Coulomb's Law:

$$F_A = k(q_Aq_C/r^2) \quad = k[(+2)(+1)/(2)^2] = k/2$$
$$F_B = k(q_Bq_C/r^2) \quad = k[(-2)(+1)/(2)^2] = -k/2$$

r = 2 m (meters) is derived by:

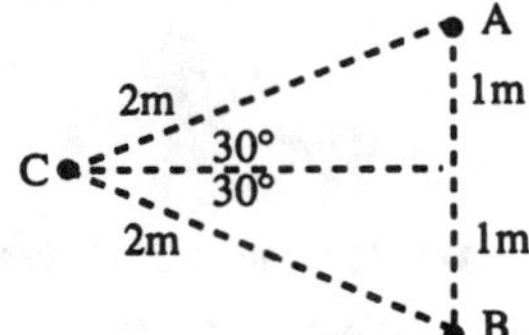

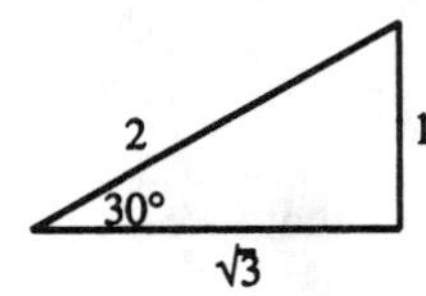

the side opposite the 30° angle is 1/2 the hypotenuse (which must then be 2 m)

The x-components still cancel and the y-components are:

$$F_{Ay} = +(1/2)F_A = -1/2(k/2) = -k/4$$
$$F_{By} = (1/2)F_B = 1/2(-k/2) = -k/4$$
$$F_y = F_{Ay} + F_{By} = -k/4 - k/4 = -k/2 \text{ nts}$$

the minus sign means F_y is directed down the y-axis.

Question #18 (Answer: C) The formula for the electric field (E) is:

$$E = F/q_0 = kq/r^2; \text{ hence, } E \propto 1/r^2.$$

Question #19 (Answer: C) Eq = force generated by E on q.

Question #20 (Answer: C). The direction of the lines of an electric field is the direction a positive charge would move if placed in it. To move a positive charge in the opposite direction requires energy, and this energy is stored as the potential energy which increases. The potential energy of the system may be used to move any charge along the direction of the field lines.

Question #21 (Answer: C). The direction of the field lines of an electric field is the direction a positive charge would move if placed in it. So, a negative charge would normally move in the opposite direction or against the field. When a charge moves in the expected direction in an electric field, the potential energy of the charge system decreases. This is like the potential energy of a rock decreasing as it falls toward earth, because this expected direction makes it move in the gravitational field.

Question #22 (Answer: C) The formula for V is:

$$V = kq/r = k(+4/1) = +4k \text{ volts.}$$

Question #23 (Answer: D). Since the electric potential (V) is a scalar, the V contribution by each charge is determined separately and added algebraically to get the net potential at point A:

For q_1: $V_1 = k(q_1/r_1) \quad = \quad k(+4/1) = +4k$ volts
For q_2: $V_2 = k(q_2/r_2) \quad = \quad k(-16/2) = -8k$ volts
Total: $V_A = V_1 + V_2 \quad = \quad +4k - 8k = -4$ k volts.

Question #24 (Answer: C). The work done in this instance can be calculated by using the following formulations:

$W = q_1 (V_B - V_A) = q_1$ (PD)

$V_B = k(q/r_B) = k(+8/3) = (+8/3)$ k volts

$V_A = k(q/r_A) = k(+8/2) = +4$ k volts

q is generating the potential for both points A and B.

PD (Potential difference) = $V_B - V_A = (8/3)k - 4k = (8\text{-}12)k/3 = -4k/3$ volts

$W = q_1 \text{ (PD)} = (-2)(-4k/3) = (+8/3)$ k joules.

The positive sign means that work must be put into (done to) the system.

Questions #25 and #26 Adequately discussed in the Section.

5.18.5 Checklist for Electrostatics and Electromagnetism

______	charges	______	paramagnetic	______	electrical dipoles
______	conductors	______	ferromagnetic	______	magnetic field
______	insulators	______	Biot and Savart law	______	Tesla
______	Coulomb's Law	______	Right-hand rule	______	Weber
______	electrical forces	______	magnetic dipoles	______	Bohr magneton
______	electric field	______	volts	______	magnetic flux
______	X-rays	______	dipole moment	______	electromagnetic induction
______	magnetotactic bacteria	______	potentials	______	Faraday's law
______	diamagnetic	______	potential differences	______	Ampere-Maxwell law

5.19 ELECTRIC CIRCUITS

5.19.1 Review of Electric Circuits

5.19.1.1 ELECTRIC CIRCUITS

The main elements in an electric (DC = direct current) circuit are the emf source (V) and the resistors (R). The current (I) results from their interaction These three quantities are interrelated in *Ohm's* Law as:

$$V = IR.$$

V, I, R are the total of each in the circuit Capacitors may also be used in electronic circuits.

Circuit elements may be in series, in parallel, or in combinations of both. Two components are in series when they have only one point in common; that is, the current traveling from one of them back to the emf source must pass through the other. In a complete series circuit, or for individual series loops of a larger mixed circuit, the current (I) is the same over each component and the total voltage (V_T is the sum of all the emf sources) is the sum of voltages across each resistor (including the internal resistances of emf sources—see below). Two components are in *parallel* when they are connected to two common points in the circuit; that is, the current traveling from one such element back to the source of emf (assume current started at source of emf) need not pass through the second component because there is an alternate path. In a parallel circuit, the total current is the sum of currents for each path (i.e., each path has a different current), and the voltage is equal for all paths and thus equals V_T Circuits can be simplified into subunits that are either series or parallel, and the above rules are applied to them.

Electromotive force (V) maintains a constant potential difference and thereby maintains a continuous current. The emf source replaces energy lost by the moving electrons. Sources of emf are batteries (conversions of chemical energy to electrical energy) and generators (conversion of mechanical energy to electrical energy). A source of emf is symbolized in a circuit as in Fig. 5.34.

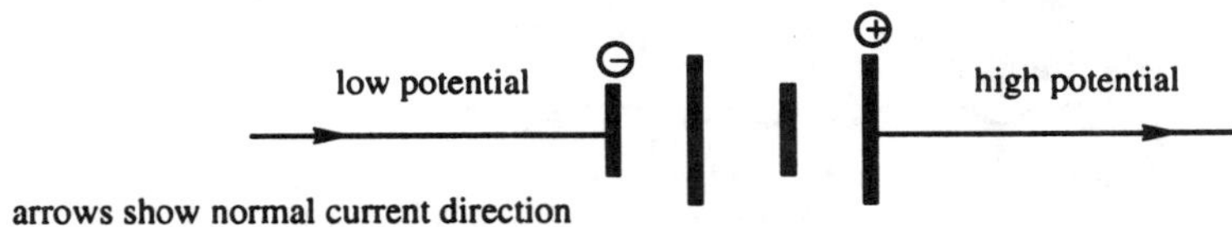

Fig. 5.34—Electromotive Force

The source of emf does work on each charge to raise it from a lower potential to a higher potential. Then as the charge flows around the circuit (naturally from higher to lower potential) it loses energy which is replaced by the emf source again, etc. Therefore work (energy) must be supplied at the rate energy is lost by the current flowing through the circuit,

$$\text{energy supplied} = \text{energy lost.}$$

Energy is lost whenever a charge (as current) passes through a resistor.

The *units of emf (E)* are volts (Section 5.18.1). The actual voltage delivered to a circuit is not equal to the V_T value of the source V_T represents the total potential difference across the external source terminals. It is also called the EMF of the source Generally $V_T = V$ unless otherwise specified.

This is reduced by Ir which represents the voltage loss by the *internal resistance (r)* of the source itself. The net voltage is called the terminal voltage (V_t) and is:

$V_t = V_T - Ir = IR$ = terminal voltage
IR = totals for the whole circuit = terminal voltage
V = maximal voltage output of emf source = $V_T = I(R + r)$
r = internal resistance
R = external resistance

The V_t is the voltage delivered to the circuit by that emf source.

Normally, a charge gains energy as it flows through a source of emf. But when two sources of emf are connected in opposition (positive pole to positive pole), the charge flows from the higher emf source to the lower emf source. In this instance, it loses energy when passing through the smaller emf because it passes in the opposite direction to normal. If there is more than one source of emf in a circuit, the *total emf* is a sum of these by taking into account the differences in polarity (i.e., reversed emf's are negative):

$$V_t\,(\text{total}) = \Sigma V_{ti},\ i = 1, 2, \ldots.$$

A voltmeter is used to measure voltages (potential differences) in circuits and is *symbolized* as:

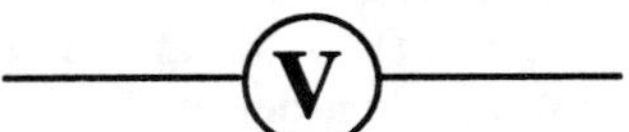

Resistance (R) is the opposition to the flow of electrons in a substance. *Resistivity* (ρ) is an inherent property of a substance and is directly related to resistance. Resistivity varies directly as resistance and cross-sectional area, and indirectly as length.

Resistance has a fixed value for a given material and depends on the size, shape and temperature but not on the emf or current Note these relations ($R \propto 1/A$):

R increases as L increases
R increases as A decreases
R increases as temperature increases.

Resistance increases with temperature because the thermal motion of atoms (molecules) increases and results in more collisions with electrons which impede their flow. The units of resistance are ohms symbolized by Ω (omega). From Ohm's Law, an ohm = volt/ampere.

When + I (current) flows across a resistor, there is a voltage decrease and an energy loss:

energy loss = Vq = VIt = joules
power loss (P) = VIt/t = VI = watts = volt-amperes = joules/sec.

The energy loss may be used to perform work. These relations hold for power (P),

$$P = VI = (IR)(I) = I^2R = V(V/R) = V^2/R.$$

Resistance in a circuit is *symbolized* by,

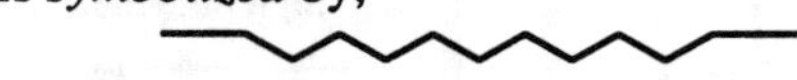

A variable resistance (as with a rheostat) is symbolized by:

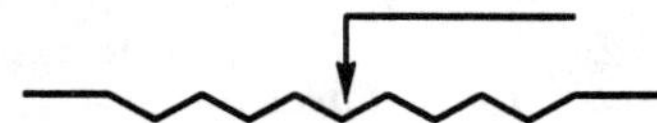

Resistance in a series circuit is:

$$R = R_1 + R_2 + R_3 + \ldots$$

Resistance in a parallel circuit is,

$1/R = 1/R_1 + 1/R_2 + 1/R_3 + \ldots$ The R's are the total resistances.

Current (I) is the amount of charge (Q) that flows past a point in a given amount of time (t),

$$I = Q/t = \text{amperes} = \text{coulombs/sec}.$$

Current is caused by the movement of electrons. The velocity of electrons is slowed by impurities in the conductor and by the thermal motion of atoms According to Ohm's Law, if specific conducting impurities are added to a semiconductor, then the resistance of the semiconductor drops. This results in increased flow of current. A transient current is set up when a capacitor discharges (below). A continuous current is set up when a source of emf is present to replace the energy lost by moving electrons (see above). The direction of current is taken as the direction a positive charge moves, by convention. It is represented on a circuit diagram by arrows. Ammeters are used to measure the flow of current and are symbolized as:

Capacitance (C) is an inherent property of a conductor and is formulated as:

$$C = \text{charge/electric potential} = Q/V = \text{farad} = \text{coulomb/volt}.$$

This means that C is the number of coulombs that must be transferred to a conductor to raise its potential by one volt. The amount of charge than can be stored is determined by the size, shape and surroundings of the conductor. A smaller conductor usually has a smaller capacitance. A greater degree of curvature (or more pointed) usually means a greater capacity to store charge. The higher the dielectric strength (i.e., the electric field strength at which a substance ceases to be an insulator and becomes a conductor) of the medium, the greater the capacitance of the conductor.

A *capacitor* is two or more conductors with opposite but equal charges placed near each other. A common example is the parallel plate capacitor. The formulas of importance for capacitors are:

(1) $C = Q/V$
V = potential difference between the plates

(2) $V = Ed$
E = electric field strength
d = distance between the plates

(3) C is directly proportional to the area of the plates
C is inversely proportional to the distance between the plates;
i.e.: $C_o = E_o A/d$ for air and vacuum (as the medium) between the plates.

(4) $K = C/C_o$ = *dielectric constant*
$K = V_o/V = E_o/E$ also
$C = KC_o$.

The *dielectric substances* set up an opposing electric field to that of the capacitor which decreases the net electric field and allows the capacitance of the capacitor to increase ($C = Q/Ed$). The molecules of the dielectric are dipoles which line up in the electric field.

Fig. 5.35—Capacitor without Dielectric

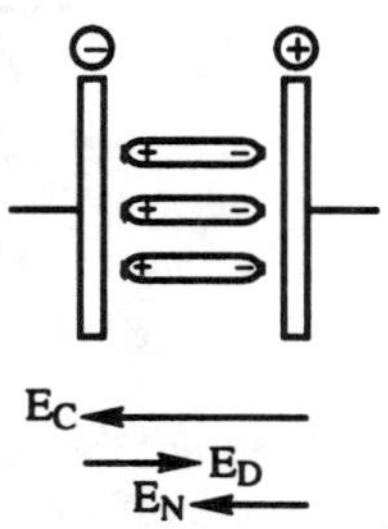

Fig. 5.36—Capacitor with Dielectric

E = electric field
D = dielectric
C = capacitor
N = net

The C's are the total capacitances (See also 5.19.1.2)

The *energy associated with each charged capacitor* is:

$V_{avg} = 1/2\ V$
Potential Energy (PE) = $W = (1/2V)(Q) = 1/2\ QV = 1/2\ (CV)(V) = 1/2CV^2$
$= 1/2\ Q(Q/C) = 1/2Q^2/C.$

The *symbol for a capacitor* is:

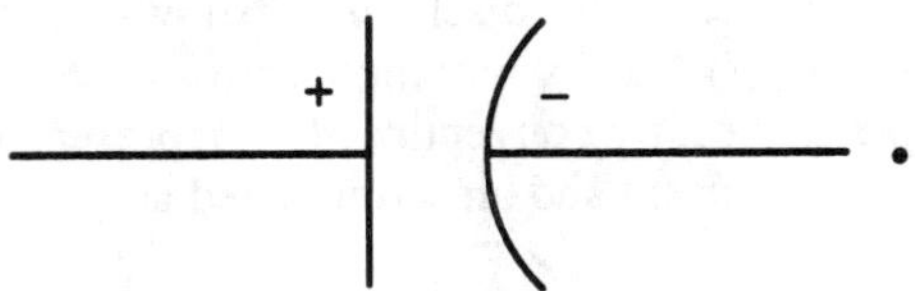

In an *electric circuit, the capacitor* charges up until the charge (Q_{max}) equals V_t C and then the current stops. If the V_t is then removed, the capacitor will discharge. In an *alternating electric circuit* (AC), there is an alternating surge of charge onto and off the capacitor, and a current exists there even though there is no transfer of charge between the plates. The behavior of a capacitor in a circuit is summarized below to show some key results:

(1) When a C is combined in series with an R:
$V_t = IR + Q/C$
(2) RC = capacitive time constant τ = (ohms)(farads) = seconds
(a) The capacitor takes about 5τ to become fully charged ($Q_{max} = CV_t$).
(b) In one τ, the capacitor is 63% charged and has 37% of its final current (V_t/R) delivered to it (these numbers arise from the solution and the base of the natural logs which is e = 2.7183, $\therefore$ 1/e = 0.37, 1 – 1/e = 0.63)
(c) The capacitor will be nearly fully discharged after 5τ.
(d) The capacitor will have discharged down to 37% of Q_{max} after one τ.

5.19.1.2 ALTERNATING ELECTRIC CIRCUITS

AC (alternating current) electricity constitutes 99% of that used in the U.S. It is made by converting mechanical energy to electrical energy An armature, which is a loop of wire, is rotated in a magnetic field using mechanical energy. A current is induced (see inductance below) in the wire of the armature. This current changes direction because the direction of the velocity of the loop and the magnetic field changes. Slip rings are fused to each end of the wire loop and rotate with it. Since the direction of the current alternates, the slip rings alternate in conducting the current away from the loop (hence AC). Graphite brushes are on the slip rings and these brush against conducting materials which carry away from the generator AC looks like a sine wave.

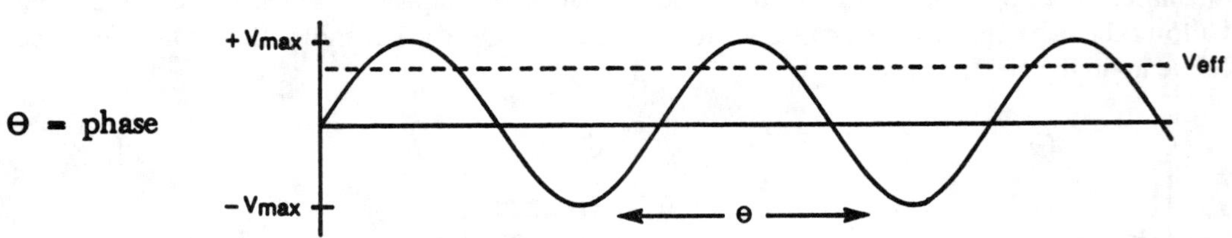

Fig. 5.37—EMF or Alternating Voltage Curve

Note that the maximum voltages (V) are not the same as V_{eff} (effective voltage, or root-mean square voltage). Similarly, the maximum current is not the effective (root-mean square) current delivered (I_{eff}). These relations are,

$V_{eff} = 0.707\ V_{max}$
$I_{eff} = 0.707\ I_{max}$.

One effective volt of AC will develop one effective ampere of current through a resistance of one ohm. The frequency of alternation of the cycle is also important in determining the V and I values. A typical frequency is 60 cycles/second. Note: $\omega = 2\pi f$ = angular frequency In a capacitive circuit the capacitive reactance is defined as $X_C = 1/(\omega C)$ and in an inductive circuit the inductive reactance is defined as $X_L = \omega L$.

The combined effect of a resistance and an inductive reactance is known as apparent resistance or *"impedance"*. The letter Z is generally used to indicate impedance. Thus, in an AC circuit, we can write

Ohm's Law as:

$$I\ (\text{amperes}) = \frac{V(\text{volts})}{(\text{Ohms})}$$

Impedance can be represented vectorially as the hypotenuse of the right triangle whose two sides are the ohmic resistance and the reactance, thus:

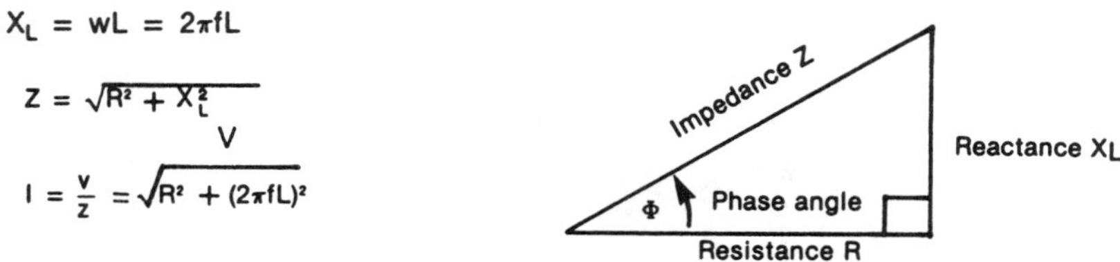

Fig. 5.38—Vector Triangle Relating Resistance, Reactance, and Impedance

The angle ϕ between R and Z is called the phase angle and is equal to the lag of the current behind the voltage, in electrical degrees.

Concept of Capacitance

The capacitance C of the capacitor is defined as the ratio of the charge Q on either conductor to the potential difference V_{ab} between the conductors.

$$C = \frac{Q}{V_{ab}}$$

The net charge on the capacitor as a whole is zero and "the charge on a capacitor" is understood to mean the charge on either conductor, without regard to sign. From the definition, note that capacitance is expressed in coulombs per volt. Since one volt is equivalent to one joule per coulomb, one coulomb per volt is equivalent to one $coul^2$/joule. A capacitance of one coulomb per volt is called one farad (for Faraday). That is, the capacitance of a capacitor is one farad if one coulomb is transferred from one conductor to the other, per volt of potential difference between the conductors.

Capacitors find many applications in electrical circuits. A capacitor is used to eliminate sparking when a circuit containing inductance is suddenly opened. The ignition system of the automobile engine contains a capacitor for this purpose. Capacitors are used in radio circuits for tuning, and for "smoothing" the rectified current delivered by the power supply. The efficiency of alternating current power transmissions can often be increased by the use of large capacitors.

Dielectric Coefficient

Most capacitors utilize a solid, nonconducting material or dielectric between their plates. A common type is the paper and foil capacitor, in which strips of metal foil form the plates and a sheet of paper impregnated with wax is dielectric. By rolling up such a capacitor, a capacitance of several microfarads can be obtained in a relatively small volume. The "Leyden jar," constructed by cementing metal foil over a portion of the inside and outside surfaces of a glass jar, is essentially a parallel-plate capacitor, with the glass forming the dielectric.

Electrolytic capacitors utilize as their dielectric an extremely thin layer of nonconducting oxide between a metal plate and a conducting solution. Because of the small thickness of the dielectric, electrolytic capacitors of relatively small dimensions may have a capacitance of the order of 50 μF.

5.19.2 Questions to Review Electric Circuits

1. In a DC circuit if the resistors are:

   A. in series, the currents are different for each component.
   B. in series, the voltages are the same for each component.
   C. in parallel, the currents are equal for all paths (of the circuit).
   D. in parallel, the voltages are equal for all paths.

2. The following graph represents which type of current(s)?

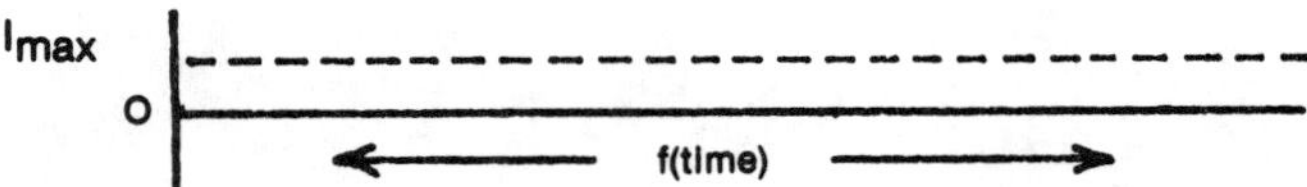

   A. AC only
   B. DC only
   C. AC or DC
   D. neither AC nor DC

3. Ohm's Law is:
   (V = potential difference, I = current, R = resistance, C = capacitance, Q = charge, L = inductance, t = time):

   A. $C = Q/V$
   B. $L = -\Delta V/\Delta I/\Delta t)$
   C. $V = IR$
   D. $V = QLt$

4. The actual voltage output of an electromotive source:

   A. may be equal to, less than, or greater than the expected voltage of the source.
   B. is always equal to the expected voltage.
   C. is always more than the expected voltage.
   D. is always less than the expected voltage.

5. All of the following statements concerning electromotive force (emf) are correct except:

   A. units are microfarads.
   B. maintains constant potential differences in a circuit.
   C. replaces energy lost by the moving electrons in a circuit.
   D. sources include both batteries and generators.

6. A source of emf (electromotive force):

   A. generates positive and negative charges.
   B. decreases the resistance an electron faces in moving through a circuit.
   C. does work on each charge to raise it from a lower potential (electrical) to a higher potential.
   D. changes the sign of the charge during each transit of the circuit.

7. Normally, a charge gains energy as it moves through a source of emf, but it can lose energy if:

   A. the emf source has an internal resistance.
   B. the emf source has a reversed polarity.
   C. the emf source is a generator.
   D. the emf source is of low voltage.

8. Resistance, as used in electricity, is:

   A. the opposition to flow of electrons in a substance.
   B. the opposition to the generation of emf.
   C. the location of storage of energy of electrons.
   D. in the units of farads.

9. Resistance, as used in electricity, is:

   A. inversely proportional to the density of the conductor.
   B. inversely proportional to the resistivity of the conductor.
   C. directly proportional to the cross-sectional area of the conductor.
   D. directly proportional to the length of the conductor.

10. Resistance (electrical) has a fixed value for a given material and depends on all except:

   A. size of a conductor.
   B. current in a conductor.
   C. shape of a conductor.
   D. temperature.

11. The resistance of a substance can be expected to increase for all the following situations except:

   A. increasing cross-sectional area.
   B. increasing length.
   C. increasing temperature.
   D. increasing resistivity of materials.

12. The unit of electric power is the:

   A. joule.
   B. volt.
   C. ampere.
   D. watt.

13. Current is:

   A. time/charge.
   B. charge/time.
   C. (charge)(time).
   D. none of these.

14. An ampere is:

   A coulombs/secs.
   B. (coulombs)(secs).
   C. (volts)(ohms).
   D. ohms/volts.

15. Current is:

   A. caused by the movement of positive charge.
   B. increased by the thermal motion of atoms.
   C. increased by impurities in the semiconductor.
   D. all of the above.

16. To set up a continuous current, as opposed to a transient current, in a circuit, one may use a:

   A. source of emf.
   B. capacitor.
   C. capacitor and resistor.
   D. capacitor and inductor.

17. Capacitance is:

A. charge/potential.
B. (charge)(potential).
C. (resistance)(current).
D. charge/resistance.

18. The farad is a unit of capacitance and is equal to:

A. coulombs/volts.
B. (volts)(coulombs).
C. amperes/ohms.
D. (amperes)(ohms).

19. All of the following are associated with increased capacitance of a conductor except:

A. increased inducibility.
B. increased size.
C. increased curvature.
D. increased dielectric strength of the medium.

20. In a parallel plate capacitor:

A. both plates carry the same charge.
B. capacitance is directly proportional to the distance between the plates.
C. capacitance is independent of the medium between the plates.
D. capacitance is directly proportional to the area of the plates.

21. A capacitor will charge up to a certain point and then will cause the current to stop in a(n):

A. DC circuit.
B. AC circuit.
C. both DC and AC circuits.
D. neither DC nor AC circuits.

22. In an AC circuit a capacitor is placed in series with a resistor. The voltage of the AC generator (neglecting internal resistance) is:

A. (capacitor voltage)(resistor voltage).
B. voltage across the capacitor minus voltage across the resistor.
C. voltage across the resistor minus voltage across the capacitor.
D. voltage across the resistor plus voltage across the capacitor.

23. If total resistance is 9 ohms and total voltage is 3 volts the current is:

A. $^1/_{27}$ ampere
B. $^1/_3$ ampere
C. 3 amperes
D. 27 amperes

24. A current of 2 amperes and a resistance of 8 ohms requires what voltage (in a circuit):

A. $^1/_{16}$ volt
B. $^1/_4$ volt
C. 4 volts
D. 16 volts

25. If it requires 20 volts to cause a current of 5 amperes in a wire, the resistance of the wire is:

A. $^1/_{100}$ ohm
B. $^1/_4$ ohm
C. 4 ohms
D. 100 ohms

26. Assuming internal resistances of circuit elements is negligible, a charge would lose the most energy when it passes through a(n):

A. capacitor.
B. inductor.
C. resistor.
D. battery.

27. A battery has a voltage of 6V marked on it and an internal resistance of 0.5 ohm. If it is placed in the circuit below, what is the actual voltage it is producing in that circuit?

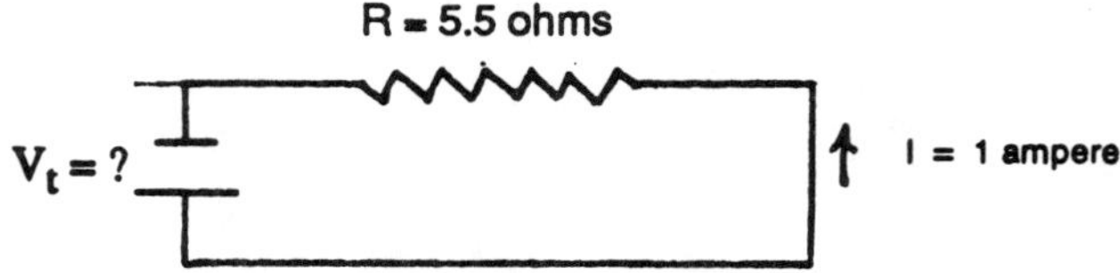

A. 10 volts
B. 8.5 volts
C. 5.5 volts
D. 5 volts

28. Calculate the internal resistance of the 20-volt battery in the following circuit:

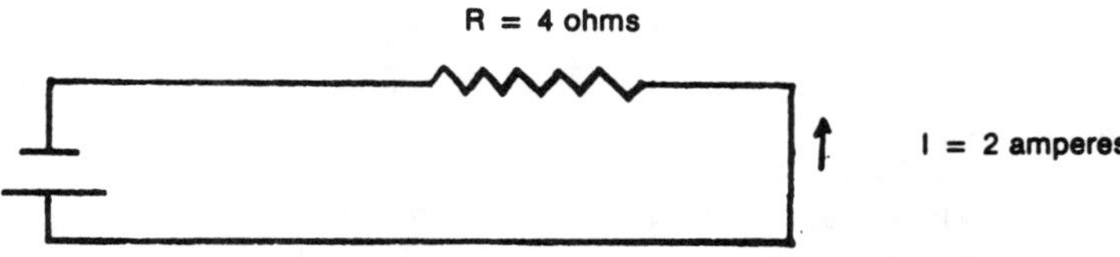

A. 16 ohms
B. 10 ohms
C. 6 ohms
D. 2 ohms

29. Determine the total emf (electromotive force) in the following circuit:

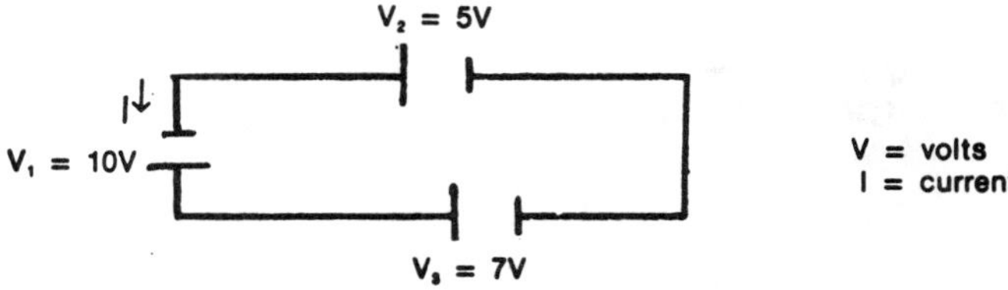

A. 2 volts
B. 8 volts
C. 12 volts
D. 22 volts

30. All are formulations of power (P) in a circuit with an emf (V) source and a resistor (R) with a current (I), except:

A. $P = VI$
B. $P = IR/V$
C. $P = I^2R$
D. $P = V^2/R$

31. A circuit has a current of 2 amperes and a resistance of 4 ohms. The maximum power that can be delivered is:

A. 16 watts
B. 8 watts
C. 2 watts
D. $^1/2$ watt

32. If the cross-sectional area of a conductor is quadrupled ($\times$ 4), the resistance:

A. increases 16 times.
B. increases 4 times.
C. decreases to $^1/4$.
D. decreases to $^1/16$.

33. If the length of a conductor is doubled, the resistance:

A. is not affected.
B. decreases to 50% of original resistance.
C. decreases to 25% of original resistance.
D. doubles.

34. In a circuit with a voltage of 10 volts and a resistance of 10 ohms and a current passing for 10 secs, the maximum possible number of joules of heat produced is:

A. 100 joules.
B. 1000 joules.
C. 1 joule.
D. 10 joules.

35. Determine the current (I) in the following circuit:

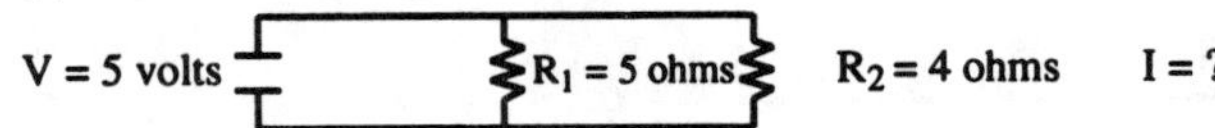

A. $^5/9$ amperes
B. 1.8 amperes
C. 2.25 amperes
D. 45 amperes

36. The voltage (V) of the following battery is (neglect internal resistance of battery):

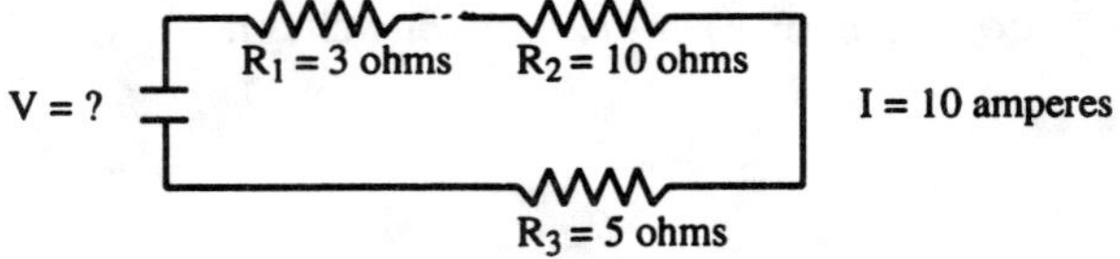

A. 180 volts
B. 18 volts
C. 1.8 volts
D. 0.55 volts

37. A current of 8 amperes will deliver what charge in 4 seconds?

A. 2 statcoulombs
B. 2 coulombs
C. 32 statcoulombs
D. 32 coulombs

38. If 10 coulombs pass a point in 2 seconds, the current is:

A. 0.20 amps.
B. 5 amps.
C. 20 amps.
D. 200 amps.

39. A conductor discharges (i.e., cannot hold any more charge) when 40 coulombs is placed on it at a voltage of 10 volts. What is its capacitance?

A. 4000 farads
B. 400 farads
C. 0.25 farads
D. 4 farads

40. The capacitance of a parallel plate capacitor in air is 20 farads. This capacitor is placed in a medium with a dielectric constant equal to 5. What is the capacitance now?

A. 20 farads
B. 4 farads
C. 400 farads
D. 100 farads

41. In air, a parallel plate capacitor has a capacitance of 4 farads. In medium A, the capacitance is 32 farads. What is the dielectric constant of medium A?

A. $^{1}/_{8}$
B. 8
C. 128
D. need the dielectric constant of air

42. The units of resistance times capacitance is:

A. voltage.
B. amperes.
C. henries.
D. seconds.

43. Convert the following circuit into a simple single equivalent resistance

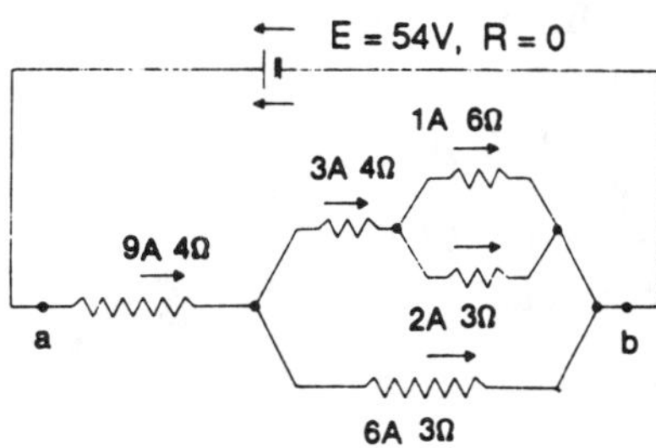

44. In an AC circuit, the effective value of the current is:

A. equal to the maximum value of the AC current.
B. greater than the maximum value of the AC current.
C. less than the maximum value of the AC current.
D. greater than the maximum value of the DC current.

45. When a coil whose resistance is 15Ω is connected to a 120V, 60 Hz source, it draws 2.5A. Find (i) the impedance and (ii) the inductance of the coil.

A. 17.5Ω, 12.5H
B. 8Ω, 0.92H
C. 48Ω, 0.12H
D. 24Ω, 22.8H

5.19.3 Answers to Questions in Section 5.19.2

(1) D	(2) B	(3) C	(4) D	(5) A	(6) C	(7) B	(8) A	(9) D	(10) B
(11) A	(12) D	(13) B	(14) A	(15) C	(16) A	(17) A	(18) A	(19) A	(20) D
(21) A	(22) D	(23) B	(24) D	(25) C	(26) C	(27) C	(28) C	(29) B	(30) B
(31) A	(32) C	(33) D	(34) A	(35) C	(36) A	(37) D	(38) B	(39) D	(40) D
(41) B	(42) D	(43) See discussion of answer to question #43.					(44) C	(45) C	

5.19.4 Discussion of Answers to Questions in Section 5.19.2

Questions #1 to #22: Adequately discussed in the Section.

Question #23 (Answer: B) From Ohm's Law:

$$V = IR$$
$$I = V/R = 3 \text{ volts}/9 \text{ ohms} = 1/3 \text{ amp.}$$

Question #24 (Answer: D) Solve using Ohm's Law:

$$V = IR = (2 \text{ amps})(8 \text{ ohms}) = 16 \text{ volts.}$$

Question #25 (Answer: C) Use Ohm's Law:

$$V = IR$$
$$R = V/I = \frac{20 \text{ volts}}{5 \text{ amps}} = 4 \text{ ohms}$$

Question #26 (Answer: C). Energy is lost when a charge passes through a resistance.

Question #27 (Answer: C). The terminal voltage (V_t) of an emf source is determined by taking into account the internal resistance:

$r = 0.5$ ohms
$R = 5.5$ ohms
$V_T = 6$ volts

$$V_t = V_T - Ir = IR$$
$$V_T = I(R + r)$$
$$6 = I(5.5 + 0.5)$$
$$I = 1 \text{ amp}$$
$$\text{Hence, } V_t = V_T - Ir = 6 - 1(0.5)$$

Question #28 (Answer: C). See Section for an explanation of the formula:

$V_T = 20$ volts $r = ?$
$R = 4$ ohms
$I = 2$ amps

$$V_T = I(R + r)$$
$$20 = 2(4 + r)$$
$$20 - 2r = 8$$
$$r = 6 \text{ ohms}$$

Question #29 (Answer: B). The total emf's around the loop of the circuit is:

$$V_{total} = \Sigma V = V_1 + V_2 - V_3 = 10 + 5 - 7 = 8$$

V_3 is negative because the current is moving through it in the reverse direction.

The internal resistances of the batteries have been neglected.

Question #30 (Answer: B). Try to remember how to convert it to the others using Ohm's Law

Question #31 (Answer: A). The appropriate formula is:

$$P = I^2 R = (2)^2(4) = 16 \text{ watts}$$

The units are arrived at as follows:

$$P = (\text{amperes})^2(\text{ohms}) = (\text{amps})^2(\text{volts/amps}) = (\text{amps})(\text{volts})$$
$$= (\text{coulomb/sec})\text{volts} = \text{volt}\cdot\text{coulomb/sec} = \text{joules/sec} = \text{watts}$$

Remember: joule = volt·coulomb.

Question #32 (Answer: C) Resistance (R) $\propto$ 1/Area(A). Then if A increases by a factor of 4, the R decreases to 1/4 of the original value.
OR:

$R_2/R_1 = (\rho l/A_2)/(\rho l/A_1) = (1/A_2)/(1/A_1) = (1/A_2)(A_1/1) = A_1/A_2$
$= A_1/(4A_1) = 1/4 \qquad (A_2 = 4A_1)$
$\therefore R_2 = 1/4\ R_1$.

Question #33 (Answer: D). Resistance (R) $\propto$ length (l). So, if length doubles, the R is doubled.
OR:

$R_2/R_1 = (\rho l_2/A)/(\rho l_1/A) = (l_2/l_1) = 2l_1/l_1 = 2$
$\therefore R_2 = 2R_1. \qquad (l_2 = 2l_1)$

Question #34 (Answer: A) $P = V^2/R$ (see Section)

$P = (10)^2/10 = 10$ watts
(Power)(time) = joules = (10)(10) = 100 joules.

Question #35 (Answer: C) R_1 and R_2 are in parallel Then:

$1/R_T = 1/R_1 + 1/R_2 = 1/5 + 1/4 = 4/20 + 5/20 = 9/20$
$\therefore R_T = 20/9$ ohms.

Then using Ohm's Law: V = IR

$I = V/R = 5$ volts/(20/9 ohms) = 5(9/20) = 9/4 = 2.25 amps.

Question #36 (Answer: A) This is a series circuit because the current (I) *must* pass through each resistor (R) before returning to the voltage source (V). The total resistance (R_T):

$R_T = R_1 + R_2 + R_3 = 3 + 10 + 5 = 18$ ohms.

Calculate V using Ohm's Law: V = IR = (10 amps) (18 ohms)
= 180 volts.

Question #37 (Answer: D)

I = q/t
q = (I)(t) = (8 amps)(4 seconds) = 32 coulombs.

Question #38 (Answer: B)

I = q/t = 10 couls/2 secs = 5 amps

Question #39 (Answer: D) C = q/V = 40 coulombs/10 volts = 4 farads

Question #40 (Answer: D) $C = K\,C_o$, C_o = capacitance of air
C = (5)(20) = 100 farads.

Question #41 (Answer: B) $C = K\,C_o$
$K = C/C_o = 32/4 = 8$.

Question #42 (Answer: D)

resistance (R) = ohms = volts/amperes = volts/(coulombs/sec) = (volt-sec)/couls
capacitance (C) = farads = couls/volt

Then: (R)(C) = (volt-sec/coul)(coul/volt) = secs.

Question #43

Use principles of parallel/series resistors

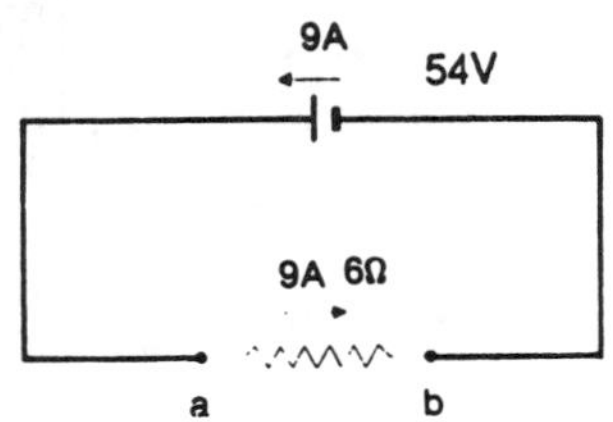

Question #44 Adequately discussed in the Section.

Question #45 Solution:

(a) First solve for the impedance of the circuit.

$$Z = \frac{V}{I} = \frac{120\text{ V}}{2.5\text{ A}} = 48\Omega.$$

(b)

$$Z^2 = R^2 + X_L^2$$
$$X_L = \sqrt{Z^2 - R^2} = \sqrt{(48\Omega)^2 - (15\Omega)^2} = 45.6\Omega$$

But since $X_L = 2\pi fL$, or $L = X_L/2\pi f$,

$$L = \frac{45.6\Omega}{6.28 \text{ x } 60 \text{ cycles/sec}} = 0.1210\text{H}$$

5.19.5 Checklist for Electric Circuits

_____ current
_____ battery
_____ internal resistance
_____ Ohm's law
_____ resistors
_____ resistivity
_____ resistance
_____ capacitors
_____ capacitance
_____ impedance
_____ root mean-square current/voltage
_____ capacitive resistance
_____ DC electricity
_____ series circuits
_____ parallel circuits
_____ emf
_____ volts
_____ farad
_____ ohm
_____ dielectric constant
_____ dielectrics
_____ AC circuits
_____ AC electricity
_____ inductive reactance

5.20 WAVE CHARACTERISTICS AND PERIODIC MOTION

5.20.1 Review of Wave Characteristics and Periodic Motion

A *wave* is a disturbance in a medium such that each particle in the medium vibrates about an equilibrium point in a simple harmonic motion (below). If the direction of vibration is perpendicular to the direction of propagation of the wave, the wave is called a *transverse wave* (e.g., light). If the direction of vibration is in the same direction as propagation of the wave, the wave is called *a longitudinal wave* (e.g., sound). Longitudinal waves are characterized by condensations (regions of crowding of particles) and rarefactions (regions where particles are far apart) along the wave in the medium See Fig. 5.39(b).

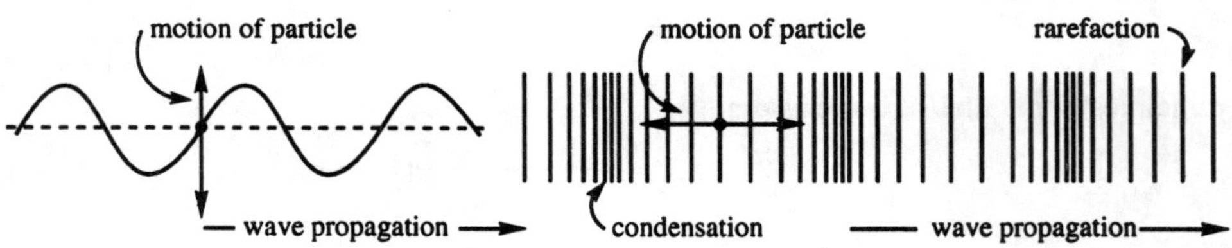

Fig. 5.39(a)—Transverse Wave　　*Fig. 5.39(b)—Longitudinal Wave*

The *wavelength* (λ) is the distance from crest to crest (or valley to valley) of a transverse wave. It may also be defined as the distance between two particles with the same displacement and direction of displacement. In a longitudinal wave, the wavelength can be taken as the distance from one rarefaction (or condensation) to another. The *amplitude* (A) is the maximum displacement of a particle in one direction from its equilibrium point. *Frequency* (f) is the number of wavelengths (cycles) that pass a point per unit time. *Period* (T) is the time required for one wavelength to pass a point. *Speed* (v) of a wave refers to its propagation through the medium. Speed increases as the inertia of the medium decreases (e.g., as density decreases). *Phase* (ϕ) is the difference in displacement and direction of a particle due to two different waves. Two waves are in phase if each particle has the same displacement and direction of motion (ϕ = 0)(Fig. 5.40):

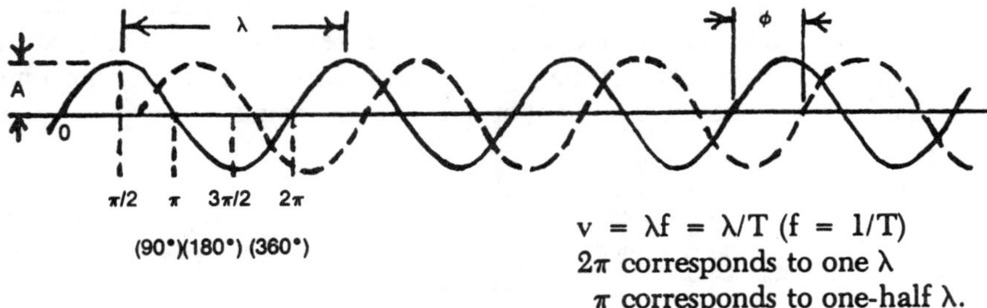

$v = \lambda f = \lambda/T$ ($f = 1/T$)
2π corresponds to one λ
π corresponds to one-half λ.

Fig. 5.40—Characteristics of Waves

The *superposition principle* states that the effect of two or more waves on the displacement of a particle are independent. This means the displacement of a particle by simultaneous waves in a medium are algebraically additive *Interference* is the summation of the displacements of different waves in a medium. *Constructive interference* is when the waves add to a larger resultant wave than either original. This occurs maximally when the phase difference (ϕ) is a whole wavelength (λ) which corresponds to multiples of 360° (2π). So, this occurs at $\phi = 0, 2\pi, 4\pi$, etc Since $\phi = 2\pi\Delta L/\lambda$, where ΔL equals the difference in path to a point of two waves (of equal wavelength), these waves interfere constructively when ΔL = 0, λ, 2λ, 3λ, etc. *Destructive interference* is when the waves add to a smaller resultant wave than either original wave. This occurs maximally when $\phi = \pi, 3\pi, 5\pi$, etc., which are multiples of one-half wavelengths (180° = π corresponds to $^1/_2\lambda$). This occurs when ΔL = λ/2, 3 λ/2, 5 λ/2, etc.

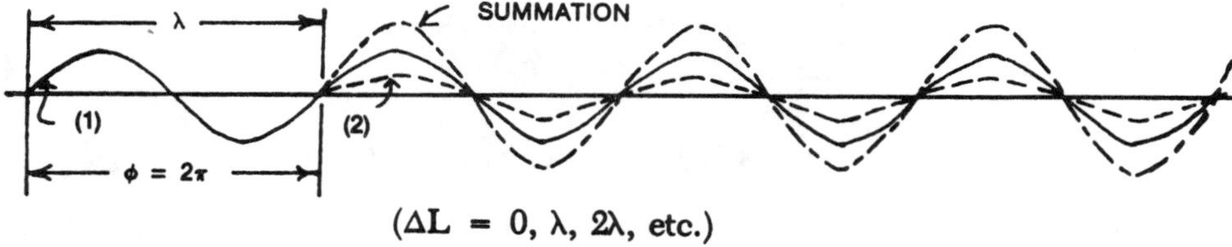

(ΔL = 0, λ, 2λ, etc.)

Waves (1) and (2) begin at the points shown, have the same λ but different A's.
The summation wave is maximal since ΔL = λ in this example.

Fig. 5.41—Maximal Constructive Interference

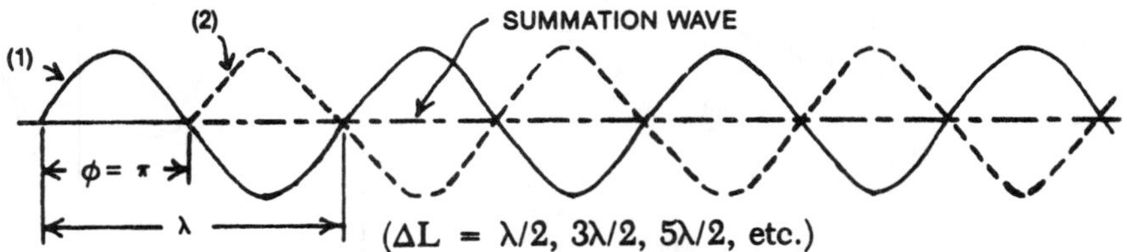

(ΔL = λ/2, 3λ/2, 5λ/2, etc.)

Waves (1) and (2) begin as shown, have the same λ and the same A's.
The summation wave is the horizontal line (or the minimum) since ΔL = λ/2 in this example.

Fig. 5.42—Maximal Destructive Interference

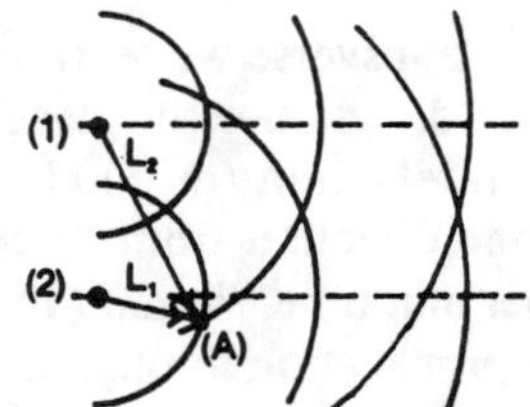

L_1, L_2 are distances from origins of waves to point A
$\Delta L = |L_2 - L_1|$ (absolute value).

Fig. 5.43—Schematic for ΔL

Standing waves result when waves are reflected off a stationary object back into the oncoming waves of the medium, and superimposition (see above) results. *Nodes* are points where there is no particle displacement, which are similar to points of maximal destructive interference (above). Nodes occur at fixed end points (points that cannot vibrate). *Antinodes* are points that undergo maximal displacements and are similar to points of maximal constructive interference. Antinodes occur at open or free end points.

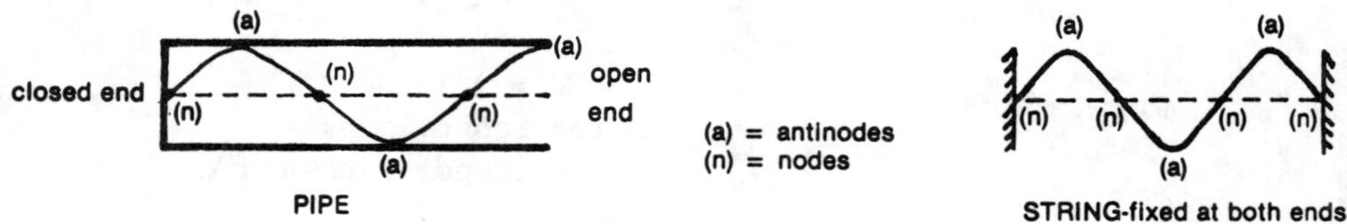

Fig. 5.44—Standing Waves

The particles that are undergoing displacement when a wave passes through a medium undergo motion called simple harmonic motion (SHM) and are acted upon by a force described by Hooke's Law. SHM is caused by an inconstant force (called a restoring force) and as a result has an inconstant acceleration. The force is proportional to the displacement (distance from the equilibrium point) but opposite in direction,

$F = -kx$	*Hooke's Law*
k = constant	x = displacement from equilibrium

Fig. 5.45(a)—Simple Harmonic Motion

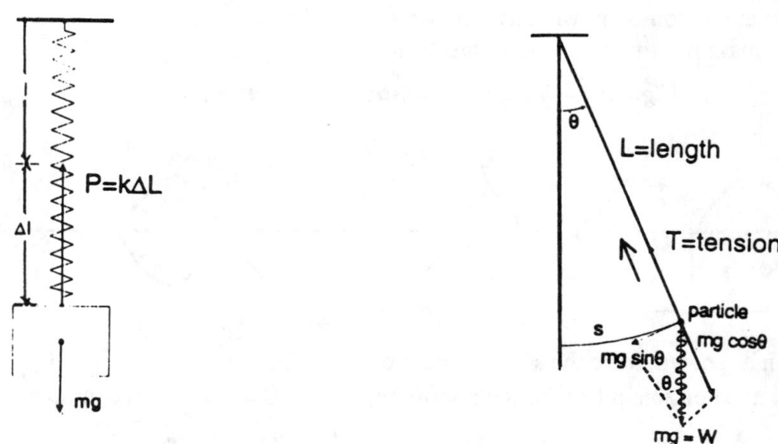

Fig. 5.45(b)—Simple Harmonic Motion (Oscillator) *Fig. 5.45(c)—Simple Harmonic Motion (Pendulum)*

Features of SHM and Hooke's Law are:

(1) Force and acceleration are always in the same direction.
(2) Force and acceleration are always in the opposite direction of the displacement.
(3) Force and acceleration have their maximal values at + A and – A; they are zero at the equilibrium point.
(4) Velocity direction has no constant relation to displacement or acceleration.
(5) Velocity is maximum at equilibrium and zero at A and – A.

The *electromagnetic spectrum* has the sequence below from long wavelength (λ) and low frequency (f) to short wavelength and high frequency Many regions overlap,

Long λ *Short λ*

radiowaves/microwaves/infrared/visible/ultraviolet/X-rays/gamma rays

Low f *High f*

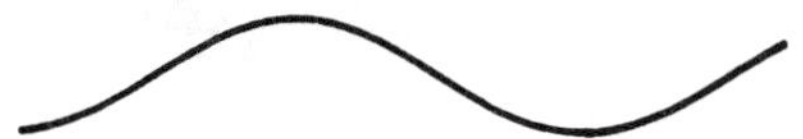

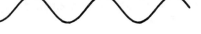

Fig. 5.46(a)—Long Waves ***Fig. 5.46(b)—Short Waves***

The visible light is broken down into colors remembered by the mnemonic, ROY G. BIV:

Red, Orange, Yellow, Green, Blue, Indigo, Violet

Planck developed the relation between energy (E) and the frequency (f) of electromagnetic radiation,

$$E = hf$$

h = Planck's Constant

Since, $f \propto 1/\lambda$, then, $E \propto 1/\lambda$. That is, high frequencies but short wavelengths correspond to high energy and vice versa. See Section 5.21.1 for resonance and beats.

5.20.2 Questions to Review Wave Characteristics and Periodic Motion

1. If the direction of vibration of particles of a medium is in the direction of propagation of a wave, the wave is called:

A. longitudinal.
B. transverse.
C. both.
D. neither.

2. Condensations and rarefactions would be found in:

A. light waves.
B. water waves.
C. transverse waves.
D. longitudinal waves.

3. "The effects of two or more waves on the displacement of a particle are independent" is a statement of:

A. Interference Principle.
B. Huygens' Principle.
C. Correspondence Principle.
D. Superposition Principle.

4. At the node of a wave:

 A. the displacement is maximal.
 B. there is no displacement.
 C. there may be an open or a free point.
 D. both (A) and (C) are true.

5. Select the *incorrect* relationship between the energy (E) of a wave and the parameters given: (f = frequency, λ = wavelength, A = amplitude)

 A. $E \propto f$
 B. $E \propto A^2$
 C. $E \propto 1/\lambda$
 D. all are correct

6. The restoring force that causes an object to undergo simple harmonic motion is:

 A. a constant force.
 B. inversely proportional to the displacement (from equilibrium) and in the same direction.
 C. directly proportional to the displacement but opposite in direction.
 D. both (A) and (B).

7. All of the following are true about simple harmonic motion *except*:

 A. force and acceleration have their maximum values at the equilibrium point.
 B. force and acceleration are always in the same direction.
 C. velocity direction has no constant relation to displacement or acceleration direction.
 D. velocity is maximal at the equilibrium point.

8. Which of the following colors of visible light has the shortest wavelength?

 A. green
 B. blue
 C. yellow
 D. red

9. Which of the following colors of visible light has the longest wavelength?

 A. yellow
 B. orange
 C. blue
 D. green

10. If f = frequency and λ = wavelength of light, then the speed of light (c) is:

 A. $c = 1/f$
 B. $c = \lambda/f$
 C. $c = f/\lambda$
 D. $c = f\lambda$

11. The relation, $E = h\upsilon$ was put forth by:

 A. Planck.
 B. Einstein.
 C. Newton.
 D. Maxwell.

12. Constructive interference occurs when:

 A. phase differences are 0, 2π, 4π, etc.
 B. path differences are 0, λ, 2λ, 3λ, etc.
 C. neither (A) nor (B) are correct.
 D. both (A) and (B) are correct.

13. If the frequency of a wave is 10,000 hertz and it is traveling at 5000 m/sec, then its wavelength is:

A. 5 m
B. 2m
C. 0.5 m
D. 0.2 m

14. The speed of light (c) is 3.0×10^{10} cm/sec If the wavelength of (λ) of red-light is approximately 400 nm (nm = 10^{-9}m), then the frequency (f) of red-light is:

A. 7.5×10^{12}/sec
B. 7.5×10^{14}/sec
C. 1.2×10^{4}/sec
D. 1.2×10^{6}/sec

15. Electromagnetic radiation (e.g., light) with frequency (f) of 50,000 hertz (hertz = 1 cycle/sec) would have a wavelength (λ) of:

A. 1/50,000 cms
B. 6.0×10^{-5} cms
C. 6.0×10^{5} cms
D. cannot be determined

16. In a vibrating column of air:

A. open ends can only have nodes.
B. nodes can occur at open or closed ends.
C. open ends can only have antinodes.
D. antinodes may only occur at closed ends.

Use the following data for Questions #17 through #22

The particle of mass = 2 kg below is oscillating about the fixed point O as shown. Given are some values of the force on the particle at different values of displacement (x) from O. The maximal displacement from O in any one direction is ± A and A = 5 m.

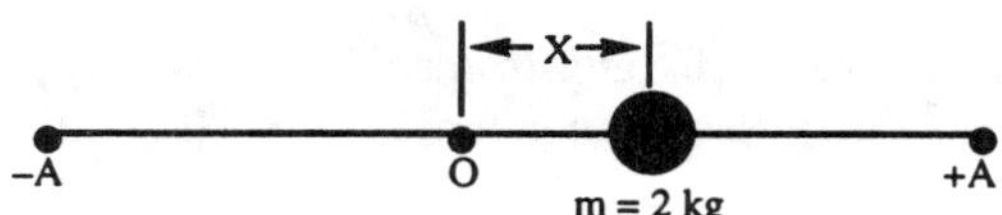

x (meters)	+3	+1	–2	–4
F (newtons)	–0.6	–0.2	+0.4	+0.8

17. This type of motion is called:

A. rigid body translation.
B. simple harmonic motion.
C. projectile motion.
D. free fall motion.

18. The force is described by:

A. Faraday's Law.
B. Newton's First Law.
C. Hooke's Law.
D. none of the above.

19. If the above motion and force follow Hooke's Law, the value of k (neglect the units) is:

A. 0.1
B. 0.2
C. 0.5
D. 1.0

20. The value of F at A = – 5m is:

A. 0.2 nts
B. 0.5 nts
C. 1.0 nts
D. 5 nts

21. The force has a value of zero at x = ?

A. 0 m
B. + 5 m
C. – 5 m
D. ± 2m

22. At x = – 2 m, the acceleration (a) is (in m/sec^2):

A. 4.0
B. 2.0
C. 1.0
D. 0.2

23. A standing wave is established in a string fixed at both ends between two points 1m apart. Which of the following is not a possible wavelength for this system?

A. 4 m
B. 2 m
C. 1.0 m
D. 0.5 m

24. A standing wave is established in a pipe which is open at one end and is 2m long. All of the following are possible wavelengths for this system except:

A. 8 m
B. 6 m
C. 2 2/3 m
D. all are possible

25. The wavelength of ultraviolet waves is 10^3 angstroms. Find the energy of the ultraviolet waves, given Planck's constant = 6.626×10^{-34} joule-sec (1 angstrom = 1Å = 10^{-10}m)

A. 6.626×10^{-31}J
B. 6.626×10^{-41}J
C. 2×10^{18}J
D. 2×10^{-18}J

5.20.3 Answers to Questions in Section 5.20.2

(1) A (2) D (3) D (4) B (5) D (6) C (7) A (8) B (9) B (10) D (11) A (12) D (13) C (14) B (15) C (16) C (17) B (18) C (19) B (20) C (21) A (22) D (23) A (24) B (25) D

5.20.4 Discussion of Answers to Questions in Section 5.20.2

Questions #1 to #11, #16 Adequately discussed in the text.

Question #12 (Answer: D) It takes one whole cycle (2 π = 360°) for a sine wave to completely repeat itself. For two waves to add constructively at every point, their phase must differ by multiples of 2π, i.e.,

2nπ where n = 0, 1, 2, 3, etc.

The phase difference (ϕ) for any given path difference to a given point is $\phi = 2\pi(\Delta L/\lambda)$ for a given wave with wavelength = λ. This is reasoned from the graph below:

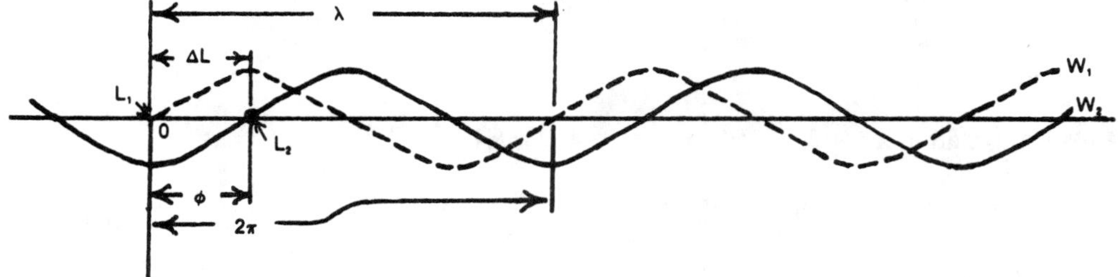

W_1 and W_2 are two waves out of phase.
L_1, L_2 are distances from O (origin).
the phase difference is ϕ
the path difference is ΔL
the following ratio holds because the corresponding distances are equal in the diagram above:
part/whole = $\phi/2\pi \quad \Delta L/\lambda$
then: $\phi = 2\pi(\Delta L/\lambda)$

For constructive interference:

$\phi = 2n\pi = 2\pi(\Delta L/\lambda)$
$n = \Delta L/\lambda$
$\Delta L = n\lambda$ where n = 0, 1, 2, 3 etc.

Question #13 (Answer: C)

$v = \lambda f$
$\lambda = v/f = 5{,}000/10{,}000 = 0.5$ m

Question #14 (Answer: B)

$c = f\lambda$
$f = c/\lambda = (3.00 \times 10^{10}\text{cm/sec})/4 \times 10^{-5}\text{cm} = 0.75 \times 10^{15}/\text{sec} = 7.5 \times 10^{14}/\text{sec}$
$(\lambda = 400 \times 10^{-9}\text{m} = 4.0 \times 10^{-7}\text{m} = 4 \times 10^{-5}\text{cm})$

Question #15 (Answer: C)

$c = f\lambda = 3.00 \times 10^{10}$cm/sec
$f = 50{,}000/\text{sec} = 5.0 \times 10^4/\text{sec}$
$\lambda = c/f = 3.00 \times 10^{10}/5.0 \times 10^4 = 0.60 \times 10^6$ cms
$\lambda = 6.0 \times 10^5$ cms.

Question #17 (Answer: B). The particle is oscillating about a fixed point (O) which is called simple harmonic motion.

Question #18 (Answer: C). The force is a restoring force and the motion is SHM. Hooke's Law as $F = -kx$, determines the restoring force.

Question #19 (Answer: B). The motion follows Hooke's Law: $F = -kx$.
So, to find the k, any set of F and x may be substituted in the equation:

$k = -(F/x) = -(-0.6 \text{ nts}/+3\text{m}) = +0.2$ nt/m
$k = -(F/x) = -(-0.2 \text{ nts}/+1\text{m}) = +0.2$ nt/m

Question #20 (Answer: C). Use the data from #19:

$F = -kx$
$F = -(0.2)(-5) = +1.0$ nts

Note at $\pm A$, F has its maximal value.

Question #21 (Answer: A)

$$F = -kx = 0$$
$$-kx = 0$$
$x = 0$ because k is not equal to zero.

Question #22 (Answer: D)

$F = +0.4$ nts from chart at $x = -2$, $a = F/m = 0.4/2 = 0.2\ m/s^2$

or, $F = -kx$ from Hooke's Law

$F = ma$ from Newton's 2nd Law (Section 5.14.1)

$$ma = -kx$$
$$a = -kx/m = -(0.2)(-2)/2 = +0.2 m/sec^2.$$

Question #23 (Answer: A). If the string is fixed at both ends, then only nodes can occur at these points. Then the smallest part of a wave than can exist between these points is $^1/2\lambda$ which then equals 1 m:

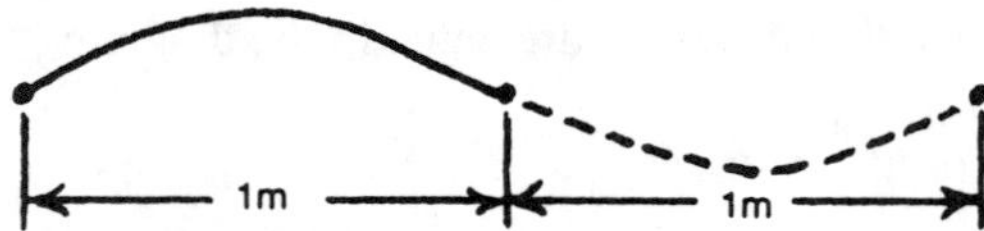

Then the λ of the above situation is 2 m as shown. This is the maximal allowed λ for this set-up. Other λ's are possible as follows:

the next node after $^1/2\lambda$ is $^1/2\lambda$ away and the next node after that is another $^1/2\lambda$ away. These then are $n(^1/2\lambda)$ where n = 0, 1, 2, 3 etc., are the possible $^1/2\lambda$'s that can fit into the distance (l = lm)

then: $n(^1/2\lambda) = lm = l$

$$n\lambda/2 = l$$
$$\lambda = 2l/n = \text{allowable } \lambda\text{'s}$$

Then, the 1.0 m and 0.5m are allowable λ's:

$$n = 2\ l/\lambda = (2)(1)/0.5 = 4 \text{ for } \lambda = 0.5m$$
$$n = 2\ l/\lambda = (2)(1)/1 = 2 \text{ for } \lambda = 1.0m$$

Also, the λ = 4m is not allowable because it does not give a value of n that is a whole number:

$n = 2l/\lambda = (2)(1)/4 = 0.5$ which is not acceptable.

Note that the allowable frequencies (f) are:

$$f = v/\lambda = v/(2l/\lambda) = nv/2l$$
v = velocity of wave propagation.

Question #24 (Answer: B) At the closed end of the pipe there must be a node and at the open end there must be an antinode. The shortest fraction of a wave that has a node and antinode in sequence is $^1/4\lambda$ which must equal the 2m:

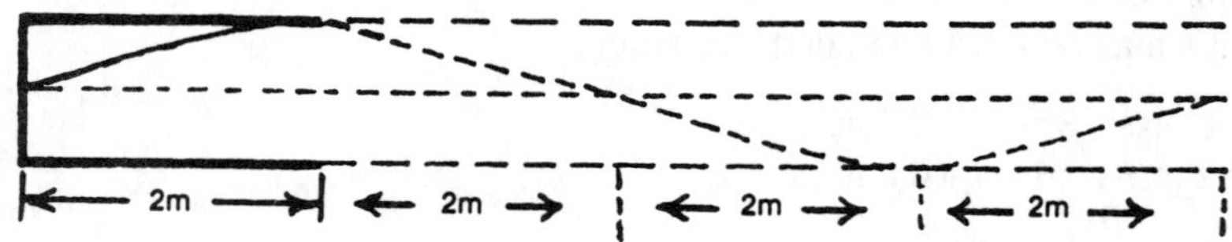

$^1/4\lambda = 2m$

λ = 8 m as the longest possible allowable. The next antinode occurs $^1/2\lambda$ beyond $^1/4\lambda$ and then the next is $^1/2\lambda$ beyond that, etc. (Only worry about the next antinode because these go at the open end of the pipe.) The sequence of possible fractions of λ's for this system is:

$^1/_4\lambda$
$^1/_4\lambda + {}^1/_2\lambda = {}^3/_4\lambda$
$^3/_4\lambda + {}^1/_2\lambda = {}^5/_4\lambda$
$^5/_4\lambda + {}^1/_2\lambda = {}^7/_4\lambda$ etc.

or to generalize this: $n\lambda/4$ where n = 1, 3, 5, 7, 9 etc.
(note that only the odd numbers are possible.)

Then each of these fractional λs must fit into the 2m = *l*:

$n\lambda/4 = 2m = l$
$n\lambda/4 = l$
$\lambda = 4l/n \quad n = 1, 3, 5, 7$ etc.

Then any λ is possible as long as it gives n = 1, 3, 5, 7, etc., when substituted in the above equation:

$n = 4l/n$

for $\lambda = 8m$: $n = (4)(2)/8 = 1$ ∴ possible
for $\lambda = 6m$: $n = (4)(2)/6 = {}^4/_3$ ∴ not possible
for $\lambda = {}^8/_3$ m: $n = (4)(2)/({}^8/_3) = 8(3/8) = 3$ ∴ possible

Note that the frequencies (f) in this case are
$f = v/\lambda = v/(4l/n) = vn/4l \quad n = 1, 3, 5$
v = velocity of wave propagation.

Question #25 (Answer: D)

$E = hf,\ v = f\lambda$
$v = 2.998 \times 10^8$ m/sec
$1J = 1$ Newton-meter
$\lambda = 10^3 Å = 10^3 10^{-10} = 10^{-7}$m
$$f = \frac{v}{\lambda} = \frac{2.998 \times 10^8}{10^{-7}} = 2.998 \times 10^{15} \text{ Hz}$$
E = Planck's Constant × f = hf
$= 6.626 \times 10^{-34} \times 2.998 \times 10^{15}$
$= 1.99 \times 10^{-18}$ joules

5.20.5 Checklist for Wave Characteristics and Periodic Motion

______ simple harmonic motion
______ constructive interference
______ destructive interference
______ frequency
______ velocity
______ amplitude
______ transverse waves
______ longitudinal waves
______ superposition of waves
______ electromagnetic radiation
______ energy of waves
______ gamma rays
______ phase
______ period
______ Hooke's Law
______ wavelength
______ standing waves
______ nodes
______ antinodes
______ radiowaves
______ microwaves
______ infrared
______ visible
______ ultraviolet
______ x-rays
______ E = hf

5.21 SOUND

5.21.1 Review of Sound

Sound is a longitudinal (Section 5.20.1) mechanical wave which travels through an elastic medium. Sound is thus produced by vibrating matter. There is no sound in a vacuum (because there is no matter). Compressions (condensations) are regions where particles (of matter) are close together and are high pressure regions. Rarefactions are regions where particles are sparse and are low pressure regions of sound waves.

The *speed* (v) of sound is proportional to the square root of the elastic restoring force and inversely proportional to the square root of the inertia of the particles (e.g., density, ρ, is a measure of inertia),

$$v \propto \sqrt{F}$$
$$v \propto 1/\sqrt{\text{inertia.}}$$

The speed in various substances is calculated as follows (Also see Section 5.11.1):

solid wire or rod:	$\sqrt{Y/\rho}$	Y = Young's modulus
fluid (gas or liquid)	$\sqrt{B/\rho}$	B = bulk modulus

The speed of sound in solids and liquids is considerably higher than the speed in air. The speed of sound in air at 0°C is 331.5 m/s and it increases with temperature at approximately 0.6 m/s per degree celsius. The speed of sound in water at 0°C is 1402 m/s and is 6000 m/s in granite.

Forced vibrations occur when a series of waves impinge upon an object and cause it to vibrate. Natural frequencies are the intrinsic frequencies of vibration of a system. If the forced vibration causes the object to vibrate at one of its natural frequencies, the body will vibrate at maximal amplitude. This situation is called *resonance*. Note also that energy and power are proportional to the amplitude squared, so these two are also at a maximum.

Hearing is subjective but its characteristics are closely tied to the physical characteristics of sound. These relations are:

SENSORY:		PHYSICAL:	
	loudness		intensity (I)
	pitch		frequency (f)
	quality		waveforms

The *quality* depends on the number and the relative intensity of the overtones of the waveforms. Frequency, and, therefore, *pitch*, are perceived by the ear from 20 to 20,000 Hz (Hertz = cycles/second). Frequencies below 20 Hz are called infrasonic. Frequencies above 20,000 Hz are called ultrasonic. *Sound intensity* (I) is the rate of energy (power) propagation through space:

$$I = \text{Power/area} \propto f^2A^2$$
f = frequency and A = amplitude

5.21.1.1 THE HUMAN EAR

The human (Fig. 5.47) ear is divided into an *external ear* (pinna and auditory canal), the *middle ear* (the tympanic membrane and the three bones—malleus or hammer, incus or anvil, and stapes or stirrup), and the *internal ear* (the cochlea, the semicircular canals, and the origin of the vestibulocochlear nerve). The *tympanic membrane* (eardrum) is attached to the *malleus* which attaches to the *incus* which attaches to the *stapes* which attaches to the *oval window* of the cochlea. The outer and middle ear function to match the impedance of the air outside and the fluid of the cochlea inside. This mechanism results in more efficient transmission of sound. Sound waves are transmitted from the stapes via the oval window to the fluid in the *cochlea.* This fluid sets up vibrations in the *basilar membrane* which causes special hair cells to send impulses to the auditory part of the vestibulocochlear (VIII) nerve which transmits them to the auditory cortex in the temporal lobe of the cerebrum. The *basilar membrane*, tectoral membrane, and hair cells run the full length of the cochlea and together constitute the *organ of Corti.* The distance from the oval window that the vibration of the basilar membrane is at maximum determines the *frequency (pitch)* of the sound—highest frequencies are closest to the oval window. The *round window*, at the other end of the cochlea, serves as a release of pressure imparted to the cochlear fluid by the stapes.

The *vestibular system* is continuous anatomic :lly but not functionally with the cochlea. The system is filled with fluid (endolymph) and contains the sacculus, the utricle and three perpendicular *semicircular* canals. Each *semicircular canal* has an *ampulla* region which contains hair cells sensitive to changes in angular acceleration. The *utricle* and *sacculus* contain a special sensory region called the *macula* which has crystals of calcium carbonate on it. These regions are sensitive to changes in gravity (position) and linear acceleration. Impulses travel from these special regions via the vestibular portions of the vestibulocochlear nerve (Cranial Nerve VIII) to the central nervous system. The vestibular system helps maintain posture, balance, spatial orientation, and stabilization of eye movements. This section should also be used in solving Biological Sciences problems.

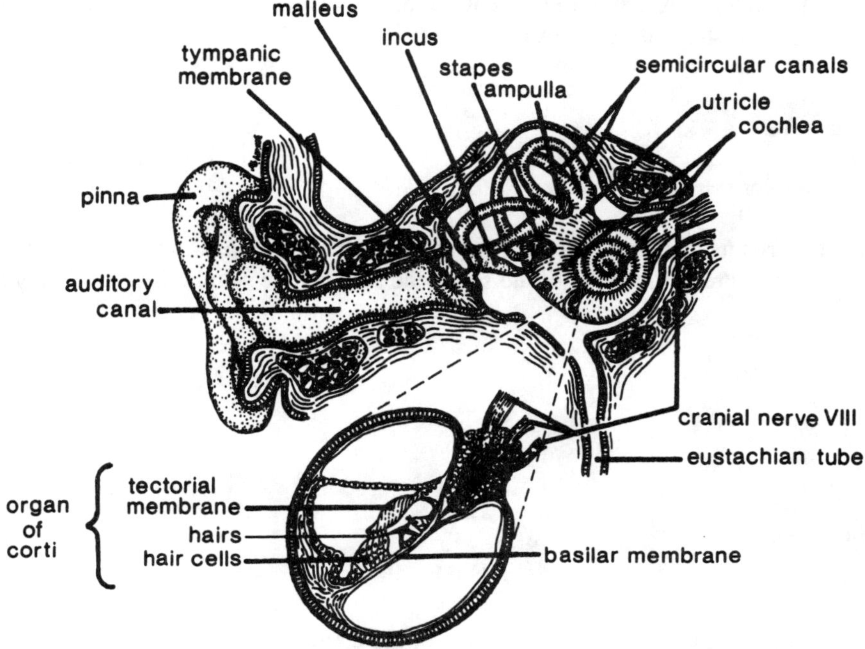

Fig. 5.47—The Human Ear

The *loudness* varies with the amplitude. The ears are most sensitive (hear sounds of lowest intensity) at approximately 2,000 to 4,000 Hz. I_o, taken to be 10^{-12} watts/m^2, is barely audible and is assigned a value of 0 (zero) dB (decibels).

Then the intensity level (I) of a sound wave in dB is,

$$dB = 10 \log (I/I_o)$$

I = intensity at a given level

I_o = threshold intensity.

Examples of some values of dB's are: whisper (20), normal conversation (60), subway car (100), pain threshold (120) and jet engine (160). Continual exposure to sounds greater than 90 dB can lead to hearing impairment.

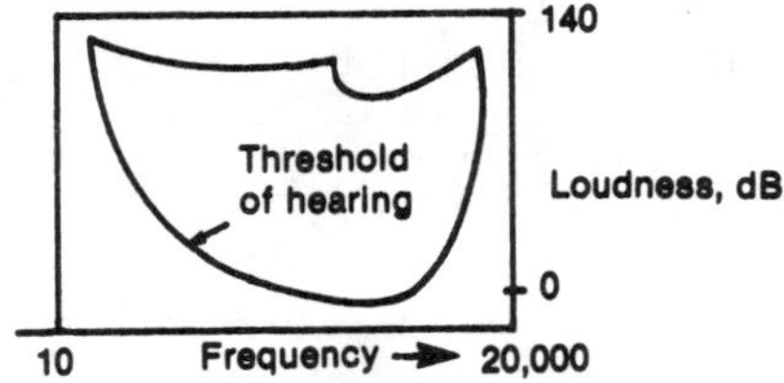

Fig. 5.48—Audible Sound Intensities

When sounds of different frequencies are heard together, they interfere (Section 5.20.1). Constructive interference results in *beats*. The number of beats per second is the absolute value of the difference of the frequencies ($|f_1 - f_2|$). Hence, the new frequencies heard include the original frequencies and the absolute differences between them.

The *Doppler Effect* is the effect upon the observed frequency caused by the relative motion of the observer (o) and the source (s). If the distance is decreasing between them, there is a shift to higher frequencies and shorter wavelengths, (to higher pitch for sound and toward the blue-violet for light). If the distance is increasing between them, there is a shift to longer wavelengths and lower frequencies (to lower pitch for sound and toward red for light). The summary equation of the above in terms of frequency (f) is:

$f_O/(V \pm v_O) = f_S/(V \pm v_S)$
$f_O = f_S(V \pm v_O)/(V \pm v_S)$
V = speed of wave
v = speed of observer (o) or source (s).

Choose the (+) or (−) such that the frequency varies as you would predict. If the o or s is moving toward the other the f should increase and vice versa. Predict the results and select the sign for the s and o independently of the motion of the other.

5.21.2 Questions to Review Sound

1. Sound waves:

A. are transverse waves.
B. are produced by vibrating matter.
C. may be transmitted in a vacuum.
D. are all of the above.

2. The speed of sound is:

A. proportional to the square root of the elastic restoring force of the medium.
B. inversely proportional to the square root of the inertia of the particles of the medium.
C. neither (A) nor (B).
D. both (A) and (B).

3. The speed of sound is ________ by an increase of temperature and is ________ in denser media.

A. decreased, lower
B. increased, higher
C. decreased, higher
D. increased, lower

4. When an object is forced to vibrate at one of its natural frequencies of vibration:

A. resonance exists.
B. energy is a minimum.
C. work is a minimum.
D. the amplitude of vibration is a minimum.

5. Which sensory (as interpreted by the brain) aspect of sound is incorrectly paired with its physical correlate of sound?

A. loudness-intensity
B. pitch-frequency
C. quality-waveforms
D. all are correctly paired

6. A human with normal hearing probably could not hear sound at:
   - A. 100,000 Hz
   - B. 20,000 Hz
   - C. 5,000 Hz
   - D. 20 Hz

7. The intensity (power per unit area) of a sound is:
   - A. inversely proportional to the square of the frequency.
   - B. directly proportional to the square of the frequency.
   - C. inversely proportional to the frequency.
   - D. directly proportional to the frequency.

8. Decibels are used in describing:
   - A. light.
   - B. sound.
   - C. electricity.
   - D. magnetism.

9. The effect upon the frequency of sound observed when the source of the sound is moving relative to the observer is explained by the:
   - A. Doppler Effect.
   - B. Compton Effect.
   - C. Theory of Relativity.
   - D. combination of Compton and Doppler effects.

10. If the density of a gas is quadrupled ($\times$ 4), the speed (v) of sound through it is:
    - A. decreased by $^1/2$ of its initial value.
    - B. multiplied by a factor of 2.
    - C. multiplied by a factor of 4.
    - D. decreased to $^1/4$ of its initial value.

11. If the elasticity (restoring force) of medium #1 is four times the elasticity of medium #2, then the sound will travel:
    - A. twice as fast in #1 as in #2.
    - B. twice as fast in #2 as in #1.
    - C. four times as fast in #1 as in #2.
    - D. four times as fast in #2 as in #1.

12. If the tension (F) in a string is increased by a factor of 4, the speed (v) of a wave in that string will be:
    - A. quadrupled ($\times$ 4).
    - B. doubled.
    - C. reduced by $^1/2$.
    - D. reduced to $^1/4$ the original.

13. Three notes of 128, 256, and 512 are sounded; the frequencies heard are:
    - A. 128, 256, 384, 512, 640, 768
    - B. 512, 640, 768
    - C. 128, 256, 384, 512
    - D. 128, 256, 512

14. A sound has an intensity 100 times that of the standard intensity. How many decibels is it?
    - A. 10
    - B. 20
    - C. 50
    - D. 100

15. If a source which is emitting sound is moving toward an observer, the frequency of sound heard by the observer is _______ the frequency emitted by the source, caused by _______ _______.

A. the same as, Doppler effect
B. less than, mutual interference
C. greater than, Doppler effect

16. If a source which is emitting light is moving away from an observer, the wavelength of light seen by the observer is _______ the wavelength emitted by the source, due to _______ _______.

A. the same as, Planck's constant
B. shorter than, increased frequency
C. longer than, decreased frequency

17. An observer is moving toward a source at 170 m/sec. The source is moving toward the observer at 130 m/sec and is emitting sound at a frequency of 10,000 hertz. The frequency of sound heard by the observer (assume speed of sound is 330 m/sec) is:

A. 15,000 hertz
B. 7,500 hertz
C. 25,000 hertz
D. 5,000 hertz

18. The threshold of human hearing lies between:

A. 20 Hz – 20,000 Hz.
B. 10 Hz – 10,000 Hz.
C. 18 Hz – 8,000 Hz.
D. 12 Hz – 1,200 Hz.

19. Given $I_o = 10^{-12}$ watts/m^2, find the intensity in watts/m^2 of sound, given the intensity in dB = 100.

A. 100 W/m^2
B. 1000 W/m^2
C. 10^{-10} W/m^2
D. 10^{-2} W/m^2

20. Determine loudness in decibels at the threshold of human hearing:

A. 0 dB
B. 20 dB
C. 200 dB
D. 2,000 dB

21. Given the intensity of sound of a subway car (I_1) is 100 dB and the intensity of sound of a whisper (I_2) is 20 dB. Compare their intensities in watts/cm^2.

A. $I_1 = 10^8 I_2$
B. $I_1 = {}^1/_5 I_2$
C. $I_1 = 5I_2$
D. $I_2 = 5I_1$

22. An ambulance, traveling 24m/sec, is moving towards an approaching car which is traveling at a speed of 14m/sec. The siren emits a frequency of 1,000 Hz, what is the frequency heard by the driver of the car? Speed of sound = 350m/sec.

A. 1,000 Hz
B. 1,116 Hz
C. 1,350 Hz
D. 1,038 Hz

23. Frequency (pitch) of sound is determined in the ear by the:

A. oval window.
B. basilar membrane.
C. tympanic membrane.
D. medial geniculate body.

24. Which structure is not found in the middle ear of humans?

A. cochlea
B. tympanic membrane
C. anvil
D. incus

25. $CaCO_3$ crystals are found on:

A. sacculus.
B. malleus.
C. macula.
D. ampulla.

26. Hearing is localized in which lobe of the cerebral cortex?

A. frontal
B. parietal
C. temporal
D. occipital

27. All are components of the vestibular system except:

A. semicircular canals.
B. sacculus.
C. organ of Corti.
D. utricle.

28. Semicircular canals are sensitive to:

A. linear acceleration.
B. angular acceleration.
C. magnetic repulsion.
D. all of the above.

29. The vestibular system is important for all of the following except:

A. balance.
B. posture.
C. spatial orientation.
D. voluntary movement.

5.21.3 Answers to Questions in Section 5.21.2

(1) B (2) D (3) B (4) A (5) D (6) A (7) B (8) B (9) A (10) A (11) A (12) B
(13) C (14) B (15) C (16) C (17) C (18) A (19) D (20) A (21) A (22) B (23) B (24) A
(25) C (26) C (27) C (28) B (29) D

5.21.4 Discussion of Answers to Questions in Section 5.21.2

Questions #1 to #9 Adequately discussed in the Section.

Question #10 (Answer: A)

$$v \propto 1/\sqrt{\rho} \quad \rho = \text{density}, \rho_2 = 4\rho_1$$

$$\frac{v_2}{v_1} = \frac{1/\sqrt{\rho_2}}{1/\sqrt{\rho_1}} = \frac{1}{\sqrt{\rho_2}} \cdot \frac{\sqrt{\rho_1}}{1} = \frac{\sqrt{\rho_1}}{\sqrt{\rho_2}} = \sqrt{\frac{\rho_1}{\rho_2}} = \sqrt{\frac{\rho_1}{4\rho_1}} = \sqrt{1/4} = 1/2$$

$$\frac{v_2}{v_1} = 1/2$$

$$v_2 = 1/2 v_1.$$

Question #11 (Answer: A)

Speed of sound (v) $\propto \sqrt{\text{restoring force}} = F, F_1 = 4F_2$

$$\frac{v_2}{v_1} = \frac{1/\sqrt{F_2}}{1/\sqrt{F_1}} = \sqrt{\frac{F_2}{F_1}} = \sqrt{\frac{F_2}{4F_2}} = \sqrt{1/4} = 1/2$$

$$\frac{v_2}{v_1} = 1/2$$

$$2v_2 = v_1.$$

Question #12 (Answer: B)

$$v \propto \sqrt{F}$$

$$F_2 = 4F_1$$

$$v_2/v_1 = \sqrt{F_2}/\sqrt{F_1} = \sqrt{F_2/F_1} = \sqrt{4F_1/F_1} = \sqrt{4} = 2$$

$$v_2 = 2v_1$$

Question #13 (Answer: C) The frequencies heard are the original frequencies plus all new frequencies resulting from the differences of the original frequencies:

512 – 128 = 384 (This is the only new frequency.)

Question #14 (Answer: B)

$$dB = 10 \log I/I_o = 10 \log (100/1)$$

$$= 10 \log 100 = 10(2) = 20$$

$$(\log 100 = 2).$$

Question #15 (Answer: C) As the observer and source move together the observed frequency increases.

Question #16 (Answer: C) If the distance between observer and source is increasing, the wavelength observed increases as the frequency decreases.

Question #17 (Answer: C) Use Doppler's relation as given in the Section:

$$f_o = f_s (V \pm v_o)/(V \pm v_s).$$

Since the source (s) is moving toward the observer (o), this tends to increase the f_o over the f_s; for the $f_o > f_s$ you must use $V - v_s$ because as the denominator decreases the fraction increases and this makes $f_o > f_s$. Since the o is moving toward the s, this tends to increase the f_o over the f_s; for the $f_o > f_s$ you must use $V + v_o$ because as the numerator increases the fraction increases and this makes $f_o > f_s$.

$f_o = f_s(V + v_o)/(V - v_s)$ for this problem

$$f_o = (10{,}000)(330 + 170)/(330 - 130) = (10{,}000)(500/200) =$$

$f_o = (10{,}000)(5/2) = 25{,}000$ hertz.

Question #18 (Answer: A) Review the loudness-frequency graph, Fig. 5.48.

Question #19 (Answer: D)

$$dB = 10 \log \frac{I}{I_o}$$

$$100 = 10 \log \frac{I}{10^{-12}}$$

$$10 = \log I + \log 10^{12} = \log I + 12$$

$$-2 = \log I \qquad I = 10^{-2} \text{ watts/m}^2$$

Question #20 (Answer: A) $I = I_o$ for threshold hearing

$$dB = 10 \log \frac{I}{I_o}$$

$$= 10 \log \frac{I_o}{I_o} = 0$$

Question #21 (Answer: A)

For subway car, 100 $= 10 \log \frac{I_1}{I_o}$

For the whisper, 20 $= 10 \log \frac{I_2}{I_o}$

$10 = \log \frac{I_1}{I_o}$ and $2 = \log \frac{I_2}{I_o}$

$10 = \log I_1 - \log I_o$ and $2 = \log I_2 - \log I_o$

$10 - \log I_1 = -\log I_o$ and $2 - \log I_2 = -\log I_o$

$10 - \log I_1 = 2 - \log I_2$

$8 = 10 - 2 = \log I_1 - \log I_2 = \log \frac{I_1}{I_2}$

$10^8 = \frac{I_1}{I_2}$ which is answer (A)

In other words, the subway car is 100 million times louder than the whisper or the sound level of the subway car is 100 million times that of the whisper.

Question #22 (Answer: B) v = sound speed

$$f_o = f_s \left(\frac{v + v_o}{v - v_s}\right)$$

$$= 1000 \frac{(350 + 14)}{(350 - 24)}$$

$$= 1000 \frac{(364)}{(326)} = 1{,}116 \text{ Hz}$$

Questions #23 to #29 Adequately discussed in Section.

5.21.5 Checklist for Sound

______ production of sound
______ intensity
______ speed of sound
______ beats
______ loudness
______ middle ear
______ outer ear
______ tympanic membrane
______ basilar membrane
______ pitch
______ decibel scale
______ resonance
______ Doppler Effect
______ inner ear
______ utricle
______ stapes
______ cochlea
______ round window

5.22 LIGHT AND GEOMETRICAL OPTICS

5.22.1 Review of Light and Geometrical Optics

5.22.1.1 THE HUMAN EYE

Anatomically, the eye is separated by the lens into an anterior region filled by the *aqueous humor* and a posterior region filled by the *vitreous humor*. There are three layers in the eye. The *sclera* (dense connective tissue) is the outermost. It is covered anteriorly by the conjunctiva (whites of the eyes). It is continuous with the clear portion called the *cornea* which is important in focusing light. Inside the sclera is the *choroid* which contains the blood vessels and black pigment to prevent light scattering. Continuous with the choroid in front are the *iris* (which gives the eye its color and opens and shuts to let light in through the *pupil*) and the *ciliary muscle* (which controls the shape of the lens and helps to focus or accommodate the eye to distance). The innermost layer is the retina which is the light sensitive layer containing a mixture of rods and cones. *Rods* are concentrated more peripherally in the eye, are concerned with vision in dim light and peripheral vision, and contain *rhodopsin* (retinal from Vit A and a protein called opsin). Light converts retinal from a *cis* to a *trans* form which causes rhodopsin to fall apart and somehow sets up an impulse which is eventually transmitted to the optic nerve (Cranial Nerve II). Cones are concentrated more centrally, are more sensitive to bright light and are responsible for color vision, contain *iodopsin* (light sensitive substance) and are maximally concentrated at the *fovea* (or macula area) which has the highest visual acuity (ability to see clearly points that are close together).

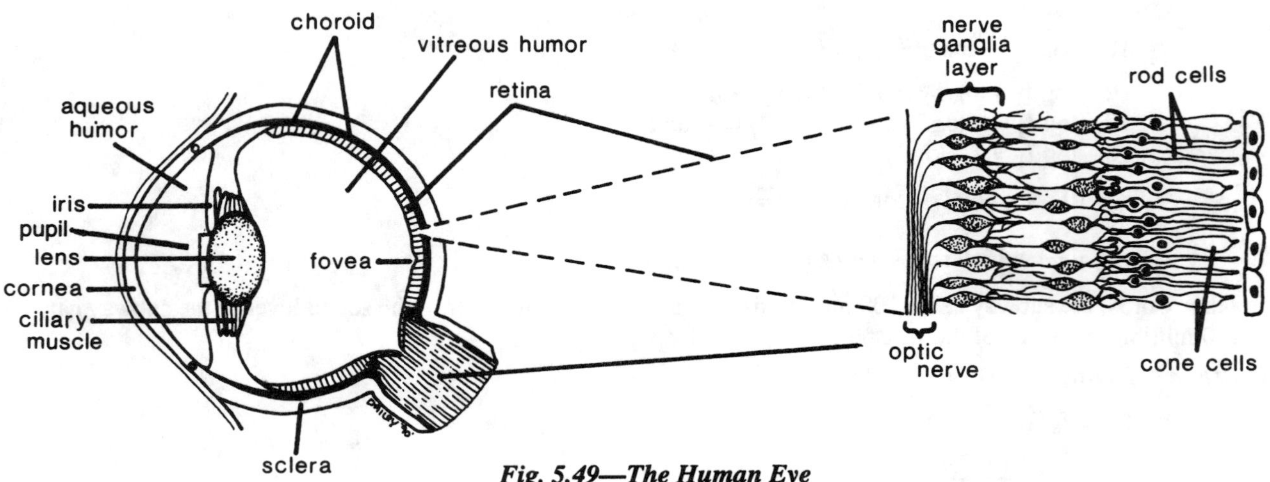

Fig. 5.49—The Human Eye

Light passes through the cornea where it is refracted (bent). It then passes through the aqueous humor and then through the pupil. The pupil size is regulated by the iris which is regulated by the parasympathetic (causes pupil to get smaller) and the sympathetic (causes pupil to get larger) systems. Next, the light passes through the lens where it is refracted further and focused upon the retina (after it passes through the vitreous humor). The lens is flat for objects far away (ciliary muscle relaxed), and it is rounded for objects nearby (ciliary muscle contracted—parasympathetic). Light then stimulates the cones and rods of the retina. From here nerve impulses are transmitted via the Ocular nerve (II) to the visual center in the occipital cortex of the cerebrum. This section should also be used in Solving Biological Sciences problems.

Emmetropia means that light is focused on the retina (by the cornea-lens system) when objects are near or far. *Myopia* (near-sightedness) means light is focused on the retina only when objects are near but not when objects are far away. A cause may be an eyeball that is too long and correction is by diverging (concave) glasses (i.e., lens). *Hypermetropia* (far-sightedness) means light is focused on the retina when objects are far away and not when they are near. A cause may be an eyeball that is too short and correction is by converging (convex)glasses. To *summarize* (Fig. 5.50) the problem in myopia is a cornea-lens system that refracts light relatively (for the eyeball length) too strong and focuses light in front of the retina when the object is far away. In hypermetropia, the problem is a cornea-lens system that refracts light relatively too weak and focuses light behind the retina when objects are near.

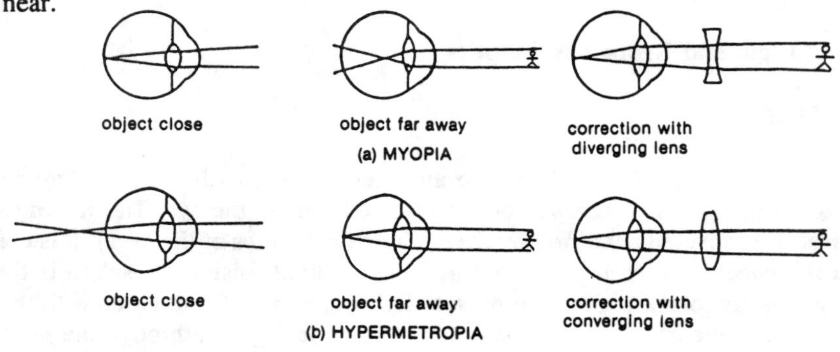

Fig. 5.50—Myopia (a) and Hypermetropia (b)

5.22.1.2 REFLECTION

Reflection is the process by which light rays (imaginary lines drawn perpendicular to advancing wave fronts) bounce back into a medium from a surface with another medium (versus being refracted or absorbed). The *Laws of Reflection* are: (1) The angle of incidence (I) equals the angle of reflection (R) at the normal (N, perpendicular to surface), and (2) the I, R, N all lie on the same plane.

Mirrors may have a plane surface or a curved surface; only spherical curved mirrors will be discussed. For a plane mirror, all incident light is reflected in parallel off it and therefore all images seen are virtual, erect, left-right reversed and appear to be just as far (perpendicular distance) behind the mirror as the object is in front of the mirror. A *virtual image* has no light rays passing through it and cannot be projected upon a screen. A *real image* has light rays passing through it and can be projected upon a screen.

Spherical mirrors may have the reflecting surface convex (diverges light) or concave (converges light). Note the images formed by a converging mirror (concave) are like those for a converging lens (convex); and diverging mirrors (convex) and diverging lens (concave) also form similar images. The terminology for spherical mirrors (see Fig. 5.51) is:

R = radius of curvature
C = center of curvature
F = focal point
V = vertex (center of mirror itself)
axis = line through C and V
f = focal length (distance from F to V)
i = image distance (distance from V to image along axis)
o = object distance (distance from V to object along axis)
AB = linear aperature (chord connecting ends of mirror, larger aperature means better resolution)
s, s′ = object distance from spherical mirror and image distance from spherical mirror (See fig. 5.52 (b))

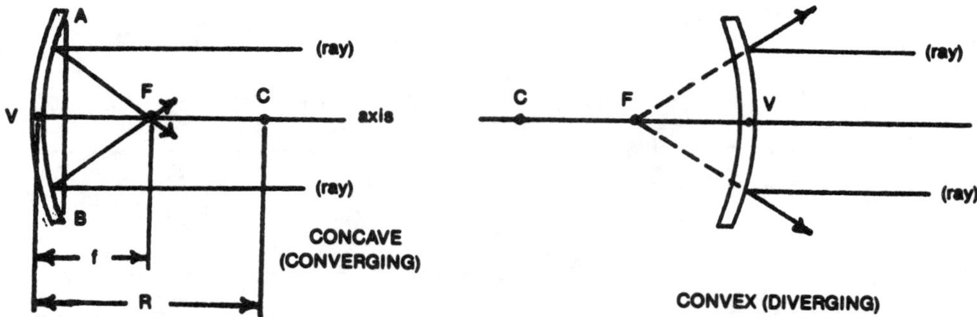

Fig. 5.51—Reflection by Spherical Mirrors

With *concave mirrors (spherical)* the incident light is converged (toward the axis). The path of light rays is as follows:

(1) incident rays parallel to the axis reflect through F;
(2) incident rays along a radius (of curvature) reflect back on themselves (rays through C);
(3) incident rays through F reflect parallel to the axis.

The image formed by an object depends on the position of the image relative to F and C (or f and R). General rules for image formation are:

(1) if $o < f$, then image is virtual and erect;
    if $o > f$, then image is real and inverted;
(2) if $o = f$, then no image is formed;
(3) if $o < R$, then image is enlarged in size;
    if $o > R$, then image is reduced in size;
    if $o = R$, then image is same size.

These relations are similar to those for a converging lens (convex).
With *convex (spherical) mirrors*, the incident light is diverged (from the axis) after reflection. It is the backward extension (dotted lines above) that may pass through the F. The path of light rays are as follows:

(1) incident rays parallel to the axis have backward extension of their reflections through F (see above);
(2) incident rays along a radius (that would pass through C if extended) reflect back along themselves;
(3) incident rays that pass through F (if extended) reflect parallel to the axis.

The image formed for a convex mirror is always virtual, erect and smaller than the object.
The *mirror equation* and derivations from it allow the above relations between object and image to be calculated instead of memorized. The equation is valid for convex and concave mirrors:

$1/i + 1/o = 1/f$

$f = R/2$

$M = \text{magnification} = -i/o$

conventions: for i and o, positive values mean real, negative values mean virtual,
for R and f, positive means converging, negative is diverging,
for M, positive means erect, negative is inverted.

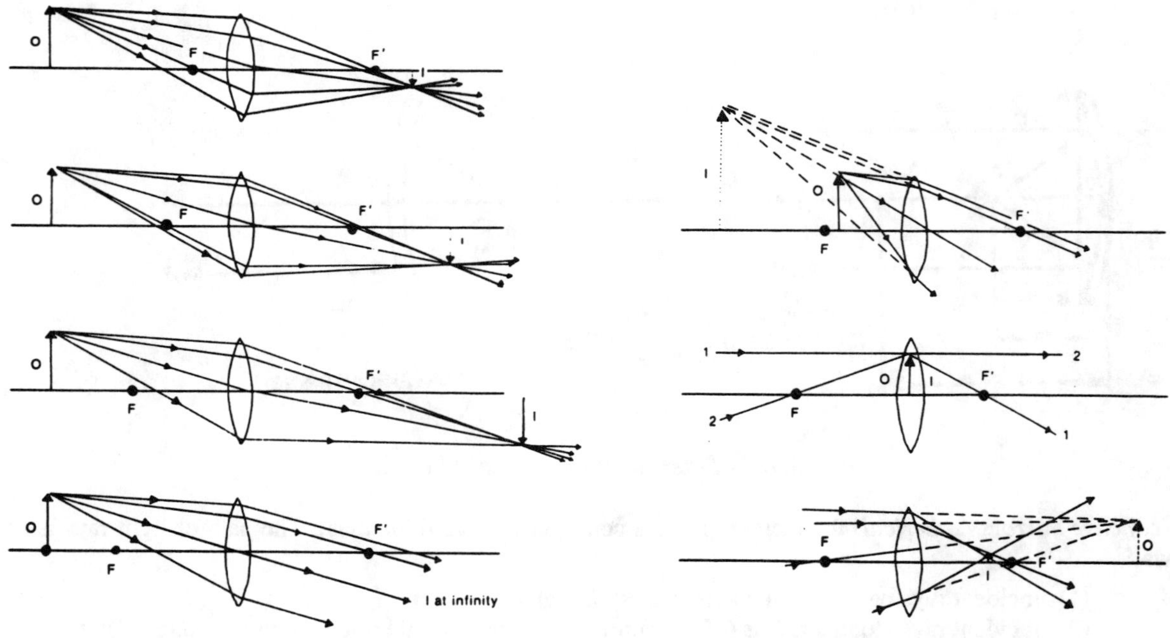

Fig. 5.52(a)—Refraction through Convex Lens

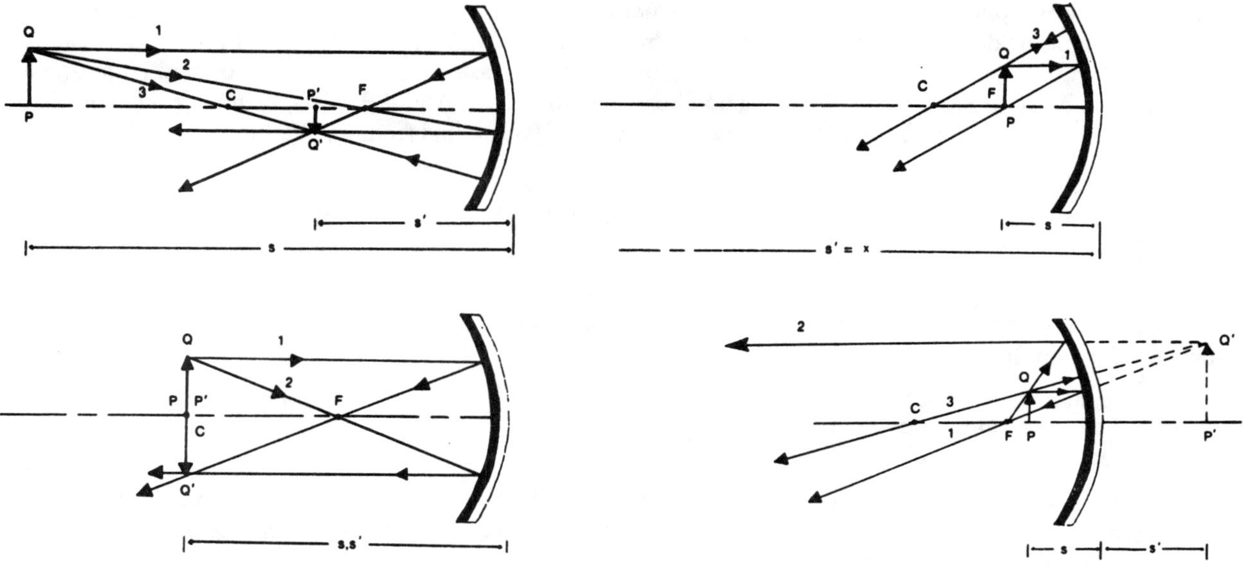

Fig. 5.52(b)—Reflection from Concave Mirrors

5.22.1.3 REFRACTION

Refraction is the bending of light as it passes from one transparent medium to another and is caused by the different speeds of light in the two media. If θ_1 is taken as the angle (to the normal) of the incident light and θ_2 is the angle (to the normal) of refracted light, where 1 and 2 represent the different media, the following relations hold (*Snell's Law*)(Fig. 5.53):

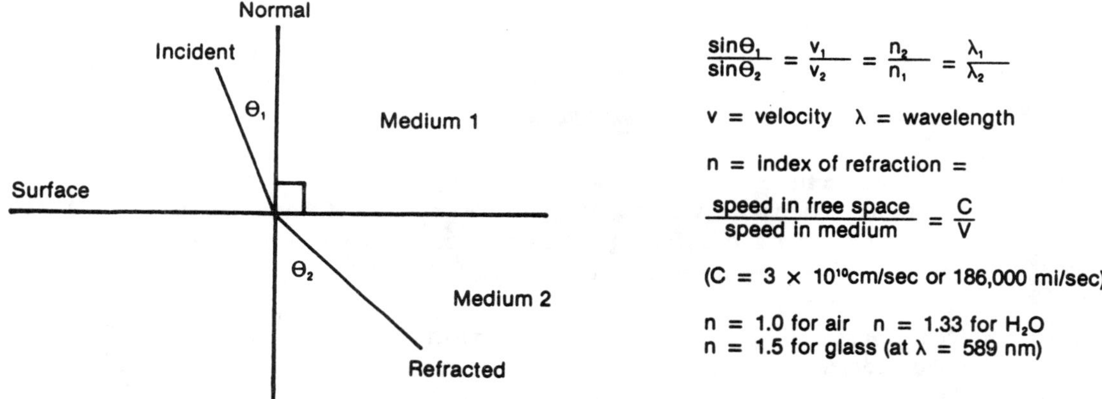

Normal
Incident
θ_1
Medium 1
Surface
θ_2
Medium 2
Refracted
$\frac{\sin\theta_1}{\sin\theta_2} = \frac{v_1}{v_2} = \frac{n_2}{n_1} = \frac{\lambda_1}{\lambda_2}$
v = velocity λ = wavelength
n = index of refraction =
$\frac{\text{speed in free space}}{\text{speed in medium}} = \frac{C}{V}$
(C = 3×10^{10}cm/sec or 186,000 mi/sec)
n = 1.0 for air n = 1.33 for H_2O
n = 1.5 for glass (at λ = 589 nm)

Fig. 5.53—Refraction

Note that the θ is smaller (closer to the normal) in the more optically dense (higher n) medium. Also the smaller the wavelength of the incident light (i.e., toward the violet end), the closer is θ_2 to the normal (i.e., it is smaller than θ_1. This means longer wavelengths travel faster in a medium than shorter wavelengths. This leads to dispersion which is the separation of white light (all colors together) into the individual colors by this differential refraction. For example, a prism disperses white light. The *Laws of Refraction* are:

(1) The incident ray, the refracted ray and the normal ray all lie in the same plane.
(2) The path of the ray (incident and refracted parts) is reversible.

When light passes from a more optically dense (higher n) medium into a less optically dense medium, there exists an angle of incidence such that the angle of refraction θ_2 is 90°. This special angle of incidence is called the critical angle θ_C. This is because when the angle of incidence is less than θ_C, refraction occurs. If the angle of incidence is equal to θ_C, then neither refraction nor reflection occur. And if $\theta_1 > \theta_C$, then *internal reflection* (ray is reflected back into the more dense medium) occurs. The \θ_C is found from Snell's Law.

$n_1 \sin \theta_C = n_2 \sin \theta_2$.
$n_1 \sin \theta_C = n_2(1)$ (Since $\theta_2 = 90°$ and $\sin 90° = 1$)
$\sin \theta_C = n_2/n_1$
e.g., $\theta_C = 42°$ for glass and air.

When looking at an object under water from above the surface, the object appears closer than it actually is. This is due to refraction. In general:

apparent depth/actual depth = n_2/n_1
n_2 = medium of observer
n_1 = medium of object.

A *lens* is a transparent material which refracts light. Converging lenses refract light toward the axis, and diverging lenses refract the light away from the axis. A converging lens is wider at the middle than at the ends, and a diverging lens is thinner at the middle than at the ends (Fig. 5.54).

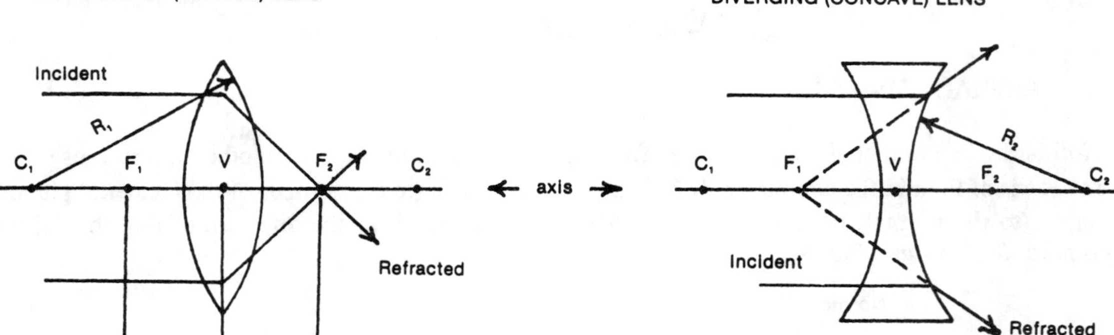

Fig. 5.54—Lens

R = radius of curvature
If the surface (note) is convex, then R is positive (R_1, e.g.). If the surface is concave then R is negative (R_2, e.g.). Subscript $_1$ refers to m incident side, subscript $_2$ refers to the refracted side.
C = center of curvature
F = focal point
V = optical center of the lens
axis = line through C and V

f = focal length is distance between V and F
i = image distance (from V to image)
o = object distance (from V to object).

The path of rays through a lens is:

(1) incident rays parallel to the axis refract through F_2 of a converging lens, and appear to come from F_1 of a diverging lens (backward extensions of the refracted ray, see dotted line on diverging diagram);
(2) an incident ray through F_1 of a converging lens or through F_2 of a diverging lens (if extended) are refracted parallel to the axis;
(3) incident rays through V are not deviated (refracted).

For a *converging lens* (biconvex, e.g.) the image formed depends on the object distance relative to the focal length (f). The relations (note similarity to a converging mirror) are:

(1) if $o < f_1$, the image is virtual and erect,
if $o > f_1$, the image is real and inverted,
(2) if $o = f_1$, no image is formed,
(3) if $o < 2f_1$ (R), image is enlarged in size,
if $o > 2f_1$, image is reduced in size,
if $o = 2f_1$, image is the same size.

For a *diverging lens* (biconcave, e.g.), the image is always virtual, erect and reduced in size as for a diverging mirror.

The above relations can be calculated rather than memorized by the use of the *lens equation* (similar to the mirror equation) and derivations from it,

(1) $1/o + 1/i = 1/f$ (lens equation, same as mirror equation)
(2) *dioptres* (D) = $1/f$ where f is in meters
Measures the refractive power of the lens, the larger the dioptres (D) the stronger the lens. It has a + D for converging lens and a – D for diverging lens. To get the refractive power (D) of lenses in series just add the dioptres which can then be converted into focal length:

$$D_T = D_1 + D_2 = 1/f_T.$$

(3) Note that you cannot add focal lengths except as reciprocals:
$1/f_T = 1/f_1 + 1/f_2$.
(4) M = magnification = $-i/o$
$M = M_1M_2$ for lens in series.

Conventions:

(1) for i and o, positive values are real, negative values are virtual;
(2) for R, see above;
(3) for f, positive means converging, negative is diverging;
(4) for M, positive means erect, negative is inverted.

The lens equation holds only for thin lenses—the thickness is small relative to other dimensions.
For a combination of lenses not in contact with each other, the image is found for the first lens (nearer the object) and then this image is used as the object of the second lens to find the image formed by it (see questions for examples).

5.22.2 Questions to Review Light and Geometrical Optics

1. Using the diagram below, select the *incorrect* statement of the Laws of Reflection of light from surfaces

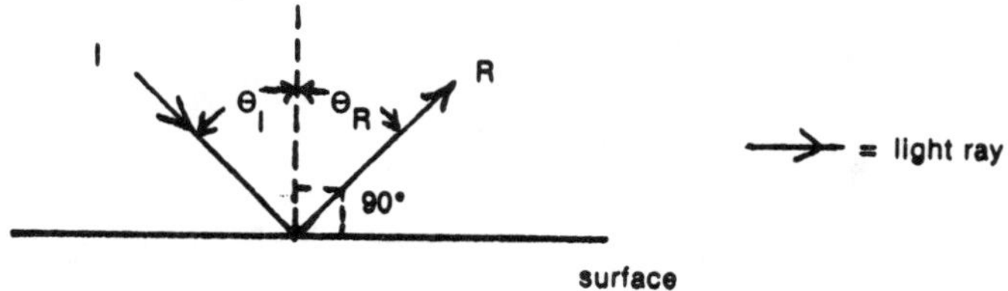

A. $\theta_I = \theta_R$
B. $\theta_I + \theta_R = 90°$
C. I, N and R all lie in the same plane
D. both (A) and (C)

2. All are true of images seen in plane (flat) mirrors *except*:

A. they are always virtual.
B. they appear at a distance behind the mirror equal to the distance (perpendicular) of the object in front of the mirrors.
C. they are right-left reversed.
D. they are inverted.

3. A virtual image:

   A. cannot be projected onto a screen.
   B. has light rays passing through it.
   C. cannot be formed by plane (flat) mirrors.
   D. has all of the above characteristics.

4. The reflected light rays from a smooth concave mirror:

   A. converge.
   B. diverge.
   C. are parallel.
   D. are diffused.

5. The reflected rays from a convex mirror:

   A. diverge.
   B. converge.
   C. are parallel.
   D. are diffused.

6. In terms of the reflected light and images, concave mirrors are most like:

   A. triangular prisms.
   B. square prisms.
   C. concave lens.
   D. convex lens.

7. In terms of reflected light and images, a convex mirror is most like a(n):

   A. convex lens.
   B. concave lens.
   C. triangular prism.
   D. square prism.

8. For the spherical convex mirror below:
   ($f_1 = f_2$; $R_1 = R_2$; f = focal length; R = radius of curvature)

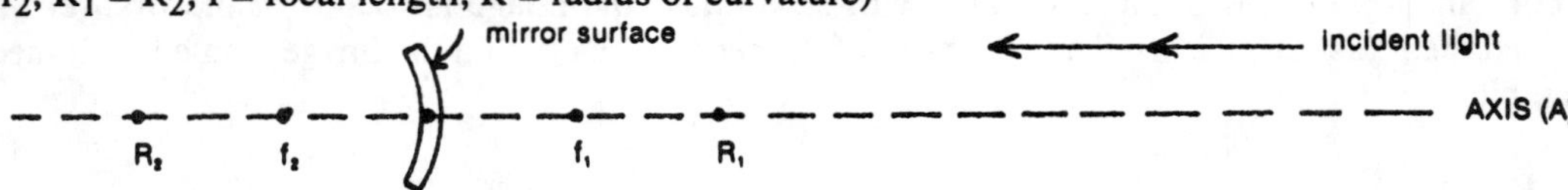

   A. incident rays parallel to A reflect through f_1.
   B. incident rays passing through R_1 reflect through R_2.
   C. the forward extensions of incident rays that reflect through f_2 pass through f_1.
   D. the backward extensions of reflected rays that result from incident rays parallel to A pass through f_2.

9. For the spherical concave mirror below:

mirror surface

R = radius of curvature

f = focal point

AXIS (A)

   A. incident rays parallel to A reflect through f.
   B. incident rays passing through R reflect parallel to A.
   C. incident rays through f reflect through R.
   D. all of the above are correct.

10. For a convex mirror with f = focal length, R = radius of curvature, and o = object distance (along the axis) from the mirror, then:

   A. the image is always virtual, erect and reduced in size.
   B. if $o > f$, the image is virtual and inverted.
   C. if $o = R$, the image and object are the same size.
   D. if $o > R$, the image is larger than the object.

11. For a concave mirror with f = focal length, R = radius of curvature and o = distance (along the axis) of the object from the mirror, then:

A. if $o < f$, then the image is real and inverted.
B. if $o = f$, then no image if formed.
C. if $o > f$, then the image is virtual and erect.
D. if $o > R$, then the image is larger than the object.

12. The mirror equation is:
(f = focal length, o = object distance, i = image distance)

A. $f = o + i$
B. $f = 1/o + 1/i$
C. $1/f = o + i$
D. $1/f = 1/o + 1/i$

13. If f = focal length, R = radius of curvature of a spherical mirror, then:

A. $f = 2R$
B. $f = R/2$
C. $f = R^2$
D. $f = \sqrt{R}$

14. If i = image distance and o = object distance from a mirror, then linear magnification (m) is:

A. $m = -i/o$
B. $m = (i)(o)$
C. $m = -o/i$
D. $m = 1/(i)(o)$

15. The phenomenon of refraction ("bending" of light rays) is attributable to:

A. the particle character of light.
B. the varying speeds of light in different media.
C. the longitudinal wave character of light.
D. none of the above.

16. Given the diagram below for refraction of light, the correct relationship between the angles (Θ) shown and the indices of refraction (n) in the media is:

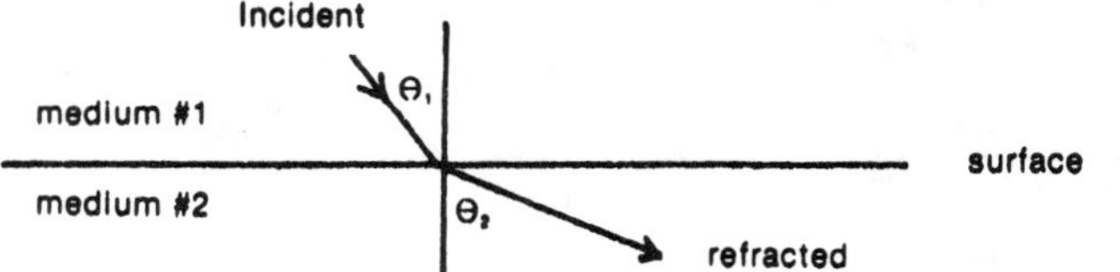

A. $n_2 \sin\theta_1 = n_1 \sin\theta_2$
B. $n_1 \theta_1 = n_2 \theta_2$
C. $\sin\theta_1 / \sin\theta_2 = n_2/n_1$
D. $\theta_1/\theta_2 = n_1/n_2$

17. The index of refraction of a medium is:

A. the speed of light in free space divided by the speed of light in that medium.
B. the density of the medium divided by the density of air.
C. the absorption of light in the medium divided by the absorption of light in water.
D. none of the above.

18. Dispersion of white light into its component colors (as in a prism) occurs by the process of:

A. diffraction
B. polarization
C. refraction
D. reflection

19. A critical angle of incidence (θ_C):

A. is reached when light passes from a lower optically dense medium into a higher optically dense medium.
B. means that the angle of refraction is 90°.
C. means that at all angles of incidence less than θ_C, light is reflected.
D. is all of the above.

20. A converging lens should be:

A. of equal width at the middle and ends.
B. wider at the ends than at the middle.
C. wider at the middle than at the ends.
D. any of the above.

21. A concave lens:

A. diverges light.
B. converges light.
C. performs both functions.
D. performs neither function.

22. Select the correct statement concerning the lens below:
V = vertex; F = focal point; C = center of curvature

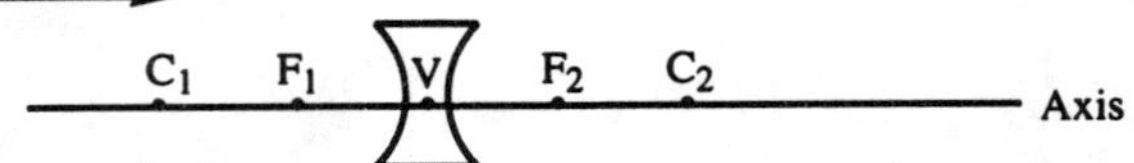

A. If the incident rays are parallel to the axis, the backward extensions of the refracted rays pass through C_1.
B. If the forward extension of an incident ray would pass through F_2, then the backward extension of the refracted ray would pass through F_1.
C. Incident rays through V are not refracted.
D. All of the above are correct.

23. Select the correct statement concerning the lens below:
F = focal points; C = center of curvature; V = vertex

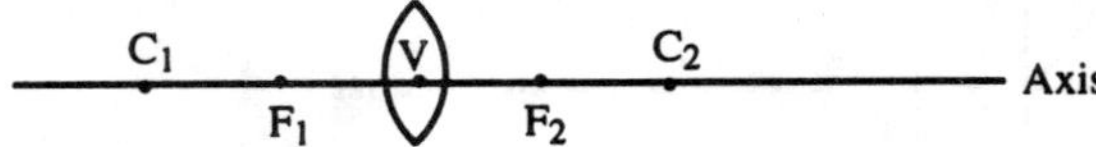

A. Incident rays parallel to the axis refract through C_2.
B. Incident rays through F_1 refract parallel to the axis.
C. Incident rays through V refract along the axis.
D. All of the above are correct.

24. Concerning the image formed by a converging lens, select the incorrect statement:
(f = focal length, o = object distance)

A. If $o < f$, the image is virtual and erect.
B. If $o = f$, no image is formed.
C. If $o > f$, the image is real and inverted.
D. If $o < 2f$, the object is reduced in size.

25. Select the correct statement concerning the image formed by a diverging lens:
(f = focal length, o = object distance)

A. If $o > f$, the image is virtual and inverted.
B. If $o < 2f$, the image is real and reduced.
C. All images are virtual, erect and reduced.
D. All images are real, inverted and enlarged.

26. Dioptres are:

A. the number of degrees of visual acuity.
B. a type of lens that corrects astigmatism.
C. the refractive power of a lens.
D. the reflective power of a mirror.

27. A concave mirror with a focal length (f) = 4 cms forms an image (i) of an object (o) placed 10 cms from it. The magnification (M) of this image is:

A. 1/3 of the object.
B. 2/3 of the object.
C. 5/2 times the object.
D. 3 times the object.

28. An object (o) is placed 10 cms from a concave mirror with focal length (f) = 2 cms. The image is:

A. real, inverted, reduced and 2.50 cms from the mirror.
B. virtual, erect, enlarged and 8 cms from the mirror.
C. virtual, erect, enlarged and 20 cms from the mirror.
D. real, erect, enlarged and 2.50 cms from the mirror.

29. An image formed by a concave mirror is 5 cms from the mirror, erect and virtual. If the focal length of the mirror is 2 cms, the object is how far from the mirror?

A. 5/3 cms
B. 2 cms
C. 10/7 cms
D. 3/5 cms

30. Optically dense media have high indices of refraction. From the diagram below, select the correct statement:

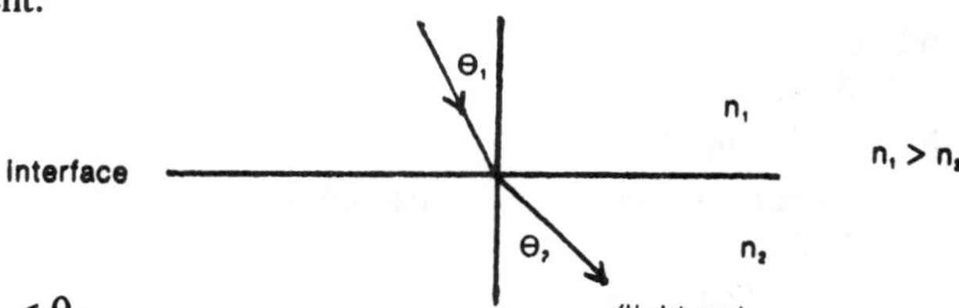

A. $\theta_1 < \theta_2$
B. $\theta_1 = \theta_2$
C. $\theta_1 > \theta_2$
D. need more information

31. The index of refraction (n) for water is 1.5. The speed of light in water is:

A. 4.5×10^{10}cm/sec.
B. 2×10^{10}cm/sec.
C. 3×10^{10}cm/sec.
D. indeterminable without the frequency of light in water.

32. If violet light and red light both have the same angle of incidence, which statement is correct concerning the angles of refraction?

A. The angles of refraction are equal.
B. The angle of refraction of the violet light is larger than that of the red light.
C. The angle of refraction of the red light is larger than that of the violet light.
D. The velocities in the media are needed to evaluate the angles of refraction.

33. A ray of light passing from a type of glass into air has a critical angle (Θ_c) of: (n = index of refraction, n of air = 1.00 and n of glass = 2.00)

A. 5°
B. 15°
C. 30°
D. 45°

34. A fish is 8 meters from the surface in a tank of water. Looking from the air surface, the fish would appear to be how deep?
(n of air = 1.00, n of water = 1.33)

A. 6 m
B. 8 m
C. 10.67 m
D. The angles of incidence and refraction are needed to determine the correct answer.

35. An object is 15 cms from a converging lens with a focal length of 5 cms. The image formed is:

A. virtual, erect, enlarged
B. virtual, erect, reduced
C. real, erect, enlarged
D. real, inverted, reduced

36. An object is placed 8 cms from a biconcave lens with a focal length of 10 cms. The image formed is:

A. virtual, erect, reduced
B. real, inverted, reduced
C. real, erect, enlarged
D. virtual, inverted, reduced

37. An object is placed 5 cms from a diverging lens with a focal length of 10 cms. The image formed is:

A. virtual, inverted, enlarged
B. virtual, erect, reduced
C. real, inverted, enlarged
D. real, erect, reduced

38. A 20 cm tall object is placed 5 cms from a convex lens with a focal length of 10 cms. The image is:

A. real, erect, 2.5 cms from lens and 10 cms tall.
B. virtual, erect, 10 cms from lens and 40 cms tall.
C. real, inverted, 10 cms from lens and 40 cms tall.
D. virtual, inverted, 2.5 cms from lens and 10 cms tall.

39. An object 10 cms tall is placed 20 cms from a concave lens with a focal length of 5 cms. The image is:

A. virtual, inverted, 40 cms from lens and 20 cms tall.
B. virtual, erect, 4 cms from lens and 2 cms tall.
C. real, inverted, 40 cms from lens, 20 cms tall.
D. real, erect, 4 cms from lens and 4 cms tall.

40. A lens with a focal length of 10 cms is how many dioptres?

A. 0.10
B. 1
C. 10
D. 100

41. A lens of 2 dioptres has a focal length equal to:

A. 50 cms.
B. 25 cms.
C. 4 cms.
D. 0.5 cms.

42. A diverging lens of focal length (f_1) 20 cms is placed in contact with a converging lens of focal length (f_2) 10 cms, the focal length (f_T) of the combination is:

A. $^{10}/_{3}$ cms.
B. 10 cms.
C. 20 cms.
D. 30 cms.

43. Which of the following is not a converging lens?

A. B. C. D.

44. Which structure is anterior to the lens in the human eye?

A. aqueous humor
B. vitreous humor
C. retina
D. choroid

45. From the outside in, the sequence of layers of the eye is:
(C = choroid, R = retina, S = sclera)

A. S,C,R
B. C,R,S
C. R,S,C
D. S,R,C

46. Select the incorrect association of structure and function in the eye:

A. cornea—scatters light
B. choroid—prevents light scattering
C. iris—regulates amount of light that enters eye
D. ciliary muscle—controls shape of the lens

47. Select the *incorrect* statement concerning rods and cones of the eye:

A. Rods are for vision in dim light.
B. Rods are located peripherally in the eye.
C. Cones are for color vision.
D. Cones contain rhodopsin.

48. All are functions or properties of cones of the eye except providing for:

A. high visual acuity.
B. peripheral vision.
C. color vision.
D. vision in bright lights.

49. Select the correct path of light through the eye (anterior to posterior):

A. cornea, aqueous humor, lens, vitreous humor, retina
B. lens, aqueous humor, cornea, vitreous humor, retina
C. cornea, vitreous humor, lens, aqueous humor, retina
D. retina, cornea, aqueous humor, lens, vitreous humor

50. Select the incorrect statement:

A. Converging lenses will correct for myopic eyes.
B. Light is focused in front of the retina when objects are distant in myopic eyes.
C. Light is focused behind the retina.
D. A convex lens will correct hypermetropic eyes.

5.22.3 Answers to Questions in Section 5.22.2

(1) B (2) D (3) A (4) A (5) A (6) D (7) B (8) D (9) A (10) A (11) B (12) D
(13) B (14) A (15) B (16) C (17) A (18) C (19) B (20) C (21) A (22) C (23) B (24) D
(25) C (26) C (27) B (28) A (29) C (30) A (31) B (32) C (33) C (34) A (35) D (36) A
(37) B (38) B (39) B (40) C (41) A (42) C (43) D (44) A (45) A (46) A (47) D (48) B
(49) A (50) A

5.22.4 Discussion of Answers to Questions in Section 5.22.2

Questions #1 to #26 Adequately discussed in the Section.

Question #27 (Answer: B) Use the mirror equation:

$$1/f = 1/o + 1/i$$
$$f = +4 \text{ cm because of converging mirror}$$
$$1/4 = 1/10 + 1/i$$
$$20i(1/4) = 20i(1/10) + 20i(1/i)$$
(note 20i is the least common denominator)
$$5i = 2i + 20$$
$$3i = 20$$
$$i = 20/3 \text{ cms from the mirror and is real}$$

$$m = -i/o = (-20/3)/10 = (-20/3)(1/10) = -2/3 \text{ of the object}$$

The image is inverted (because it is negative).

Question #28 (Answer: A) Use the mirror equation:

$$1/f = 1/o + 1/i$$
$$f = +2\text{m because of converging mirror}$$
$$1/2 = 1/10 + 1/i$$
$$10i(1/2) = 10i(1/10) + 10i(1/i)$$
$$5i = i + 10$$
$$4i = 10$$
$$i = 10/4 = +5/2 = 2.50 \text{ cms from the mirror}$$

Since, o (10 cms) > f (2cms), the image is real and inverted.
Since, o (10 cms) > R (4cms), the image is reduced

$$R = 2f = 2 \cdot 2 = 4.$$

Question #29 (Answer: C) Use the mirror equation:

$$1/f = 1/o + 1/i$$
$$i = -5\text{cm because it is virtual}$$
$$f = +2\text{cm because the mirror is converging}$$
$$1/2 = 1/o - 1/5$$
$$10o(1/2) = 10o(1/o) - 10o(1/5)$$
$$5o = 10 - 2o$$
$$7o = 10$$
$$o = 10/7 \text{ cms.}$$

Question #30 (Answer: A) The angle to the normal is smaller in the more optically dense medium for refraction of light.

Question #31 (Answer: B)

$$n = \text{speed in free space/speed in medium (s)}$$
$$1.5 = (3.0 \times 10^{10} \text{ cm/sec})/s$$
$$s = (3.0 \times 10^{10})/1.5 = (2)(10^{10} \text{ cm/sec}) = 2 \times 10^{10} \text{ cm/sec.}$$

Question #32 (Answer: C) For light, the smaller the wavelength, the closer the refracted ray to the normal. Since violet light has a shorter wavelength than red, red light will be refracted through a larger angle.

Question #33 (Answer: C)

$$\sin \theta_c = n_2/n_1 = 1.00/2.00 = 0.5$$
$$n_2 = \text{less optically dense (air)}$$
$$n_1 = \text{more optically dense (glass)}$$
$$\theta_c = 30°$$

You should remember that sin 30° = 1/2 or recall that in a 30°–60° right triangle the following is true:

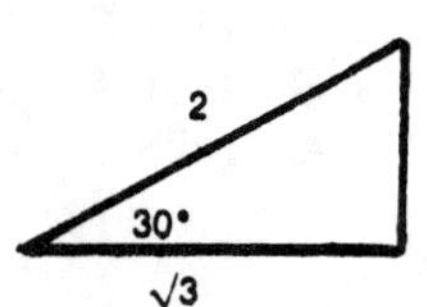

Question #34 (Answer: A) apparent depth (D_a)/actual depth = n_2/n_1

$n_2 =$ of observer = 1.00
$n_1 =$ of object = 1.33
$D_a/8 = 1.00/1.33 = 1/(4/3) = 3/4$
$D_a = (3/4)(8) = 6$ meters.

Question #35 (Answer: D) Since the object distance is greater than the focal length, the image is real and inverted. Since the object distance is more than twice the focal length, the image is reduced in size.

Question #36 (Answer: A) A biconcave lens is a diverging lens. The image is always virtual, erect and reduced in size.

Question #37 (Answer: B) All images formed by diverging lenses are virtual, erect and reduced.

Question #38 (Answer: B) Use the lens equation:

$1/f = 1/o + 1/i$
$f = +10$cm because of converging lens
$1/10 = 1/5 + 1/i$
$10i(1/10) = 10i(1/5) + 10i(1/i)$
$i = 2i + 10$
$-i = 10$
$i = -10$ cm
this means the object is virtual (negative sign) and 10 cms from the mirror
$M =$ magnification $= -i/o = -(-10)/5 = +2$
$\therefore$ the image is erect (positive sign) and is 2(20) = 40 cms tall.

Question #39 (Answer: B) A concave lens is a diverging lens. Use the lens equation:

$1/f = 1/o + 1/i$
$f = -5$cms because of converging lens
$1/-5 = 1/20 + 1/i$
$20i(1/-5) = 20i(1/20) + 20i(1/i)$
$-4i = i + 20$
$-5i = 20$
$i = -4$ cms (negative means virtual)
$M =$ magnification $= -i/o = -(-4)/20 = 4/20 = 1/5$
positive M means the object is erect; the image is $(1/5)(10) = 2$ cms tall.

Question #40 (Answer: C)

dioptres = 1/focal length in meters $= 1/(1/10) = (1)(10/1) = 10$
10 cms = $1/10$ meter

Question #41 (Answer: A)

dioptres (d) = 1/focal length in meters (f)
$d = 1/f$
$f = 1/d = 1/2$m
$1/2$m = $(1/2$m$)(100$ cms/1m$) = 50$ cms.

Question #42 (Answer: C) The focal length of lenses in contact is found by:

dioptres: lens #1: 20 cm = $1/5$m
$D_1 = -5$ (because diverging)
lens #2: 10 cm = $1/10$m
$D_2 = 10$

Total dioptres: $D_T = D_1 + D_2 = -5 + 10 = +5$
Then $f_T = f = 1/D_T = 1/5$m or 20 cm

Question #43 (Answer: D) A converging lens is smaller at the edges than the middle—this holds for (A), (B) and (C). The lens in (D) is larger at the ends than in the middle.

Question #44 to #50: Adequately discussed in the Section.

5.22.5 Checklist for Light and Geometrical Optics

- ______ reflection
- ______ virtual image
- ______ real image
- ______ combination of lenses
- ______ spherical mirror
- ______ Snell's Law
- ______ total internal reflection
- ______ center of curvature
- ______ aqueous humor
- ______ sclera
- ______ choroid
- ______ pupil
- ______ ciliary muscle
- ______ rods
- ______ retinal
- ______ cones
- ______ fovea
- ______ hypermetropia
- ______ diverging lens
- ______ dioptres
- ______ plane mirror
- ______ lens equation
- ______ mirror equation
- ______ focal length
- ______ converging lens
- ______ vitreous humor
- ______ cornea
- ______ iris
- ______ lens
- ______ retina
- ______ rhodopsin
- ______ opsin
- ______ iodopsin
- ______ emmetropia
- ______ myopia

5.23 NUCLEAR AND ATOMIC STRUCTURE

5.23.1 Review of Nuclear and Atomic Structure

5.23.1.1 REVIEW OF NUCLEAR STRUCTURE

An atom is made of a *nucleus* containing protons (mass = 1 a.m.u., charge + 1) and neutrons (mass = 1 a.m.u., charge = 0). The *atomic number (AN)* is the number of protons in the nucleus of an atom. An *element* is a group of atoms with the same AN; i.e., it is the number of protons that make elements different from each other. The *mass number (MN)* is the sum of protons and neutrons in a given atom (not element!). *Isotopes* are atoms of the same element with different MNs, i.e., they have the same number of protons but different numbers of neutrons. The *atomic weight* (AW) is the weighted average of all naturally occurring isotopes of an element. Note that it is the number of protons that distinguishes one element from another, and it is the electron configuration (Section 5.1.1) of a given element that determines its chemical reactivity.

Coulomb repulsive forces (between protons) in the nuclei are overcome by *nuclear forces*. The nuclear force is a nonelectrical type of force that binds nuclei together and is equal for protons and neutrons. The *nuclear binding energy* (E_b) is a result of the Coulomb and nuclear binding forces. Einstein derived the relation between energy and mass changes associated with nuclear reactions,

$\Delta E = \Delta mc^2$ = ergs if m = grams and c = cm/sec
ΔE = energy released or absorbed
Δm = mass lost (*mass deficit*) or gained, respectively
c = speed of light = 3.0×10^{10} cm/sec

conversions:

1 gram = 9×10^{20} ergs
1 amu (atomic mass unit) = 931.4 MeV
1 amu = 1/12 the mass of C_6^{12}

The above is a statement of the *Law of Conservation of Mass and Energy*. The value of E_b depends upon the mass number (MN) as follows,

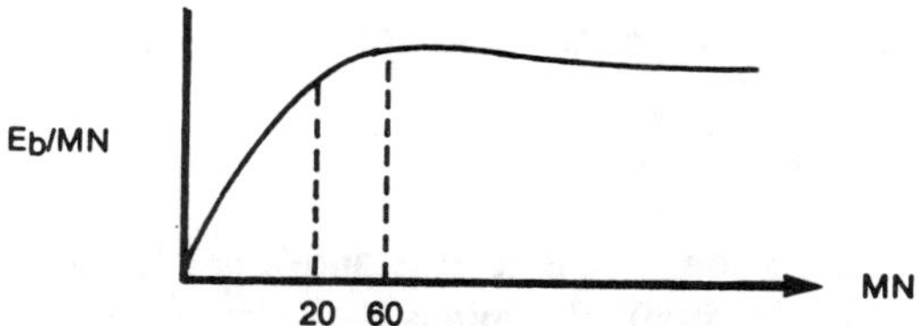

E_b/MN = binding energy per nucleon; this is the energy released by the formation of a given nucleus.

Fig. 5.55—Binding Energy Diagram

Note that the peak E_b/MN is at MN = 60. Also, the E_b/MN is relatively constant after MN = 20. *Fission* is when a nucleus splits into smaller nuclei. *Fusion* is when small nuclei combine to form a larger nucleus. Energy is released from a nuclear reaction (see diagram above) when nuclei with mass number » 60 undergo fission or nuclei « 60 undergo fusion.

Not all combinations of protons are equally likely or stable. An even number of protons or an even number of neutrons, in general, means the nuclei are more stable. The *most stable* nuclei are those with an even number of protons and an even number of neutrons. The *least stable* nuclei are those with an odd number of protons and an odd number of neutrons. Also, as the atomic number (AN) increases, there are more neutrons (N) needed for the nuclei to be stable (Fig. 5.56).

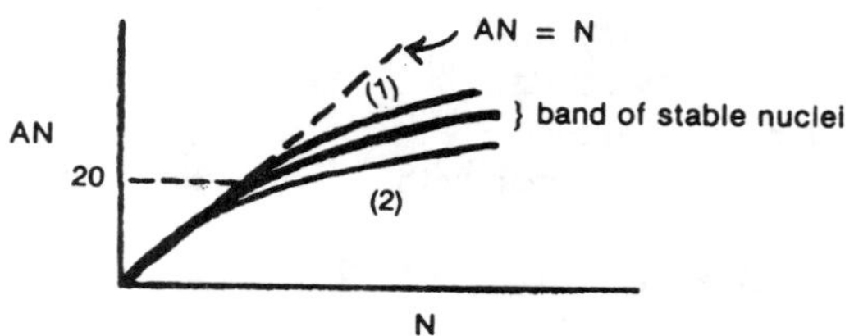

Fig. 5.56—Stability of Atoms

Up to AN = 20 (Calcium) the protons equal the neutrons, after this there are more neutrons. If an atom is in region #1 above, it has too many protons or too few neutrons and must decrease its protons or increase its neutrons to become stable. The reverse is true for region #2. Also all nuclei after AN = 84 (Polonium) are unstable.

Unstable nuclei can become stable nuclei by fission (splitting) to smaller nuclei or by absorbing or emitting small particles. Spontaneous fission is rare. *Spontaneous radioactivity* (emitting particles) is common. The common particles are (1) *alpha (α) particle* ${}_2He^4$ (helium nucleus); (2) *beta (β) particle* $-{}_1e^o$ (an electron); (3) a *positron* $+{}_1e^o$; (4) gamma (γ) ray—no mass, just energy; and (5) *orbital electron capture*—nucleus takes electrons from K shell and converts a proton to a neutron. If there is a flux of particles such as neutrons (${}_on^1$), the nucleus can absorb these also.

Nuclear reactions are reactions in which changes in nuclear composition occur. An example of nuclear reactions and the terminology is:

$${}_{92}U^{238} + {}_1H^2 \rightarrow {}_{93}Np^{238} + 2{}_on^1$$

Note: $U^{238} \leftarrow$ mass number $\rightarrow {}^{238}U$

$92 \leftarrow$ atomic number $\rightarrow 92$

the sum of the lower (higher) numbers on one side of the equation equals the sum of the lower (higher) numbers on the other side.

Another way of writing the above reaction is:

$${}_{92}U^{238}({}_1H^2, 2{}_on^1){}_{93}Np^{238}$$

Each type of radioactive atom (radioisotope) is characterized by its own specific fractional decay rate. Radioactivity (A) is directly proportional to the number of atoms available for decay (N). The rate of decay, $\Delta N/\Delta t$, can be expressed as:

$$A = \Delta N/\Delta t = -\lambda N$$

A is the radioactivity in nuclear disintegrations per unit time and λ is a proportional factor called the decay constant (a specific constant for each radioisotope). The minus (–) sign is used to indicate that the total number of radioactive atoms is decreasing with time. Integrating the above equation yields:

$$A = N_0 e^{-\lambda t},$$

where N_0 is the number of atoms present at t = 0, and e is the base of the natural logarithm.
To compare relative strengths of radioactivity, the basic unit of activity, the curie (Ci), is used, which equals 3.7×10^{10} disintegrating atoms per second (dps). A millicurie (mCi) is therefore 3.7×10^{7} dps, a microcurie (μCi) is 3.7×10^{4} dps. Since each radioisotope has a specific decay constant, a useful way of comparing relative isotope activity is called the *half-life*, the time required for the radioactivity to decrease to one-half of its initial value or, $t_{1/2} = 0.693/\lambda$. Note: time can be expressed in any unit (seconds, minutes, hours, days, years).

Although not exactly correct, the amount left after n half-lives is:

amount left = $(^1/2)^n A$
A = activity began with
n = number of half lives = elapsed time/$T_{1/2}$

Or, the amount that has disappeared can be calculated using k from equation #2 and is:

amount decayed = $\Delta A = (k)(\Delta t)(A)$
k = decay constant
Δt = elapsed time
A = activity began with.

5.23.1.2 REVIEW OF ATOMIC STRUCTURE

The energy that an electron contains is not continuous over the whole range of possible energies. Rather, electrons in an atom may contain only discrete energies and occupy certain orbits. Electrons of each atom are restricted to these discrete energy levels. These levels have an energy below zero. This means energy is released when an electron moves from infinity into these energy levels. A representative set of energy levels of an electron in an atom may be:

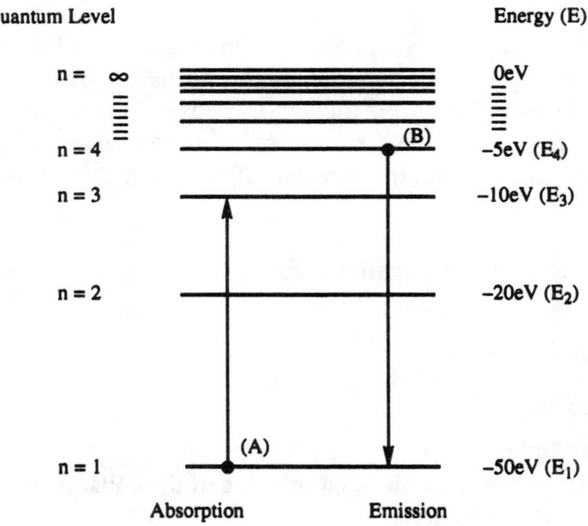

Fig. 5.57—Absorption and Emission Spectra

If there is one electron in the atom above, its *ground state* will be in the n = 1, or lowest energy level available. Any other energy level, n = 2 or n = 3, e.g., is considered an *excited state* for that electron. The difference in energies (E) between the levels gives the energy and, hence, frequency (f) of light necessary to cause the excitation (absorption, electron A):

$$E_3 - E_1 = hf$$

E_1 = energy level one
E_3 = energy level three
h = Planck's Constant
f = frequency of light absorbed.

So, if light is passed through a substance (gas, e.g.), certain wavelengths (since $\lambda = c/f$, c = speed of light, λ = wavelength) will be absorbed, which correspond to the energy needed for the electron transitions. An *absorption spectrum* will result that has dark lines against a light background. Multiple lines result because there are possible transitions from all quantum levels occupied by electrons to any unoccupied levels (e.g., n = 1 to n = 2, n = 3, etc., n = 2 to n = 3, n = 4, etc.).

An *emission spectrum* results when an electron is excited to a higher level by another particle or by an electric discharge, for example. Then, as the electron falls from the excited state to lower states, light is emitted that has wavelength (frequency) corresponding to the energy differences between the levels. As an example (emission, electron B):

$$E_1 - E_4 = hf$$

The resulting spectrum will have light lines against a dark background.

The absorption and emission spectrums should have the same number of lines but often will not. This is because in the absorption spectrum, there is rapid radiation of the absorbed light in all directions, and transitions are generally from the ground state initially. These factors result in fewer lines in the absorption than in the emission spectrum.

Fluorescence is an emission process that occurs after light absorption excites electrons to higher electronic and vibrational levels. The electrons spontaneously lose excited vibrational energy to the electronic level and then emit light as they fall to the ground vibrational and electronic states. There are certain molecular types that possess this property, e.g., some amino acids (tryptophan).

The *fluorescence* process is depicted as follows:

Step 1 — absorption light
Step 2 — spontaneous deactivation of vibrational levels to zero vibrational level for electronic state
Step 3 — fluorescence with light emission (longer wavelength than absorption.)

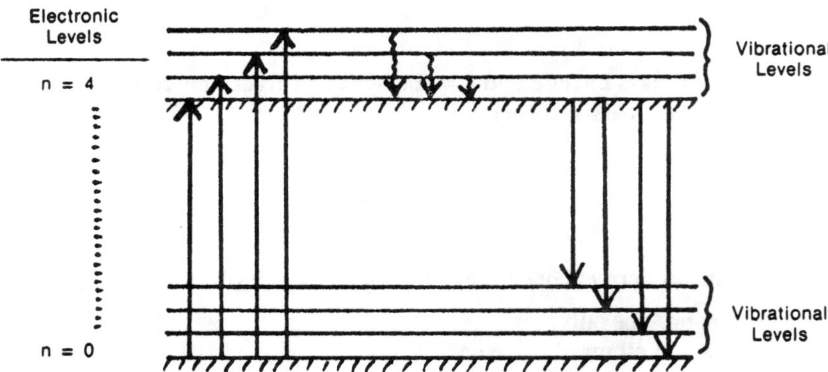

Fig. 5.58—Fluorescent Emission

5.23.2 Questions to Review Nuclear and Atomic Structure

1. A proton is ________ charged and has a mass of ________ amu(s).
   - A. positively, one
   - B. negatively, $^1/_{1845}$
   - C. neutral, one
   - D. None of the above are correct.
2. The sum of protons and neutrons in a nucleus is called the:
   - A. electron number.
   - B. atomic number.
   - C. atomic weight.
   - D. mass number.
3. Isotopes have the _______ atomic numbers and _______ mass numbers.
   - A. same, same
   - B. same, different
   - C. different, same
   - D. different, different
4. The particles that distinguish one element from another are the:
   - A. neutrons.
   - B. protons.
   - C. electrons.
   - D. mesons.
5. The subnuclear particle that has mass and is neutral is called the:
   - A. neutron.
   - B. proton.
   - C. neutrino.
   - D. meson.
6. Which particle has no mass?
   - A. neutron
   - B. meson
   - C. neutrino
   - D. electron
7. The nuclear binding energy of nuclei depends on:
   - A. coulomb forces.
   - B. nuclear forces.
   - C. both forces.
   - D. neither force.
8. If ΔE = the energy change, Δm = mass change and c = the speed of light, the correct relation between these for describing the conversion of mass and energy is:
   - A. $\Delta E = \Delta m/c$.
   - B. $\Delta E = c^2/\Delta m$.
   - C. $\Delta E = \Delta mc$.
   - D. $\Delta E = \Delta mc^2$.
9. Which of the following statements is correct concerning binding energy (E_b)?
   - A. Binding energy depends on protons only.
   - B. Binding is relatively constant at all mass numbers.
   - C. The peak in binding energy per nucleon is at mass number = 60.
   - D. None of the above are correct.

10. Which of the following particles is emitted by nuclei in spontaneous radioactivity?

   A. α-particle
   B. β-particle
   C. γ-ray
   D. all of the above

11. The particle composed of two protons and two neutrons is the:

   A. γ-ray.
   B. α-particle.
   C. neutrino.
   D. positron.

12. The rate of radioactive decay:

   A. is independent of the radioactive atoms.
   B. is inversely proportional to the radioactive atoms present.
   C. varies unpredictably but does depend on the amount of radioactive atoms present.
   D. is directly proportional to the amount of radioactive atoms present.

13. The radioactive decay constant:

   A. is the fraction of radioactive atoms that decay in a given amount of time.
   B. is the number of radioactive atoms that decay in one half-life.
   C. is not related to the half-life.
   D. is none of the above.

14. The atomic number is the number of ______ contained in the nucleus.

   A. neutrons
   B. electrons
   C. protons
   D. positrons

15. The atomic weight of an element is:

   A. the weighted average of naturally occurring isotopes.
   B. the sum of protons and neutrons.
   C. twice the number of protons.
   D. none of the above.

16. Carbon has an atomic number (AN) of 6. One of its isotopes has a mass number (MN) of 13. The number of neutrons in this isotope is:

   A. 6.
   B. 7.
   C. 13.
   D. 19.

17. An isotope of boron has 5 protons and 6 neutrons. The atomic number (AN) of boron is:

   A. 11.
   B. 10.
   C. 6.
   D. 5.

18. Suppose the natural abundance of the isotopes of berylium (atomic number = 4) is 90% of mass number = 8; 10% of mass number = 9. The atomic weight (AW) is:

   A. 9.00.
   B. 8.50.
   C. 8.10.
   D. 8.00.

19. An atom has an atomic number (AN) = 18 and a mass number (MN) = 38. Letting P = # of protons and N = # neutrons, which atom below is an isotope of this atom?

A. P = 18, N = 20
B. P = 20, N = 19
C. P = 19, N = 18
D. none of the above

20. A nuclear reaction proceeds with a mass deficit (mass loss) of 5×10^{-5} gms. The amount of energy released is:

A. 1.5×10^{6} ergs.
B. 4.5×10^{16} ergs.
C. 9.0×10^{20} ergs.
D. none of the above.

21. A radioactive substance has a half-life ($T_{1/2}$) of 10 secs; the decay constant (k) is:

A. 1.4 $secs^{-1}$.
B. 0.069 $secs^{-1}$.
C. 6.9 $secs^{-1}$.
D. none of the above.

22. After 20 days, how much of a substance with a half-life of 5 days is left if there were 10 mCi initially?

A. 2.50 mCi
B. 2 mCi
C. 5/8 mCi
D. none of the above

23. How much of 5 mCi of radioactive substance with a half-life of 10 secs has decayed in 2 seconds?

A. 1.38 mCi
B. 1.0 mCi
C. 0.69 mCi
D. none of the above

24. What is the missing particle in the following reaction? ${}_{27}Co^{59} + ? \rightarrow {}_{27}Co^{60}$

A. proton
B. electron
C. neutron
D. none of the above

25. What is the missing particle in the following reaction? ${}_{92}U^{238} + ? \rightarrow {}_{94}Pu^{239} + 3\ n$

A. β-particle
B. proton
C. γ-ray
D. none of the above

26. Determine the amount of phosphorus left after 4 weeks if we start with 100 mCi of ${}^{32}_{15}P$ (half-life = 14 days).

A. 50 mCi
B. 37.5 mCi
C. 25 mCi
D. 12.5 mCi

27. The half-life of a substance called JUNKIUM is 11.5 hrs. How much time will it take to lose 25% of its original starting mass?

A. 2.88 hrs
B. 46 hrs
C. 5.75 hrs
D. 4.77 hrs

5.23.3 Answers to Questions in Section 5.23.2

(1) A (2) D (3) B (4) B (5) A (6) C (7) C (8) D (9) C (10) D (11) B (12) D
(13) A (14) C (15) A (16) B (17) D (18) C (19) A (20) B (21) B (22) C (23) C (24) C
(25) D (26) C (27) D

5.23.4 Discussion of Answers to Questions in Section 5.23.2

Question #1 to #15 Adequately discussed in the Section.

Question #16 (Answer: B)

MN = protons (P) + neutrons (N)
13 = 6 + N (AN = P)
7 = N.

Question #17 (Answer: D) AN is the number of protons in an atom.

Question #18 (Answer: C) AW is the weighted average of the naturally occurring isotopes. This is simply found by multiplying the percent abundance (as a decimal) of each isotope times the mass number of that isotope and adding all of these together:

$$AW = (0.90)(8) + (0.10)(9) = 7.2 + 0.9 = 8.1$$

Question #19 (Answer: A) AN = the number of protons and this must be the same because isotopes are of the same element. Therefore, the answer is (A).

Question #20 (Answer: B)

$$\Delta E = \Delta mc^2 = (5 \times 10^{-5} \text{ gms})(3.0 \times 10^{10} \text{ cm/sec})^2$$
$$= (5 \times 10^{-5})(9 \times 10^{20}) = 45 \times 10^{15} = 4.5 \times 10^{16} \text{ ergs.}$$

Question #21 (Answer: B)

$$k = 0.693/T_{1/2} = 0.693/10 \text{ secs} = 0.0693 \text{ secs}^{-1}$$

Question #22 (Answer: C)

$$\text{amount decayed} = (1/2)^n A = (1/2)^{20/5}(10) = (1/2)^4(10)$$
$$= (1/16)(10) = 10/16$$
$$= 5/8 \text{ mCi}$$

Question #23 (Answer: C) One may use $T_{1/2}$ or k to find the amount left. In this case it is easier to use k:

$$k = 0.693/T_{1/2} = 0.693/10 \text{ secs} = 0.069 \text{ secs}^{-1}$$
$$\text{amount left} = (k)(\Delta t)(A)$$
$$= (0.069)(2)(5) = (0.069)(10) = 0.69 \text{ mCi}$$

Question #24 (Answer: C) Adding the top numbers (the sum of protons and neutrons):

59 + x = 60
x = 1

Adding the bottom numbers (the number of protons):

27 + y = 27
y = 0.

The particle is then: $0^{?1}$, which fits the neutron: 0^{n1}.

Question #25 (Answer: D) See question #30 for steps:

top numbers
238 + x = 239 + 3(1) = 242
x = 242 – 238 = 4
bottom numbers
92 + y = 94 + 3(0) = 94
y = 94 – 92 = 2.

The particle is: $2^{?4}$, which fits the α-particle (or helium nucleus): 2^{He4}.

Question #26 (Answer: C)

$$\frac{A}{A_0} = (1/2)^{t/t_0}$$

$A_0 =$ 100 mCi

$t_0 =$ 14 days = half-life

$t =$ 4 weeks = 28 days

$A =$ activity left $= A_0(1/2)^{t/t_0}$

$= 100(1/2)^{28/14}$

$= 100(1/2)^2 = 25$ mCi.

Question #27 (Answer: D)

$t_0 =$ 11.5 hrs

$A_0 =$ starting activity

activity lost = $0.25\ A_0$

activity left = $A = A_0 - 0.25\ A_0 = 0.75\ A_0$

$$\frac{A}{A_0} = (1/2)^{t/t_0}$$

$$\frac{0.75A_0}{A_0} = (1/2)^{t/11.5}$$

$$0.75 = (1/2)^{t/11.5}$$

$$\log 0.75 = \left(\frac{t}{11.5}\right) \log (1/2)$$

$$\log 3 - \log 4 = \left(\frac{t}{11.5}\right) (\log 1 - \log 2)$$

$$4771 - 0.6021 = \left(\frac{t}{11.5}\right) (0 - 0.3010)$$

$$-0.1249 = \left(\frac{t}{11.5}\right) (-.3010)$$

$t =$ 4.77 hrs.

5.23.5 Checklist for Nuclear and Atomic Structure

- ______ atomic number
- ______ atomic weight
- ______ binding energy (nuclear)
- ______ neutrons
- ______ protons
- ______ half-life
- ______ decay constant
- ______ mass deficit
- ______ $\Delta E = \Delta mc^2$
- ______ mass number
- ______ isotopes
- ______ electrons
- ______ β-particle
- ______ nuclear reactions
- ______ α-particle

5.24 REFERENCES

Applied Physics, 3rd or latest ed., Paul E. Tippens. New York: McGraw-Hill Book Company.

Chemical Principles, with Qualitative Analysis, 6th or latest ed. W. L. Masterson and E.J. Slowinski. Philadelphia: Saunders College Publishing.

Fundamentals of Physics, 3rd or latest ed. D. Halliday and R. Resnick. New York: John Wiley & Sons, Inc.

General Chemistry with Quantitative Analysis, 2nd or latest ed. Ralph H. Petrucci and Robert K. Wismer. Ed. by Peter Gordon. Philadelphia: Saunders College Publishing.

Introductory Applied Physics, 4th or latest ed. N. C. Harris and E. M. Hemmerling. New York: McGraw-Hill Book Co.

University Chemistry, 4th or latest ed. B. Mahan. Redwood City, Calif.: Benjamin-Cummings Publishing Co.

Chapter 6:

The MCAT Writing Sample

6.1 WRITING SKILLS AND COMMUNICATION

The addition of a scored writing module in the MCAT is a clear message on the importance of communication in medicine and the need for effective writing. This is a strong statement that medical education involves more than acquiring facts. It is affirmation that one must be able to acquire information, consider it critically, and then communicate it to patients, medical team members, and professional colleagues. Science majors who have not written much during their college years may find this a disturbing prospect.

Language serves as the mediator for thought processes. It provides a mechanism for structuring thoughts, expressing relationships, and working with abstraction. Writing is a record of one's thought processes and a means of enhancing one's thinking skills.

In order to assess your ability to develop and express ideas in a logical and organized manner, you will be asked to write two essays for the MCAT. The essay topics are based upon quotations from well-known authors or observations from such fields as history, literature, ethics, business, politics, or art. The topic will be followed by a three-part task. The first task will ask you to provide an explanation of what you think the statement means. The second task will ask you to demonstrate your understanding of the statement by describing an example or a situation which might negate the statement. And finally, the third task will require you to demonstrate your understanding by discussing the topic's broader aspects, which might resolve the conflict between the original statement and the contradictory example that you provided. The subtest is 60 minutes long with 30 minutes allowed to complete each essay.

According to the AAMC, you will be evaluated for your skills in:
- developing a central idea,
- synthesizing concepts and ideas,
- presenting ideas cohesively and logically,
- writing clearly, observing the accepted practices of grammar, syntax, punctuation, and spelling consistent with timed, first-draft compositions.

The informational materials available from the AAMC further state that the MCAT essay will <u>not</u> include:
- a demonstration of technical or scientific knowledge,
- topics based upon religious issues,
- a duplication of the AMCAS essay which you submit with your application to medical school,
- questions designed to prove your character, morality, or personality,
- topics based upon "social or cultural issues not in the general experience of MCAT examinees."

6.2 WRITING SKILLS ASSESSMENT

How will you do on the essay test? The following writing exercise is similar to the one which you will be given on the MCAT. Read the quotation and respond to the directions. After you have written your essay, evaluate your work using the Writing Sample Analysis form that follows in section 6.2.2. Ask a study partner or an English composition instructor to evaluate your work and discuss it with you. Compare your evaluation to theirs to see what improvements may be in order.

6.2.1 Essay Topic

Consider the following statement:

Essay Topic: "Often the test of courage is not to die but to live." (Alfieri)

Write a unified essay in which you perform the following tasks:

- Explain what you think the above statement means.
- Describe a specific situation in which dying rather than living is a test of courage.
- Discuss what you think determines the qualities of a courageous human.

At the end of this chapter we provide examples of this essay written under actual MCAT conditions.

6.2.2 Writing Sample Analysis Form

Evaluate your essay using the following form. Variable points are given for all questions except 2, 3, and 4 so that you can judge your performance within the range provided. For numbers 2, 3, and 4, record the total points only if you can identify the item in your essay. Total the points and use the score to compare your performance on this essay to other essays you will write as part of your writing preparation. You may want to make copies of this sheet.

ELEMENTS OF WRITING	POINTS	ESSAY #1	ESSAY #2	ESSAY #3	ESSAY #4
Preparation: Before writing, was the topic outlined either formally by jotting notes or by establishing the purpose?	1 to 5				
Organization: Underline the main idea statement and label it MI in the margin.	0 or 5				
Underline the statements of detail that support the main idea and label them by number in margin.	0 or 5				
Underline the topic sentence in concluding paragraph and label it SS (summary statement).	0 or 5				
Content: Judge the effectiveness of the main idea statement. Does it comprehensively cover the supporting details?	1 to 5				
Do the details follow in a logical sequence? Is there a direct relationship to the main idea?	1 to 5				
Are there statements of transition between the paragraphs?	1 to 5				
Is the evidence persuasive? Is there use of examples, authorities, comparison and contrast, or cause and effect?	1 to 5				
Is there a balance in presenting both sides of the issue before a stance is taken?	1 to 5				
Is there clear differentiation between opinions and statements of fact?	1 to 5				
Is the summary statement directly related to the details presented?	1 to 5				
Does the conclusion go beyond the superficial to show some insight into the topic?	1 to 10				
Vocabulary: Is the range of word choice good?	1 to 5				
Mechanics: Is the sample free of grammatical errors?	1 to 20				
Spelling: Is spelling correct?	1 to 10				
Total	**100**				

How well did you do? In addition to the specific criteria on the checklist, did you note that the essay question has three parts? You were asked to demonstrate your understanding of the statement by providing an explanation of its meaning. Then you were asked to apply your understanding of the concept to a specific example or situation that would negate the statement. Finally, you were asked to discuss what you think determines the qualities of a courageous human. As a writer, did you conclude your essay by resolving the conflict between the original statement and its contradiction?

Have you noticed that the elements discussed in the Verbal Reasoning chapter can be directly applied to your writing performance? Remember that analysis considers structural elements of writing such as: main idea, details, etc. However, you also need to determine whether premises led to the appropriate conclusions and whether there were any fallacies in the logical reasoning process used to present your argument. You may want to re-evaluate your essay to determine if you included any of the following fallacies:

- appeal to authority
- appeal to tradition
- argument from analogy
- begging the question
- either-or
- equivocation
- hasty generalization
- non sequitur
- semantical ambiguity
- slippery slope

Writing this essay may have been particularly difficult or relatively manageable. No matter what your writing skills are, they can always be improved. The following sections offer many suggestions for improving your writing. As you work through this chapter, pay particular attention to those areas you recognized as weak on your Writing Sample Analysis form.

6.3 GETTING STARTED

Like an athlete, you must be in shape before you can exercise your writing skills and perform them well. What if you are really unfit and find it difficult to get started? This may create problems for you since you will have only 30 minutes on each essay to analyze the task, formulate and organize your ideas, and get them down on paper. If you are intimidated by a blank sheet of paper, there are ways to break your writer's block and begin to develop writing fluency.

This is also a good time to remind you that the MCAT is a paper and pencil exam. Your essay writing practice should also be on paper and not on computer with word-processing software.

The following strategy should be part of your long-term plan for developing writing fluency. In order to write, you must have something to say. Prepare yourself by reading newspapers, editorials (such as the *USA Today* Debate section), and magazines such as *Time, Newsweek,* etc. Read about current issues to find suitable writing topics. Even when you lack time to write a reactive essay, spend some time formulating an opinion and synthesizing your thoughts about it. Find the time to enrich your perspective by thinking about philosophical and social issues. Writing is easier if you feel strongly about the subject matter.

6.3.1 Pressure Writing

Picking up a pen and staring at a blank sheet of paper is enough to cause anyone to develop writer's block regardless of how much one knows about a topic. If this is true for you, then you may need to pressure yourself into writing. Prepare a list of topics so that you will be less likely to put off writing practice for lack of something to write about.

Begin by gathering topics that you find uncomfortable, e.g., short quotations, philosophical sayings, proverbs, etc. Writing about an intimidating subject makes the subject more approachable because you probably have an opinion about it. List the topics that fit into this category and use the list to get started.

LIST OF WRITING TOPICS

____

____

____

____

____

Writing with your course work in mind may provide additional incentives. Anytime after class (but on the same day) write for ten minutes on everything you remember from class without looking at your notes. Using this approach, you will have a ready source of information to serve as the content of your writing. Attend seminars and meetings in social sciences to become more aware of current issues in those fields.

Your studies also benefit from this approach, since it will provide timely review and an opportunity to try to break the information down into its component parts (analyze) and then put it back together again in your own words (synthesize). Unless you can explain in your own words something you have learned, you have not really learned it. Timely review will reinforce learning and increase long-term retention.

6.3.2 The Ten-Minute Exercise

After you decide upon a topic, time yourself and write on the topic for no more than ten minutes. Even if you become involved in what you are writing, stop at the ten-minute time limit. Next time you can always pick up where you stopped if the topic still seems compelling. Your goal on this task is to initiate and sustain the active process of writing on a topic for a ten-minute period without stopping.

Although you should be writing in complete sentences, do not worry about syntax, grammar, spelling, or organization. Rather, work to keep your ideas flowing and your hand moving steadily across the page. Do not spend time pondering word choice: substitute and move on. Keep in mind that your finished product should not be a list of what you did on a given day, but rather ideas relating to a single event, topic, or issue.

This simple ten-minute writing exercise should be done each day. Do not postpone this exercise until a day when you can write for fifty minutes, since this will not accomplish your goal. If you regularly jog a mile a day, you would not postpone all of your jogging until Friday because on that day you can run five miles at a stretch. The same is true of writing.

Try the ten-minute exercise described above. If you easily covered two pages in ten minutes, go directly to the next section. However, if you wrote less than two pages, continue working to improve your writing fluency. Keep pushing yourself to write a little more in each ten-minute period. After a week or so, you should begin to see an improvement in your writing fluency and an increase in the amount you can write in the given time.

6.4 WRITING FOR THE MCAT

Based on the given statement, each essay you write should have three parts: (1) an introduction (one paragraph), (2) a body (two to four paragraphs), and (3) a conclusion (one paragraph). The content of each of these parts will be evaluated for the depth, clarity, and precision of your argument.

I In the introduction use no factual examples, but write your own explanation or interpretation of the given statement. Think of the introduction to the essay as:

- an explanation of your understanding of the given statement,
- a restatement of the main idea with a paraphrase of the given statement, or
- a declaration of what the given statement means to you.

II Using new information for the body of the essay, state whether you agree or disagree with the given statement. Think of the body of the essay as:

- establishing whether you judge the statement to be contradictory,
- providing a concrete example of how you evaluate the contradictions in the given statement (where do you come down on it and why), and
- describing a specific situation (real or hypothetical) that illustrates the contradiction in the statement.

III The conclusion of the essay should address the conflict in the given statement. Think of the ending in these terms:

- identify a problem (of principle, choice, judgement, or evaluation) illustrating the contradiction in the statement,
- explain how the contradictory statement applies to the problem identified, and
- conclude by resolving the conflict inherent in the given statement.

6.4.1 Writing for Quality

Once you have achieved writing fluency, you are ready to address writing for quality. Many people find that essay exams are primarily tests of whether or not you can write "correctly." Writing effectively, however, is a more complex task than simply writing correctly. It involves putting one's thoughts into a logical written form for the purpose of making them intelligible to the reader. Although many people think first about writing correctly, mechanical considerations should be preceded by other considerations.

There are many books available to help students develop effective writing skills. Many of them are quite good, especially if you are interested in developing more than just basic skills. They offer a systematic approach that builds upon a sequence of steps ranging from brainstorming to writing drafts, revising, and ultimately polishing the finished product.

Writing for the MCAT, however, requires special consideration since it confines you to a very limited time period. You do not have the luxury of time to develop, revise, and refine multiple drafts. You must achieve a finished product in fewer steps. Therefore, it is crucial to use a systematic approach when writing your essay. The following provides suggestions and guidelines for the writing section of the MCAT. Once again, practice is required to improve quality.

6.4.2 The Four Writing Stages

Following are additional instructions for developing a good writing sample. MCAT writing consists of four stages: analysis, organization, writing, and editing. Specific guidelines are given here for effectively accomplishing the goal at each stage.

1. ANALYSIS

   Rule 1: Understand the essay topic

   Analyze the topic statement carefully to be sure you understand it and follow the directions carefully. Do not rush through the analytical stage. It could result in misdirected efforts based on an initial misunderstanding of the statement.

   Rule 2: Interpret the topic as serious, not frivolous

   MCAT topics tend to ask questions with broad philosophical implications. This means that topics presented are serious ones. The comparisons you make and the examples you provide should therefore be serious as well.

2. ORGANIZATION

   Rule 3: Organize your ideas

   A random list of ideas is difficult to work with. Try grouping related ideas together and organizing your material according to introduction, body, and conclusion. Construct a key word outline or a relational map of your ideas. As long as you limit your notes to single words or even abbreviations, this should take only a few minutes. Time invested at this stage will make your actual writing go faster. As you group ideas, eliminate anything that does not seem relevant to the development of the topic.

   Rule 4: Organize your time

   Take time to think and organize. Do not be put off by those test-takers around you who start to write furiously a minute after the essay portion of the test begins. In general, thinking and note-taking should take up to half of your time on the essay portion or about 10-15 minutes. This leaves another 10-15 minutes for actual writing and about 5 minutes to proofread.

3. WRITING

   Rule 5: Respond directly to the quotation

   Expand your outline into fully-developed ideas that respond directly to the quotation. Keep your writing relevant to the topic. As you elaborate on your ideas, be sure that you are developing and clarifying the main idea and not digressing. To maintain focus, eliminate anything that is NOT relevant to the main idea. This can be difficult because it is tempting to try to demonstrate everything you know about a topic. Keep in mind that your goal is not to showcase your range of information but to develop specific aspects of the topic that were requested.

Rule 6: Understand essay format

Standard essay format consists of an opening paragraph, two or more supporting paragraphs, and a concluding paragraph. Writing in standard format makes the task easier because it frees your energies for thinking through the problem and for expressing your thoughts in a coherent manner. It also makes it easier for your reader who has certain expectations. The figure illustrates standard essay format.

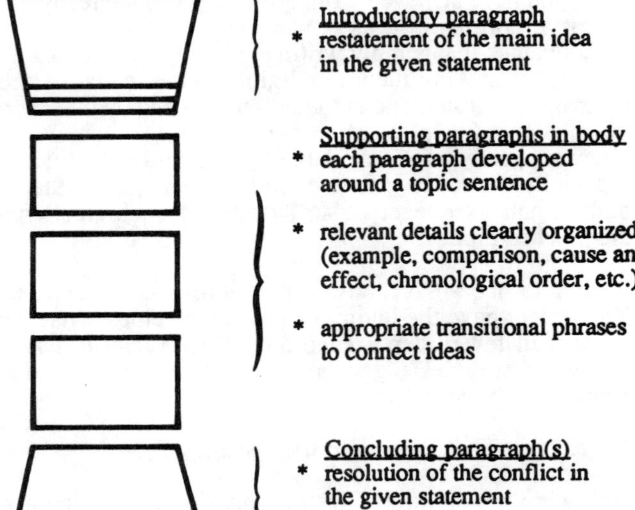

Introductory paragraph
* restatement of the main idea in the given statement
Supporting paragraphs in body
* each paragraph developed around a topic sentence
* relevant details clearly organized (example, comparison, cause and effect, chronological order, etc.)
* appropriate transitional phrases to connect ideas
Concluding paragraph(s)
* resolution of the conflict in the given statement

Rule 7: Focus your essay in the introduction

In the first paragraph, begin your essay by restating the main idea of the quote. It will not only orient the reader, but also serve as a reminder of the main elements that you need to develop. A secondary benefit is that it gives you an immediate beginning and provides an early feeling of control.

The restatement of the main idea of the quote should lead to your thesis statement, i.e., the controlling idea. This statement is one of the most important sentences of your essay. A carefully written thesis statement will greatly facilitate the writing of the rest of the essay since it provides the guideline for what should be included in the body of the essay. The thesis statement should be broad enough to cover the theme of the essay as a whole, but focused enough to delineate whatever aspect of the topic you will cover or position on the subject you will take.

Rule 8: Use your thesis statement to guide the development of the body of the essay

With supporting paragraphs, the body of the essay expands upon the thesis statement in the opening paragraph. The number of paragraphs in the body is determined by the number of main ideas needed to fully develop your thesis statement. Each paragraph should have a main idea statement that tells the reader what the paragraph is about. Keep in mind that each paragraph should develop only one point. For example, if you are directed on the MCAT essay to explain both what a statement means and how a situation or example might negate its premise, your first paragraph of the body would deal only with the meaning of the statement.

Rule 9: Show the relationship among details in the paragraph

Once you have determined the information to be included in the paragraph, present it in an organized form. In the Verbal Reasoning chapter, patterns of organization were discussed in terms of the role they play in validating reading comprehension. In writing an essay, your job shifts from identifying organizational structure to constructing it and providing appropriate examples.

Rule 10: Present information in a logical progression

Information should follow a logical progression, usually in either ascending or descending order of importance. The order that you choose depends upon the kind of effect you hope to make. If you want the reader's immediate attention, then begin with your most important point. The less important points that follow are used to add additional confirmation. If you would rather build gradually to a climax in order to lock in reader's attention toward the end, save the most important point for last.

Rule 11: Provide a smooth transition between paragraphs

Since most essays have more than one paragraph, it is important that you provide a good transition to move the reader from one idea to the next. Your essay as a whole should have unity. When paragraphs appear to be disjointed, some of the meaning is lost. Without transitional words or phrases, one understands each paragraph individually, but not the way the paragraphs are connected. Examples of transitions are:

Words and Phrases. Moreover, then, however, accordingly, besides, therefore, nevertheless, on the other hand, and on the contrary.

Statements. "Although the author's comments resulted from a very specific situation, one can see broader implications." "After considering the essence of what this statement means, it is important to consider the potential outcomes that arise from this philosophy."

Rule 12: Provide the reader with a summary

Your essay should end with a summary paragraph. The summary should include a restatement of the thesis sentence and provide a resolution of the conflict between the original statement and its contradiction. This paragraph should not include any new information.

4. EDITING

Rule 13: Assess the content of your essay first

After you have completed your essay, reread it to evaluate content. Have you answered all parts of the question? Is there a well-formulated thesis statement? Are your ideas serious? Are they broad enough? Do you support them with adequate details or examples?

Check your concluding paragraph. Does it relate back to your thesis? Have you changed your mind in the course of writing? If so, it is quicker to modify your thesis than it is to rewrite the body of the paper. What about the body of the paper? Do the middle paragraphs support the thesis, that is, are there logical connectors provided or implied? Are your details specific enough?

Rule 14: Correct for mechanical errors

The test-makers and evaluators expect you to quickly proofread and correct your essay for mechanical errors (grammar, spelling, and word choice) when you have finished writing. They do not give you enough time to recopy your essay and they do not expect you to do so. They do, however, expect you to correct errors. Using an erasable pen can greatly aid you in this process.

As you proofread, look for errors that you commonly make. You will want to direct extra effort toward improving these areas, since repeated errors are a sign of careless preparation. Specifically, you will want to proofread for the following:

- Sentence fragments: especially check for sentences beginning with "and," " or," " but," etc.
- Run-on sentences: can be corrected either by changing a comma into a semi-colon or by splitting the sentence into two separate sentences. The latter can be done by changing the comma to a period, crossing out the connecting word, and capitalizing the first letter of the word that begins the new sentence.
- Subject-verb agreement errors: watch especially for the third person singular.
- Verb tense errors: a sentence may begin in one tense and shift to another.
- Common spelling errors: most often these are ones you tend to repeat, e.g., mathmatics vs mathematics, recieve vs receive, comparible vs comparable, seperate vs separate.
- Confusion with homophones: words that sound alike but have different spelling and meaning, e.g., there vs their, to vs too or two, all vs awl, etc.
- Common punctuation errors: its vs it's, inappropriate use of commas, etc.

Rule 15: Include good writing techniques

In addition to avoiding certain error types, evaluate your essay to be sure that it does contain the following:

- Careful and precise word choice: "junction" is a better choice than "gap" if you are defining "synapse."
- Mixture of long, short, and midlength sentences: a short sentence coming at the end of a paragraph can sometimes provide an effective finish.
- Mixture of simple, compound, and complex sentences: a simple sentence at the end of a paragraph or essay can be very powerful.

- Use of active rather than passive voice: practice to avoid this problem; read old essays and underline every passive form of the verb "to be." Revise the essays by exchanging what you underlined with an active verb (e.g., "In 1909 the Futurist manifesto was written by the poet Marinetti" becomes "In 1909 the poet Marinetti wrote the Futurist manifesto").

6.5 PRACTICE ESSAYS

As you practice, try to simulate the real test situation by writing according to the instructions below. Then practice your writing skills by developing an essay for each of the topics that follow. After you have finished your essay, evaluate it using the Writing Sample Analysis form in section 6.2.2. Conclude by reviewing the essays at the end of this chapter. These essays are several responses from students who have completed them under MCAT testing conditions. Note the differences in quality of organization, thought, etc., among the responses.

Instructions

1. Limit yourself to 30 minutes for the planning and writing of each essay.
2. Spend at least 10 minutes of the allotted time considering the given statement. Write notes in the margin or on the back of your paper, but do not start to write until you have thought through the definitions, formulated the thesis, and decided not only on what supporting information you are going to use, but also on the organizational structure.
3. Allow at least 5 minutes at the end of the period to proofread and make corrections.

Essay Topic

"Education is the cheap defense of nations." (Edmond Burke)

- Write a cohesive essay in which you address the following. Explain what you think the statement means. Describe a situation in which education might not prevent more expensive solutions. Discuss whether education is always the solution to problems of national importance.

Note that there are three parts to the essay directions. In the first, you are asked to demonstrate your specific understanding of the given statement; in the second part, you are asked to move from this specific understanding to an application of the concept; and in the third part, you are asked to discuss the topic in a broader context.

When you have finished writing your essay, take a few moments to proofread what you have written. Correct the spelling, punctuation, and grammar where necessary. You can even add a sentence or change a word, but make your corrections as neatly and legibly as possible so that the reader can follow your changes.

Essay topic

"Every calling is great when greatly pursued." (Oliver Wendell Holmes)

- Write a cohesive essay in which you do the following. Explain what you think the statement means. Describe a situation in which a calling was greatly pursued but did not result in greatness. Discuss those elements which you think comprise a great calling.

Essay topic

"What we need is not more government in middle America but more middle America in government." (George Bush)

- Write a cohesive essay in which you do the following. Explain what you think the statement means. Describe a situation in which having more middle American involvement would not improve the functioning of government. Discuss what you think is the ideal working relationship between citizens and government.

Essay Topic

"Many readers judge the power of a book by the shock it gives their feelings." (Henry Wadsworth Longfellow)

- Write a cohesive essay in which you address the following. Explain what you think the statement means. Describe a book that might have a strong impact upon one's feelings but might not be considered a powerful book. Discuss whether impact upon feelings is the key indicator of a powerful book.

Essay Topic

"Fine art is that in which the hand, the head, and the heart of man go together." (John Rankin)

- Write a cohesive essay in which you address the following: Explain what you think the statement means. Describe a piece of art or an art form which you did not feel reflected the unity of hand, head, and heart. Discuss the definitional components which you think are important in defining "fine art."

Essay Topic

"(In business,) the chairperson of the team should be someone with an easy conversational access to the very top management." (Philip B. Crosby)

- Write a cohesive essay in which you address the following: Explain what you think the statement means. Describe a situation in which a person with easy conversational access to the top management should not be the team leader. Discuss criteria for selecting an effective team leader.

Essay Topic

"What is essential is invisible to the eye." (Saint-Exupery)

- Write a cohesive essay in which you do the following: Explain what you think the statement means. Describe a situation in which something essential is visible to the eye. Discuss whether essential things are perceived to be invisible or really are invisible.

6.6 PRACTICE ESSAY WITH EXAMPLES

Essay Topic

"Often the test of courage is not to die but to live." (Alfieri)

- Write a unified essay in which you preform the following tasks: explain what you think the above statement means, describe a specific situation in which dying rather than living is a test of courage, discuss what you think determines the qualities of a courageous human.

SAMPLE: KEY WORD OUTLINE FOR ESSAY TOPIC

I. what does mean:
One test of courage is not to die but to live

- Test - indicator
- Courage - strength
- Fighting an illness; accident

II. Dying Rather Than Living test of Courage

Young men willing to die for abolishment of slavery

III. Courageous Human

- Someone who is strong, fearless, undaunted

- will stand if he must stand alone
- will not cower in the face of iniquity
- will not yield to temptation
- inner strength

SAMPLE: SENTENCE OUTLINE FOR ESSAY TOPIC

Being courageous is associated with the will to live rather than accepting defeat and accept death. A test of courage means that a person wants to fight for their life it means that they realize how precious time on this earth really is.

There are some instances in which a person is courageous by giving up his right to live and accepts death. An example would be the soilders lost during the Vietnam War. These soilders that put themselves in a situation where saving a country from dictatorship was more important then their own life. Soilders are taught to think this way in an effort to benefit another.

Qualities of a courageous human

- Accepts what lies ahead and gives his best shot to succeed.
  - A door to door salesperson takes each new customer as a challenge
- Takes one day at a time and cherishes every min of that day.
  - A person with a terminal illness learns the value of life and cherishes what others might consider small and ____.
- Letting guards down
  - Emotionally speaking a courageous person is one who will allow themselves to be vulnerable espically in a relationship were feeling are concerned.
- Accepting defeat as a last resort

communism

Being courageous is antiquated with the will to live rather then to accept death. A test of courage to live means that a person wants to fight for his life and realizes how precious time is on this earth and how there is so much to live for. All of life's challenges are right at a person's fingertips as long as they are courageous enough to live.

There are some instances in which a person is courageous by giving up the right to live and will accept death as his duty to mankind. For example, the brave soldiers that fought in the Vietnam War. These soldiers fought so that they could defeat communistic views and set a country free from communisim. These soldiers were very brave to place their lives in jeporady for the sake of principles, that they believed to be right.

Qualities of a courageous person are often found in people who have gotten over the hurdles of lifes experiences such as what life holds ahead and determination to see any obstacle through. For instance the salesman that takes each new customer as a new challenge. Or the individual that takes life one day at a time and cherishes every minute. A person with a terminal illness would display this sort of courage.

An individual who drops his guard and reveals his emotions might also be described as having courage.

A final component of courage is knowing when to accept defeat and realizing that there will be times

IF YOU NEED MORE SPACE, PLEASE CONTINUE ON THE BACK OF THIS PAGE.

like ~~these~~ this but that life is full of unexpetencie and as a human ~~[illegible]~~ learning to deal with defeat is also a brave ordeal.

In conclusion, it is ~~[illegible]~~ more courageous to deal with the challenges of life then to accept death so willingly.

Often the test of courage is not to die but to live.

A test is a tool which challenge's a persons level of knowledge about a particular subject, skill or a reaction to a situation. Courage is having the ability to take on a task that entails doing something one normally would not do and the task also has a level of risk. When one states, "Often the test of courage is not to die but to live, he means that living courageous does not mean to be a show off.

Heroism tasks that are done without thought and do not unnecessarily place oneself in a situation to die because that's not courageous; that's foolish.

An example of a situation in which dying rather than living is a test of courage is when a seven year old female is about to die in a week and decides to donate her lungs to an eight year old female in need of a lung transplant. The aspect which is courageous is that the donor will give up her lungs before her week to die is up. This is extraordinary because although she knows she is going die her time is up. She has decided to leave a place filled with her loved one's, go

IF YOU NEED MORE SPACE, PLEASE CONTINUE ON THE BACK OF THIS PAGE.

to a place (Heaven) which she knows nothing about and most importantly, She's giving up her life. Most people try to hold on to life as long as they can because they feel safe and it's familiar therefore, many of them would not have donated their lungs although they were going to die anyway. This is definitely an example of when dying rather than living is courageous because it will allow someone else to lead a normal healthy life.

The qualities that exemplify a courageous human being are: having the ability to take a stand when others may not agree, be willing to sacrifice for others, take risks that will enhance the other person but not pull the courageous person down and one into desires to help others by any means but can also recognize when things are out of his control.

Therefore, the test of courage is not to die but to live implies that it's okay to be courageous but don't jump into unnecessary situations or situations that are beyond ones control because that is not courageous; it's foolish.

Alfieri's statement "Often the test of courage is not to die but to live" presents the vehicle in which the courage of people, real or fictional can be describe and, to some degree, qualitatively examined. One must also look at examples to the contrary and the factors defining courageousness.

The statement means the true courage is not only to battle against your antagonists, struggling through difficulties, one should survive in the process. People find it easier, at times, to just give up the battle and thus dying. This easy way out does not constitute true courage despite the battle waged before surrender. Alfieri says that to fight and survive defines courage. Suicide and surrender ~~are not~~ do not find a place in courage; only the continued fight against all enemies constitutes courage.

Alfieri's quotation does leave room, however, for courage through death by qualifying it with "often." Indeed there exist in life and literature examples of dying with courageousness. I feel that one such example can be found in Victorian literature. One novel, A Tale of Two Cities, tells us of courage in death. The courageous man has loved a woman from afar for many years; she refuses his love. He remains in love after her marriage to another man. ~~His~~ Her new husband receives the sentence of death by a tribunal of the French revolution, but his life is spared when the courageous man decides to demonstrate his love by dying in the place of his love's husband. The courage and bravery ~~exhibit~~ exhibited in his death outweighs any that he could have achieved by living.

IF YOU NEED MORE SPACE, PLEASE CONTINUE ON THE BACK OF THIS PAGE.

Several factors determine courageousness in our society. Among the many factors exist the quality of the challenge, the resolve to fight, and the hope maintained throughout. For courage to Manifest itself, a challenge of significant proportion must be faced. Battling and defeating many without real threat to yourself, without risk, may be glamorous but not courageous. Courage can be seen when someone fails to succumb to the challenge of the overwhelming. The courage maintains itself when the resolve to continue to fight does not receive significant damage. The desire to battle further must be present to avoid falling into submission. Finally hope should burn within the courageous. Hope bolsters the resolve to continue; without it, people teeter on the edge of submission.

To fight and live remains the test of courage.

War is a devistating time that effects the entire being. Those who have participated, can tell stories which express the most explicit, catastrophic scenes possible to man. When self esteem, moral and self identity is low, self confidence and courage is most important. During these time, living means the most to solders. If one was to engage in a particular battle, and return alive, intact and sane, he or she would be glorified for their courage and self commitment. Alfieri's statement would now hold true. The test of courage, during war time, is measured by one's ability to survive, and returns alive and well. This experience confirms that he or she was sucessful, determined and extremely committed

Though a person's performance during war can be based on his courage of survival, ones will to die can be compared as courage in certain situations. For instance, an individual who has been

IF YOU NEED MORE SPACE, PLEASE CONTINUE ON THE BACK OF THIS PAGE.

diagnosed for terminal cancer or one who is on a life support system after a devistating accident. There entire exsistance has been placed at a halt. In these cases, if that individual or his/her family can comes to terms with dying, then that is a courageous choice. When one can be frank with reality and say to one self that "My life is comming to a close and I am brave enough to contend with it" then it is just to say that this person can be placed in the same category as the surviving war hero.

Never the less, courage is a personal discription that can be use to define an array of situations. Though time, one can be involved in several situations, each with their own unique flavor and quality, and still that person can be called courageous. Courage is when a man can sincerly utilize his mind to come to a honest conclusion. He must use his confidence with in self, and weigh and judge the senerio well. If he is sucessful

IF YOU NEED MORE SPACE, PLEASE CONTINUE ON THE NEXT PAGE.

in his endevers, then he canbe classified as being coraragous.

6.7 SCORING THE MCAT ESSAY

On the MCAT, your essay will be evaluated by two trained evaluators of writing who will score it using a holistic approach. This means that the essay will be evaluated as a total unit rather than scored according to separate components of essay writing. Each rater will score your essay on a scale from 1 to 6. After the second reader has completed the evaluation, if there is more than one point difference between their scores, a third reader will evaluate it and assign a final score. The scores from both essays will be combined and averaged. The numerical score will be converted to an alphabetic score, ranging from J (lowest) to T (highest). In order to interpret the meaning of the scores, they will be accompanied by a description of the elements of writing represented in the essays.

According to the *MCAT Student Manual* published by the Association of American Medical Colleges, the six levels of essay writing will be described as follows:

6 Addresses all three tasks; presents a complete exploration of the topic; demonstrates depth and complexity of thought; shows coherent organization; expresses ideas with superior clarity and precision.

5 Addresses all three tasks; presents substantial treatment of the topic, shows adequate organization but not at a 6 level; demonstrates some depth of thought; expresses ideas with clarity and precision.

4 Addresses all three tasks; presents only moderate treatment of the topic; demonstrates clarity of thought but may have some lack of complexity; has coherent organization with possible digressions; expresses most ideas with clarity and precision.

3 Lacks or distorts one or more of the writing tasks; shows some clarity of thought but with possible simplistic treatment; demonstrates problems in organization; has fluency but language may not communicate ideas effectively.

2 Shows serious neglect or distortion of one or more of the tasks; demonstrates problems with organization and analysis; may have recurrent mechanical problems making the essay difficult to read.

1 Fails to address the tasks entirely or demonstrates marked difficulty with mechanics and organization.

6.8 REFERENCES

Elements of Composition, 1985..Joseph A. Alvarez. San Diego: Harcourt Brace Jovanovich

Responding to Prose: A Reader for Writers, 1982. Judith Fishman. New York: Bobbs-Merrill (Macmillan)

Shaping College Writing: Paragraph and Essay, 1979. Joseph D. Gallo and Henry W. Rink. San Diego: Harcourt Brace Jovanovich

Getting it Down: How to Put Your Ideas on Paper, 1983. Judi Kesselman-Turkel and Franklynn Peterson. Chicago: Contemporary Books

1 1 1 1 1

IF YOU NEED MORE SPACE, PLEASE CONTINUE ON THE BACK OF THIS PAGE.

IF YOU NEED MORE SPACE, PLEASE CONTINUE ON THE BACK OF THIS PAGE.

1 1 1 1 1

IF YOU NEED MORE SPACE, PLEASE CONTINUE ON THE BACK OF THIS PAGE.

IF YOU NEED MORE SPACE, PLEASE CONTINUE ON THE BACK OF THIS PAGE.

1 1 1 1 1

IF YOU NEED MORE SPACE, PLEASE CONTINUE ON THE BACK OF THIS PAGE.

1 1 1 1 1

IF YOU NEED MORE SPACE, PLEASE CONTINUE ON THE BACK OF THIS PAGE.

TIPS FOR ACTIVE LEARNING OF ADVANCED CONCEPTS IN BIOLOGICAL SCIENCES

As a student getting ready to take the MCAT, acquiring advanced concepts (premedical concepts that link your knowledge in biological sciences to clinical situations using basic medical terminology) should be a part of your daily routine. Active learning of advanced concepts requires your interaction with laboratory equipment, research tools, discussing clinical data with a nurse or lab technician and combining it with your daily MCAT review. The following tips give you specific techniques to acquire advanced concepts from various resources.

1. Relate the advanced concepts to your knowledge base in biology, chemistry, physics and mathematics.
2. Visit a biological or physical sciences laboratory at your school and review some of the designs of various instruments and equipment; try to remember various experiments you performed in the past.
3. From your lab notes, recall the data you collected, graphs you plotted, and the conclusions you drew from your work in the laboratory.
4. Obtain permission from your county or state hospital to see various pieces of equipment and, if possible, watch them being used.
5. Find an opportunity to speak to a nurse or laboratory technician and ask someone to explain a few of the clinical procedures for which the equipment is used.
6. Request permission from a medical school to visit the anatomy lab, microbiology and histology lab, and the audiovisual aids center. If possible, watch slides or videotapes of medical lectures, medical procedures and other medical research topics. You may be able to arrange this through a premedical club or by working with your preprofessional advisor.
7. Become informed about medical specialties in allopathic and osteopathic medicine.
8. Learn organic chemistry of medical compounds through your own experimentation. The pedagogical chart in organic chemistry demonstrates that experimental work is done separately and linked to theoretical concepts. Organic chemistry laboratory techniques are tested on the MCAT. No prior knowledge of pharmacy or internal medicine is required. Elementary techniques are usually learned by experimentation and research. Review your organic chemistry lab and course notes and your own experimental work. Challenge each and every principle and reaction, including those in your textbooks and lab manuals, to master experimental methodologies. Learn the following about each experiment:

   - Propose hypotheses, testing each hypothesis by using experimental techniques.
   - Compare hypotheses in order to understand various approaches to investigation.
   - Explain and evaluate the organic reactions behind each experiment.
   - Understand mechanisms, including stereoselectivity of organic reactions.
   - Learn physical, chemical, and biological effects of common medical compounds.
   - Review procedures to perform modern experimental analyses of medical compounds.

Correlate advanced concepts with books and journals in the library. Your specialized reading, laboratory experience, and hospital visits will provide insight into advanced materials beyond the scope of this book and will prepare you for any new information you may encounter in the MCAT.

Chapter 7:

Problem Solving in the Biological Sciences

EXPANDED TABLE OF CONTENTS FOR BIOLOGICAL SCIENCES

Introduction to Problem Solving in the Biological Sciences 7–5
Biology-related Chemistry 7–9
7.1 **Molecular Structure of Organic Compounds** 7–9
7.1.1 Introduction to Molecular Structure of Organic Compounds 7–9
7.1.1.1 Sigma Bonds and Pi Bonds 7–9
7.1.1.2 Stereochemistry of Covalently Bonded Molecules 7–9
7.1.2 Questions Related to Molecular Structure of Organic Compounds 7–14
7.1.3 Answers to Questions in Section 7.1.2 7–16
7.1.4 Discussion of Answers to Questions in Section 7.1.2 7–16
7.1.5 Advanced Concepts 7–17
7.2 **Bioorganic Molecules** 7–18
7.2.1 Introduction to Bioorganic Molecules 7–18
7.2.1.1 Amino Acids 7–18
7.2.1.2 Proteins 7–20
7.2.1.3 Carbohydrates 7–22
7.2.1.4 Lipids 7–25
7.2.2 Questions Related to Bioorganic Molecules 7–28
7.2.3 Answers to Questions in Section 7.2.2 7–33
7.2.4 Discussion of Answers to Questions in Section 7.2.2 7–33
7.2.5 Advanced Concepts 7–34
Biology 7–35
7.3 **DNA and RNA (Molecular Biology)** 7–35
7.3.1 Introduction to DNA and RNA 7–35
7.3.1.1 Nucleic Acid Structure 7–35
7.3.1.2 DNA Structure 7–36
7.3.1.3 RNA Structure 7–36
7.3.2 Questions Related to DNA and RNA 7–37
7.3.3 Answers to Questions in Section 7.3.2 7–39
7.3.4 Discussion of Answers to Questions in Section 7.3.2 7–39
7.3.5 Advanced Concepts 7–39
7.4 **Protein Synthesis (Molecular Biology)** 7–39
7.4.1 Introduction to Protein Synthesis 7–39
7.4.1.1 Genetic Code-Transcription and Translation 7–40
7.4.2 Questions Related to Protein Synthesis 7–42
7.4.3 Answers to Questions in Section 7.4.2 7–43
7.4.4 Discussion of Answers to Questions in Section 7.4.2 7–43
7.4.5 Advanced Concepts 7–43
7.5 **Prokaryotic and Eukaryotic Cells (Microbiology)** 7–43
7.5.1 Introduction to Prokaryotic and Eukaryotic Cells 7–43
7.5.1.1 Cytoplasm and Cytoplasmic Organelles 7–44
7.5.1.2 Prokaryotic and Eukaryotic Cells 7–45
7.5.1.3 Cell Membrane and Transport 7–46
7.5.1.4 Viruses 7–48
7.5.1.5 AIDS 7–49
7.5.1.6 General Characteristics of Fungi and Their Life Cycle 7–50
7.5.2 Questions Related to Prokaryotic and Eukaryotic Cells 7–51
7.5.3 Answers to Questions in Section 7.5.2 7–54
7.5.4 Discussion of Answers to Questions in Section 7.5.2 7–55
7.5.5 Advanced Concepts 7–56

7.6 Enzymes (Molecular Biology) 7–56
7.6.1 Introduction to Enzymes 7–56
7.6.1.1 Structure and Function 7–56
7.6.2 Questions Related to Enzymes 7–58
7.6.3 Answers to Questions in Section 7.6.2 7–60
7.6.4 Discussion of Answers to Questions in Section 7.6.2 7–60
7.6.5 Advanced Concepts 7–61
7.7 Cellular Metabolism (Molecular Biology) 7–61
7.7.1 Introduction to Cellular Metabolism 7–61
7.7.1.1 Biochemical Energy Production 7–62
7.7.1.2 Biochemical Processes 7–62
7.7.2 Questions Related to Cellular Metabolism 7–66
7.7.3 Answers to Questions in Section 7.7.2 7–67
7.7.4 Discussion of Answers to Questions in Section 7.7.2 7–67
7.7.5 Advanced Concepts 7–67
7.8 Reproductive System 7–68
7.8.1 Introduction to Reproductive System 7–68
7.8.1.1 Female and Male Anatomy (Gonads and Genitalia) 7–68
7.8.1.2 Gametogenesis 7–69
7.8.1.3 Mitosis 7–70
7.8.1.4 Meiosis 7–71
7.8.1.5 Menstrual Period 7–72
7.8.2 Questions Related to Reproductive System 7–73
7.8.3 Answers to Questions in Section 7.8.2 7–76
7.8.4 Discussion of Answers to Questions in Section 7.8.2 7–76
7.8.5 Advanced Concepts 7–76
7.9 Developmental Mechanisms (Embryology) 7–77
7.9.1 Introduction to Developmental Mechanisms 7–77
7.9.1.1 Development of Human Embryo 7–77
7.9.2 Questions Related to Developmental Mechanisms 7–79
7.9.3 Answers to Questions in Section 7.9.2 7–81
7.9.4 Discussion of Answers to Questions in Section 7.9.2 7–82
7.9.5 Advanced Concepts 7–82
7.10 Genetics and Evolution 7–82
7.10.1 Introduction to Genetics and Evolution 7–82
7.10.1.1 Genetic Variability 7–82
7.10.1.2 Mendel's Laws 7–83
7.10.1.3 Chromosomal Mutations 7–84
7.10.1.4 Pedigree Charts 7–85
7.10.1.5 Punnett Squares 7–87
7.10.1.6 Hardy-Weinberg Principle with Applications 7–88
7.10.1.7 Gene Mapping 7–89
7.10.1.8 Population Growth 7–90
7.10.1.9 The Mechanism of Evolution 7–92
7.10.1.10 Consequences of Evolution (Species Concepts and Speciation) 7–92
7.10.1.11 Taxonomy 7–93
7.10.1.12 Comparative Anatomy 7–93
7.10.2 Questions Related to Genetics and Evolution 7–94
7.10.3 Answers to Questions in Section 7.10.2 7–101
7.10.4 Discussion of Answers to Questions in Section 7.10.2 7–102
7.10.5 Advanced Concepts 7–104
7.11 Nervous System 7–104
7.11.1 Introduction to Nervous System 7–104
7.11.1.1 Neural Cells (Specialized Eukaryotic Cells) 7–104
7.11.1.2 Structure and Function 7–106
7.11.1.3 Afferent and Efferent Neurons 7–108
7.11.1.4 Classification Chart of Cranial Nerves 7–109
7.11.1.5 Sensory Reception and Processing 7–110
7.11.2 Questions Related to Nervous System 7–110
7.11.3 Answers to Questions in Section 7.11.2 7–112
7.11.4 Discussion of Answers to Questions in Section 7.11.2 7–112
7.11.5 Advanced Concepts 7–112
7.12 Endocrine System 7–113
7.12.1 Introduction to Endocrine System 7–113

7.12.1.1 Major Endocrine Glands 7–114
7.12.1.2 Major Hormones of Endocrine Glands 7–115
7.12.1.3 Mechanisms of Hormone Action 7–117
7.12.2 Questions Related to Endocrine System 7–117
7.12.3 Answers to Questions in Section 7.12.2 7–119
7.12.4 Discussion of Answers to Questions in Section 7.12.2 7–119
7.12.5 Advanced Concepts 7–119
7.13 Circulatory System 7–120
7.13.1 Introduction to Circulatory System 7–120
7.13.1.1 Functions and Principles 7–120
7.13.1.2 Human Heart and Types of Circulation 7–121
7.13.1.3 Blood Vessels 7–122
7.13.1.4 Composition of Blood 7–123
7.13.1.5 Hemoglobin Binding Sites 7–124
7.13.2 Questions Related to Circulatory System 7–124
7.13.3 Answers to Questions in Section 7.13.2 7–128
7.13.4 Discussion of Answers to Questions in Section 7.13.2 7–128
7.13.5 Advanced Concepts 7–128
7.14 Lymphatic and Immune Systems 7–129
7.14.1 Introduction to Lymphatic and Immune Systems 7–129
7.14.1.1 Structure and Function 7–129
7.14.2 Questions Related to Lymphatic and Immune Systems 7–132
7.14.3 Answers to Questions in Section 7.14.2 7–132
7.14.4 Discussion of Answers to Questions in Section 7.14.2 7–132
7.14.5 Advanced Concepts 7–132
7.15 Digestive System 7–133
7.15.1 Introduction to Digestive System 7–133
7.15.1.1 Structure and Function 7–133
7.15.1.2 Digestive Functions of Bioorganic Molecules 7–135
7.15.2 Questions Related to Digestive System 7–136
7.15.3 Answers to Questions in Section 7.15.2 7–139
7.15.4 Discussion of Answers to Questions in Section 7.15.2 7–139
7.15.5 Advanced Concepts 7–139
7.16 Excretory System 7–140
7.16.1 Introduction to Excretory System 7–140
7.16.1.1 Body Fluid Composition 7–140
7.16.1.2 Kidney: Structure and Function 7–141
7.16.1.3 Role of the Excretory System in Body Homeostasis 7–143
7.16.1.4 Physiologic Buffers in Body Fluids 7–144
7.16.2 Questions Related to Excretory System 7–144
7.16.3 Answers to Questions in Section 7.16.2 7–146
7.16.4 Discussion of Answers to Questions in Section 7.16.2 7–146
7.16.5 Advanced Concepts 7–146
7.17 Muscle System 7–146
7.17.1 Introduction to Muscle System 7–146
7.17.1.1 Basic Muscle Types and Functions 7–147
7.17.1.2 Voluntary and Involuntary Muscle Control 7–149
7.17.2 Questions Related to Muscle System 7–149
7.17.3 Answers to Questions in Section 7.17.2 7–151
7.17.4 Discussion of Answers to Questions in Section 7.17.2 7–151
7.17.5 Advanced Concepts 7–152
7.18 Skeletal System 7–152
7.18.1 Introduction to Skeletal System 7–152
7.18.1.1 Connective Tissue (Specialized Eukaryotic Cells and Tissues) 7–152
7.18.1.2 Bone Types and Structure 7–152
7.18.1.3 Skeletal and Cartilage Structure 7–153
7.18.2 Questions Related to Skeletal System 7–154
7.18.3 Answers to Questions in Section 7.18.2 7–156
7.18.4 Discussion of Answers to Questions in Section 7.18.2 7–156
7.18.5 Advanced Concepts 7–156
7.19 Respiratory and Skin Systems 7–157
7.19.1 Introduction to Respiratory and Skin Systems 7–157
7.19.1.1 Function of Respiratory System 7–157
7.19.1.2 Breathing Structures and Mechanisms 7–157

7.19.1.3 Structure and Function of Skin System 7–159
7.19.1.4 Thermoregulation (Skin System) 7–160
7.19.2 Questions Related to Respiratory and Skin Systems 7–161
7.19.3 Answers to Questions in Section 7.19.2 7–163
7.19.4 Discussion of Answers to Questions in Section 7.19.2 7–163
7.19.5 Advanced Concepts 7–163
Organic Chemistry 7–164
7.20 Hydrocarbons 7–164
7.20.1 Introduction to Hydrocarbons 7–164
7.20.1.1 Alkanes (Saturated Hydrocarbons) 7–164
7.20.1.2 Alkenes, Dienes, Alkynes (Unsaturated Hydrocarbons) 7–169
7.20.1.3 Benzene (Aromatic Hydrocarbons) 7–176
7.20.2 Questions Related to Hydrocarbons 7–181
7.20.3 Answers to Questions in Section 7.20.2 7–188
7.20.4 Discussion of Answers to Questions in Section 7.20.2 7–189
7.20.5 Advanced Concepts 7–190
7.21 Alcohols, Aldehydes and Ketones (Oxygen-Containing Compounds) 7–190
7.21.1 Introduction to Oxygen-Containing Compounds 7–190
7.21.1.1 Alcohols 7–191
7.21.1.2 Aldehydes and Ketones 7–197
7.21.2 Questions Related to Alcohols, Aldehydes and Ketones 7–200
7.21.3 Answers to Questions in Section 7.21.2 7–204
7.21.4 Discussion of Answers to Questions in Section 7.21.2 7–204
7.21.5 Advanced Concepts 7–205
7.22 Carboxylic Acids and Derivatives, Ethers and Phenols 7–206
7.22.1 Introduction (See Section 7.21.1) 7–206
7.22.1.1 Carboxylic Acids (Oxygen-Containing Compounds) 7–206
7.22.1.2 Amides (Carboxylic Acid Derivatives) 7–209
7.22.1.3 Esters (Carboxylic Acid Derivatives) 7–209
7.22.1.4 Ethers (Oxygen-Containing Compounds) 7–210
7.22.1.5 Phenols (Oxygen-Containing Compounds) 7–211
7.22.2 Questions Related to Carboxylic Acids and Derivatives, Ethers and Phenols 7–212
7.22.3 Answers to Questions in Section 7.22.2 7–218
7.22.4 Discussion of Answers to Questions in Section 7.22.2 7–218
7.22.5 Advanced Concepts 7–219
7.23 Amines (Nitrogen-Containing Compounds) 7–219
7.23.1 Introduction to Amines 7–219
7.23.1.1 Nomenclature and Stereochemistry 7–219
7.23.1.2 Important Properties and Reactions 7–220
7.23.2 Questions Related to Amines 7–221
7.23.3 Answers to Questions in Section 7.23.2 7–223
7.23.4 Discussion of Answers to Questions in Section 7.23.2 7–223
7.23.5 Advanced Concepts 7–224
7.24 Separations and Purifications 7–224
7.24.1 Introduction to Separations and Purifications 7–224
7.24.1.1 Solvent Extraction 7–224
7.24.1.2 Chromatography 7–225
7.24.1.3 Distillation 7–228
7.24.1.4 Recrystallization 7–230
7.24.2 Questions Related to Separations and Purifications; Chromatography 7–231
7.24.3 Answers to Questions in Section 7.24.2 7–233
7.24.4 Discussion of Answers to Questions in Section 7.24.2 7–233
7.24.5 Advanced Concepts 7–233
7.25 Use of Spectroscopy in Structural Identification 7–234
7.25.1 Introduction to Use of Spectroscopy in Structural Identification 7–234
7.25.1.1 Infrared Spectroscopy 7–234
7.25.1.2 Proton Magnetic Resonance Spectroscopy 7–235
7.25.1.3 Systematic Approach to Spectroscopy Problems 7–239
7.25.1.4 Sample Spectral Interpretation Problem Solution 7–240
7.25.2 Questions Related to Use of Spectroscopy in Structural Identification 7–242
7.25.3 Answers to Questions in Section 7.25.2 7–245
7.25.4 Discussion of Answers to Questions in Section 7.25.2 7–245
7.25.5 Advanced Concepts 7–246
7.26 References 7–246

Introduction to Problem Solving in the Biological Sciences

Review chapters 4 and 5 before beginning to work in this chapter. According to the MCAT Student Manual, problem solving in the biological sciences focuses on application and understanding of basic premedical concepts. Chapter 7 has been divided into 3 parts: Biology-related Chemistry, Biology and Organic Chemistry. Each section should be reviewed to develop a *conceptual understanding* of scientific facts and their application to medically or health-related situations.

MEDICAL KNOWLEDGE AND TECHNOLOGY IN AAMC PUBLICATIONS

The MCAT is based on premedical concepts and problem solving strategies according to AAMC guidelines. Review these statements to get a clearer picture of the nature of the MCAT.

1. The knowledge base and technologies of medicine are rapidly changing and expanding.
2. The basic concepts and principles of medicine are applied to the solution of scientific and clinical problems.
3. Applicants are encouraged to broaden their undergraduate education.
4. Students are encouraged to investigate a wide variety of course offerings outside the natural sciences.
5. If you need to retake the MCAT, it may be that course work was inadequate for the materials included in the test.
6. While passages may discuss advanced level topics, the questions accompanying the passages will not require knowledge of these topics.
7. The content outline focuses primarily on areas necessary for the study of medicine.
8. Some of the topics included in the outline may not have been emphasized in your school's introductory undergraduate courses.
9. The materials assume the appropriate background knowledge, but they also contain new information or new uses of information.
10. Research studies are incorporated in passages, documenting all or part of the rationales, methods, and results of research projects. The questions test your understanding of the projects and are designed to convince the reader that particular perspectives, methodologies, pieces of evidence, or products are correct.
11. The content outline may differ in several important ways from the content of your introductory biological sciences courses.
12. Topics may focus on some aspect of the structure or function of a given body system, on the interaction of two or more body systems, or on the effects of an external factor (for example, a disease or an environmental influence) on the total physiology of an organism.
13. These concepts include basic principles of molecular biology, cellular structure and function, and genetics and evolution.
14. The passages call upon your knowledge of organic compounds and reactions and ask you to explain results, arguments and experimental procedures in terms of reactions or principles of organic compounds.
15. The passages require you to solve basic chemistry problems and evaluate research in general chemistry.
16. The questions may deal with situations or problems you have not previously encountered.
17. You should be prepared to apply your knowledge of these concepts to experimental situations.
18. Check course descriptions in catalogues and syllabi, review class notes and laboratory exercises.
19. If you find that the basic science courses at your school do not address the required skills and content, then you may need additional course work or outside reading. Supplemental activities might include reading selected parts of basic science texts, reading science journals or working in labs where you can be involved in research planning or analysis.

ADVANCED CONCEPTS LINKED TO MEDICAL KNOWLEDGE AND TECHNOLOGY

Each section in this chapter presents new material called Advanced Concepts, a listing of medically-related concepts not usually covered in a college curriculum or in traditional science courses. These concepts provide a window into medical school and aspects of medical practice, such as a medical laboratory, medical equipment, medical experiments, and clinical research. It provides exposure to scientific concepts used by medical professionals and specialists.

The topics covered include biochemistry, immunology, human physiology, human and vertebrate anatomy, microbiology, and genetic engineering. Vocabulary in medical literature is covered in these concepts as it appears in journal articles, research reports and data collection. Once you encounter these advanced concepts in the lists in this chapter, it will help you to continue your learning of new medical knowledge and technology.

PROBLEM SOLVING IN THE BIOLOGICAL SCIENCES USING THIS BOOK

Chapter 7 is structurally different from chapter 5, "Problem Solving in the Physical Sciences." Each section in chapter 7 begins with an introduction to the topic. There is no vocabulary checklist in chapter 7. In its place at the end of each section is a checklist of advanced concepts in which modern and sophisticated instruments, medical terms, and related medical disorders are briefly mentioned. Biological sciences and medical research are changing rapidly and this checklist provides a brief overview of these current changes.

The checklist of advanced concepts lists medical procedures and experiments, medical principles, theories and laws. Do not memorize these concepts for the MCAT. You may encounter them in the biological or physical sciences, but not in a way that expects you to understand them factually. The advanced concepts included in MCAT passages are usually defined. Recognition of these concepts adds to your understanding of the passage and this recognition factor is why the advanced concepts checklist was written.

The biological sciences include problems both in applied biology and applied organic chemistry. Review the section on "Integrating Intellectual Tools" at the beginning of chapter 5 (physical sciences). This will prepare you to use reading, critical reasoning, graphical interpretations, and problem solving tools to answer problems in the biological sciences as well. MCAT problems are based on concepts and on research and experiment situations. The concept based problems are direct and cover mastery of knowledge in biology or organic chemistry. The experiment/research situation problems are more difficult and indirect. To solve these problems you must apply not only your fundamental knowledge, but also your specialized reading skills, interpretation skills, and reasoning skills. In your review you should practice these various intellectual skills by integrating them with your problem solving practice. And remember to review chapter 8 to understand how biological sciences are tested using integrated subject matter.

It is fairly easy to relate topics in biology and organic chemistry, e.g., molecular structure and spectroscopy of ACTH or PTH (organic chemistry of a biological compound), or biological structure and function of lipids or proteins (biology of an organic compound). As a premedical student, you should relate various biologically important compounds—molecular structure and biological function. This permits you to understand scientific articles related to medicine, to review laboratory experiments and to become a better problem solver who is well equipped to read long passages and make appropriate connections.

The arrangement of subtopics within a major topic in this book is based on interdisciplinary and sequential learning. Biology is presented in four levels: molecular, cellular, tissues, and systems. Organic chemistry is presented first at a molecular level followed by complex biological molecules. This arrangement of subject matter covers the entire MCAT outline, but not in the same order as shown in pages 85–95 of the MCAT Student Manual. All sections in A Complete Preparation for the MCAT are related to the AAMC MCAT Student Manual to better organize your review. In order to help make your learning process easier, complete pedagogical flow charts are included below.

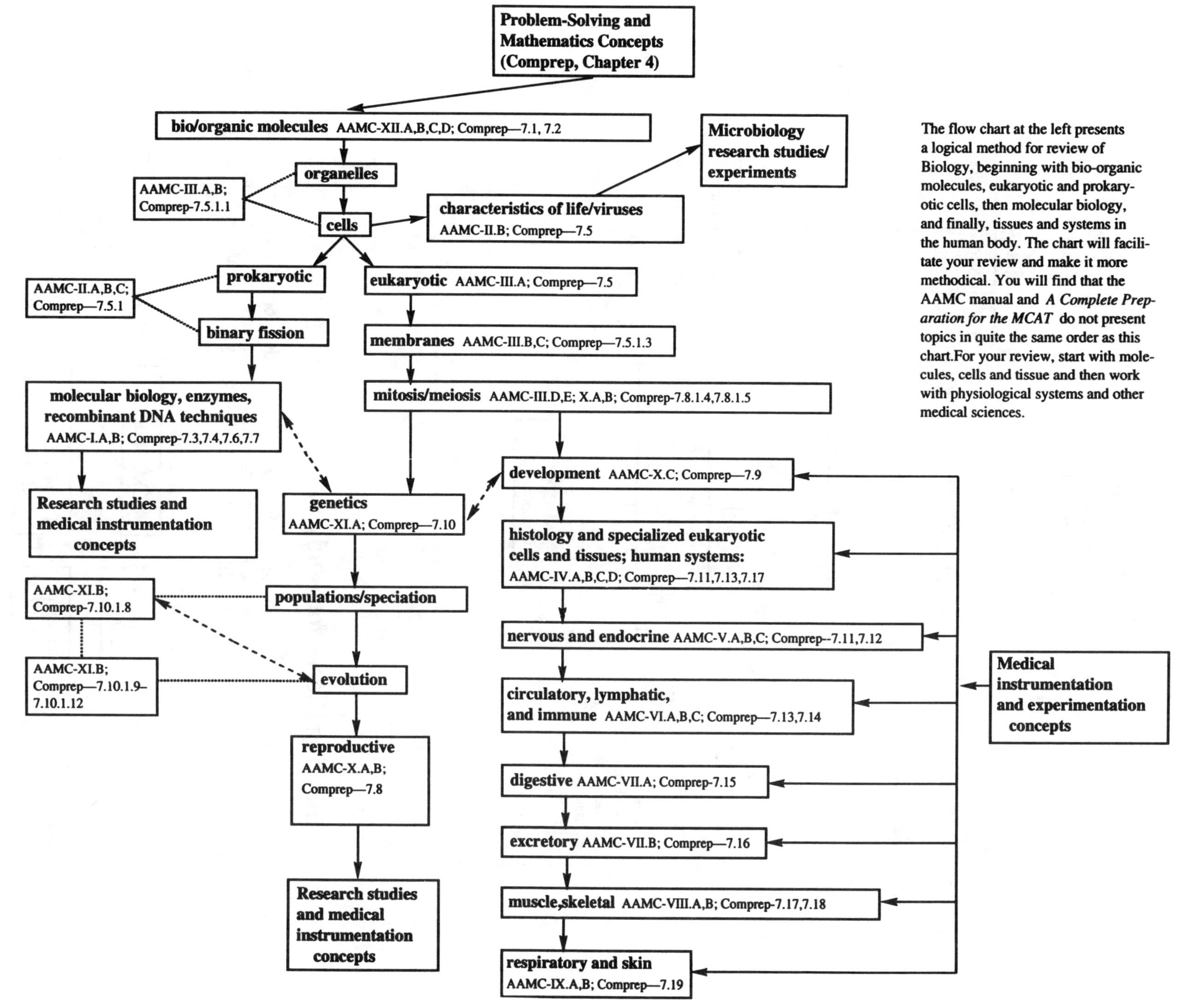

The flow chart at the left presents a logical method for review of Biology, beginning with bio-organic molecules, eukaryotic and prokaryotic cells, then molecular biology, and finally, tissues and systems in the human body. The chart will facilitate your review and make it more methodical. You will find that the AAMC manual and *A Complete Preparation for the MCAT* do not present topics in quite the same order as this chart.For your review, start with molecules, cells and tissue and then work with physiological systems and other medical sciences.

Building Blocks for Studying MCAT Organic Chemistry

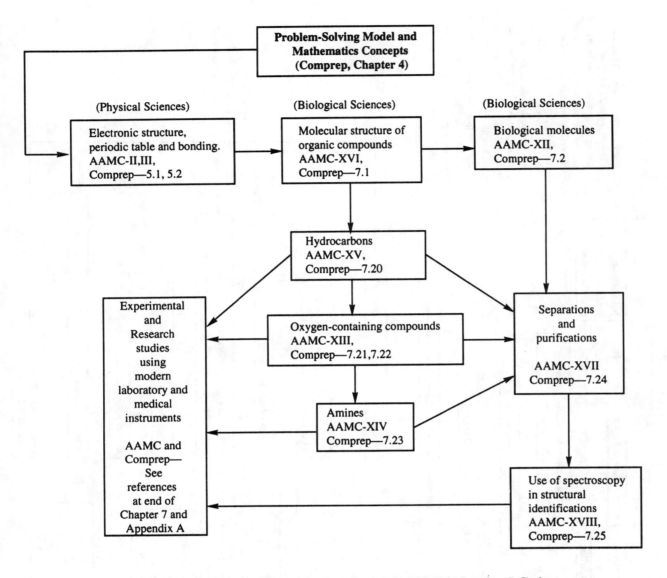

Problem-Solving Model and Mathematics Concepts (Comprep, Chapter 4)

(Physical Sciences)

Electronic structure, periodic table and bonding. AAMC-II,III, Comprep—5.1, 5.2

(Biological Sciences)

Molecular structure of organic compounds AAMC-XVI, Comprep—7.1

(Biological Sciences)

Biological molecules AAMC-XII, Comprep—7.2

Hydrocarbons AAMC-XV, Comprep—7.20

Experimental and Research studies using modern laboratory and medical instruments

AAMC and Comprep— See references at end of Chapter 7 and Appendix A

Oxygen-containing compounds AAMC-XIII, Comprep—7.21,7.22

Separations and purifications

AAMC-XVII Comprep—7.24

Amines AAMC-XIV Comprep—7.23

Use of spectroscopy in structural identifications AAMC-XVIII, Comprep—7.25

Building Blocks for Studying MCAT Biological Sciences

Following are major topics according to the AAMC Student Manual that form the learning structure for Biological Sciences. When visiting the library, find books in the following subject areas and try to interrelate various topics within each subject. (DO NOT TAKE ADVANCED COURSES IN THE FOLLOWING SUBJECTS.)

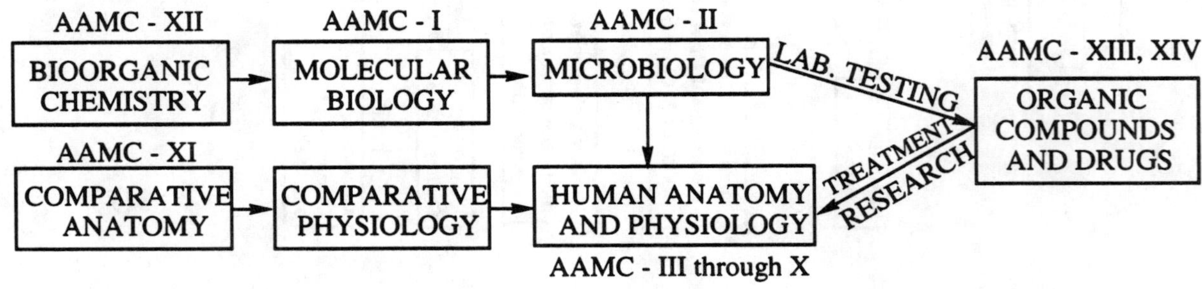

BIOLOGY-RELATED CHEMISTRY

7.1 MOLECULAR STRUCTURE OF ORGANIC COMPOUNDS

7.1.1 Introduction to Molecular Structure of Organic Compounds

The physical and chemical properties (including chemical reactions) of organic and biological compounds are connected to the molecular structure, the types of bonds and the strengths of chemical bonds. This section presents classification and nomenclature (how to name an organic molecule) techniques for organic compounds. These nomenclature techniques include a brief discussion of hybrid orbitals, resonance in bonds and chemical rigidity. Students should learn six to eight basic rules in naming organic compounds. Learn these rules with at least 3 to 5 applications of each rule. Molecular structure is also determined using: 1) laboratory instruments such as various types of polarimeters (working and design of polarimeters is required for the MCAT) and 2) special laboratory procedures such as preparing racemic mixtures.

7.1.1.1 SIGMA BONDS AND PI BONDS

Refer to Section 5.3 (Chemical Bonding) in this book under the chapter: "Problem Solving in the Physical Sciences."

7.1.1.2 STEREOCHEMISTRY OF COVALENTLY BONDED MOLECULES

Isomers are compounds which have the same molecular formula but different structural formulas. The structural formulas may differ in the arrangement of atoms and bonds (structural isomers) or the arrangement of the atoms in space (stereoisomers). For example, ethanol and dimethyl ether are structural isomers, but cis-2-butene and trans-2-butene are stereoisomers. In the pair of structural isomers, the carbon and oxygen atoms are arranged differently: C-C-O and C-O-C; in the pair of stereoisomers, the carbon atoms are arranged identically: C-C = C-C.

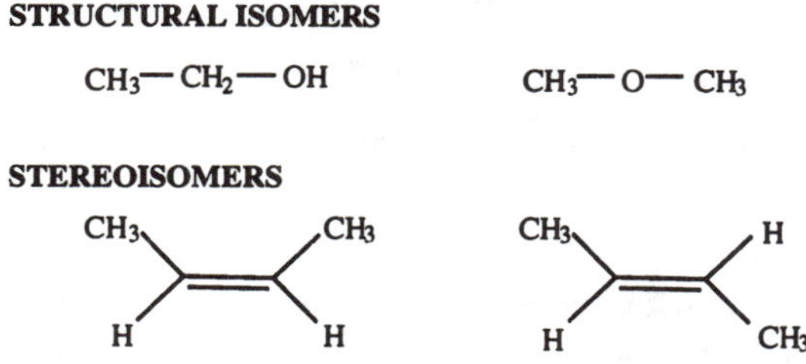

Fig. 7.1—Isomer Comparisons

Stereoisomers are divided into two categories; enantiomers and diastereomers. Stereoisomers which are non-superimposable mirror images of each other are called enantiomers. If any object is not super-imposable on its mirror image, for example, a hand or shoe, the object is chiral or it displays chirality. A pair of gloves is a pair of chiral objects; the chirality of each glove is designated by "left" or "right". Enantiomers are chiral molecules whose chirality is designated by different notations which are described below. A useful method to see if an object or molecule is chiral is to see if it possesses a plane of symmetry: an object with a plane of symmetry cannot be chiral (not chiral = achiral).

> A left ear has no plane of symmetry: it is chiral; it has an enantiomer—a right ear.
> A nose has a plane of symmetry bisecting it vertically: it is achiral; it has no enantiomer.

A tetrahedron has several planes of symmetry: it is achiral. However, a tetrahedron whose corners are painted four different colors does not have a plane of symmetry. There are two different permutations for the corners of a tetrahedron with four different colors: these painted tetrahedrons are enantiomers. Because carbon atoms with single bonds have tetrahedral geometry, a molecule in which a carbon atom is attached to four different groups is a chiral molecule, and there are two stereoisomers (enantiomers) of the molecule. [In the drawings, a heavy line means the bond is coming towards you, and a broken line means the bond is going away from you.]

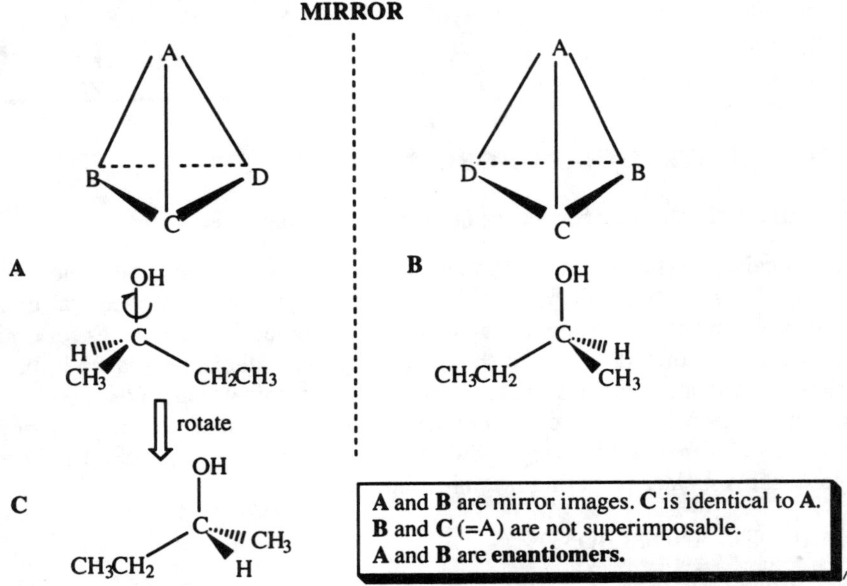

Fig. 7.2—Enantiomers

Designation of chirality: The chirality of a compound may be specified in one of two ways: absolute configuration, which requires a set of rules that are applied to the substituents on the chiral carbon, and relative configuration where the configuration is compared to a standard reference compound.

I. Absolute Configuration: To determine the absolute configuration it is necessary to assign priorities to the four groups attached to the chiral carbon according to the sequence rules. In general, the higher atomic number gets priority over the lower. When two atoms have the same atomic number, continue down the chain until there is a difference.

examples: Br>Cl>O>N>C>H $\quad CH_2CH_3>CH_3 \quad CCl_3>CH_2Cl$

Double bonds are treated as two substituents, and triple bonds as three substituents: C = O is counted as

C–O and, C≡N is counted as N–C–N.
| |
O–C   N

Consider $CH{=}O>CH_2OCH_3>CH_2OH$. After the priorities have been assigned to the groups, the molecule must be oriented so that the group of lowest priority (4) is pointed away from you. When the molecule has been oriented in this way, groups 1, 2 and 3 will be toward you and the direction which turns 1 into 2 into 3 is determined. If that direction is clockwise, the chiralty designation is **R**; if it is counterclockwise, the chirality designation is **S**. One enantiomer will always have the **R** configuration and the other will have the **S** configuration. It is easy to determine the configuration with a model of the molecule, but it takes more effort to determine R or S from a drawing. In the compounds shown below for 2-butanol (**A** and **B**), the priorities are OH = $1>CH_2CH_3 = 2>CH_3 = 3>H = 4$. The molecules are oriented with the H pointing away from you, as shown in the figure, and the direction of rotation of the groups is noted. From this it is determined that enantiomer A has the R configuration and enantiomer **B** has the **S** configuration. Any other drawing of 2-butanol which indicates stereochemistry must be treated as **A** or **B** and its configuration will be **R** or **S**. For example, structure **D** is rotated as shown on the following page to determine its configuration.

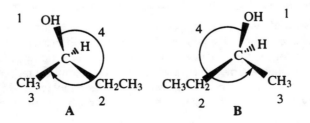

1 OH, 4 H, CH3 3, CH2CH3 2 — **A**

OH 1, 4 H, CH3CH2 2, CH3 3 — **B**

Compound **A** has the **R** configuration; compound **B** has the **S** configuration
A is R-2-butanol; **B** is S-2-butanol.

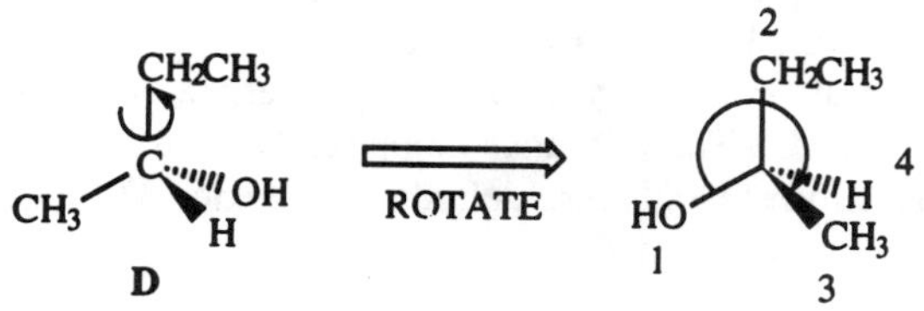

CH_2CH_3 / CH_3—C—OH / H — **D** — ROTATE ⟹ 2 CH_2CH_3 / HO 1 / H 4 / CH_3 3

D must be oriented so group 4 is away from you, which can be done by rotating around the bond between the chiral carbon and the ethyl group. The correct orientation leads to the **R** configuration, which means that **D** and **A** are different drawings of the same compound.

Fig. 7.3—Absolute Configurations

Fischer projections: The stereochemistry around a chiral carbon may be represented in a useful shorthand way developed by Emil Fischer. The groups are written at the ends of a cross or plus sign with groups on the vertical axis going away from you and groups on the horizontal axis coming toward you. There is no rule for representing a molecule like 2-butanol as a specific Fischer projection; that is, there are several projections for the R enantiomer and several for the S enantiomer. Several useful rules for Fischer projections with one chiral carbon:

1. Turning the drawing 180° retains the configuration (**R** stays **R**)
2. Turning the drawing 90° inverts the configuration (**R** becomes **S**)
3. Interchanging any two groups inverts the configuration.

Rules to determine absolute configuration (**R** or **S**) from Fischer projections:

1. Determine order of priority as before
2. Determine direction (clockwise or counterclockwise) of 1→2→3
3. See if group 4 is on a horizontal or vertical axis

Then use chart below:

1→2→3	axis of group 4: vertical	horizontal
clockwise	**R**	**S**
counterclockwise	**S**	**R**

The figure shows several Fischer projections of 2-butanol and their absolute configurations.

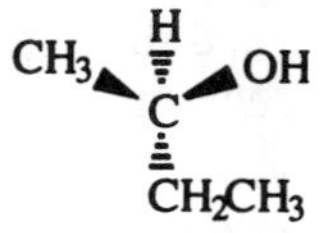

CH_3, H, OH, C, CH_2CH_3 EQUIVALENT TO CH_3—+—OH (H top, CH_2CH_3 bottom) FISCHER PROJECTION

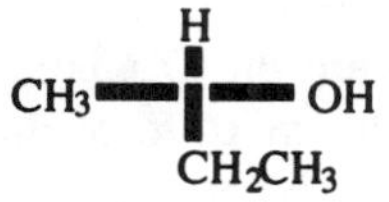

DETERMINATION OF ABSOLUTE CONFIGURATION FROM FISCHER PROJECTION

④ H ① / ③ CH_3 — OH / ET ②   H / HO — CH_3 / ET   H / HO — ET / CH_3 ET / HO — H / CH_3 OH / H — CH_3 / ET

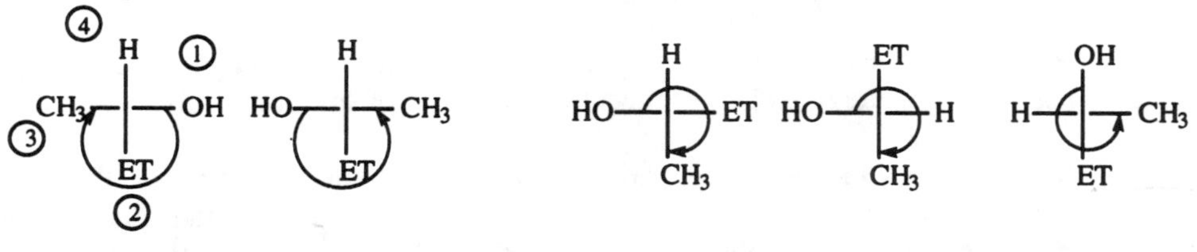

ABBREVIATIONS: ET = C_2H_5 CW = clockwise CCW = counterclockwise
H = horizontal V = vertical

1→2→3	CW	CCW	CW	CW	CCW
4 AXIS	V	V	V	H	H
CONFIG	R	S	R	S	R

Fig. 7.4—Fischer Projections and Their Absolute Configurations

II. Relative Configuration: Before rules for absolute configuration were adopted, chemists used standard compounds and related other configurations to the standards. At the time, the actual configurations of the standards were not known, but they are known now. The relative configuration system is still used extensively in carbohydrate and amino acid chemistry. The symbols used to denote configuration in the relative system are dextrorotatory (**D**) and levorotatory (**L**). The reference compounds are the enantiomers of glyceraldehyde. Other compounds whose structure are similar to glyceraldehyde are labeled **D** or **L**, as shown in Fig 7.5. Note for MCAT: The relative configuration is determined by the chiral carbon farthest from the carbonyl group.

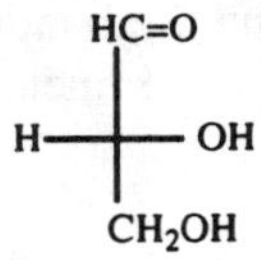

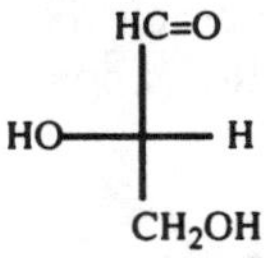

HC=O / H—C—OH / CH_2OH HC=O / HO—C—H / CH_2OH CO_2H / H—C—OH / CH_3 CO_2H / NH_2—C—H / CH_2OH

D-glyceraldehyde   **L**-glyceraldehyde   **D**-lactic acid   **L**-serine

(all configurations are related to glyceraldehyde)   (almost all naturally occurring amino acids have the L configuration)

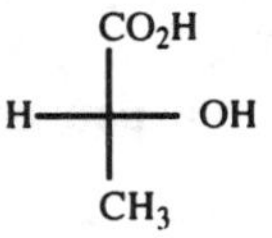

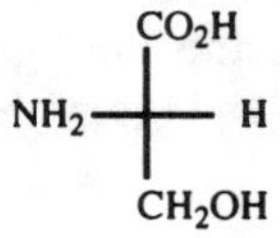

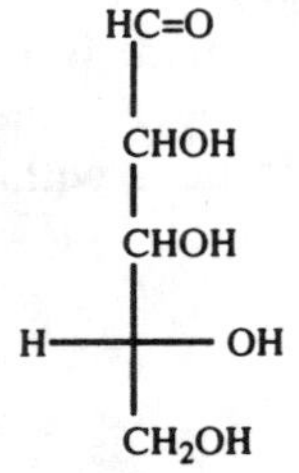

HC=O / CHOH / CHOH / H—C—OH / CH_2OH CH_2OH / C=O / CHOH / CHOH / HO—C—H / CH_2OH CH=O / H—C—OH / HO—C—H / H—C—OH / H—C—OH / CH_2OH

a **D**-aldopentose 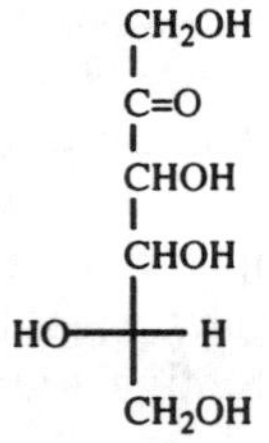   a **L**-ketohexose 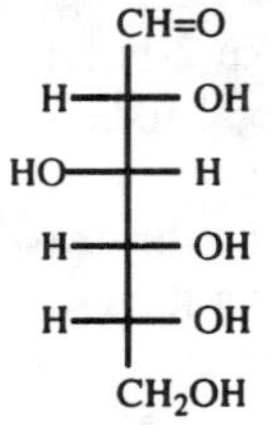   **D**-glucose

Figure 7.5—Relative Configurations and Carbohydrates

III. Optical Activity as related to enantiomers: Structural isomers usually have different physical properties, such as melting points, boiling points, and solubilities. Enantiomers have the same physical properties with one important exception: they rotate the plane of polarized light to an equal and opposite extent. Because of this property, which is an optical effect, enantiomers are called optical isomers, and the ability to rotate the plane of polarized light is called optical activity. The instrument used to measure the rotation of polarized light by an optical isomer is a polarimeter. Rotation is measured in degrees, either positive [clockwise (+), dextrorotatory (**D**)] or negative [counterclockwise (–), levorotatory (**L**)]. There is no correlation between direction of rotation of polarized light and absolute configuration. That is, a molecule with **R** configuration may have either + or – observed rotation. There is no correlation between the relative configuration (**D** or **L**) and the observed rotation (+ or –), except for glyceraldehyde where the D enantiomer has the + rotation. Because enantiomers have opposite and equal rotations, an equimolar mixture of the two enantiomers does not show rotation: this is a racemic mixture or racemate. Racemization is the process in which an optically active compound loses optical activity because of a chemical reaction.

To find the observed rotation use the equation

$a = [a] (l \times C)$, where a = observed rotation (degrees), [a] = specific rotation (degrees), l = path length (decimeters), and C = concentration (g/mL of solution).

IV. Diastereomers: Stereoisomers which are not enantiomers are diastereomers. That means that geometric (cis-trans) isomers are diastereomers, whether in alkenes or in cyclic compounds, but other diastereomers are the result of more than one chiral atom in a molecule. An example is 3-chloro-2-butanol, which has two chiral carbons and has four stereoisomers, whose Fischer projections are shown. The absolute configuration is determined for each chiral center as described above, giving the following stereoisomers:

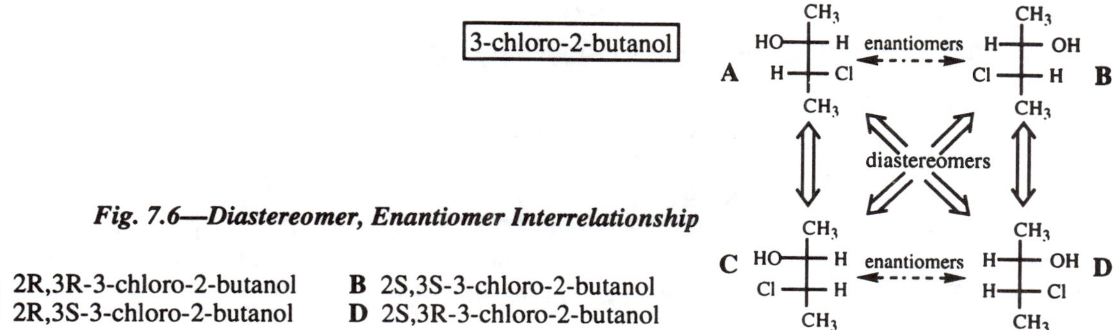

Fig. 7.6—Diastereomer, Enantiomer Interrelationship

A 2R,3R-3-chloro-2-butanol **B** 2S,3S-3-chloro-2-butanol
C 2R,3S-3-chloro-2-butanol **D** 2S,3R-3-chloro-2-butanol

If compounds have more than one chiral center, enantiomers will have opposite configurations at every chiral center; diastereomers will have at least one chiral center with the same configuration. The figure shows the relationships between the stereoisomers.

Epimers are diastereomers which have several chiral carbons, but have opposite configurations at only one chiral center. Epimers are commonly found in carbohydrates, but may apply to any kind of compound. Meso compounds are compounds that have more than one identically substituted chiral carbons, which are symmetrically arranged (plane of symmetry in molecule) so that the molecule is achiral. Meso compounds do not have enantiomers (they are superimposable on their mirror images) and are not optically active. Meso compounds do have diastereomers, which may be optically active. Examples of stereoisomers which include enantiomers, diastereomers and a meso compound are shown for 2,3-butanediol.

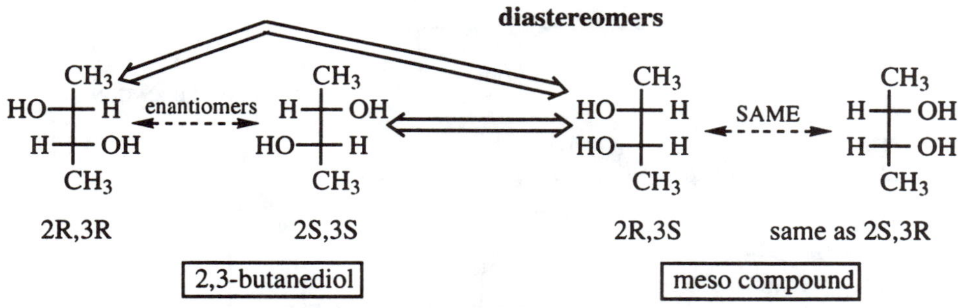

Fig. 7.7—Meso Compounds

Fischer projection rules for diastereomers:

1. Rotation 180° retains configuration
2. Interchanging any two groups on one chiral carbon converts to another diastereomer.
3. Interchanging two groups on every chiral carbon converts to the enantiomer.

V. Separation of stereoisomers: Because diastereomers have different physical properties, they may be separated by physical means used to separate any compounds; e.g., fractional distillation, chromatography, crystallization. Special techniques must be used to separate enantiomers because their physical properties are identical. The separation of a racemic mixture into pure enantiomers is called resolution.

VI. Reactions of chiral stereoisomers: Chiral centers may be formed or destroyed in chemical reactions. A molecule which has no chiral carbon may be converted to a racemic mixture (pair of enantiomers), or an enantiomer may be converted into a pair of diastereomers in a reaction.

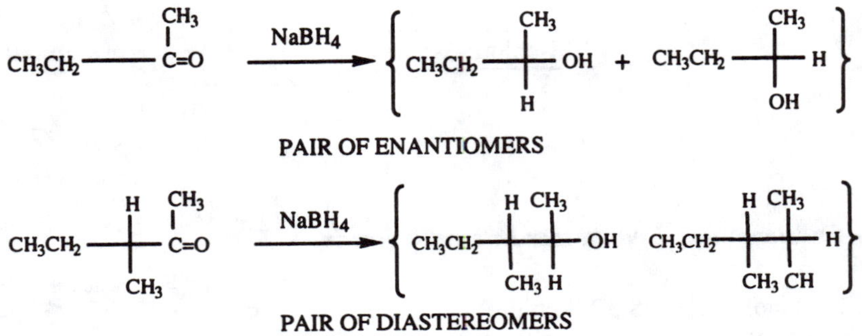

$$CH_3CH_2—C(CH_3)=O \xrightarrow{NaBH_4} \{CH_3CH_2—C(CH_3)(H)—OH + CH_3CH_2—C(CH_3)(OH)—H\}$$

PAIR OF ENANTIOMERS

$$CH_3CH_2—C(H)(CH_3)—C(CH_3)=O \xrightarrow{NaBH_4} \{CH_3CH_2—C(H)(CH_3)—C(CH_3)(H)—OH \quad CH_3CH_2—C(H)(CH_3)—C(CH_3)(OH)—H\}$$

PAIR OF DIASTEREOMERS

Fig. 7.8—Chiral Stereoisomer Reactions I

A pure enantiomer with a single chiral carbon may undergo a reaction in which the configuration is unchanged (retention) or inverted or racemized. If the chiral carbon is not at the reaction center, the configuration is retained. In an S_N2 reaction (bimolecular nucleophilic substitution), the configuration is inverted. In a reaction in which a trivalent carbon species (carbocation, free radical, carbanion) is an intermediate, the product is racemic.

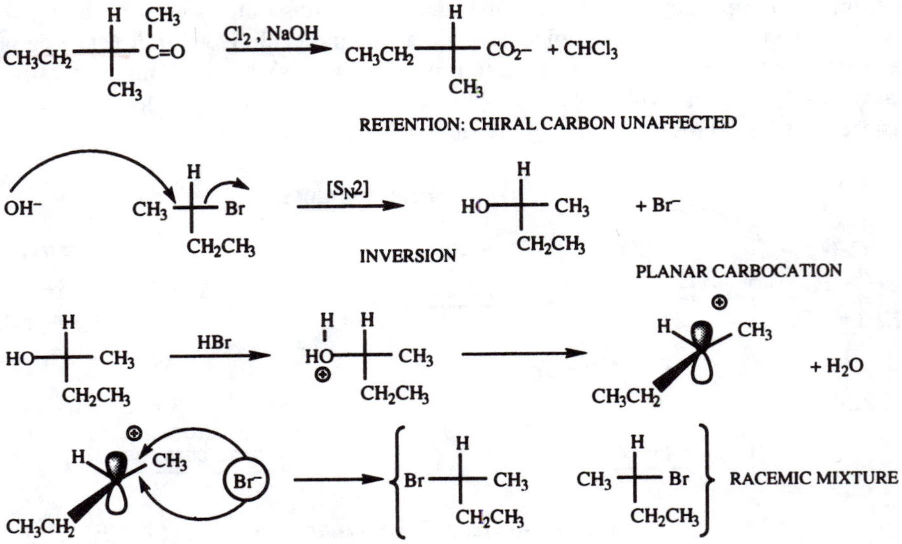

$$CH_3CH_2—C(H)(CH_3)—C(CH_3)=O \xrightarrow{Cl_2,\ NaOH} CH_3CH_2—C(H)(CH_3)—CO_2^- + CHCl_3$$

RETENTION: CHIRAL CARBON UNAFFECTED

$$OH^- \quad CH_3—C(H)(CH_2CH_3)—Br \xrightarrow{[S_N2]} HO—C(H)(CH_2CH_3)—CH_3 + Br^-$$

INVERSION

PLANAR CARBOCATION

$$HO—C(H)(CH_2CH_3)—CH_3 \xrightarrow{HBr} H(H)O^{\oplus}—C(H)(CH_2CH_3)—CH_3 \longrightarrow [H, CH_3, CH_3CH_2]C^{\oplus} + H_2O$$

$$[H, CH_3, CH_3CH_2]C^{\oplus} \quad Br^- \longrightarrow \{Br—C(H)(CH_2CH_3)—CH_3 \quad CH_3—C(H)(CH_2CH_3)—Br\}$$ RACEMIC MIXTURE

Fig. 7.9 —Chiral Stereoisomer Reactions II

7.1.2 Questions Related to Molecular Structure of Organic Compounds

1. cis-2-pentene and trans-2-pentene are:
   A. structural isomers.
   B. optical isomers.
   C. enantiomers.
   D. diastereomers.

2. Which compound may be optically active?
   A. 2-methyl-2-pentanol
   B. 2-methyl-3-pentanol
   C. 2-methyl-3-pentanone
   D. 3-methyl-3-pentanol

3. Which is the enantiomer of compound A?

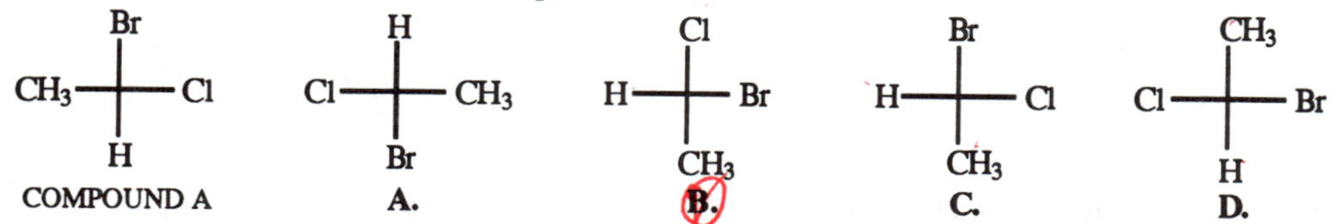

4. Which structure(s) represent(s) 2R, 3R-3-bromo-2-pentanol?

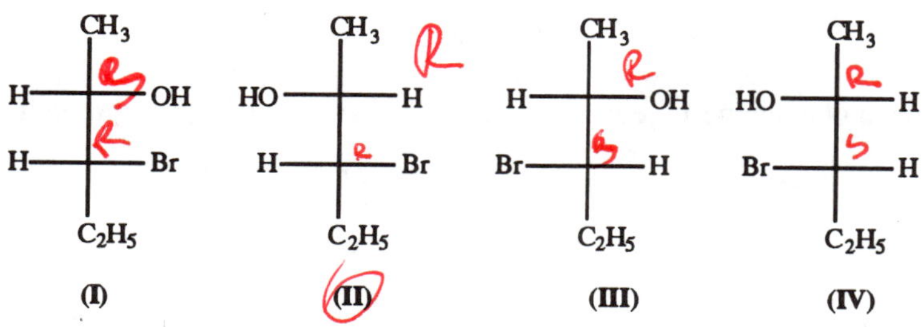

A. I and II only
B. I and III only
C. II and IV only
D. II and III only

5. Compounds (I) and (III) in question 4 are:
A. enantiomers.
B. diastereomers.
C. structural isomers.
D. racemic.

6. Compounds (II) and (III) in question 4 are:
A. enantiomers.
B. diastereomers.
C. structural isomers.
D. meso compounds.

7. The specific rotation of compound W is –37°.

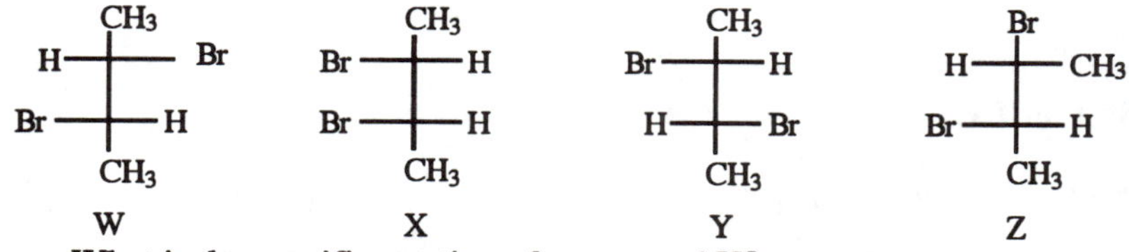

What is the specific rotation of compound X?
A. + 37°
B. – 37°
C. 0°
D. cannot be determined

8. In question 7, what is the specific rotation of compound Y?
A. + 37°
B. – 37°
C. 0°
D. cannot be determined

9. In question 7, what is the specific rotation of compound Z?
A. + 37°
B. – 37°
C. 0°
D. cannot be determined

10. 2-methylcyclohexanol has ____ stereoisomers, and ____ of these are optically active.
   A. 2; 0
   B. 2; 2
   C. 4; 2
   D. 4; 4

11. 4-methylcyclohexanol has ____ stereoisomers, and ____ of these are optically active.
   A. 2; 0
   B. 2; 2
   C. 4; 2
   D. 4; 4

12. If a single, pure stereoisomer of 2-methylcyclohexanone is reduced to 2-methylcyclohexanol, the product will be:
   A. a single enantiomer.
   B. a racemic mixture.
   C. a pair of diastereomers.
   D. a mixture of four stereoisomers.

13. Two grams of an amino acid is dissolved in 10 mL water. The solution is placed in a polarimeter tube which is 5 cm long, and shows an observed rotation of – 12°. What is the specific rotation of the amino acid?
   A. – 1.2°
   B. – 12°
   C. – 120°
   D. some other value

14. D-lyxose is an aldopentose. We know that in the Fischer projection of D-lyxose:
   A. the OH on carbon 2 is on the right.
   B. the OH on carbon 3 is on the right.
   C. the OH on carbon 4 is on the right.
   D. all the OH groups are on the right.

15. A reaction produces a mixture of amino acids D-alanine and L-alanine. One could obtain the pure D-alanine by:
   A. fractional crystallization.
   B. electrophoresis.
   C. biological separation.
   D. ultracentrifugation.

7.1.3 Answers to Questions in Section 7.1.2

(1) D (2) B (3) C (4) B (5) B (6) A (7) C (8) A (9) D (10) D (11) A (12) C (13) C (14) C (15) C

7.1.4 Discussion of Answers to Questions in Section 7.1.2

Question #1 (Answer: D) Cis/trans isomers are a type of diastereomer.

Question #2 (Answer: B) Only (B) has a chiral carbon (carbon-3).

Question #3 (Answer: C) From the rules concerning configuration of Fischer projections, compound A has the R configuration [Br>Cl>CH_3>H], as do all the others except (C).

Question #4 (Answer: B) Assign configurations to each chiral carbon. For carbon-2, the order is OH>carbon-3>CH_3>H, and for carbon-3 the order is Br>carbon-2>CH_3>H. From the rules, (I) is 2R, 3R (II) is 2S, 3R (III) is 2R, 3R (IV) is 2S, 3R.

Question #5 (Answer: B) Options (I) and (III) have the same configuration at carbon-2, and opposite configurations at carbon-3; therefore they are diastereomers.

Question #6 (Answer: A) They have opposite configurations at each chiral carbon atom.

Question #7 (Answer: C) Compound X is a meso compound (plane of symmetry) and shows no optical activity.

Question #8 (Answer: A) Compound Y is the enantiomer of W, and must have opposite specific rotation.

Question #9 (Answer: D) Compound Z is the diastereomer of W because two groups on the top chiral carbon have been interchanged. In this case, the diastereomer of W is Z (not a meso compound), so the rotation cannot be determined. If the diastereomer was also a meso compound, the rotation will be 0°.

NOTE FOR QUESTIONS 10–12, FOLLOWING: Two possible configurations at each chiral carbon R and S produces 2^n possible stereoisomers and 2^{n-1} enantiomers for n chiral carbon atoms if all chiral carbons have different substituents. If some carbons have identical substituents, meso compounds will exist (i.e., $< 2^n$ stereoisomers).

Question #10 (Answer: D) There are two non-identical chiral carbons, so there are $2^2 = 4$ stereoisomers; all of them are chiral.

CH_3 OH OH CH_3 CH_3 OH OH CH_3

cis enantiomers trans enantiomers

Question #11 (Answer: A) There is a plane of symmetry through the molecule, and there are NO chiral carbons. There is a cis and a trans form, neither optically active.

OH CH_3 OH CH_3

cis isomer trans isomer

Question #12 (Answer: C) The products will have the same configuration at the carbon bearing the methyl, and opposite configurations at the alcohol; they are diastereomers.

CH_3 O → CH_3 OH + CH_3 OH

cis trans

Question #13 (Answer: C) Observed rotation = Specific rotation × (Concentration of solid or density of liquid) × Length of polarimeter tube (1 dm = 10 cm), $\alpha = [\alpha]Cl$. From formula: observed rotation = $-12°$; C = 2g/10mL = 0.2; L = 5 cm = 0.5 dm spec. rot. = $(-12°)/(0.2)(0.5) = -120°$.

Question #14 (Answer: C) From convention about relative configuration of carbohydrates.

Question #15 (Answer: C) Organisms will metabolize L isomer, ignore D isomer.

7.1.5 Advanced Concepts

- Relate chirality of molecules to the formation of enzyme-substrate complexes and to hormonal action and feedback inhibition
- Examine laboratory methods and research techniques in developing racemic mixtures for biological hormones, steroids and complex molecules. Understand properties of organic and biologic compounds as related to varying percentages of components in a racemic mixture. Review stereoselective reactions

- Review the historical work done by Louis Pasteur on using a polarimeter to study the structure of tartaric acid—appraise the experimental evidence and decide whether the research was valid (use various reasoning patterns provided in chapter 4 of this manual)
- Learn the naming conventions of rectus (R) and sinister (S) forms of enantiomers. Check your understanding of conventions by applications to biologically important enantiomers.

7.2 BIOORGANIC MOLECULES

7.2.1 Introduction to Bioorganic Molecules

Review the chemical composition of structures present in eukaryotic cells and constituents of body fluids. Proteins, amino acids, phospholipids and carbohydrates have complex classification techniques and experimental analysis techniques. Study this section with a biological focus to understand types and configurations of biologically significant molecules. Memorize the twenty-two α-amino acids and their structures along with the RNA genetic code showing base sequence. Note all possible distinctions between anomers and epimers as well as phospholipids and sphingolipids. The MCAT requires learning of classification and experimentation techniques for bioorganic molecules, e.g., how are steroids classified? how are steroids tested in the laboratory to determine pK_{a1}, pK_{a2} and isoelectric points?

7.2.1.1 AMINO ACIDS

Biologically important macromolecules (proteins, nucleic acids and polysaccharides) are composed of repeating monomeric subunits, often referred to as "building blocks," that polymerize to form these compounds. Amino acids are the building blocks of proteins. There are 20 different amino acids, each found at least once in the vast majority of proteins. Those "rare" amino acids found in proteins in excess of 20 are formed by modification of one or more of the "standard" 20 after the protein has been formed, a change usually referred to as a post-translational modification.

All of the amino acids found in proteins are α-amino substituted carboxylic acids (in this system of nomenclature the Greek alphabet is used to designate the position of a substituent . . . the α-carbon is the first substitutable carbon adjacent to the functional group for which the compound is named, i.e., an acid, the β-carbon is next, etc.). In all but one of the 20 amino acids commonly found in proteins the α-carbon is chiral. Glycine is the exception since it contains 2 hydrogens on the α-carbon. Only the L-isomers are found in proteins. These compounds are therefore optically active (will rotate plane polarized light). With only one exception (proline) the amino acids all conform to the structure given below in a perspective formula, differing only in the R-group. Note that when written in the projection formula the chiral carbon by convention is considered in the plane of the page. The vertical bonds project behind the sheet and the horizontal bonds project in front of the page. If the structure is rotated 90°, the bonds must be changed because of this difference, if the absolute configuration of the chiral center is to be represented.

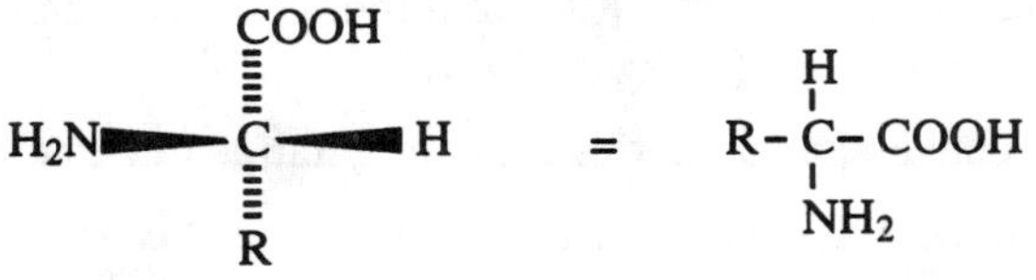

```
          COOH
           ⋮                      H
                                  |
  H2N ◄── C ──► H       =     R - C - COOH
           ⋮                      |
           R                     NH2
```

The types and sequences of AA's in proteins determine their structural properties and acid-base behavior. The following AA's have R groups that are hydrocarbon in nature, are hydrophobic and are found in the interiors of proteins:

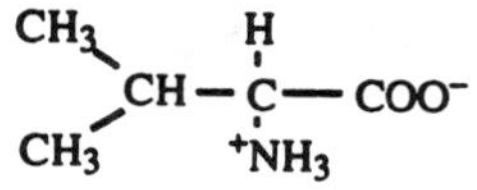

$(CH_3)_2CH-CH(NH_3^+)-COO^-$

Valine

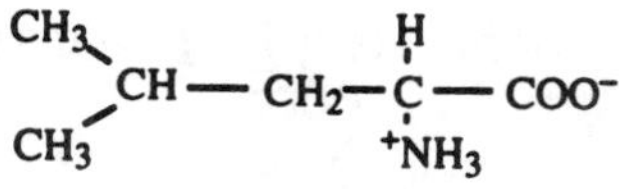

$(CH_3)_2CH-CH_2-CH(NH_3^+)-COO^-$

Leucine

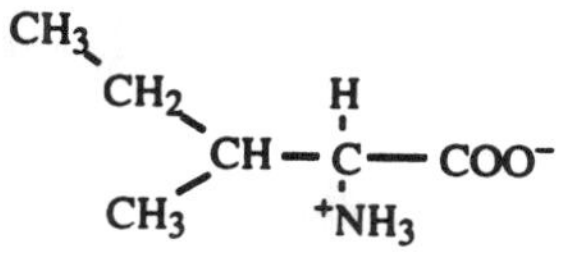

$CH_3-CH_2-CH(CH_3)-CH(NH_3^+)-COO^-$

Isoleucine

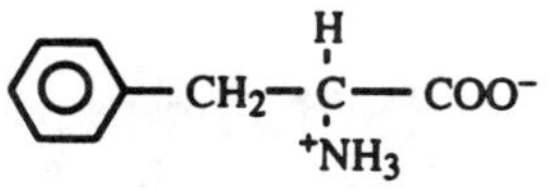

$C_6H_5-CH_2-CH(NH_3^+)-COO^-$

Phenylalanine

$CH_3-S-CH_2-CH_2-CH(NH_3^+)-COO^-$

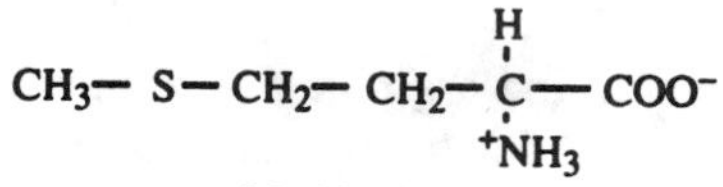

Methionine

Ionic and/or polar AA's are hydrophilic and tend to be found on the exterior of proteins:

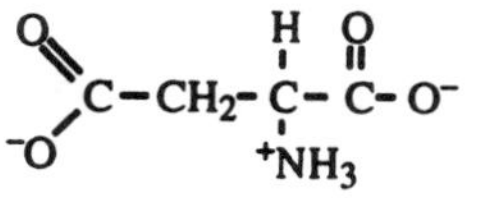

$^-O-C(=O)-CH_2-CH(NH_3^+)-C(=O)-O^-$

Aspartic Acid (and its amide)

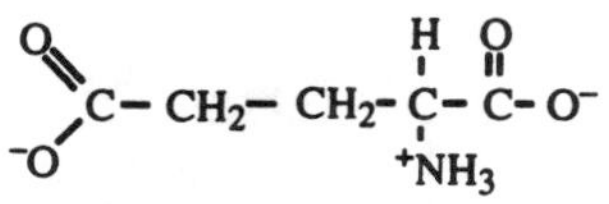

$^-O-C(=O)-CH_2-CH_2-CH(NH_3^+)-C(=O)-O^-$

Glutamic Acid (and its amide)

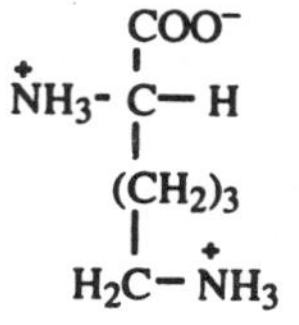

$H_3\overset{+}{N}-CH(COO^-)-(CH_2)_3-H_2C-\overset{+}{N}H_3$

Lysine

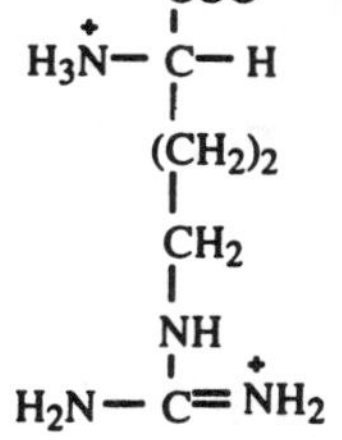

$H_3\overset{+}{N}-CH(COO^-)-(CH_2)_2-CH_2-NH-C(H_2N)=\overset{+}{N}H_2$

Arginine

$(^+NH, NH \text{ imidazole ring})-CH_2-CH(NH_3^+)-COO^-$

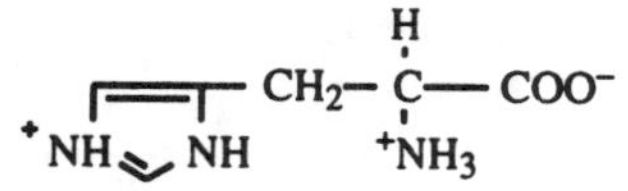

Histidine

Certain amino acids can be found on the exterior or interior of proteins (these are polar also):

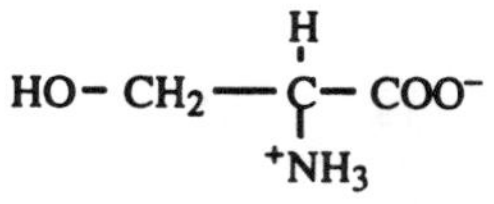

$HO-CH_2-CH(NH_3^+)-COO^-$

Serine

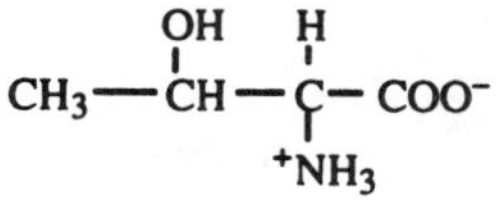

$CH_3-CH(OH)-CH(NH_3^+)-COO^-$

Threonine

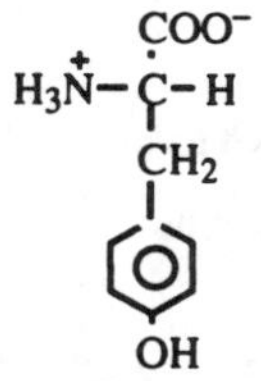

$H_3\overset{+}{N}-CH(COO^-)-CH_2-C_6H_4-OH$

Tyrosine

$(\text{indole, N-H})-CH_2-CH(NH_3^+)-COO^-$

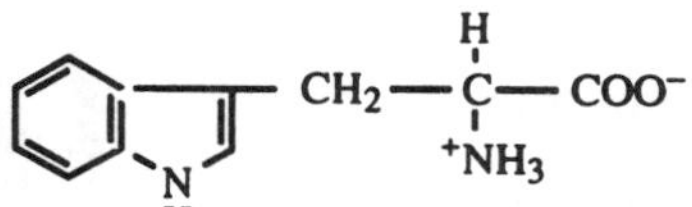

Tryptophan

Cysteine forms sulfur-sulfur covalent bonds with itself to stabilize the tertiary structure of proteins:

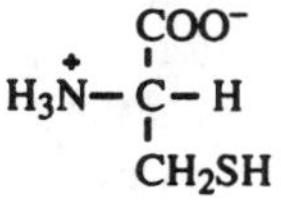

$H_3\overset{+}{N}-CH(COO^-)-CH_2SH$

Cysteine

$H_3\overset{+}{N}-CH(COO^-)-CH_2-S-S-CH_2-CH(COO^-)-\overset{+}{N}H_3$

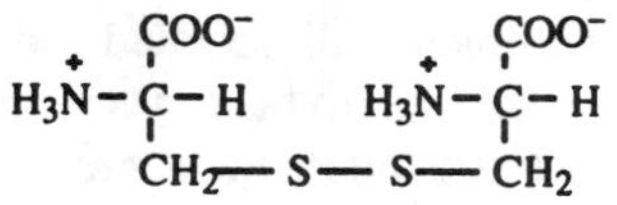

Cystine

Glycine, the smallest AA and the only one that is not optically active, is often found at the "corners" of proteins:

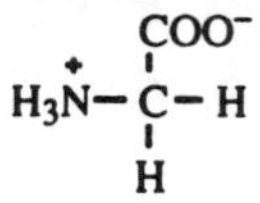

$H_3\overset{+}{N}-CH(H)-COO^-$

Glycine

Proline breaks the α-helix structure of proteins:

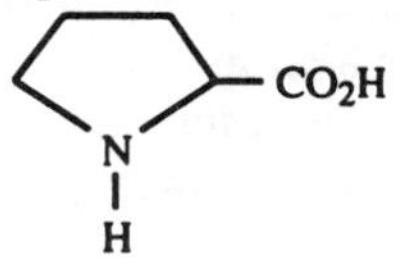

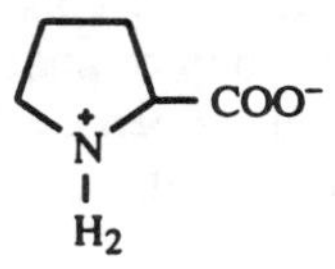

$(\text{pyrrolidine ring, N-H})-CO_2H \qquad (\text{pyrrolidine ring}, \overset{+}{N}H_2)-COO^-$

Proline

Alanine, being small, is usually found on the surface of proteins even though it is hydrophobic:

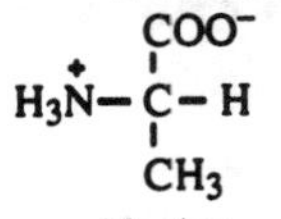

$$\begin{array}{c} COO^- \\ | \\ H_3\overset{+}{N}-C-H \\ | \\ CH_3 \end{array}$$

Alanine

The basic amino acids are lysine and arginine due to their extra amino ($-NH_2$) groups. The acidic amino acids are aspartic acid and glutamic acid due to their extra carboxyl ($-CO_2H$) groups. Histidine can act as a base or an acid depending upon the pH, and it is the best physiologic buffer of the AA's. All of the others are considered neutral amino acids.

Amino acids exist as dipolar ions due to the presence of both a basic part (the $-NH_2$) and an acidic part (the $-CO_2H$):

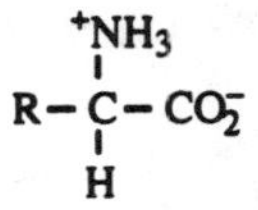

$$\begin{array}{c} {}^+NH_3 \\ | \\ R-C-CO_2^- \\ | \\ H \end{array}$$

dipolar ion

The charge on the amino acid varies with the pH and the isoelectric point. The isoelectric point (pI) of an AA is the pH where the AA has no net charge:

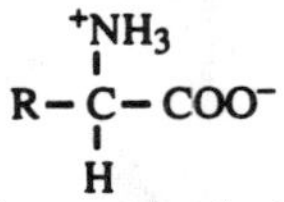

$$\begin{array}{c} {}^+NH_3 \\ | \\ R-C-COO^- \\ | \\ H \end{array}$$

no *net* charge at isoelectric points

If the pH is above the isoelectric point, AA's have a net negative charge (anions):

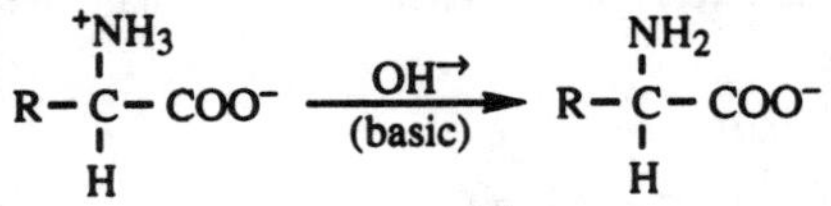

$$\begin{array}{c} {}^+NH_3 \\ | \\ R-C-COO^- \\ | \\ H \end{array} \xrightarrow[\text{(basic)}]{OH^-} \begin{array}{c} NH_2 \\ | \\ R-C-COO^- \\ | \\ H \end{array}$$

uncharged form   anionic form

If the pH is below the isoelectric point or very acidic, AA's have a net positive charge (cations):

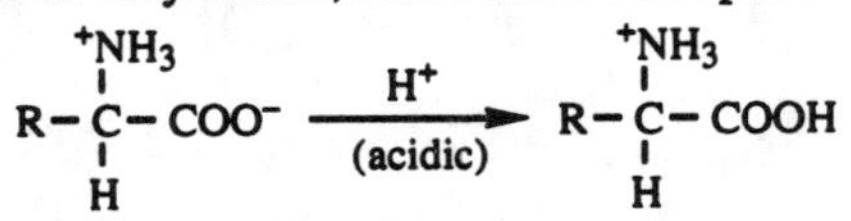

$$\begin{array}{c} {}^+NH_3 \\ | \\ R-C-COO^- \\ | \\ H \end{array} \xrightarrow[\text{(acidic)}]{H^+} \begin{array}{c} {}^+NH_3 \\ | \\ R-C-COOH \\ | \\ H \end{array}$$

uncharged form   catatonic form

At neutral pH the free amino acid is polar since these molecules exist as zwitterions (there is a full negative charge on the carboxyl since it is completely dissociated and a full positive charge on the amino group since it is protonated). Once protonated the amino group becomes a proton donor (in the reverse direction), hence it is the conjugate acid of the base. (Amino acids follow the same rules of dissociation as weak acids; review section 5.8 in the physical sciences chapter for their behavior at differing pHs). These charges are not present when the amino acids are polymerized into a polypeptide chain, hence the R-groups largely determine the properties of the protein.

7.2.1.2 PROTEINS

In proteins or fragments of proteins (oligopeptides), the α-amino acids are linked through peptide bonds into a linear sequence. These bonds are formed by a condensation reaction in which water is removed from the α-carboxyl of one acid and the α-amino group of another, which makes them chemically similar to a substituted amide. These peptide bonds have special properties due to the resonance structures that exist across the peptide bond, giving partial double bond character to the C-N bond, as follows:

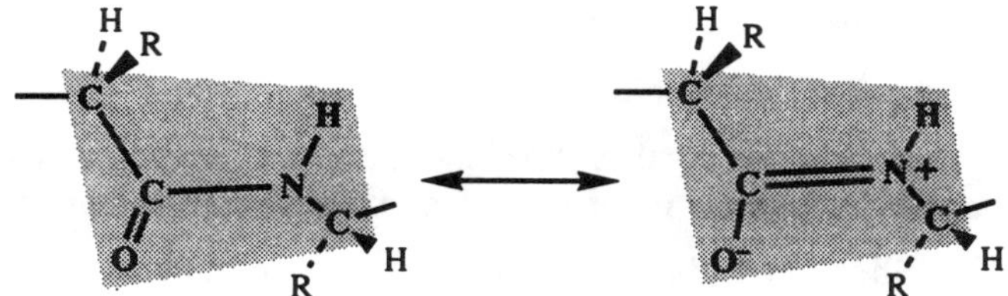

Fig. 7.10—Peptide Bond Characteristics

Due to the partial positive charge on the amino nitrogen in a peptide bond, these amino nitrogens do not bind protons. These amino nitrogens are not completely charged even in the presence of high proton concentrations. This partial double bond character of the peptide bond also makes it rigid and planar. It is unable to rotate as a typical single bond, for the bond has the characteristics of an sp^2 hybrid orbital. The illustration above shows the planar nature of the peptide bond. The six atoms in the shaded area all lie within the same plane.

In a peptide chain only the free amino group and the free carboxyl can contribute to the charge of the peptide (see Fig. 7.10) except for the R-groups. These side chains or R-groups therefore determine the charge on a polypeptide chain. If there is a high concentration of nonpolar amino acids (based strictly on the polarity of the side chain), the protein will be insoluble. If the protein contains a high concentration of polar amino acids it will usually be soluble in water. Basic proteins have more basic amino acids than acidic amino acids; acidic proteins have a preponderance of aspartic and glutamic acids.

By convention peptides are written with the free amino group to the left and the free carboxyl group to the right (they are also numbered and named left to right). A tetrapeptide illustrates this principle:

$$H_3\overset{+}{N}-\underset{R_1}{\underset{|}{CH}}-\overset{O}{\overset{\|}{C}}-NH-\underset{R_2}{\underset{|}{CH}}-\overset{O}{\overset{\|}{C}}-NH-\underset{R_3}{\underset{|}{CH}}-\overset{O}{\overset{\|}{C}}-NH-\underset{R_4}{\underset{|}{CH}}-COO^-$$

Fig. 7.11—Peptide Illustration

To determine the total charge for an oligopeptide it is usually easy to write the amino acid, including the amino-terminal and the carboxyl-terminal group, at a given pH then determine the net charge by simply taking the algebraic sum of the charged groups. The changes that occur when amino acids are polymerized is seen in the fact that the amino-terminal group of a protein usually has a pKa near 8.0 and the carboxyl-terminal will be near 3.0.

Proteins are destroyed by hydrolysis (water is added) of the peptide bond. There are many enzymes that will hydrolyze the peptide bond, including trypsin, chymotrypsin, pepsin, carboxypeptidase, and aminopeptidase, which are found in the gastrointestinal tract of higher animals. Their normal function is to hydrolyze ingested proteins to their constituent amino acids so that they may be absorbed across the intestinal wall and into the bloodstream. These enzymes and certain chemicals such as cyanogen bromide are used by protein chemists to experimentally hydrolyze proteins so as to determine their amino acid sequence.

$$H_2N-\underset{R_1}{\underset{|}{\overset{H}{\overset{|}{C}}}}-\overset{O}{\overset{\|}{C}}-NH-\underset{R_2}{\underset{|}{\overset{H}{\overset{|}{C}}}}-CO_2H+H_2O\xrightarrow{H^+}H_2N-\underset{R_1}{\underset{|}{\overset{H}{\overset{|}{C}}}}-\overset{O}{\overset{\|}{C}}-OH+NH_2-\underset{R_2}{\underset{|}{\overset{H}{\overset{|}{C}}}}-CO_2H$$

Fig. 7.12—Hydrolysis of a Peptide Bond

Proteins are classified according to *biological function,* shape, chemical composition or the number of constituent peptide chains. Proteins function as transport proteins, contractile proteins, structural proteins, storage proteins, regulatory proteins, protective proteins or enzymes. Proteins may be globular (usually soluble and biologically active) or fibrous (highly asymmetric and often insoluble). Some proteins are simple (contain only amino acids), others are conjugated (contain other non-amino acid components such as metals, phosphates, heme, flavin, or sugars). Some proteins are monomeric (contain only one polypeptide chain) or are oligomeric (contain 2 or more peptide chains, e.g., dimers, trimers, tetramers).

I. Protein structure. These may be described at several different levels of organization and are:

1) Primary (1°) structure—the sequence of amino acids within a chain.

2) Secondary (2°) structure—describes the regular, repeating pattern of folding that is stabilized primarily by hydrogen bonds between groups close together in the sequence (examples are α-helix and β-pleated sheet).

3) Tertiary (3°) structure—describes the folding of the chains in three dimensions, stabilized by interactions between segments far apart in sequence.

4) Quaternary (4°) structure—describes interactions between different polypeptide chains in an oligomeric protein, stabilized solely by noncovalent bonds.

Biologically active proteins spontaneously assume a unique structure that is referred to as the native *conformation*. Renaturation experiments have demonstrated that the information necessary to correctly fold into the proper 2° and 3° structure that will yield a biologically active molecule resides in the sequence of amino acids in the chain. A number of different forces stabilize globular proteins, including: 1) hydrogen bonds, 2) electrostatic interactions, 3) hydrophobic interactions, 4) van der Waals forces, and 5) disulfide bonds. Individually many of these forces are relatively weak, but since they act cooperatively, the structure of proteins is relatively stable.

Most proteins with intense biological activity are globular and they are active in aqueous solution. The folding of the polypeptide chain that results in 2° and 3° structure will bring certain functional groups (side chains) into close proximity even though they may be separated by long distances in the sequence of amino acids. Interaction of these side chains may create the active site of enzymes, antibodies, or toxins, in a cleft or pocket on the protein. The active site occupies only a small part of the total volume of the molecule. It has been found that globular proteins exclude water from the internal structure, and that the nonpolar side chains tend to aggregate in this nonpolar environment, while the polar amino acid side chains tend to be found on the surface of the protein in contact with water.

Stability of the 2°, 3°, 4° structure can be disrupted by heat, extremes of pH, detergents, urea, acetone, and ethanol. Such agents are termed *denaturing agents.* Denaturation results in changes in conformation, which causes the native proteins to unfold and results in loss of the shell of water surrounding the molecule. Denatured proteins often precipitate from solution. For example, when an enzyme unfolds, the active site is thus distorted so that biological activity is lost.

7.2.1.3 CARBOHYDRATES

Carbohydrates is the name given to the family of organic molecules that is composed of sugars (saccharides). The basic units are *monosaccharides,* given general names ending in -ose according to (a) the number of carbons (e.g., pentose, hexose), (b) the nature of the carbonyl group (aldose or ketose), or a combination of both, e.g., ribose is an aldopentose (five-carbon aldehyde), fructose is a ketohexose (six-carbon ketone). Chemically, they are polyhydroxyaldehydes or ketones of the formula $(CH_2O)n$, with a hydroxy group on each carbon other than the carbonyl.

Monosaccharides are frequently drawn as *Fischer projections* to emphasize stereochemical relationships, with the aldehyde (C-1) at the top. Examples of hexoses are:

CHO	CHO	CHO	CH_2OH	CHO
H–OH	HO–H	H–OH	$=O^2$	HO–H
HO–H	HO–H	HO–H	HO–H	H–OH
H–OH	H–OH	HO–H	H–OH	HO–H
H–OH	H–OH	H–OH	H–OH	HO–H
CH_2OH	CH_2OH	CH_2OH	CH_2OH	CH_2OH
D-Glucose	D-Mannose	D-Galactose	D-Fructose	L-Glucose

I. Stereoisomerism: Aldohexoses contain four asymmetric centers (carbons 2-5), so there are $2^4 = 16$ stereoisomers, or eight pairs of enantiomers. Each of the eight has a distinct common name. The sugars found in nature are pure enantiomers, optically active. Stereochemical descriptors common in carbohydrates include:

1) D and L—These symbols refer to the absolute configuration of the highest numbered asymmetric center, i.e., the bottom asymmetric carbon in the Fischer projection (C-5 in glucose). When the OH lies on the right, the sugar is D; if the OH is on the left, the sugar belongs to the L-series. Most common sugars of nature have the D-configuration. Note that L-glucose, the enantiomer of D-glucose, must have the opposite configuration at every asymmetric center.

The simplest chiral carbohydrate is the aldotriose *glyceraldehyde*, and the higher sugars can be considered as homologs of either D- or L-glyceraldehyde.

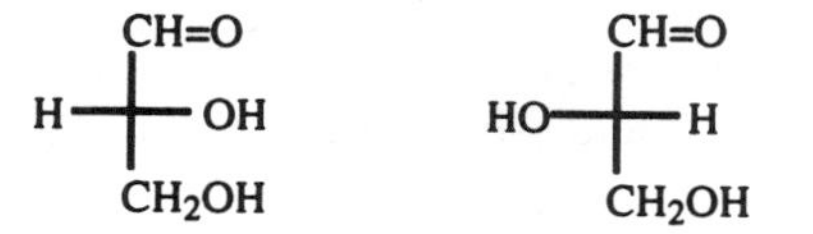

CH=O
H—+—OH
CH_2OH

CH=O
HO—+—H
CH_2OH

D-Glyceraldehyde L-Glyceraldehyde

2) Epimers—Two sugars that differ in configuration at only one of several asymmetric centers are called *epimers*, a kind of diastereomer. Glucose and mannose are epimers at C-2, glucose and galactose are C-4 epimers.

II. Cyclic Structures: Hydroxyl groups suitably situated can add intramolecularly to the carbonyl group, forming cyclic hemiacetals or hemiketals. Indeed, these cyclic structures predominate at equilibrium, and monosaccharides exist almost totally in ring forms. Two relatively unstrained ring sizes are possible, five-membered (named *furanose*) and six-membered (named *pyranose*). They are drawn in several ways, illustrated for the pyranose form of glucose:

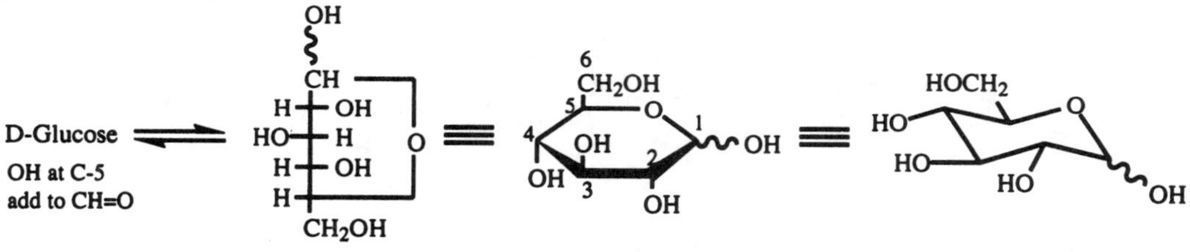

D-Glucose
OH at C-5
add to CH=O

Fischer Haworth Conformation

Fischer projections clearly show the relationship to the aldose structure, but are awkward in representing the configuration at C-1. *Haworth formulas* depict the ring as a planar hexagon, with substituents oriented either on the top or bottom of the ring. The most geometrically accurate representation is a *conformational drawing*, showing the six-membered ring in the familiar chair conformation with substituents either equatorial or axial. Aldopentoses (e.g., arabinose) are usually drawn as Haworth formulas.

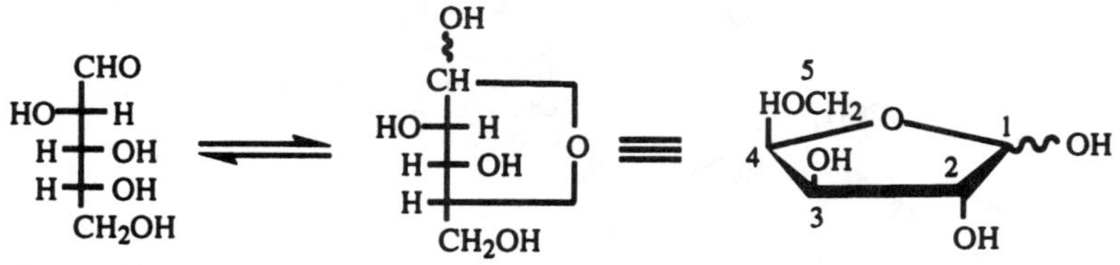

D-Arabinose Furanose structure Haworth

III. Cyclic hemiacetal equilibria: 1) The cyclic hemiacetals possess a new asymmetric center at C-1, in addition to the four already present in the aldohexoses, so two diastereomers (called α and β *anomers*) are possible. In the conventional Haworth or conformational drawings, the C-1 OH is down in the α-anomer, up in the β-anomer. A wavy bond indicates that the OH may be either α or β. The cyclic structure of β-D-glucose is easy to remember as the one in which all substituents are equatorial in the chair conformation.

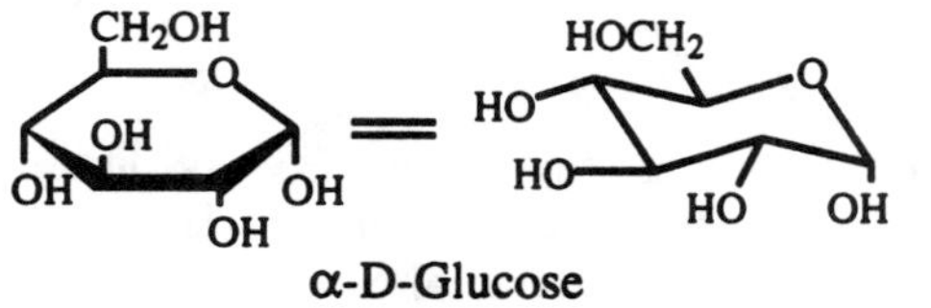

α-D-Glucose 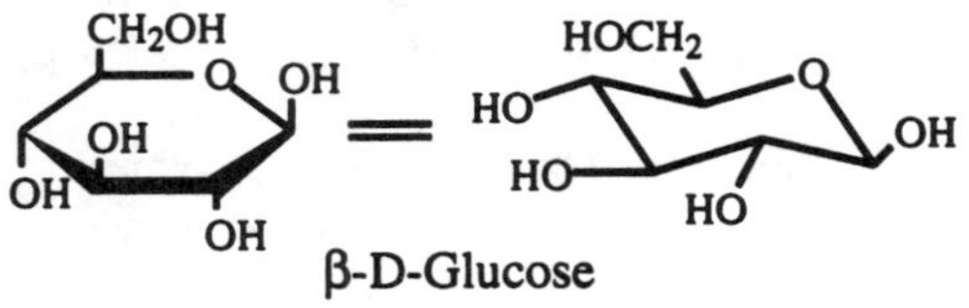 β-D-Glucose

(2) Even though the cyclic structures predominate and can be crystallized as pure solids, in aqueous solution they are in equilibrium with the open-chain carbonyl forms. The structural formulas of cyclic hemiacetals do not show an aldehyde group, but they exhibit all the characteristic aldehyde reactions, such as the Fehlings test (see below). Experimental evidence for this equilibrium comes from the phenomenon of *mutarotation*; the opticalrotation of a freshly prepared solution or pure α- or β-D-*glucose* changes with time until an equilibrium value is reached starting from either anomer.

$$\underset{[a]_D + 112°}{\alpha\text{-D-Glucose}} \rightleftharpoons \underset{[a]_D + 52.7°}{\text{Equilibrium mixture}} \rightleftharpoons \underset{[a]_D + 19°}{\beta\text{-D-Glucose}}$$

At equilibrium in aqueous solution D-glucose exists as about 39% of the α-pyranose anomer, 61% as the β-pyranose anomer, about 0.15% each of the α and β-furanose rings, but no detectable aldehyde.

IV. Periodate cleavage: HIO_4 (periodic acid) cleaves the carbon-carbon bond between vicinal hydroxyl groups to leave carbonyl groups. It also cleaves α-hydroxy aldehydes and ketones (imagine the carbonyl group as its hydrate). The examples show how this oxidation can be used to determine the ring size in methyl glucoside: periodate cleavage of the pyranoside gives one equivalent of formic acid, while cleavage of the furanoside gives one equivalent of formaldehyde:

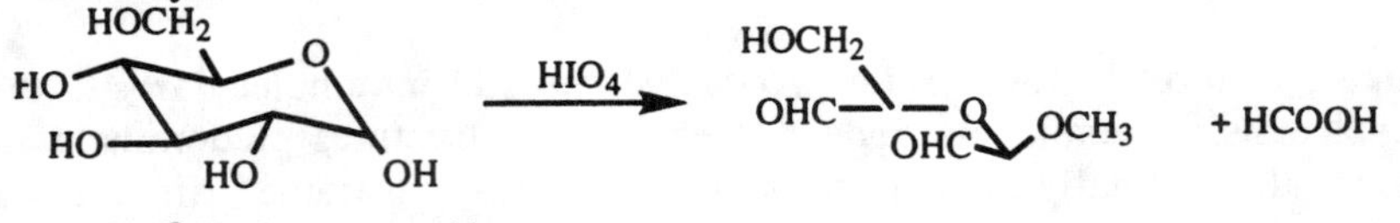

Methyl β-D-glucopyranoside

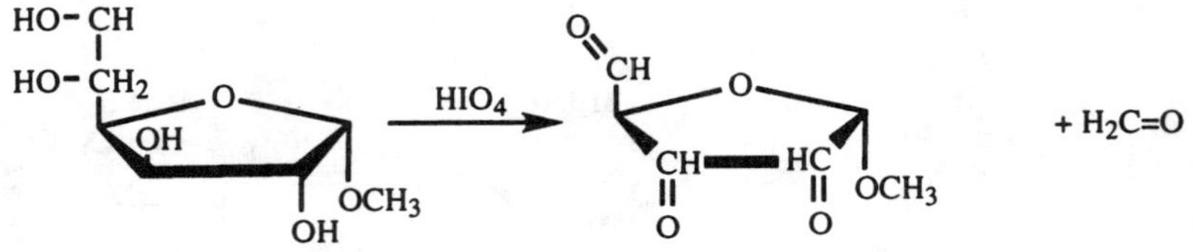

Methyl α-D-glucofuranoside

V. Disaccharides: are molecules composed of two monosaccharides connected by an acetal bond; one of the five OH groups of one hexose, e.g., is used to bond to the carbonyl carbon (usually C-1) of a second hexose in its cyclic form. Examples of three common disaccharides are shown:

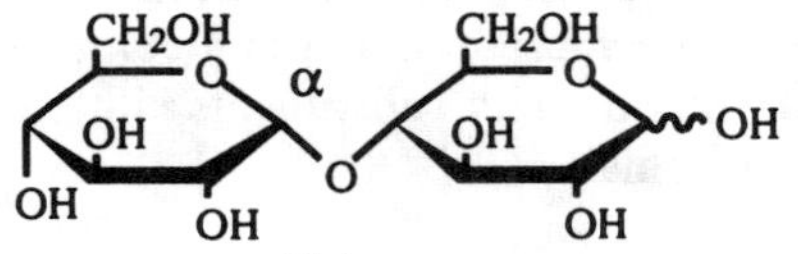

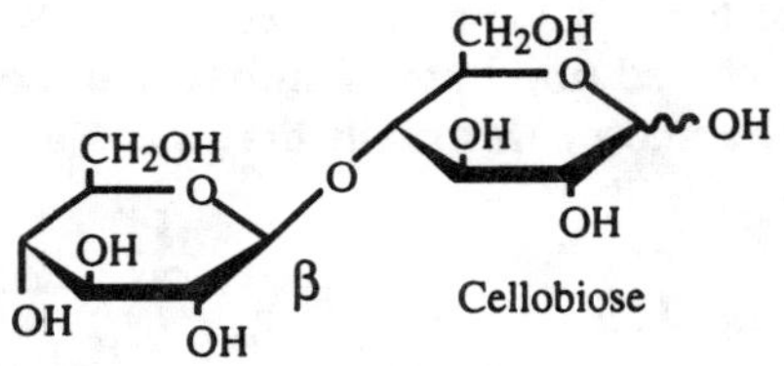

VI. Maltose: the repeating unit of starch, and *cellobiose*, the repeating unit of cellulose, are both composed of two D-glucose units, the second attached by the hydroxyl at C-4. The sole difference is the configuration at the anomeric carbon C-1, maltose being α (α-1,4 bond) and cellobiose β (β-1,4 bond). While the oxygen which links the rings is part of an acetal group, the right-hand ring in each is still a cyclic hemiacetal, in equilibrium with an aldehyde, so that maltose and cellobiose are reducing sugars. *Sucrose*, on the other hand, is a non-reducing sugar; the bridging oxygen atom connects an acetal carbon (C-1) in a D-glucose unit with a ketal carbon (C-2) in a fructose unit. The right-hand ring is an example of a ketose in its cyclic furanose structure. Lactose (milk sugar) is made of galactose and glucose (β-1,4 bond).

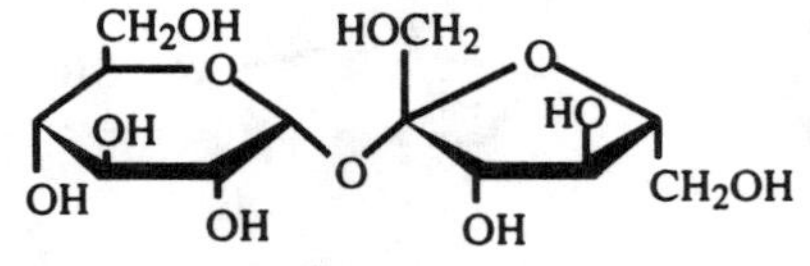

VII. Polysaccharides: These are large polymeric molecules, containing as many as hundreds or thousands of repeating monosaccharides linked together by acetal (glycoside) bonds. The most important are starch, glycogen, and cellulose. Cellulose, the most abundant organic compound and the main structural component of vegetable matter, is a 1,4-β-polymer of glucose (or cellobiose). Starch and glycogen, also 1,4-polymers of glucose but with α-links, are ways of storing glucose to meet energy needs; both are relatively insoluble but can be hydrolyzed on demand by enzymes (a-glycosidases) to release soluble glucose units. When more glucose is available than needed, animals store it in the liver as glycogen. Starch, the polysaccharide found in plants, is a mixture of amylose, an unbranched polymer, and amylopectin, which has branching chains formed by acetal formation with the C-6 hydroxyl.

VIII. Natural monosaccharides: L-Ascorbic acid (vitamin C) is a natural monosaccharide found in citrus fruits and many vegetables, important for the prevention of scurvy. It is a lactone in which C-1 of a hexose has been oxidized to the carboxylic acid level, and with a double bond between carbons 2 and 3. This enediol moiety is easily oxidized, and vitamin C is believed to serve a protecting role by reducing some biological oxidants; e.g., free radicals and hydroperoxides.

Ribose is the aldopentose unit in ribonucleic acid (RNA), and 2-*deoxyribose* is the sugar unit in deoxyribonucleic acid (DNA). The related ketopentose *ribulose* plays a crucial role in photosynthesis as the acceptor of carbon dioxide.

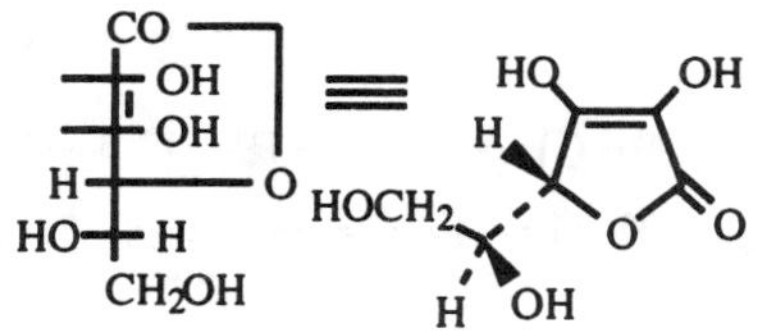

Ascorbic acid (Vitamin C) 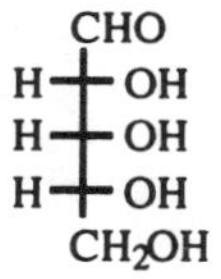 D-Ribose 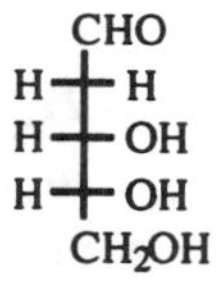 2-Deoxyribose 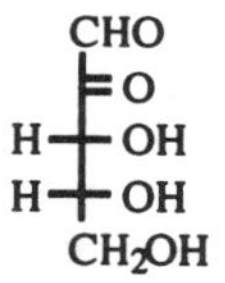 D-Ribulose

7.2.1.4 LIPIDS

The term lipids denotes several types of organic compounds of biological origin. Almost all lipids are soluble in organic solvents and insoluble in water. They are unlike carbohydrates and proteins that have specific chemical structures. Important classes of lipids are fats and oils, steroids, prostaglandins, terpenes, glycolipids and phospholipids. Simple lipids do not undergo hydrolysis reactions (examples: steroids and terpenes), whereas complex lipids may be hydrolyzed (examples: fats and oils, phospholipids). Lipids are obtained from plant or animal tissue by extraction with organic solvents.

Fatty acids (carboxylic acids) do not usually occur in the free state. They are bound as esters of glycerol (triacyl glycerols, see below). The common fatty acids are straight-chain (non-branched) carboxylic acids that contain an even number of carbons between 12 and 20. The acids may be saturated (no double bonds) or unsaturated (contain double bonds). The saturated fatty acids have higher melting points than the unsaturated acids that have cis double bonds. This is due to irregularity in the geometry of the unsaturated molecule. This leads to difficulty in stacking in the crystal. Compare stearic acid with oleic acid:

$CH_3(CH_2)_{16}COOH$
stearic acid mp 70°
(saturated)

(cis) $CH_3(CH_2)_7CH = CH(CH_2)_7COOH$
oleic acid mp 4°
(unsaturated)

The biosynthesis of fatty acids involves a series of reactions in which the chain is built from acetate; i.e., two carbons at a time. Acetate is derived from pyruvate in carbohydrate metabolism, or from metabolism of fats. Some fatty acids are called *essential fatty acids*, because mammals cannot synthesize them from acetate and must obtain them from plants. An important essential fatty acid is linoleic acid (9, 12-octadecadienoic acid), which is converted by mammals to arachidonic acid (5, 8, 11, 14-icosatetraenoic acid). Arachidonic acid, obtained from human fat, is the starting compound in the biosynthesis of prostaglandins, which have important physiological functions.

Soaps are sodium or potassium salts of fatty acids, obtained from basic hydrolysis of triacyl glycerols. Soaps solubilize dirt and grease particles because the hydrocarbon chain of the molecule (hydrophobic) interacts with the organic grease while the carboxylate anion end of the molecule (hydrophilic) interacts with the water solvent. The soap thereby emulsifies the grease and brings it into the water where it may be disposed of.

[grease]- - - - -/\/\/\/\/\/\/\/\/\/\/\/\/\ CO_2^- - - $[H_2O]$

soap micelles

Hard water contains metal ions (Fe^{3+}, Ca^{2+}) which form insoluble salts with fatty acid anions, and precipitate the soap. Synthetic detergents substitute the sulfonic acid anion SO_3^{--} for the carboxylate anion CO_2^-. Detergents are soluble in hard water.

Triacyl glycerols (triglycerides, glycerides, glyceryl trialkoanoates) are triesters of fatty acids. *Fats* are solid triacyl glycerols that contain mostly saturated fatty acids, and *oils* are liquid triacyl glycerols that contain mostly unsaturated fatty acids. Two commercial reactions of triacyl glycerols are *hydrogenation* and *saponification*. In hydrogenation, unsaturated fatty acid groups in oils are converted to saturated groups, thereby raising the melting point and producing fats used in shortening.

$$\begin{array}{l} R-CH=CH-R'-CO_2-CH_2 \\ \qquad\qquad\qquad\qquad\quad | \\ R-CH=CH-R'-CO_2-CH \\ \qquad\qquad\qquad\qquad\quad | \\ R-CH=CH-R'-CO_2-CH_2 \end{array} \xrightarrow{\text{excess } H_2\text{, catalyst}} \begin{array}{l} R-CH_2-CH_2-R'-CO_2-CH_2 \\ \qquad\qquad\qquad\qquad\qquad | \\ R-CH_2-CH_2-R'-CO_2-CH \\ \qquad\qquad\qquad\qquad\qquad | \\ R-CH_2-CH_2-R'-CO_2-CH_2 \end{array}$$

In saponification, a triacyl glycerol (triester) is hydrolyzed with base to give the sodium salts of the fatty acids and glycerol. The salts are soaps (see below).

$$\begin{array}{l} RCO_2-CH_2 \\ \qquad\quad | \\ RCO_2-CH \\ \qquad\quad | \\ RCO_2-CH_2 \end{array} \xrightarrow{3\ NaOH} \underset{\text{soap}}{3\ RCO_2Na} + \underset{\text{glycerol}}{HOCH_2-CH(OH)-CH_2OH}$$

Triacyl glycerols (fats) are used to store chemical energy. Twice as much energy per gram is released when fats are oxidized to CO_2 and water than when carbohydrates are oxidized. The major cause is the hydrocarbon nature of the fats (many C-H bonds).

Steroids are complex tetracyclic molecules of physiological significance. The general steroid structure consists of four rings designated A, B, C and D. The most significant biological steroid is *cholesterol*, which is most abundant in humans. It is the starting compound for other steroids. Other steroids include *bile acids*, which assist in the digestion of fats, *corticosteroids*, such as cortisone, and sex hormones, which are secreted by endocrine glands. *Ergosterol* is a steroid derived from yeast which may be converted to vitamin D by irradiation. Synthetic steroids are used as oral contraceptives and for other medicinal purposes. The structure of cholesterol is shown, with the numbering system used for steroids.

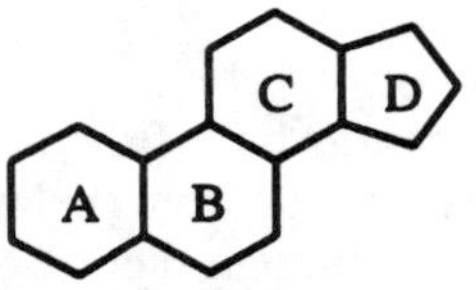

STEROID STRUCTURE

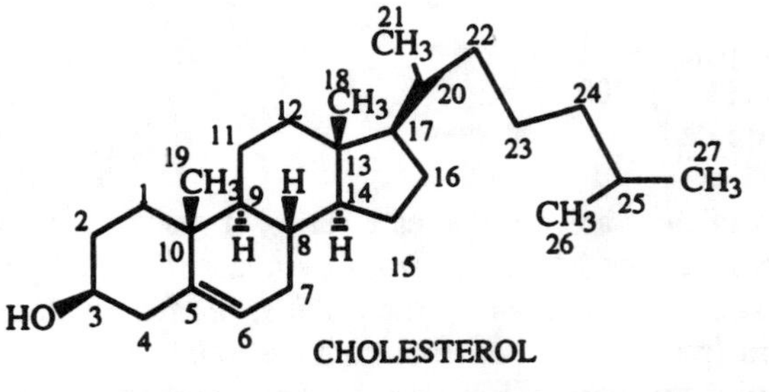

CHOLESTEROL

Stereochemistry of steroids is complex. Cholesterol has eight chiral carbon atoms, which means 256 possible stereoisomeric forms are possible. Cholesterol has unique stereochemistry as shown in the formula. Studies on conformation of steroids show that cyclohexane rings have the chair conformation, with substituent groups on axial or equatorial positions. Cholesterol is almost a planar molecule, and the face on the same side as the methyl substituent (19 in the formula) is the β face; the side opposite the methyl group is the α face. The OH group on carbon 3 is cis to the reference methyl group: it is referred to as 3-β-hydroxy. The conformational structure of cholesterol is shown as follows:

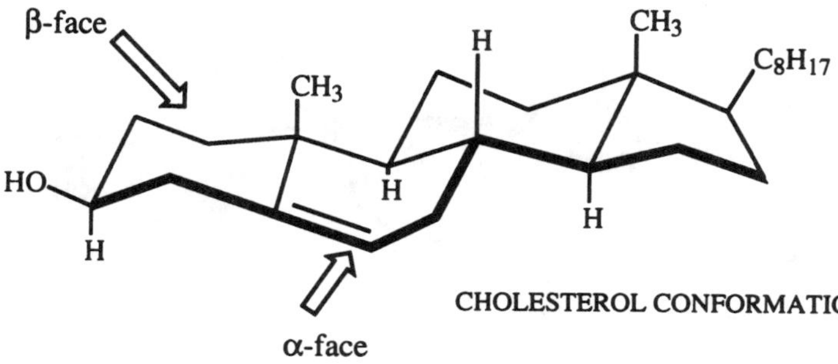

β-face

CH_3 H CH_3 C_8H_{17}

HO H H H

CHOLESTEROL CONFORMATION

α-face

PHOSPHOROUS COMPOUNDS

Some bioorganic compounds are derivatives of phosphoric acid. Organic esters of phosphoric acids are compounds where one or more of the acid hydrogens are replaced by an organic group.

HO HO-P = O HO	RO HO-P = O HO	RO RO-P = O HO	RO RO-P = O RO
phosphoric acid	alkyl phosphate	dialkyl phosphate	trialkyl phosphate

Organic phosphate esters are hydrolyzed to phosphoric acid and the corresponding alcohol in acid solution. Only trialkyl phosphates are hydrolyzed in basic solution, and only one alkyl group is removed. The acidic hydrogens are removed by base and the resulting anions are not susceptible to basic hydrolysis:

$$(RO)_3PO + H_3O^+ \rightarrow 3\ ROH + (HO)_3PO$$
$$(RO)_3PO + OH^- \rightarrow ROH + (RO)_2PO_2^-$$

Phosphorous esters are important in the biosynthesis of triacyl glycerols. Two fatty acid residues are joined to L-glycerol-3-phosphate:

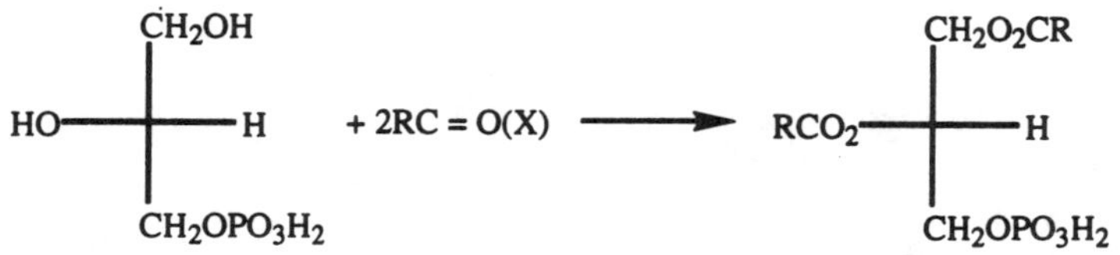

CH_2OH / HO—C—H / $CH_2OPO_3H_2$ + $2RC = O(X)$ → CH_2O_2CR / RCO_2—C—H / $CH_2OPO_3H_2$

phosphatidic acid

The produce is called phosphatidic acid. Phosphatidic acid is hydrolyzed to give a diacyl glycerol, which is then acylated to give the triacyl glycerol.

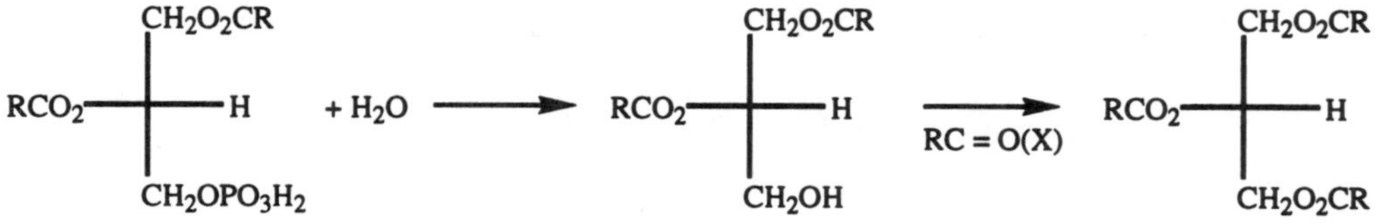

CH_2O_2CR / RCO_2—C—H / $CH_2OPO_3H_2$ + H_2O → CH_2O_2CR / RCO_2—C—H / CH_2OH —($RC = O(X)$)→ CH_2O_2CR / RCO_2—C—H / CH_2O_2CR

diacyl glycerol triacyl glycerol

Phosphatidic acids are also precursors to another class of compounds called *phosphatides*. These compounds are dialkyl phosphates where one alkyl group is diacyl glycerol and the other contains an amino group, as an ammonium ion. These compounds are present in cell membranes, nerve, and brain tissue. In addition to esters of phosphoric acids, organic groups may be bonded to phosphoric acid anhydrides, as in the compounds ADP and ATP, which are involved in energy transfer in metabolism [SEE SECTION 7.7]. The structures are shown below. At physiological pH, phosphorus esters and anhydrides are converted to their corresponding anions, and are inert to hydrolysis. However, enzymes catalyze the hydrolysis in living cells.

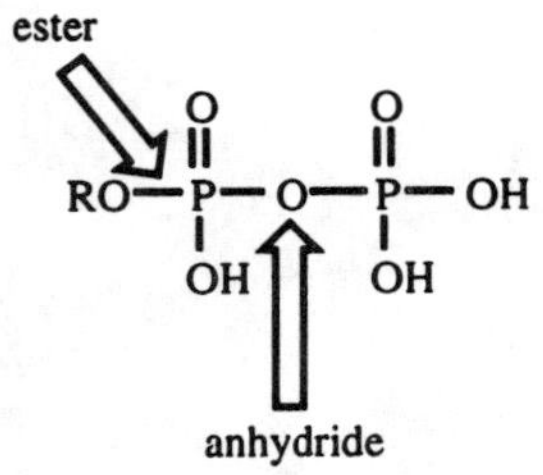

ester

RO—P(=O)(OH)—O—P(=O)(OH)—OH

anhydride

ADP

R has the structure

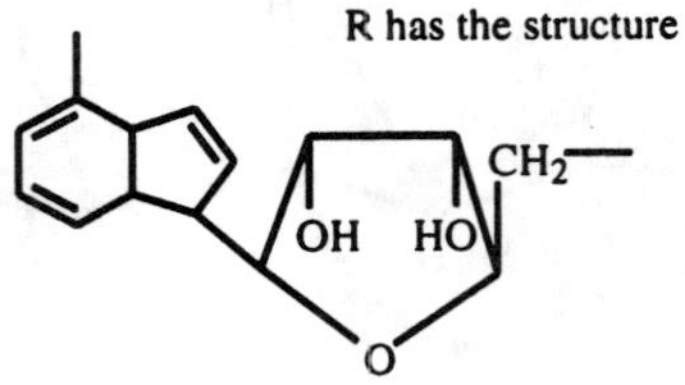

R

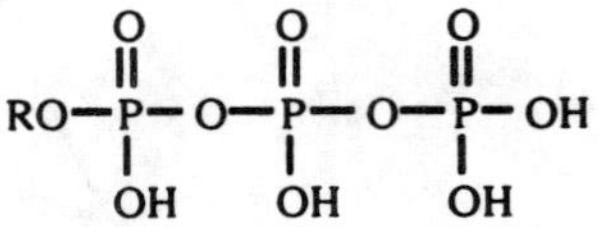

RO—P(=O)(OH)—O—P(=O)(OH)—O—P(=O)(OH)—OH

ATP

7.2.2 Questions Related to Bioorganic Molecules

1. What characteristics of amino acids determine the primary structure of proteins?
   A. acid-base properties
   B. side chain composition
   C. hydrogen bonding properties
   D. sequence in proteins

2. Which is an α-amino acid?

   A. 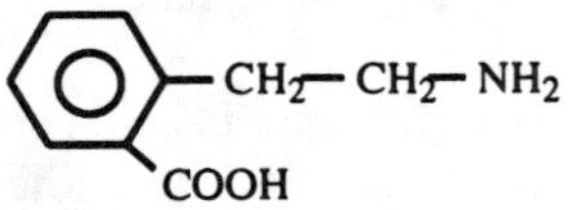 (benzene ring with COOH)—CH_2—CH_2—NH_2

   B. 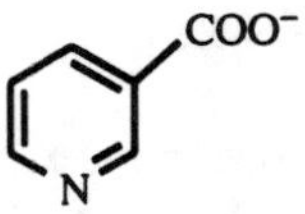 (pyridine ring with COO^-)

   C. 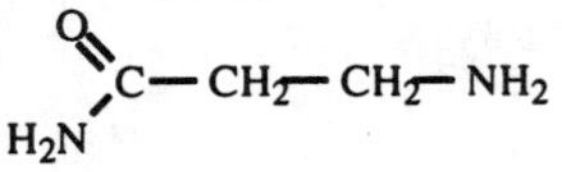 H_2N—C(=O)—CH_2—CH_2—NH_2

   D. 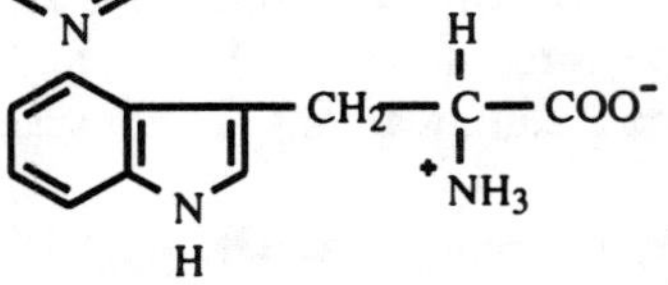 (indole ring, N–H)—CH_2—C(H)($^+NH_3$)—COO^-

3. The peptide bond would be described chemically as which type of bond?
   A. ester
   B. amide
   C. ether
   D. anhydride

4. When a peptide bond is hydrolyzed (split):
   A. water is released from the peptide bond.
   B. water is added to the peptide bond.
   C. oxidation of the peptide bond occurs.
   D. reduction of peptide bond occurs.

5. Primary structure of amino acids is:
   A. the sequence of amino acids.
   B. not found in quaternary proteins.
   C. coded for by DNA.
   D. all of the above.

6. Secondary structure of proteins is associated with:
   A. sequence of amino acids.
   B. not in globular proteins.
   C. coded for by DNA.
   D. α-helix.

7. Select the type(s) of bonding important in maintenance of tertiary structure of proteins:
   A. hydrophobic
   B. van der Waals
   C. covalent
   D. all are important

8. The highest level of protein structure found in monomeric globular proteins is:
   A. primary.
   B. secondary.
   C. tertiary.
   D. quaternary.

9. Which of the following would be considered a hydrophilic amino acid?

   A. 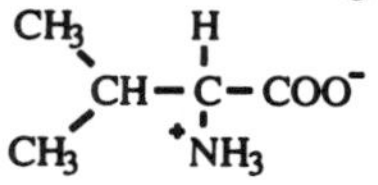 $(CH_3)_2CH{-}CH(\overset{+}{N}H_3){-}COO^-$

   B. 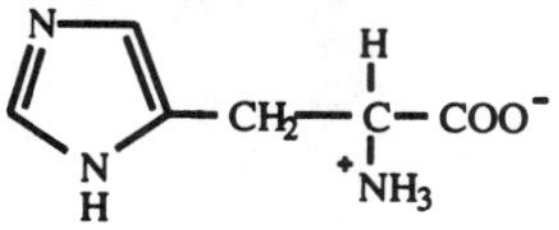 (imidazolyl, N / N–H ring)$-CH_2{-}CH(\overset{+}{N}H_3){-}COO^-$

   C. 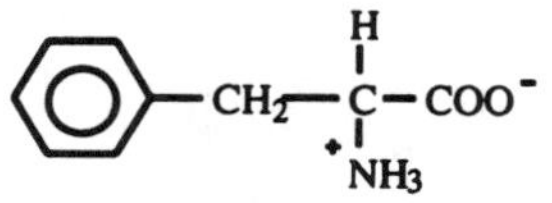 $C_6H_5{-}CH_2{-}CH(\overset{+}{N}H_3){-}COO^-$

   D. none of the above

10. Select the basic amino acid:

    A. 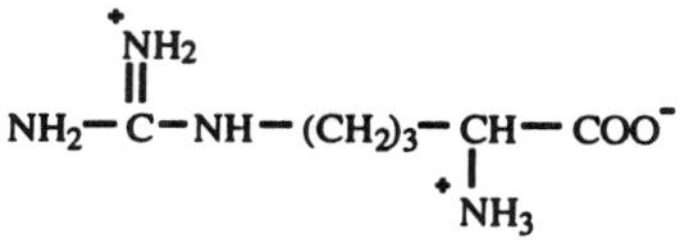 $NH_2{-}C(={\overset{+}{N}H_2}){-}NH{-}(CH_2)_3{-}CH(\overset{+}{N}H_3){-}COO^-$

    B. $^-OOC{-}CH_2{-}CH(\overset{+}{N}H_3){-}COO^-$

    C. $CH_3{-}S{-}CH_2{-}CH_2{-}CH(\overset{+}{N}H_3){-}COO^-$

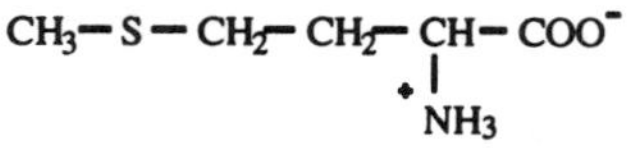

    D. none of the above

11. Select the acidic amino acid:

    A. 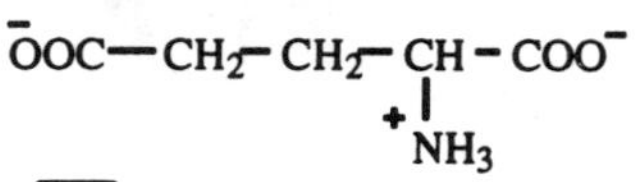 $^-OOC{-}CH_2{-}CH_2{-}CH(\overset{+}{N}H_3){-}COO^-$

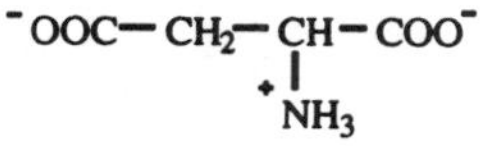

    B. 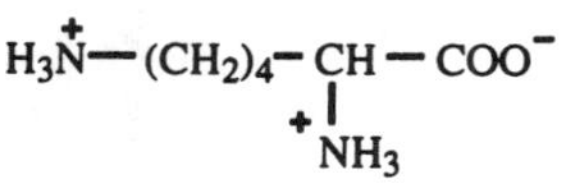 $H_3\overset{+}{N}{-}(CH_2)_4{-}CH(\overset{+}{N}H_3){-}COO^-$

    C. 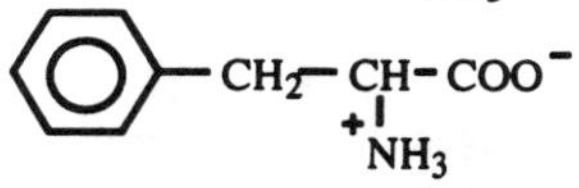 $C_6H_5{-}CH_2{-}CH(\overset{+}{N}H_3){-}COO^-$

    D. none of the above

12. Which amino acid in question #11 will most likely be found on the interior of globular proteins?
    A.
    B.
    C.
    D.

13. Which of the following peptides has the highest pI?

    A. 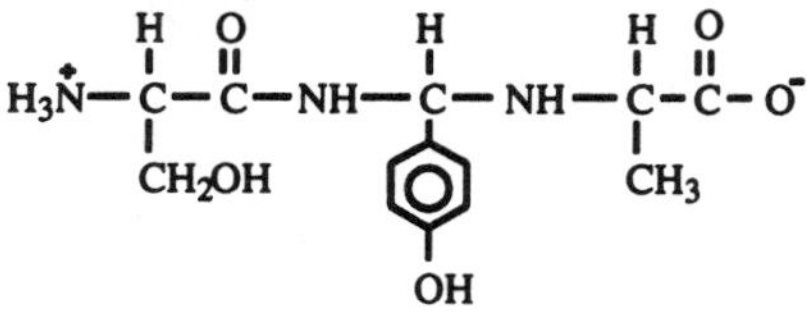 $H_3\overset{+}{N}{-}CH(CH_2OH){-}C(=O){-}NH{-}CH(C_6H_4OH){-}NH{-}CH(CH_3){-}C(=O){-}O^-$

    B. $H_3\overset{+}{N}{-}CH(CH_2COO^-){-}C(=O){-}NH{-}CH(CH_2CH_2COO^-){-}C(=O){-}NH{-}CH(CH_2{-}\text{imidazolyl}){-}C(=O){-}O^-$

    C. $H_3\overset{+}{N}{-}CH(CH(CH_3)_2){-}C(=O){-}NH{-}CH(CH(OH)CH_3){-}C(=O){-}NH{-}CH(CH_2OH){-}C(=O){-}O^-$

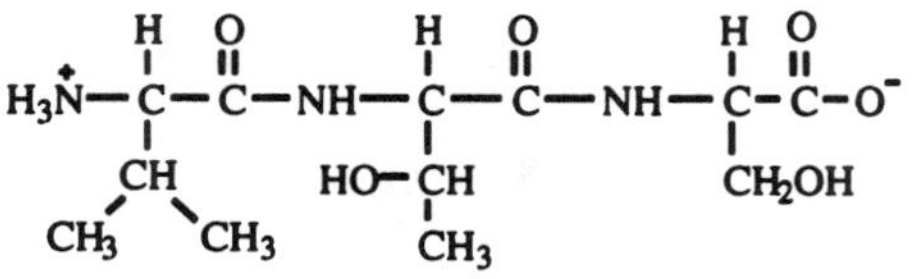

    D. 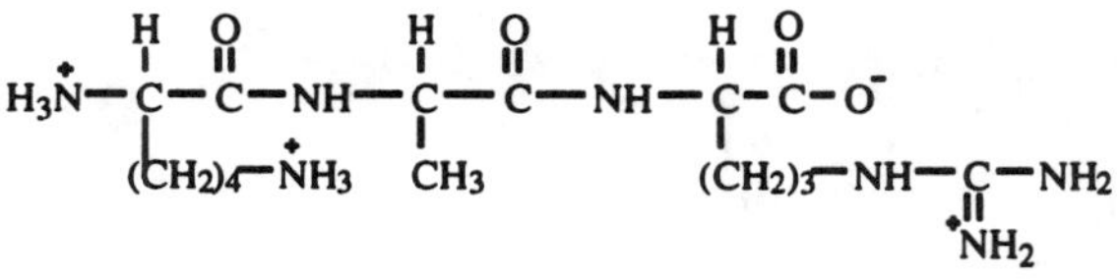 $H_3\overset{+}{N}{-}CH((CH_2)_4{-}\overset{+}{N}H_3){-}C(=O){-}NH{-}CH(CH_3){-}C(=O){-}NH{-}CH((CH_2)_3{-}NH{-}C(={\overset{+}{N}H_2}){-}NH_2){-}C(=O){-}O^-$

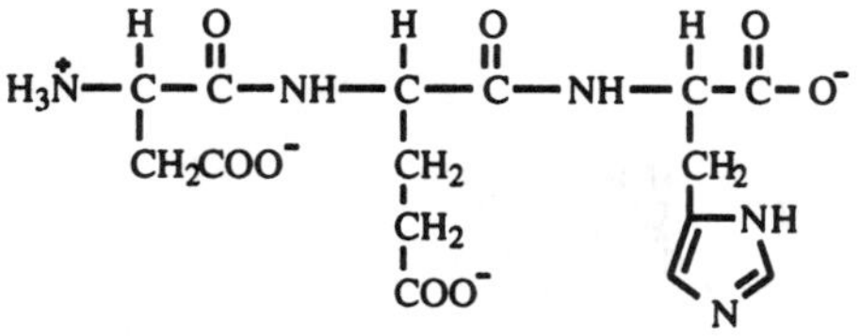

14. Which of the peptides in #13 will migrate to the cathode at pH = 7.0?
   A.
   B.
   C.
   D.

15. Which of the peptides in #13 will migrate to the anode at pH = 7.0?
   A.
   B.
   C.
   D.

16. Which disaccharide has the *incorrect* monosaccharide components listed by it?
   A. maltose—mannose and glucose
   B. lactose—galactose and glucose
   C. sucrose—fructose and glucose
   D. cellobiose—two glucoses

17. Which of these is not a monosaccharide?
   A. ribose
   B. galactose
   C. maltose
   D. mannose

18. Which compound is the reference for the relative configuration of sugars and amino acids?
   A. D-glucose
   B. D-glyceraldehyde
   C. L-glycine
   D. D-alanine

19. Both glycogen and cellulose are polymers of glucose. The main factor that makes them different is:
   A. cellulose has more glucose units.
   B. glycogen has more branch points.
   C. glycogen has α-1,4 bonds and cellulose has β-1,4 bonds between glucose units.
   D. cellulose has more glucose units and more branch points.

20. For monosaccharides, the ring forms (pyranose or furanose) are:
   A. acetals.
   B. hemiacetals.
   C. carbonyls.
   D. esters.

Use the following structures for questions #21–#27:

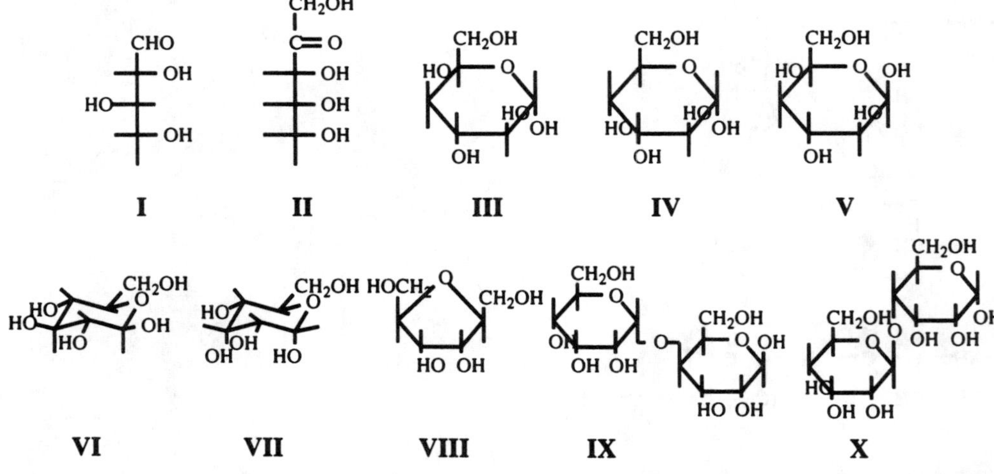

21. Which structure is a furanose?
  A. III
  B. VI
  C. VIII
  D. IX

22. Which structure is a ketose?
  A. I
  B. II
  C. III
  D. VI

23. Which structure is the anomer of III?
  A. I
  B. IV
  C. V
  D. none of these

24. Which structure is an epimer of IV?
  A. III
  B. V
  C. VI
  D. none of these

25. Which conformation is more stable?
  A. VI
  B. VII
  C. Both conformations are equally stable.
  D. Both conformations are unstable.

26. Which compound is a pentose?
  A. I
  B. II
  C. III
  D. VIII

27. Which compound has an α-1,4 glycosidic bond?
  A. IX
  B. X
  C. both IX and X
  D. neither IX nor X

28. A triacyl glycerol (TG-1) is hydrolyzed and the only fatty acid obtained has molecular formula $C_{16}H_{33}CO_2H$. The molecular formula of TG-1 is:
  A. $C_{53}H_{100}O_6$
  B. $C_{51}H_{100}O_6$
  C. $C_{56}H_{102}O_6$
  D. $C_{54}H_{104}O_6$

29. The most likely structural formula of the fatty acid from TG-1 is:
  A. $CH_3(CH2)_{15}CO_2H$
  B. $CH_3(CH_2)_6CH = CH(CH_2)_7CO_2H$
  C. $CH_3(CH_2)_6CH(CH_3)(CH_2)_7CO_2H$
  D. not determinable from the above information.

30. A second triacyl glycerol (TG-2) is hydrolyzed and yields only one fatty acid whose molecular formula is $C_{16}H_{27}CO_2H$. In comparing the melting points of the acids from TG-1 and TG-2, melting point of TG-1 would be:
A. higher.
B. lower.
C. about the same as the acid from TG-2.
D. unpredictable; any result is possible.

31. The infrared spectrum of TG-1 would show absorption at which frequencies (cm^{-1})?
A. 3500 and 1700
B. 3500 and 2900
C. 2900 and 1700
D. 3500, 2900, and 1700

32. TG-1 is allowed to undergo partial hydrolysis to give a mixture of monoacyl and diacyl glycerols (R is $C_{16}H_{33}$) as follows:

$RCO_2CH_2CH(OH)CH_2OH$ I	$HOCH_2CH(O_2CR)CH_2OH$ II
$RCO_2CH_2CH(O_2CR)CH_2OH$ III	$RCO_2CH_2CH(OH)CH_2O_2CR$ IV

Which of the glycerides can exist in enantiomeric forms?
A. I and II
B. III and IV
C. I and III
D. II and IV

33. The principal constituent of beeswax is $CH_3(CH_2)_{14}CO_2(CH_2)_{29}CH_3$. This compound is a lipid because it:
A. has the ester functional group.
B. is obtained from an animal.
C. has a high molecular weight.
D. can be extracted by organic solvents.

34. The hydroxyl group on carbon-3 of cholesterol is on an equatorial bond. If cholesterol is oxidized to a ketone and the ketone is reduced to an alcohol with an axial hydroxyl on carbon-3, what is the relationship between the isomeric alcohols?
A. enantiomers
B. diastereomers
C. anomers
D. meso compounds

35. The structures of the male hormone testosterone and the female hormone estradiol are shown below. Which statement is true about the chemistry of these hormones?

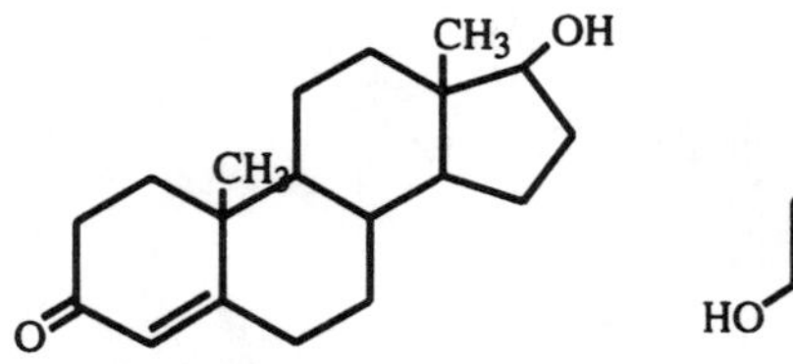

A. Testosterone is the stronger acid; it has more stereoisomers than estradiol.
B. Testosterone is the weaker acid; it has more stereoisomers than estradiol.
C. Testosterone is the stronger acid; it has fewer stereoisomers than estradiol.
D. Testosterone is the weaker acid; it has fewer stereoisomers than estradiol.

36. Which conditions are most favorable for the hydrolysis of an alkyl phosphate?
A. strongly acidic
B. strongly basic
C. neutral pH
D. strongly acidic or strongly basic

37. In a phosphorylation reaction ATP reacts with an alcohol:
ATP + ROH → ADP + $ROP(OH)_2$
In this reaction phosphorous is transferred from:
A. an anhydride to an anhydride.
B. an anhydride to an ester.
C. an ester to an anhydride.
D. an ester to an ester.

7.2.3 Answers to Questions in Section 7.2.2

(1) D (2) D (3) B (4) B (5) C (6) D (7) D (8) C (9) B (10) A (11) A (12) C
(13) D (14) D (15) B (16) A (17) C (18) B (19) C (20) B (21) C (22) B (23) C (24) A
(25) A (26) B (27) A (28) D (29) A (30) A (31) C (32) C (33) D (34) B (35) B (36) A
(37) B

7.2.4 Discussion of Answers to Questions in Section 7.2.2

Questions #1 to #8 None.

Questions #9-#11 Look at the R groups to determine the neutrality, basicity, acidity or hydrophilicity. Refer to Section if necessary.

Question #12 (Answer: C) Hydrophobic AA's are found on the interior. The AA in option (C) with the phenyl group is hydrophobic.

Question #13 (Answer: D) (A) and (C) have only polar or hydrophobic AA's, so its pI is around 7. (B) has two acidic AA's and one AA that may be basic or acidic; therefore, its pI is less than 7. (D) has two basic amino acids and, therefore, has a pI greater than 7. See Section for discussion.

Question #14 (Answer: D) The cathode attracts the positive ion. Therefore, the peptide must be positively charged at pH = 7.0. This means that the pI must be greater than 7, which means it must contain basic AA's.

Question #15 (Answer: B) The anode attracts the negative ion. Therefore, the peptide must be negatively charged at pH = 7.0. This means that the pI must be less than 7. Therefore, there must be an excess of acidic AA's. See discussion in Section.

Questions #16 to #20 None.

Question #21 (Answer: C) A furanose is a ring form which contains four carbon atoms and one oxygen atom.

Question #22 (Answer: B) A ketose is a sugar which has ketone functional grouping. (Section 7.26.1).

Question #23 (Answer: C) Anomers are compounds in the ring that differ in configuration only at the former carbonyl carbon:

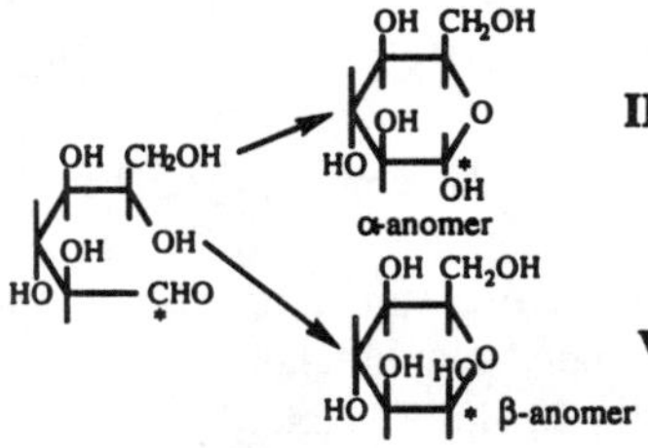

III α-anomer

V β-anomer

Question #24 (Answer: A) Epimers are stereoisomers that are different in configuration at a carbon other than the anomeric. III differs from IV at Carbon #4.

Question #25 (Answer: A) The more stable conformation is that in which the maximum number of substituents, especially the larger substituents, are in equatorial positions.

Question #26 (Answer: B) A pentose has a total of five carbons.

Question #27 (Answer: A) The acetal oxygen at C-1 is down in an a-bond.

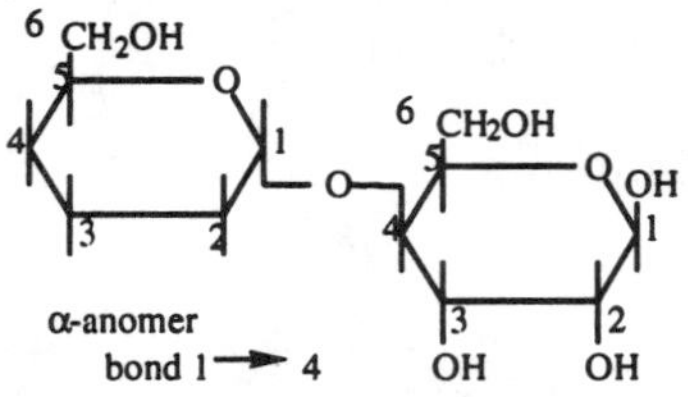

α-anomer bond 1→4

Question #28 (Answer: D) The triacyl glycerol contains three $C_{16}H_{33}CO_2$ units and one CH_2CHCH_2.

Question #29 (Answer: A) The common fatty acids are unbranched chains.

Question #30 (Answer: A) The acid from TG-2 has three double bonds. Saturated acids have higher melting points.

Question #31 (Answer: C) The infrared spectrum will show absorption for C-H (2900) and C = O (1700).

Question #32 (Answer: C) The second carbon atoms are chiral in I and III only.

Question #33 (Answer: D) Definition of a lipid.

Question #34 (Answer: B) Only one chiral center is changed, others are unchanged.

Question #35 (Answer: B) The phenol in estradiol is more acidic than the alcohol in testosterone; testosterone has more chiral carbon atoms.

Question #36 (Answer: A) Base or neutral conditions change the esters to anions which cannot be hydrolyzed.

Question #37 (Answer: B) ATP is an anhydride (also ADP); the alcohol is converted to an ester of phosphoric acid.

7.2.5 Advanced Concepts

Read research papers and journals to familiarize yourself with new bioorganic molecules, their current physiological applications and recent experimental procedures to study structure and chemical reactions. Advanced concepts are arranged by type of compound (A = Amino acids, C = Carbohydrates, L = Lipids).

- Electrophoresis showing difference between anionic and dicationic ions; racemic resolutions of amino acids; role of globular proteins as antibodies; ninhydrin reaction to produce colors with special understanding of reliability and error analysis of ninhydrin test (Compound type A).
- A complete theory, design, functions and reactions in the automatic amino acid analyzer; 2-D gel scanner; DNA sequencer and synthesizer; protein sequencer; chromatography of amino acids (only paper chromatography (Compound type A).
- Theory, design, functions of thin-layer chromatography applied to polypeptides, e.g., hemoglobin, insulin. Section 7.24 explains various types of chromatography (Compound type A).
- Measuring mutarotation of D-Glucose using a polarimeter and determining equilibrium constant and relation between α-D-glucose and β-D-glucose; understanding of thin-layer chromatography of saccharides and working with Benedict's test accuracy, Barfoed's test accuracy both linked to special anomers and epimers (Compound type C).
- Compare and contrast: Ruff degradation (make chain shorter) and Fischer synthesis (make chain longer) (Compound type C).
- Role of cellulose, cellobiose, glycogen, lactose and starch in cellular metabolism; using stereochemistry of each of these carbohydrates to illustrate metabolic biochemical reactions (Compound type C).
- Biological functions and stereochemistry of lipids, e.g., cholesterol, reproductive hormones, phospholipids and sphingolipids (Compound type L).

7.3 DNA AND RNA (MOLECULAR BIOLOGY)

7.3.1 Introduction to DNA and RNA

This section provides an insight into the structure and function of DNA and RNA as complex biomolecules. The Watson-Crick model (traditionally proposed as a right-handed double helix) for DNA was challenged and a new Z-DNA model (considered as a left-handed double helix) was suggested. Compare the old and new DNA models with special focus on assumptions (given and implied), molecular biology applications and current research trends. Understand terms such as target and vehicle DNA, plasmids, genomes, modern DNA cloning techniques and genetic repair. The specific roles of mRNA, tRNA and rRNA should be linked to translation and transcription mechanisms. Review Okasaki fragments for enzymes involved in semiconservative replication.

7.3.1.1 NUCLEIC ACID STRUCTURE

Nitrogen bases (NB) combine with five-carbon sugars (S) to form *nucleosides* which combine with *inorganic phosphate* (P) to form *nucleotides* which polymerize to form *nucleic acids* (Fig. 7.13).

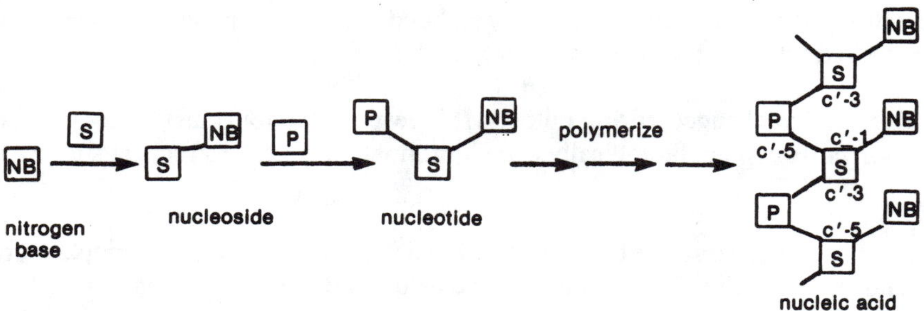

Fig. 7.13—Relation of Nucleotides, Nucleosides, and Nucleic Acids

An example of a nucleotide is deoxyadenylic acid:

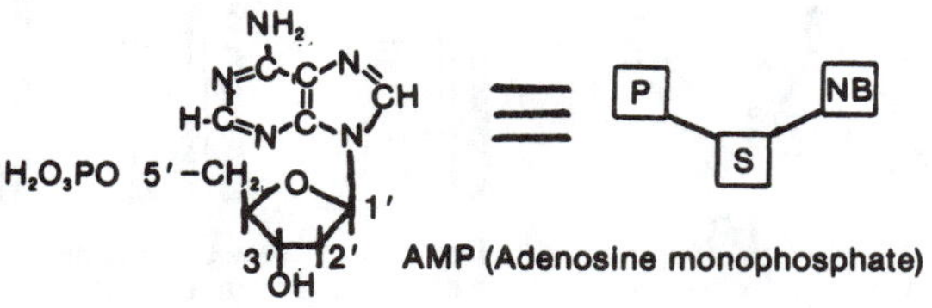

AMP (Adenosine monophosphate)

The *nitrogen bases* are the substituted *purines* (two rings) and *pyrimidines* (one ring), see Fig. 7.14. *Guanine (G)* and *adenine (A)* are purines. *Thymine (T), cytosine (C),* and *uracil (U)* are pyrimidines.

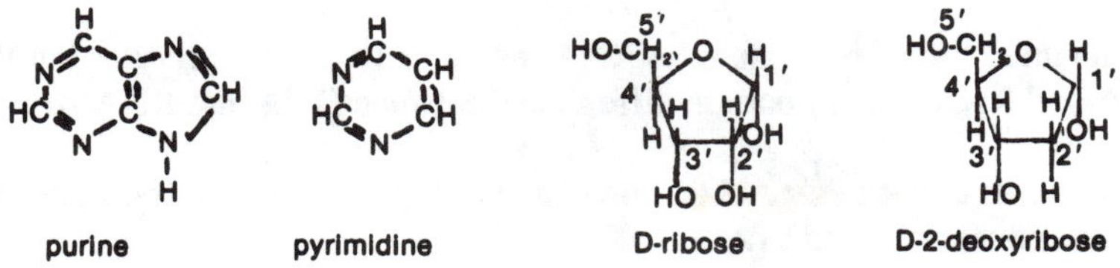

purine pyrimidine D-ribose D-2-deoxyribose

Fig. 7.14—Components of Nucleotides

The sugars are *ribose* and *2-deoxyribose* (Fig. 7.14) The nitrogen bases bond at C'-1 of the sugar to form nucleosides. Then one, two, or three phosphates attach at C'-5 of the sugar and nucleotides result (figs. 7.13 and 7.14).

The triphosphate nucleotides then polymerize to form nucleic acids by eliminating two phosphates in the process. The phosphate of one nucleotide is bound to the C'-3 hydroxyl of the sugar of the next. If the sugar is ribose, then the nucleic acid is *ribonucleic acid (RNA).* If the sugar is deoxyribose, then the nucleic acid is *deoxyribonucleic acid (DNA).*

7.3.1.2 DNA STRUCTURE

DNA has a *helical structure* with sugar-phosphates as the backbone with the nitrogen bases sticking off at more-or-less right angles (Fig. 7.15). It is composed of two strands of nucleic acids running in antiparallel fashion (i.e., one strand goes 5' → 3' and the other 3' → 5'). The nitrogen bases pair by hydrogen bonding and this holds the strands together. The nitrogen bases that pair are dictated by the matching up of hydrogen bonding sites and by space limitations in the double helix (proposed by Watson-Crick), which require a purine (two rings) and pyrimidine (one ring) to bond to each other. Adenine and thymine pair forming two hydrogen bonds. Guanine and cytosine pair forming three hydrogen bonds. Uracil replaces thymine in RNA which may occasionally have pairing of strands. The more hydrogen bonds, the more stable the nucleic acid. Hydrophobic bonds between the stacked nitrogen bases also stabilize the double helix.

DNA remains constant and unchanged during mitosis. It is responsible for transmitting genetic and hereditary information. DNA molecules contain biologically coded information which instruct cells to perform polypeptide synthesis.

DNA is *duplicated* in a semi-conservative fashion. That is, each strand serves as the template upon which a new complementary strand is made (Fig. 7.16). Note that the actual process is very complicated and may occur at multiple sites along the DNA strand simultaneously

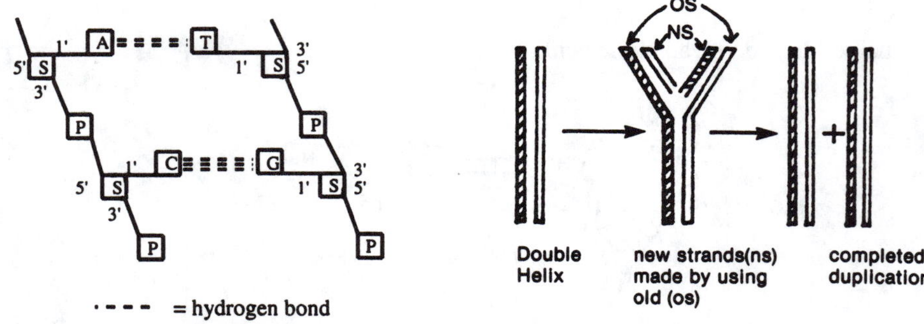

Fig. 7.15—Base Pairing

Fig. 7.16—Semiconservative Replication

7.3.1.3 RNA STRUCTURE

RNA is involved in the manufacture of proteins. The RNA molecules are much shorter but there are structural similarities between DNA and RNA. The important differences between DNA and RNA structures are:

(a) RNA usually has only *one* strand of nucleotides. The strand does not bond to a complementary strand as in a DNA molecule and hence does not form a helix.

(b) The four bases in RNA are *uracil, guanine, cytosine,* and *adenine*. The base *thymine* is not found in RNA. Instead, uracil forms a complementary pair with adenine.

(c) RNA nucleotides contain ribose sugars instead of deoxyribose sugars. The ribose sugars contain an extra oxygen atom.

There are three different types of RNA:

1. *mRNA:* Messenger RNA transfers the DNA code from the eukaryotic nucleus to the ribosomes.
2. *rRNA:* Ribosomal RNA makes up a part of the ribosomes.
3. *tRNA:* Transfer RNA carries amino acids to the messenger RNA at the ribosomes.

7.3.2 Questions Related to DNA and RNA

1. Which of the pairs below do not normally hydrogen bond in nucleic acids?

A. adenine-thymine
B. adenine-guanine
C. guanine-cytosine
D. adenine-uracil

2. Both DNA and RNA contain all the nitrogen bases except:

A. guanine.
B. adenine.
C. cytosine.
D. thymine.

3. The sugar found in DNA is:

A. deoxyribose.
B. ribose.
C. dextrose.
D. deoxyglucose.

4. Nucleic acids are composed of repeating units of:

A. nucleotides.
B. nucleosides.
C. nitrogen bases.
D. adenines.

5. Which is not a pyrimidine?

A. guanine
B. thymine
C. cytosine
D. uracil

6. DNA always differs from RNA by:

A. forming hydrogen bonds between strands.
B. having thymine and not uracil.
C. being found only in the nucleus.
D. having a sugar-phosphate backbone.

7. The following is one strand of a double helix of DNA (showing only nitrogen bases). What is the structure of its complementary strand? (A = adenine, G = guanine, T = thymine, C = cytosine, U = uracil)

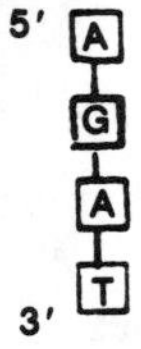

5′ A
G
A
T 3′

A. 5′ A
G
A
T 3′

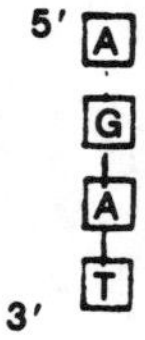

B. 5′ T
A
G
A 3′

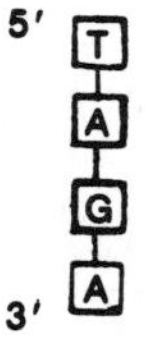

C. 3′ T
C
T
A 5′

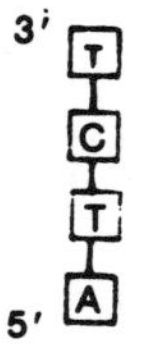

D. 3′ T
A
G
A 5′

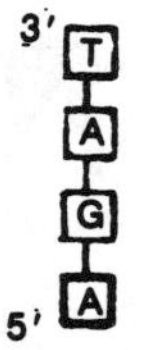

8. Given the following data, which organism *probably* has the most heat stable DNA?

Organism	(A + T) / (G + C) ratio
Mycobacterium phlei	0.49
Escherichia coli	1.02
Calf thymus	1.29
Bacteriophage T2	1.90

A. *Mycobacterium phlei*
B. *Escherichia coli*
C. *Calf thymus*
D. *Bacteriophage T2*

9. Methods to differentiate between DNA and RNA might involve all of the following except:

A. reaction of ribose with orcinol under suitable conditions.
B. ultraviolet absorption by nitrogen bases at 260nm.
C. chromatography to separate the different nitrogen bases.
D. ^{14}C labeled uracil.

7.3.3 Answers to Questions in Section 7.3.2

(1) B (2) D (3) A (4) A (5) A (6) B (7) C (8) A (9) B

7.3.4 Discussion of Answers to Questions in Section 7.3.2

Questions #1 to #6 Discussed in Section 7.3.1.

Question #7 (Answer: C) The complementary DNA strand is the opposite of the given strand and must be 3' → 5'. The base pairing is as discussed in the reference.

Question #8 (Answer: A) The higher the percentage of G + C pairs, the higher the heat stability because more hydrogen bonds (three per G + C pair vs. two per A + T pair) are present making it more difficult to disrupt the double helix. This means the smaller the ratio $\frac{A+T}{G+C}$ the larger the G + C so the answer is (A).

Question #9 (Answer: B) One must look for chemical differences between DNA and RNA and exploit them. (A) uses the fact that RNA contains ribose and DNA contains deoxyribose. (C) and (D) use the fact that RNA contains uracil and DNA doesn't. The selection (B) measures nitrogen bases, in general, and does not distinguish between them and, therefore, could not distinguish between RNA and DNA. This method does distinguish between proteins and nucleic acids.

7.3.5 Advanced Concepts

Read laboratory reports, research findings and current literature in addition to your college textbooks in this field. Genetic engineering is an ever-changing field with new findings almost everyday. The following concepts should be learned and applied:

- The major differences between highly and moderatively repetitive DNA
- DNA replication (biosynthesis) connected to DNA gyrase, ligase, polymerase (α and β) and topoisomerase—review terminology
- Fundamental research methods in modifications and repair of DNA as applied to genetic engineering and gene splicing
- Application of Chargaff's rules to the genetic code including biochemical genetics and viral genetics
- Viral mutations related to the functions and structural compositions of DNA and RNA
- Current designs, methods and evaluation of various genetic tests and special medical instruments to obtain: electronmicrographs, x-ray diffraction, NMR techniques, ultracentrifugation, autoradiographs; denaturing and renaturing of DNA

7.4 PROTEIN SYNTHESIS (MOLECULAR BIOLOGY)

7.4.1 Introduction to Protein Synthesis

Protein synthesis (also called biosynthesis) is made of two subprocesses: translation and transcription. Link biological molecules (structure and chemistry) to the mechanics of translation and transcription. Each process (translation and transcription) consists of three major steps: initiation, elongation and termination or release of the biochain. The emphasis is to comprehend Crick's law of molecular biology. The law states, "DNA information is passed onto the RNA which in turn transfers it to the proteins". Focus on: How is information passed from DNA to RNA? How is information passed from RNA to proteins? How is experimental research done to prove the law?

7.4.1.1 GENETIC CODE—TRANSCRIPTION AND TRANSLATION

DNA has the information that is the key of life. This information codes for the sequence of amino acids in proteins and is the sequence of nucleotides (see Section 7.3.1) in DNA. The *genetic code (triplet code)* is 64 sets of sequences of three nucleotides each. Sixty-one of these code for amino acids and three are punctuation marks (terminate protein chains). Some amino acids have only one triplet (methionine, tryptophan) while others have six (leucine).

The *genetic code is universal* (all living organisms have the same code). A *gene or cistron* is the sequence of triplets that codes for a single polypeptide chain. DNA is *duplicated* semiconservatively (using each strand as a template for the new DNA strand) by DNA polymerase from 5′ to the 3′ end (see Section 7.3.1). Information on DNA is passed to mRNA (messenger RNA) by the process called *transcription.* Only one of the DNA chains is used, the enzyme is called RNA polymerase, and the direction of synthesis is 5′to 3′.

Once the mRNA is synthesized from DNA, it moves out of the nucleus (eukaryotes) through nuclear pores and into the cytoplasm where the process called *translation* occurs, (as shown in Fig. 7.18). The mRNA attaches to the *small subunit* of the ribosome (composed of rRNA and protein). The large subunit is then attached and a complete ribosome is formed. Meanwhile, an amino acid in the cytoplasm is being activated by phosphorylation with ATP by an *activating enzyme* (there is one enzyme for each amino acid). Another type of RNA called tRNA (transfer RNA), specific for the amino acid (AA) and activating enzyme (AE) is first bound by the enzyme, and then the amino acid is transferred to it by enzymatic action (Fig. 7.17). The tRNA ~ AA dissociates from the enzyme and moves to a specific position on the large subunit. Another position on the large subunit is occupied by the last tRNA to attach and which binds the carboxyl end of the growing peptide chain. The tRNA molecule has at least three recognition regions, one for the activating enzyme, and, hence, the AA, one for the ribosome, and a sequence of three nucleotides called the anticodon which pairs (hydrogen bonds) with the codon of the mRNA. So, the *anticodon* of tRNA pairs with the *codon* of mRNA and the next AA is in position for *peptide bond formation* which causes a transfer of the growing peptide to this new tRNA. After the peptide bond is formed, a *translocation* occurs moving the newly attached tRNA peptide into the position previously occupied by the old tRNA-peptide. This latter tRNA is now displaced. A new codon is exposed on the mRNA for another tRNA~AA to attach and the process is repeated. The protein is made from the free amino end to the free carboxyl end. More than one ribosome may "read" a mRNA at a time—this creates polyribosomes (polysomes). Synthesis stops when one of the punctuation mark codons is reached. *Note* that a gene (three nucleotides in this case) is on DNA, a codon is on mRNA and an anticodon is on tRNA.

$$\text{AA} + \text{AE} \rightarrow \text{AE} - \text{AA} \sim \text{Pi} \xrightarrow{+\text{RNA}} \text{AE}\begin{smallmatrix}\diagup\text{AA} \sim \text{Pi} \\ \diagdown\text{tRNA}\end{smallmatrix} \xrightarrow{-\text{AE}} \text{t-RNA} \sim \text{AA}$$

~ = energy bond

Fig. 7.17—Activation of Amino Acid (AA) by Activating Enzyme (AE)

Protein Synthesis and the DNA Code:

Cells manufacture the proteins they need. The making of proteins is called protein synthesis. The sequence of DNA bases determines the code for protein synthesis. The bases of one chain attach to those of the other according to the "base-pairing rule". The base-pairing rule states that:

(1) Adenine always pairs with thymine (A:T or T:A)
(2) Cytosine always pairs with guanine (G:C or C:G)

Scientists found that at least 20 different amino acids are used to make proteins. The following reasoning was used to justify that each codon is made up of 3 bases. If a codon was only 1 base long, messenger RNA could code for only 4 amino acids (both DNA and RNA have 4 bases). If a codon was 2 bases long, only $4^2 = 16$ amino acids could be coded. However, if a codon is 3 bases, $4^3 = 64$ arrangements are possible. Review in this book the math section on permutations, combinations, and probability to understand the fundamental principles of arranging 4 letters, 3 at a time. Scientific experiments also support the concept of a 3-base codon.

List of Amino Acids and DNA Codons

1. Termination Codons:	ATT, ATC, ACT
2. Valine:	CAA, CAG, CAT, CAC
3. Tyrosine:	ATA, ATG
4. Tryptophan:	ACC
5. Threonine:	TGA, TGG, TGT, TGC
6. Serine:	AGA, AGG, AGT, AGC, TCA, TCG
7. Proline:	GGA, GGG, GGT, GGC
8. Phenylalanine:	AAA, AAG
9. Methionine:	TAC
10. Lysine:	TTT, TTC
11. Leucine:	AAT, AAC, GAA, GAG, GAT, GAC
12. Isoleucine:	TAA, TAG, TAT
13. Histidine:	GTA, GTG
14. Glycine:	CCA, CCG, CCT, CCC
15. Glutamine:	GTT, GTC
16. Glutamic Acid:	CTT, CTC
17. Cysteine:	ACA, ACG
18. Aspartic Acid:	CTA, CTG
19. Asparagine:	TTA, TTG
20. Arginine:	TCT, TCC, GCA, GCG, GCT, GCC
21. Alanine:	CGA, CGG, CGT, CGC

THE GENETIC CODE DICTIONARY

5' end Ist position	U Uracil IInd position	C Cytosine IInd position	A Adenine IInd position	G Guanine IInd position	3' end IIIrd position
U Uracil	UUU Phe UUC Phe UUA Leu UUG Leu	UCU Ser UCC Ser UCA Ser UCG Ser	UAU Tyr UAC Tyr UAA STOP UAG STOP	UGU Cys UGC Cys UGA STOP UGG Trp	U C A G
C Cytosine	CUU Leu CUC Leu CUA Leu CUG Leu	CCU Pro CCC Pro CCA Pro CCG Pro	CAU His CAC His CAA Gln CAG Gln	CGU Arg CGC Arg CGA Arg CGG Arg	U C A G
A Adenine	AUU Ile AUC Ile AUA Ile AUG Met	ACU Thr ACC Thr ACA Thr ACG Thr	AAU Asn AAC Asn AAA Lys AAG Lys	AGU Ser AGC Ser AGA Arg AGG Arg	U C A G
G Guanine	GUU Val GUC Val GUA Val GUG Val	GCU Ala GCC Ala GCA Ala GCG Ala	GAU Asp GAC Asp GAA Glu GAG Glu	GGU Gly GGC Gly GGA Gly GGG Gly	U C A G

STOP = nonsense codons (UAA, UAG, UGA)

Ist IInd IIIrd

Index: Gly = glycine, Phe = phenylalanine, Leu = leucine, Ile = isoleucine, Met = methionine, Val = valine, ser = serine, Pro = proline, Thr = threonine, Ala = alanine, Tyr = trysone, His = histidine, Gln = glutamine, Asn = asparagine, Lys = lysine, Asp = aspartic acid, Glu = glutamic acid, Cys = cysteine, Trp = tryptophan, Arg = arginine

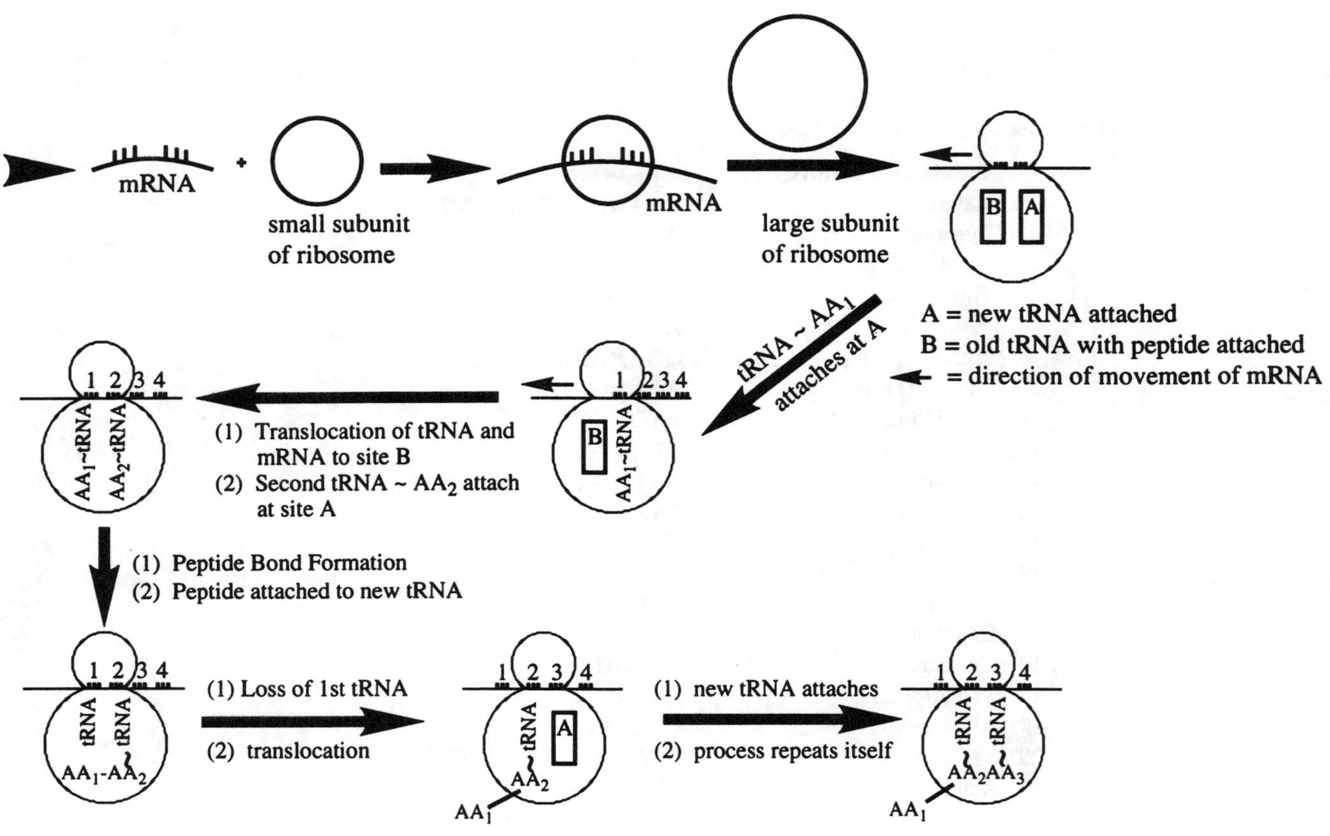

Fig. 7.18—Protein Synthesis on Ribosome (Translation)

7.4.2 Questions Related to Protein Synthesis

1. The genetic code is composed of sequences of:

   A. three nucleotides.
   B. three nucleosides.
   C. three amino acids.
   D. two amino acids.

2. The genetic code (triplet code) consists of 64 sets of three nucleotides each. Which statement is *incorrect* concerning the triplet code?

   A. The code is universal (i.e., all living organisms have the same code).
   B. All 64 triplets code for amino acids.
   C. More than one triplet can code for the same amino acid.
   D. A triplet may code for only one amino acid or termination codon.

3. Select the *correct* association:

   A. duplication-synthesis of DNA using DNA as a template
   B. transcription-synthesis of RNA using DNA as a template
   C. translation-synthesis of proteins using information on RNA
   D. all of the above associations are correct

4. Translation of the genetic code does *not directly* require:
   - **A.** activated tRNA ~ AA.
   - **B.** ribosomes.
   - **C.** mRNA.
   - **D.** DNA.
5. Select the *incorrect* association:
   - **A.** DNA-codon
   - **B.** mRNA-anticodon
   - **C.** tRNA-gene
   - **D.** all of the above associations are incorrect
6. Translation is the synthesis of proteins using mRNA as a guide. All are correct concerning translation *except:*
   - **A.** mRNA initially binds to the small ribosomal subunit.
   - **B.** the codon of tRNA pairs with the anticodon of mRNA.
   - **C.** protein synthesis is from the free amino to the free carboxyl end of the protein chain.
   - **D.** more than one ribosome may read a given mRNA at a time.
7. All of the following processes occur on the ribosome *except:*
   - **A.** binding of mRNA to be "read" by tRNAs.
   - **B.** activation of tRNA and its amino acid.
   - **C.** peptide bond formation.
   - **D.** binding of AUG codon with formyl methionine tRNA.

7.4.3 Answers to Questions in Section 7.4.2

(1) A (2) B (3) D (4) D (5) D (6) B (7) B

7.4.4 Discussion of Answers to Questions in Section 7.4.2: None

7.4.5 Advanced Concepts

- Using the genetic code dictionary as a guideline, study the definitions and usage of introns, exons, operons, template binding, super coiled DNA, RNA polymerase, mutagen chemistry, nonsense suppressions as tRNA mutations.
- Understand the organic structure and function of various antibiotics such as tetracycline, streptomycin and how does one molecule of these antibiotics suppress the protein synthesis process?
- Reading research reports and journals related to protein biosynthesis, molecular biology, relationship of protein biosynthesis to cytology will provide advanced terminology resources

7.5 PROKARYOTIC AND EUKARYOTIC CELLS (MICROBIOLOGY)

7.5.1 Introduction to Prokaryotic and Eukaryotic Cells

This section is medically important. Microbiology of prokaryotic cell and fungus is compared to the microbiology of the eukaryotic cell. Learn with emphasis the structures, life history and sources of disease for bacteria, bacteriophage, virus and fungus. Learn the detailed structure and functions of eukaryotic cells. Connect the study of generalized eukaryotic cells to specialized eukaryotic cells such as neural cells (neurons), contractile cells (sarcomeres), epithelial cells and connective cells. Evaluate the physical and chemical aspects of cell membrane transport models, ion channels, chromosome movement mechanics, cellular adhesion and membrane receptors.

7.5.1.1 CYTOPLASM AND CYTOPLASMIC ORGANELLES

Cytoplasm is a watery millieu containing membrane-bound organelles, centrioles and storage molecules (e.g., lipid droplets and glycogen). Enzymatic activity takes place in the cytoplasm, i.e., glycolysis. (See Fig. 7.19 below.)

Endoplasmic reticulum (ER) is a double membrane system running throughout the cell. It probably breaks up and re-forms and is continuous with the cell membrane and nuclear envelope. In this way it is probably a precursor for other membrane systems and peroxisomes. Rough (granular) ER contains ribosomes on its surface and is concerned with protein synthesis. Smooth ER (SER) is devoid of ribosomes and may serve several functions, a primary one being steroid synthesis. In the liver, SER plays an important role in the metabolism of endogenous small organic molecules, exogenous drugs, and toxins. In muscle, SER is called the sarcoplasmic reticulum and plays a role in impulse conduction and muscle contraction via calcium regulation. It may also serve a storage function—starch in plants, glycogen in animals.

Golgi complex is a collection of smooth membranes probably continuous with the SER. Its primary function is in packaging and secretion of proteins and polysaccharides. It also plays a role in synthesis of complex polysaccharides.

Mitochondria are double membraned organelles which produce ATP. The inner membrane is folded into cristae which contain the enzyme systems of electron transport and oxidative phosphorylation. The matrix contains a circular DNA molecule, prokaryotic type ribosomes, elementary bodies (ionic crystals), and enzymes of the Kreb's Cycle. Mitochondria replicate independently of the cell.

Lysosomes are single membraned organelles containing acid hydrolases (digestive enzymes). Functions of lysosomes include digestion of the cell at death (autolysis), digestion of substances within the cell, and digestion of substances taken in by phagocytosis (heterolysis). Storage diseases result when one or more of the hydrolytic enzymes are absent or defective. Lysosomes are produced in the rough ER and packaged in the Golgi apparatus.

Peroxisomes are single membraned, are part of a group of organelles formerly called microbodies and contain enzymes for the metabolism of oxygen and/or hydrogen peroxide. They are found in large numbers in the liver.

Cilia (see also Fig. 7.19) are long extensions of the plasma membrane that contain a highly ordered and coordinated set of microtubules. The cilia function to move mucus and debris from passageways (e.g., trachea) in humans and to provide locomotion in protozoans. At the cell surface cilia are bound to the cell by centrioles (basal body or kinetosome). *Microvilli* are shorter, more numerous extensions of the plasma membrane found primarily in absorptive cells to increase the surface area of the cells.

Flagella are longer than cilia, are used for locomotion, and are composed of a cylinder of nine paired microtubules with two unpaired centrally. They contain ATPase.

Microfilaments are aggregated proteins with no lumen and may be important for maintenance of cell structure and cytoplasmic streaming.

Microtubules are aggregated proteins with a lumen, may be important for intracellular transport and structure, and are inhibited by colchicine.

Ribosomes are important in protein synthesis, composed of rRNA and protein, and are divisible into a large subunit and a small subunit (see Section 7.4.1).

Cells are held together in tissues by *junctional complexes*. There are several types, but the most important are the *tight junction* (zonula occludens), *desmosome* (macula adhaerens or spot weld) and *gap junction* (electronic couple). The tight junction is a zone of fusion between adjacent cells and precludes the passage of most molecules between cells (e.g., lining of the gut, kidney tubule cells). The desmosome is a small point of contact; there may be numerous desmosomes joining two adjacent cells (e.g., spinous layer of skin). Gap junctions are actual microchannels between adjacent cells that provide passage of ions and small molecules (e.g., smooth muscle liver cells).

7.5.1.2 PROKARYOTIC AND EUKARYOTIC CELLS

Eukaryotes differ from prokaryotes (see Section 7.5.1) primarily by virtue of membrane bound structures in the former. The eukaryote is, thus, conveniently divided into a cell membrane, cytoplasmic region, and nuclear region.

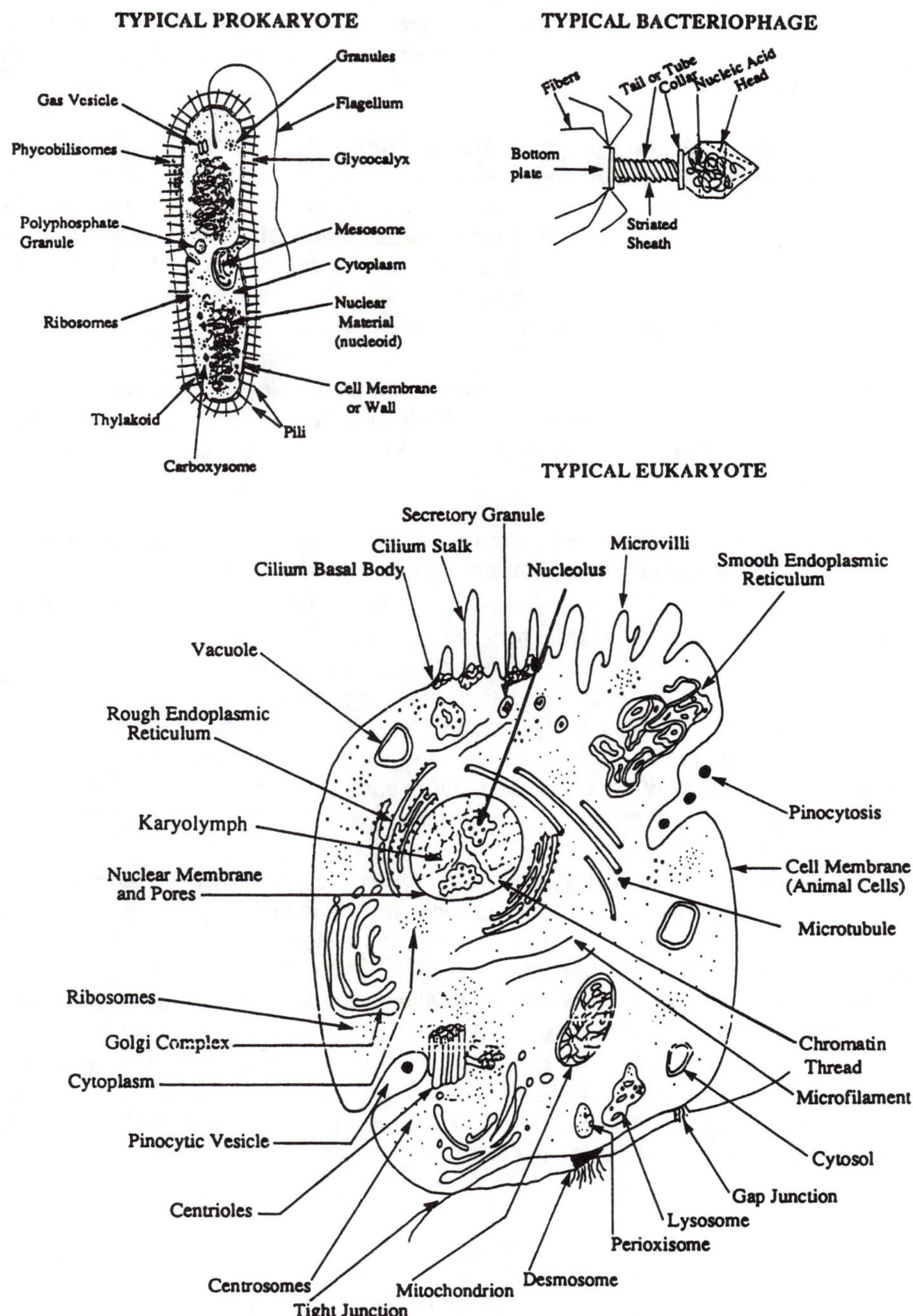

Fig. 7.19—Typical Prokaryote, Eukaryote and Bacteriophage

Prokaryotes differ from *eukaryotes* (Section 7.5.1) by the latter having (1) genetic material in a nucleus and DNA conjugated with proteins, (2) organelles bound within membranes, (3) subcellular structural units to carry out specific functions, e.g., ATP production, photosynthesis, and (4) presence of cell walls made of cellulose or chitin versus murein (amino sugars and amino acids) as in prokaryotes. The DNA of prokaryotes is found in a non-membrane region called the nucleoid. Enzymes for metabolism and energy production are either free in the cytoplasm or bound to the cell membrane, and the ribosomes are smaller than in eukaryotes. Viruses are not prokaryotes or eukaryotes but constitute a group unto themselves. Prokaryotic cells have *no* well-defined nucleus. Examples are bacteria and cyanobacteria (blue-green algae). They are subdivided into four groups: 1) *Gracilicutes* (gram-negative bacteria), 2) *Firmicutes* (gram-positive bacteria), 3) *Tenericutes* (Mycoplasmata), and 4) *Mendosicutes* (Archaeobacteria).

The general characteristics of bacterial *structure* were discussed above under prokaryotes. More specifically, from outside in, a bacterium may have a *capsule* which is usually made of a polysaccharide mucoid material and protects the bacterium from phagocytosis. Inside the capsule is the cell wall, which prevents a hypertonic bacterium from bursting. Inside the cell wall is the cell membrane which may contain invaginations called *mesosomes* where localization of enzymes concerned with similar functions may be found. The cytoplasm and nucleoid are as described above. The DNA is circular and is haploid. Some bacteria contain flagella for locomotion—these are structurally different from their eukaryotic counterparts.

Bacteria have three common *shapes: Cocci* (spherical or ovoid), *bacilli* (cylindrical or rod-like), and *spirillia* (helically coiled). The cocci are often found in clusters: diplococci (two bacteria together), *streptococci* (linear chains of cocci), or *staphylococci* (grape-like clusters of cocci). All of these are made up of individual bacteria with distinct cell walls.

Metabolically, bacteria are aerobic or anaerobic. Anaerobic bacteria may use fermentation (where an organic molecule such as pyruvate or lactate is the final electron acceptor) or inorganic substances as final electron receptors (such as $S \rightarrow H_2S$). An *obligate anaerobe* is one that is killed if exposed to oxygen. This is usually because they cannot handle the peroxides (very toxic) produced in oxidative metabolism. A *facultative anaerobe* can survive in the presence or absence of oxygen. Bacteria may use a great variety of molecules as nutrients. Some are photosynthetic, others heterotrophic (using organic molecules made by other organisms) and others are chemosynthetic (making organic molecules and energy from inorganic precursors). The last group are important in fixation of nitrogen for use by all organisms. The variety of metabolic nutrients required and products produced are extremely important in studying basic questions of genetics, as well as biochemistry, and also in differentiating between the different types of bacteria.

Most bacteria *reproduce asexually* by the process of *binary fission* which produces two identical haploid daughter cells by the simple process of mitosis. Genetic recombination,(e.g., transfer and rearrangement of genetic information) may occur by three distinct means: transformation, transduction, and conjugation. *Transformation* involves a bacterium picking up free DNA from a medium, the free DNA being from a different bacterium. *Transduction* is the transfer of parts of DNA between bacteria by bacteriophages. In *conjugation* there is pairing of "male" and "female" forms. DNA is passed sequentially between them via structures called pili. All or a fraction of the DNA may be passed in this way. The above three genetic mechanisms allow extraordinary adaptability and variability of bacteria. Since bacteria can reproduce in a span as short as twenty minutes, a new trait such as drug resistance can spread rapidly in a given population. A typical bacterial cell (about 1 micrometer in diameter) is shown in Fig. 7.19.

7.5.1.3 CELL MEMBRANE AND TRANSPORT

Cell membranes are composed of lipids (*cholesterol, phospholipids,* etc.) and many types of proteins with distinctive functions (e.g., receptors, ion transporters, second messengers, enzymes, cell coat). Cell membranes vary greatly in composition depending upon the cell type and their function. In general the lipids form a bilayer (two molecules thick) in which the polar ends of the lipid molecules (particularly phospholipids) extend outward and the non-polar extend inward, adjoining each other. The *lipid bilayer* is interrupted by *integral proteins* that penetrate the width of the lipid bilayer. Smaller protein molecules may decorate the outer and inner sides of the lipid bilayer in very large numbers (e.g., molecules and enzymes of the electron transport chain in mitochondria) or relatively small numbers (e.g., membrane receptors and antigen recognition molecules on white blood cells).

Cell membranes may be quite fluid (membrane molecules readily flow—*fluid mosaic model*) or, conversely, relatively rigid. The membrane becomes more rigid when cholesterol is substituted for phospholipids, when fatty acid chains of lipid molecules are saturated and/or when there are a large number of protein molecules present on the inner and outer surface of the lipid bilayer. Even greater rigidity is possible when closely packed sheets of cells are held together by junctional complexes, microfilaments or microtubules. Surface membrane coats such as the basal lamina further restrict membrane movement.

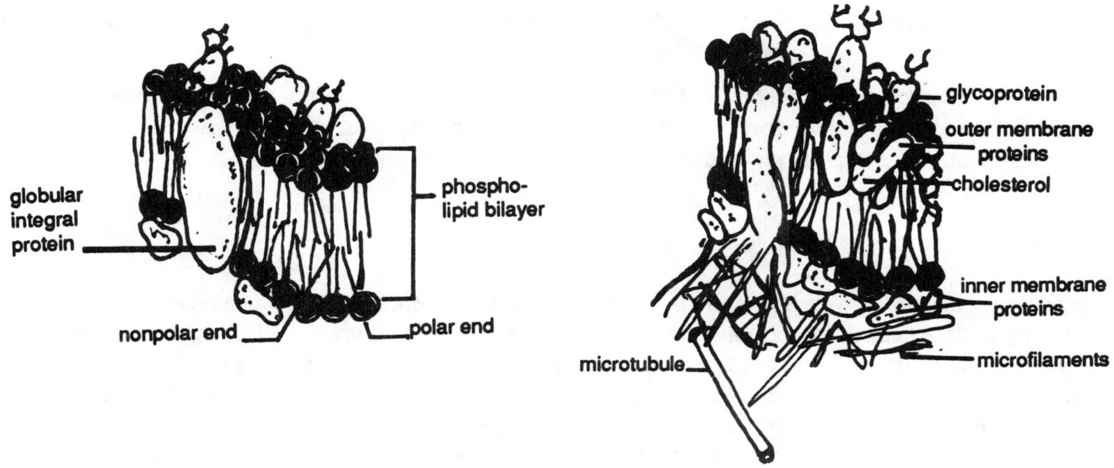

Fig. 7.20—Fluid Mosaic Membrane Model

Fig. 7.21—Rigid Membrane Model

Substances move through the membrane by diffusion, osmosis, facilitated diffusion, active transport, endocytosis, or exocytosis. *Diffusion* is the random movement of free molecules or ions or particles in solution or suspension under the influence of thermal motion toward a uniform distribution throughout the available volume. This can occur through cell membranes if the substance diffuses through the cell "pores." In diffusion, the net movement of solute is from the region of higher concentration to that of lower concentration. Small organic molecules (ethanol, glycerol) and some ions (Cl^-) and H_2O are moved by diffusion.

Osmosis is diffusion through a semi-permeable membrane. In osmosis, a solute cannot cross the membrane in order to equalize its concentration on both sides. This then creates a concentration difference for water across the membrane and the water diffuses in response to this to the side with the lower concentration of water (which is the side with the highest concentration of solute). *Tonicity* refers to relative concentrations of solute in two solutions. *Isotonic* means the two are equal. A *hypertonic* solution has more solute per unit volume than the reference. Osmosis (flow of solvent) occurs from hypotonic to hypertonic solution. If an RBC is placed in a solution less concentrated than itself (RBC is hypertonic), it swells until it hemolyzes (bursts). If it is placed in a solution more concentrated than itself, it crenates (shrinks). *Osmotic pressure* is the hydrostatic pressure needed to oppose the movement of the solvent.

Facilitated diffusion is a process by which substances insoluble in a membrane are carried across the membrane with the concentration gradient by means of a carrier substance. Saturation kinetics are observed; that is, as the substrate concentration rises relative to the number of carrier molecules, the rate of transport levels off. Some sugars and amino acids are transported in this fashion.

Active transport is the process of moving molecules uphill against an electrochemical gradient. A carrier molecule is involved as well as the expenditure of energy (ATP). This system exhibits saturation kinetics and inhibition by inhibitors of energy production (e.g., cyanide or 2,4-DNP). An important active transport system is the Na-K pump which is responsible for maintaining the electrical gradient of various membranes and neurons.

neurons. Other locations of active transport include the gut (for sugars and amino acids) and the kidney tubules (for secretion and reabsorption of ions and small molecules).

Endocytosis is a process by which large molecules are surrounded by plasma membrane and brought into the cell. Exocytosis is a reverse process whereby molecules are exported out of the cell. Endocytosis occurs as: phagocytosis, pinocytosis or receptor-mediated endocytosis.

Phagocytosis, also called "cell eating", is a process by which large particulate matter, bacteria, or even cells, are engulfed by the cell membrane through invagination forming a vesicle which is internalized. The vesicle then may combine with a primary lysosome becoming a secondary lysosome (phagosome). The enzymes digest its contents. This is an energy-requiring process.

Pinocytosis is similar to phagocytosis but on a smaller scale. It occurs in response to proteins or strong solutions of electrolytes. It involves the uptake of liquids and for this reason is also called "cell drinking." This is an energy requiring process.

Receptor-mediated endocytosis is carried out by the plasma membrane containing protein receptors that have ligand binding sites. Vesicles are formed between receptors and ligands, which in turn form endosomes. Ligands separate from the receptors and move to various points in the cell.

7.5.1.4 VIRUSES

Viruses are usually called "non-living" and *differ from bacterial and other "living" organisms* because they (1) don't contain both DNA and RNA, (2) have no metabolic machinery for energy production or protein synthesis, (3) do not develop from other viruses but depend on the host's metabolic machinery to synthesize them, and (4) have no membranes to regulate exit and entry of substances. *Structurally*, most viruses consist of a protein coat (*capsid*) surrounding a core (center) of nucleic acids, which are encoded with genetic information and composed of either DNA or RNA. A *virion* is the form of a virus existing *outside* of a host cell. A *viroid*, similar to a virus, infects plants, and contains only a single strand of RNA and no protein coat. The process by which a virus causes disease is *pathogenesis* and its capacity to produce illness or death is known as *virulence*. *Tropism* is the capacity of a virus to selectively enter and infect cells.

There are many variations of the basic *life cycle* of a virus. A cell may have a special receptor or region that is recognized by the virus and to which the virus attaches. It should be noted that although receptor binding of virus to cell may be exhibited, subsequent steps in the viral life cycle also must be successful for infection to occur. The virus may enter the cell via a process similar to phagocytosis. In the cell, the central core of DNA or RNA and occasionally special enzymes or proteins take over the host's metabolic machinery to produce new coat proteins and new viral DNA or RNA. This may occur in the nucleus or the cytoplasm or both. The viral coat and viral core (DNA or RNA) then combine to form complete viral particles. At a certain point, the host cell lyses (bursts) and releases the new viral particles as well as uncombined viral coats and viral cores. Sometimes the viral particles exit by a process similar to reverse phagocytosis and incorporate part of the host's cell membrane onto their protein coat in doing so. The above is typical of a virus that attacks an animal or plant cell. Once inside the animal host, the primary methods by which viruses reach target organs are via the lymphatic system, the blood stream, or through nerves. The presence of the virus in the blood is called *viremia*. Continued viral infection depends on the balance between ongoing viral replication and host defense mechanisms (i.e., viral clearance and neutralizing antibodies). Antiviral treatment in man is designed to disrupt viral binding or entry into the cell or to interfere with DNA or RNA replication.

Some viruses specifically attack bacteria and are called *bacteriophages* (see Fig. 7.19). Bacteriophages, in general, consist of a *head* made of a protein coat and a core as before, and they also contain a *tail* made of protein which is specialized for attaching to bacteria. A bacteriophage attaches to the surface of a bacteria, the core of RNA or DNA is injected into the bacteria, and the protein coat remains on the surface. Then the cycle may proceed as described for viruses above and is called *lytic* or *virulent*.

However, the bacteriophage nucleic acid may become combined with the bacterial nucleic acid and remain as such for long periods before new bacteriophages are produced and cell rupture occurs. In this case, the bacteriophage is called *lysogenic* or *temperate*. The nucleic acid from the bacteriophage is called a *prophage*. Newly released bacteriophages may contain some bacterial nucleic acid which may be passed on to other bacteria when they are attacked by these bacteriophages. This is the mechanism of transduction.

Rickettsiae multiply by binary fission, contain both RNA and DNA, and have both synthetic and energy-producing enzyme systems; they are now classified as bacteria.

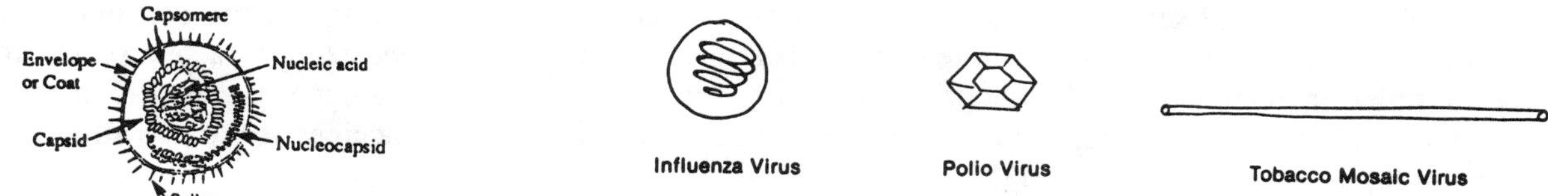

Fig. 7.22—Typical Virus

Fig. 7.23—Several Common Viruses (about 100 nanometers in diameter)

7.5.1.5 AIDS

The *Acquired Immune Deficiency Syndrome (AIDS)* is transmitted by the *human immunodeficiency virus (HIV)*. Two forms of HIV have been identified, HIV-1 and HIV-2. HIV-1 is the more common form. The primary modes of transmission include sexual transmission, parenteral exposure, and perinatal transmission. Individuals at highest risk for HIV infection include homosexual/bisexual men, persons with hemophilia, blood transfusion recipients, IV drug abusers, sex partners of individuals carrying the virus, and children born to mothers with HIV. All patients with HIV do not have AIDS. According to Center for Disease Control (CDC) definition, a person is characterized as having AIDS if s/he has the HIV virus and exhibits one of 23 specific symptoms, such as specific types of pneumonia, cancer, or fungal or parasitic infections. This definition is disease-based, while a new definition, which is currently undergoing a period of public comment, is laboratory-based. Under the new definition, patients would be considered to have AIDS if their *T4 lymphocytes* (white blood cells whose levels are reflective of immune system function) are less than 200 (normal levels are about 1000). The acute stage of infection with HIV may be associated with a mononucleosis-like illness (fever, lymphadenopathy, sweats, myalgia, rash, sore throat, nausea, headache). However, symptoms are generally nonspecific, cause little discomfort, and pass unnoticed. T4 levels are normal at the time of infection. During the early stage, the patient may be asymptomatic, have persistent generalized *lymphadenopathy* (enlargement of the lymph nodes), have aseptic meningitis, have dermatologic manifestations, and T4 levels greater than 400. During the middle stage, the patient may continue to be asymptomatic, have persistent generalized lymphadenopathy, thrush, hairy leukoplakia, or idiopathic thrombocytopenic purpura. At this stage, T4 levels range from 200 to 400. During the late stage the patient develops *opportunistic infections* (infections seen primarily in individuals with an impaired immune system), malignancy (e.g., *Kaposi's sarcoma*), wasting, and dementia; T4 levels are below 200.

HIV is an RNA *retrovirus* in the *"lentivirus"* family. Lentiviruses are characterized by slow progression of infection and persistence of the virus despite the host's immune response. They frequently have a lengthy incubation period before symptoms develop. The interval from the time of infection with HIV to development of the clinical disease averages about 10 years. However, the HIV *antigen* (foreign material to which the body's immune system reacts) can be detected within 1 to 4 weeks and HIV *antibodies* (molecules formed to fight specific antigens) within 3 to 12 weeks following infection.

Structurally, the HIV has a dense cylindrical core that encases two molecules of the viral RNA. The core is surrounded by a spherical lipid envelope that is acquired as the virion buds from the surface of an infected cell. HIV contains three structural genes—one for the viral core, one for the enzymes involved in viral replication, and one for the envelope proteins. The outer envelope of the HIV binds to the *CD4 molecule*, which is expressed on the surface of *T4 cells* and monocyte-macrophages (these cells are essential components of the human immune system; T4 cells activate other T cells, natural killer cells, macrophages, and B cells, which produce antibodies). When the virus invades a human cell, it makes copies of its genes and splices them into the genes of the cell. The infection may enter a latent phase until cellular activation occurs. Upon activation, the genes force the cell to complete the formation of a new HIV and to release a mature virion from the surface of the cell via budding. The ultimate result of HIV infection is a profound immunosuppression caused by depletion and functional abnormalities of the CD4 + T-cell, which leads to the development of opportunistic infections. The immune system normally responds to a viral infection by sensing the protein coat of an invading virus and attacking the invader. In the case of AIDS, the immune system successfully controls the infection for years but, for unknown reasons, is unable to clear it. Over time there is a progressive decline in the quality and function of the CD4 + population and the infection ultimately progresses. As a result, immunity cannot be generated against opportunistic pathogens to which the patient ultimately succumbs. Therapy for AIDS includes antiretroviral agents that inhibit HIV replication (e.g., zidovudine [AZT], ddI, ddC) or interfere with the binding of HIV to CD4 + cells. But it is unlikely that antiretroviral treatment will eradicate the virus in an infected person because it exists in a dormant state for an indefinite period. Therefore vaccines may be the best approach to preventing HIV transmission, infection, and disease progression. Vaccines that stimulate the immune system after infection with HIV but before the development of AIDS are under evaluation, as are vaccines for administration to patients at high-risk of exposure to HIV.

7.5.1.6 GENERAL CHARACTERISTICS OF FUNGI AND THEIR LIFE CYCLE

Fungi are composed of *eukaryotic cells*, are plant-like, but contain *no chlorophyll.* They are *unicellular* (e.g., yeast) or *multicellular* (e.g., molds, mushrooms) with little differentiation into tissue types. They are *parasitic* (survive upon living organisms) or *saprophytic* (survive upon dead organic matter), and they can *digest food* extracellularly by the excretion of digestive enzymes before absorbing them or can *absorb* already digested foods. Multicellular fungi tend to be filamentous with individual filaments called *hyphae.* Masses of hyphae are called mycelia. Fungi are important as causes of disease, in spoilage of food and materials, as decomposers of dead organic matter, as sources of food (mushrooms), in food production (bread yeast, cheese molds), and in alcohol production.

Reproduction is by *sexual* and/or *asexual* means with the latter predominating. The specific cycles vary among the different groups of fungi. Various *sexual stages* include ascus formation (has haploid spores), basidium (2n) formation, or just fusion of special cells to form zygotes (2n). *Asexual structures* or stages include the spores (n), the sporangium (n), and the conidia (n). These are either spores or give rise to spores. The sporangium and conidia arise from specialized hyphae. A general scheme for the life cycle of a typical fungus is in Fig. 7.24.

(Note that the spores can result from sexual or asexual reproduction.)

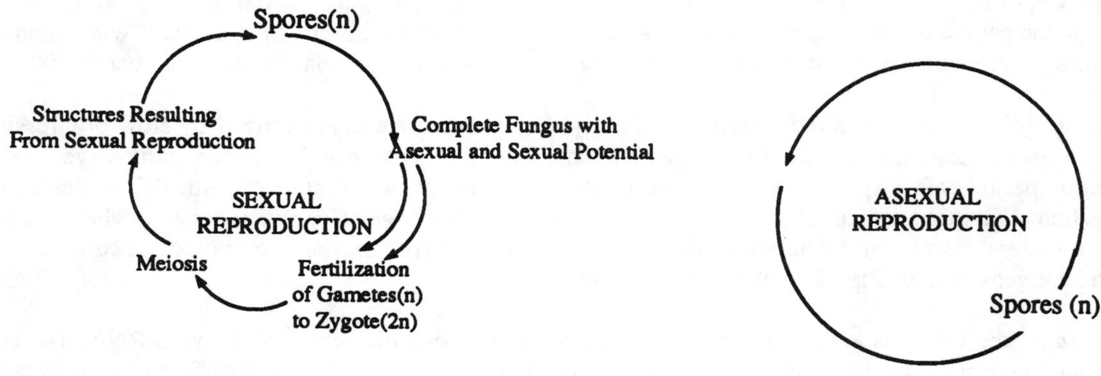

Fig. 7.24—Life Cycle of a Typical Fungus

7.5.2 Questions Related to Prokaryotic and Eukaryotic Cells

1. Bacteriophages:
   - **A.** cause disease in humans.
   - **B.** are viruses.
   - **C.** are bacteria.
   - **D.** can reproduce by binary fission.
2. Select the substance not ordinarily found in viruses:
   - **A.** carbohydrates
   - **B.** proteins
   - **C.** RNA
   - **D.** DNA
3. Viruses:
   - **A.** are considered to be living organisms.
   - **B.** consist of protein, lipids, and carbohydrates only.
   - **C.** do not arise from other viruses directly.
   - **D.** have an incomplete metabolic machinery for energy production.
4. Eukaryotes are characterized by all of the following except:
   - **A.** genetic material within a nuclear envelope.
   - **B.** organelles bound within membranes.
   - **C.** presence of cell walls made of murein.
   - **D.** subcellular structural units to carry out specific functions.
5. "Contains DNA or RNA, no means of energy production, cannot reproduce self directly" would be a description of a (an):
   - **A.** animal cell.
   - **B.** plant cell.
   - **C.** bacteria.
   - **D.** virus.
6. In the replication of a virus in a host cell:
   - **A.** the virus directs the metabolic machinery of the host.
   - **B.** the host directs synthesis of new viral particles.
   - **C.** viral particles are made as a single unit (i.e., coat and core).
   - **D.** coat and core structures are released from the host and then combined.
7. Structurally, bacteriophages differ from the usual virus by:
   - **A.** having a protein coat.
   - **B.** having a core of DNA or RNA.
   - **C.** being able to replicate independently of a host cell.
   - **D.** having a tail region made of protein for attaching to cells.
8. The part of the cycle of a bacteriophage that may be different from that of a typical virus is:
   - **A.** taking over of host cell's metabolic machinery.
   - **B.** incorporation of its nucleic acid into the host cell's nucleic acid.
   - **C.** lysis of host cell.
   - **D.** synthesis by host cell of coat and core separately and then combining to form complete particle.
9. Which structure may protect a bacteria from phagocytosis by white blood cells?
   - **A.** mesosome
   - **B.** capsule
   - **C.** nucleoid
   - **D.** cell wall

10. Select the incorrect association:

A. *cocci*-spherical
B. *bacilli*-rod-like
C. *diplococci*-two cocci
D. *staphylococci*-linear combinations of cocci

11. The process whereby a bacterium picks up DNA from a medium and incorporates it into it's own DNA is called:

A. binary fission.
B. conjugation.
C. transformation.
D. transduction.

12. Bacteria transfer (exchange) genetic information between themselves by all except:

A. transformation.
B. transduction.
C. budding.
D. conjugation.

13. Methods used to distinguish between various bacteria types may include all of the following except:

A. shape.
B. nutrient requirements.
C. products of metabolism.
D. antiseptic surgery.

14. A form of hepatitis (inflammation of the liver) is caused by a virus. The serum of patients with hepatitis may contain antigens from the virus, HB_SAg (hepatitis B surface antigen) and HB_CAg (hepatitis B core antigen). (An antigen is a substance foreign to the body capable of eliciting an immune response.) Select the correct statement:

A. This information is inconsistent with what is known about modes of viral replication.
B. The HB_CAg is probably a lipid.
C. The HB_SAg is probably a protein.
D. Enzymes found in liver cells probably do not increase in the serum during the acute disease.

15. Which of the following agents would block the replication of a virus? Assume all agents can only affect the host cell and its contents.

A. an agent that blocks synthesis of lipids
B. an agent that blocks synthesis of carbohydrates
C. an agent that blocks synthesis of proteins
D. an agent that blocks synthesis of bioorganic molecules

16. In the treatment of viral infections, a drug is discovered that directly blocks the synthesis of the viral protein coat. This drug:

A. probably adversely affects protein synthesis by the host cell and hence may cause side affects in the host.
B. probably does not affect host protein synthesis.
C. probably causes naked virions to fall off because they are not slightly bound to the cell's surface.
D. probably allows coronaviruses, picornaviruses and sometimes togaviruses to function as non-mRNA molecules.

17. Given a bacterial population without resistance to a certain drug, all of the following may cause introduction of bacterial resistance except (excluding mutations):

A. transformation.
B. binary fission.
C. transduction.
D. conjugation.

18. Which is not a feature of the unit membrane model of the cell membrane?

   A. continuous lipid bilayer present
   B. globular proteins floating in lipids
   C. hydrophobic ends of lipids not in contact with water
   D. continuous protein bilayers outside lipid layer

19. The concept of "cell drinking" refers to:

   A. phagocytosis.
   B. pinocytosis.
   C. both phagocytosis and pinocytosis.
   D. neither phagocytosis nor pinocytosis.

20. The substance not ordinarily found in cell membranes is (are):

   A. globular proteins.
   B. phospholipids.
   C. DNA.
   D. cholesterol.

21. Active Transport is due to:

   A. thermal diffusion.
   B. concentration gradient variations.
   C. phagocytosis.
   D. Na-K-ATPase pump.

22. Which of the following is *not* a function of smooth endoplasmic reticulum?

   A. metabolism of drugs and toxins in the liver
   B. synthesis of proteins
   C. conduction of impulses in muscle
   D. synthesis of steroids

23. Chloroplasts are:

   A. found only in prokaryotes.
   B. vestigial structures in animal cells.
   C. responsible in producing negative ions.
   D. used during photosynthesis.

24. Mitochondria are responsible for:

   A. transport of molecules.
   B. protein synthesis.
   C. cell replication.
   D. energy production.

25. Synthesis of proteins occurs in the:

   A. lysosomes.
   B. Golgi bodies.
   C. mitochondria.
   D. rough endoplasmic reticulum.

26. Centrioles:

   A. exist in the nucleus.
   B. constitute chromosomes.
   C. make microvilli.
   D. form spindle fibers during cell division.

27. Facilitated diffusion:

A. enables carrier substances to carry molecules across the membrane.
B. can go against a concentration gradient.
C. requires energy.
D. is a result of saturation kinetics.

28. If container A has a higher concentration of a solute than container B, and they are separated by a semipermeable (to solute) membrane, then:

A. nothing happens because the membrane is only semipermeable.
B. solute particles move from B to A.
C. solvent moves from B to A.
D. solvent moves from A to B.

29. What probably limits the size a cell may attain?

A. surface area
B. volume of a cell
C. balance of surface area and volume
D. specialization of the cell

30. Which structure below is found in eukaryotes but not prokaryotes?

A. ribosomes
B. mesosomes
C. cell walls
D. mitochondria

31. Which structure or molecule is *not* found or made in the nucleus of eukaryotes?

A. nucleolus
B. microsomes
C. tRNA
D. chromatin

32. If red blood cells are put into a hypertonic solution, they will:

A. remain the same size.
B. hemolyze.
C. swell up.
D. shrink.

33. Which structure does not play a part in motion of cells?

A. microvilli
B. cilia
C. flagella
D. pseudopods

34. Which of the following substances probably would not cross a membrane by simple diffusion?

A. ethanol
B. chloride ion
C. glucose
D. water

7.5.3 Answers to Questions in Section 7.5.2

(1) B (2) A (3) C (4) C (5) D (6) A (7) D (8) B (9) B (10) D (11) C (12) C
(13) D (14) C (15) C (16) A (17) B (18) B (19) B (20) C (21) D (22) B (23) D (24) D
(25) D (26) D (27) A (28) C (29) C (30) D (31) B (32) D (33) A (34) C

7.5.4 Discussion of Answers to Questions in Section 7.5.2

Questions #1 to #13 Discussed in Section.

Question #14 (Answer: C) From the knowledge about viral replication, the coat (protein) and core (nucleic acid) are synthesized separately and then combined. When cell lysis occurs, complete viral particles as well as coat (e.g., HB_sAg) and core (HB_cAg) may be released. Since the cells do lyse, their contents would also appear (e.g., the liver enzymes). And, since the antigens are found in the serum, it is not unreasonable to expect the liver enzymes to be there also. In fact, a rise in certain liver enzymes are key to the diagnosis of hepatitis. Also, since incomplete viral particles are liberated into the serum, it might be expected that other viral products might also appear as antigens. Some do, for example the "e"-antigen and viral DNA-polymerase.

Question #15 (Answer: C) Viruses need the synthesis of proteins by the host cell machinery to make their protein coats as well as enzymes necessary to make nucleic acids.

Question #16 (Answer: A) It is the host's metabolic machinery that makes viral protein. Therefore, if the synthesis of viral coat protein is blocked, it is likely, not absolutely necessary, that this is due to a blockage of host protein synthesis.

Question #17 (Answer: B) Without new mutations, binary fission can only produce identical non-resistant daughter cells. The other mechanisms allow the introduction of new nucleic acid which may contain drug resistant genes.

Question #18 to #27 Discussed in Section.

Question #28 (Answer: C) The solvent moves across the semipermeable membrane from the side *it* is more concentrated, and the solute is less concentrated (which is side B), to the side where it is less concentrated (and the solute is more concentrated) which is side A. This is osmosis.

Question #29 (Answer: C) This is not discussed in the Section. The reasoning is as follows: the nutritional and energy requirements and waste production are proportional to the volume of the cell. The volume of a cell is proportional to a linear dimension (l = length) cubed, i.e., l^3. The flux (i.e., the exchange rates) of materials in (nutrients) and out (wastes) is proportional to the surface area of a cell. The surface area is proportional to a linear dimension squared, i.e., l^2. As the cell increases in size (as volume increases), the requirements, given by l^3, increase much more rapidly than supply and waste removal, given by l^2. Hence, a balance between surface area and volume is required such that supply (and waste removal) can keep in balance with cell requirements.

Question #30 (Answer: D) Membrane-bound organelles are not found in prokaryotes, e.g., the mitochondrion. The cell walls (also in plants) and mesosomes (invaginations of cell membrane) are found in prokaryotes. Ribosomes are found in both, although the structures are different.

Question #31 (Answer: B) Microsomes are artifacts produced from the endoplasmic reticulum during cell homogenization and centrifugation. Nucleolus and chromatin are parts of DNA. All RNA, including tRNA, are made from the DNA template in the nucleus.

Question #32 (Answer: D) This is discussed in the Section. The solvent (water) flows from the hypotonic (red cells) to the hypertonic solution by osmosis.

Question #33 (Answer: A) Microvilli and pseudopods were not discussed in the Section. The latter are cytoplasmic extensions that aid in motion as found in amoeba. Microvilli are evaginations (out pouches) of the cell membrane which increase its surface area. Its function is to permit more area for flux of materials in and out of cells, as in the gut.

Question #34 (Answer: C) This is alluded to in the Section. Some ions, lipid soluble substances, and very small molecules (such as ethanol, glycerol, urea) can diffuse through membranes. Polar molecules, ions (especially cations), and larger molecules must enter by other processes.

7.5.5 Advanced Concepts

- Recognize and understand the following terms:
  - — specificity, saturation and competition in mediated transport
  - — cell inclusions e.g., glycogen, melanin pigment and hemoglobin
  - — problems in basic physiology related to tonicity (isotonic, hypotonic, hypertonic) and calculation of osmolarity and osmolality
  - — integral and peripheral proteins (compare/contrast), cristae, cisternae (trans, medial and cis), nucleosome, microtrabeculae, autophagy, hyaluronic acid, metastasis, autocrine motility factor (AMF), megakaryocytes, macrophages, polypeptide growth factor, interleukin, fibrils, connective tissue (embryonic, adipose, reticular, vascular)
  - — random growth of cancer cells, malignant tumors, chemotherapy procedures
- Understand the significance of bacteria in medicine (size of bacteria, gram + or gram – bacteria and multiplying ratio and rate) such as: *pseudomonadales, eubacteriales, spirochaetales, actinomycetales, rickettsiales, mycoplasmatales* etc.
- Recognize and understand the following terms: bacterial cytoplasm, movement of bacterial DNA (intercellular movement by conjugation, transduction and transformation), endospores, auxotrophs, bacterial surface analysis (study of extracellular gels and slimes causing stickiness to surfaces), bacterial infections (laboratory procedures such as incubation and basic treatment methods of salmonellosis, shigellosis, staphylococcal and streptococcal infections)
- Understand the medical usage of terms such as: specific immunity; cellular immunity (T-lymphocytes, and humoral immunity (B-lymphocytes); cytotoxic T-cells; heterophilic antigens; agglutination (Weil-Felix test); opsonization; IgA, IgD, IgE, IgG, IgM; allergies and hypersensitivities; Coombs test; immuno-hematology Ouchterlony test; radial immunodiffusion procedure; viroids, prions, and virusoids.
- Read more to conceptualize energy; T-cells and how 2 signals are used before they attack an invading virus (applications in renal transplants, hay fever, etc.) hybridomas (how are cells created in the laboratory?)
- Introductory interpretation with comparison and contrast of DNA viruses (herpesviruses, poxviruses, rhabdoviridae, togaviridae). Go over the laboratory cultivation and analysis techniques e.g., inoculation techniques, electron microscope analysis of biopsies and darkfield microscope analysis
- Study the life cycles and current research papers on viral cancer, Epstein-Barr virus, papilloma virus, human T-cell leukemia-lymphoma-virus-1 and life history of fungi substantiating blastomycosis, histoplasmosis and rhinosporidiosis.
- Identify the basic sterilization and disinfection tests such as: phenol coefficient test, tissue toxicity test, use-dilution test; air and liquid filtration systems; ultraviolet radiation sterilization and physical sterilization (ultra-high heat) methods.

7.6 ENZYMES (MOLECULAR BIOLOGY)

7.6.1 Introduction to Enzymes

Focus on the molecular structure and functions of enzymes for the human body. Understand that enzymes are chiral molecules and behave as stereospecific or geometry specific biochemicals. Remember classification of enzymes as isomerases, ligases, oxidoreductases, transferases, hydrolases and lyases. Review the molecular structure and special functions of elastase, plasmin, trypsin, urease, α-amylase, enterokinase and bovine pancreatic ribonuclease. Recognize allosteric effectors and the role they play in enzymology. Identify important coenzymes such as biotin, nicotinamide and lipoic acid.

7.6.1.1 STRUCTURE AND FUNCTION

Enzymes are the agents by which organisms make (anabolism) needed molecules or are involved in biosynthesis. Enzymes also break down complex molecules (catabolism) into simpler ones thus producing energy, and, in general, maintain homeostasis (e.g., by regulating entry and exit of molecules and ions). A key aspect of their function is that they can be regulated to function as needed.

The total enzyme (holoenzyme) may be composed of a protein (apoenzyme) part with or without an associated molecule called a *prosthetic group* (nonprotein organic molecule) also called a *cofactor or coenzyme* or a *metal ion*. The enzyme molecule *catalyzes* (by lowering the activation energy) chemical reactions at the conditions found in living organisms—conditions under which these reactions would not ordinarily occur. Note that the protein part passes through the reaction unchanged (like a true catalyst), but the prosthetic groups, etc., which function as donors or acceptors of chemical groups, may or may not pass through the reaction unchanged. Some enzymes exist as zymogens and need to be activated by the cleaving of certain peptide bonds. A portion of the molecule may or may not be lost, but a conformational change usually occurs to expose the active site of the enzyme. An example is the conversion of trypsinogen to trypsin by enterokinase.

A key feature of enzyme function is its *specificity*. This means that enzymes are able to recognize certain molecules and not others due to minor chemical differences between them. A microenvironment is created by the tertiary structure of the protein that creates distinctive requirements of spatial and electrical organization (distribution of positive/negative charges or polar groups) that a molecule must possess in order to be bound by the molecule. This microenvironment need not be rigid as in the lock (enzyme) and key (molecule or substrate) idea, but may be inducible in the enzyme by the substrate as in the "induced fit hypothesis." Specificity may be *absolute* (only one molecule acceptable to the enzyme) or *relative* (a series of molecules acceptable, but some more than others). Note that since enzyme reactions are reversible, an enzyme can still have absolute specificity by reacting with one molecule in one direction and with another molecule in the opposite direction. The bonding is of a non-covalent type (hydrogen, ionic, van der Waals, hydrophobic).

Another key aspect of enzyme function is the *active site* idea. The substrate (molecule) is bound as discussed under specificity above. The appropriate chemical reaction is then catalyzed by structures in this active site. Note that for a reaction to occur the molecule bound must be able to undergo the reaction catalyzable by the enzyme. It is doubtful that the active site functions by causing mechanical bond strain in appropriate bonds, such that they are broken and new ones are made. Rather, the active site has the appropriate side groups of the amino acids, appropriate prosthetic groups, etc., and a microenvironment all conducive to lowering the activation energy of the reaction. The combination required varies with the type of reaction being catalyzed. For example, a reaction that involves a hydrolysis reaction of an ester may have serine (with its – OH group) to displace the alcoholic part of the ester, aspartic acid (with its $-CO_2H$) and/or histidine (acts as acid or base) for acid-base catalysis, and a hydrophilic microenvironment (versus a hydrophobic one) because ions are produced during the reaction.

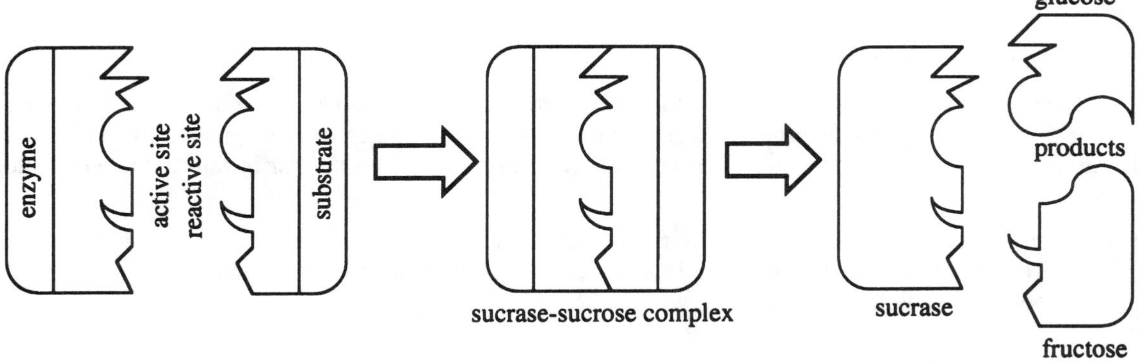

Fig. 7.25—Enzyme and Substrate Model
(Two parts of a jigsaw puzzle)

In 1958, the induced fit theory was introduced. This theory states that the active site of an enzyme must adjust to fit the reactive site of the substrate. As the enzyme and the substrate join, the enzyme may change slightly in shape to fit the substrate better. In both the lock and key hypothesis and the induced fit theory, a specific interaction occurs between the enzyme's active site and the substrate's reactive site. During the interaction, the enzyme and the substrate are joined by weak chemical bonds that are made and broken easily. Look at the equation for the breakdown of sucrose by sucrase, shown below:

sucrase + sucrose → sucrase-sucrose complex → sucrase + glucose + fructose
enzyme + substrate → enzyme – substrate complex → enzyme + product.

In conclusion, the discussion above shows that the lock and key model provides a rigid conformation of the enzyme, whereas the induced fit model provides a flexible configuration. In addition, the lock and key model does not consider the effects of allosteric ligands (molecules that bind to the enzyme at a place other than the active site to cause a conformational change in the enzyme).

Enzyme Activity Control (Feedback Inhibition)

Enzymes are controlled in a number of ways. *Feedback inhibition* (FI) is a basic and effective method of enzyme control. In FI, the product of the enzyme reaction feeds back and blocks the enzyme from converting more substrate to product. In this manner, excessive product is not produced. Similarly, when the product is present in low amounts, there is no enzyme inhibition and the enzyme is converting substrate to product. Graphically:

Enzyme Reaction:	**Substrate (S) $\xrightarrow{\text{Enzyme (E)}}$ Product (P)**
Excess Product:	**(1) Excess product present: $S \xrightarrow{E} P$**
	(2) Enzyme binds product: E······P
	(3) Reaction is blocked: $S \overset{E \cdots P}{\nrightarrow}$
Insufficient Product:	**(1) Low amounts of product: $S \xrightarrow{E} P$**
	(2) Enzyme does not bind product
	(3) Reaction proceeds: $S \xrightarrow{E} P$

Names of Enzymes

Enzymes are usually named for the reaction they cause or for their substrate. A substrate is the substance upon which the enzyme acts. Most enzyme names end in the letters -ase. The enzyme sucrase is named for the substrate sucrose. Some enzymes are named for the reaction they cause and their substrate, such as the enzyme DNA polymerase, which helps make the molecules of DNA.

Enzyme Cofactors or Coenzymes

Many enzymes are made up of protein and a nonprotein part. A nonprotein molecule found in some enzymes is called a coenzyme. Coenzymes are organic molecules that work with enzymes. A coenzyme binds weakly to the protein part of an enzyme, and can join and leave it easily. Coenzymes are needed for certain chemical reactions to take place.

Some coenzymes are made of vitamins or their parts. Organisms cannot make most vitamins and must take them in as part of their food. If vitamins are lacking, certain coenzymes cannot be made and the organism's metabolism does not function normally.

7.6.2 Questions Related to Enzymes

1. Enzymes probably play a direct role in all of the following except:

A. maintenance of resting membrane potential by extrusion of Na^+ from cells.
B. synthesis of mRNA from DNA.
C. storage of hereditary information.
D. production of ATP.

2. Since enzymes are proteins, they are affected by the same factors that affect proteins. An enzyme is "designed" to function under a certain set of conditions. Which of the following conditions would be most conducive to the normal function of a human cellular enzyme?

   A. Temperature = 25° C
   B. Temperature = 37° C
   C. pH = 1.0
   D. pH = 10.0

3. NAD^+ is a non-covalently bound coenzyme for the enzyme α-glycerol-phosphate dehydrogenase. NAD^+ picks up an H^{-1} (hydride) and becomes NADH; the enzyme is not affected by the reaction. The activation energy was lowered by the system.

   A. This is not true catalysis because the NAD^+ was changed in the reaction.
   B. This is true catalysis because the NAD^+ was not covalently bound to the enzyme.
   C. This is true catalysis because the activation energy of the reaction was lowered by the enzyme which was unchanged in the reaction.
   D. None of the above are correct.

4. Succinate dehydrogenase catalyzes the following reaction:

   succinate ⇌ fumarate.

   The specificity of the enzyme is:
   A. relative because it binds more than one substrate.
   B. absolute because it catalyzes only one reaction of one pair of substrates.
   C. absolute because it has only one substrate, succinate.
   D. none of the above.

5. D-amino acid oxidase catalyzes the following reaction:

$$\underset{\underset{\text{HNR}'}{|}}{\text{R–}\overset{(1)}{\text{C}}\text{H–}\overset{(2)}{\text{C}}\text{O}_2\text{H}} + 1/2\ O_2 \longrightarrow \text{R–}\underset{\underset{\text{O}}{\|}}{\text{C}}\text{–CO}_2\text{H} + \text{R}'\text{NH}_2.$$

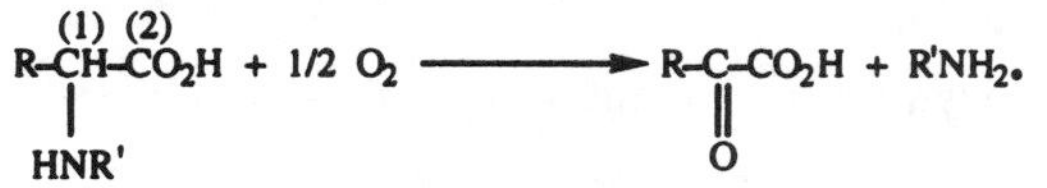

Following are some relative rates of reaction of various substrates with this enzyme.

Substrate	Relative Rate	R	R'
D-Tyrosine	13.6	$-C_6H_4-OH$	H
D-Alanine	4.6	$-CH_3$	H
D-Isoleucine	1.6	$-CH(CH_3)-CH_2-CH_3$	H
D-Leucine	1.0	$-CH_2-CH(CH_3)_2$	H
L-Tyrosine	0	$-C_6H_4-OH$	H
L-Leucine	0	$-CH_2-CH(CH_3)_2$	H
D-Leucylalanyltyrosine	0	$-C_6H_4-OH$	$-C(=O)-CH(CH_3)-NH-C(=O)-CH(NH_2)-CH_2-CH(CH_3)_2$

Fig. 7.26—Relative Rates of Substrate Reactions

The above information implies that:

   A. the specificity of D-amino acid oxidase is absolute because D-tyrosine has a much higher rate of reaction than other substrates.
   B. the configuration of carbon #1 is not important for the reaction to occur.
   C. from the data given, the group at R has more effect on the outcome of the reaction than the group at R′.
   D. the specificity of the enzyme is relative because several molecules may react with the enzyme.

6. Enzymes usually combine readily with substrates in order for a reaction to occur. When the reaction is over, the product (derived from the substrate) usually readily dissociates from the enzyme. This is in spite of only minor changes in the substrate. A reason for this might be that (the best of those given):

   A. although the site of attachment for the substrate has not changed, the overall conformation of the enzyme may be made unfavorable to the product by the reaction.
   B. minor differences in spatial or electrical organization of a molecule are all that are required to make a molecule unacceptable to the enzyme.
   C. the enzyme is forced into an unnatural conformation and this causes it to forceably expel the product.
   D. the substrate is covalently bound to the enzyme because of the enzyme's specificity, whereas the product is not.

7. Malonate blocks (inhibits) the catalysis of the following reaction by succinate dehydrogenase:

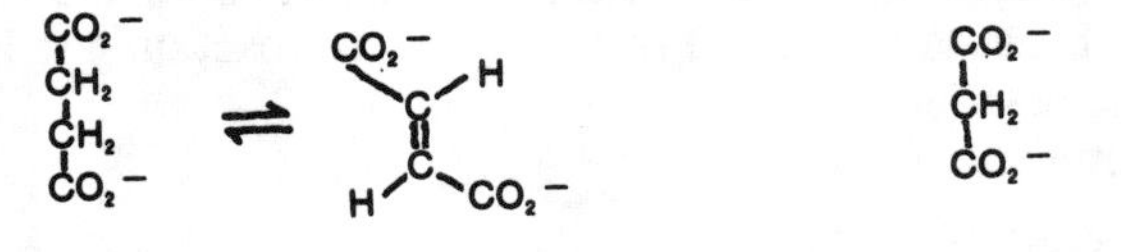

Fig. 7.27—Catalytic Inhibitors

Diethyl malonate will not block the reaction. Nor will the diethyl esters of succinate or fumarate undergo the reaction. The above information implies that:

   (I). inhibition of the enzyme may be brought about by molecules that resemble the substrate but cannot undergo the reaction.
   (II). the active site of the enzyme may contain positive ions or at least require the presence of $-CO_2^-$ on the substrate.
   (III). monoethyl malonate will not inhibit the reaction.

   A. (I) only
   B. (II) and (III) only
   C. (I) and (II) only
   D. all are implied by the data

7.6.3 Answers to Questions in Section 7.6.2

(1) C (2) B (3) C (4) B (5) D (6) B (7) C

7.6.4 Discussion of Answers to Questions in Section 7.6.2

Question #1 (Answer: C) The storage of hereditary information is a function of DNA, enzymes play no direct role in this. All of the other processes require direct involvement of enzymes.

Question #2 (Answer: B) The function of a cellular enzyme should be maximal at those conditions found in the internal milieu of a cell or a particular compartment of a cell. This would generally be conditions similar to the whole organism. The temperature of 37° C is the normal body temperature and the normal pH of blood is 7.40. The other conditions are extreme, but there are enzymes that can function at or near most of these—some in the human, some not.

Question #3 (Answer: C) True catalysis occurs when the activation energy is lowered and this lowering is accomplished by the enzyme's active site environment. Coenzymes serve the accessory function of transferring chemical groups.

Question #4 (Answer: B) Nearly all enzymatic reactions are truly reversible. The product occupies the same site occupied by the substrate, so the enzyme can recognize it, and the substrate-product can be considered as a pair.

Question #5 (Answer: D) The relative specificity of the enzyme should be clear from the several different substrates undergoing the reaction. A case might be made for the "absolute" specificity for D-amino acids which is supported by the data. The configuration of carbon #1 is essential to the reactivity of the substrate because this is the carbon about which the *D* or *L* configuration is determined (see α-amino acids in Section 7.2.1.1). The *R* group represents the side chains of the various amino acids, if the configuration is D at the α-carbon (#1 in diagram), the reaction can still occur although variable. The R′ could represent a second amino acid (or more), as in D-leucylalanyltyrosine, which does not react at all. Hence, with the limited information given, the presence of a group (other than H) appears critical in the reaction.

Question #6 (Answer: B) Although the other options may sound reasonable, the simplest reason is as in (B) which serves to emphasize that only small differences in substrate structures can affect enzyme recognition and reaction.

Question #7 (Answer: C) The structures not given are

O = C-O-CH_2-CH_3
CH_2
O = C-O-CH_2CH_3
Diethyl malonate

O=C-O⁻
CH_2
O=C-O-CH_2CH_3
Monoethyl malonate

O = C-OCH_2CH_3
CH_2
CH_2
O = C-OCH_2CH_3
Diethyl succinate

CH_3CH_2O-C(=O)-CH=CH-C(=O)-OCH_2CH_3
Diethyl fumarate

Statement (I) is reasonable given that malonate and succinate are similar and since specificity is based upon similarity in structure. Also this reaction requires the group,

$$-CH_2-CH_2- \longrightarrow -CH=CH- + H^+ ; H:^-$$

for the reaction to occur and malonate does not have this. So, malonate will bind at the active site and block succinate; but it will just sit there and not react. It appears that only molecules with two (or one?) $-CO_2^-$ (which is negative) are attracted to the active site. There is no evidence one way or the other about a molecule with one $-CO_2^-$ and one $-CO_2CH_2CH_3$.

7.6.5 Advanced Concepts

- Identify basic comparative relationships among catalytic mechanisms (cationic, acid-base, electrostatic, nucleophilic covalent and electrophilic covalent).
- Describe the structure and functions of digestive enzymes such as carboxypeptidase, aminopeptidase, pepsin, maltase and sucrase.
- Familiarize yourself with enzyme kinetics (but *not* in too much detail) emphasizing: assumptions in various models; Michaelis-Menten equation forms and how to graph them; catalytic efficiency; competitive and uncompetitive inhibitors; pH effect on rate of enzymatic reaction; bibi reactions (bisubstrate reactions such as Ping Pong Bi Bi reactions and Rapid equilibrium random Bi Bi reactions).
- Learn various applications of biocatalyst electrodes to: biofuel cells, bioreactors, clinical integrated microbiosensors (amperometric) and the electropolymerization process.

7.7 CELLULAR METABOLISM (MOLECULAR BIOLOGY)

7.7.1 Introduction to Cellular Metabolism

Cellular metabolism consists of a series of complex biochemical reactions. These reactions are of four types: (1) Carbon bond reactions (making and breaking of C bonds), (2) Isomerization, substitution and reorganizing reactions, (3) oxidation and reduction reactions and (4) electrophilic group-transfer reactions (nucleophile to nucleophile). Learn to apply and integrate these four reactions with the four major biochemical processes of glycolysis, citric acid cycle, electron transport chain and oxidative phosphorylation. Understand various mechanisms which determine and control biochemical synthesis of lipids, fatty acids, lipoproteins, amino acids and urea. Relate biochemical synthesis to basal metabolic rate. Carefully review Gibbs free energy linked to cellular metabolism. In doing so, compare and contrast exergonic, isogonic and endergonic reactions related to $\Delta G = \Delta G° + RT (\ln[P_1][P_2]/[R_1][R_2])$. P_1, P_2 are the biochemical products and R_1, R_2 are the biochemical reactants. Understand Lipmann's law as it applies to eukaryotes and prokaryotes. Lipmann's law states that "The ADP-ATP coupling is the receptor and distributor of biochemical energy in *all* living organisms (or more complex systems)."

7.7.1.1 BIOCHEMICAL ENERGY PRODUCTION

Energy production involves the step-wise degradation of organic molecules *from more reduced to more oxidized states* (reduced means abundance of hydrogen atoms and lack of, or few, oxygen atoms). The process may be *aerobic* (in the presence of oxygen) or *anaerobic* (without the presence of oxygen). *Fermentation* is a type of anaerobic respiration where the final acceptor of electrons is an organic molecule. In aerobic respiration, O_2 is the final acceptor of electrons producing H_2O (the fate of hydrogens in organic molecules being oxidized) and CO_2 is also produced (the fate of carbon). (See Section 7.16.1 for the fate of nitrogen.)

Key organic molecules in energy production are:

(1) *ATP* (adenosine triphosphate). The bonds between the inorganic ortho phosphates (P_i) are high energy (P~P), and when hydrolyzed (split by adding water), this energy (about 7-8 kcals/mole) is released. ATP is the main short term energy storage molecule. ADP (adenosine diphosphate) and P_i combine to form ATP.

(2) *NAD* $^+$ *and NADP* $^+$ (nicotinamide adenine dinucleotide and nicotinamide adenine dinucleotide phosphate). These carry two electrons and one hydrogen to form, respectively, NADH and NADPH (reduced forms of coenzymes NAD and NADP respectively). NADH transfers its electrons to the electron transport system. NADPH is used for synthetic purposes and is the major product of the Pentose Shunt in which glucose-6-phosphate dehydrogenase is a key enzyme. ($NADH_2$ is also a reduced form of the coenzyme NADP.) Niacin is a part of NAD^+ and $NADP^+$.

(3) *FAD* (flavin adenine dinucleotide). FAD carries two electrons and two hydrogens as $FADH_2$ (reduced form of coenzyme FAD) to the electron transport chain. Its most important role is in the breakdown of fatty acids. Riboflavin is a component of FAD.

(4) *Cytochromes* (b, c, a). They transfer electrons (which are attached to iron) and they are part of the electron transport chain. The iron is in a porphyrin ring (together called heme) which is bound by a protein.

7.7.1.2 BIOCHEMICAL PROCESSES

The *four key processes* of energy production are glycolysis, the citric acid cycle (Krebs cycle, Tricarboxylic Acid Cycle or TCA cycle), the electron transport system (ETS), and oxidative phosphorylation. Gluconeogenesis and glycogen synthesis should be studied after glycolysis to understand the differences.

Glycolysis (Figs. 7.28, 7.29) takes glucose (C_6) and converts it to two pyruvates (C_3). This produces 2ATPs and 2NADHs. If no oxygen is around, the NADH converts pyruvate to lactic acid (as in exercise) which may be converted to alcohol (as in a type of fermentation). The latter process is *anaerobic glycolysis*. In the presence of oxygen, the pyruvate (C_3) is converted to acetyl CoA (C_2) and CO_2 with 2NADHs produced per original glucose. CoA (Coenzyme A) is an acyl carrier and the vitamin pantothenic acid is a key component. Acetyl CoA may also arise from fatty acid and amino acid breakdown. The acetyl CoA (C_2) enters the *citric acid cycle* (Fig. 7.30) by combining with oxaloacetic acid (C_4) to form citrate (C_6). This is degraded step-wise to oxaloacetic acid again producing 3NADHs, $1FADH_2$, and 1ATP (from GTP, guanosine triphosphate) for each cycle (must double to get production per original glucose) as well as CO_2 and H_2O. The NADH and $FADH_2$ enter the *ETS* (Fig. 7.31) in this sequence:

$$\begin{array}{ccc} (1) & (2) & (3) \end{array}$$
$$NAD \rightarrow FAD \rightarrow \text{ubiquinone (CoQ)} \rightarrow \text{Cyt b} \rightarrow \text{Cyt c} \rightarrow \text{Cyt a} \rightarrow O_2$$

Each intermediate is first reduced (receives electrons from) by the preceding and oxidized (gives electrons to) by the following, with oxygen as the final acceptor being converted to water. ATPs are produced at 1, 2, and 3 by the process called *oxidative phosphorylation* (Fig. 7.32). Each NADH produces 3ATPs and each $FADH_2$ produces 2ATPs. Malonate is a potent inhibitor of the citric acid cycle. Cyanide is a potent inhibitor of the ETS at Cyt a. An exception is the NADH produced outside the mitochondria from glycolysis. The electrons of NADH are transported by a shuttle to ubiquinone and only 2ATPs per NADH (of glycolysis) are produced.

Glycolysis occurs in the cell cytoplasm. The citric acid cycle occurs in the matrix of the mitochondrion. Electron transport and oxidative phosphorylation occur on the inner membrane of the mitochondrion. The transfer of electrons down the respiratory chain from NADH to molecular oxygen is the primary source of the energy utilized for the formation of ATP by the coupling of ADP phosphorylation.

The net product in the linking of electron transport and oxidative phosphorylation can be expressed by,

$$NADH + H^+ + 3ADP + 3P_i + 1/2\, O_2 \rightarrow$$
$$NAD^+ + 3ATP + 4H_2O$$

Anaerobic glycolysis yields a net of 2ATPs per glucose. *Aerobic glycolysis* (because it proceeds to the citric acid cycle and ETS) yields a total of 38ATPs per glucose. Of the 686 kcals (for glucose $\rightarrow$ $CO_2 + H_2O$), aerobic processes store 308 kcals (for 45% efficiency) as ATP; anaerobic efficiency is much less. Fats store the most energy (9.1 kcals/gm), whereas proteins (about 4.1) and carbohydrate (approximately 4) are about the same.

Gluconeogenesis and Glycogen Synthesis

In animals the primary site for gluconeogenesis or formation of glucose is the liver. The involvement of oxaloacetate in the initial steps of gluconeogenesis provides a connection between this process and the Krebs cycle. All of the intermediates of the Krebs cycle may thus serve as precursors of glucose.

Gluconeogenesis requires a supply of pyruvate. In animals the primary source is the lactate and pyruvate produced by the glycolysis occurring in active skeletal muscle. Lactate and pyruvate can easily penetrate cell membranes and enter the blood for transport to the liver. Glycogen, a glucose polymer and storage form of glucose in animals is required for the expenditure of energy (UTP, uridine triphosphate) in animals.

Glycogen
Glycogenolysis ↓↑ Glycogenesis
Glucose
Glycolysis ↓↑ Gluconeogenesis
Lactate

STEP	Molecules Produced	ATP Yield
Glycolysis	2ATP	2ATP
	2NADH	4ATP + 2ATP*
Pyruvate to acetyl CoA	2NADH	6ATP
Citric Acid Cycle (2 turns)	2ATP	2ATP
	6NADH	18ATP
	$2FADH_2$	4ATP
* These 2ATPs are used up in transporting the electrons across the mitochondrial membranes.		38ATP

Fig. 7.28—Glycolysis

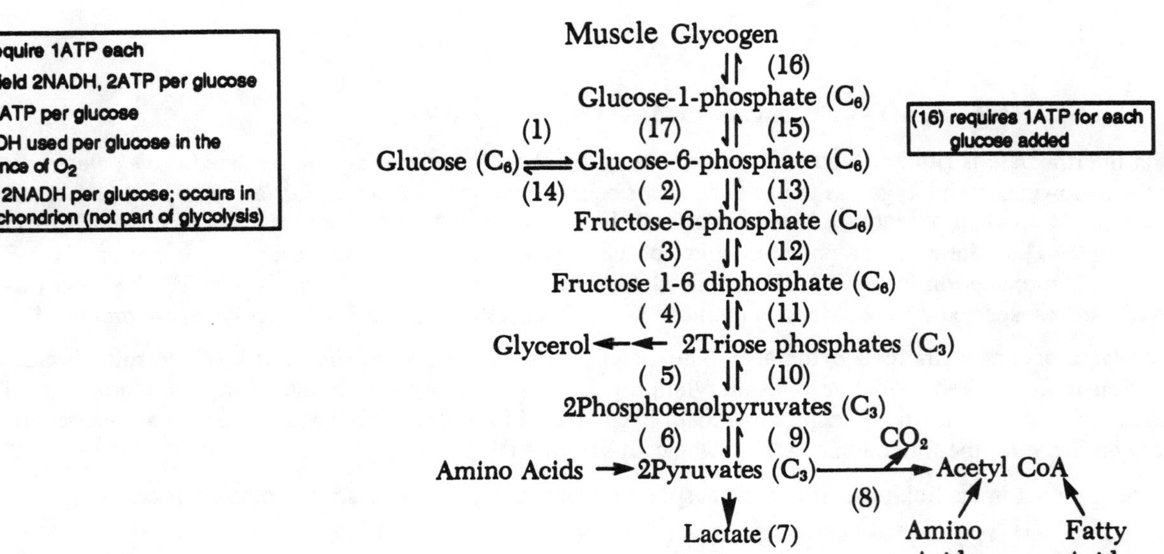

Fig. 7.29—Glycolysis (1-8), Gluconeogenesis (9-14), Glycogenesis (15-16)

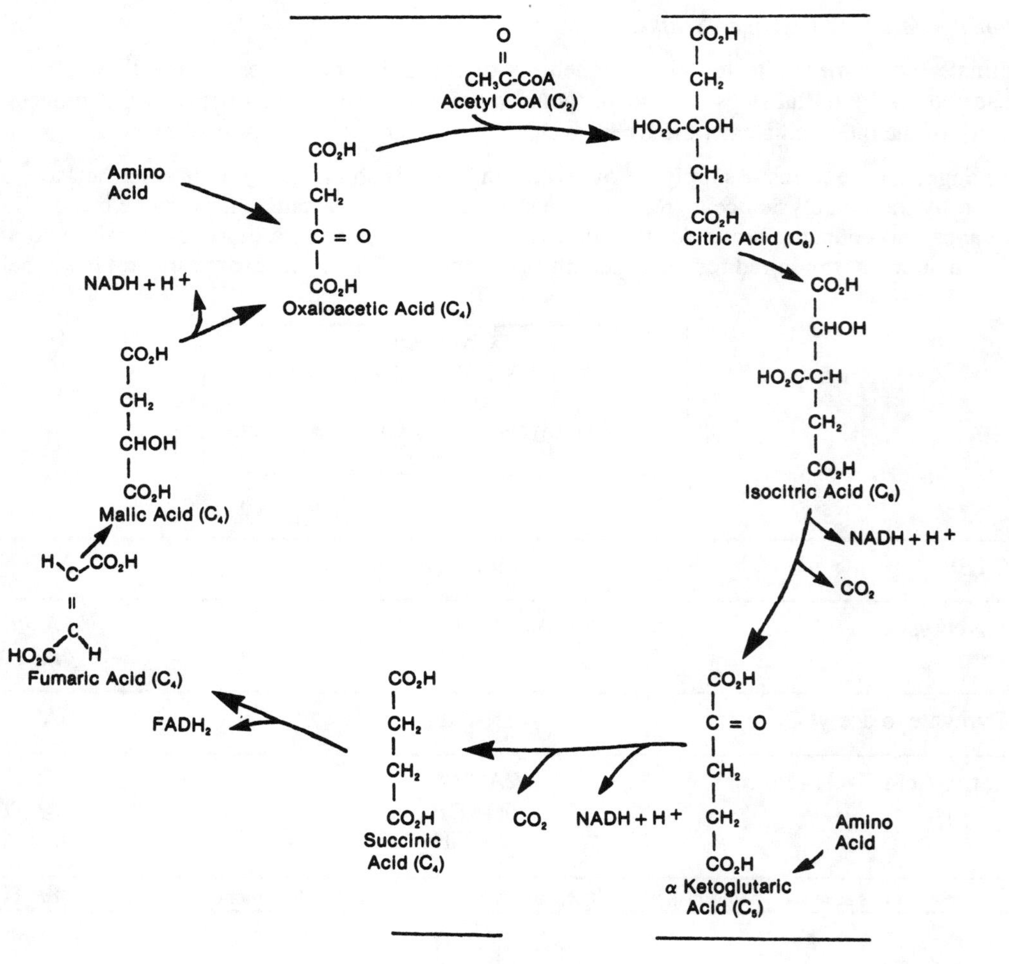

Fig. 7.30—Citric Acid Cycle

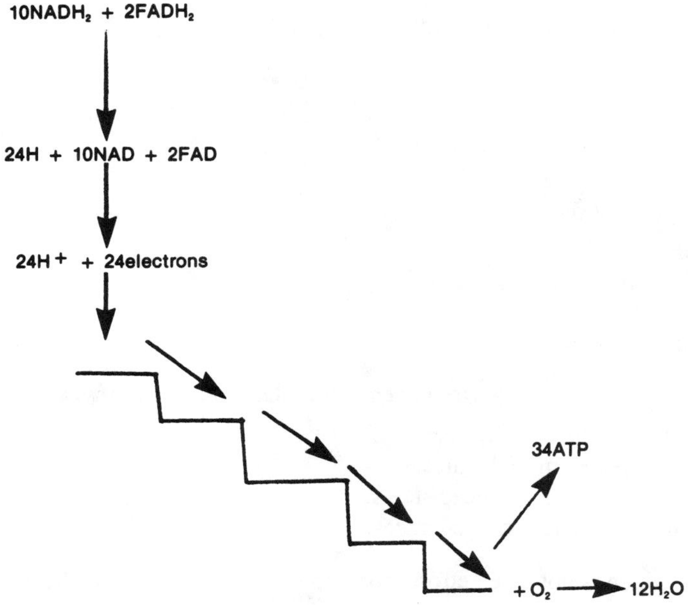

Fig. 7.31— Electron Transport Chain

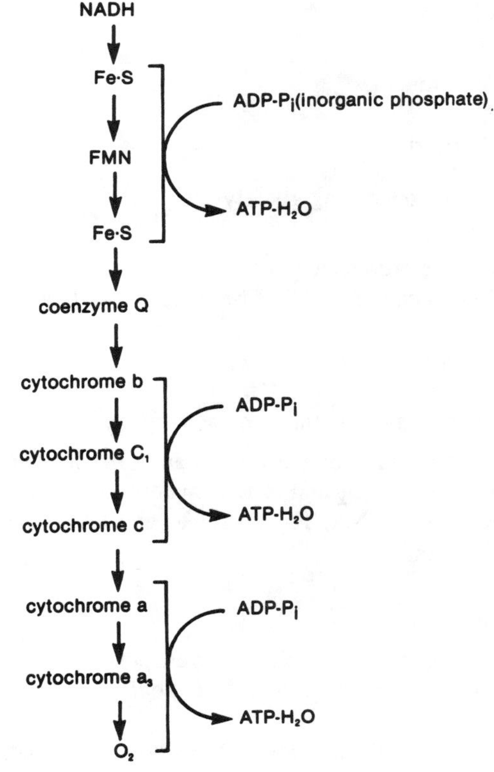

Fig. 7.32—Oxidative Phosphorylation

7.7.2 Questions Related to Cellular Metabolism

1. Which substance has the highest energy content per gram?

A. proteins
B. fats
C. carbohydrates
D. phospholipids

2. The cytochromes are part of the:

A. citric acid cycle.
B. oxidative phosphorylation.
C. glycolysis.
D. electron transport system.

3. In the biological production of energy from chemical molecules, the step-wise degradation is:

A. by addition of hydrogens to molecules.
B. by removal of oxygen from molecules.
C. from more oxidized to more reduced states.
D. from more reduced to more oxidized states.

4. Select the substance which is not an electron carrier in cellular energy production:

A. NAD^+
B. ATP
C. FAD
D. ubiquinone

5. Select the *incorrect* association:

A. ATP - adenine
B. NAD - nicotinamide or niacin
C. FAD - folic acid
D. cytochromes - porphyrin ring

6. Select the *incorrect* statement concerning glycolysis:

A. end product may be lactate
B. if anaerobic, no ATPs are produced
C. if aerobic, the ATP yield can be 36ATPs because its products enter the citric acid cycle and electron transport system
D. it occurs in the cytoplasm

7. Select the *incorrect* statement regarding the citric acid cycle:

A. The first step is the combination of acetyl CoA and oxaloacetate to form citrate.
B. It is not a true cycle because CO_2 and H_2O are net products of it.
C. Each turn of the cycle yields 3NADHs, 1$FADH_2$, and 1ATP (from GTP).
D. It occurs in the mitochondrion.

8. Select the *incorrect* statement:

A. The final receptor of electrons in the electron transport system is oxygen.
B. Oxidative phosphorylation (production of ATPs) occurs only at certain steps in the electron transport system.
C. The electron transport system can produce ATPs without oxidative phosphorylation occurring.
D. Both electron transport and oxidative phosphorylation occur on the inner membrane of the mitochondrion.

9. At which stage does cyanide block cellular production of energy?

   A. glycolysis
   B. citric acid cycle
   C. electron transport system
   D. oxidative phosphorylation

10. Below are structures of a typical fatty acid and a hexose:

$$\begin{array}{c} HO\diagdown C{=}O \\ | \\ (CH_2)_4 \\ | \\ CH_3 \end{array} \qquad\qquad \begin{array}{c} H\diagdown C{=}O \\ | \\ H-C-OH \\ | \\ H-C-OH \\ | \\ H-C-OH \\ | \\ H-C-OH \\ | \\ CH_2OH \end{array}$$

Fatty Acid

Hexose

If equal weights of both were degraded bioenergetically to CO_2 and H_2O, the fatty acid would yield:

   A. more energy because it is more reduced than the hexose.
   B. less energy because it is more oxidized than the hexose.
   C. less energy because it is more reduced than the hexose.
   D. more energy because it is more oxidized than the hexose.

7.7.3 Answers to Questions in Section 7.7.2

(1) B (2) D (3) D (4) B (5) C (6) B (7) B (8) C (9) C (10) A

7.7.4 Discussion of Answers to Questions in Section 7.7.2

Questions #1 to #9 Discussed in the Section.

Question #10 (Answer: A) A reduced compound has all (or mostly) hydrogens and not oxygens. The fatty acid has many more hydrogens and fewer oxygens so it is more reduced. The more reduced a compound, the higher the energy that can be released when it is oxidized to CO_2 and H_2O. The factor of the number of atoms in each molecule is eliminated by considering the substances on a weight basis.

7.7.5 Advanced Concepts

- Learn usage and application of terms such as: metabolites, catabolism, anabolism, amphibolism, Mitchell's chemiosmotic theory (proton gradient and proton motive force similar to electromotive force), phototrophs, chemotrophs, metabolic inhibitors, zymase, enolase, irreversibility of metabolic pathways
- Understand the causes and effects for the following diseases: Cori, Anderson, McArdle's, Krabbe and Tay-Sachs (enzyme deficiency) and Beriberi disease
- Develop a more indepth understanding of glycolysis especially glucose catabolism or Embden-Meyerhof glycolytic pathway; pentose phosphate pathway, muscle glycolysis and glycogen metabolism in maintaining blood glucose levels through glucagon production
- Review concentration cells and electrochemical cells (see complete discussion in chapter 5) with applications to Nernst equation for aerobic metabolism (both for prokaryotes and eukaryotes)
- Identify experimental methods and techniques used in metabolite pathways research such as: isotopic labeling of metabolites, NMR and mass spectrometer techniques, Geiger counters, liquid scintillation counters, autoradiographs, cell storing, organ perfusion techniques and tissue slice techniques. Review papers in mitochondrial research using freeze-fracture and freeze-etch micrographs
- Compare and contrast glycolysis, gluconeogenesis, glycogenesis, and glycogenolysis for muscle glycogen and liver glycogen

7.8 REPRODUCTIVE SYSTEM

7.8.1 Introduction to Reproductive System

Review reproductive system essentials as they link to the endocrine system, Mendelian genetics (sex-linked characteristics) and major differences and similarities between embryogenesis and gametogenesis. Obtain permission to visit your area hospital or clinic and talk to nurses or doctors in the obstetrics and gynecological wards. Observe and analyze sonograms, rooms where newborns are kept and special infant instrumentation. Familiarize yourself with current issues and problems related to the reproductive systems of females and males, e.g., in-vitro fertilization and embryo transfer technology.

7.8.1.1 FEMALE AND MALE ANATOMY (Gonads and Genitalia)

Female anatomy The *labia* are composed of the *major folds* or *labia majora*, and the *minor folds* or *labia minora*. The *clitoris* (located between the minor folds ventrally) is very sensitive. The *vagina*, the passage from the external genital opening, terminates in the *cervix* (part of the uterus), which has an *os* (opening) to the uterine cavity (where the fertilized egg implants). The *placenta* derives from the uterus and the developing embryo. Connected to the uterus are the *Fallopian tubes* that lead to the *ovaries* (but are not connected to them).

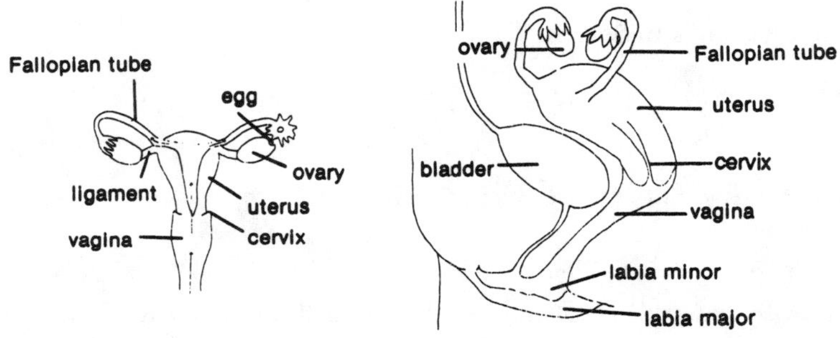

Fig. 7.33—Female Reproductive System

The female gonads, the ovaries, lie behind (retroperitoneally to) the abdominal cavity. They produce female hormones. They also produce the female gametes. Each female gamete is called an egg, or ovum. An ovum is huge compared to a sperm. Ova (plural of ovum) are produced by meiosis. Even before a female is born, egg-producing cells in the ovary have developed into primary oocytes. At birth, all the primary oocytes for a life-time are present. Primary oocytes are diploid.

Male anatomy The *testicles* are located outside the body because spermatogenesis requires a temperature lower than body temperature. The *scrotum* is the sack that contains the testicles. Sperm travels from the testis to the *epididymis* (where sperm maturation is completed) to the *vas deferens* to the *ejaculatory duct* to the *penile urethra* to the exterior. The *seminal vesicles* and *prostate gland* contribute fluid to the ejaculate (which averages 1-2cc). The *penis* consists of a *glans penis* (very sensitive) and a shaft (consisting of cavernous tissue for blood engorgement). *Penile erection* (mostly parasympathetic stimulation) results from veins of the penis clamping down and, hence, holding blood in the penis. Ejaculation is a reflex mediated by the sympathetic nervous system. Males continue to produce sperm from puberty onwards.

The sperm is produced by the process of meiosis, which results in haploid gametes. Gametes have only half the number of chromosomes contained in the body cells. Human body cells contain 46 chromosomes. Gametes contain only 23 chromosomes. It may be noted that before a male is born, the testes develop retroperitoneally to the abdominal cavity.

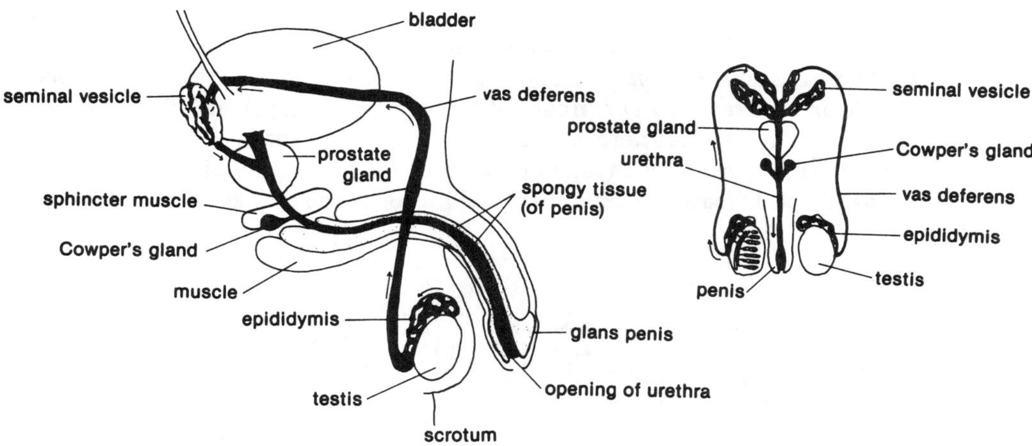

Fig. 7.34—Male Reproductive System

7.8.1.2 GAMETOGENESIS

Gametogenesis in Females (Fig. 7.35) The ovary contains *oogonia* (2n) which replicate their DNA and differentiate (before birth) into *primary oocytes* (46 chromosomes each made up of two chromatids, DNA = 2n) which become surrounded by *follicular cells* (from the mesenchymal stroma), and together constitute the *primordial follicle*. The primary oocytes are arrested in the prophase of the first meiotic division, and they may remain as such from birth to menopause. There are about 5 million oogonia, but only 1 million primary oocytes at birth and about 40,000 at puberty—the remainder degenerate (become *atretic follicles*). Beginning at puberty, a group of primordial follicles begin differentiation to *Graffian follicles*. The primary oocyte divides unevenly to form the secondary oocyte and a polar body, each cell having the haploid number of chromosomes (23) but containing DNA in their duplicated (daughter) chromatids. The secondary oocyte is surrounded by the *zona pellucida* (a gel-like substance), this is surrounded by follicular cells, and these are surrounded by *thecal cells* (which secrete estrogens). Next, *ovulation* occurs by expelling the secondary oocyte and zona pellucida plus some follicular cells (*corona radiata*) into the *Fallopian tubes*. If fertilization occurs in the Fallopian tubes (the usual location), the secondary oocyte completes meiosis to become an ovum and a *polar body* (both 1n—the replicated chromatids uncouple at their centromeres). The ovum fuses with the sperm. If it is not fertilized, the ovum degenerates. The follicular and thecal cells left behind become the *corpus luteum*, a main source of progesterone, which maintains pregnancy. The other follicles that began to develop degenerate because only one follicle completes development and is ovulated from one ovary during each cycle. The *polar bodies* that result from the division of the primary oocyte, the secondary oocyte, and possibly the first polar body are nonfunctional. Polar bodies have nuclear material but no cytoplasm. Hence, each primary oocyte (2n) produces only one gamete (1n).

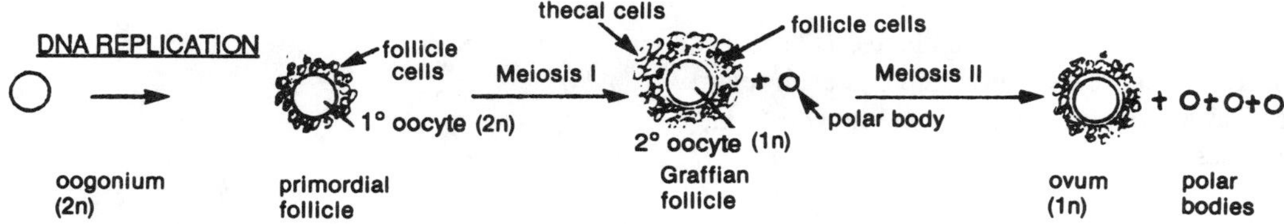

Fig. 7.35—Gametogenesis in Females

Gametogenesis in Males (Fig. 7.36) The first step is a differentiation of *spermatogonia* (2n), which includes DNA replication into *primary spermatocytes* (2n). Primary spermatocytes divide reductionally to form two secondary spermatocytes, both functional haploid cells (23 chromosomes) having duplicated chromosomes (daughter chromatids) and DNA. Secondary spermatocytes divide equally and at the centromeres of their duplicated chromosomes to form spermatids (1n and 23 individual chromosomes). The second step is called *spermiogenesis* in which spermatids (1n) are transformed into *sperm* (1n). A sperm consists of a head, a middle part and a tail. The head contains an *acrosome* (contains digestive enzymes to penetrate egg, derived from the Golgi apparatus) and *nuclear material (DNA)* surrounded by very little cytoplasm. The midpiece contains mitochondria for power. The tail has the structure of a centriole and provides locomotion. *Leydig or interstitial cells* (produce testosterone) and *Sertoli cells* (support sperm development) are also in the testis. Sperm deposited in the vagina by the penis reach the cervix within 90 seconds and migrate up the Fallopian tubes to fertilize the ovum there.

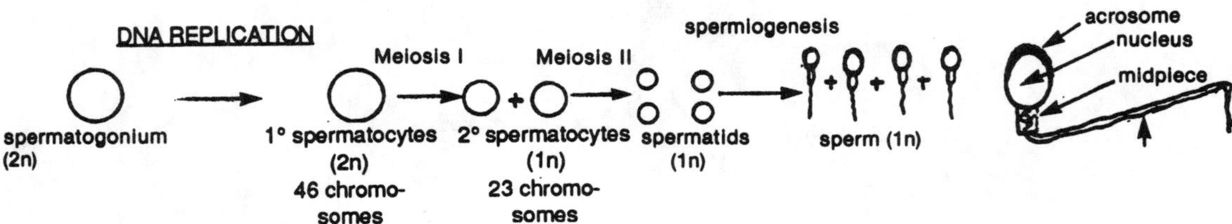

Fig. 7.36—Gametogenesis in Males

7.8.1.3 MITOSIS

The nucleus is surrounded by a nuclear envelope that consists of two *membranes* interrupted regularly by pores. Inside the nucleus is DNA in a form called *chromatin* (DNA, histones, non-histone protein) which becomes visible as *chromosomes* during cell division. A specific region of the chromatin is called the nucleolus where rRNA is made. Cells that are dividing or that have flagella or cilia have centrioles (basal bodies).

Mitosis occurs to maintain an optimal nucleus to cytoplasm volume ratio, allow growth, cell replacement, differentiation, and specialization of cells in a multicellular organism. All human somatic cells are diploid and 2n. They contain twice as many chromosomes (46) and twice (2n) the haploid amount of DNA (n) to express the entire genome (i.e., 23 chromosomes—a set from each parent gamete).

This cell division involves the processes of *cytokinesis* (division of the cytoplasm, not discussed) and *karyokinesis* (division of the nucleus). When a cell becomes *specialized,* it generally loses its ability to divide or reproduce itself (nerve cells, muscle cells, red blood cells, e.g.). Therefore, most cell division occurs in *"stem cells"* which are highly undifferentiated, multipotential cells with a high rate of cell division (e.g., bone marrow stem cells, crypt cells of the gut).

The *cell cycle* is divided into four phases. G_1 (Gap) is the fist period of cell growth. It immediately follows cell division and precedes DNA replication (Synthesis phase). G_2 follows DNA replication and precedes the M phase. M *(mitosis)* is the period of separation of the chromatids. The cycle is thus:

Prior to each mitosis the DNA is replicated (Phase S) so that when mitosis occurs the daughter cells each retain 2n number of chromosomes as in the parent cell (e.g., 46 chromosomes in humans).

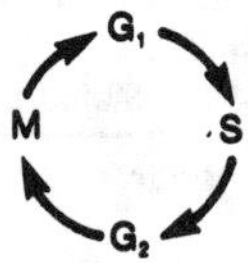

Interphase comprises, G_1, S, and G_2. Prophase, metaphase, anaphase, and telophase are part of the M phase. *Prophase* — the DNA coils tightly and becomes visible as chromosomes. The nuclear envelope may disappear. The *centrioles* consist of a cylinder of nine sets of three tubules each, found near the nucleus in a region called the centrosome. The centrosome contains two copies of a pair of centrioles at right angles to each other. A pair of centrioles move to opposite poles of the nucleus and spindle fibers (microtubule structure) are formed from a region near them. *Metaphase* — the chromosomes arrange radially along the equatorial plane of the cell and the spindle fibers are attached to the centromeres of each chromosome (now being composed of two chromatids, each of which becomes a new chromosome after the centromere uncouples). *Anaphase* — individual chromosomes divide at their centromeres and each new resulting chromosome migrates to the opposite pole being guided by the spindle fibers. Note that each chromatid of the chromosome at metaphase gives rise to a complete new chromosome after the centromeres uncouple. *Telophase* — the chromosomes uncoil, the nuclear envelope reforms, cytokinesis occurs, and the centrioles replicate themselves. The cell now enters *interphase*. See Section 7.8.1.4 to contrast mitosis and meiosis. The above concepts are diagrammed in Fig. 7.37.

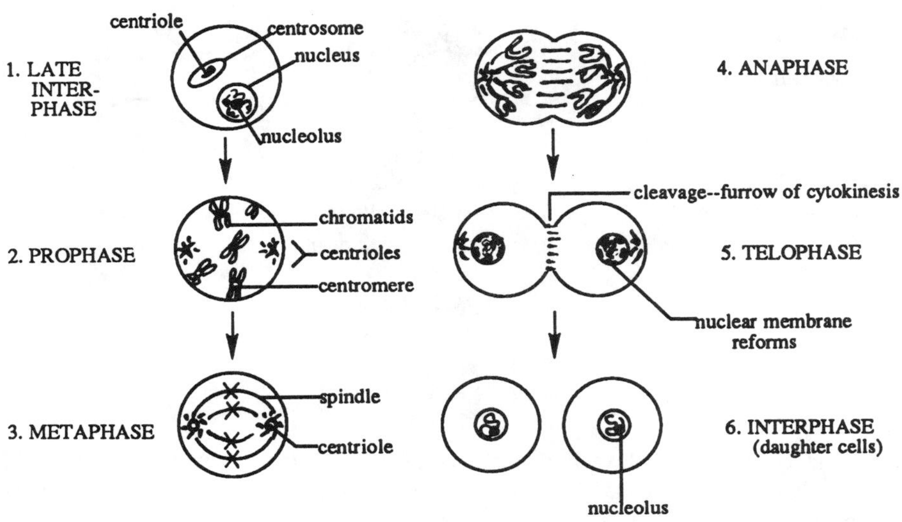

Fig. 7.37—Mitosis

7.8.1.4 MEIOSIS

Meiosis (Fig. 7.38) Meiosis has two phases. The first, a *reductional division* is different from mitosis (Section 7.8.1.3). *Prophase I*—the replicated DNA coils to become the chromosome, and there is *exact pairing (synapsis)* of the pairs of homologous chromosomes allowing crossing-over to occur. The nuclear envelope disintegrates, and the centrioles migrate to opposite poles of the nucleus. *Metaphase I*—the two members of the *homologous pair align* along the equatorial plane. The disposition of the maternal and paternal members of the pair toward either pole is random. The spindle fibers attach to the centromere of only one member of each homologous pair. *Anaphase I*—chromosomes of each homologous pair *separate* by moving toward opposite poles, and the *centromeres do not uncouple*. *Telophase I*— cytokinesis occurs. In spermatocytes the distribution of the cytoplasm is equitable giving two cells of equal size. In oocytes, the division is unequal giving one secondary oocyte and one polar body. *Interphase I*—a short period in which chromosomes may uncoil somewhat and the nuclear membrane may be partially reconstituted. The daughter cells now contain the haploid number of chromosomes each composed of two daughter chromatids. *Prophase II*, *metaphase II* and *anaphase II* are all like the corresponding mitosis phases. *Telophase II* is like mitosis but has haploid cells.

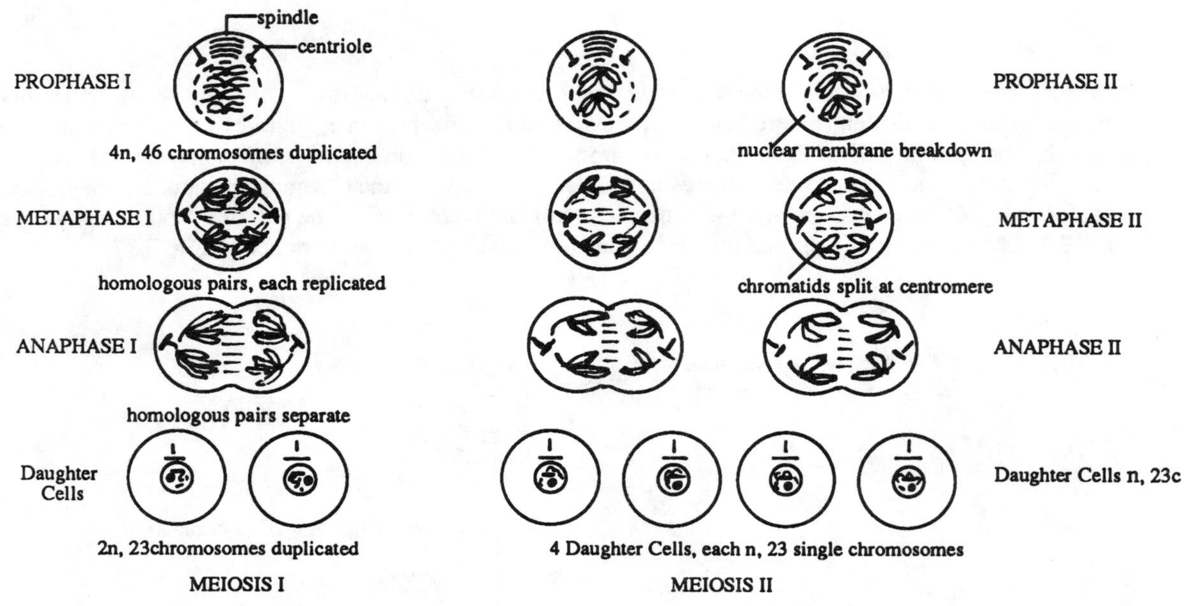

Fig. 7.38—Meiosis

7.8.1.5 MENSTRUAL PERIOD

The female period is typically 28 days and consists of a menstrual flow (mensus), a *follicular phase (ovary)/proliferative phase (uterus), ovulation,* and a *luteal phase (ovary)/secretory phase (uterus)* in that order. The first day of mensus is conveniently taken as the first day of the cycle. Shedding of the uterine lining occurs during the menstrual flow. Development of the follicle under the stimulation of *FSH* (Follicle Stimulating Hormone) and proliferation of the cells of the uterine lining under the stimulation of *estrogen* (from the ovary) occurs in the follicular/proliferative phase. A rapid increase of estrogen triggers a surge of *LH* (Luteinizing Hormone) at midcycle which causes ovulation to occur (at about 14 days *prior to* the first day of mensus). Just before ovulation, there is a slight dip in body temperature which then rises with ovulation—the progesterone is responsible for the temperature rise. During the luteal/secretive phase, the corpus luteum secretes progesterone, which, with estrogen, readies the uterine wall for the acceptance of the fertilized egg. If fertilization and implantation occur, the corpus luteum continues to secrete progesterone under the stimulation of *HCG* (Human Chorionic Gonadotropin) from the placenta. If implantation does not occur, the corpus luteum degenerates and there is no progesterone to support the uterus, and mensus (shedding of the uterine lining) occurs. Then the cycle repeats itself as FSH and estrogen concentrations rise. Menstrual cycles occur until nearly all the oocytes are depleted—this results in menopause. (Fig. 7.39)

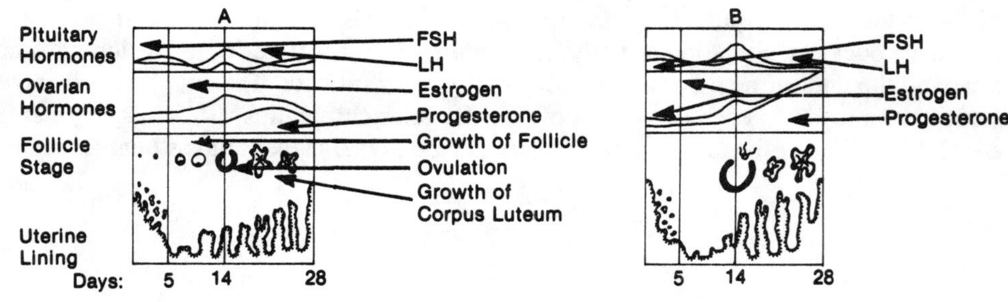

Fig. 7.39—Menstrual Cycle: (A) Without Pregnancy, (B) With Pregnancy

7.8.2 Questions Related to Reproductive System

1. The testicles are located outside the body because:
   - A. that is the normal embryologic location.
   - B. there is direct connection from the epididymis to the penile urethra.
   - C. there is a need for automatic peripheral nerves.
   - D. spermatogenesis requires a temperature lower than body temperature.

2. Sperm travels through all of the following structures except the:
   - A. ureter.
   - B. urethra.
   - C. vas deferens.
   - D. epididymis.

3. What structure is directly attached to the ovary?
   - A. vagina
   - B. uterus
   - C. Fallopian tubes
   - D. none of the above

4. The placenta of humans is composed of tissue derived from the:
   - A. uterus and developing embryo.
   - B. uterus only.
   - C. developing embryo only.
   - D. fallopian tubes.

5. The menstrual period (total cycle) is typically closest to:
   - A. 2 weeks.
   - B. 4 weeks.
   - C. 2 months.
   - D. 1 year.

6. The sequence of stages of the menstrual cycle (in reference to the ovary) following the menstrual flow is: (F = follicular phase, L = luteal phase, O = ovulation)
   - A. F, O, L
   - B. L, O, F
   - C. O, F, L
   - D. F, L, O

7. Ovulation usually occurs:
   - A. 1-3 days after menses (blood flow).
   - B. 14 days before menses.
   - C. 1-3 days before menses.
   - D. during menses.

8. The corpus luteum secretes:
   - A. progesterone.
   - B. LH.
   - C. FSH.
   - D. HCG.

9. The organ in the female analogous to the glans penis in the male is the:
   - A. vagina.
   - B. labia minora.
   - C. labia majora.
   - D. clitoris.

10. Which hormone below is found primarily during the first half (follicular/proliferative phase) of the menstrual cycle?

A. FSH
B. progesterone
C. prolactin
D. HCG

11. Synapsis and crossing over of chromosomes occur in which phase of meiosis?

A. Interphase I
B. Prophase I
C. Prophase II
D. Metaphase I

12. When do the centromeres divide in meiosis?

A. Anaphase I
B. Anaphase II
C. Telophase I
D. Telophase II

13. Which substance is not secreted by the fetus or placenta in a pregnant female?

A. FSH
B. HCG
C. progesterone
D. estrogen

14. In males, gametes are formed in the:

A. vas deferens.
B. Leydig cells.
C. epididymis.
D. seminiferous tubules.

15. Polar bodies:

A. are the poles of magnets.
B. result from gametogenesis in the male.
C. result from gametogenesis in the female.
D. form dipoles.

16. Fertilization of the ovum by the sperm usually occurs in the:

A. ovary.
B. Fallopian tubes.
C. uterus.
D. vagina.

17. Select the incorrect association:

A. oogonium—1n
B. primary oocyte—2n
C. secondary oocyte—1n
D. ova—1n

18. Corpus luteum:

A. results from mature ovum.
B. contains no hormones.
C. degenerates before ovulation.
D. degenerates after ovulation.

19. Tissue/cells not found in the testis are:

A. seminiferous tubules.
B. Leydig cells.
C. spermatogonia.
D. seminal vesicles.

20. The primary oocyte remains arrested in what phase of meiosis from birth to puberty?

A. Prophase I
B. Prophase II
C. Metaphase I
D. Metaphase II

21. Which of the following contains no developing ovum?

A. Graffian follicle
B. primordial follicle
C. corpus luteum
D. oocytes

22. Select the incorrect association:

A. spermatogonia—2n
B. primary spermatocytes—2n
C. spermatids—1n
D. spermatozoa—2n

23. Which is not associated with the male reproductive system?

A. epididymis
B. Leydig cells
C. thecal cells
D. Sertoli cells

24. The number of mature gametes resulting from meiosis of the primary oocyte in the female:

A. 1
B. 2
C. 3
D. 4

25. The number of mature gametes resulting from meiosis in the male:

A. 1
B. 2
C. 3
D. 4

26. The key difference(s) in anaphase I of meiosis and anaphase of mitosis is:

A. crossing over occurs in anaphase I of meiosis.
B. centromeres divide in anaphase I of meiosis.
C. homologous chromosomes move to opposite poles in anaphase I of meiosis.
D. all of the above.

27. The correct sequence of steps in mitosis is:

A. Prophase, Metaphase, Interphase, Anaphase, Telophase
B. Interphase, Anaphase, Metaphase, Prophase, Telophase
C. Interphase, Prophase, Metaphase, Anaphase, Telophase
D. Anaphase, Prophase, Interphase, Metaphase, Telophase

28. Which is not true about the cell cycle?
   A. There are typically four phases, G_1, G_2, S, and M.
   B. Interphase corresponds with the M phase.
   C. S is the phase of DNA synthesis.
   D. M is the phase of cell division.

29. Which is not true about mitosis?
   A. It can maintain an optimal nucleus to cytoplasm volume ratio.
   B. It can allow growth of organisms.
   C. It has phases of karyokinesis and cytokinesis.
   D. It results in haploid daughter cells when the parent cells are diploid.

30. The chromosomes become coiled and visible and the nuclear membrane disintegrates. This is what phase of mitosis?
   A. interphase
   B. prophase
   C. metaphase
   D. telophase

31. A key difference in the mechanism of mitosis and meiosis is that:
   A. mitosis has crossing over of homologous chromosomes during prophase.
   B. meiosis has a second duplication of DNA during interphase I.
   C. meiosis has alignment of homologous chromosomes in metaphase I and separation of homologous chromosomes in anaphase I.
   D. mitosis has a reductional division.

32. The main difference in the outcome of mitosis versus meiosis is that:
   A. meiosis produces identical daughter cells and mitosis produces different daughter cells.
   B. mitosis occurs only in vertebrates.
   C. meiosis produces somatic cells.
   D. meiosis results in haploid cells and mitosis results in diploid cells when the parent cells are diploid.

7.8.3 Answers to Questions in Section 7.8.2

(1) D (2) A (3) D (4) A (5) B (6) A (7) B (8) A (9) D (10) A (11) B (12) B
(13) A (14) D (15) C (16) B (17) A (18) D (19) D (20) A (21) C (22) D (23) C (24) A
(25) D (26) C (27) C (28) B (29) D (30) B (31) C (32) D

7.8.4 Discussion of Answers to Questions in Section 7.8.2: None

7.8.5 Advanced Concepts

- Focus more on the functions of various parts of the reproductive systems in females and males. Understand the cellular and molecular physiology of each gland or organ, e.g., development of follicles in the ovary, function of spermatocytes and the physics of ultrasound tests in a pregnant woman.
- Understand the chemical and endocrinal relationship among FSH, LH (defined in 7.8.1.6) and Gonadotropin releasing hormone (GnRH) as released in the female and inhibition by male hormones such as testosterone and inhibin.
- Distinguish between terms such as: spermatogenesis, spermatids, spermatocytes, spermiogenesis; progesterone, follicular fluid, testosterone (interstitial Leydig cells), amniotic fluid, teratogen, oocytes and oogonia; syncytiotrophoblasts and osteoblasts, allantois.
- Determine the fundamental causes and effects of the following and develop a system to remember them: vasectomy, episiotomy, oophorectomy, lumpectomy, mastectomy, cryptorchidism, mittelschmerz, endometriosis, amenorrhea, and dysmenorrhea.

- Understand various factors linked to parturition including uterine contraction frequency and the role of oxytocin during labor.
- Understand the instrumentation and objectives of various tests such as: pap smear test, semen analysis (pH, volume, count, fertility, etc.), colposcopy, dilation and curettage, computed tomography and mammography, ultrasound cancer test, prostate gland cancer test, ectopic pregnancy test, tubal ligation sonograms (to determine fetal position and development, etc.) and amniocentesis.
- Recognize the chemicals used and functions of birth control pills, IUD, condoms, diaphragms, sponges and tampons. Which of these devices cause the toxic shock syndrome and how can it be prevented?
- Investigate and understand the technology behind induced abortion techniques such as use of suction, saline solution and basic scraping.
- Most home pregnancy tests are inaccurate tools to predict pregnancy. The basic test tube is used to test HCG in urine. Particle clumping in a ring like form indicates positive testing of HCG and no clumping/no ring indicates negative testing of HCG. Realize why these tests are not reliable depending on type of pregnancy and stage of pregnancy. Blood tests are more accurate.
- Understand the concept of natural titrants such as semen (alkaline with a pH of 7.5) and vaginal secretions (acidic with a pH of about 3.5-4.0) and how various hormonal releases affect their biochemical nature.
- Recognize modern fetal surgery techniques (done on unusual tissues or organs), development of Graffian follicles, new fetal ultrasonography tests, artificial insemination methods (in vitro and embryo transfer) and karyotyping.
- Understand the abnormal inheritance traits and diseases: sickle-cell anemia, Huntington's chorea, Turner's Syndrome, Klinefelter's syndrome and Down's syndrome. Determine the specific chromosomal abnormality causing the abnormal traits and learn the use of karyotyping techniques to photograph chromosomes (birth defects are usually caused by various factors related to centromeres, e.g., shape, size).
- Learn the definitions (including structure and function) of the following mitotic and meiotic terminology: mitotic spindle, cleavage furrow, astril fibrils, asters, telomeres, kinetochores and nuclear membrane breakdown. Learn mechanistic differences between mitosis (somatic cell division) and meiosis (reproductive cell division) e.g., stages in prophase which are leptonema, zygonema, pachynema, diplonema and diakinesis.

7.9 DEVELOPMENTAL MECHANISMS (EMBRYOLOGY)

7.9.1 Introduction to Developmental Mechanisms: None

7.9.1.1 DEVELOPMENT OF HUMAN EMBRYO

Embryogenesis: Embryogenesis can be broken down into fertilization, cleavage, blastulation, gastrulation and neurulation. *Fusion of the gametes* produced by meiosis (see Section 7.8.1 for details) involves first the penetration of the ovum by the sperm. The acrosome (part of sperm that contains hydrolytic enzymes) dissolves the *corona radiata* (collection of follicle cells) and zone pellucida around ovulated ovum, and only the head of the sperm (contains the DNA) penetrates the ovum. Upon penetration, a reaction in the ovum occurs preventing additional sperm from entering. The ovum now completes meiosis II (see Section 7.8.1.4). Then the male (n) and female (n) pronuclei fuse and cleavage of the fertilized egg (zygote = 2n) begins.

Growth, differentiation, and morphogenesis occur together after the first few cleavages. The amount of yolk in the egg is an important determinator of the cleavage pattern but will not be discussed. Note, though, that the egg has polarity (i.e., is asymmetrical) by virtue of the yolk distribution. The first few cleavages (4-5) result in a grape-like cluster of cells called the *morula*. There is no morula in humans. These divisions occurred without cell growth, and, hence, the morula is not much larger than the zygote.

The morula develops into a *blastula* which is a hollow sphere one-cell thick with a cavity called the blastocoel. From this point *morphogenesis* (movements of cells to delineate shape and function) begins with the invagination of the blastula. What results is a two-layered structure with a new cavity called the *archenteron* that opens to the outside via the *blastopore* (site of invagination): this structure is the *gastrula*. Cells from the lip of the blastopore migrate between the two layers of cells to form a third layer. The *gastrula* then becomes a three-layered structure composed of *ectoderm* (outside), *mesoderm* (middle), and *endoderm* (inside). The blastopore cells induce the overlying ectoderm to form a neural groove and the embryo is now called a *neurula.* The neural groove forms the *neural tube.* At the margins of the neural tube detachment are a group of cells called the *neural crest* cells which form the adrenal medulla, melanocytes, and myelin sheaths among other tissues. The neural tube develops into the central nervous system (spinal cord and brain). Ventral to the neural tube, mesodermal tissue forms somites which gives rise to the vertebral column (formed on, but not from, the notochord) and associated muscles. The *ectoderm develops into* the nervous system, the epidermis of the skin and its derivatives, the lens of the eye, and the linings of the mouth and anus. The *endoderm will develop into* the gut (esophagus, stomach, intestines), associated organs (liver, gallbladder, pancreas), the lung, and the thyroid gland. The *mesoderm develops into* the skeleton, muscles, kidney, circulatory system (heart and vessels), blood, and dermis of skin. A schematic summary of the sequence above is in Fig. 7.40.

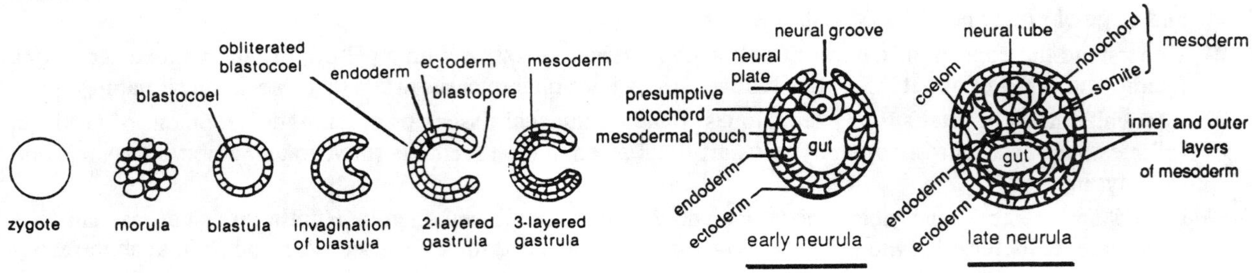

Fig. 7.40—Early Development of Frog Embryo (Embryogenesis)

Developmental Mechanisms: The question of how a single egg develops into a complex organism is not completely answered. The concepts of differentiation, determination and induction are integral to understanding the changes which occur.

Differentiation is the process whereby a cell can change into more specialized cells to become a tissue. A *tissue* is a set of similar cells which carries out a specific function, such as muscle. The magnitude of this process is appreciated when one realizes that all the varied cells of the human body (muscle, bone, skin, nerve, etc.) arise from the same zygote. What is it about the zygote that allows this differentiation to occur? It is generally accepted that *all cells in an organism contain the same genetic information* (sequences of genes on DNA). What probably makes one cell different from another is which of these genes is activated. The *set of activated genes is responsible for each cell's characteristics*—the structural components, metabolic machinery, and general composition of the cell. So, in some way, after gastrulation, different tissues *must have different sets of genes activated.* No activation of genes occurs in blastula or late gastrula. Induction turns on protein synthesis.

Differentiation is not brought about by the daughter cells having different genes (i.e., different sets of genetic material), in general. If the cytoplasm of the zygote was totally homogeneous, then each daughter cell, resulting from the cleavage, would be identical with regard to the nucleus and the cytoplasm and would remain undifferentiated. But, if there were an asymmetrical distribution of cytoplasmic constituents, and the cleavage results in daughter cells with different distributions of these constituents, then the daughter cells would be different. That is, a small amount of cytoplasmic differentiation would have occurred. If these cytoplasmic differences led to the activation of different sets of genes in their respective nuclei, differences between the cells would be perpetuated in their daughter cells, and some degree of true differentiation (production of daughters different from parent cells) will have occurred. So, asymmetrical distribution of cytoplasmic constituents is one way differentiation may be brought about. Then, in general, if a factor can affect the cell's cytoplasmic composition (which can affect the set of activated genes) or if it can affect the nucleus directly to activate (or inactivate) genes, and this effect is unevenly distributed among the cells, differentiation of the cells along different lines can be brought about.

Other factors which cause cells to differentiate are: (1) *Neighboring cells* (by contact inhibition of growth by secreting a diffusible chemical that stimulates or inhibits the cytoplasm or nucleus). An example is tissue **induction** in which a given tissue can induce cells in contact with it to develop along a certain line. For example, the dorsal lip of the blastopore induces the overlying ectoderm to become neural tissue as mentioned above. (2) *Physical environment* (by differences in light, temperature, pressure, humidity, pH, etc.). As the embryo develops, some cells are internal, some are on the surface, some have lots of yolk, some a little yolk, etc., so more opportunities occur for agents to act on cells in a differential manner. In general, the more specialized a cell becomes (i.e., the more differentiated), the less likely it is to differentiate to perform other functions or even divide. Certain cells remain at low levels of differentiation such that they may differentiate as they are needed. Examples are the mesenchymal cell found throughout the body and the bone marrow stem cell which can give rise to all the blood elements. Occasionally, a cell may dedifferentiate (i.e., revert to a less differentiated form), and, thus, its potential to divide increases. This is what happens in many cancers.

The concept of **determination** is related to that of differentiation in that, as a cell differentiates, fewer options become available. That is, at certain points a cell or tissue may be "determined" to become one of a certain set of cells and not others. For example, the surface cells of the gastrula are "determined" to become ectodermal structures and not endodermal or mesodermal structures. So, although in the blastula all the cells were surface cells and, apparently, had the option of becoming ectodermal cells, only those that did not invaginate became so. The mechanism of determination is probably also related to the environmental differences of cells and their interaction with preset sequences of gene activation and inactivation. Occasionally, the cells resulting from cleavage of a zygote are not "determined" until after 3 divisions (8 cells). Up to this point each cell can develop into a complete organism. After this point, only incomplete organisms would develop from each cell. Cleavages up to this point are called indeterminate because each cell has all the options available. The next cleavage is called determinate because the daughter cells no longer have all options available. In some instances the first cleavage may be determinate.

7.9.2 Questions Related to Developmental Mechanisms

1. The blastula is generally preceded by the:

A. gastrula.
B. morula.
C. neurula.
D. gastrula and morula.

2. The three germ layers—the ectoderm, the mesoderm and the endoderm—are found at which stage?

A. morula
B. gastrula
C. blastula
D. neurula

3. Select the one that is not derived from the ectoderm germinal layer:

A. nerve
B. muscle
C. lens of eye
D. epidermis of skin

4. Select the organ/tissue not derived from the mesodermal germinal layer:

A. muscle
B. kidney
C. intestines
D. bones

5. Select the organ/tissue derived from the endodermal germinal layer:
   A. intestines
   B. muscle
   C. kidney
   D. bones

6. The individual cells resulting from the cleavage of a fertilized egg may occasionally give rise to complete organisms up to the *third* cleavage. Select the correct statement:
   A. Cleavages prior to the *third* were determinate cleavages.
   B. The number of cells resulting from the third cleavage is 16.
   C. Determinate cleavages cannot occur, in general, prior to the third cleavage.
   D. The cells resulting after the next cleavage are probably different in cytoplasmic composition.

7. Once the sperm head penetrates the __________, a reaction ensues that __________.
   A. corona radiata; causes the pronuclei to fuse.
   B. corona radiata; prevents the penetration of additional sperm.
   C. ovum; causes the pronuclei to fuse.
   D. ovum; prevents the penetration of additional sperm.

8. All of the following processes occur during the process of fertilization of the egg by the sperm except that:
   A. the acrosome dissolves the corona radiata.
   B. only the head of the sperm enters the ovum.
   C. the sperm nucleus completes its second meiotic division.
   D. the ovum nucleus completes its second meiotic division.

9. The correct sequence of the early states of development is:
   A. morula, gastrula, blastula, neurula
   B. morula, blastula, gastrula, neurula
   C. blastula, morula, gastrula, neurula
   D. neurula, blastula, gastrula, morula

10. Which of the following stages is essentially the same size as the zygote?
    A. gastrula
    B. blastula
    C. morula
    D. all are larger

11. The first stage of development in which a cavity appears is the:
    A. neurula.
    B. morula.
    C. gastrula.
    D. blastula.

12. Morphogenesis begins at which stage?
    A. morula
    B. blastula
    C. gastrula
    D. neurula

13. Factors important in the differentiation of cells include:
    A. cytoplasmic composition and distribution of constituents.
    B. characteristics of neighboring cells.
    C. physical environmental agents.
    D. all of the above.

14. As a cell becomes more specialized for a particular function, the opportunity for it to become specialized for other functions:

A. decreases.
B. increases.
C. remains the same.
D. increases steadily and decreases exponentially.

15. A cell found in the middle layer of the three-layered gastrula has probably lost the option to become:

A. epidermis.
B. kidney.
C. muscle.
D. blood.

16. Select the following situation(s) that have the best likelihood of leading to differentiated daughter cells after a cleavage occurs:

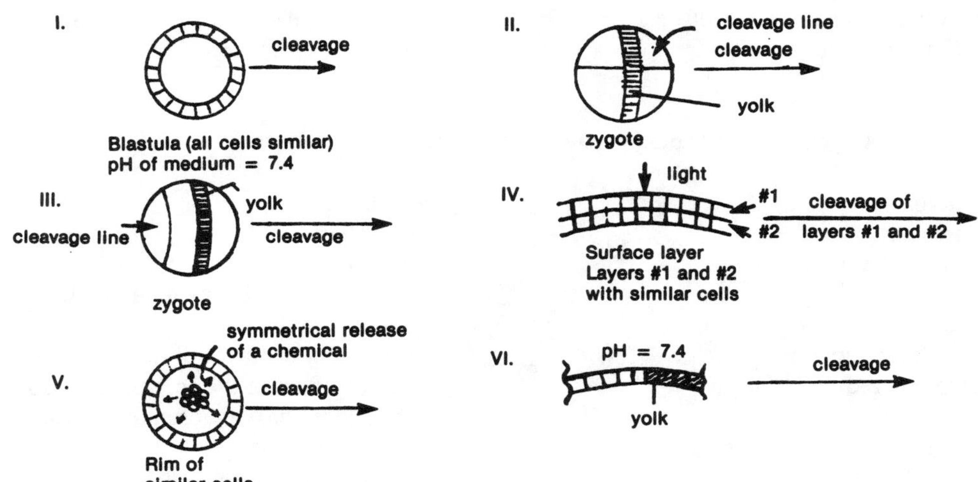

A. III, IV, VI
B. II, IV, V, VI
C. II, III, IV, V, VI
D. all of them

17. Which of the following cells or cell types is the most differentiated?

A. mesenchymal cell
B. nerve cell
C. cancer cell
D. bone marrow stem cell

7.9.3 Answers to Questions in Section 7.9.2

(1) B (2) B (3) B (4) C (5) A (6) D (7) D (8) C (9) B (10) C (11) D (12) B (13) D (14) A (15) A (16) A (17) B

7.9.4 Discussion of Answers to Questions in Section 7.9.2

Questions #1 - #5, #7-#15, #17 Discussed in Section.

Question #6 (Answer: D) This is discussed in the Section. The implication of the question being that the divisions after the third are determinate and result in cells that have different cytoplasmic components. The cells resulting from the nth cleavage is 2^n assuming at each cleavage all cells divide (not always true). Then $2^3 = 2 \cdot 2 \cdot 2 = 8$ and not 16 as in option (B).

Question #16 (Answer: A) The point stressed in the Section was that differentiation is possible if a factor can affect a group of similar cells in an unsymmetrical or unequal manner. In (I), the pH affects all the similar cells equally. In (II), the cleavage results in two cells with similar yolk distributions. In (III), the cleavage results in different yolk distributions so the daughter cells are different cytoplasmically and this can lead to differentiation. In (IV), the light may either affect the surface layer only or affect the surface layer (#1) more strongly than the underlying layer (#2). This can potentially affect gene activation and can lead to differentiation between the cell layers. In (V), the rim of similar cells are probably affected similarly by the symmetrically diffusing chemicals, and the daughter cells will probably be similar. In (VI), although the pH is constant, this can have different effects on cells with and without yolks, and, hence, result in potentially differentiated daughter cells.

7.9.5 List of Advanced Concepts (as covered in text) See list below:

_______ acrosome
_______ morula
_______ archenteron
_______ ectoderm
_______ neurula
_______ tissue induction
_______ corona radiata
_______ blastula
_______ blastopore
_______ mesoderm
_______ neural tube
_______ cleavages
_______ blastocoel
_______ gastrula
_______ endoderm
_______ neural crest
_______ fertilization of the ovum and related changes in the egg
_______ sequences of stages of development
_______ development of the ectoderm, mesoderm, endoderm into organs and/or organ systems
_______ morphogenesis
_______ concept of determination
_______ concept of differentiation
_______ concept of induction

7.10 GENETICS AND EVOLUTION

7.10.1 Introduction to Genetics and Evolution

Molecular genetics, mutations and comparative chordate anatomy should be studied as parts of the large-scale evolution process. The history and mechanisms controlling evolution (for various organisms) should be directly applied to problem solving in gene flow, genetic drift and genetic (chromosomal) mapping. Recognize and appraise this section as a series of hypotheses, explanations and conclusions and determine how current information is used to solve special mathematical problems in genetics. Review Chapter 4 (sections on problem solving and probability mathematics) before learning this section.

7.10.1.1 GENETIC VARIABILITY

Each organism has a set of chromosomes. *Chromosomes* of eukaryotes are a complex of DNA, *histone* (basic protein), and non-histone protein. The normal complement of chromosomes is called *diploid (2n)* as occurs in somatic cells. Gametes (male and female) are *haploid (1n)*. Gametes combine to form the diploid cell. The complement of chromosomes may be divided into *autosomes* and *sex chromosomes* (having to do with sex determination). Humans have 22 pairs of autosomes and 1 pair of sex chromosomes (X, Y) for a total of 46. The female is XX, and the male is XY. Either the whole set of chromosomes can be in some multiple of n which is called *polyploidy*, e.g., 4n = *tetraploidy*, or one or more chromosomes may be missing or in excess, which is called *aneuploidy*, e.g., *monosomy* (only one of a chromosome type is present) or trisomy (three representatives of a given chromosome). Down's Syndrome (Mongolism) is caused by trisomy 21 (i.e., there are three of the chromosomes numbered 21 instead of two).

On each chromosome there is a sequence of *genes*. For this section, a gene is a specific trait. Hence, each *locus* (or position) on a chromosome is for a specific trait. In the diploid (2n) cell, there is a pair of *homologous chromosomes* (which pair in meiosis). Homologous chromosomes are similar by having the same sequence of trait loci (except the pair X and Y, see below); hence they are the same size. For any given general trait (e.g., eye color), there are many alternative genes (e.g., blue, brown) for its determination. The alternative genes for a general trait constitute a set of *alleles* for that trait. Since there is only one locus (usually) for a simple trait on a chromosome, there can be only one allele of that trait per homologous chromosome. Then, for any given trait, there is a maximum of two alleles per diploid cell (one on each homologous chromosome). But the total number of different alleles for a given trait can be greater than two (e.g., there are many different alleles for types of hemoglobin—normal adult, fetal, sickle, hemoglobin C, hemoglobin Milwaukee, etc.). For an individual, the specific alleles present is called the genotype. If the alleles for a given trait on each homologous chromosome are identical, the genotype is called *homozygous*. If the alleles for a given trait on each homologous chromosome are different, the genotype is called *heterozygous*. The term genotype can refer to the alleles of a specific trait or the total genetic makeup (all of the alleles) of an individual. Each of the alleles (genes) of a given trait will attempt to express itself via its protein product. If one allele of a pair expresses itself over another (e.g., eye color with brown over blue), that allele is said to be *dominant* and the other *recessive*. (Note that these terms go together like oxidation-reduction in chemistry.) If both alleles express themselves, they are called *codominant*. The expression (what is seen as the trait of the individual) of the genotype is called the *phenotype*.

7.10.1.2 MENDEL'S LAWS

Gametes (haploid) are formed during meiosis by the separation of homologous chromosomes (diploid state). This results in the separation of each of the alleles of a homolog into a different gamete. This is *Mendel's First Law of Segregation* (of alleles of the same trait). Different traits (i.e., loci) may be on the same chromosome or on different chromosomes. If the traits are on different chromosomes, the alleles of these different traits should separate independently of each other into gametes. This is *Mendel's Second Law of Independent Assortment* (of alleles of different traits). But if different traits are on the same chromosome, they may be far apart or close together. Traits far apart on the same chromosome separate into gametes as if they were on separate chromosomes. This is possible because of *crossing-over* (reciprocal exchange of parts of homologous chromosomes) during *synapsis* in the first meiotic prophase. The farther apart two different traits are on a chromosome, the easier it is for cross-over to occur. Alleles of traits which are close together do not separate frequently by the mechanism of crossing-over into different gametes because they tend to remain on the same chromosome. So they cannot independently (of each other) assort, do not follow Mendel's Second Law, and are called *linked traits* (or genes). (Fig. 7.41)

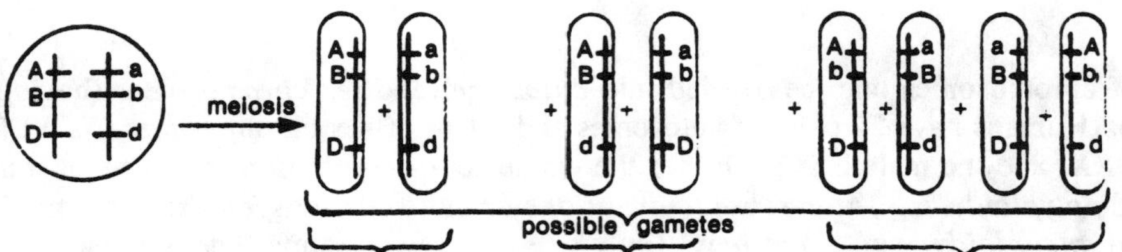

Diploid (2n) cell showing a pair of homologous chromosomes with loci for three different traits with alleles A,a and B,b and D,d. Traits A,a and B,b are linked. Traits A,a and D,d and traits B,b and D,d are not linked.	Mendel's 1st Law: Each allele of a given trait (A vs. a, B vs. b, and D vs. d) segregate independently of each other.	Mendel's 2nd Law: Consider A,a vs. D,d. These alleles of different traits assort independently of each other (also for B,b vs. D,d). Not true for A,a vs. B,b because these are linked.	Recombination of the linked genes A,a vs. B,b. A,a and B,b do not assort independently of each other because they are so close together. One would normally expect A & B or a & b to be together in gametes. But by crossing over, Ab and aB also are possible but at frequencies less than expected.

Fig. 7.41—Mendel's Law; Crossing-over; Recombination; Gamete Formation

Recombination is the process of separating alleles of linked traits into different gametes, i.e., onto different homologous chromosomes. *Linkage (recombination)* studies and cytogenetics (study of markings, e.g., band on chromosomes) are used to map chromosomes as to the loci of traits. Another of Mendel's great contributions to genetics was his recognition that genes are *particulate* (i.e., not indivisible or blendable). Mendel's mechanisms of assortment and segregation and the later discovered ideas of recombination illustrate mechanisms of *genetic variability* which can be viewed as the passage to offspring, via gametes, of different combinations of alleles than existed in the parent.

7.10.1.3 CHROMOSOMAL MUTATIONS

Another set of mechanisms responsible for genetic variability is *mutations*. A mutation may be considered a stable heritable change in genetic material (DNA). Changes, or structural changes, in chromosomes are called chromosomal aberrations that may occur at the level of the chromosome (see Fig. 7.42) are:

(1) *inversion*—sequence of genes on the chromosomes is reversed
(2) *translocation*—a part of one chromosome attaches to another
(3) *deletion*—a part of the chromosome is missing
(4) *duplication*—part of the chromosome is repeated.

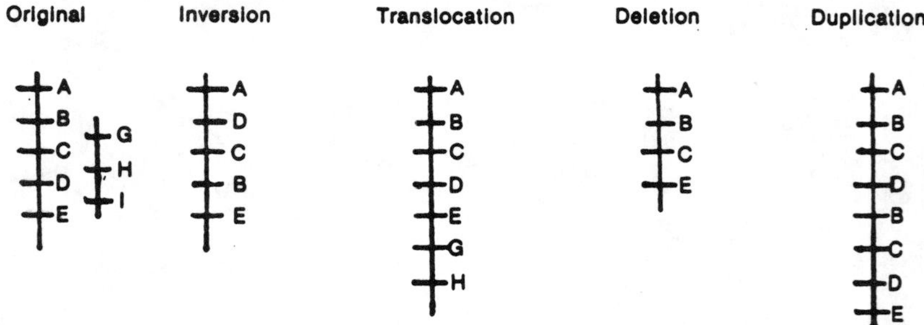

Fig. 7.42—Chromosomal Aberrations

Mutations (section 7.10.1.1) are the ultimate source of all new genes in the population, and as such, they are the raw material for all evolutionary changes. Genes mutate forward to new genes and backward to the old gene. The *mutation pressure* is the net change of these two processes. Genes arising by mutation tend to be recessive, and since they are rarely homozygous, they tend to be carried silently, i.e., not expressed, in the population for long periods of time. Stable alleles are those with low mutation rates and they tend to increase in frequency. This contrasts with unstable alleles which have high mutation rates and tend to decrease in frequency. This process results in a slow shift in gene frequencies in the population. It seems reasonable that mutation alone could cause evolutionary change. The major reason that mutation per se does *not* cause evolutionary change is that *mutation is random* and, consequently, usually is in a direction away from the organism's evolutionary trend. So mutation alone has a slow and non-directional effect on evolution with the exception of polyploidy (section 7.10.1.1) *Polyploidy* is the doubling (e.g., 2n $\rightarrow$ 4n), of the set of chromosomes usually by nondisjunction during meiosis. What results is an organism with a larger set of chromosomes which result in pheontypic differences in them. Also, note that mutations in somatic cells have no effect on evolution because they are not passed on to the offspring.

In the sex chromosomes, the X is larger than the Y (i.e., has more loci for traits), and hence, traits on the X may not appear on the Y. Traits of this type are called *sex-linked traits.* Examples in humans are hemophilia, color blindness, and glucose-6-phosphate dehydrogenase deficiency. The X and Y chromosomes are homologous because they can pair (synapse) in meiosis. Sex-linked traits are unique in their inheritance because the male (with only one X chromosome) can express (phenotypes) recessive alleles because there is only one allele present. The female requires both recessive alleles to be present for expression of the recessive trait. Also note that transmission to the male occurs usually only from the mother. Whereas if the daughter is diseased, both mother and father must have passed on the allele. As an aside, *Barr bodies* are inactivated "excess" X chromosomes (only one X remains active). This phenomenon is referred to as the *Lyon* or *Lyon-Russel* hypothesis. The above concepts are illustrated in Fig. 7.43.

Given a trait with alleles A = dominant, a = recessive and phenotypes A and a.

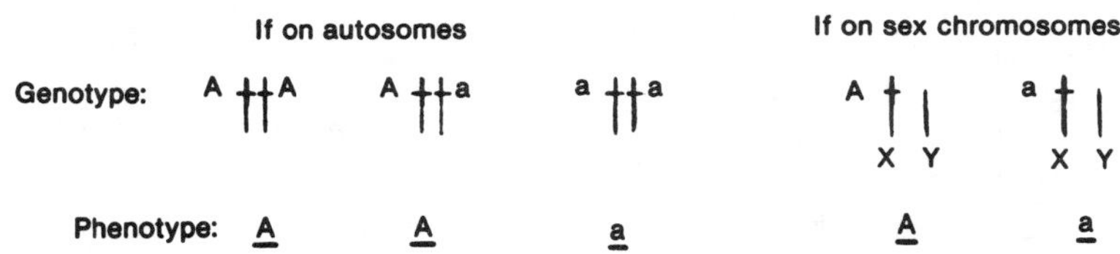

Note that the *a* allele can only be expressed when it is present on both chromosomes (i.e., it is homozygous).

Note that *a* (the allele) is alone and is expressed.

Fig. 7.43—Autosomal and Sex Chromosomes: Phenotype Expressions

Cytoplasmic inheritance is the determination of genetic traits by constituents of the cytoplasm rather than the nucleus. This inheritance does not follow Mendelian Laws. The mother (most of the cytoplasm of the zygote comes from the ovum) plays the major role in this type of inheritance. Chloroplasts (contain DNA), mitochondria (contain DNA), centrioles, and basal bodies of flagella and cilia are examples of structures that replicate without input from the nucleus.

7.10.1.4 PEDIGREE CHARTS

Pedigrees are convenient diagrams for showing phenotypic appearance of traits in a family. The basic nomenclature is given in Fig. 7.44.

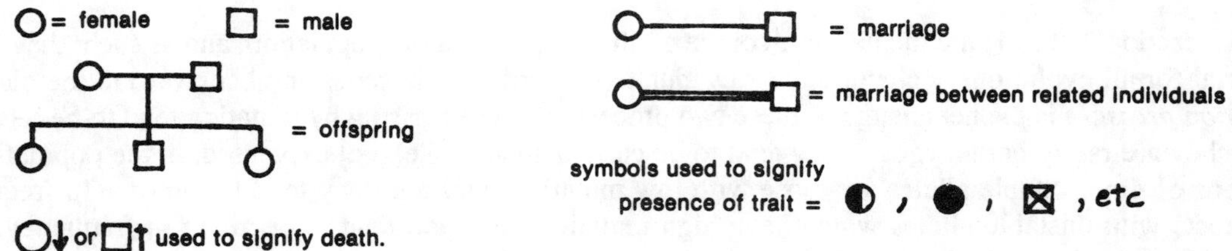

7.44—Pedigree Terminology

A dominant autosomal trait, with complete *penetrance* (i.e., the trait appears in all with the allele), will have a pedigree that shows both sexes affected, many individuals affected, passage of trait from affected parent to children even if heterozygous. (Fig. 7.45).

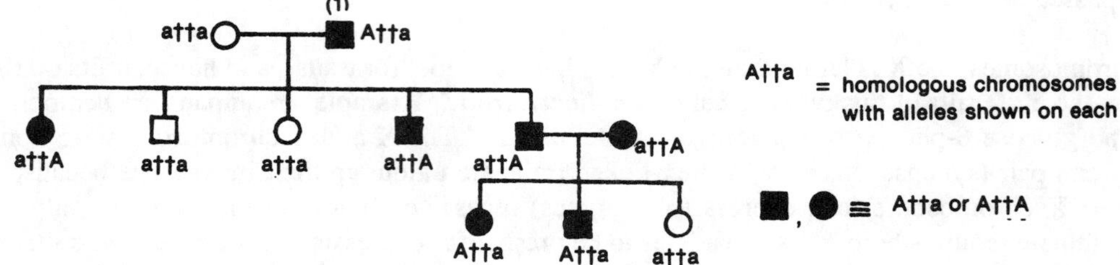

Case (1) is probably heterozygous for the trait because if homozygous then all offspring would be affected.

7.45—Dominant Pedigree

An autosomal recessive trait will also show both sexes affected, but fewer individuals will be affected and passage may be from an unaffected parent (because heterozygous) to an affected offspring (Fig. 7.46).

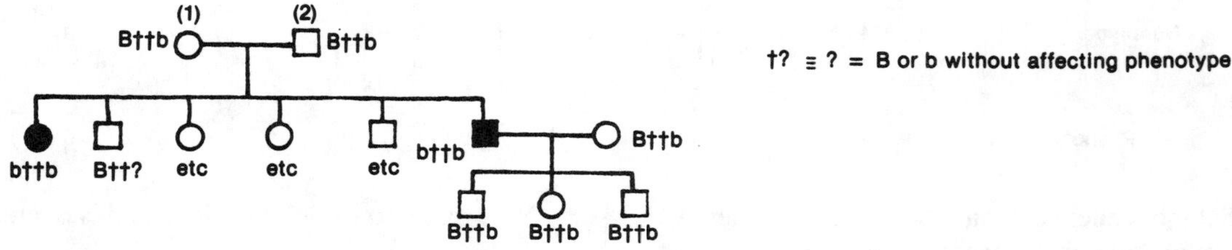

Both parents are heterozygous for the recessive allele

Fig. 7.46—Recessive Pedigree

A sex-linked recessive trait usually shows only males affected and passage of the trait from an unaffected mother to a son. A daughter can get the trait only if the father has it and the mother is, at least, heterozygous (Fig. 7.47).

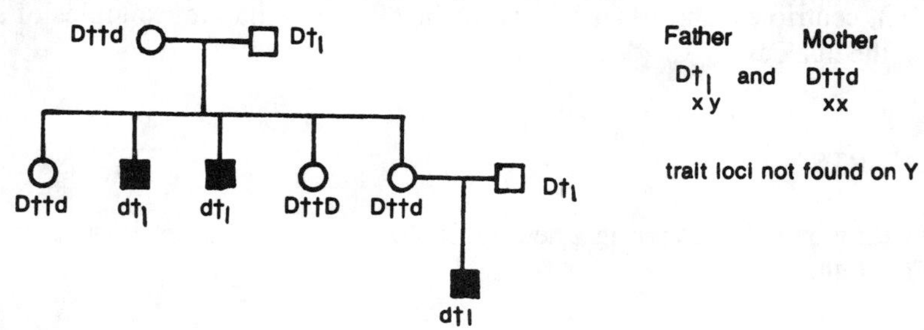

Fig. 7.47—Sex-Linked Pedigree

7.10.1.5 PUNNETT SQUARES

Punnett squares are useful ways of determining the genotypes possible from the mating of two individuals with known genotypes. First the possible gametes are determined (Fig. 7.48), then these are combined in all possible ways. Then by knowing dominant-recessive relationships, the frequency of phenotypes can be ascertained. The Punnett square gives expected ratios only. Fig. 7.49 and Fig. 7.50 are examples.

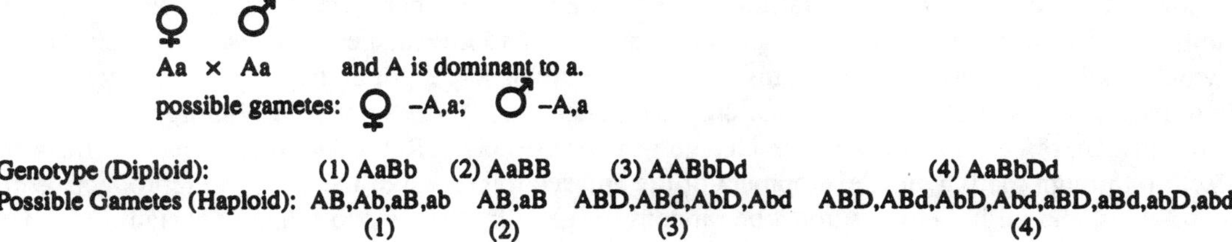

7.48—Gamete Formation by Example

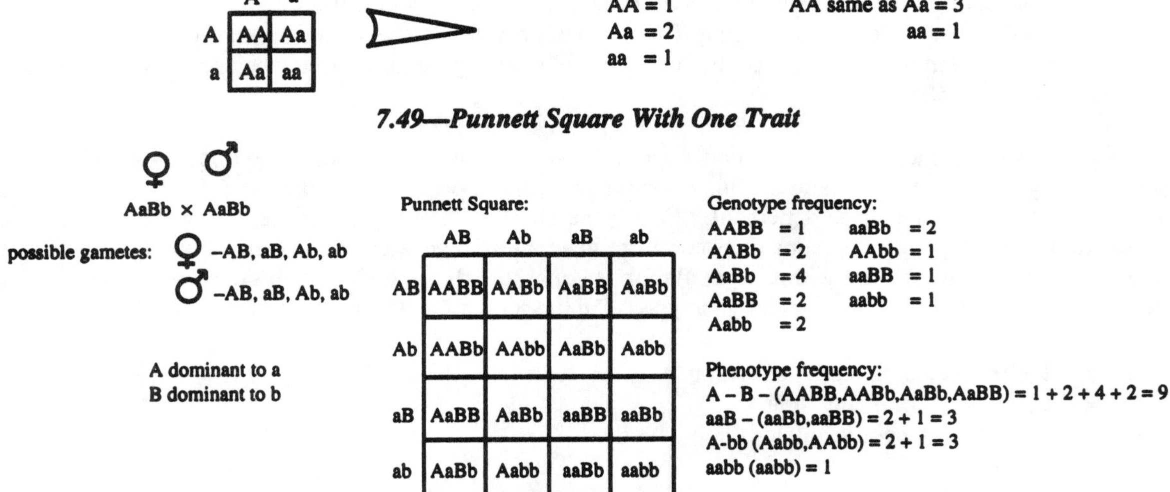

7.49—Punnett Square With One Trait

Fig. 7.50—Punnett Square With Two Traits

Mutations produce a small but important change in the gene frequencies of the *gene pool* (section 7.10.1.3) of a population. These gene frequencies determine the genotypic ratios which determine the distribution of phenotypes in the population. *Genotypic ratios* (i.e., numbers and types of genotypes) can be determined from the gene frequencies and the Punnett square method as shown in Fig. 7.51.

allele B = 0.8, allele b = 0.2 as frequencies in the population

Punnett Square to determine genotypes:

	B (0.8)	b (0.2)
B (0.8)	BB (0.64)	Bb (0.16)
b (0.2)	Bb (0.16)	bb (0.04)

Fig. 7.51—Genotypic Frequencies

genotypic frequencies BB = 0.64, Bb = 2(0.16) = 0.32, bb = 0.04.

7.10.1.6 HARDY-WEINBERG PRINCIPLE WITH APPLICATIONS

The *Hardy-Weinberg Law* states that under certain conditions the above gene frequencies and genotypic frequencies remain constant from generation to generation in sexually reproducing populations. This means no evolution would occur under *these conditions* which are: (1) large populations, (2) no mutations or the existence of mutation equilibrium (3) no immigration or emigration of the population, and (4) random reproduction. The reason large populations (#1) are required is that gene frequencies undergo random fluctuations called *genetic drift*. In a small population, these random changes may cause an increase in certain alleles which leads to homozygosity. This effect is small in large populations (e.g., greater than 10,000 breeding individuals). As noted above, mutations always occur so #2 does not hold. Immigration or emigration leads to loss or gain of certain alleles which change gene frequencies. Reproduction includes all the steps from mate selection through mating and development of the embryo to growth of the young to reproductive maturity. All of these steps, and all in between, must be random for gene frequencies to remain constant (#4). But in all populations, non-random reproduction exists, and this non-random reproduction is called *natural selection* as set forth by *Darwin*. The reason reproduction is non-random is because phenotypes vary, and different phenotypes result in differences in reproductive capabilities. Natural selection does change gene frequencies by causing new combinations of genes which result in new phenotypes. Additionally, recombination and gene mutation, if left alone, can destroy favorable gene combinations and substitute unfavorable combinations for them. Natural selection also serves a conservative function by eliminating these unfavorable combinations. Note that natural selection can act on gene frequencies only when the genetic variation is expressed as phenotypic variation, and that phenotypic variation can lead to changes in gene frequencies only when it reflects underlying genetic variation.

The Hardy-Weinberg principle states that under certain random mating conditions, gene frequencies will remain constant from generation to generation. This principle is useful in population genetics. Gene frequencies may be expressed as a decimal or as a percent. Under the Hardy-Weinberg principle, the gene frequency of dominant and recessive alleles remains the same from generation to generation. In other words, the sum of all the allele frequencies for a gene within a population is equal to 1.0, or 100%. Each genotype is made of two alleles. The chance of getting a particular genotype is the product of the probabilities of the two alleles.

The Hardy-Weinberg equation states, $p^2 + 2pq + q^2 = 1$.

p = frequency of dominant allele

q = frequency of recessive allele

As a simple example, consider a population of dogs, 16 percent are white. The gene for white is recessive. In order to find the frequency of the dominant gene (dominant = W, recessive = w), apply Hardy-Weinberg principle as shown:

	p +	q
p +	WW	Ww
q	Ww	ww

WW = homozygous dominant

2Ww = heterozygous dominant

ww = homozygous recessive

	p +	q
p +	p^2	pq
q	pq	q^2

$$(p + q)(p + q) = 1$$
$$p^2 + 2pq + q^2 = 1$$
$$p + q = 1$$

In the population of dogs provided, 16% are white (these are the homozygous recessive dogs). Hence, $q^2 = 0.16$, $q = 0.4$, $p = 1 - 0.4 = 0.6$. The frequency of the dominant gene W = p = 0.6.

In order to determine the frequency of heterozygosity for whiteness/non-whiteness for the dog population, determine $2pq = 2(0.6)(0.4) = 0.48$.

$$
\begin{aligned}
\text{Finally, } p &= 0.6 = 60\% \\
q &= 0.4 = 40\% \\
2pq &= 0.48 = 48\% \\
p^2 &= (0.6)^2 = 0.36 = 36\% \\
q^2 &= (0.4)^2 = 0.16 = 16\% \\
p^2 + 2pq + q^2 &= 36\% + 48\% + 16\% = 100\%
\end{aligned}
$$

The above examples should be studied and applied to various population genetics problems.

7.10.1.7 GENE MAPPING

Simple gene mapping is done utilizing recombinant techniques. This is done with viral and bacterial DNAs. The map is a linear, one-dimensional structure. The map units indirectly represent the percent recombination between various traits (genetic loci). The traits must be measurable in some manner (e.g., nutrient utilization, products produced, temperature dependence, etc.). The combination of traits in the offspring, as compared with the parents, helps determine the recombinant frequencies (percentages) that help determine the gene map. An example of a two-factor (trait) cross:

Parents			**Offspring**	
a		a^+	a / b^+	—35%
	×		a^+ / b	—35%
b^+		b	a / b	—15%
			a^+ / b^+	—15%

- — the original genotypes are in the highest frequency.
- — the larger percentage of recombinants, the farther apart are the traits on the map. Consequently, the traits are linked less tightly.
- — the trait loci (a *or* a^+ and b *or* b^+) are linked (see below).

A series of two-factor crosses may be used to sequence the gene loci. The maximal possible frequency of any recombinant is 50%. If the frequency of recombination between the loci is near 50%, then there is no linkage. The smaller the recombination frequency between the two loci, the stronger the linkage (i.e., the closer together the traits). Triple factor (i.e., three traits at three loci) are used to order gene loci. The (original) parental genotypes will appear in the highest frequency, single recombinants next, and double recombinants in the lowest frequency. The probability of the central locus recombining with both outside loci (double recombination) is equal to the products of the probability of it combining with each individually (single recombination).

Example: **Parents**

x	x^+
y	y^+
z	z^+

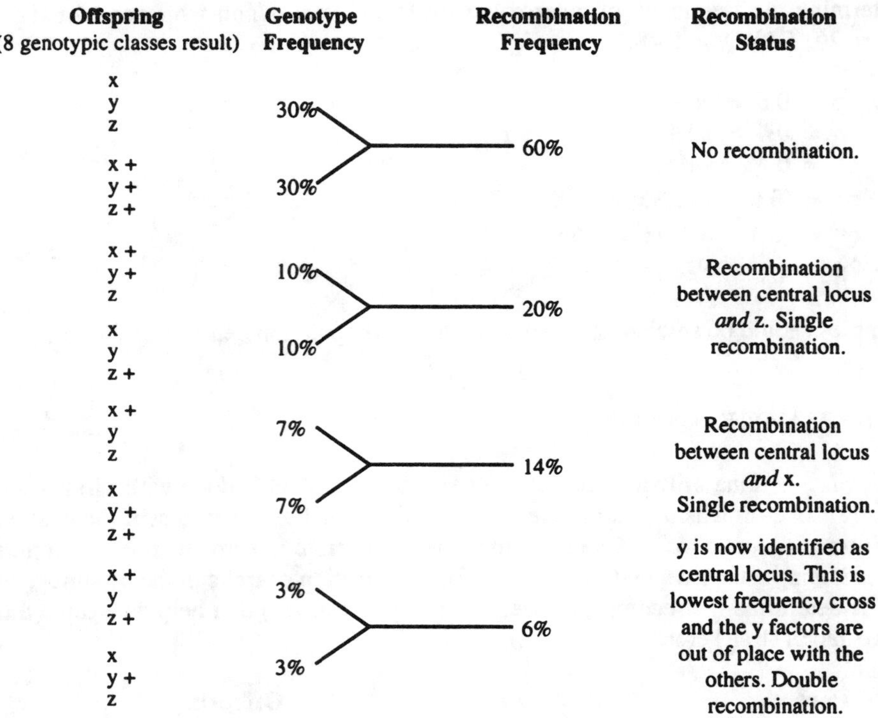

Note that y is closer to x than to z (lower recombination frequency for x than for z above).

There are factors that modify the percentage distributions of the offspring and may affect the analysis. Besides the probability factor (i.e., each cross will not lead to exact ratios, just as in Mendelian crosses), conditional lethal mutations may occur and cause some genotypes not to survive, and therefore, not to be counted.

7.10.1.8 POPULATION GROWTH

Although many factors affect the ultimate growth of a population (species), four factors can be used to describe the growth rate (R). These are the birth rate (B), the death rate (D), the carrying capacity (C), and the number of individuals in the population (N). B is the rate of live births per unit population (e.g., 5/1000 means 5 live births per 1000 individuals). D is similarly defined. Both are dependent on the age of the population and the reproductive capacity of the population. Very old or young populations will have high D. C represents the number of individuals the environment is able to support. C is independent of the R of the population, but over time the total N can affect its value (e.g., by using up the food supply). The maximum growth rate may vary as the C of particular environments varies. The equation linking these four factors is:

$$R = (B - D) \times \left(\frac{C - N}{C}\right) \times N.$$

Note that B − D is the intrinsic growth rate (IGR) of the population. The key points to remember are:

(1) R is directly proportional to IGR;
(2) R is directly proportional to N;
(3) when N is small, the term (C-N)/C is about one and growth is exponential;
(4) when N approaches and equals C, the term (C-N)/C is zero and the population is in zero growth (mild fluctuations may occur);
(5) the (C-N)/C factor results in the logistic (S shaped) growth curve for populations.

Growth curves are:

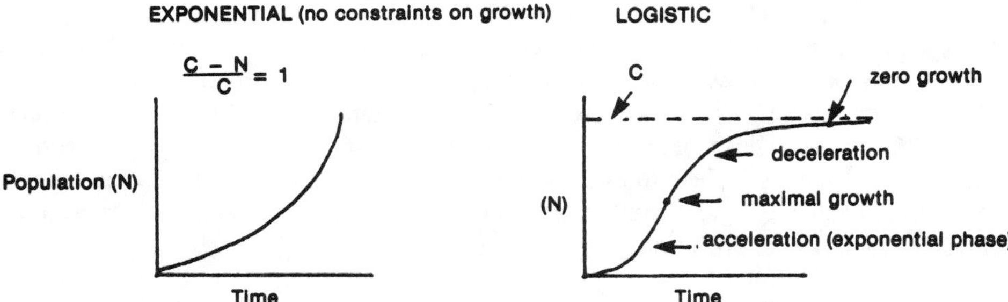

Note the maximal growth rate occurs in approximately the center of the curve (logistic). The maximal growth rate of the exponential growth curve is not reached as it is always increasing (and is never realized except for very short periods and then the logistic curve will intervene). The point of maximal growth is also the point of optimal yield of a population. This means to get the greatest number of individuals (including more mature) out of a population, the population size (N) should be kept near this point. It is always near the center of the logistic growth curve.

Age distributions of populations are important in understanding and predicting changes in population growth. Age distribution curves may be done in many different graphic representations. One example is (with different distributions):

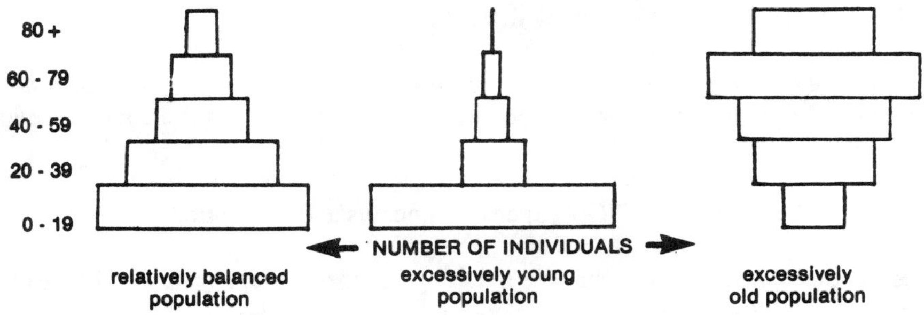

Survivorship of the population may also be graphically represented as:

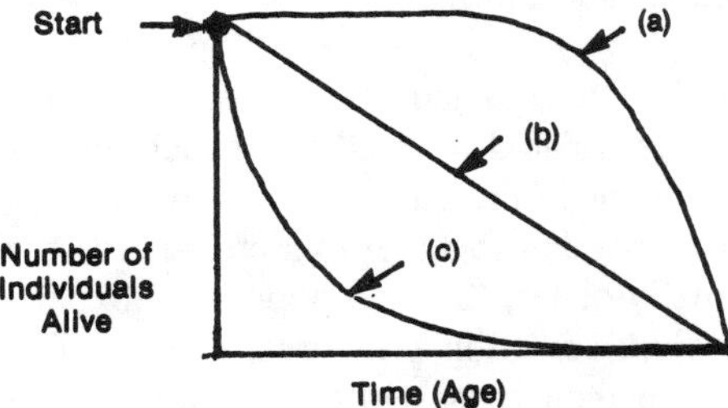

(a) individuals live to older ages, many younger and older
(b) death rates same at all ages, equal representation of all ages
(c) younger die at high rates, few older in population

The factors limiting population growth may be divided into density dependent (DD) and density independent (DI) effects. DD effects (as population grows, these are more important) include space, food, diseases, predation, and other competitive factors. DI effects include weather, natural disasters, and aging. The limitations on population growth can be overcome by emigration (relocation to alleviate DD effects), migration (relocating annually to maximize environments), evolution of different characteristics, or undergoing population cycles (increases and decreases in population size on a regular basis by mechanisms unknown, e.g., the lemmings). If unsuccessful, the population may become extinct.

7.10.1.9 THE MECHANISM OF EVOLUTION

Evolution is the study of the changes that occur in organisms, how the changes occur, and the results of the changes. These changes may be minor and lead to better adaptation to an environment, or they may be major and lead to a totally different species. Changes come about when organisms are *"selected"* to survive on the basis of *phenotypic differences.* These phenotypic differences must be based upon underlying *genetic differences,* as found in the germ cells, to lead to evolutionary change. The survival of selected organisms leads to *changes in the gene frequencies and gene combinations* in the population, which in turn leads to *changes in phenotypic characteristics* and, hence, evolution.

Phenotypic differences are in a distribution in any population. The distribution is often an approximation of the bell shaped curve.

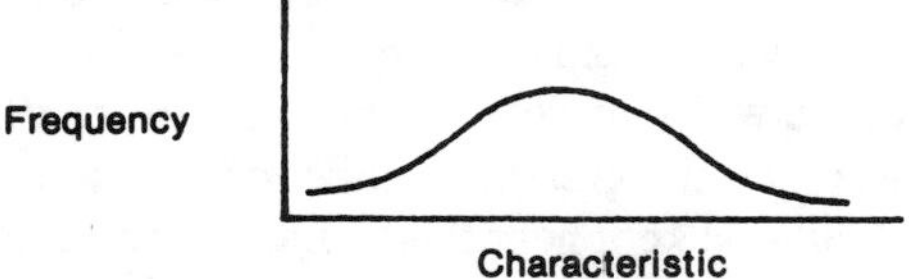

An example is the distribution of height in humans. *Environmental factors* (meteorologic, geographic, physical, or biologic) also vary greatly. It is a small step to infer that certain characteristics are better suited for certain environments. Or, to look at it differently, environments may select organisms with certain phenotypic characteristics that are most likely to survive in them. As above, if these phenotypic characteristics reflect genetic differences then a change in gene frequencies and evolution can occur. Environmental factors and reproductive factors (i.e., natural selection) interact with each other.

In summary, mutations provide the raw material for evolution. But it is the *selection pressure* for certain phenotypes exerted by natural selection and environmental factors that determines the course of evolution.

7.10.1.10 CONSEQUENCES OF EVOLUTION (Species Concepts and Speciation)

The consequences of evolution are seen in the changes that may occur in a given species. These changes can be minor and reflected as *clines.* Clines are gradual variations in a species due to geographic (environmental) variations such as altitude or latitude. *Subspecies (races)* result when an abrupt environmental change is associated with an abrupt change in characteristics. Finally, the evolutionary changes may be so great as to result in a totally new species—a process called speciation.

A *species* is viewed as a set of genetically distinct organisms that share a common gene pool (i.e., gene flow is possible between them) and are reproductively isolated from all other such groups. The first step in *speciation* is usually *geographic isolation* of two populations of the same species. A *barrier* (e.g., rivers, oceans, canyons, mountains, etc.) prevent the populations from coming together to mate. The two separate populations will tend to differ because: (1) gene frequencies usually differ, (2) each population experiences different mutations, (3) the different environments will exert different selection pressures, and (4) if small, genetic drift can cause differences. The second factor in speciation then comes into play; it is *reproductive isolation.* The two populations will begin to differ such that gene flow between them is no longer possible even if they are brought together. This is brought about by *intrinsic reproductive isolating mechanisms* which act at all the steps of reproduction discussed earlier. These are: (1) *ecogeographic isolation* (organisms can no longer survive in each other's environment), (2) *habitat isolation* (organisms may occupy only certain, but different, habitats within the same range), (3) *seasonal isolation* (the breeding periods may be at different times of the year), (4) *behavioral isolation* (mating rituals differ), (5) *mechanical isolation* (nonfitting of genitals), (6) *gametic isolation* (fertilization cannot occur), (7) *hybrid unviability* (the offspring cannot reproduce), and (8) *developmental isolation* (fertilization can occur, but the embryo dies). So, by geographic isolation followed by reproductive isolation, the mechanisms of evolution lead to new species.

General *patterns* of evolution are *divergent* (moving from one species to different species, the usual pattern), *convergent* (moving from separate to common species), or *parallel* (two species resulting from one but evolving in a parallel fashion). *Adaptive radiation* is the gradual divergent differentiation of a species, usually as a response to environmental variations. *Homologous* structures are those that arose from a common structure even though functions may be different. *Analogous* structures have common functions but arose from different structures.

7.10.1.11 TAXONOMY

A hierarchical classification that exists for organisms was due primarily to *Linnaeus*. Organisms are grouped at each level on the basis of similarities. As the hierarchy is ascended (shown below), the similarities become more general. A well-known mnemonic is given with the hierarchy:

Kings	Kingdom
Play	Phylum
Chess	Class
On	Order
Fine	Family
Grain	Genus
Sand	Species

All organisms are given a two-component Latin name. The first is the genus (capitalized), and the second is the species (not capitalized), e.g., *Homo sapiens.*

7.10.1.12 COMPARATIVE ANATOMY

The major adaptive evolutionary changes are discussed for chordates. *Chordates* are distinguished by (1) a dorsal, hollow nerve cord, (2) gill slits in the throat region, and (3) a notochord. Chordates are divided into invertebrate chordates (tunicates, acorn worms, cephalochordates or amphioxus) and vertebrates. *Vertebrates* have a vertebral column, closed circulatory system (enabling large growth), a better developed nervous system and improved sensory apparatus. *Fish* include the Agnatha (jawless, e.g., lampreys), Chondrichthyes (e.g., sharks, all cartilage except inner ears) and Osteichthyes (bony fish). The pectoral fins, pelvic fins and lateral line system are important for balance. Lobe fin fish (or crossopterygians, e.g., latimeria) invaded land, had lungs, had stubby fins (bones into fins—was a crucial step for land invasion) and gave rise to the amphibians. *Amphibians* (frogs, toads, salamanders) are still tied to water because their eggs are easily dessicated. *Reptiles* (snakes, turtles, lizards, crocodiles and alligators) arose from amphibians. Total land life was possible because of the amniotic egg which wouldn't dessicate and which had a sufficient food supply. Reptiles are also advanced beyond amphibians by (1) internal fertilization by copulation, (2) ventricle of heart is partly divided to separate oxygenated and unoxygenated blood, (3) ribs aid in respiration, and (4) the brain has small cerebral hemispheres. The pterosaurs (extinct) gave rise to the birds. *Aves* (birds) can fly because of special feathers (modified reptile scales, large quills for flying surface, fanlike tail feathers for stabilization, contour and down feathers for insulation), light skeleton and a special breastbone for flight muscles, warm-blooded, efficient respiration with the four-chambered heart, advanced sight and muscular coordination by the brain. *Mammals* arose from a different type of reptile than did the birds. Key distinguishing features of mammals are: (1) internal development of young and nutrition by mammary glands, (2) jaw is strengthened and teeth are differentiated, (3) a diaphragm is present to separate thorax and abdomen and is used in breathing, (4) legs are swung underneath the body, and (5) the brain is greatly enlarged.

Evolutionary Timetable

GEOLOGIC ERA	PERIOD	TIME (in millions of years ago)	FEATURES
Precambrian	--------	2,700	Marine invertebrates; protozoans
Paleozoic	Cambrian	600	Trilobites; brachiopods
	Ordovician	500	First fish
	Silurian	430	First air-breathing animals; first insects
	Devonian	410	First amphibians; sharks; sea lilies
	Carboniferous	350	First reptiles; insects
	Permian	275	Mammal-like reptiles; emergence of modern insects
Mesozoic	Triassic	225	First dinosaurs
	Jurassic	175	First birds, flying reptiles; dinosaurs; first mammals
	Cretaceous	130	Primitive mammals; first modern birds; dinosaurs become extinct
Cenozoic	Tertiary	60	Rapid development of higher mammals and birds
	Quaternary	2	Appearance of modern humans; extinction of giant mammals

7.10.2 Questions Related to Genetics and Evolution

1. Which of the following is correct for gene mapping?

A. Only three-factor crosses may be used to sequence gene loci.
B. The recombination frequencies are always representative of the recombination rates of the gene loci.
C. The recombination frequency is equal to the map units.
D. Viral DNAs are used for gene mapping.

2. Cytoplasmic inheritance:

A. does not follow Mendelian Laws.
B. is due to maternal cytoplasm playing the dominant role.
C. is represented by replication of mitochondria.
D. is characterized by all of the above statements.

3. Homozygous refers to:

A. similar types of chromosomes.
B. having similar functions on an evolutionary basis.
C. particles in a solution not being separable microscopically.
D. identical alleles for a given trait.

4. Which statement is *incorrect* concerning X and Y chromosomes?

A. X is larger than Y.
B. X and Y are not homologous.
C. XY is a genotypic male.
D. Traits appearing on X but not on Y are called sex-linked traits.

5. Select the *incorrect* statement:

A. Genotype is the alleles for a given trait in an individual.
B. Phenotype is the expression of the genotype.
C. A given genotype will give rise to different phenotypes.
D. Different genotypes may give rise to the same phenotype.

6. Crossing-over of chromosomes:
   - A. involves reciprocal exchanges of segments of homologous chromosomes.
   - B. occurs in Metaphase I of meiosis.
   - C. is more frequent between traits located close together.
   - D. prevents independent assortment of traits on the same chromosome.

7. Genetic recombination:
   - A. occurs by exchange of chromosomes between gametes.
   - B. is the exchange of similar alleles between gametes.
   - C. is the mixing of alleles of various traits between homologous chromosomes.
   - D. is not used to make chromosome maps.

8. An allele for a trait:
   - A. is a gene.
   - B. can be different on homologous chromosomes in a given cell.
   - C. is both (A) and (B).
   - D. is neither (A) nor (B).

9. Barr bodies:
   - A. are densities associated with desmosomes.
   - B. are crystals of enzymes seen in lysosomes.
   - C. are inactivated X-chromosomes seen in certain cells.
   - D. represent a synonym for polar bodies resulting during oogenesis.

10. Which of the following is an example of aneuploidy?
    - A. 4n
    - B. trisomy 21
    - C. XO (no Y chromosome)
    - D. both (B) and (C)

11. Select the *incorrect* statement about the number and type of chromosomes in the normal human male:
    - A. there are 44 autosomal chromosomes
    - B. there are 46 chromosomes total
    - C. there are two X chromosomes
    - D. there is one Y chromosome

12. In the typical somatic cell, the number of chromosomes is symbolized as:
    - A. 1n.
    - B. 2n.
    - C. 3n.
    - D. 4n.

13. Chromosomes (eukaryotes) are composed of all except:
    - A. histones.
    - B. non-histone protein.
    - C. DNA.
    - D. RNA.

14. Select the *incorrect* statement:
    - A. A recessive allele is only expressed when it is homozygous.
    - B. A dominant allele can be expressed when heterozygous.
    - C. A codominant allele may express itself completely or partially when homozygous or heterozygous, respectively.
    - D. Dominant alleles may not be expressed.

15. Mendel's First Law states that:

   A. alleles of the same trait segregate (separate on homologous chromosomes) in the formation of gametes.
   B. alleles of different traits separate independently of each other in the formation of gametes.
   C. genes are particulate in nature.
   D. genes are indivisible (i.e., cannot be subdivided and yet produce a given trait).

16. Select the *incorrect* statement regarding homologous chromosomes:

   A. Except for X and Y, they are the same size.
   B. They have identical sequences of genes.
   C. They snynapse in meiosis.
   D. Except for X and Y, they have the same sequence of loci as traits.

17. Sex-linked traits:

   A. are found more in females than in males.
   B. are found on the X and Y chromosomes.
   C. allow recessive alleles to be expressed when one such allele is present in the male.
   D. in males have a 50% chance of receiving sex-linked alleles from the father.

18. If the genotype for a trait is Aa (A dominant to a), possible gametes are:

   A. Aa only.
   B. AA and aa.
   C. A, a.
   D. Aa, A, and a.

19. Given the following pedigree, select the correct explanation assuming that the pedigree is representative of the inheritance patterns (blackened symbols mean trait is present):

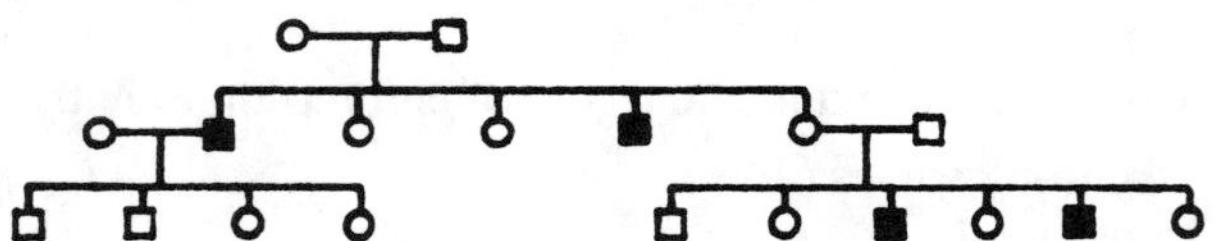

   A. autosomal dominant
   B. autosomal recessive
   C. sex-linked dominant
   D. sex-linked recessive

20. Given the following representative pedigree, select the most likely pattern of inheritance (blackened symbols mean the trait is present):

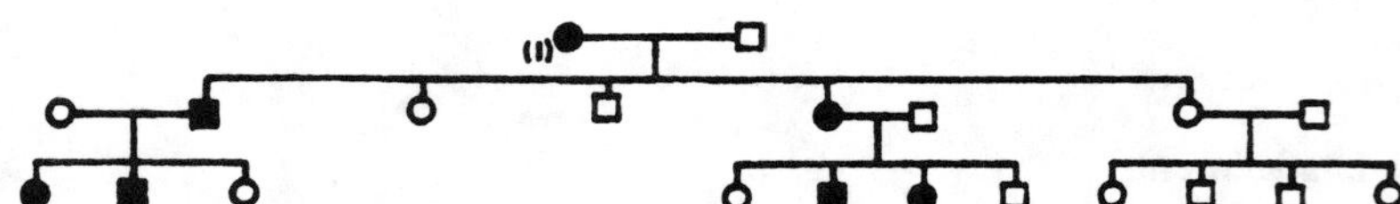

   A. autosomal dominant
   B. autosomal recessive
   C. sex-linked dominant
   D. sex-linked recessive

21. Given the following representative pedigree, what is the most likely pattern of inheritance (blackened symbols mean trait is present)?

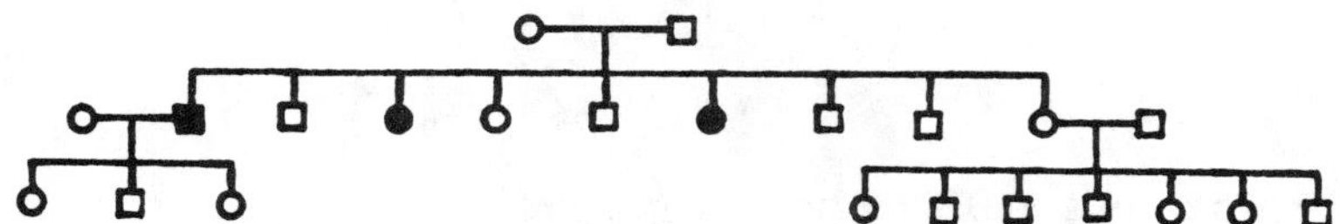

A. autosomal dominant
B. autosomal recessive
C. sex-linked recessive
D. mutation

22. If brown eyes (B) is dominant to blue eyes (b), the parents have what genotype for eye color (open symbol: brown eyes; blackened symbol: blue eyes)?

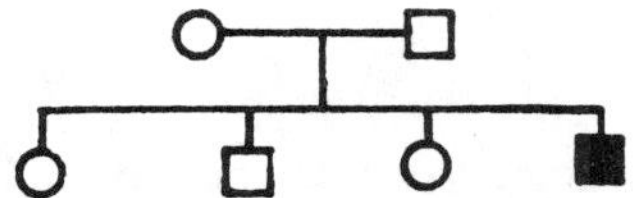

A. father Bb, mother BB
B. father BB, mother Bb
C. father Bb, mother Bb
D. cannot be determined from information given

23. Suppose gray (G) is dominant to white (g) coat color for rats. Given the following representative pedigree, what are the most likely genotypes of the parents (open symbol: white; blackened symbol: gray)?

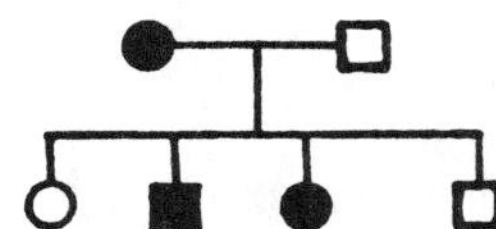

A. father GG, mother gg
B. father Gg, mother Gg
C. father gg, mother Gg
D. cannot be determined from the information given

24. Suppose round peas (R) are dominant to wrinkled peas (r) and green peas (G) are dominant to yellow peas (g). The following cross is made:

RrGg × RrGg

What are the expected phenotypes and their frequencies in the offspring (assume the traits are not linked)?

A. 3 round, green: 1 wrinkled, yellow
B. 2 round, green: 1 round, yellow: 1 wrinkled, green
C. 9 round, green: 3 wrinkled, green: 3 round, yellow: 1 wrinkled, yellow
D. all round, green

25. If red (R) is dominant to white (r) and parents with genotypes RR(male) and rr(female) are crossed, what are the colors and their expected frequencies in the offspring?

A. 1 red: 3 white
B. 1 red: 1 white
C. 3 red: 1 white
D. all red

26. If the offspring from Question #25 are crossed with each other, what are the colors and their frequencies in the offspring from this second cross?

A. 1 red: 2 pink: 1 white
B. 3 red: 1 white
C. 1 red: 1 white
D. all red

27. If the genotype for two traits is AaBB, the possible gametes are:

A. Aa, BB.
B. AB, aB.
C. A, a, B, B.
D. Ab, ab, AB, aB.

28. Mendel's Second Law states that:

A. alleles of the same trait segregate (separate on homologous chromosomes) in the formation of gametes.
B. alleles of different traits separate independently of each other in the formation of gametes.
C. genes are particulate in nature.
D. genes are indivisible.

29. Suppose the only alleles that determine blood type are A and B, and that they are codominant. If parents, both with Type AB, have children, what are the ratios of the childrens' expected blood types? Type A = AA, Type B = BB, Type AB = AB (genotypes of each type)

A. 1 Type A: 2 Type AB: 1 Type B
B. 1 Type A: 1 Type B
C. 3 Type AB: 1 Type A: 1 Type B
D. all Type AB

30. The following three-factor cross is done. Which answer is correct?

Parent Genotypes:	Offspring Genotypes	Percentage of Total
r r+ s+ s t t+	r s+ t	26%
	r+ s t+	26%
	r s+ t+	16%
	r+ s t	16%
	r+ s+ t+	6%
	r s t	6%
	r+ s+ t	2%
	r s t+	2%

A. The genotypes representing the double recombination are (r s t) and (r+ s+ t+).
B. The s locus is farthest from the central locus.
C. The map distance between the three loci is 16 units.
D. The r locus is the central locus.

31. Select the correct statement:

A. Phenotypic differences alone serve as a basis for evolution.
B. Phenotypic differences serve as a basis for evolution when they reflect somatic cell genetic differences.
C. Phenotypic differences serve as a basis for evolution when they reflect germ cell genetic differences.
D. None of the above are correct.

32. The ultimate source of all new genes in a population is due to:

A. mitosis.
B. mating.
C. meiosis.
D. mutation.

33. Mutations tend to be:

A. recessive.
B. dominant.
C. codominant.
D. corecessive.

34. Mutations do not affect evolutionary change primarily because they are:

A. expressed.
B. recessive.
C. too rare.
D. random.

35. "Under certain conditions the gene frequencies and genotypic frequencies remain constant from generation to generation in sexually reproducing populations" was put forth by:

A. Dalton.
B. Hardy-Weinberg.
C. Mendel.
D. Mendeleev.

36. All of the following are conditions under which evolution would *not* occur except:

A. large populations.
B. nonrandom reproduction.
C. no mutations.
D. no immigration or emigration.

37. Genetic drift may lead to evolution in populations that are:

A. any size.
B. large.
C. small.
D. divergent.

38. Which is *not* considered as part of the evolutionary concept of the reproductive process?

A. mate selection and mating behavior
B. embryo development
C. growth of young to reproductive maturity
D. all of the above are part of the reproductive process

39. Darwin's idea of natural selection is the same as:

A. polyploidy.
B. mutation pressure.
C. genetic drift.
D. nonrandom reproduction.

40. Natural selection results in:

A. increased favorable gene combinations.
B. decreased unfavorable gene combinations.
C. both A and B.
D. neither A nor B.

41. Selection pressure depends on:

A. nonrandom reproduction.
B. environmental factors.
C. both A and B.
D. neither A nor B.

42. The first step in the formation of a new species is:

A. reproductive isolation
B. geographic isolation
C. reproductive and geographic isolation.
D. genetic isolation.

43. Populations that are separated by geographic barriers will tend to differ because:

A. gene frequencies usually differ between them.
B. mutations vary between populations.
C. there are different environmental pressures.
D. of all of the above factors.

44. Structures that have different functions but arose from a common structure are called:

A. convergent.
B. divergent.
C. analogous.
D. homologous.

45. Assuming all other factors are constant, which situation will not result in an increase in the population growth rate?

A. increase in the total individuals in the population near the carrying capacity
B. decrease in the death rate
C. increase in the birth rate
D. increase in the intrinsic growth rate

46. Important features in the development of mammals are:

I. internal development of young.
II. that jaw is strengthened and teeth differentiated.
III. diaphragm development.
IV. legs underneath body.
V. a greatly enlarged brain.

A. I, III, V
B. I, III, IV, V
C. I, II, III, V
D. all of the above

47. A factor which would be detrimental to the flight of birds is:

- **A.** a light skeleton.
- **B.** advanced sight and muscle coordination.
- **C.** a three-chambered heart.
- **D.** large quill feathers or fan-like tail feathers.

48. Reptiles differ from amphibians by all of the following except:

- **A.** amniotic egg.
- **B.** internal fertilization by copulation.
- **C.** a complete four-chambered heart.
- **D.** ribs that aid in respiration.

49. The primary reason amphibians are still tied to the water is:

- **A.** their lungs are inadequate.
- **B.** they are cold blooded.
- **C.** their eggs are easily dessicated.
- **D.** they need to breathe through moist skin.

50. A fish manager wants to increase the productivity of a lake. He desires greater catches of fish and larger sized fish. He wants to maintain this over a long period of time. This increase will be accomplished best by:

- **A.** increasing the bait (food) available to the fish.
- **B.** keeping the fish population near the maximal growth rate point.
- **C.** restricting the number of fish caught for several years.
- **D.** stocking the lake with reproductive size fish this year.

51. Which type of heart can separate oxygenated and deoxygenated blood completely?

- **A.** two chambered.
- **B.** three chambered.
- **C.** four chambered.
- **D.** five chambered.

52. Diaphragms are muscles used in the act of breathing. Which of the following utilizes a diaphragm to breathe?

- **A.** amphibians
- **B.** reptiles
- **C.** birds
- **D.** none of the above

53. What is the correct hierarchy (from highest to lowest) of the given levels of taxonomy?

- **A.** class, order, family, genus
- **B.** order, family, genus, class
- **C.** family, genus, class, order
- **D.** family, class, order, genus

54. Organisms are given a two-component scientific name. The first part is the:

- **A.** class.
- **B.** order.
- **C.** species.
- **D.** genus.

7.10.3 Answers to Questions in Section 7.10.2

(1) D (2) D (3) D (4) B (5) C (6) A (7) C (8) C (9) C (10) D (11) C (12) B
(13) D (14) A (15) A (16) B (17) C (18) C (19) D (20) A (21) B (22) C (23) C (24) C
(25) D (26) B (27) B (28) B (29) A (30) D (31) C (32) D (33) A (34) D (35) B (36) B

(37) C (38) D (39) D (40) C (41) C (42) B (43) D (44) D (45) A (46) D (47) C (48) C (49) C (50) B (51) C (52) D (53) A (54) D

7.10.4 Discussion of Answers to Questions in Section 7.10.2

Question #1 to #9, #15, #28 — Discussed in Section.

Question #10 (Answer: D) Aneuploidy is the loss (Y is lost in XO) or addition (an extra #21 is added in trisomy 21) of one or more individual chromosomes. Polyploidy means a multiplication of the whole set of chromosomes as in 4n.

Question #11 (Answer: C) The normal male has 44 autosomes, one X and one Y chromosome. The normal female has 44 autosomes and two X chromosomes.

Question #12 (Answer: B) 2n = diploid. Gametes are haploid (1n). Occasionally, somatic cells will be triploid (3n) or tetraploid (4n).

Question #13 (Answer: D) RNA is made using the DNA of chromosomes as a template; it is not an integral part of a chromosome.

Question #14 (Answer: A) Recessive alleles may be expressed when sex-linked. Dominant alleles may not have penetrance.

Question #16 (Answer: B) A gene is a specific sequence of nucleotides with codes for a specific protein which may be expressed as a phenotypic variation (blue, brown) of a given trait (eye color). Homologous chromosomes do not usually have an identical sequence of genes; they do have a set sequence of loci for the alleles (contrasting genes) for a given trait.

Question #17 (Answer: C) This is possible because only the X chromosome carries the trait and the Y is the homologous chromosome in the male.

The allele, a, will express itself because it is the only allele present for the trait.

X Y

Allele, a

Question *#18* (Answer: C) The genotype Aa produces the gametes with A and a separately by Mendel's First Law of Segregation of alleles of the same trait. Note that A and a are on different but homologous chromosomes.

Question #19 (Answer: D) Note that the trait appears only in males, can be carried by females, and the males apparently inherit it only from their mothers.

Question #20 (Answer: A) There is no sex preference and no skipped generations. It (the trait) is only passed from those parents expressing the disease, and many individuals are affected. All of this is characteristic of a highly penetrated autosomal dominant allele. The initial mother (1) is heterozygous for the allele; because if she were homozygous, every one of her children would have the trait.

Question #21 (Answer: B) There is no sex preference, and since the initial father did not have the disease, it would be improbable that his daughters would have it if it was sex-linked recessive. A mutation is unlikely (but possible) because three offspring have the trait, few people are affected, and the trait is not passed by affected individuals. Autosomal recessive is the most likely, and the initial parents must have been heterozygous for the recessive allele.

Question #22 (Answer: C) Since both parents have brown eyes, their genotype must be at least B – for each. Since one child has blue eyes (bb), one b allele must have come from each parent. Therefore, each parent must be Bb.

Question #23 (Answer: C) The father must be gg because he is white. The mother is gray and she is, at least, G –. Since the pedigree is representative, white offspring do appear. Since each white offspring must get one g from the father, they must also get a g from the mother—otherwise there would be no white offspring. Therefore, the mother must be Gg.

Question #24 (Answer: C) Use the Punnett square to get genotypic frequencies (gametes are RG, Rg, rG, rg for each parent):

	RG	Rg	rG	rg
RG	RRGG	RRGg	RrGG	RrGg
Rg	RRGg	RRgg	RrGg	Rrgg
rG	RrGG	RrGg	rrGG	rrGg
rg	RrGg	Rrgg	rrGg	rrgg

Then, based on the dominance-recessive relationships given, the phenotypes and their ratios are:

all R-G- are round, green (RRGG-1, RRGg-2, RrGG-2, RrGg-4) = 9
all rrG- are wrinkled, green (rrGG-1, rrGg-2) = 3
all R-gg are wrinkled, yellow (RRgg-1, Rrgg-2) = 3
rrgg is wrinkled, yellow (rrgg-1) = 1

Question #25 (Answer: D) Since the gametes will be r (female) and R (male) only, all offspring will be Rr or red. See Question #26.

Question #26 (Answer: B) Using the genotype Rr derived in Question #25, determine the genotypes of the new offspring by using a new Punnett Square (gametes are R,r for both parents):

Rr = red

♂ \ ♀	r	r
R	Rr	Rr
R	Rr	Rr

for #25

	R	r
R	RR	Rr
r	Rr	rr

for #26

Then using the dominance-recessive relationship given, the phenotypes and their ratios are determined:

R- is red (RR-1, Rr-2) = 3
rr is white (rr) = 1.

Question #27 (Answer: B) Each gamete will contain one allele of each trait in all possible combinations with each other. Then each gamete can have an A or a, and it must have a B. This gives AB, aB.

Question #29 (Answer: A) Use the Punnett Square to determine the genotypes (gametes of each parent are A,B):

	A	B
A	AA	AB
B	AB	BB

Using the information relating phenotypes to genotypes given in the question:

Type A (AA = 1) = 1
Type B (BB = 1) = 1
Type AB (AB = 2) = 2

Question #30 (Answer: D) The lowest frequency recombinant is r+ s+ t and r s t+. The locus out of line with the parents is the r locus. The r must be the central locus. The t is farther from r (32% recombination frequency) than the s (12% recombination frequency). Map units are not recombination frequency units.

Questions #31 to #49 Discussed in Section.

Question #50 (Answer: B) The point of optimal yield is at the maximum growth rate (MGR). If the MGR can be determined and the population kept at this level, the lake will produce the greatest yield.

Increasing the food (that is, the carrying capacity) will not increase the yields per se. If the amount of fish caught is restricted, the lake will approach the carrying capacity and zero growth rate, and the yield will decrease. Adding more fish may overload the carrying capacity, and, of itself, may not increase the yield. Arguments for each choice may be made; the best answer is (B).

Questions #51 - #54 Discussed in Section.

7.10.5 Advanced Concepts

- Review evolution and genetics—especially the weaker points in scientific hypotheses and theories. Identify possible assumptions (implicit and explicit) in current research methodology
- Conceptualize the following terms as related to genetics:
  Molecular genetics using replica plating or enrichment techniques (limited, penicillin or delayed); episomes: merozygotes; interrupted bacterial mapping; transductional bacteriophage mapping; cis-trans test; transfection; cytogenetics and chromosome mapping; pleiotropic effects; mutant types (sterile, semilethal or lethal); epistatic and nonepistatic genetic interaction
- Understand the following evolution related terms: fossils (trilobite); comparative anatomy genetics (comparing structural similarities and differences among closely related animals, e.g., fish, amphibians, reptiles and birds); homology and homologous structures: natural selection; isolating mechanisms (Galapagos islands); polyploidy; Oparin's hypothesis; Miller's amino acid apparatus; genetic drift using Hardy-Weinberg principle (e.g., Founder principle); splitting evolution and phyletic evolution.

7.11 NERVOUS SYSTEM

7.11.1 Introduction to Nervous System

The complexity of this system is partly due to current and ongoing research efforts linking it to the enormous details associated with sensory reception and processing. Review the four major parts of the nervous system, i.e., central nervous system, peripheral nervous system, autonomic nervous system (sympathetic and parasympathetic) and the sense organs (eyes, nose, ears, tongue and skin). The central nervous system is the command center (messages or impulses arrive there and are sent to various glands, organs and muscles). Understand the similarities and differences between the motor (efferent) and the sensory (afferent) systems. The efferent system is then divided into the autonomic and somatic nervous systems. The most efficient way to review the nervous system is to understand the biological (structural or anatomical) aspects (functions of each part, physiological role of each part including dimensions and equations related to optics, sound, fluids) of the four major parts. Understand the concepts behind the labeled-line law which states, "Each type of sensory nerve fiber transmits only one modality of sensation."

7.11.1.1 NEURAL CELLS (Specialized Eukaryotic Cells)

Histologically, the nervous system is composed of neurons and glial cells. Neurons conduct impulses, and *glial cells* provide some sort of supportive function. There are many kinds of neurons and glial cells—only a typical neuron will be discussed. A *neuron* has a cell body or soma that is characterized by having *Nissl bodies* (ribosomes), one or more short branched projections of the body called *dendrites*, and, usually, one long projection called an *axon*. Although impulses can travel in either direction in a dendrite or an axon, dendrites usually convey impulses toward the soma, and axons usually convey impulses away from the soma. Do not confuse "impulse travel direction" with "ion-transport direction." The nervous system contains approximately 150 billion neurons. This directionality is achieved by the presence of *synapses* between adjacent neurons or a neuron and an effector (muscle or gland). Synapses typically include an axon ending with *transmitter substance*, a synaptic cleft, and a dendrite or muscle or gland with receptors for the transmitter substance.

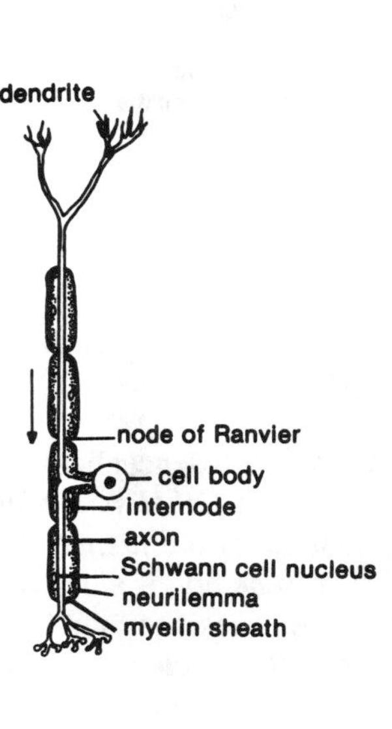

Fig. 7.52(a)—Neuron (Type I)

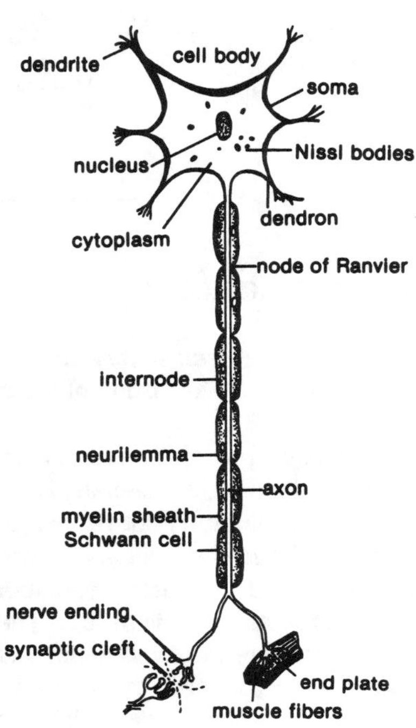

Fig. 7.52(b)—Neuron (Type II)

There are three special types of neurons: sensory, motor, and association. *Sensory neurons* transfer impulses from the various sense organs to the spinal cord or brain, e.g., picking up a hot frying pan with your hand. *Association neurons* transfer and connect the messages between the sensory neurons and the motor neurons. They are located in the brain and spinal cord. Association neurons transfer impulses similar to a switching station at a telephone exchange. In case of the hot frying pan, the impulse travels from the spinal cord to motor neurons, with the help of association neurons. *Motor neurons* transfer impulses to various muscles and glands. For the hot frying pan, the impulse travels along motor neurons to muscles in the arm. This causes the muscles in the arm to retract. This results in your hand dropping the frying pan. After you drop the frying pan, the brain receives this impulse, causing pain.

An impulse causes the axon to release the chemical transmitter; this diffuses across the cleft to the receptors and induces an impulse there which is then transmitted. An *impulse or action potential* is set up in a neuron when the *potential difference* (voltage) across its membrane reaches a *threshold potential.* The *resting potential* of a neuron is determined by the balance of Na^+ (most outside) and K^+ (most inside) on each side of the cell membrane—the outside is positive relative to the inside. An impulse or transmitter substance can disturb the ionic balance in such a way that Na^+ moves inside and K^+ moves outside (only Na^+ moves in the early phase of the action potential). This causes the cell potential to move toward the threshold potential. Once the threshold potential is reached, the action potential is initiated and this moves down the neuron to the axon end, releases transmitter and the process repeats in the next neuron. The *refractory period* is that time during which the nerve cannot respond to a stimulus. See figure below. A *Na-K ATPase* maintains the concentration across the nerve membrane by active transport of the ions. *Myelin sheaths* (tightly wrapped insulators made of cell membranes of glial cells) around axons increase the speed of conduction (saltatory conduction).

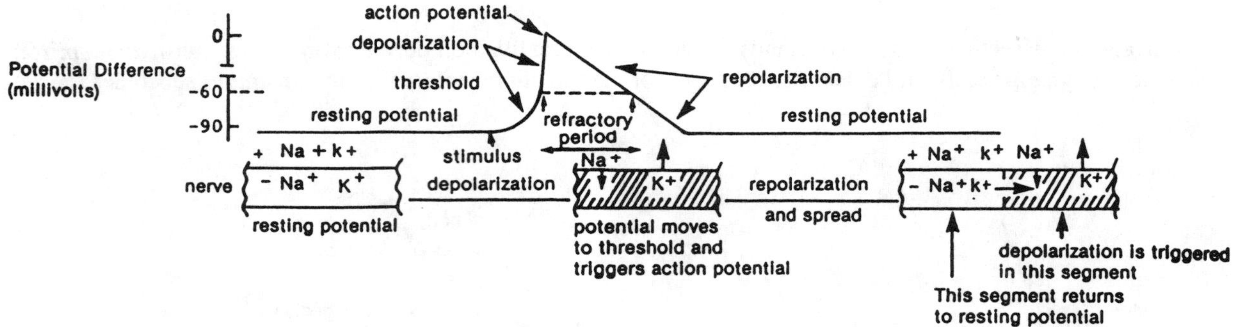

Fig. 7.53—Various Potentials of a Nerve

7.11.1.2 STRUCTURE AND FUNCTION

The nervous system is divided into the *central nervous system (CNS),* consisting of the brain and spinal cord, and the *peripheral nervous system (PNS),* consisting of the cranial nerves (CN) and peripheral nerves (PN).

In the CNS the hindbrain (rhombencephalon), midbrain (mesencephalon), and forebrain (prosencephalon) are the gross divisions of the *brain* and most are bilateral. The *hindbrain* consists of the *myelencephalon (medulla)* and *metencephalon (pons).* The midbrain is not further divided. The forebrain consists of the *diencephalon* (hypothalamus and thalamus) and the *telencephalon* (the *cerebral hemispheres*). The *cerebellum* is a derivative of the metencephalon. Respiratory and circulatory regulation, coughing, and vomiting reflexes, are functions of the medulla. Note that these are functions basic to life. The cerebellum is concerned with muscle coordination (e.g., balance). No general functions are localized in the midbrain or pons; they serve important relay functions. The hypothalamus is the important regulator of the internal environment (controls hormones of the pituitary via releasing factors, thirst and hunger centers, water balance, temperature regulation) and also behavior (sexual, aggressive). The thalamus is the relay center for nearly all sensory input. The cerebrum (especially the cerebral cortex, i.e., surface) is the integrating and interpretation center for all sensory input and voluntary motor activity. In addition, memory, learning, emotions, etc., are also located here (Fig. 7.54(a) and (b)).

The *spinal cord (SC)* has an interior of *gray matter* (neuron cell bodies) surrounded by *white matter* (myelinated axons). Serving as a path between the brain and the periphery (senses and muscles or glands) is the primary function of the SC. *Descending tracts* (from the brain to the SC) and *ascending tracts* (from SC to brain) are in the white matter. *Sensory nerves* (afferent—toward the CNS) enter dorsally and *motor nerves* (efferent—away from the CNS) exit ventrally. Several *reflexes* are at the SC level, e.g., the knee jerk (Fig. 7.55).

The PNS is divided into an *afferent sensory system* (ASS) and an *efferent motor system* (EMS). The PNS consists of the *autonomic nervous system* (ANS) and the *somatic nervous system* (SNS). The ANS is entirely motor, consisting of two motor neurons fastened together. The cell body of the first neuron is located in the CNS (SC or brain stem) and the second neuron cell body is clustered with other similar neuron cell bodies into ganglia. The ANS is divided into the sympathetic system (arising from the thoraco-lumbar levels of the SC) and the *parasympathetic system* (PS), originating in the cranio-sacral levels of the CNS.

The *sympathetic system* (SS) peripherally consists of a chain of ganglia called the sympathetic chain, which is parallel to and adjacent to the spinal cord. These ganglia receive axons from the neurons located in the CNS and themselves send out much longer axons to many organs and tissues. The SS may affect all organs they innervate simultaneously (i.e., in a diffuse manner). In general, the SS moves the organism away from homeostasis as in the "fight or flight" phenomenon. Sympathetic discharges cause the heart rate to increase, digestive process to stop, circulation to the skin to decrease, and blood flow to the heart and muscles to increase. The ganglia of the *parasympathetic system (PS)* are located near the end-organ, and receive long axons from the first neuron whose cell body is in the CNS. The ganglia of the PS generally exert specific effects directed at one organ or tissue. The PS tends to maintain homeostasis and, in general, opposes actions of the SS. Actions of the PS include slowing of the heart rate and increasing the digestive processes. The *Vagus nerve* is a very important parasympathetic nerve to the heart and abdominal viscera. *Acetylcholine* is the postganglionic (after the synapses in the ganglia discussed above) transmitter in the PS. *Norepinephrine* is the postganglionic transmitter for the SS.

There are 31 *spinal nerves* (SN). They are classified according to the level of their connection with the spinal cord—8 cervical, 12 thoracic, 5 lumbar, 5 sacral, 1 coccygeal. Each nerve contains motor and sensory components. The motor neurons are located in the ventral portion of the cord and the sensory neurons in ganglia (dorsal root ganglia) immediately adjacent to the SC. The peripheral nerves are myelinated for most of their length by the Schwann cell.

There are 12 *cranial nerves* (CN). Some are sensory only, some motor only and some carry both. In addition, motor neurons of the parasympathetic system may also be present. The medical functions and related disorders for the 12 nerves are shown in 7.11.1.4. The brain and spinal cord are covered by *meninges*. These are, from the outside in: the *dura mater* (tough fibrous layer), the *arachnoid* (vascular and nutrient layer), and the *pia mater* (fragile layer directly attached to nervous tissue). See Fig. 7.56 for summary of the above information.

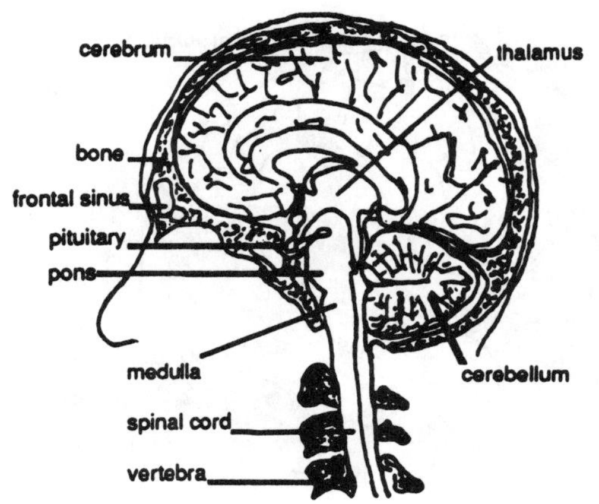

Fig. 7.54(a)—Sagittal Section of Brain and Spinal Cord

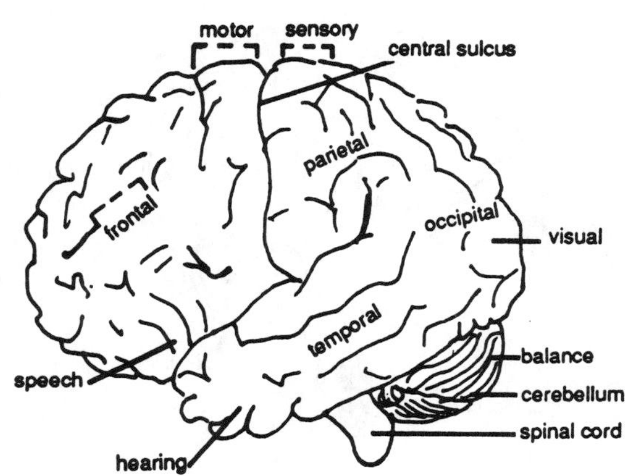

Fig. 7.54(b)—Brain (Lateral View)

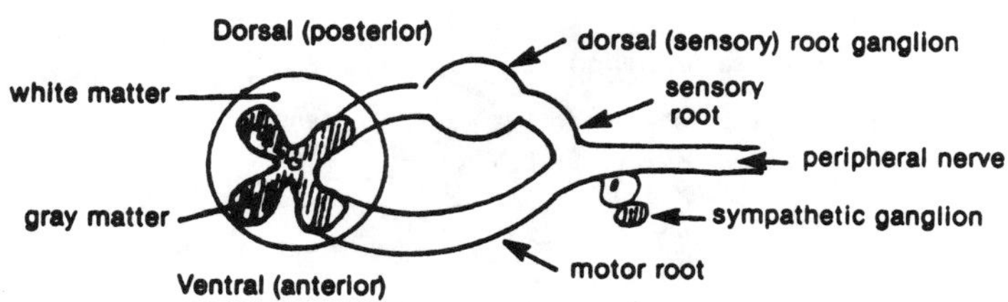

Fig. 7.55—Spinal Cord

Divisions of the Nervous System

<table>
<tr><td colspan="11">Nervous System</td></tr>
<tr><td colspan="8">CNS</td><td colspan="3">PNS</td></tr>
<tr><td colspan="7">Brain</td><td>SC</td><td colspan="2">ANS</td><td rowspan="2">S N S</td></tr>
<tr><td colspan="3">Hindbrain</td><td>Midbrain</td><td colspan="3">Forebrain</td><td></td><td>PS</td><td>SS</td></tr>
<tr><td>Myelen-cephalon</td><td colspan="2">Metencephalon</td><td>"</td><td colspan="2">Diencephalon</td><td>Telencephalon</td></tr>
<tr><td>Medulla</td><td>Pons</td><td>Cere-bellum</td><td>"</td><td>Thal-amus</td><td>Hypo-thalamus</td><td>Cerebral Hemispheres</td></tr>
</table>

Fig. 7.56—Chart of CNS Organization

the synapses in the ganglia discussed above) transmitter in the PS. *Norepinephrine* is the postganglionic transmitter for the SS.

There are 31 *spinal nerves* (SN). They are classified according to the level of their connection with the spinal cord—8 cervical, 12 thoracic, 5 lumbar, 5 sacral, 1 coccygeal. Each nerve contains motor and sensory components. The motor neurons are located in the ventral portion of the cord and the sensory neurons in ganglia (dorsal root ganglia) immediately adjacent to the SC. The peripheral nerves are myelinated for most of their length by the Schwann cell.

There are 12 *cranial nerves* (CN). Some are sensory only, some motor only and some carry both. In addition, motor neurons of the parasympathetic system may also be present. The medical functions and related disorders for the 12 nerves are shown in 7.11.1.4. The brain and spinal cord are covered by *meninges*. These are, from the outside in: the *dura mater* (tough fibrous layer), the *arachnoid* (vascular and nutrient layer), and the *pia mater* (fragile layer directly attached to nervous tissue). See Fig. 7.56 for summary of the above information.

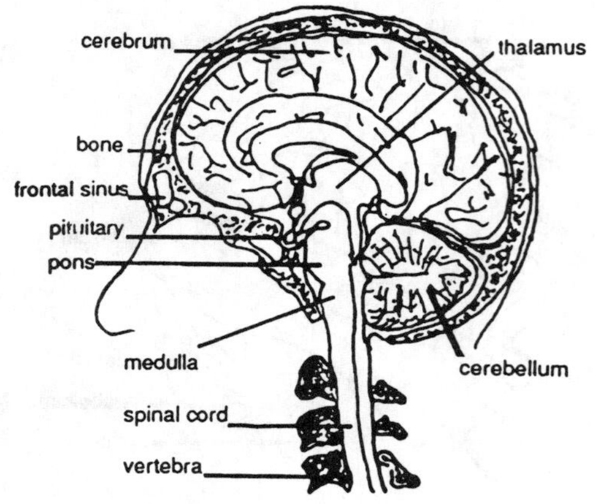

Fig. 7.54(a)—Sagittal Section of Brain and Spinal Cord

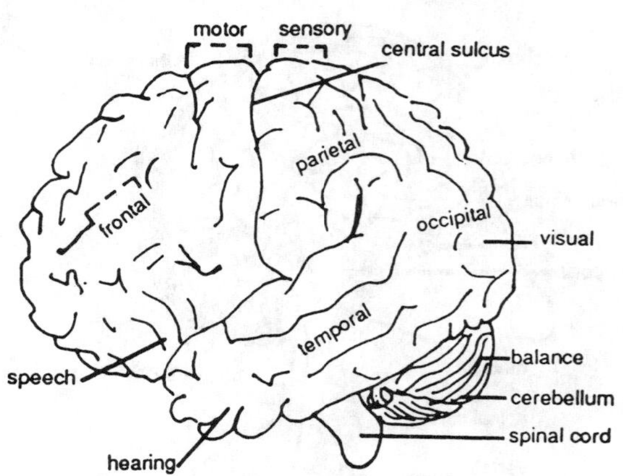

Fig. 7.54(b)—Brain (Lateral View)

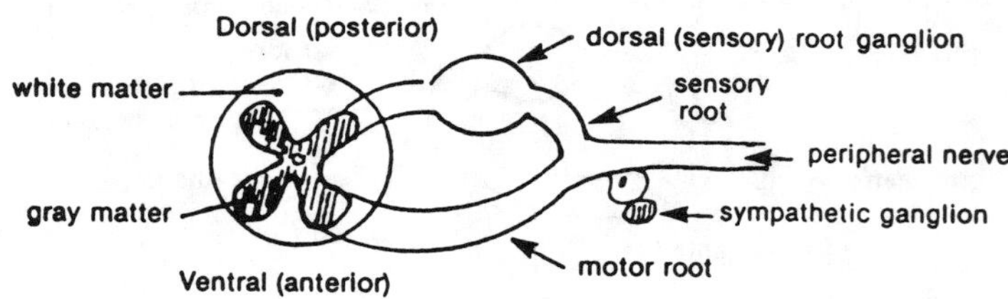

Fig. 7.55—Spinal Cord

Divisions of the Nervous System

<table>
<tr><td colspan="8">← Central Nervous System →</td></tr>
<tr><td colspan="7">Brain</td><td rowspan="4">Spinal Cord</td></tr>
<tr><td colspan="3">Hindbrain</td><td>Midbrain</td><td colspan="3">Forebrain</td></tr>
<tr><td>Myelencephalon</td><td colspan="2">Metencephalon</td><td>Midbrain</td><td>Diencephalon</td><td colspan="2">Telencephalon</td></tr>
<tr><td>Medulla</td><td>Pons</td><td>Cerebellum</td><td>Midbrain</td><td>Thalamus</td><td>Hypothalamus</td><td>Cerebral Hemispheres</td></tr>
</table>

<table>
<tr><td colspan="3">← Peripheral → Nervous System</td></tr>
<tr><td>Afferent Sensory System</td><td colspan="2">Efferent Motor System</td></tr>
<tr><td colspan="2">Autonomic Nervous System</td><td rowspan="2">Somatic Nervous System</td></tr>
<tr><td>Parasympathetic Nervous System</td><td>Sympathetic Nervous System</td></tr>
</table>

Fig. 7.56—Chart of CNS Organization

7.11.1.4 CLASSIFICATION CHART OF CRANIAL NERVES

The twelve cranial nerves can be either sensory or motor or both. They can be memorized by an acronym: Oh, Oh, Oh, to touch and feel very green vegetables—AH! (this order is followed around the ventral surface of the brain). Their dysfunctions are also provided.

Memorizing Symbol	Name of nerve (connection)	Type of nerve	Medical dysfunctions and disorders
Oh	Olfactory I (smell)	Sensory	Anosmia (loss of smelling sensation)
Oh	Optic II or Ocular II (sight)	Sensory	Anopsia (loss of visual acuity)
Oh	Oculomotor III (proprioceptive)	Motor	Diplopia (double vision) and squinting (Strabismus)
to	Trochlear IV (proprioceptive)	Motor	Diplopia (double vision) and squinting (Strabismus)
touch	Trigeminal V (proprioceptive)	Sensory (face and head), motor (mastication muscles)	trigeminal neuralgia (muscle paralysis)
and	Abducens VI (starts in pons)	Motor	eyeball movements
feel	Facial VII motor (facial expression and salivation)	Sensory (taste), control	Bell's palsy (loss of taste) and facial muscle
very	Vestibulocochlear VIII (Organ of Corti, medulla)	Sensory	vertigo (rotational balance) and tinnitus (ringing of ears)
green	glossopharyngeal IX (connected to medulla and taste buds in tongue)	Sensory (taste), motor (swallowing and salivation)	loss of taste, loss of saliva secretion
vegetables	Vagus X, (connected to medulla and jugular foramen)	Sensory (larynx), motor (voice, swallowing, slowing of heart, peristalsis of upper GI tract and stimulating endocrine glands, e.g. pancreas)	interrupts sensations from many organs. More research papers should be read to keep current
A	Spinal accessory XI (cranial and spinal connections)	Motor	swallowing actions, head rotations and shoulder movements are prevented
H	Hypoglossal XII, (connected to medulla and tongue muscles)	Motor	swallowing and speech control by tongue movements

7.11.1.5 SENSORY RECEPTION AND PROCESSING

The anatomy and sensory processing performed by the eyes (sight) and ears (hearing) has been presented in Chapter 5—Physics. The eyes are introduced in the section on optics and the ears are introduced in the section on sound. The integration of concepts of biological sensory receptors (ears and eyes) with Physics is required for the new MCAT.

7.11.2 Questions Related to Nervous System

1. Select the incorrect statement concerning the spinal cord:
   - **A.** Gray matter is central.
   - **B.** White matter is peripheral.
   - **C.** Sensory nerves enter ventrally.
   - **D.** Motor nerves exit ventrally.
2. Which is (are) not part of the central nervous system?
   - **A.** thalamus
   - **B.** hypothalamus
   - **C.** spinal cord
   - **D.** cranial nerves
3. Glial cells are found in the:
   - **A.** muscular system.
   - **B.** endocrine system.
   - **C.** nervous system.
   - **D.** skeletal system.
4. All are specifically associated with a neuron except:
   - **A.** lack of a nucleus.
   - **B.** Nissl bodies.
   - **C.** dendrites.
   - **D.** axons.
5. What entity of neurons allow for one-way conduction of impulses in the nervous system?
   - **A.** axons
   - **B.** dendrites
   - **C.** synapses
   - **D.** somas
6. Which of the following can usually conduct impulses away from the neuron cell body or toward it?
   - **A.** axon
   - **B.** dendrite
   - **C.** both
   - **D.** neither
7. When the potential difference across a nerve membrane equals the threshold, what results?
   - **A.** an action potential
   - **B.** synthesis of transmitter substances
   - **C.** destruction of transmitter substances
   - **D.** nothing until the resting potential is exceeded
8. What ion(s) determine the resting potential of a nerve cell?
   - **A.** sodium
   - **B.** potassium
   - **C.** calcium
   - **D.** both (A) and (B)

9. The concentrations of ions across the cell membrane is maintained by:
   - **A.** diffusion.
   - **B.** active transport.
   - **C.** osmosis.
   - **D.** facilitated transport.

10. Myelin sheaths are found:
    - **A.** surrounding tendons.
    - **B.** covering the brain.
    - **C.** covering muscles.
    - **D.** around axons of neurons.

11. During the early phase of the action potential:
    - **A.** only Na^+ moves.
    - **B.** only K^+ moves.
    - **C.** Na^+ moves into the cell and K^+ moves out.
    - **D.** Na^+ moves out of the cell and K^+ moves in.

12. The refractory period occurs:
    - **A.** before threshold is exceeded.
    - **B.** before the action potential.
    - **C.** after the action potential.
    - **D.** roughly during the action potential.

13. The peripheral nervous system includes:
    - **A.** spinal nerves.
    - **B.** cranial nerves.
    - **C.** the spinal cord.
    - **D.** both (A) and (B).

14. The autonomic nervous system includes:
    - **A.** the sympathetic system.
    - **B.** the parasympathetic system.
    - **C.** the somatic nervous system.
    - **D.** both (A) and (B).

15. The hindbrain contains the:
    - **A.** thalamus.
    - **B.** medulla.
    - **C.** cerebrum.
    - **D.** spinal cord.

16. All are associated with the forebrain except the:
    - **A.** diencephalon.
    - **B.** telencephalon.
    - **C.** myelencephalon.
    - **D.** hypothalamus.

17. All are functions of the medulla except:
    - **A.** voluntary movements.
    - **B.** respiratory regulation.
    - **C.** circulatory regulation.
    - **D.** cough reflex.

18. The cerebellum:

A. regulates respiration.
B. is the site of memory.
C. coordinates motor activity.
D. is the site of behavior.

19. Select the *incorrect* statement concerning the sympathetic nervous system (SNS):

A. Sympathetic ganglia are near the spinal cord.
B. The SNS causes the heart rate to increase.
C. The SNS increases blood flow in certain tissues.
D. The SNS moves the organism toward homeostasis.

20. Select the *incorrect* statement concerning the parasympathetic nervous system (PNS):

A. Ganglia are located near the end-organ.
B. The PNS increases the heart rate.
C. The PNS maintains homeostasis.
D. The PNS increases digestive actions.

21. Vagus Nerve:

A. is linked heterogeneously to the parasympathetic system.
B. is linked to the gut and the heart through specialized skeletal muscles.
C. is not a cranial nerve.
D. has afferent fibers that transmit information from receptors in the thorax.

22. Select the correct sequence of the meninges from outside inward: (A = arachnoid, D = dura, P = pia)

A. A, D, P
B. D, P, A
C. P, A, D
D. D, A, P

7.11.3 Answers to Questions in Section 7.11.2

(1) C (2) D (3) C (4) A (5) C (6) C (7) A (8) D (9) B (10) D (11) A (12) D
(13) D (14) D (15) B (16) C (17) A (18) C (19) D (20) B (21) D (22) D

7.11.4 Discussion of Answers to Questions in Section 7.11.2: None

7.11.5 Advanced Concepts

- Identify the following technical terms, learn their definitions (both structural and functional) and apply them to study the nervous system: Soma of neuron; stretch reflex; reverberating circuit; somasthetic area; enterioceptive and proprioceptive systems; cochlear biosensors; Meissner's corpuscle; Wernicke's area (impulse velocities are around 300 fps); cholinergic nerves; brain microphages; astrocytes; voltage-sensitive Na^+ and K^+ channels; spinal tap (to extract cerebrospinal fluid); and ependymocytes.
- Distinguish between excitatory (epinephrine, enkephalin, norepinephrine) and inhibitory (dopamine, glycine and Gamma aminobutyric acid—GABA) transmitters; excitatory postsynaptic potential (EPSP) with their receptor sites; and preganglionic fiber and postganglionic fiber.
- Understand the major (different) receptor sites such as: kinesthetic receptors; muscarinic (cholinergic) receptors; nicotinic (cholinergic) receptors; dopaminergic receptors; adrenergic receptors; opiate receptors; and other neuronal receptors.

- Understand light receptors in the eye such as iodopsin, lumirhodopsin, metarhodopsin, parathodopsin, photopsin, rhodopsin, luminous-rhodopsin and scotopsin (to see images)
- Recognize the scope, design and relevance of the following procedures and instruments: tonometry; opthalmoscopy; myelography; cavitron ultrasonic surgical aspirator (to shatter brain tumors); positron emission tomography (PET); electroencephalogram; audiometer (if 0-25 dB can be heard easily, probably no hearing loss has occurred); artificial ear implants and thin filament biosensor technology
- Recognize the effects and causes for diseases such as: cataracts; glaucoma; deafness; trachoma; shingles; sciatica; cerebral diseases (epilepsy, dyslexia, Tay-Sachs disease, Alzheimer's disease, Parkinson's disease)

7.12 ENDOCRINE SYSTEM

7.12.1 Introduction to Endocrine System

Learn the cellular mechanisms of hormone action to understand specificity and target tissues connected to each hormone. Review and memorize the organic structure, physical and some chemical properties (mol. weight, density, melting/boiling point, interaction with other body hormones or chemicals) of various hormones. The chemical structures of a few hormones are shown below:

(a) Oxytocin (OT)

S —— S

Cys - Tyr - Lle - Gln - Asn - Cys - Pro - Leu - Gly - NH_2

(b) Progesterone

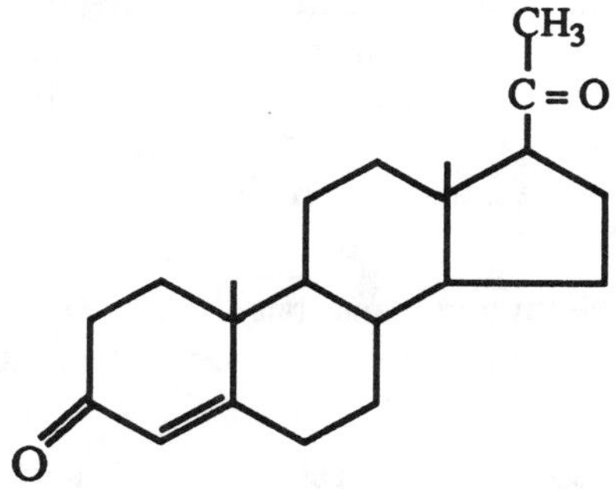

(d) Epinephrine (EP)

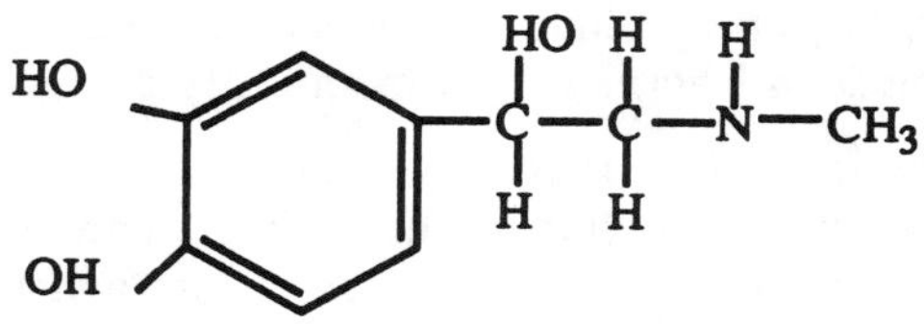

(c) Testosterone

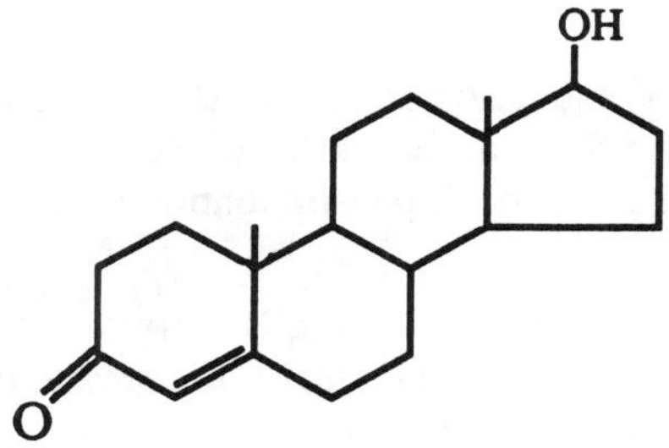

(e) Norepinephrine (NP)

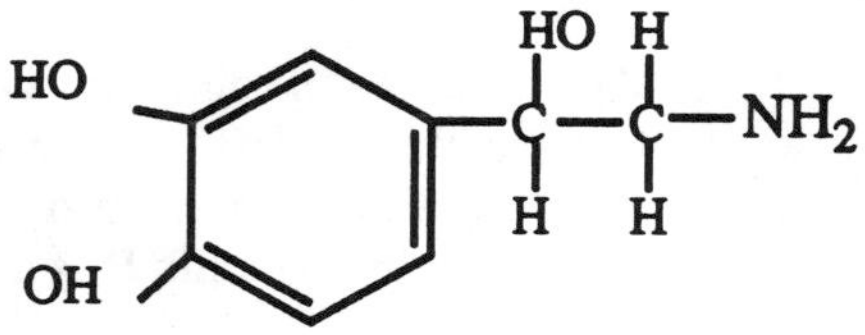

7.12.1.1 MAJOR ENDOCRINE GLANDS

Hormones are substances released from special secretory tissues, called endocrine glands, *into the blood.* From there they circulate to their target tissue(s), combine with the target receptor and exert their effect. Hormones are regulators, not catalysts (as enzymes are), of organism homeostasis. The *major glands* are the hypothalamus, pituitary, thyroid, parathyroid, adrenal, pancreas, gut ovaries, testis, liver, kidney, pineal gland, thymus gland, skin and placenta. *Gut hormones* (gastrin, secretin, cholecystokinin-pancreozymin) are discussed in Section 7.15. Ovarian, placental and testicular hormones and FSH, LH and prolactin are discussed in Section 7.8.

The *hypothalamus* synthesizes releasing factors (RF), inhibiting factors (IF), vasopressin (antidiuretic hormone—ADH) and oxytocin. *Vasopressin* causes the kidney to retain water, i.e., makes the urine more concentrated. *Oxytocin* causes contraction of certain smooth muscles and plays a role in uterine contractions of labor and milk ejection in lactation. Oxytocin and vasopressin are stored in the posterior pituitary until released. RFs and IFs act upon the anterior pituitary (AP). RFs cause the corresponding hormones of the AP to be synthesized and released from it. IFs inhibit release of the corresponding hormones. All of the hormones of the hypothalamus are peptides or proteins. Examples are TRF (THS Releasing Factor) and PIF (Prolactin Inhibiting Factor).

The *anterior pituitary* (AP) synthesizes and releases several trophic (growth stimulating and supporting) hormones among others. Hormones secreted are *thyroid stimulating hormone (TSH), adrenal cortex stimulating hormone (ACTH), follicle stimulating hormone (FSH)*, and *luteinizing hormone (LH)* which are all trophic hormones to the glands indicated by their names. The AP also secretes growth hormone (GH) and prolactin (also called lactogenic hormone). GH functions via somatomedins (produced in the liver) to stimulate the growth of many tissues in the body. Oversecretion of GH results in *giantism* (if before adolescence) or *acromegaly* (if as an adult). All of the AP hormones are proteins or glycoproteins. *MSH* (melanocyte stimulating hormone) is secreted by the intermediate lobe of the pituitary gland.

The *thyroid gland* produces thyroxin and calcitonin. *Thyroxine,* which is a modified tyrosine with iodine attached, works by increasing the rate of metabolism. *Calcitonin* decreases the calcium in the blood by causing it to move into the bones.

The *adrenal gland* is composed of a cortex and medulla. The *cortex* is stimulated by ACTH to synthesize *glucocorticoids* (the primary one being *cortisol*) which perform many functions including regulation of blood sugar (increases it) and fighting stress (e.g., infections). *Mineralocorticoids* (primary one is *aldosterone*) are also synthesized by the cortex but usually as a result of stimulation by angiotensin II (see below). Aldosterone causes the kidney to retain sodium (and hence water) and secrete potassium. The *medulla* synthesizes *epinephrine* which is a sympathetic stimulant (see Section 7.17). The cortical hormones are steroids. The medullary hormones are modified tyrosines.

Parathyroid glands (pea-sized and four in number) are located on the thyroid gland, but are not part of it; they secrete parathyroid hormone (PTH, a protein) which regulates calcium and phosphorus metabolism. Calcium and phosphate are resorbed from bone under the influence of PTH.

The islet cells of the *pancreas* secrete insulin (from β-cells) and glucagon (from α-cells). *Insulin* acts to lower blood glucose by causing cells to take up glucose, it also causes amino acid and fatty acid uptake. *Glucagon* works to increase blood glucose by stimulating *glycogenolysis* (glycogen breakdown) and *gluconeogenesis* (synthesis of glucose from amino acids) by the liver. Insulin and glucagon are both proteins. Diabetes mellitus is due to a deficiency of insulin.

Vitamin D is taken in as a nutrient, then goes through a series of activation steps. First, it is activated by ultraviolet light in the skin, then it is hydroxylated successively in the liver and kidney and becomes a true hormone. Its main role is to increase absorption of calcium by the gut through the stimulation of the synthesis of a calcium binding protein. Vitamin D is a steroid.

The *kidney* secretes renin, erythropoietin, and helps in the synthesis of active Vitamin D (above). *Renin* is an enzyme molecule that splits a small peptide called angiotensin I off the *renin substrate* (produced in the liver). Angiotensin I is further split by enzymes in the lung or blood to yield *angiotensin II* which is a potent constrictor of blood vessels and also stimulates synthesis and release of aldosterone from the adrenal. *Erythropoietin* is a protein hormone which stimulates the bone marrow to synthesize more red blood cells.

The *pineal gland* probably produces a host of hormones, but the best known is melatonin which is a modified tryptophan. The pineal gland suppresses pituitary, gonadal (ovary and testis), adrenal and thyroid function. These effects may be mediated via the hypothalamus.

Thymosin is produced by the *thymus gland* and plays a role in the immunologic system.

7.12.1.2 MAJOR HORMONES OF ENDOCRINE GLANDS

Memorize this chart in the order presented. Understand the major functions and actions of each hormone mechanistically (visualize and analyze mechanics of hormone production in a gland, observe the chemical structure of the hormone), i.e., what possible factors determine functions and actions of a specific hormone? On the MCAT, be better prepared to address some minor functions as well. These minor functions or actions may still be in an advanced research stage or not significant enough. Analyze each question and response for correctness and validity according to experimental information provided in the passage. Do not expect to find minor functions or actions in classic biology or physiology textbooks. Try recognizing new hormonal actions or functions by reading research journals and reports (as additional material).

Hormone Secreting Gland	Hormone (biological name)	Chemical Structure or Functional Group	(Major) Functions and actions
Pituitary (anterior) or Adenohypophysis	• Prolactin (PRL)	protein	• stimulates secretion of milk by the mammary glands
	• Growth hormone (GH)	protein (hypothalamic)	• regulates growth of bones
	• Adrenocortico-tropin (ACTH)	polypeptide (hypothalamic)	• stimulates secretion of adrenal cortex hormones, e.g., glucocorticoids
	• Thyroid-stimulating hormone (TSH)	glycoprotein (hypothalamic)	• stimulates activity of thyroid gland to release hormones
	• Follicle-stimulating hormone (FSH)	glycoprotein (hypothalamic)	• stimulates ovarian follicle maturity and spermatogenesis
	• Luteinizing hormone (LH)	glycoprotein (hypothalamic)	• stimulates ovulation and corpus luteum formation
Pituitary (posterior) or Neurohypophysis	• Oxytocin (OT)	peptide (neurosecretory, hypothalamic)	• stimulates uterine contractions (muscular) and milk secretion by mammary glands
	• Antidiuretic hormone or Vasopressin (ADH)	peptide (hypothalamic) neurosecretory	• regulates water reabsorption by kidneys and raises blood pressure by constricting arterioles

Hormone Secreting Gland	Hormone (biological name)	Chemical Structure or Functional Group	(Major) Functions and actions
Thyroid	• Thyroxine and triidothyronine (T_4 and T_3)	Amino acids (TSH)	• increase in thyroxine production increases metabolic rate
	• Calcitonin	peptide (calcium in blood)	• retains calcium in the bones, lowers blood calcium levels
Parathyroid	• Parathyroid hormone	peptide (calcium in blood)	• increases release of calcium from bone, raises blood calcium levels
Adrenal cortex	• Glucocorticoids	steroids (ACTH)	• multiple carbohydrate metabolism causes increase in blood sugar, anti-inflammatory
	• Mineralocorticoids (Aldosterone)	steroids (Potassium in blood)	• reabsorption of Na^+ and excretion of K^+ in kidneys
	• Gonadocorticoids	steroids	• maintain male sexual characteristics
Adecenal Medulla	• epinephrine or adrenaline (EP)	catecholamine (autonomic nervous system)	• glycogen to glucose conversion, increases blood sugar and blood vessel constriction
	• norepinephrine or noradrenaline (NP)	catecholamine (autonomic nervous system)	• cardiac muscle contraction, blood vessel constriction, increases heart rate
Pancreas	• Glucagon	polypeptide (blood glucose and amino acids)	• glycogen to glucose conversion in liver,
	• Insulin	polypeptide (blood glucose)	• lowers blood sugar, leads to hypoglycemia
	• Somatostatin	peptide (growth hormone feedback)	• inhibits release of insulin and glucagon
Ovaries (follicles & corpus luteum)	• Estrogen	steroid (FSH & LH)	• enhances female sexual characteristics
	• Progesterone	steroid (FSH & LH)	• growth of uterine lining
	• Inhibin	FSH & LH	• inhibits secretion of FSH
Testes	• Testosterone (androgen)	steroid (FSH & LH)	• enhances male sexual characteristics
	• Inhibin	(FSH & LH)	• inhibits secretion of FSH
Thymus	• Thymosin and thymopoietin	peptide	• stimulates growth of T-cells
Pineal	• Melatonin	Catecholamine	• inhibits reproductive activities (is produced in darkness, not produced with light)

7.12.1.3 MECHANISMS OF HORMONE ACTION

Hormones regulate themselves by means of a process called *feedback inhibition*. A gland produces a hormone and this hormone, or a product, feeds back at some level to shut off its synthesis. This is illustrated in Fig. 7.57. Note the following points:

(1) *Long Loop*—the specific hormone feeds back on the hypothalamus to inhibit release of the RF. This then prevents release of the trophic hormone which prevents the synthesis of the specific hormone. As this decreases, its inhibition on the hypothalamus decreases and more of the RF is released which causes more trophic hormone to be released, etc. This cycle can continue as such or be modified positively or negatively by factors outside of the axis (hypothalamus-pituitary-gland) shown.

(2) & (3) *Short Loops*—Mechanisms as above, but the hormones feed back on the gland that stimulated their synthesis (i.e., the pituitary) instead of a point farther removed (i.e., the hypothalamus).

For a given hormone all combinations of the above may exist.

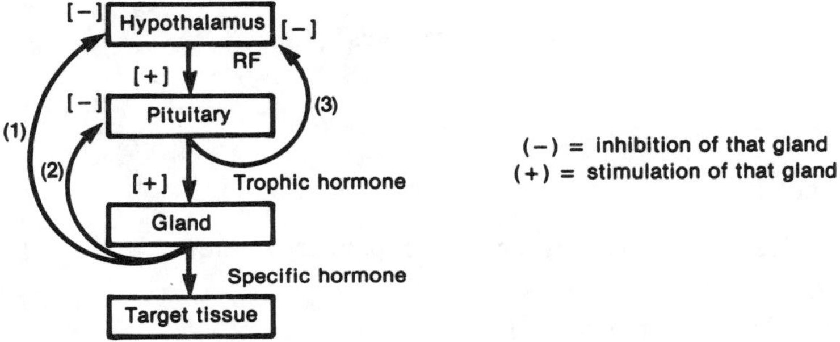

Fig. 7.57—Feedback Loops

Hormones *exert their actions* in many ways (some still unknown). Some protein hormones seem to act via cAMP by combining with specific receptors on the target cell membrane. Some steroids exert their effect by combining with receptors in the target cell cytoplasm (they diffuse through the lipid cell membrane). They then move into the nucleus to interact with DNA to cause synthesis of mRNA, which makes specific proteins (usually enzymes).

7.12.2 Questions Related to Endocrine System

1. Insulin is:

A. secreted by the pancreas.
B. a protein.
C. involved in the metabolism of glucose, amino acids, fats.
D. all of the above.

2. Vitamin D:

A. is actually a hormone after modification in the body.
B. increases absorption of calcium from the gut.
C. requires metabolic changes in the skin, liver, and kidney to function.
D. is all of the above.

3. Select the *incorrectly* paired hormone and disease or deranged process associated with an excess or deficiency of it:

A. growth hormone—acromegaly
B. insulin—diabetes mellitus
C. cortisol—enhances inflammation
D. thyroxine—altered metabolic rate

4. All of the following hormones are correctly paired with one of its major functions except:
   A. thyroxine—increases metabolic rate
   B. glucocorticoids—increases blood sugar levels
   C. aldosterone—role in "fight or flight" sympathetic response
   D. parathyroid hormone—regulation of calcium/phosphorous metabolism

5. Select the endocrine gland that is *incorrectly* paired with its hormone product:
   A. adrenal cortex—cortisol
   B. adrenal medulla—aldosterone
   C. adrenal medulla—epinephrine
   D. adrenal cortex—mineralocorticoids

6. Select the hormone *incorrectly* paired with its target tissue:
   A. TSH—thyroid glands
   B. ACTH—anterior pituitary
   C. LH—ovary or testis
   D. MSH—melanocytes

7. Which hormones are synthesized by the hypothalamus?
   A. releasing factors
   B. vasopressin
   C. oxytocin
   D. all of the above

8. Hormones synthesized and released by the anterior pituitary is (are):
   A. Thyroid Stimulating Hormone (TSH).
   B. Follicle Stimulating Hormone (FSH).
   C. Growth Hormone.
   D. all of the above.

9. Which of the following tissues secrete hormones?
   A. pancreas
   B. ovaries
   C. gastrointestinal tract
   D. all of the above

10. All of the following are general characteristics of hormones except:
    A. hormones are secreted into the blood.
    B. hormones are regulators, not initiators of homeostatic processes.
    C. hormones are all proteins.
    D. hormones do not function like enzymes.

11. All of the following are general characteristics of hormones except that:
    A. hormones regulate themselves by feedback inhibition.
    B. hormones may be proteins, peptides, steroids, or modified amino acids.
    C. some protein hormones act via cAMP.
    D. most steroid hormones act via cAMP.

12. Melatonin is produced by the:
    A. pineal gland.
    B. skin.
    C. liver.
    D. pituitary gland.

13. Thymosin is concerned with:
   - **A.** metabolic rate.
   - **B.** immunologic competence.
   - **C.** calcium/phosphate.
   - **D.** none of the above.

14. Calcitonin:
   - **A.** decreases serum calcium.
   - **B.** has no effect on serum calcium.
   - **C.** is made in the parathyroid gland.
   - **D.** is a steroid.

15. All of the following are true about glucagon except that it:
   - **A.** causes glycogenolysis.
   - **B.** is a steroid.
   - **C.** causes gluconeogenesis.
   - **D.** is made in the pancreas.

16. In the hypothalamic-pituitary-adrenal axis, if the long feedback loop holds then:
   - **A.** ACTH inhibits the production of ACTH-RF by the hypothalamus.
   - **B.** cortisol inhibits the production of ACTH by the pituitary.
   - **C.** cortisol inhibits the ACTH-RF produced by the hypothalamus.
   - **D.** none of the above are correct.

7.12.3 Answers to Questions in Section 7.12.2

(1) D (2) D (3) C (4) C (5) B (6) B (7) D (8) D (9) D (10) C (11) D (12) A (13) B (14) A (15) B (16) C

7.12.4 Discussion of Answers to Questions in Section 7.12.2: None, except

Question #16 (Answer: C) In the long feedback loop, the specific hormone (cortisol) of the gland (adrenal) feeds back past the pituitary to the hypothalamus.

7.12.5 Advanced Concepts

- Learn important terms such as: intracellular mediators (cyclic AMP and GMP), neurosecretory cells, somatomedins and major differences between stimulatory and inhibitory hormones
- Understand the basic hormonal disorders (causes and effects), e.g., adrenal disorders (Cushing's syndrome, Addison's disease); pituitary disorders (gonadal failure in both males and females); thyroid disorders (hypothyroidism and hyperthyroidism); parathyroid disorders (hypoparathyroidism and hyperparathyroidism); and pancreatic disorders (diabetes mellitus)
- Learn the fundamental structure and functions of new hormones, e.g., growth factors such as tumor angiogenesis factors; platelet derived growth factors; epidermal growth factors; nerve growth factors; lymphokines and fibroblast growth factor. Relate these to distress, eustress, resistance as it links to the immune system inhibition.
- Learn major differences between autocrine, endocrine and paracrine hormones; functional aspects of pheromones and identify probable causes for their action
- Understanding experimental design of radioimmunoassays to measure hormone molarities

7.13 CIRCULATORY SYSTEM

7.13.1 Introduction to Circulatory System

Identify the complex structure and working of contractile cells and tissues with emphasis on the cardiac muscle. Identify the thermoregulatory function of the cardiovascular system and its components: heart, blood and arterial/venous systems. Visit a hospital or clinic if permitted, to understand heart transplants, artificial heart machine and blood bank operations. Learn the following laws and their limitations (do *not* forget both stated and unstated assumptions behind these laws) as applied to the circulatory system: (i) *Marey's Law:* If blood pressure *falls* the heart beats *faster* (an inversely proportional relationship); (ii) *Starling's Law:* relates length of stretched cardiac muscle fibers to strength of contraction (a directly proportional relationship, the longer the stretched fiber, the stronger the contraction); and (iii) *Frank-Starling Law:* The heart automatically adjusts its pumping capability depending on blood volume to be pumped by it (a directly proportional relationship, the more the blood volume to be pumped, the higher the pumping capability). Understand why these laws are true for the cardiovascular system and under what conditions they are valid. Remember, cardiac muscle is *not* plastic; the tone of the heart makes it contract continuously.

7.13.1.1 FUNCTIONS AND PRINCIPLES

The function of the circulatory system is to maintain tissue oxygenation, supply nutrients and remove wastes. This function is compromised when the heart, blood vessels, or blood fail to perform as intended. Also, the lungs are critical in O_2 and CO_2 homeostasis. Malfunction in these systems can lead to a decreased flow of suitable blood (e.g., enough O_2) to tissues and this can lead to their death. Also, a fall in blood pressure or loss of blood volume can have similar effects.

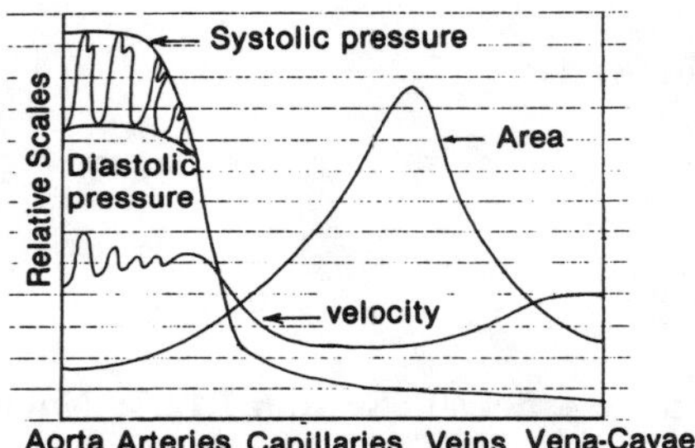

Fig. 7.58—Fundamental Principles of Blood Circulation

As shown in Fig. 7.58, generally the velocity of blood flow in any segment of the cardiovascular system is inversely proportional to the total cross-sectional area of the vessels of the segment. Efficient circulation requires an adequate volume of circulating blood. Blood encounters resistance as it flows through blood vessels. Resistance to blood flow is affected by physical and biological variables such as viscosity, temperature, diameter, etc. Four equations are provided below for studying the relationships among various circulation variables.

1. $\text{Resistance (R)} = \dfrac{\text{Pressure Gradient } (\Delta P)}{\text{Flowrate (Q)}}$

   This equation is analogous to Ohm's law in electric circuits,

$$R = \frac{V}{I} = \frac{\text{Voltage}}{\text{Current}}$$

2. $\text{Ejection fraction (EF)} = \dfrac{\text{Stroke Volume (SV)}}{\text{End-Diastolic Volume (EDV)}}$

The ventricles eject only a portion of their contained blood with each beat. The ejection fraction is that fraction of the end-diastolic volume that is ejected during systole.
Normally EF > 0.5.

3. Critical velocity (v_c) = $\frac{R\eta}{\rho r}$

R = Reynolds number
η = blood viscosity
ρ = blood density
r = tube or vessel radius

This equation is used to study heart murmurs (vibrations set up within the heart and great vessels by turbulent blood flow).

4. Cardiac output (CO) = $\frac{60I}{Ct}$

I = indicator or dye in mg
$C = \frac{I}{V}$ the mean concentration in mg/l
V = Volume of liquid in which dye is injected in liters
t = Passage time in seconds

7.13.1.2 HUMAN HEART AND TYPES OF CIRCULATION

The elements of the circulatory system in humans are the heart, the blood vessels, blood and the lymphatics. The circulatory system can be subdivided into three types based on the anatomy of the blood vessels. These are: (1) *Systemic circulation* supplies blood to the head, extremities and trunk; the main artery is the aorta and the main veins (includes lymphatic drainage) are the inferior and superior vena cavas. (2) *Pulmonary circulation* supplies blood to the lungs. (3) *Coronary circulation* supplies blood to the heart. The coronary arteries arise at the base of the aorta at the aortic valve. The arteries give rise to the coronary veins that enter the coronary sinus (on the atria), which empties into the RA.

The *heart* consists of two *atria* (left-LA and right-RA) and two *ventricles* (LV and RV). Between the RA and RV is the *tricuspid valve* (TV, 3 leaflets). Between the RV and the pulmonary artery (PA) is the *pulmonary valve* (PV). Between the LA and LV is the *mitral* (bicuspid) *valve* (MV, 2 leaflets). Between the LV and the aorta is the *aortic valve* (AV). The PV and AV valves are called *semilunar valves* (3 half-moon shaped leaflets) that prevent reflux of blood back into their respective ventricles during diastole. See Fig. 7.59. The TV and MV are attached via *chordae tendinae* to *papillary muscles* on their respective ventricles to prevent reflux into the corresponding atria during systole. Improper functioning of the valves, particularly in the mitral valve, is one of the causes of heart murmurs. A schematic of the heart and circulation is:

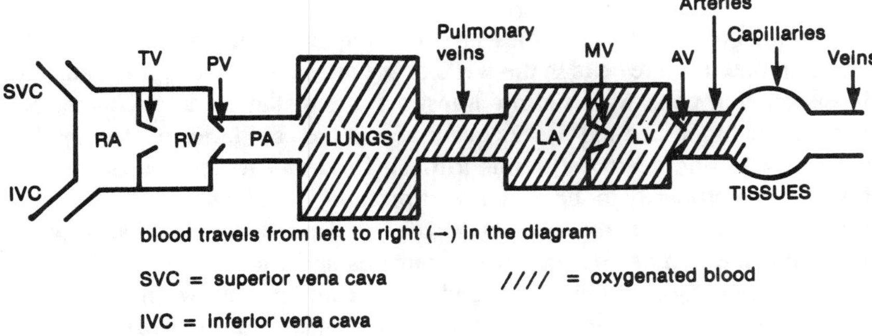

Fig. 7.59—Schematic of the Circulatory System

Cardiac Muscle (Specialized eukaryotic cells)

The heart is made of cardiac muscle. This differs from skeletal muscle (Section 7.17) by: (1) being made of branching, uninuclear cells, (2) having specializations of cell membranes called *intercalated discs* that both join cells together and decrease resistance to impulse conduction, (3) being able to initiate beats without the need of a nerve impulse, and (4) being largely involuntary. The microscopic structures are similar (see Section 7.17).

Systole and Diastole

Heart beats are divided into systole (contraction) and diastole (relaxation) on the basis of the state of the ventricles. *Beats* originate in the *sinus node* which is considered the pacemaker of the heart. Impulses from here activate the atria to contract (diastole), then pass to the *atrioventricular (AV) node.* From this point, impulses pass down the *bundle of His* to the left and right branch bundles to the *Purkinje fibers* which activate the left and right ventricles causing them to contract (systole). Beats can originate in other parts of heart if the sinus node fails. Also, some of the bundles or fibers may become injured so that they cannot conduct impulses—then the impulses find alternate paths. *Sympathetic* nerves serve to increase the heart rate and force of contraction. *Parasympathetic* nerves (e.g., the *Vagus nerve)* decrease the heart rate. During *systole* the ventricles are ejecting blood into the large vessels (PA, aorta), and during *diastole* the ventricles are being filled with blood from the atria. Note that the RV pumps blood to the lungs and the LV pumps blood to the rest of the body.

7.13.1.3 BLOOD VESSELS

Blood vessels consist of arteries, arterioles, capillaries, and veins. Vessels are made of (to different degrees), from the inside out, an *intima* (endothelial cell lining), a *media* (consisting of muscle and elastic tissue), and an *adventitia* (connective tissue covering). *Arteries* contain a lot of smooth muscle and/or elastic tissue and carry blood from the heart (not always oxygenated blood). The contraction of the ventricles in systole imparts energy and pressure to the blood as they enter the arteries. This causes expansion (elastic nature) of the arteries during systole which stores the energy part. During diastole the elastic recoil converts the stored energy to pressure and maintains the pressure. The blood pressure is higher during systole than diastole in the arteries. But because of the recoil of the arteries and the effect of the arterioles (see below) the diastolic blood pressure remains well above zero in the arteries. An average blood pressure is 120/80 (systolic/diastolic) measured in mm Hg. *Arterioles* connect arteries and capillaries and are the location of the greatest *resistance* to blood flow. Blood pressure varies directly as the flow of blood (amount of blood pumped by the heart) and directly as the resistance to flow.

$$\text{blood pressure} \propto (\text{heart output}) \times (\text{resistance}).$$

Resistance to flow varies inversely as the fourth power of the radius (r) of the vessel: resistance $\propto 1/r^4$

Arterioles can change their radii greatly and arterioles are very important determinants of blood pressure. Sympathetic nerves stimulate smooth muscle cells in the walls of the arterioles, that is, make the radius smaller. *Capillaries* contain only endothelial cells which allow transport of substances across them. Nearly all the transfer of substances between the blood and the tissues occur across the capillaries or the small venules. The *hydrostatic pressure*, generated by the heartbeat, tends to push fluid and molecules (not cells) out of the capillary. The *oncotic pressure*, due primarily to the presence of proteins like albumin in the blood, tends to pull fluid and molecules into the capillary. Hence, the *net transfer of fluid* depends on the balance of these two. On the arterial side of the capillary, the hydrostatic pressure dominates and fluid, etc., leaves the capillary and enters the tissue space (not cells directly). At the venule end of the capillary and within the venule itself, the oncotic pressure dominates and this draws fluid, etc. (different substances than exited), back into the blood stream (Fig. 7.60). Not all the fluid and proteins are pulled back in; some are returned to the blood vessels via the lymphatics (Section 7.14.1).

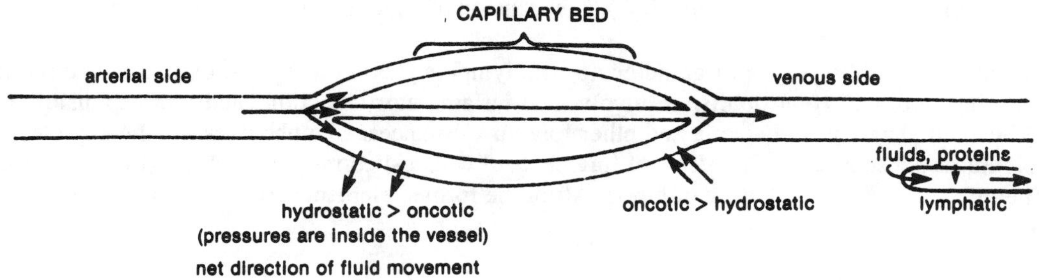

Fig. 7.60—Capillary Fluid Exchange

The *veins* have less muscle and elastin than arteries, some have valves to prevent backward flow of blood, and they carry blood to the heart (heart valves also prevent backward movement). Veins can contain a lot of blood under low pressure, i.e., they have a high capacitance (can act as a reservoir). Veins are assisted by the action of skeletal muscle contractions to move blood forward. In addition to veins, the lymphatic vessel system is an auxiliary system of vessels that carries both white blood cells and extracellular fluids (including blood proteins) back into the general circulation. The two largest lymph vessels, the right lymphatic duct and the thoracic duct, empty into the venous system (generally into the subclavian veins) in the root of the neck. Inflammation of the lymphatic vessels can cause severe retention of fluids particularly in the extremities (e.g., elephantitis).

Flow of molecules and cells into and out of the vascular system is aided by the structure and activity of endothelial cells that make up the walls of capillaries. Three types of capillaries—closed, fenestrated and discontinuous (Fig. 7.61, a-c)—handle molecules and cells in three distinctive ways. Closed capillaries transport molecules to and from the blood stream by using pinocytotic vesicles (e.g., muscle); fenestrated capillaries have circular openings that facilitate transport of larger molecules (e.g., kidney glomeruli, hormonal glands); discontinuous capillaries, including venules (e.g., bone marrow, liver, spleen), facilitate the movement of cells in addition to molecules. The basal lamina, a secreted connective tissue membrane on which the endothelial cells rest and to which they are attached, also facilitate or diminish transport depending on their thickness. In uncontrolled diabetes mellitis the basal lamina increases, slowing transport. In the kidney the basal lamina is the primary filter of the blood, inasmuch as the glomerular capillaries are fenestrated.

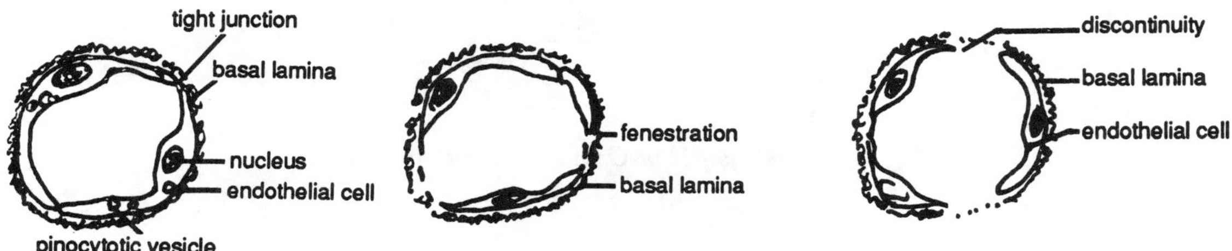

Fig. 7.61(a)—Closed Capillary *Fig. 7.61(b)—Fenestrated Capillary* *Fig. 7.61(c)—Discontinuous Capillary*

7.13.1.4 COMPOSITION OF BLOOD

Blood consists of *formed elements:* (1) red blood cells (RBC or erythrocytes), (2) white blood cells (WBC), and (3) platelets; and many *non-formed elements:* proteins, lipids, hormones, dissolved gases, ions, carbohydrates. RBCs contain hemoglobin (made of four polypeptide chains called globin, and heme, which is a porphyrin ring, and iron—II) and are biconcave discs ( ).

The *hematocrit* is the percentage of whole blood that is RBCs. The *plasma* is whole blood minus the formed elements. *Serum* is plasma after clotting has occurred. *Hemoglobin* (Hb) carries oxygen (O_2) attached to iron

(Fe). O_2 is picked up slowly by Hb at low O_2 tension, but this rapidly accelerates as O_2 tension increases, and it eventually levels off at high O_2 tension (Fig. 7.62). (The tension of a gas is the pressure of the gas.)

WBCs are mostly neutrophils (a type of granulocyte) and lymphocytes. Eosinophils, basophils and monocytes are also found in the blood. Neutrophils are involved in inflammatory reactions and are responsible for pus formation. They can phagocytize bacteria and other foreign substances. Lymphocytes are the key elements in the immunologic response system. *Platelets* are fragments of cells called megakaryocytes (located in the bone marrow). They play a part in the clotting of blood. All of the formed elements arise from precursor cells in the bone marrow.

Proteins in the blood are albumin (maintains oncotic pressure and acts as a nonspecific carrier protein) and globulins. Globulins include the immunoglobulins which are antibodies, carrier proteins, and the coagulation factors (fibrinogen, prothrombin, etc.). Calcium is also required for clotting; agents like EDTA and oxalate complex calcium and may prevent clotting. *Vitamin K* is responsible for formation of some of the clotting factors, and, thus, the clotting of blood.

7.13.1.5 HEMOGLOBIN BINDING SITES

The percent oxygen saturation of Hb is due to the allosteric nature of the Hb molecule (see Fig. 7.62). The first subunit binds O_2 slowly, but once bound, the bound O_2 causes a conformational change in the second subunit which causes it to pick up the next O_2 faster. This is repeated in the third and fourth subunits until the Hb is saturated. Hb releases O_2 more readily at low pH than at high pH—the *Bohr effect.* Hb picks up O_2 in the lung and releases it in the tissues. Release and uptake is primarily a function of O_2 tension (pressure) gradients, but pH and other factors play a role. Carbon dioxide is transported from the tissues to the lungs dissolved in blood, as bicarbonate, and bound to Hb and some other proteins. Its uptake (at tissues) by blood and release (in the lungs) by blood is also a function of CO_2 pressure gradients. Gases diffuse from regions of higher pressure to regions of lower pressure.

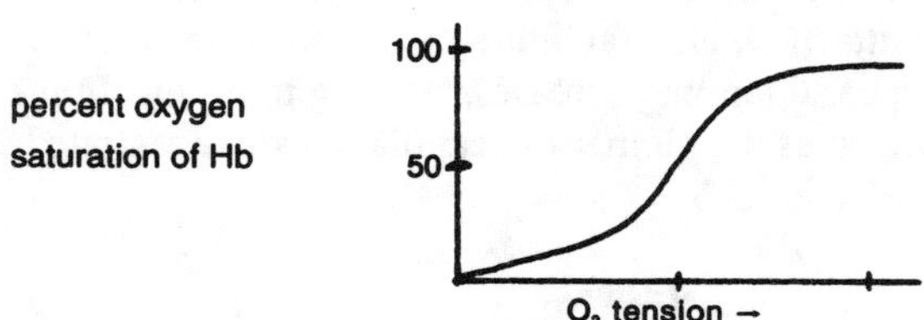

Fig. 7.62—Hemoglobin-Oxygen Saturation Curve

7.13.2 Questions Related to Circulatory System

1. Which statement(s) is(are) correct?

   A. Veins and arteries carry both oxygenated and deoxygenated blood.
   B. Veins carry only deoxygenated blood.
   C. Arteries carry only oxygenated blood.
   D. Both (B) and (C) are correct.

2. Which of the following is not part of the conduction system of the heart?

   A. atrioventricular node
   B. chordae tendinae
   C. Bundle of His
   D. Purkinje fibers

3. Cells in the blood are normally derived from precursor cells in the:

   A. liver.
   B. spleen.
   C. bone marrow.
   D. connective tissue.

4. All are types of white *blood* cells except:

   A. megakaryocytes.
   B. neutrophils.
   C. eosinophils.
   D. lymphocytes.

5. The mitral valve is located between the:

   A. left atrium and left ventricle.
   B. left and right ventricles.
   C. left and right atria.
   D. superior vena cava and the heart.

6. Which agent below chelates calcium and may prevent clotting of blood?

   A. Vitamin D
   B. EDTA
   C. Vitamin K
   D. NH_3

7. All of the following are true about albumin except that it:

   A. is found in the plasma.
   B. plays a role in immunologic reactions.
   C. is made in the liver.
   D. plays a role in maintaining the colloid oncotic pressure of the blood.

8. The beats of the heart are initiated by:

   A. the brain.
   B. the sympathetic nerves.
   C. the parasympathetic nerves.
   D. the sinoatrial node.

9. Chordae tendinae:

   A. hold muscles to bones.
   B. hold muscles to muscles.
   C. hold bones to bones.
   D. are found in the heart.

10. The Bohr Effect on hemoglobin function:

    A. makes electrons in the hemoglobin easier to ionize.
    B. is to make it a CO_2 carrier.
    C. is to increase the affinity of hemoglobin for oxygen at higher altitudes.
    D. causes it to release oxygen more readily at lower pH values.

11. What is a hematocrit?

    A. the number of red blood cells in the blood
    B. the percentage of blood that is red blood cells
    C. the amount of hemoglobin
    D. the total amount of blood in the body

12. Hemoglobin:

A. does not carry carbon dioxide.
B. is normally free (not in cells) in the blood.
C. is composed of protein, porphyrin, and iron.
D. is normally found in the plasma portion.

13. Which statement is correct concerning the heart?

A. The right ventricle pumps blood to the body excluding the lung.
B. The right ventricle pumps blood to the lung.
C. The left ventricle pumps blood to the lung.
D. The left ventricle pumps blood to the body including the lung.

14. Which is the correct sequence of blood passing through the heart? (R = right, L = left, A = atrium, V = ventricle, SVC = Superior Vena Cava, IVC = Inferior Vena Cava)

A. RA to RV to SVC/IVC to LA to LV to lungs to aorta to RA
B. SVC/IVC to LA to LV to lungs to RA to RV to aorta to SVC/IVC
C. SVC/IVC to RA to RV to lungs to LA to LV to aorta to SVC/IVC
D. RA to RV to LA to LV to lungs to aorta to IVC/SVC to RA

15. Systole refers to:

A. the contraction phase of the atria.
B. the relaxation phase of the atria.
C. the contraction phase of the ventricles.
D. the relaxation phase of the ventricles.

16. Heart muscle differs from skeletal muscle in all the following except:

A. having striations.
B. being made of distinct cells.
C. having intercalated discs.
D. having the capacity to originate beats without nervous impulses.

17. Sympathetic impulses:

A. increase the heart rate.
B. decrease the heart rate.
C. do not affect the heart rate.
D. increase the heart rate and then decrease it.

18. In diastole:

A. the aortic valve is closed.
B. the tricuspid valve is closed.
C. the mitral valve is closed.
D. the ventricles are contracting.

19. Layers of blood vessels include all of the following except:

A. tendinae.
B. media.
C. adventitia.
D. intima.

20. Arteries:

A. conduct blood toward the heart.
B. help maintain blood pressure due to their elastic recoil properties.
C. always carry oxygenated blood.
D. contain a large media, a small adventitia, and no intima.

21. The greatest resistance to blood flow is in the:

A. capillaries.
B. veins.
C. arteries.
D. arterioles.

22. All of the following might increase blood pressure except an:

A. increase in sympathetic tone of vessels.
B. increase in the radius of a vessel.
C. increase in blood output by the heart.
D. increase in resistance of vessels.

23. Exchange of substances between tissues and the blood occurs in the:

A. veins.
B. capillaries.
C. arterioles.
D. arteries.

24. The oncotic pressure of blood:

A. has no effect on the movement of fluid.
B. causes fluid to move into the tissues from the blood vessels.
C. causes fluid to move into the blood vessels from the tissues.
D. causes fluid to move from higher pressure to lower pressure.

25. On the venous side of the capillary:

A. hydrostatic pressure exceeds oncotic pressure and causes fluid to move into the tissues.
B. oncotic pressure exceeds hydrostatic pressure and causes fluid to move into the tissues.
C. hydrostatic pressure exceeds oncotic pressure and causes fluid to move into the blood vessel.
D. oncotic pressure exceeds hydrostatic pressure and causes fluid to move into the blood vessel.

26. Regarding the fluid that escapes from the blood on the arterial side of the capillaries:

A. some of the fluid and proteins is carried off by lymphatics.
B. all of the fluid is returned to the blood at the venous end of the capillary.
C. the fluid normally contains red blood cells.
D. none of the above are correct.

27. The coronary circulation supplies the:

A. brain.
B. heart.
C. lungs.
D. trunk.

28. Select the following which is most likely a red blood cell:

A.

B.

C. 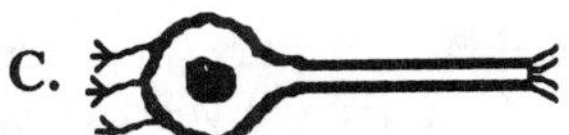

D. 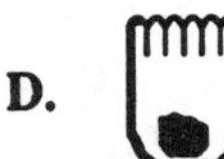

29. Hemoglobin:

A. binds O_2 uniformly at all O_2 tensions.
B. binds O_2 rapidly at low O_2 tensions.
C. binds O_2 slowly at low O_2 tensions.
D. does not become saturated at high O_2 tensions.

30. Which of the following is involved in the immune response?

A. neutrophils
B. lymphocytes
C. platelets
D. basophils

31. Clotting is caused by:

A. platelets.
B. neutrophils.
C. lymphocytes.
D. eosinophils.

7.13.3 Answers to Questions in Section 7.13.2

(1) A (2) B (3) C (4) A (5) A (6) B (7) B (8) D (9) D (10) D (11) B (12) C
(13) B (14) C (15) C (16) A (17) A (18) A (19) A (20) B (21) D (22) B (23) B (24) C
(25) D (26) A (27) B (28) A (29) C (30) B (31) A

7.13.4 Discussion of Answers to Questions in Section 7.13.2: None, except

Question #22 (Answer: B) Sympathetic tone means there is a decrease in the radius of the vessels. A decrease in the radius of the vessels means an increase in resistance (resistance $\propto 1/r^4$). This means that the pressure increases (pressure α resistance). An increase in radius causes a drop in blood pressure.

as radius increases, the resistance decreases
(resistance $\propto 1/r^4$).
as resistance decreases, the pressure decreases
(pressure $\propto$ resistance)

Options (C) and (D) are discussed in the Section.

7.13.5 Advanced Concepts

- Recognize the following concepts and terms with a definition, basic sketch and current medical usage: erythrocyte sedimentation rate; reticulocyte count; prothrombin time, partial thromboplastin time; vasomotion; blood osmotic pressure; filtration and reabsorption pressure in capillaries; platelet plug; pressure curves for the atria and ventricles; fourteen blood clotting factors (e.g., Stuart-Prower factor, Hageman factor); metaarteriole; barareceptors and chemoreceptors; circulation time; neurogenic and hypovolemic shocks; capillary beds and plasma analysis
- Understand the physical mechanisms and other causes leading to the following circulatory system disorders/diseases: Induced erythrocytemia in athletes; HLA antigen typing or tissue typing for transplants; causes for edema; congenital defects (dextrorotation of heart, Fallot's tetralogy; pulmonary stenosis and aortic stenosis); differences between etiology and pathogenesis of atherosclerosis; Buerger's disease or Raynaud's disease; coarctation; aneurysm or cerebral hemorrhage; aplastic anemia; atrial fibrillation; toxoplasmosis; histiocytosis; malaria, plague and HIV infection through blood.
- Identify equipment and instruments to determine various cardiovascular/blood related factors (as described in (1) above), e.g., reticulocyte count, blood osmotic pressure, pressure curves for atria and ventricles, etc. Do *not* forget to remember measurement units.
- Review the design, working and modern research techniques associated with: electrocardiograms (ambulatory, resting or stress); Holter monitor; artificial pacemaker; ultrasonic cardiogram; artificial heart monitors; cold spot mycocardial imaging; angiography; cardiac catheterization; heart-lung machine; laser angioplasty; balloon-laser welding; catheter artherectomy; balloon valvuloplasty; sphygmomanometer; construction of a blood pressure monitor

- Determine the molecular structure and side effects (in biochemical terms) of anticoagulants, antihypertensive medication, inotropic medication, antiarrhythmic medication, fibrinolytic drugs, debriding and antiplatelet drugs, and Fluosol-DA (blood substitute) drugs
- Learn the comparative relationships between Virchow's lipid infiltration theory and Rokitansky's encrustation theory

7.14 LYMPHATIC AND IMMUNE SYSTEMS

7.14.1 Introduction to Lymphatic and Immune Systems

Review the basic structures and functions of these systems. Understand the mechanisms which work in these systems to regulate various processes in the human body. Examine the composition of blood on both a physical and chemical basis and the mechanisms which control flow of lymph at various lymph nodes. Review the physical structure, physical properties, chemical properties and stereochemistry of helper T-cells, killer T-cells, suppressor T-cells and T-cell receptors. Place emphasis on auto immunity, active immunity and passive immunity in studying immunological publications and current medical literature. Examine and recognize current research involving bone marrow transplants, spleen and thymus surgical procedures. Connect your knowledge in microbiology (especially virus and bacteria life history) to immune system response time.

7.14.1.1 STRUCTURE AND FUNCTION

The lymphatic and immune system is the body's surveillance system against foreign invaders; it distinguishes between self and nonself. When properly functioning, it protects against bacteria, viruses, fungi, and parasites. When it encounters foreign (nonself) material (called an *antigen*), the immune system becomes activated. An antigen is recognized by characteristic shapes (*epitopes*) on its surface to which *antibodies* are formed in an attempt to neutralize the antigen. The organs of the immune system are called lymphoid organs and include the bone marrow, thymus, lymph nodes, spleen, tonsils, adenoids, appendix, and Peyer's patches (lymphoid tissues in the small intestine). The cells of the immune system include *lymphocytes* and *phagocytes* (*macrophages, neutrophils*), which are produced in the *bone marrow*. Phagocytes are white blood cells that devour (*phagocytize*) foreign matter such as bacteria and dead cells to clear them from the system. In addition, they mediate the presentation of antigens to lymphocytes and secrete factors that activate T-cells. Lymphocytes are classified as *B-cells* or *T-cells*. B-cells are produced continuously and mature in the bone morrow, while T-cells mature in the thymus, which is located behind the breast bone. T-cells differ from other cells of the immune system in that their pool is established during the fetal and early postnatal period and is maintained throughout life by expansion of T-cells that are located peripherally. Both B-cells and T-cells can distinguish between self and nonself and initiate an immune reaction in the presence of foreign material (antigens). The immune cells circulate throughout the body via the blood or *lymphatic vessels*.

Lymphatic vessels are widely dispersed peripherally within the connective tissues supporting the epithelium of all potential portals into the body, e.g., skin, oral cavity, urinary tract, gential tract, digestive tract, and respiratory tree. Individual cells or diffuse aggregations of cells (as large as the tonsils) can be found. Lymphatic capillaries flow into *lymph nodes* (regionally positioned fluid filters found in the neck, armpits, abdomen, and groin) and larger lymphatic vessels (an auxiliary drainage network to veins that interconnect the lymph nodes). *Lymphatic vessels* are generally one cell thick being made of endothelial cells (like the cells lining blood vessels). These vessels begin as blind pouches in all tissues of the body. They remove fluid, proteins, and particulate matter that arise in tissues directly or by extravasation from the blood vessels. Once in the lymphatics, the lymph (the above materials) is "filtered" at the lymph nodes and eventually re-enters the circulatory system by flowing into the large veins in the thorax (chest cavity) via the thoracic duct or right lymphatic duct. Lymph flow is passive and requires muscle action (acting as a pump) to move lymph along the vessels. If lymph vessels are destroyed, if lymph nodes are blocked, or if there is no muscle action, the lymph does not flow and the fluid remains in the tissues and that tissue swells up (becomes edematous). Note also that gravity would tend to retard the flow of lymph back into the blood vessels. The key *functions* of the lymphatic system are the return of fluid and proteins to the circulation from the tissues and protection against foreign materials.

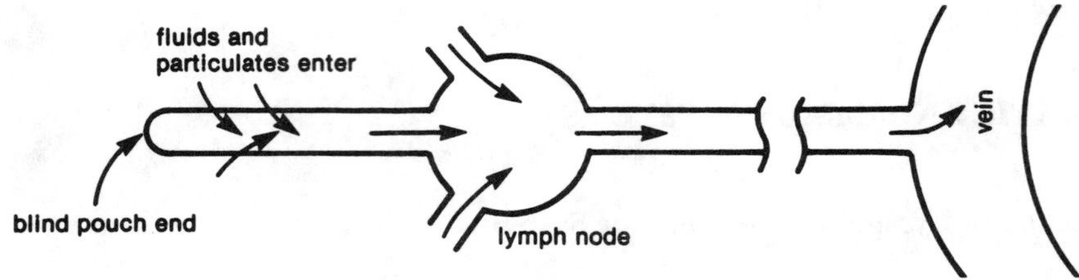

Fig. 7.63(a)—Lymphatics

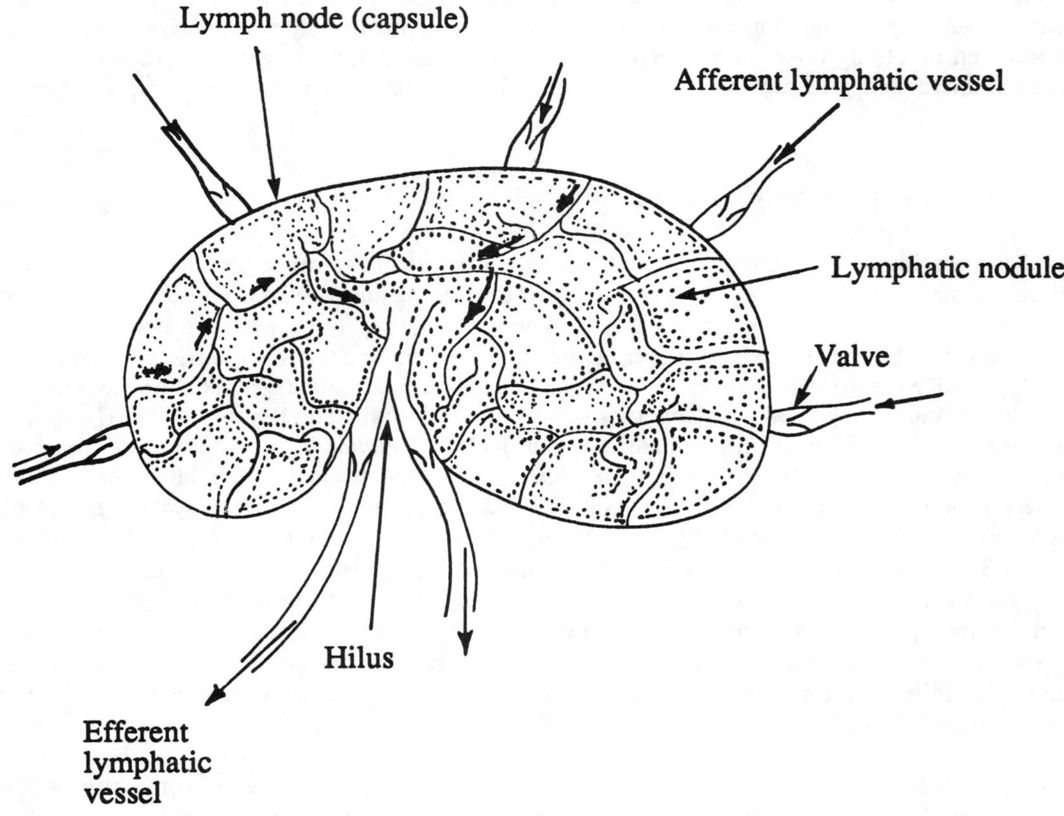

Fig. 7.63(b)—Lymph Node Schematic (*enlarged*)

Lymph nodes contain lymphocytes and macrophages. *Lymphocytes* are involved in the antibody response to antigens (foreign materials). Removing particulate (bacteria, dead cells, etc.) matter by phagocytosis and helping lymphocytes in the immune response are functions of the *macrophage* which performs a similar function all over the body (especially in the lung, liver, and spleen). Lymph nodes often swell and become tender (*lymphadenopathy*) during infection or inflammation due to this function. There are more cells, both macrophages and lymphocytes, in a swollen lymph node. Although the lymph node has some capacity for cell division, large influxes of cells presenting during periods of inflammation are transported into the lymph nodes through the vascular system and exit into the nodule through the walls of the venules. The location of the swollen node (e.g., at the angle of the jaw) is important in localizing the infection (e.g., the throat or tooth) or even a cancer (i.e., metastasis from the primary cancer) because nodes drain lymphatic vessels from given regions of the body. The spleen is the major lymphoid organ of the general circulation and as such is a key organ in fighting systemic infections. It is located in the abdominal cavity behind the stomach and is the size of a small fist. The spleen also doubles as a destruction and storage center for red blood cells.

Antigen-Antibody Reactions: B-cells control *humoral immunity* by secreting antibodies. Antibodies interact with antigens such as bacteria or viruses, but cannot penetrate living cells. Each B-cell makes an antibody that is specific for a given antigen, just as keys are made to open specific locks. When a B-cell interacts with its antigen, *plasma cells* are formed that manufacture and release the specific antibody. Antibodies belong to one of several classes of *immunoglobins* (Ig): IgG, IgA, IgM, IgE, or IgD. Each Ig class has unique characteristics. All immunoglobulins are made up of two heavy and two light chains which form the shape of a Y (see below). The ends of the Y contain the epitopes to which the antigen binds and are known as the variable (V) region. The stem end of the Y is called the constant (C) region and is the same in all antibodies of the same class. As a result of antigen-antibody binding, the antibody may disable the antigen, coat (*opsonize*) the antigen (e.g., bacteria), cause the release of *complement*, or block virus entry into cells. Complement consists of a series of proteins that assist antibodies in attacking antigens. T-cells control *cellular immunity*. *Cytotoxic T-cells* attack host cells that have been invaded by bacteria or malignancy. *Helper/inducer T-cells* (identified by the T4 marker) regulate other T-cells, natural killer cells, macrophages, and B-cells (without T-cell intervention, B-cells cannot form antibodies). T-cells work by secreting *cytokines* (e.g., interferon, tumor necrosis factor, interleukin), which are powerful chemical messengers. Cytokines initiate a wide variety of protective responses, including the inflammatory response.

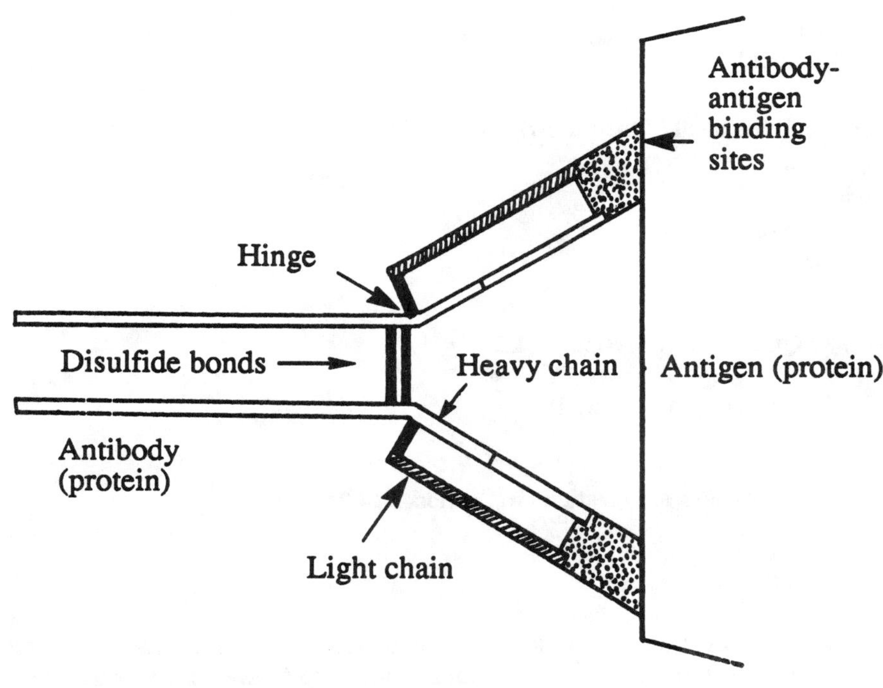

Fig. 7.63(c)—Basic Structure of an Antibody Molecule

7.14.2 Questions Related to Lymphatic and Immune Systems

1. The lymphatic system:
   - **A.** returns fluid and proteins to blood vessels.
   - **B.** has a direct connection to the heart.
   - **C.** consists of vessels only.
   - **D.** is not integral to the function of the body.
2. Lymph nodes:
   - **A.** are found in veins.
   - **B.** contain lymphocytes only.
   - **C.** may contain lymphocytes and macrophages.
   - **D.** are not directly important in protecting the body against disease.
3. Macrophages:
   - **A.** are found in lymph nodes only.
   - **B.** are phagocytic cells.
   - **C.** are the lining cells of lymphatic vessels.
   - **D.** are all of the above.
4. An enlarged lymph node may mean:
   - **A.** infection.
   - **B.** inflammation.
   - **C.** cancer.
   - **D.** all of the above.
5. Lymph moves toward the veins due to:
   - **A.** tissue pressure.
   - **B.** muscle action.
   - **C.** pumping action of heart.
   - **D.** gravity.
6. T-lymphocytes are found in all of the following EXCEPT:
   - **A.** lymphoid tissues.
   - **B.** the spleen.
   - **C.** the thymus gland.
   - **D.** bone marrow.

7.14.3 Answers to Questions in Section 7.14.2

(1) A (2) C (3) B (4) D (5) B (6) B

7.14.4 Discussion of Answers to Questions in Section 7.14.2: None

7.14.5 Advanced Concepts

Review newspaper articles, research reports and current periodicals to understand research trends, new instrumentation and experimentation techniques in immunology. The following terms and concepts are to be emphasized:

- Determine from *your* knowledge in inorganic chemistry and biology the structures and mechanisms associated to immunoglobulin homology units (IgA, IgD, IgE, IgG and IgM) and develop visual understanding of Fab and Fc fragments of IgG molecules (linked to the stereochemistry of heavy and light chains)

- Identify the following terms with definitions and sketches: Hassall's corpuscles, Malphigian corpuscles, Billroth's cords, wandering macrophages, tonsils, hyaluronic acid, phagocytic margination, spleen and thymus glands
- Review background information and arguments on the strength, applications and soundness (based on credibility of scientific analysis) of antibody diversity hypotheses: both on somatic mutation and somatic recombination. Review hypothesis concerning membrane attack complex in the immune system.
- Understand the causes, research experimentation and basic medical techniques related to: Hodgkin's disease; leukocytosis; blood transfusion problems; lymphangiography (to detect lymphomas and various lymphatic tissue tumors); and experimental procedure to produce the HAT (hypoxanthine, amethopterin, thymine) medium used for producing antibodies against antigens

7.15 DIGESTIVE SYSTEM

7.15.1 Introduction to Digestive System

Understand the histology and mechanisms associated with the digestive system, e.g., The GI tract has the peritoneum and other muscular control layers such as tunica serosa, tunica muscularis, tunica submucosa and tunica mucosa. Review the microscopic structure of muscularis mucosae, lamina propria, circular and longitudinal muscle to understand the role and mechanisms of the digestive process. Review histology of the digestive system integrated with the biochemical and muscular actions within the system.

7.15.1.1 STRUCTURE AND FUNCTION

The structure and function of the digestive system will be discussed by following a bolus of food through it (see Fig. 7.65).

The *teeth* and the *tongue* are responsible for breaking food down into swallowable chunks (called boluses). Adults have 32 teeth, children have 20 (called deciduous teeth). Each quadrant (quarter) contains two *incisors* (for cutting), one *canine* (for tearing), two *premolars* (for crushing), and 3 *molars* (for grinding). *Salivary glands* secrete alkaline *saliva* to moisten food for swallowing, protect against bacteria, and begin digestion of starch. *Swallowing* is initiated voluntarily but becomes involuntary as food enters the pharynx. The *swallowing center* is located in the medulla, and the hypoglossal (XII) and glossopharyngeal (IX) nerves are responsible for the esophageal phase after the bolus passes from the pharynx. The bolus enters the *stomach* from the esophagus where it may be stored for several hours. Grinding and liquefying the food are the main functions of the stomach accomplished by its strong muscle. *Hydrochloric acid* and *intrinsic factor* (for absorption of Vit B_{12}) are secreted by parietal cells, and the hydrolytic enzyme *pepsin* (digests proteins) is secreted by the chief cells of the stomach. *Mucus* is secreted by goblet cells to protect the stomach from the acid. The acid kills many bacteria and its secretion is controlled by the vagus nerve and the hormone *gastrin*. Food (now *chyme*) is propelled to the duodenum by *peristalsis* (propulsive contractions in the gut) through a relaxed *pyloric sphincter*. Chyme entering the duodenum causes secretin (causes bicarbonate and fluid to be released from the pancreas) and *cholecystokinin-pancreozymin* (causes primarily enzymes and water to be released from the pancreas and bile to be released by the gall bladder) to be released. The *pancreas* secretes inactive enzymes called *zymogens*. One of them, *trypsinogen*, is converted to *trypsin* by the *enterokinase*, an activating enzyme located in the duodenal mucosa. Other enzymes, chymotrypsin, lipases and amylases, are also secreted. *Bile* is secreted by the liver and stored in and released from the gall bladder. *Bile salts* in bile emulsify lipids to make them more available for digestion. The duodenum has an alkaline pH. Chyme passes into the jejunum where the mucosa contains disaccharidases and peptidases for the final breakdown of nutrients before they are absorbed by active transport. The *small intestine* is composed of the *duodenum, jejunum* and *ileum* in that order. The duodenum is important for absorption of Ca^{+2} and Fe^{+3}, the jejunum for most sugars, amino acids, fats, etc., and the ileum absorbs Vit B_{12} (complexed to intrinsic factor) and bile salts. In the *colon (large intestine)* the remaining water from the small intestine is largely absorbed as are most ions—this compacts the chyme into feces. *Feces* are stored in the *sigmoid colon* and *rectum* until they are defecated. The *appendix* is a vestigial appendage of the *cecum* (first segment of the colon).

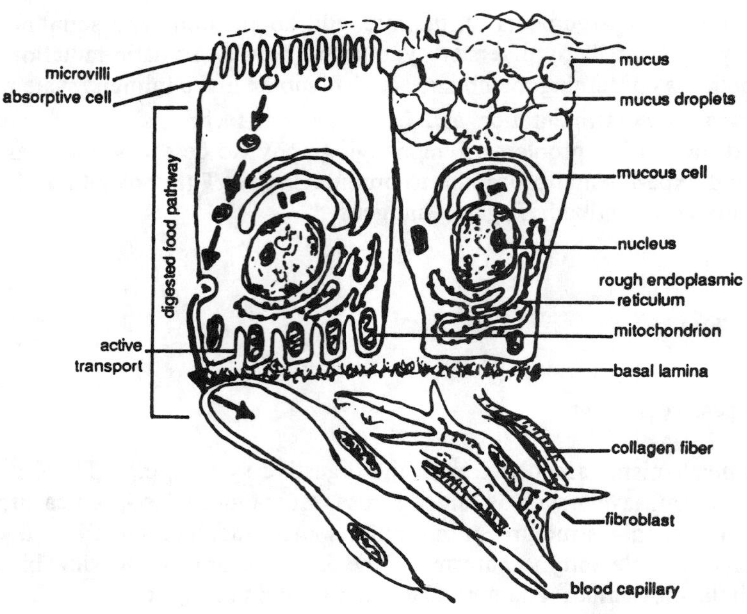

Fig. 7.64—Intestinal Lining

The small intestines have mucosal projections called *villi*. *Crypts* are regions at the base of villi where new cells are generated and digestive enzymes are synthesized by glandular cells. The simple columnar epithelium lines the intestinal tract and consists mainly of absorptive cells and goblet cells. *Absorptive cells* have thousands of microvilli, extensions of the plasma membrane, to increase the surface area of the cell and absorbed products are transported through them and released basolaterally. The microvilli are bathed by mucus (secreted by neighboring *goblet cells*) to aid in trapping digested food. The basal plasma membrane is infolded to facilitate active transport. Like all epithelial cells, absorptive and goblet cells rest on the basal lamina that separates them from the blood capillaries located in the connective tissue beneath. The connective tissue (lamina propria), surrounding the blood capillaries, is secreted by fibroblasts.

Once the products of digestion (molecules and ions) are transported across the absorptive cells, they are transported into the general circulation through the small lymphatic channels, the lacteals, as well as the small veins that coalesce to form the hepatic portal system. In the connective tissue of the ileum are housed lymphatic nodules (Peyer's patches) which are colonies of lymphocytes that provide a first line of defense against bacterial infection.

The *liver* is a vital organ reflected in its numerous functions. The major functions are: (1) *synthesis and storage of glycogen* to be converted to glucose under the stimulation of epinephrine or glucagon; (2) *gluconeogenesis*—the synthesis of glucose from amino acids stimulated by glucagon and epinephrine via cAMP; by gluconeogenesis and removal of storage glycogen the liver plays an important role in *regulation of blood glucose*; (3) *proteins*—synthesizes coagulation factors, albumin, and various others; (4) synthesizes *bile and cholesterol*; (5) contains numerous *macrophages* (called *Kupffer cells*) for defense against foreign materials (e.g., bacterial); (6) contains a system for *detoxification and degradation of* toxins, drugs, and normal metabolites; (7) *fats*—packages fats for transport, oxidizes fatty acids to ketone bodies for use by other tissues; (8) *amino acids*—deaminates (removes nitrogen), produces urea; (9) can interconvert fats, carbohydrates, and amino acids, (10) *stores* substances such as iron and vitamins, A, D, and B_{12}; and (11) red blood cells—potential site for production of RBCs in cases of severe anemia in the adult, site of destruction of old red blood cells.

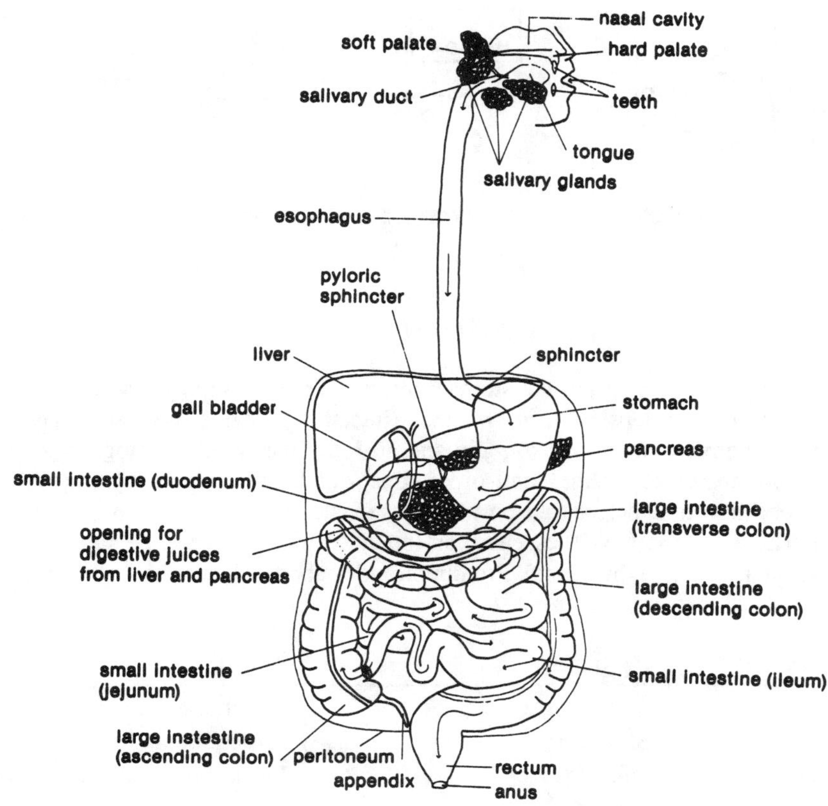

Fig. 7.65—Structure of the Digestive System

7.15.1.2 DIGESTIVE FUNCTIONS OF BIOORGANIC MOLECULES

The digestive functions will be reviewed by discussing each of the major bioorganic molecules (nutrients) in turn.

Carbohydrates (approximately 4 kcal/gm). A small amount of carbohydrate digestion occurs in the mouth (salivary *amylase*) and the stomach (acid digestion). *Pancreatic amylases* digest the starch to disaccharides (*maltose, isomaltose*) and *glucose*. These disaccharides and *sucrose* (cane sugar, sugar beets) and *lactose* (from milk) are broken down, respectively, by *maltases, sucrases*, and *lactases* located on the outer surface of *mucosal cells*. The resulting monosaccharides then enter by *active transport* (glucose and galactose) or *facilitated transport* (the above and fructose, mannose, xylose, arabinose). The active transport mechanisms involve a coupling with Na^+ via a Na-K-ATPase and a specific carrier for glucose both located in the mucosal cell. Carbohydrates are not essential (for life) to the diet. But, they normally provide (in the US) 50 + % of calories. Cellulose cannot be digested by humans.

Lipids. Triglycerides are hydrolyzed by *lipase* from the pancreas. *Bile salts* aid this by emulsifying and solubilizing the fat. Fatty acids, monoglycerides, diglycerides, and glycerol are the products of lipases. These products can diffuse across the mucosa. *Glycerol and short chain fatty acids* go directly to the liver via the venous portal system. *Long chain fatty acids, and the mono- and diglycerides* are resynthesized into triglycerides and packaged with proteins as *chylomicrons* which are absorbed into *lymphatics* and then go to the liver. In the liver, the lipids are reorganized into lipoproteins (lipid plus special proteins) and shipped to adipose cells primarily. Linolenic and linoleic acids are essential fatty acids (cannot be synthesized by humans). Fats are the long term energy storage compounds (approximately 9 kcal/gm).

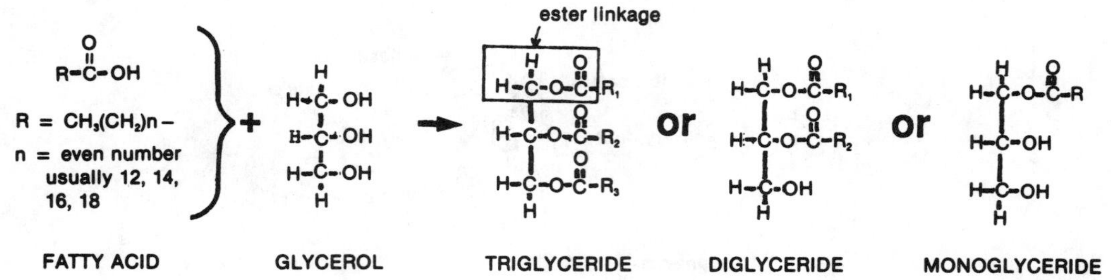

ester linkage

$R-C(=O)-OH$

$R = CH_3(CH_2)n-$

n = even number usually 12, 14, 16, 18

FATTY ACID + GLYCEROL → TRIGLYCERIDE or DIGLYCERIDE or MONOGLYCERIDE

Fig. 7.66—Lipids

Proteins. Some protein digestion occurs in the stomach by *pepsin* (secreted as inactive pepsinogen which is activated by stomach acid or other pepsins). *Enterokinase* (intestinal enzyme) converts trypsinogen to trypsin. Other activating enzymes convert *chymotrypsinogen* and all other pancreatic zymogens to active forms. The result of these digestions are oligopeptides and dipeptides which are cleaved by mucosal enzymes, e.g., carboxypeptidases. Several intestinal active transport systems exist. Absorbed amino acids go to the liver via the venous portal system. There are about 8-10 essential amino acids which have to be supplied in the diet (some are isoleucine, leucine, phenylalanine, histidine). Protein provides about 4 kcals/gm.

Enzymes	Origin	Function
Amylase	Salivary glands, pancreas	Starch breakdown
Pepsin (a protease)	Stomach	Protein breakdown
Trypsin (a protease)	Pancreas	Further breakdown of protein
Lipase	Pancreas	Fat breakdown
Peptidase	Intestinal epithelium	Breakdown of short polypeptides
Maltase	Intestinal epithelium	Maltose breakdown

7.15.2 Questions Related to Digestive System

1. Which type of tooth, in the normal adult with a full set of teeth, has the incorrect maximum number in parenthesis?
   A. incisors (4)
   B. canines (4)
   C. premolars (8)
   D. molars (12)
2. All are functions of saliva *except*:
   A. digestion of starch.
   B. digestion of protein.
   C. lubrication of food.
   D. protection against bacteria.
3. Select the incorrect association:
   A. Stomach—grinds and liquefies food
   B. Pancreas—digestive enzymes
   C. Small intestine—absorption of fluid and food
   D. Colon (large intestine)—absorption of food

4. Select the incorrect association:

   A. Chymotrypsin—protein
   B. Trypsin—carbohydrates
   C. Amylase—carbohydrates
   D. Lipases—fats

5. The correct sequence of structures in the gut is:

   A. stomach, esophagus, small intestine, large intestine.
   B. esophagus, stomach, large intestine, small intestine.
   C. esophagus, stomach, small intestine, large intestine.
   D. esophagus, small intestine, stomach, large intestine.

6. Which of the following is not a function of the liver?

   A. synthesis of insulin
   B. synthesis of carbohydrates, proteins, fats
   C. detoxifies drugs
   D. synthesis of bile

7. Most nutrients are absorbed in the:

   A. esophagus.
   B. stomach.
   C. small intestine.
   D. large intestine.

8. Digestion of carbohydrates occurs *mostly* by enzymes from the:

   A. pancreas.
   B. liver.
   C. stomach.
   D. salivary glands.

9. All of the following carbohydrates can be digested by humans except:

   A. starch.
   B. sucrose.
   C. cellulose.
   D. maltose.

10. Monosaccharides cross the intestinal wall mainly by:

    A. active transport.
    B. diffusion.
    C. facilitated transport.
    D. both (A) and (C).

11. Select the *incorrect* statement concerning bile salts:

    A. break down (digest) lipids
    B. emulsify and solubilize lipids
    C. synthesized in the liver
    D. stored in the gall bladder

12. The products of triglyceride hydrolysis by lipases in the intestine may include:

    A. fatty acids.
    B. monoglycerides.
    C. diglycerides.
    D. all of these.

13. Which is the main long-term energy storage substance in animals?
   A. carbohydrates
   B. fats
   C. proteins
   D. nucleic acids
14. All of the following enzymes are important in the digestion of proteins except:
   A. amylase.
   B. pepsin.
   C. trypsin.
   D. chymotrypsin.
15. The enzyme responsible for the activation of trypsinogen in the intestine is:
   A. pepsin.
   B. enterokinase.
   C. chymotrypsin.
   D. carboxypeptidase.
16. Swallowing is:
   A. voluntary.
   B. involuntary.
   C. both.
   D. caused by gustatory receptors.
17. Secretion of bicarbonate and fluid from the pancreas is stimulated by:
   A. secretin.
   B. cholecystokinin.
   C. enterokinase.
   D. gastrin.
18. Acid secretion from the stomach may be stimulated by:
   A. gastrin.
   B. vagus nerve.
   C. neither A nor B.
   D. both A and B.
19. Select the enzyme not made in the pancreas:
   A. Trypsin
   B. Lipase
   C. Amylase
   D. Pepsin
20. Vitamin B_{12} is absorbed in the:
   A. ileum.
   B. jejunum.
   C. duodenum.
   D. stomach.
21. Iron is absorbed in the:
   A. stomach.
   B. jejunum.
   C. ileum.
   D. duodenum.
22. The absorptive area of the small intestine is increased by structures called:
   A. crypts.
   B. villi.
   C. microvilli.
   D. villi and microvilli.

23. The liver does *not* play a role in the metabolism of:

A. fats.
B. carbohydrates.
C. proteins.
D. carboxylic acids.

24. The digestion of starch by amylase produces:

A. galactose.
B. glucose.
C. maltose.
D. both (B) and (C).

25. The digestion of small peptides and disaccharides occurs:

A. in the stomach lumen.
B. in the lumen of the bowels.
C. on the mucosal cell surface.
D. inside the mucosal cell.

26. Certain lipids, in contrast to other nutrients, leaving the intestine enter the:

A. portal system.
B. lymphatics.
C. arteries.
D. veins.

27. Chylomicrons primarily contain:

A. carbohydrates.
B. lipids.
C. proteins.
D. nucleic acids.

7.15.3 Answers to Questions in Section 7.15.2

(1) A (2) B (3) D (4) B (5) C (6) A (7) C (8) A (9) C (10) D (11) A (12) D
(13) B (14) A (15) B (16) C (17) A (18) D (19) D (20) A (21) D (22) D (23) D (24) D
(25) C (26) B (27) B

7.15.4 Discussion of Answers to Questions in Section 7.15.2: None

7.15.5 Advanced Concepts

- Understand causes, effects and research related to digestive disorders such as: peptic ulcer, gallstone, pancreatitis, hepatitis, cirrhosis, appendicitis, porphyria, regional ileitis and Chrohn's disease.
- Review the histology of pancreas and liver with emphasis on: differences between falciform and round ligaments in the pancreas and liver.
- Learn the chemical composition, pH value and average daily secretions of: saliva, gastric juice, pancreatic juice and bile.

7.16 EXCRETORY SYSTEM

7.16.1 Introduction to Excretory System

Focus on the functional unit of a kidney—the nephron. Remember there are 1 million nephrons per kidney, each nephron is made up of glomerulus and the tubule (made up of renal corpuscles, podocytes, distal and proximal tubules). Understand the histology of podocytes and examine sample electron micrographs. Identify various types of nephrons, e.g., juxtamedullary nephrons, cortical nephrons and their special functions. Review tubular reabsorption (both active and passive), definition and use of milliosmol as a concentration unit and various hydrostatic forces involved in effective filtration. Work with numerical problems to apply various concepts to experimental data on kidneys and filtration rates.

7.16.1.1 BODY FLUID COMPOSITION

Human body fluids divide conveniently into an *intracellular (IC) compartment* and an *extracellular (EC) compartment.* The EC compartment is further divided into an *interstitial (I) compartment* (outside of cells and outside of the circulation) and a *plasma (P) compartment* (circulatory component). Each compartment has a particular substance that tends to maintain its volume. Potassium (K^+) ion is the main molecule of the IC compartment. Sodium (Na^+) ion is the main molecule of the EC compartment. And protein, in addition to Na^+, is important in the plasma compartment.

In the plasma there are *cations,* Na^+ and K^+ primarily, balanced by *anions,* chloride (Cl^-) and bicarbonate (HCO_3^-) primarily. Also, there are many small organic molecules such as glucose, amino acids, etc. Larger organic molecules such as proteins and fat complexes are also present.

The *acidity,* measured by the pH, is relatively constant at pH ≈ 7.40 for the plasma. The major sources of acidity are the CO_2 (produced in tissues) and acids from the oxidation of glucose, fats, and amino acids such as pyruvate, lactate, or sulfur (from sulfur containing amino acids). Bicarbonate (basic) is produced by the kidney to balance these acids. The ratio of dissolved CO_2 and HCO_3^- is the determinator of the pH. As CO_2 increases the pH decreases and as HCO_3^- increases the pH increases:

$$pH \propto \frac{[HCO_3^-]}{PCO_2}$$

where PCO_2 is the partial pressure of CO_2. Remember that CO_2 undergoes this reaction with water,

$$CO_2 + H_2O \rightleftharpoons \underset{\text{carbonic acid}}{H_2CO_3}$$

and carbonic acid dissociates to give H^+, $H_2CO_3 \rightleftharpoons H^+ + HCO_3^-$ (remember H^+ is measured by the pH).

The plasma also contains waste products of the tissues, one of the most important being urea. *Urea,* is the result

$$O=C(NH_2)_2$$

Urea Molecule

of the breakdown of nitrogen-containing organic molecules, especially amino acids. *Creatinine* is a product of muscle metabolism and is also continuously released into the plasma. Both are excreted by the kidneys.

7.16.1.2 KIDNEY: STRUCTURE AND FUNCTION

The structure and function of the kidney will be described by following the path of blood through the kidney and the formation of urine by the kidney.

Blood from the renal artery enters the center of the kidney (*hilus*) and divides into hundreds of branches as it radiates outward into the *cortex*. At a million locations within the cortex of each kidney, the smallest of arteries, the arterioles, branch into a knotted cluster of capillaries termed the *glomerulus*, then fuse together again into an arteriole before breaking finally into the vast capillary beds of the kidney. The capillary loops of the glomerulus have small holes called fenestrae (see Section 7.13) that readily allow passage of much of the watery ions and smaller molecules, but retain the larger blood proteins, blood cells and platelets within the capillary. The actual filter of the kidney is a slightly thickened *basal lamina* of the capillary endothelial cells. The knotted glomerulus is housed in the first segment of the nephron, a long, folded tubule capped by a cellular funnel, termed *Bowman's capsule*, that wraps around the glomerulus and aids in the filtration and directs the filtrate toward the cellular tubule. In the *proximal convoluted tubule (PCT)*, proteins, amino acids, sugars and other nutrients are *reabsorbed* by active transport by the tubular cells. Most of the cells of the tubular nephron are cuboidal epithelial cells and, like those absorptive cells of the small intestine, possess both microvilli and modifications of the basal plasma membrane to aid in active transport; they rest on a basal lamina.

Sodium, potassium and bicarbonate are reabsorbed as is most of the water. Hydrogen ion and ammonium ions are *secreted* into the tubular lumen by the PCT cells. Also, toxic substances and waste molecules are secreted into the lumen by the PCT cells. The fluid remaining in the lumen continues into the *descending limb of the loop of Henle (LOH)* where Na^+ is picked up from the medulla (inside of kidney) interstitium. The filtrate continues around the LOH to the *ascending limb of the LOH* where Cl^- is being actively extruded into the medulla and Na^+ passively follows. A Cl^- pump that requires energy as ATP is responsible for this extrusion against the concentration gradient. This *countercurrent multiplier system* between the limbs of the LOH maintains a high concentration of Na^+ in the medulla. The filtrate (urine) passes on to the *distal convoluted tubule (DCT)* where Na^+ in the lumen is exchanged for K^+ (and H^+ in the cells stimulated by *aldosterone* (from the adrenal gland). The filtrate (now urine) continues to the *collecting tubule (CT)* which dips into the medulla with its large Na^+ concentration. The Na^+ in the medulla draws most of the water out of the CT into the medulla, where the water is picked up by a system of blood vessels called the *vasa rectae*. *ADH* (antidiuretic hormone; vasopressin) is synthesized in the hypothalamus and stored in and released from the posterior pituitary. It acts on the CT to increase water resorption and results in a more concentrated urine. The urine passes, in order, through the *calyces*, the *pelvices*, the *ureter*, the *urinary bladder*, and the *urethra* to the outside of the body.

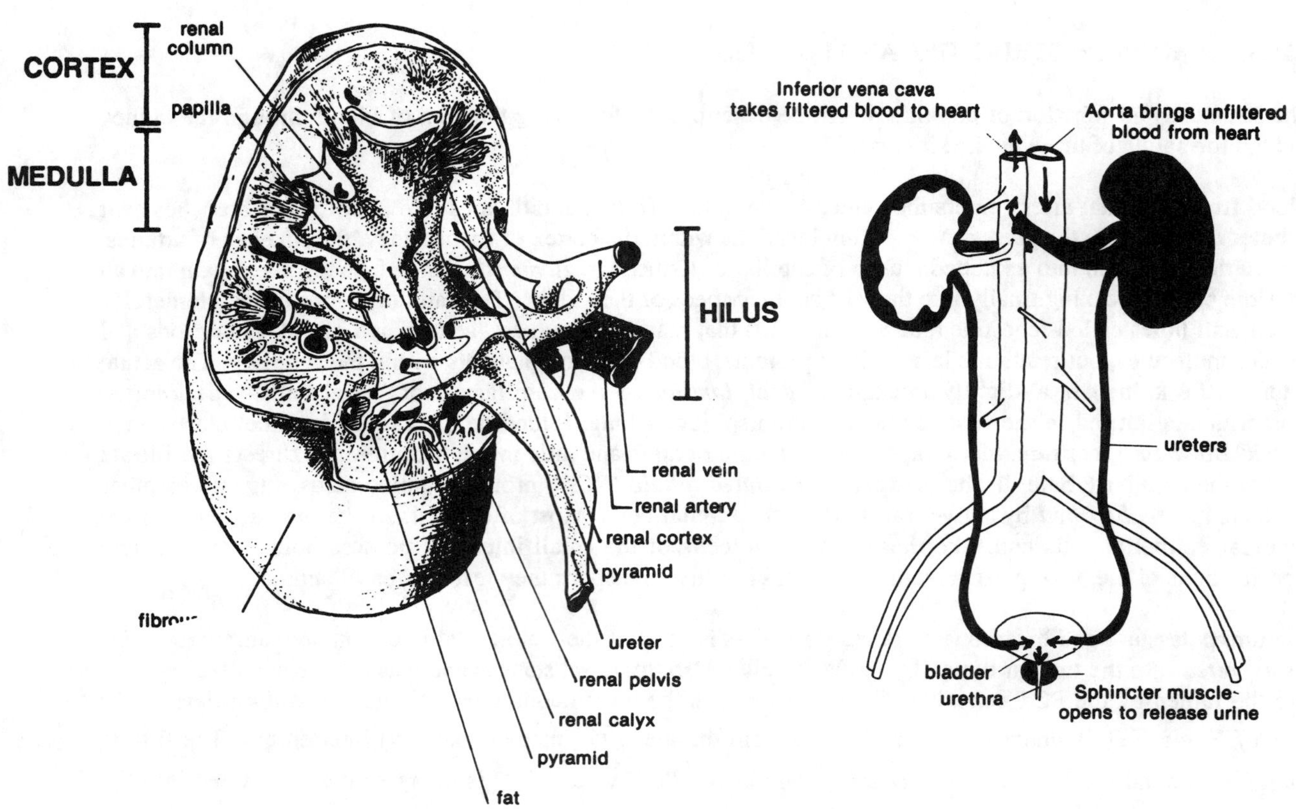

Fig. 7.67(a)—Kidney

Fig. 7.67(b)—Excretory System

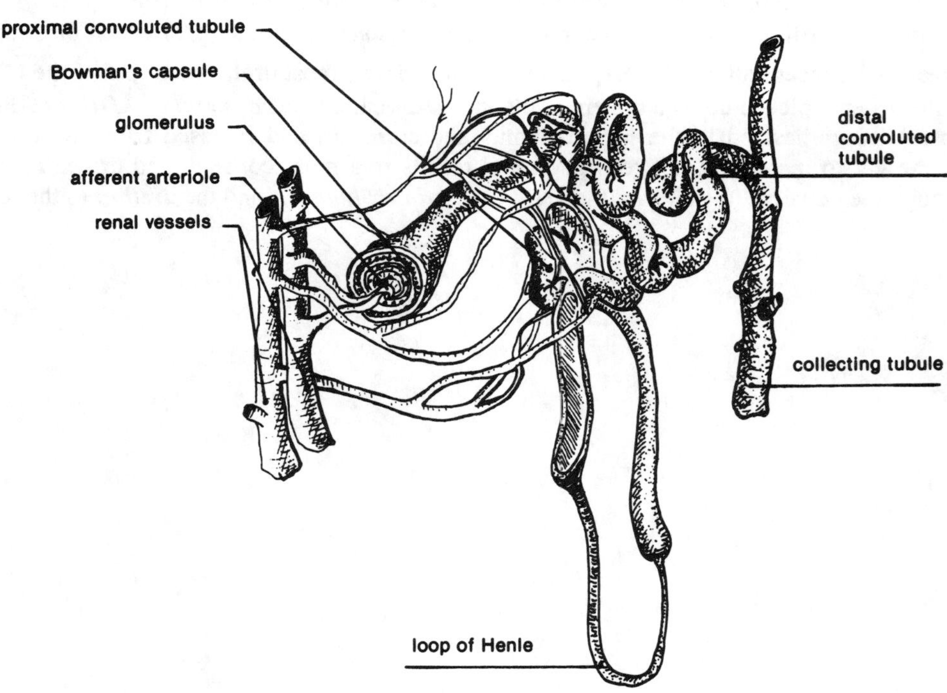

Fig. 7.67(c)—Microscopic View of the Nephron

7.16.1.3 ROLE OF THE EXCRETORY SYSTEM IN BODY HOMEOSTASIS

The body regulates the composition of its body fluids within fairly narrow limits. This is because too much or too little of most substances is toxic to cells. The kidney is the central regulator. In general, substances taken into the body (by gastrointestinal tract, lungs, skin or directly into vessels) and substances made in the tissues are in balance with substances used by the tissues and *excreted* by the body (in the lungs, gastrointestinal tract, skin, and kidneys). That is, Input = Output. This results in fairly constant levels of most substances in the blood. Changes in the function or amount of the load imposed on any of the above can destroy homeostasis and cause changes in body fluid composition.

The *heart and blood vessels* (7.13.1.2) serve their part by keeping blood flowing to all the organs and tissues. This allows a constant exchange between the tissues and the blood. If cardiovascular function decreases, fluid nutrients can't get to tissues and wastes accumulate in tissues and the blood. Also, if the heart output falls too much the kidney cannot function. The *lymphatic vessels* (7.14.1.1) return fluid and protein to the cardiovascular system to help maintain its function. When lymphatic function decreases, fluid accumulates in the tissues, and the heart has less blood to pump which compromises its function. The *lungs* (7.19.1.2) remove CO_2 from the body and supply the O_2 needed. If lung function is affected, the acidity of blood is affected as well as the production of energy (need O_2). The *skin* (7.19.1.3) plays a role in the passage of water and ions (Na^+, K^+, Cl^-) in the form of sweat. If sweating is excessive, water and ion loss can compromise the circulation. The *gastrointestinal tract* (7.15.1.1) is responsible for the intake of nutrients and excretion of certain wastes and ions (Na^+, K^+, Cl^-, HCO_3^-) and water. So, malfunctions, as in diarrhea, can lead to body fluid abnormalities.

Finally, the *kidney* serves the role of fine tuning the body fluids. After the other systems have upset or tried to correct the homeostasis, the kidney, through the mechanisms described in Section 7.16.1.2, can return the body fluids to a new (not necessarily the same) homeostasis. When kidneys malfunction, substances collect in the blood (e.g., urea) and/or are excreted (e.g., sugar, excess Na^+) that would ordinarily not be retained or excreted.

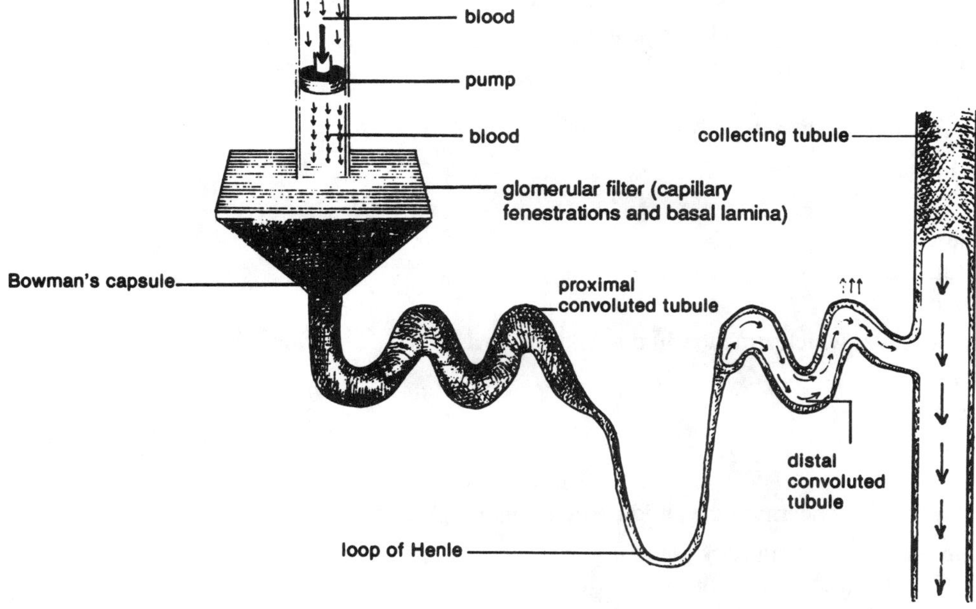

Fig. 7.67(d)—Schematic of Function of a Nephron

7.16.1.4 PHYSIOLOGIC BUFFERS IN BODY FLUIDS

The main buffer in the ECF (extracellular fluid) is bicarbonate. Its interaction with hydrogen ions has been explained earlier in 7.16.1.1. In order to use the Henderson-Hasselbalch equation,

$$pH = pK + \log\frac{\text{base}}{\text{acid}}$$

we should use actual experimental values of an average person: pK = 6.1 for the ECF.

Example: Add 10mM/L of hydrochloric acid to 1L of water and to 1L of extracellular fluid. Assume that the ECF [HCO_3^-] is 20 mM/L and the [H_2CO_3] is 1.2mM. Study pH changes.

Solution: For water, 10mM HCl contains $10mM = \frac{10}{1000} = 0.010M$ hydrogen ion.

Therefore, by definition, pH

$$= -\log[H^+]$$
$$= -\log[.010]$$
$$= 2.00$$

For ECF, $10HCl + 20NaHCO_3 \rightarrow 10NaCl + 10NaHCO_3 + 10H_2CO_3$.

As seen, bicorbonate reduces the change in pH caused by addition of H^+. Using Henderson-Hasselbalch equation, and noting that there is already 1.2 mM H_2CO_3 in the fluid,

$$pH = 6.1 + \log\frac{10}{10 + 1.2}$$

$$= 6.1 + \log\frac{10}{11.2} = 6.99$$

HCO_3^- is the most important physiologic buffer because its two components can be regulated by the kidneys and the lung.

7.16.2 Question Related to Excretory System

1. Functions of the kidneys include all except:

A. excretion of NH_3 from protein oxidation as urea.
B. regulation of fluids and electrolytes.
C. elimination of toxic substances.
D. elimination of carbon dioxide directly.

2. All are part of the human kidney except the:

A. glomerulus.
B. loop of Henle.
C. Malpighian tubules.
D. collecting ducts.

3. Filtration of *blood* occurs at which structure in the kidney?

A. loop of Henle
B. collecting ducts
C. tubules
D. glomerulus

4. Select the correct statement concerning the antidiuretic hormone (ADH):

A. synthesized in the posterior pituitary gland
B. acts on the collecting duct of the kidney
C. also called aldosterone
D. all of the above are correct

5. Select the correct sequence of filtered blood through the kidney:
   A. Bowman's capsule, glomerulus, tubules, collecting duct
   B. glomerulus, Bowman's capsule, collecting ducts, tubules
   C. Bowman's capsule, collecting ducts, glomerulus, tubules
   D. glomerulus, Bowman's capsule, tubules, collecting duct
6. The volume of fluid in the plasma is maintained by:
   A. protein.
   B. Na^+.
   C. Na^+ and protein.
   D. K^+.
7. The cations of Na^+ and K^+ are balanced in the plasma by:
   A. Cl^-.
   B. HCO_3^-.
   C. Cl^- and HCO_3^-.
   D. proteins.
8. The acidity of the plasma is caused by:
   A. oxidation of glucose and fats.
   B. metabolism of sulfur-containing amino acids.
   C. production of CO_2 by the tissues.
   D. all of the above.
9. Carbon dioxide when dissolved in water:
   A. has base properties.
   B. has acid properties.
   C. is neutral.
   D. behaves as a ketone.
10. Urea:
    A. is a product of protein metabolism.
    B. contains only carbon, hydrogen, and oxygen.
    C. is excreted by the lungs.
    D. is a product of protein regeneration.
11. The ___________ is part of the circulatory system.
    A. Bowman's capsule
    B. loop of Henle
    C. medulla
    D. glomerulus
12. All of the following substances are filtered at the glomerulus except:
    A. platelets.
    B. proteins.
    C. glucose.
    D. sodium.
13. Reabsorption of most of the water, glucose, amino acids, sodium and other nutrients occurs at the:
    A. loop of Henle.
    B. collecting duct.
    C. proximal convoluted tubule.
    D. distal convoluted tubule.

14. The high concentration of sodium in the medulla is maintained by the:
   A. proximal convoluted tubule.
   B. distal convoluted tubule.
   C. loop of Henle.
   D. collecting duct.

15. The movement of Cl^- out of the ascending limb of the loop of Henle occurs by:
   A. diffusion.
   B. active transport.
   C. osmosis.
   D. facilitated diffusion.

16. In the distal convoluted tubule:
   A. K^+ moves into the lumen.
   B. H^+ moves into the tubular cells.
   C. Na^+ moves into the lumen.
   D. Na^+ is actively extruded into the medulla.

17. Malfunction in which of the following systems might result in body fluid disturbances?
   A. heart
   B. skin
   C. lung
   D. all of them

7.16.3 Answers to Questions in Section 7.16.2

(1) D (2) C (3) D (4) B (5) D (6) C (7) C (8) D (9) B (10) A (11) D (12) A (13) C (14) C (15) B (16) A (17) D

7.16.4 Discussion of Answers to Questions in Section 7.16.2: None

7.16.5 Advanced Concepts

- Understand the basic differences between nephrology and urology and get a basic recognition of: kidney stones and methods to remove them; prostate hypertrophy in males, glomerulonephritis, cystitis, nephrosis and nephrectomy. Understand the physics of various instruments used to correct the above renal disorders
- Understand the design, construction and working of an artificial kidney and dialysis machine. Recognize the symptoms of a complete renal failure and pathological studies done to correct it or make histological recommendations to a specialist

7.17 MUSCLE SYSTEM

7.17.1 Introduction to Muscle System

The student should learn nervous control of muscles. Compare and contrast characteristics of motor and sensory control. Distinguish between the control mechanisms for voluntary and involuntary muscles. Develop a detailed understanding of the sliding filament theory and mechanisms of muscular contractions (emphasize myosin binding mechanism in contractile process). Review differences between isotonic and isometric contractions. Do *not* memorize but realize that there are 700 skeletal muscles (focus on the location, shape and size of these muscles).

7.17.1.1 BASIC MUSCLE TYPES AND FUNCTIONS

The three types of muscles are smooth, cardiac, and striated or skeletal. The cytoplasm of all three muscle types is filled with contractile proteins.

Smooth muscle is named because its contractile protein is so organized that it lacks microscopic striations; smooth muscle is composed of distinct spindle-shaped, uninucleated cells. They are innervated by the autonomic nervous system and are largely involuntary, but not every muscle cell is innervated. Therefore, smooth muscle cells are interconnected by gap junctions that propagate a wave of contraction. They can contract slowly and maintain contractions for long periods of time. This feature is useful for their function in organs where they are found, including the gut (for peristalsis and churning of food), blood vessels (for regulation of blood pressure), and many ducts (e.g., the ureter for peristalsis).

Cardiac muscle is composed of uninucleated cells joined together by a saw-toothed array of junctional complexes (including extensive gap junctions) termed the *intercalated disc* to speed impulse conduction. Microscopically, cardiac muscle appears striated. The muscle fibers are highly branched—this probably adds to their strength. Innervation is by the autonomic nervous system but beats are originated by specialized muscle cells (see section 7.13).

Skeletal muscle consists of multinucleated cells fused together to form a single cell called a *syncytium*. Skeletal muscle is distinctly striated microscopically. Skeletal muscles are innervated by the somatic nervous system and are voluntary. The control of voluntary movements originates in a portion of the *cerebral cortex* (surface of cerebrum) and are coordinated by impulses from the *cerebellum*. Skeletal muscles contract rapidly but tire easily. A simple *twitch* of a muscle involves the following steps: (1) impulse from a nerve stimulates the muscle, (2) a brief latent period, (3) then the phase of contraction, and (4) a phase of relaxation. If the muscle is stimulated during the relaxation phase it can be made to contract again. If these stimuli are in rapid succession the contractions can be made to summate to a sustained contraction called *tetanus*.

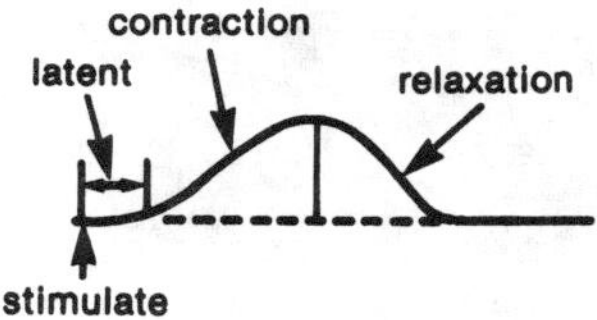

Fig. 7.68—Phases of Muscle Contraction

Muscle *tone* differs from tetanus in that groups of muscle fibers of a muscle alternatingly contract and relax. This allows form and position (at rest) to be maintained.

Skeletal muscle uses O_2 (oxygen) in aerobic metabolism (Sec. 7.7) when it is available. In the absence of O_2, the production of energy requires that there be a final electron acceptor. This electron acceptor becomes pyruvate which is converted to lactate (Fig. 7.69).

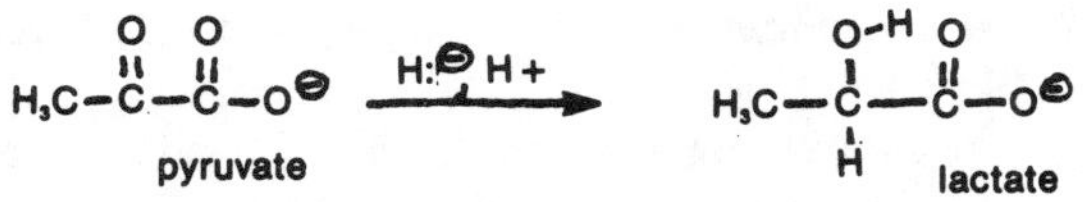

$$\underset{\text{pyruvate}}{H_3C-\overset{O}{\overset{\|}{C}}-\overset{O}{\overset{\|}{C}}-O^{\ominus}} \xrightarrow{H{:}^{\ominus}\ H+} \underset{\text{lactate}}{H_3C-\overset{O-H}{\overset{|}{\underset{H}{\underset{|}{C}}}}-\overset{O}{\overset{\|}{C}}-O^{\ominus}}$$

NADH could transfer an $H{:}^-$ and H^+ is picked up from solution.

Fig. 7.69—Formation of Lactate

The amount of lactate formed becomes a measure of the lack of O_2, (the usual electron acceptor). This is a partial measure of the *oxygen debt* that muscles incur during exercise when their rate of O_2 demand exceeds that supplied. After exercise, the lactate is converted back to pyruvate, and the electrons are passed to O_2 as O_2 is supplied to the muscles and the oxygen debt is repaid. In *summary*, during exercise the energy metabolism of muscle switches from aerobic to anaerobic and an oxygen debt is incurred which is repaid when the exercise ends.

The skeletal muscles act across joints to move body parts. Each muscle has an *origin* and an *insertion.* In general, the origin is stationary, and when the muscle contracts, the insertion (and the bone it is attached to) moves toward the origin (Fig. 7.71). The functioning unit of the striated muscle is the *myofibril* (muscle fibers or cells are composed of myofibrils). Myofibrils are composed of linearly arranged sarcomeres. A *sarcomere* is limited by regions that anchor the *actin* (thin filaments) called the *Z-lines. Myosin* (thick filaments) alternate with the actin and are not anchored. Bands are labeled as shown in Fig. 7.70.

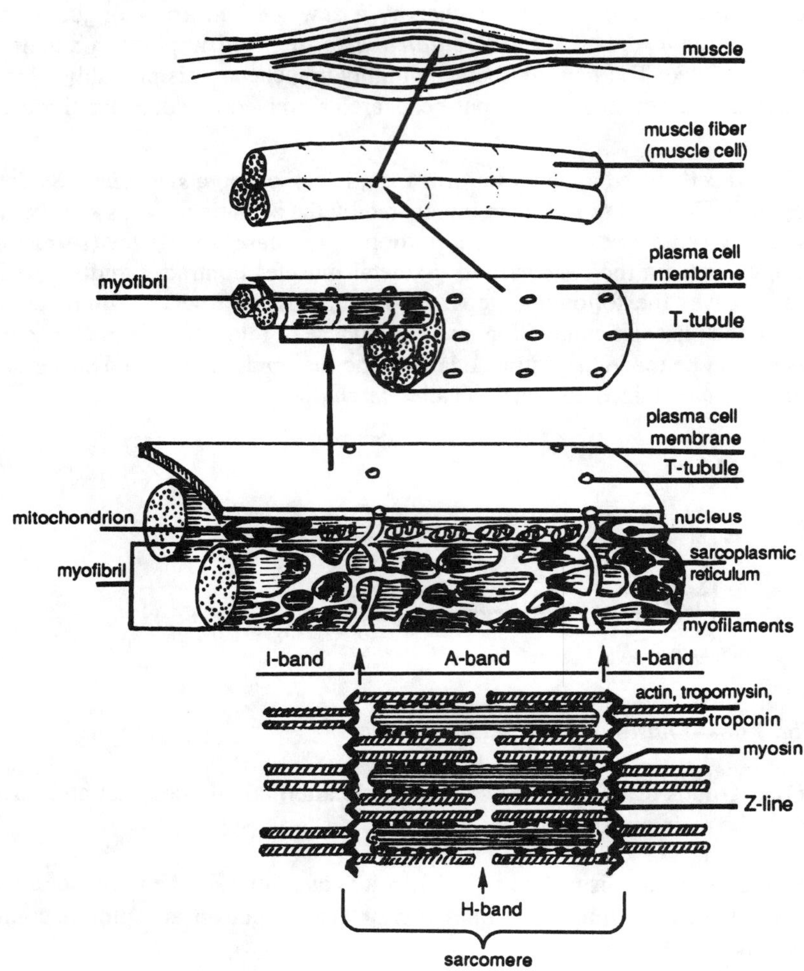

Fig. 7.70—Components of a Sarcomere (Skeletal Muscle)

When the muscle contracts, the Z-lines move together, the I and H bands decrease in size, and the A-band remains the same size. The *actin complex* is composed of actin, tropomyosin and troponin. *Actin* has sites which bind to heavy meromyosin when contraction occurs. *Tropomyosin* is an α-helical protein wound around the actin (which is two intertwined α-helical chains) and blocks the myosin binding site. *Troponin* is a regulator protein bound to tropomyosin and has a site for binding Ca^{+2} and a site that inhibits myosin's binding to actin. When there is no Ca^{+2} present, the troponin and tropomyosin prevent myosin binding and, hence, contraction. When Ca^{+2} is present, the Ca^{+2} binds to troponin causing a conformational change which in turn causes tropomyosin to shift, uncovering the actin binding region for myosin, and contraction proceeds. *Myosin* is composed of *light meromyosin* (the tail) and *heavy meromyosin* (the head). The head binds to actin and contains an ATPase to break the bonds to actin. *Contraction* is caused by the heads of myosin alternatingly binding and releasing actin in a rachet-like fashion. The *sarcolemma* (cell membrane of muscle) sends a system of membranes (T-tubules) into the muscle. When an impulse from a nerve reaches the sarcolemma, this is transmitted down the *T-tubules* which release Ca^{+2} into the sarcoplasm (muscle cell interior) for contraction. The *sarcoplasmic reticulum* (specialized smooth endoplasmic reticulum) abuts upon the T-tubules, its role is to remove the Ca^{+2} from the sarcoplasm.

Muscles work in pairs (or in more complex arrangements). For a muscle that moves a joint in one direction there is an *antagonistic muscle* that will move the joint in the opposite direction (i.e., undo that motion). There are also *synergistic muscles* that aid in the motion caused by a given muscle. At the elbow, the triceps (extension) and biceps (flexion) are examples of antagonistic muscles. At the shoulder, the deltoid (raises arm) and supraspinatous (raises arm) are examples of synergistic muscles. Complex neural pathways insure coordination of the muscle groups. A *flexor* decreases the angle of a joint. An *extensor* increases the angle of a joint. An *abductor* moves a limb away from the midline. An *adductor* moves a limb toward the midline.

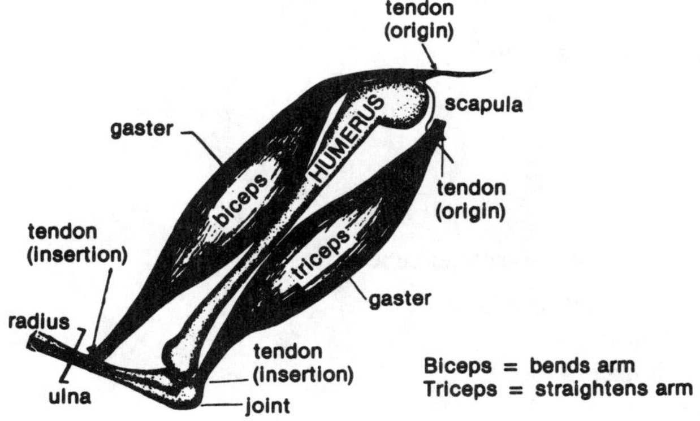

Fig. 7.71—Attachments of a Muscle

7.17.1.2 VOLUNTARY AND INVOLUNTARY MUSCLE CONTROL

During intense physical activity oxidative metabolism cannot supply all the ATP that muscles require. As soon as intense muscular activity ceases, aerobic processes must provide ATP for the resynthesis of creatine phosphate. These aerobic activities account for the deep, rapid breathing that continues after muscular activity has ceased. The elevated rate of respiration provides the oxygen required to produce ATP for the resynthesis of creatine phosphate and to convert lactic acid back to glucose and glycogen.

When skeletal muscles are not used, the muscle fibers diminish in size. Regular exercise, on the other hand, can produce increases in muscle size, endurance, and strength. Endurance exercises, such as running, produce cardiovascular and pulmonary changes, causing the muscles to be better supplied with materials such as oxygen and carbohydrates. Cramps are involuntary muscle contractions that are painful. Their precise cause is unknown—possibly a low oxygen supply causes them.

7.17.2 Questions Related to Muscle System

1. All of the following are muscle proteins except:

- **A.** actin.
- **B.** myosin.
- **C.** fibrinogen.
- **D.** troponin.

2. One of the histology muscle types has striated fibers and is involuntary. It is:

   A. smooth muscle.
   B. skeletal muscle.
   C. cardiac muscle.
   D. none of the above.

3. Select the muscle type composed of distinct cells:

   A. Smooth
   B. Skeletal
   C. Cardiac
   D. Both (A) and (C)

4. Intercalated discs are found in which type of muscle?

   A. skeletal
   B. cardiac
   C. smooth
   D. all types

5. Which type of muscle is a syncytium?

   A. skeletal
   B. cardiac
   C. smooth
   D. all types

6. All are true concerning smooth muscle except they:

   A. are composed of distinct spindle cells.
   B. are largely involuntary.
   C. have intercalated discs.
   D. are found in the gut.

7. All are true concerning cardiac muscle except:

   A. it is a syncytium.
   B. it is striated.
   C. it is involuntary.
   D. gap junctions speed conduction.

8. All are true concerning skeletal muscles except:

   A. they are a syncytium.
   B. they are involuntary.
   C. they are responsible for locomotion.
   D. they contract rapidly but tire readily.

9. Select the incorrect statement concerning muscles:

   A. Ligaments attach bone to bone.
   B. Flexors decrease the angle at a joint.
   C. Adductors move a limb away from the midline.
   D. Tendons attach muscle to bone.

10. The A-band of striated muscle represents:

    A. myosin only.
    B. actin only.
    C. both (A) and (B).
    D. neither (A) nor (B).

11. The Z-line as seen in striated muscle anchors:

A. both actin and myosin.
B. neither actin nor myosin.
C. actin.
D. myosin.

12. During muscle contraction, all of the following occur except that:

A. Z-lines move together.
B. A-band decreases in size.
C. I-band decreases in size.
D. H-band decreases in size.

13. Which of the following ions is of most importance in the mechanical contraction of muscle?

A. Na^{+1}
B. Ca^{+2}
C. K^{+1}
D. Cl^{-1}

14. Muscle tone depends upon:

A. continual low level contraction of all fibers in the muscles.
B. summation of twitches to a plateau.
C. presence of short fibers that constantly appear contracted.
D. alternating contractions of different fiber groups in a muscle.

15. During exercise:

A. muscles depend on the Kreb's Cycle for energy.
B. O_2 becomes the electron acceptor.
C. lactate levels decrease.
D. energy metabolism changes from aerobic to anaerobic.

16. Troponin:

A. binds Ca^{+2}.
B. binds to tropomyosin.
C. inhibits myosin's binding to actin.
D. performs all of the above functions.

17. The phase of contraction of a muscle occurs when:

A. tropomyosin binds and releases actin.
B. myosin alternately binds and releases actin.
C. actin alternately binds and releases myosin.
D. none of the above biochemical reactions occur.

7.17.3 Answers to Questions in Section 7.17.2

(1) C (2) C (3) D (4) B (5) A (6) C (7) A (8) B (9) C (10) C (11) C (12) B
(13) B (14) D (15) D (16) D (17) B

7.17.4 Discussion of Answers to Questions in Section 7.17.2: None, except

Question #10 (Answer: C) Technically, the band is visible as such because of the myosin, but within the limits of the band actin is also present.

7.17.5 Advanced Concepts

- Develop basic recognition of muscle twitch (slow and fast), tetanus, treppe, tic, tremor, etc.
- Understand the mechanisms associated with muscular dystrophy, cramps, muscular atrophy
- Acquaint yourself with electromyogram and instruments used to obtain it
- Understand glycogen - lactic acid system, smooth muscle contractions, and role played by calmodulin

7.18 SKELETAL SYSTEM

7.18.1 Introduction to Skeletal System

Review the skeletal system with focus on the axial skeleton, appendicular skeleton and articulations (arthrology is a medical specialty). Understand the six types of synovial joints (ball-and-socket, ellipsoidal, gliding, hinged, pivot and saddle).

7.18.1.1 CONNECTIVE TISSUE (Specialized Eukaryotic Cells and Tissues)

Bone is considered a special connective tissue. Tendons, ligaments, cartilage, vertebral discs, tooth dentin, the dermis of the skin and the mesentery of the gut, are all connective tissue. Connective tissue differs from the other three basic kinds of tissue (nervous, muscle and epithelium) in that connective tissue is largely secretory material. The secreted molecules are extremely diverse. Collagen is the most prevalent molecule in connective tissue (basically three peptides wrapped around each other like a rope). There are at least 12 different kinds of collagen (Types I to XII). Other major components of connective tissue are chondroitin sulfate proteoglycan, heparan sulfate proteoglycan, hyaluronic acid, lipoproteins, glycoproteins and phosphoproteins. In all but special connective tissues, the cell that synthesizes and secretes all these molecules is termed a fibroblast (fibro = fiber, blast = former). Other cells present in connective tissue are the endothelial cells of blood vessels, macrophages (histiocytes), lymphocytes and mast cells.

7.18.1.2 BONE TYPES AND STRUCTURE

Bones in the human are of two types, flat bones and long bones. *Flat bones* include the skull bones, ribs and vertebrae, contain red marrow (much blood cell production), are found where little movement is required, and perform protective functions in general. *Long bones* (Fig. 7.72) include the bones of the hands, feet, arms and legs, contain yellow marrow, are involved in locomotion and motion primarily.

When bone (Fig. 7.73) is laid down it may be spongy or compact. *Spongy bone* is porous like a sponge with the bone present as spicules and the spaces filled with either red or yellow bone marrow. *Compact bone* is densely packed but richly vascularized. It is very strong bone and found where great strength is required as in the cortex of long bones.

Bone is composed of a crystal part (65% hydroxyapatite which is a complex of Ca^{+2} and PO_4^{-3}, but also Na^{+}, K^{+}, Mg^{+2} and other anions) and an organic part (35% Type I collagen and other noncollagenous proteins and growth factors). Collagen molecules are arranged end-to-end and quarter-staggered side-to-side to form a collagen fibril. Collagen fibrils are coated with non-collagenous proteins that aid in the alignment and deposition of the hydroxyapatite crystals along the collagen.

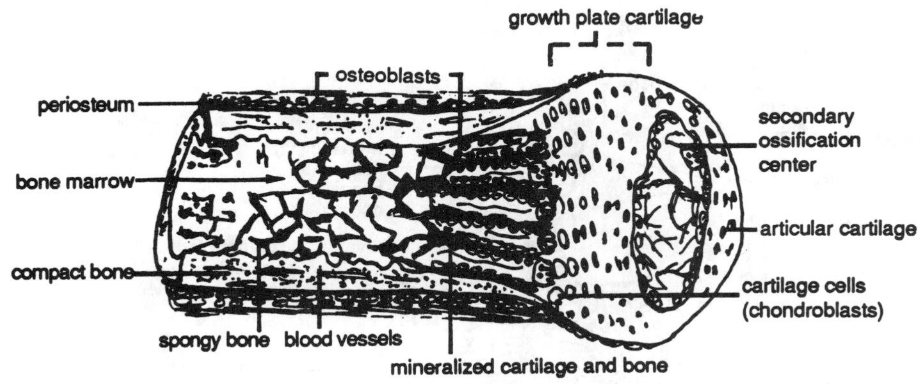

Fig. 7.72—Long Bone

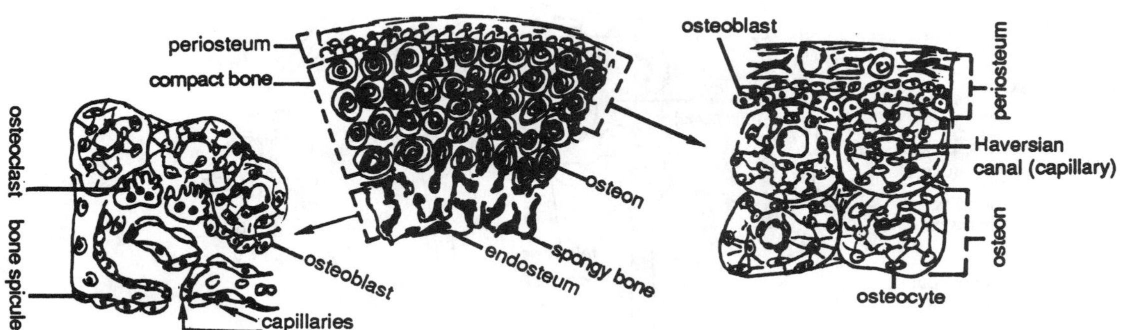

Fig. 7.73—Bone Cross Section

7.18.1.3 SKELETAL AND CARTILAGE STRUCTURE

Bone can be formed directly within primitive connective tissue (*intramembranous* bones such as skull bones) or can be formed from a cartilaginous model (*endochondral bone* formation, such as long bones). *Cartilage cells* construct a mineralized cartilage matrix scaffolding then die. The scaffolding is partially removed by multinucleated cells, *osteoclasts.* Bone forming cells (*osteoblasts*) accompanied by capillaries invade the remainder of the mineralized scaffolding and begin to secrete bone. Some osteoblasts become osteocytes (bone maintenance cells) when in the process of bone formation they become totally surrounded by secreted bone matrix. Osteoblasts and osteocytes are tethered together through gap junctions that form between their numerous cell processes. The basic functional unit in mature bone is the *osteon* (Haversian System) found in both compact bone and bony spicules. Periodically old osteons are replaced by new bone (bone turnover) throughout the lifetime of the human. Osteoclasts destroy old bone and osteoblasts replace old bone with new. About 5-10% of compact bone is replaced yearly.

Joints allow for motion between bones. The contacting and mobile surfaces between bones are covered by *cartilage. Ligaments* help hold bones together at the joint—that is, they are attached bone to bone. *Tendons* connect muscles to bones—they also help hold bones together at joints.

Parathyroid hormone (PTH) causes Ca^{+2} (and phosphate) to be removed from the bony matrix, thus causing demineralization of bone. The Ca^{+2} appears in the serum. The bone matrix serves as a storage depot for many cations (Ca^{+2}, K^+, Mg^{+2}, Na^+) and serves to buffer (help control the levels of) these in the blood (as well as an H^+ buffer). PTH is stimulated by low serum calcium. *Calcitonin* is secreted from special cells in the thyroid gland. It is stimulated by high serum calcium and causes Ca^{+2}, etc., to be deposited in bone. A schematized drawing of some of the bones of the human body is in Fig. 7.74.

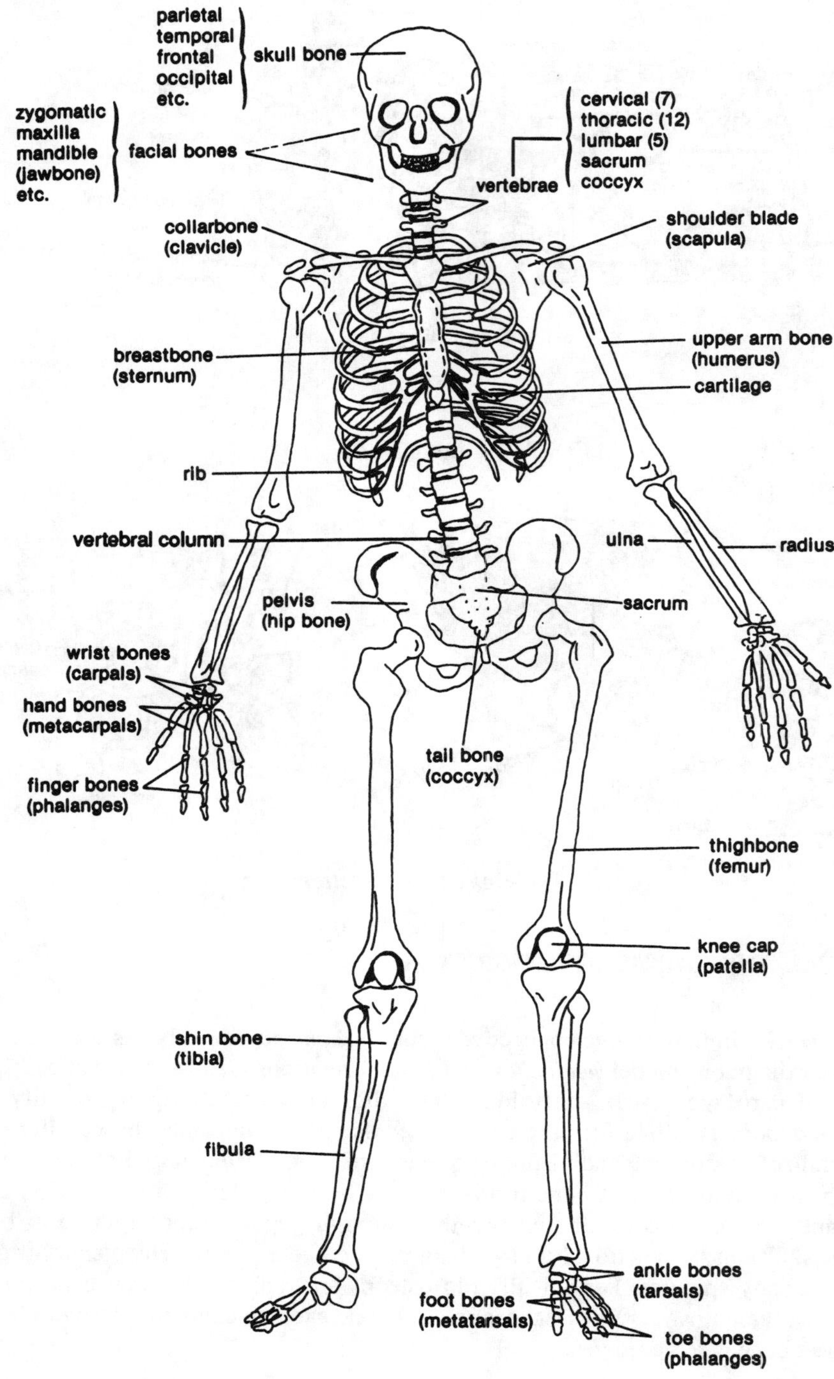

Fig. 7.74—Human Skeleton

7.18.2 Questions Related to Skeletal System

1. All bone is formed:

   A. from a cartilage model.
   B. without a cartilage model.
   C. within one to two hours.
   D. without the use of osteoblasts.

2. Parathyroid Hormone:

   A. helps in demineralization of bone.
   B. helps in mineralization of bone.
   C. increases basal metabolic rate.
   D. leads to Graves' disease when in excess.

3. Which cell makes bone?

   A. osteoblast
   B. osteocyte
   C. osteoclast
   D. all of the above

4. Haversian canals are:

   A. markings seen on Mars.
   B. nutrient systems of bone.
   C. found in the inner ear.
   D. communication between the left and right cerebral hemispheres.

5. Components of a *mature* Haversian canal system would include all except:

   A. osteoblasts.
   B. lacunae.
   C. canaliculi.
   D. blood vessels.

6. Components of the human axial skeleton include all except the:

   A. sternum.
   B. vertebral column.
   C. hips.
   D. skull.

7. Components of the appendicular human skeleton include all except the:

   A. shoulder girdle.
   B. arm bones.
   C. ribs.
   D. leg bones.

8. The humerus, radius and ulna are found in the:

   A. vertebral column.
   B. shoulder girdle.
   C. arm.
   D. leg.

9. All are parts of the vertebral column except:

   A. cervical
   B. thoracic
   C. caudal
   D. lumbar

10. The parietal and occipital bones are found in the:

   A. vertebral column.
   B. skull.
   C. hip girdle.
   D. foot.

11. The bones of the wrist are called:

A. carpals.
B. metacarpals.
C. tarsals.
D. metatarsals.

12. The hip bone connects the ________ to the ________.

A. femur, sternum
B. humerus, sacrum
C. femur, sacrum
D. humerus, sternum

13. Phalanges are found in the:

A. fingers.
B. toes.
C. fingers and toes.
D. Nissl bodies inside a neuron.

14. Bone is composed of ________ and ________.

A. calcium; phosphate
B. globular proteins; ions
C. collagen; hydroxyapatite
D. enzymes; calcium

15. ________ serves as the focus of the deposition of the crystal matrix.

A. Collagen
B. Osteocytes
C. Hydroxyapatite
D. Cartilage

16. The hormone that mobilizes Ca $+^{2}$, from bone is:

A. thyroxine.
B. parathyroid hormone.
C. calcitonin.
D. Vitamin D

7.18.3 Answers to Questions in Section 7.18.2

(1) C (2) A (3) A (4) B (5) A (6) C (7) C (8) C (9) C (10) B (11) A (12) C (13) C (14) C (15) A (16) B

7.18.4 Discussion of Answers to Questions in Section 7.18.2: None

7.18.5 Advanced Concepts

- Understand the mechanisms behind athletic injuries, e.g., pulled hamstring, runner's knee, shinsplint syndrome and Achilles tendonitis
- Understand the organic structure of polyactic acid (plastic) used for artificial ligaments
- Differentiate between gomphosis, symphysis, synchondrosis and syndesmosis in joints
- Understand the nature of the following skeletal disorders and medical procedures: bone scintigraphy, hypertrophic osteoarthropathy, osteoporosis, spondylitis, collagen's disease, bone fracture types (e.g., closed, open, greenstick, etc.), rheumatoid arthritis, Paget's disease, and piezoelectric effect in bone due to mechanical/physical stress.

7.19 RESPIRATORY AND SKIN SYSTEMS

7.19.1 Introduction to Respiratory and Skin Systems

The respiratory and skin systems are both subjected to external environmental factors. Pollution and ozone layer depletion lead to various breathing and skin problems. The health sections of newspapers and magazines are good sources for new techniques and problems as they are discovered. Students should review racing, running and other exercises which affect ventilation of lungs and sweating. The mechanisms controlling inspiration, expiration and protective actions of the skin are closely linked to the MCAT. Memorize the basic volumes and capacities shown in spirograms (remember that total lung capacity is around 5000 mL and anatomical dead space is approximately 100 mL). Review the design construction and working of a spirometer and a bronchoscope.

7.19.1.1 FUNCTION OF RESPIRATORY SYSTEM

In humans, air enters through the *mouth or nose* where it is cleaned, warmed and moistened. It then passes down the *trachea* to two main *bronchi* and then to *bronchioles* then to *alveoli* (Fig. 7.75). Gas exchange occurs in the alveoli. Incomplete cartilage rings hold the trachea, bronchi, and bronchioles open. *Mucus* (secreted by mucous cells) traps ingested particles which are then moved out of the respiratory tract by *ciliary action* (ciliated epithelial cells) of the lining cells (respiratory epithelium). This epithelium is classified as *pseudostratified ciliated columnar epithelium* and has basic features of all epithelia (i.e., avascular, with basal lamina and junctional complexes to maintain the sheet of cells). Connective tissue beneath the basal lamina supplies the cells through its microvascular supply (see Fig. 7.76). *Coughing* is a reflex action mediated by the medulla (glossopharyngeal and vagus nerve). The reflex is initiated by a stimulation (e.g., by particles) of the tracheobronchial tree, followed by expulsion of these particles and mucus as sputum (or phlegm). *Sneezing* is a reflex mediated by the medulla also, but the initial stimulation is in the nose followed by forceful expulsion of the irritating substance and naso-oral secretions.

Effects of Smoking

Tobacco smoke consists of gases such as carbon dioxide and tiny unburned carbon particles. These substances harm the *cilia* and *mucous membranes* that line the breathing passages. Many smokers cough frequently. The cough is the body's effort to clear the breathing passages. Healthy cilia and mucous membranes accomplish the cleaning process automatically. Smoke also damages the lungs. Long-term smoking can cause the walls of the alveoli to rupture, or break. As a result, the surface area for *gas exchange* decreases considerably. This condition, called *emphysema* interferes with oxygen intake.

7.19.1.2 BREATHING STRUCTURES AND MECHANISMS

The act of *inspiration* is accomplished by the contraction of the diaphragm (via impulses from the *phrenic nerve*) which moves downward and/or by certain rib muscles lifting the rib cage up. These mechanisms create a negative pressure inside the chest cavity which causes the lungs to expand and pull in air. *Expiration* is a passive process due to the elastic recoil of the chest wall and lung tissue itself. Respiration is largely *involuntary*, but some voluntary control is possible over the rate and depth of respiration. The *control center* of respiration is in the medulla of the brainstem. It causes an increase in the rate of respiration when there is a fall in pH (e.g., more acidic), an increase in CO_2 tension (which causes a drop in pH), or a decrease in oxygen tension in the blood. Also impulses from the cerebrum can affect ventilatory rate, as in anxiety, causing the rate to increase.

A key substance for the function of lungs is *surfactant* (dipalmitoyllecithin—a phospholipid). This substance coats the alveoli and creates a variable surface tension in them. As the alveoli get smaller, the surface tension decreases due to surfactant. This prevents the alveoli from collapsing during expiration, because high surface tension would cause alveoli to collapse. In the absence of surfactant, collapsed alveoli require fairly high inspiratory forces to re-expand them. This is what happens in *RDS* (Respiratory Distress Syndrom) of the newborn in whom there is an absence of surfactant. The infant is not strong enough to re-expand the collapsed alveoli.

In summary, the respiratory system functions mechanically to move air in and out of the lungs (highest O_2 and lowest CO_2 tension) and to allow diffusion of gases in and out of the body. *Oxygen* moves into the blood (lower O_2 tension and highest CO_2 tension) where it is taken up and utilized. In the tissues, *carbon dioxide* (CO_2) is produced by oxidation of nutrients. The CO_2 then diffuses into the blood where it dissolves in the serum, is converted to carbonic acid ($CO_2 + H_2O \rightarrow H_2CO_3$) and then to bicarbonate (HCO_3^-), or combines with hemoglobin. Next it circulates to the lungs where the above reactions are reversed and the CO_2 is expired. Note that in all cases the gases go from higher tensions (pressures) to lower. By regulating the amount of carbonic acid and bicarbonate in the serum, the lungs are important in the regulation of acid-base balance in the body.

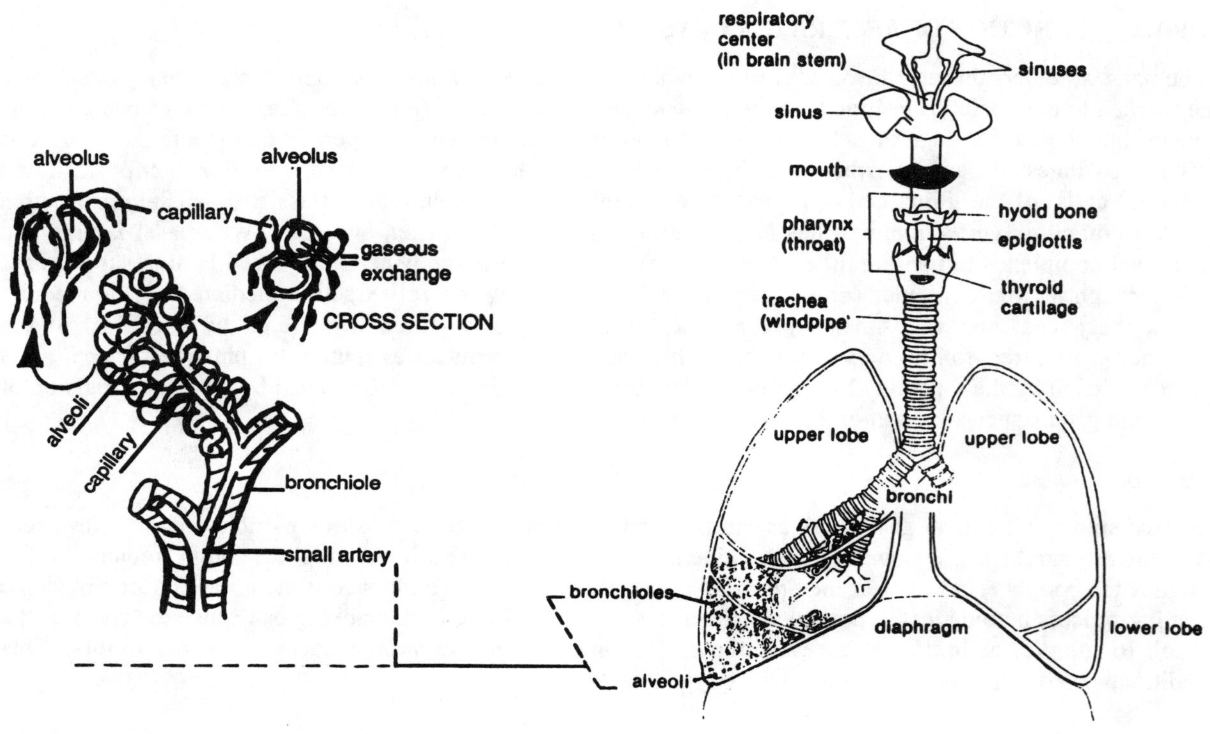

Fig. 7.75—Respiratory System; Bronchiole and Alveoli

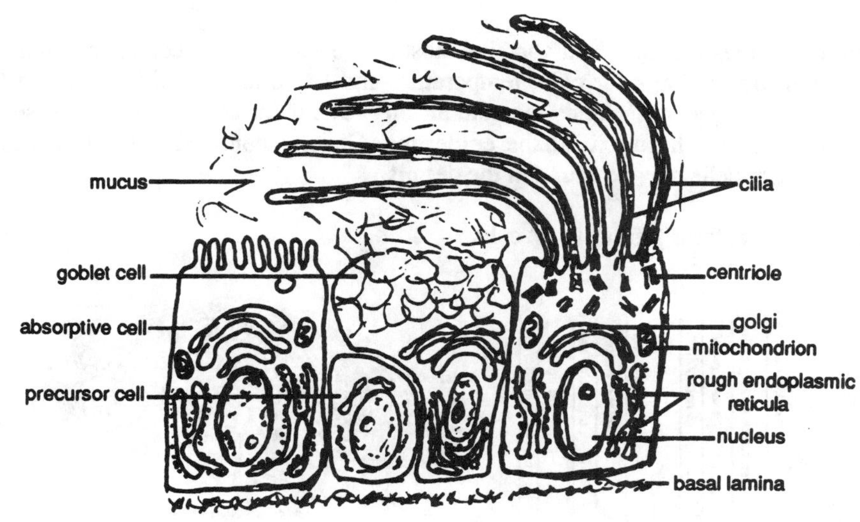

Fig. 7.76—Respiratory Epithelium (specialized eukaryotic cells)

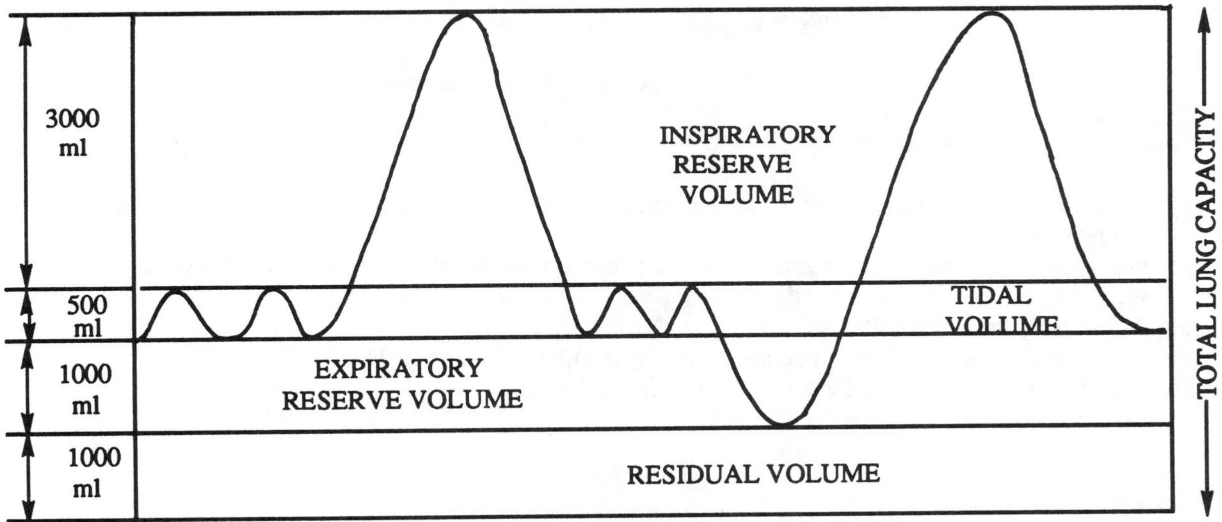

Fig. 7.77—Typical Spirogram

7.19.1.3 STRUCTURE AND FUNCTION OF SKIN SYSTEM

The skin is made of specialized eukaryotic cells and tissues. Layers of skin are epidermis, dermis, and subcutaneous tissue. The *epidermis* (stratified squamous epithelium and lamina propria) (Fig. 7.78) is a layer comprised of several types of related cells and melanocytes. The deepest layer of the epidermis, the basal layer, contains cells which are dividing. The broad middle layer of cells is termed the spinous layer and are joined together at multiple foci by the junctional complex, the desmosome. As these cells move toward the surface, they lose their nuclei and produce a protein called *keratin* (which is stable and water insoluble). At the surface, these cells have no nuclei, are dead, are essentially keratin and are called *stratum corneum* which is the scaly dry surface layer of the skin. *Melanocytes*, dendritic cells found among the basal cell layer, synthesize *melanin* (a black to dark-brown pigment) which is responsible for the color of the skin. It also responds to ultraviolet light to produce tanning of the skin. As in all epithelia, a basal lamina attaches the epithelium to all underlying connective tissue.

The *dermis* is internal to the epidermis and contains most of the accessory structures of the skin. Blood vessels end in the dermis. Sensory endings for pain, temperature and touch are found here and in the subcutaneous tissue. Hair follicles and sebaceous glands (secrete an oily fat substance; if clogged cause acne), and sweat glands originate here. All of these exit at the epidermis. General connective tissue cells, fibroblasts, and macrophages among other cells may be found in the dermis.

The *subcutaneous tissue* contains primarily fat cells.

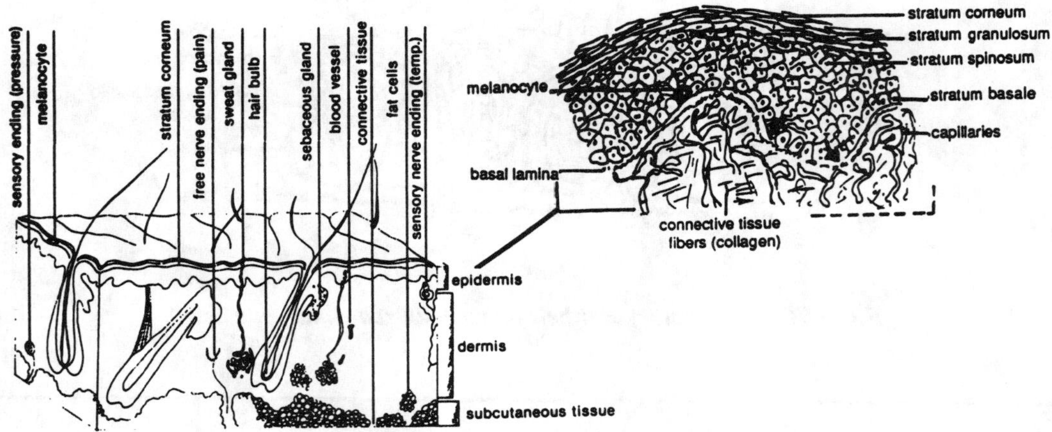

Fig. 7.78—Human Skin and Epidermis

Functions of skin system include:

(1) protection from physical agents (wind, water, etc.)—afforded by the stratum corneum and melanocytes (radiation),
(2) protection from microbial agents especially bacteria—afforded by the stratum corneum and some secretions of the sebaceous glands,
(3) thermoregulation (see 7.19.1.4),
(4) waste removal (e.g., excess water, salts, urea, others)—via the sweat glands,
(5) site of the first activation of vitamin D—by ultraviolet light,
(6) sensation—by the many nerve endings.

7.19.1.4 THERMOREGULATION (Skin System)

Thermoregulation is the regulation of the internal body temperature between the narrow limits necessary for life. Too high or low a temperature can cause proteins (enzymes especially) to become less effective or totally inactive (denatured) and cause the protoplasm to gel (become more solid).

Normally, the body temperature is a balance between heat produced by metabolism and heat loss by the various means described below. Processes that increase body metabolism increase body heat, this is especially true of muscle activity (e.g., shivering). Regulation of body temperature is centered in the *hypothalamus* (in the brain).

Pyrogens released during bacterial infections, among other causes, can affect the hypothalamus in a way that it allows the body temperature to rise higher than normal, and fever results.

The mechanisms of heat conservation include those that are always present and those called upon in emergencies: (* = most important)

(A) Mechanisms always present:
* (1) subcutaneous fat as insulation;
(2) presence of hair or fur (lower animals).

(B) Mechanisms called upon as needed:
* (1) shivering—contractions of muscles produce heat;
* (2) constriction of vessels to skin—prevents heat loss from surface;
(3) piloerection of hair on skin—traps air against skin that once warmed serves as an insulation;
(4) increase in metabolic rate.

The mechanisms of heat loss include those that are always present and those called upon in emergencies:

(A) Mechanisms always present:
(1) loss of heat by radiational cooling;
(2) low level of evaporation of moisture from skin—for a liquid to evaporate, heat must be supplied; this heat comes from the skin which is cooled.

(B) Mechanisms called upon as needed:
* (1) sweating and consequent evaporation of water—the sweat itself removes heat from the body and more is lost when this evaporates;
* (2) dilation of vessels to the skin—increases the amount of radiational cooling.

7.19.2 Questions Related to Respiratory and Skin Systems

1. The path of air into the lungs of humans is:

A. alveoli, trachea, bronchi, bronchioles
B. trachea, bronchi, bronchioles, alveoli
C. bronchi, bronchioles, trachea, alveoli
D. trachea, bronchioles, bronchi, alveoli

2. Expiration of air from the lungs:

A. is a passive process.
B. causes negative pressure in the chest cavity.
C. requires contraction of the diaphragm.
D. is an active process.

3. During inspiration of air into the lungs:

A. the chest cavity has a positive pressure.
B. the diaphragm moves upward.
C. the diaphragm contracts.
D. the rib cage moves down.

4. What structure(s) is(are) used to prevent the bronchi from collapsing?

A. cartilage rings
B. bony rings
C. fibrous tissue
D. none of the above

5. Surfactant:

A. is depalmitoyllecithin.
B. decreases surface tension.
C. deficiency may result in respiratory distress syndrome.
D. is characterized by all of the above statements.

6. Which reflex moves secretions out of the tracheobronchial tree?

A. cough
B. sneeze
C. baroceptor
D. pH

7. The control center of respiration is in the:

A. cerebrum.
B. cerebellum.
C. medulla.
D. thalamus.

8. All of the following may cause an increase in respiratory rate except:

A. increased hydrogen ion concentration.
B. increased carbon dioxide tension.
C. increased oxygen tension.
D. anxiety.

9. Carbon dioxide may be present in all of the following forms except:

A. dissolved in the blood.
B. bound to hemoglobin.
C. as dimers.
D. as bicarbonate.

10. The type of epithelium found lining the trachea is:

A. pseudostratified ciliated columnar.
B. stratified squamous.
C. simple cuboidal.
D. simple squamous.

11. Layers of the skin include all except:

A. epidermis.
B. dermis.
C. lamina propria.
D. subcutaneous tissue.

12. Dead cells are found in the:

A. subcutaneous tissue.
B. dermis.
C. epidermis.
D. carbuncle.

13. Melanocytes are found in the:

A. dermis.
B. epidermis.
C. subcutaneous tissue.
D. endoderm.

14. The dermis usually contains all of the following except:

A. hair follicles.
B. sweat glands.
C. fat cells.
D. fibroblasts.

15. All are functions of the skin except:

    A. exchange of gases.
    B. thermoregulation.
    C. activation site of Vitamin D.
    D. protection from bacteria.

16. The main effect of extremes of temperature is on the functions of:

    A. carbohydrates.
    B. phospholipids.
    C. proteins.
    D. nucleic acids.

17. Control of body temperature is localized in the:

    A. skin.
    B. heart.
    B. cerebrum.
    D. hypothalamus.

18. Select the mechanism that is *not* used to conserve heat:

    A. shivering
    B. dilation of blood vessels
    C. piloerection
    D. subcutaneous fat

19. Select the mechanism that is *not* used to lose heat:

    A. sweating
    B. increase in metabolic rate
    C. radiational cooling
    D. dilation of blood vessels

7.19.3 Answers to Questions in Section 7.19.2

(1) B (2) A (3) C (4) A (5) D (6) A (7) C (8) C (9) C (10) A (11) C (12) C
(13) B (14) C (15) A (16) C (17) D (18) B (19) B

7.19.4 Discussion of Answers to Questions in Section 7.19.2: None

7.19.5 Advanced Concepts

- Understand the biochemical structure and growth rate of fibrin; burns (first, second and third degree); acne, sunburns, and skin cancer
- Identify the biology of healing (where the edges of cut skin wounds are drawn together) and basic skin grafting techniques
- Distinguish terminology which sounds alike and is related to the same medical term: pleura (visceral and parietal), pleural cavity, pleural fluid (composition, density, pH), intrapleural pressure and pleurisy
- Understand mechanisms responsible for volume changes in thoracic cavity. Identify changes in physical and chemical properties of gases (O_2, CO_2) in liquids (volumes, partial pressures, temperature and arterial pH related to binding with hemoglobin). Review the transport and diffusion processes of gas molecules in liquids
- Understand basic cardiopulmonary resuscitation (CPR) techniques with emphasis on A, B, C (airway, breathing, and circulation)

- Recognize Bohr effect on hemoglobin structure, Haldane effect and diphosphoglycerate concentration in hemoglobin
- Recognize respiratory disorders such as: hypoxia, CO poisoning, cyanosis, bronchial asthma, bronchitis, tuberculosis, pneumonia, emphysema, common cold, hyperventilation, hypercapnia, hypoventilation and hypocapnia

ORGANIC CHEMISTRY

7.20 HYDROCARBONS

7.20.1 Introduction to Hydrocarbons

The various types of reactions and stereodifferences between alkanes, alkenes and alkynes constitute the bulk of this section. Differentiate angle strain, ring strain and torsional stain with examples. Learn various types of hydrogen binding mechanisms to carbon atoms, e.g., acetylenic, vinylic (allylic or benzylic) and aliphatic classifications of hydrogen atoms. Review inhibition mechanisms of alkanes and dehydrohalogenation reactions of haloalkanes.

7.20.1.1 ALKANES (Saturated Hydrocarbons)

I. Nomenclature:

The basic ideas of *nomenclature* for alkanes will hold for more complex molecules also. Alkanes are simple because they contain only carbon and hydrogen (also called hydrocarbons) and contain no aromatic rings. The longest straight carbon chain is determined and is named depending upon the number of carbons:

C_1-meth-, C_2-eth-, C_3-prop-, C_4-but(a), C_5-pent(a), C_6-hex(a), C_7-hept(a), C_8-oct(a), C_9-non(a), C_{10}-dec(a).

If these carbons contain only C and H the suffix -yl is added:

$$CH_3- = \text{methyl},\ CH_3CH_2- = \text{ethyl},\ CH_3CH_2CH_2- = \text{propyl, etc.}$$

There are special names for some branched chain alkanes:

$(CH_3)_2CH-$ = iso-group

$(CH_3)_2CH-$ = isopropyl

$(CH_3)_2CH-CH_2-$ = isobutyl

$CH_3-CH(CH_2CH_3)-$ = sec-butyl

$(CH_3)_3C-$ = tert-butyl

Once the longest chain is determined, the groups attached to it are numbered such that the lowest set of numbers is obtained. The side groups are placed in the molecule name in alphabetical order or in order of increasing size. The prefixes di-(two), tri-(three), tetra-(four), etc., are used when a particular group is present more than once. The suffix indicating alkanes is *-ane*. For example:

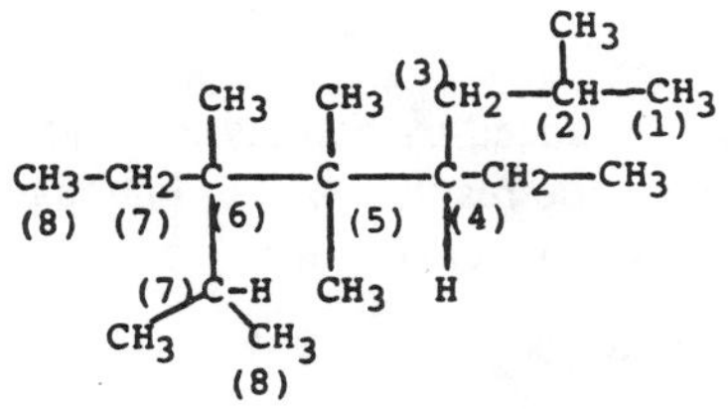

```
                              CH3
          CH3  CH3  (3)CH2—CH—CH3
                           (2) (1)
CH3-CH2-C————C————C-CH2—CH3
(8) (7)  (6)  (5)  (4)
      (7)C-H  CH3   H
      CH3  CH3
           (8)
```

2,5,5,6-Tetra methyl-4-ethyl-6-isopropyl octane or 2,5,5,6,7-Pentamethyl-4, 6-diethyl octane.

Alkanes (if no rings, C_nH_{2n+2}; and lose 2 hydrogens for each ring) may be open chains or rings. The rings are named for the number of carbons that make them up:

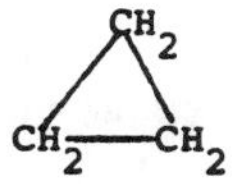

cyclo-propane

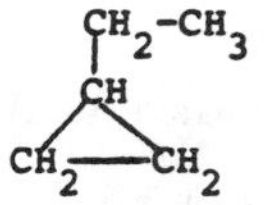

ethylcyclopropane

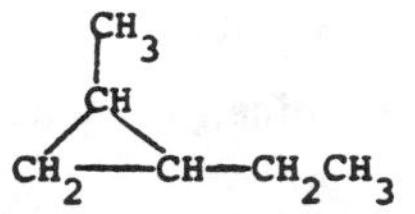

cis-1-Methyl-2-ethyl cyclopropane

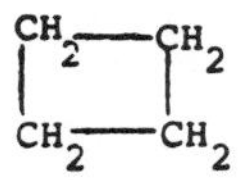

cyclobutane

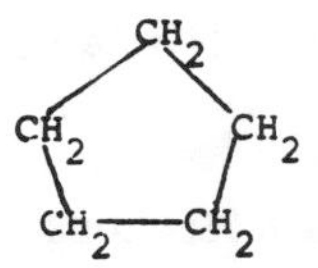

cyclopentane

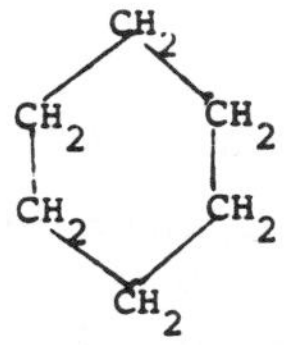

cyclohexane

The main *chemical features* are the lack of functional groupings (e.g., – OH, Br) and full saturation (no double or triple bonds). These factors cause them to be chemically unreactive except when induced by heat or light.

II. Physical Properties:

Physical properties of alkanes are fairly straightforward. Because they are nonpolar and have weak intermolecular forces, they have low boiling points and are not soluble in water. Branching makes the molecules more symmetrical and this lowers the boiling points even more, which is true for other classes of compounds as well. With increasing molecular weights, the intermolecular forces increase and the boiling point increases; this is also observed in other classes of molecules. Melting points increase as molecular weights increase. Solubility is in nonpolar solvents and not in aqueous solvents. Cycloproprane is an anesthetic used in surgical procedures. Because of its low solubility in blood, and since it is rapidly eliminated from the body, patients recover quickly.

III. Important Reactions:

The main reactions of alkanes are combustion and substitution (radical) reactions:

(1) Combustion

$$C_n + H_{2n+2} + O_2\ (\text{excess}) \xrightarrow{\text{flame}} nCO_2 + (n+1)H_2O$$

(2) Free radical substitution.

$$CH_3CH_3 + X_2 \xrightarrow{h\nu \text{ or } \Delta} CH_3CH_2X + HX$$

$$X_2 = Cl_2 \text{ or } Br_2$$

also get multiple substitutions.

$$CH_4 + Cl_2 \rightarrow CH_3Cl \rightarrow CH_2Cl_2 \rightarrow CHCl_3 \rightarrow CCl_4$$

The mechanism is:

(a) initiation-radicals are produced by homolytic bond cleavage of the halogen by the action of heat or light. Fluorine is too reactive and iodine is too unreactive to be of practical value in the laboratory without special conditions.

$$X_2 \rightarrow 2X\bullet$$

(b) propagation-generation of radicals by radicals.

$X\bullet + CH_3CH_3 \rightarrow HX + CH_3CH_2\bullet$

$CH_3CH_2\bullet + X_2 \rightarrow CH_3CH_2X + X\bullet$

The process above constitutes a chain reaction which results when one intermediate reacts with a molecule to produce a new radical which can react further, allowing the process to repeat itself.

(c) termination. Reaction of a radical with a radical to produce a stable molecule.

$$X\bullet + X\bullet \rightarrow X_2$$

$$CH_3CH_2\bullet + X\bullet \rightarrow CH_3CH_2X$$

$$2\ CH_3CH_2\bullet \rightarrow CH_3CH_2CH_2CH_3$$

IV. Chain-Reaction Mechanism

Free radical induced polymerizations are chain reactions. A source of radicals initiates the process in which one radical adds to the double bond of a molecule producing a new radical which can add again and therefore long chain polymeric molecules result.

$$R\bullet + >C{=}C{-}G \longrightarrow R{-}C{-}\dot{C}{-}G \xrightarrow[\text{etc.}]{CH_2{=}CHG} \left(C{-}\underset{G}{C}\right)_n$$

Radicals result from homolytic cleavage of chemical bonds:

$$X\text{-}Y \rightarrow X\bullet + Y\bullet$$

Note that each species is neutral (if begun neutral), and that each has a free unpaired electron. Because of the free unpaired electron, radicals are paramagnetic. Most radicals are very unstable and react rapidly.

V. Stability of Free Radicals:

The stability of free radicals depends on the presence of substituents which can localize the free electron. Alkyl groups act to stabilize a radical. Benzene rings and allylic double bonds which readily delocalize electrons are very effective.

$$C_6H_5\dot{C}H_2 > CH_2{=}CH{-}\dot{C}H_2 > (CH_3)_3\dot{C} > (CH_3)_2\dot{C}H > CH_3\dot{C}H_2 > CH_2{=}\dot{C}H$$

benzylic R• > allylic R• > 3° R• > 2° R• > 1° R• > vinylic R•

VI. Ring Strain in Cyclic Hydrocarbons:

The smaller the number of carbons in a ring, the less stable the ring is. This is due to ring strain of the bonding orbitals. The usual angle between bonds is 109.5° in the sp^3 hybridized carbon. The expected bond angles in the following ring compounds are:

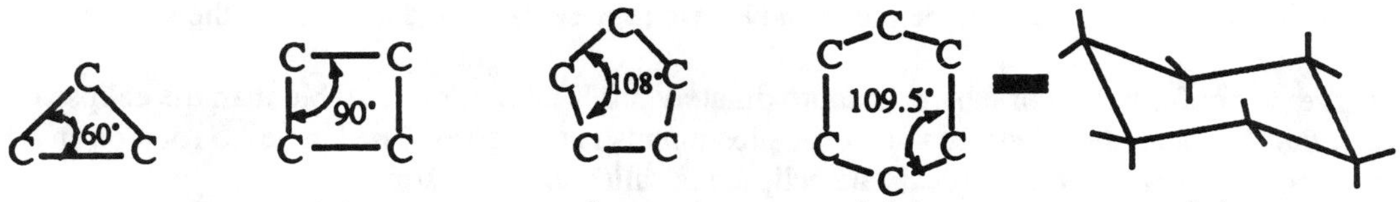

60° 90° 108° 109.5°

cyclopropane cyclobutane cyclopentane cyclohexane normal angles chair

The ring strain is very high in cyclopropane. This makes cyclopropane as reactive with H_2,Br_2 as alkenes are. Cyclobutane relieves some of the ring strain by assuming a bent conformation,

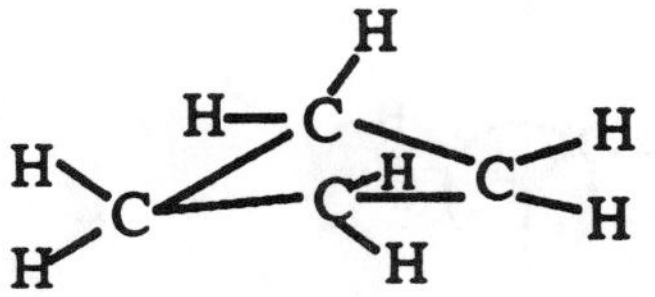

Cyclopentane is puckered to relieve the strain,

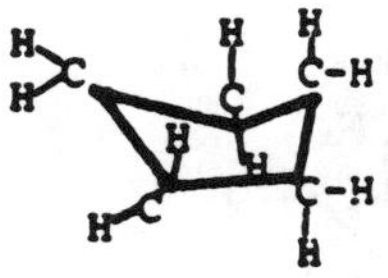

Cyclohexane has no strain in the chair form as shown above and explained below. Cyclobutane is fairly reactive, but cyclopentane or cyclohexane are not.

VII. Planar and Non-Planar Conformations:

Molecules may exist in different spacial arrangements called conformations which result from rotation about a carbon - carbon single bond. The various conformations of molecules may be represented by projection drawings known as Newman projections or wedge and dash drawings. In a Newman projection, one sights down a carbon to carbon bond and a point represents the front carbon and an open circle represents the back carbon. In the wedge and dash projection, a wedge indicates a bond coming from the plane towards the viewer. A normal line represents a bond in the plane and a dash represents a bond away from the viewer.

The staggered conformation of ethane is approximately 3.0 Kcal/mol more stable than the eclipse conformation in which the torsional angle between adjacent substituents is 0 degrees. The barrier to rotation in ethane due to electron pair repulsions when the bonds are eclipsed is called torsional strain.

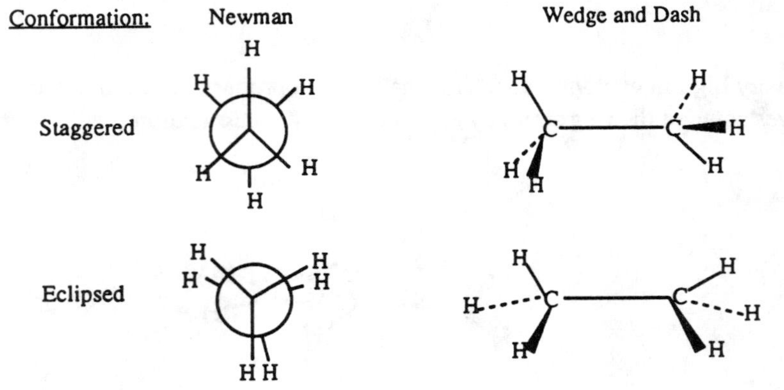

Conformation: Newman Wedge and Dash

Staggered

Eclipsed

Rotation about the C_2-C_3 bond in butane produces a number of conformations varying in energy. Rotation about a carbon to carbon bond is not completely free but the energy barrier is low and internal rotation at room temperature is very rapid. Various conformations of butane are shown below.

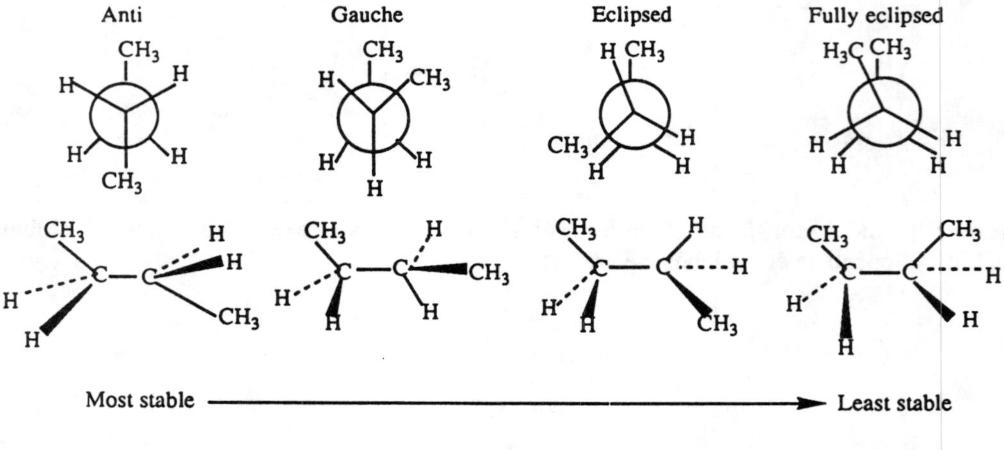

Anti Gauche Eclipsed Fully eclipsed

Most stable ⟶ Least stable

The anti and gauche forms of butane are free of torsional strain. In the gauche form, the methyl groups are closer together than the sums of their van der Waals radii resulting in van der Waals strain or steric strain due to repulsion between the methyl groups. Van der Waals strain and torsional strain are at a maximum when the methyl groups are eclipsed.

Two non-planar conformations of cyclohexane are known as the chair and boat forms. Both forms are free of bond angle strain and the chair form also is free of torsional strain. The boat form has significant torsional strain since four of its carbon atoms are eclipsed. The boat form is destabilized because of the van der Waals repulsion between the hydrogens at position 1 and 4 of the ring.

Six of the carbon to hydrogen bonds of the chair form lie perpendicular to the plane of the ring and are called axial bonds. The remaining six hydrogens are located around the circumference (equator) of the ring and are designated equatorial.

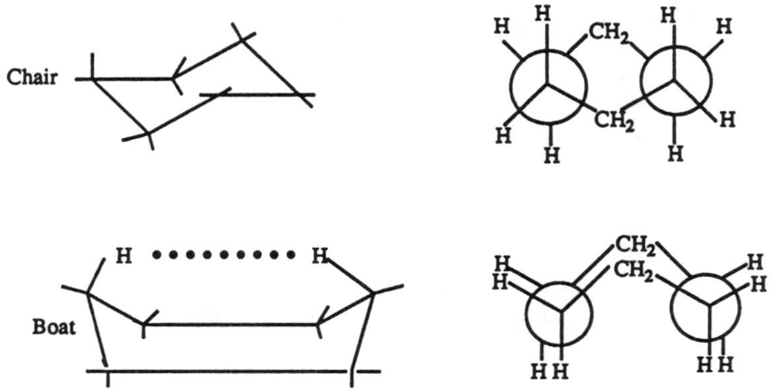

Chair

Boat

A cyclohexane ring may have substituents in the axial or equatorial positions. Cyclohexane rings are conformationally mobile and undergo ring inversion or "ring flipping." A cyclohexane ring having an axial substituent may undergo inversion to a new chair conformation in which the substituent is equatorial by passing through the boat conformation. The chair formation with the substituent group in the equatorial position generally is the more stable. The larger the substituent the greater the tendency for the group to be equatorial. Therefore methylyclohexane exists almost entirely in the chair conformation with the methyl group equatorial.

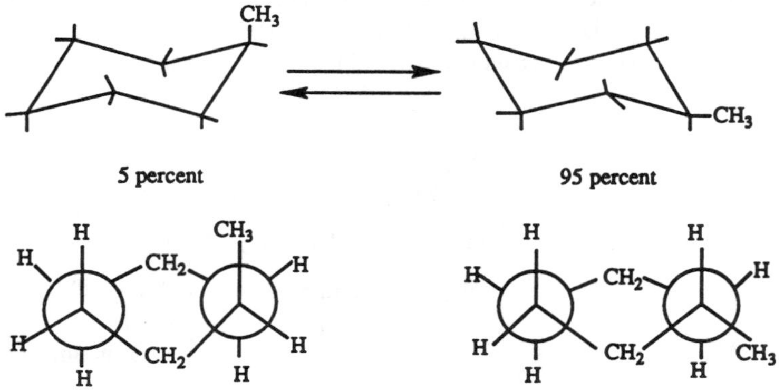

5 percent

95 percent

7.20.1.2 ALKENES, DIENES, ALKYNES (Unsaturated Hydrocarbons)

I. Nomenclature of Alkenes:

See Section 7.1 for cis-trans isomerism. See Section 7.20.1.1 for basic points on nomenclature. See Section 7.1 for composition of the double bond.

Alkenes (if no ring, C_nH_{2n}) are hydrocarbons having a double bond as the functional group. For each double bond, the molecule loses two hydrogens from the alkane formula (C_nH_{2n+2}). The IUPAC name of alkenes is obtained by replacing the -ane ending of the corresponding alkane name with -ene. The longest carbon chain contained in the double bond is used to name the alkene and the first carbon of the double bond is numbered as the lowest possible locant. Substituents are named as usual. The numbering of the double bond takes precedence over alkyl groups and halogens but not the hydroxyl group. Some of the simpler alkenes are frequently known by common names ending in -ylene which are not acceptable IUPAC names. For example:

$CH_2{=}CH_2$ ethene (ethylene)

$CH_3CH{=}CH_2$ propene (propylene)

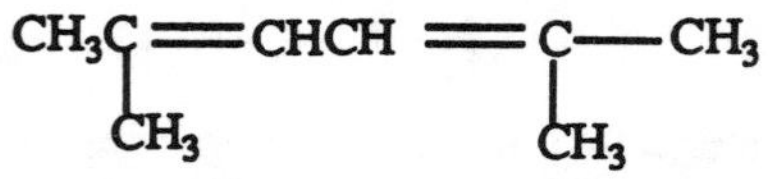

$CH_3C(CH_3){=}CHCH{=}C(CH_3){-}CH_3$ 2,5-dimethyl-2,4-hexadiene

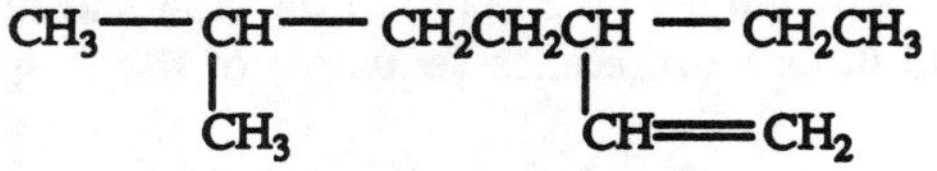

$CH_3{-}CH(CH_3){-}CH_2CH_2CH(CH{=}CH_2){-}CH_2CH_3$ 3 - ethyl - 6 - methyl - 1 - heptene

$CH_3CH_2CH{=}CHCH_2CH_2CH_2CH_2CH_2OH$ 6 - nonen - 1 - ol

Cycloalkenes are named in a manner similar to alkenes with the carbons of the double bond being carbon-1 and carbon-2:

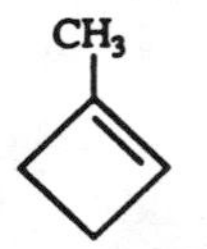

1-methylcyclobutene

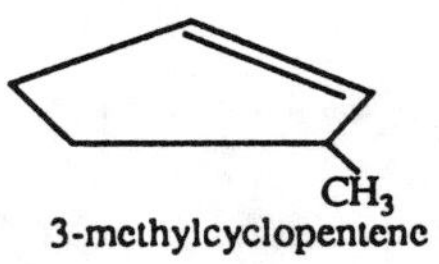

3-methylcyclopentene

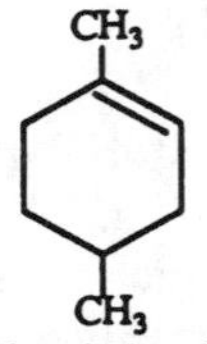

1,4-dimethylcyclohexene

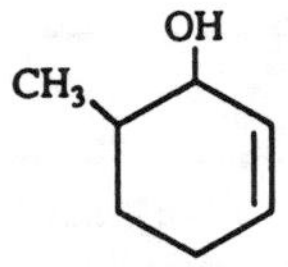

6–methyl–2–cyclohexen–1–ol

Because of the lack of rotation about the carbon double bond alkenes may exist as stereoisomers known as geometrical isomers. When an alkene has two like groups or atoms on a single carbon of a double bond this type of isomerism is not possible. Those isomers with like groups on the same side of the double bond are designated cis isomers whereas those with the groups on opposite sides of the double bond are designated trans as shown below:

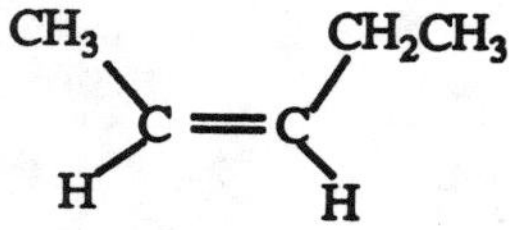

cis - 2 - pentene

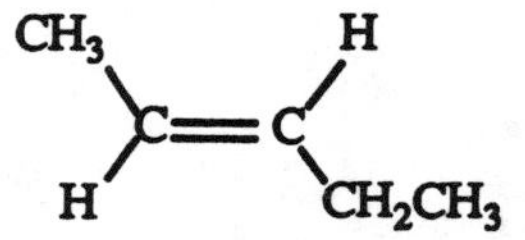

trans - 2 - pentene

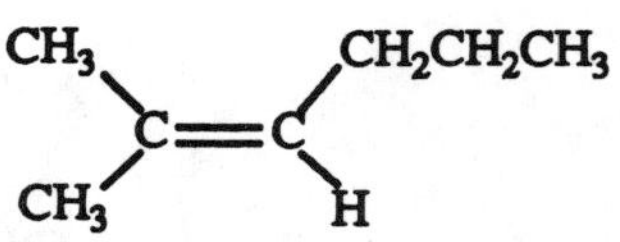

2 - methyl - 2 hexene

no geometric isomers

A hydrocarbon having two double bonds is called a diene, one with three double bonds is called a triene, and so forth.

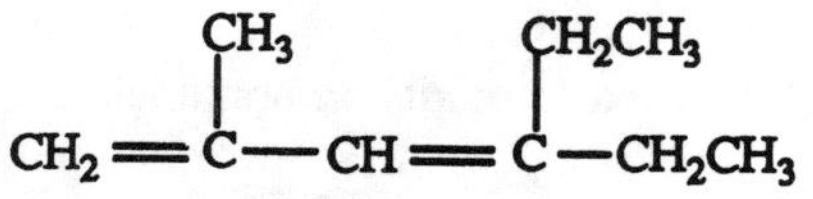

$CH_2{=}C(CH_3){-}CH{=}C(CH_2CH_3){-}CH_2CH_3$ 4 - ethyl - 2 - methyl - 1, 3 - hexadiene

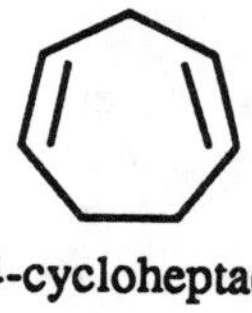

1,4-cycloheptadiene

II. Physical Properties:

The physical but not chemical properties of the alkenes are much like those of the alkanes (Section 7.20.1.1) in that those with corresponding carbon skeletons have similar boiling points. The boiling point of a homologous series of alkenes increases about 20-30°C for each methylene group ($-CH_2-$) and chain branching slightly lowers the boiling point. Alkenes are very weakly polar and are insoluble in water but soluble in nonpolar solvents such as hexane, cyclohexane, ethyl ether, dichloromethane, benzene, etc. One difference is that alkenes may be polar due to cis-trans isomers and to the nature of the double bond itself (an election withdrawer):

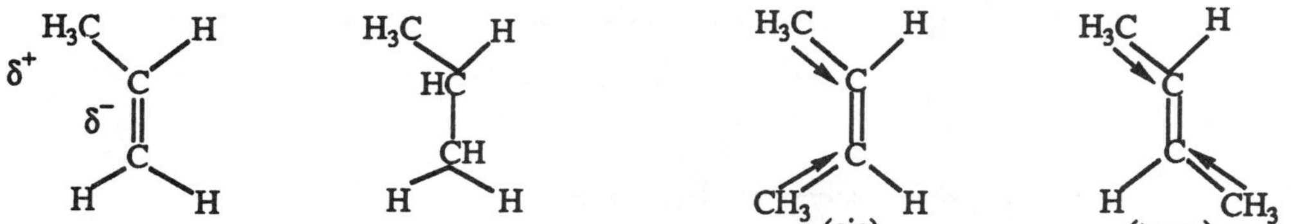

has a small dipole moment

has no dipole moment

(cis) small dipole moment

(trans) no dipole moment

Also trans compounds tend to have higher melting points (due to better symmetry) but lower boiling points (due to less polarity) than the corresponding cis compounds (see Section 5.3.1 and 5.9).

III. Chemical Properties:

Nearly all the chemistry of alkenes involve addition reactions to the double bond. The pi (π) electrons of the double bond are available for reaction with reagents capable of reacting with a pair of electrons. Protons and carbocations (carbenium ions) are Lewis acids which are electron acceptors. Carbon anions are called carbanions. Carbocations are electron-seeking reagents. They are also called electrophilic reagents or electrophiles. Alkenes, which are electron donating, are Lewis bases and are nucleophilic reagents or nucleophiles. The most important reaction of alkenes is electrophilic addition to the double bond. A general reaction is as follows:

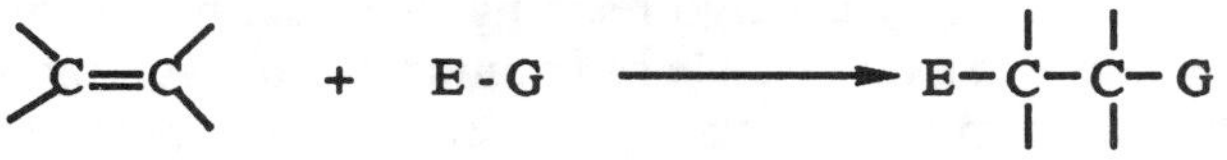

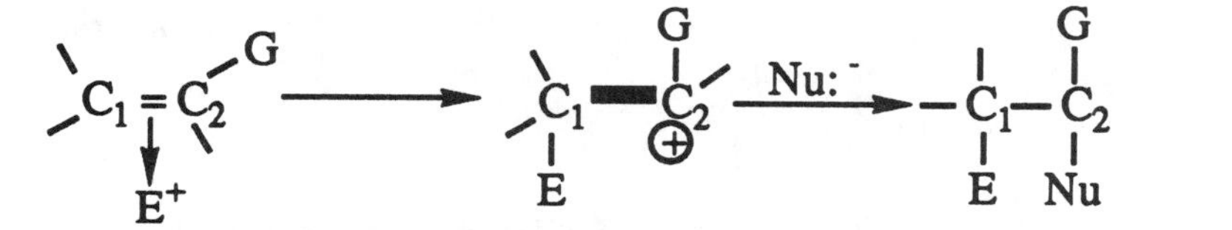

$$>C=C< \; + \; E\text{-}G \longrightarrow E-\overset{|}{\underset{|}{C}}-\overset{|}{\underset{|}{C}}-G$$

E = electrophile

Carbenium ion

Nu = nucleophile

Examples of addition reactions:

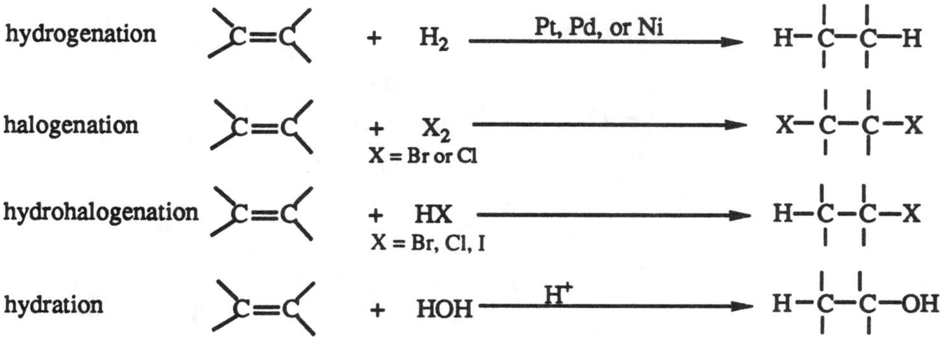

hydrogenation $>C=C< \; + \; H_2 \xrightarrow{\text{Pt, Pd, or Ni}} H-\overset{|}{\underset{|}{C}}-\overset{|}{\underset{|}{C}}-H$

halogenation $>C=C< \; + \; X_2 \longrightarrow X-\overset{|}{\underset{|}{C}}-\overset{|}{\underset{|}{C}}-X$
X = Br or Cl

hydrohalogenation $>C=C< \; + \; HX \longrightarrow H-\overset{|}{\underset{|}{C}}-\overset{|}{\underset{|}{C}}-X$
X = Br, Cl, I

hydration $>C=C< \; + \; HOH \xrightarrow{H^+} H-\overset{|}{\underset{|}{C}}-\overset{|}{\underset{|}{C}}-OH$

IV. Electrophilic Addition Reactions:

Halogenation, hydrohalogenation and hydration of alkenes are examples of electrophilic addition reactions. The electrophilic addition reactions of HX and HOH to unsymmetrical alkenes are regioselective and follow Markovnikov's rule. This rule states that in the addition of HX and HOH reagents to unsymmetrical alkenes, the hydrogen adds to the carbon of the double bond which has the greater number of hydrogens.

Mechanism (general)

$$R-CH=CH_2 + H-X \longrightarrow R-\overset{+}{C}H-CH_3 + X^-$$

$$R-\overset{+}{C}H-CH_3 + X^- \longrightarrow R-\underset{X}{\underset{|}{C}H}-CH_3$$

Hydration

$$H_2SO_4 + HOH \longrightarrow H_3O^+ + HSO_4^-$$

$$R-CH=CH_2 + H_3O^+ \longrightarrow R-\overset{+}{C}H-CH_3 + HOH$$

$$R-\overset{+}{C}H-CH_3 + HOH \longrightarrow R-\overset{OH_2^+}{\overset{|}{C}H}-CH_3$$

$$R-\overset{OH_2^+}{\overset{|}{C}H}-CH_3 + HOH \longrightarrow R-\overset{OH}{\overset{|}{C}H}-CH_3 + H_3O^+$$

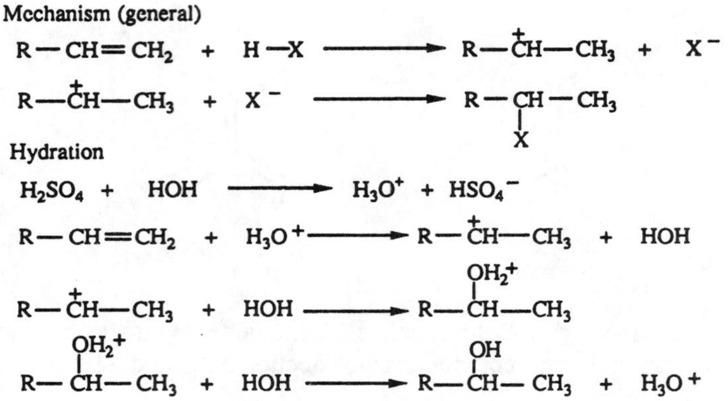

Markovnikov's rule holds because the addition of the proton to the carbon having the greater number of hydrogens yields the more stable carbocation which is formed via a lower energy transition state. In the above example a secondary carbocation (carbenium ion) is formed, whereas the alternate mode of addition would yield the less stable primary carbocation.

$$R-CH=CH_2 + H^+ \longrightarrow R-\overset{+}{C}H-CH_3 \quad \text{rather than } RCH_2CH_2^+$$

$$R_2C=CH-R + H^+ \longrightarrow R_2\overset{+}{C}-CH_2R \quad \text{rather than } R_2CH\overset{+}{C}HR$$

The carbon skeleton of an alkene may undergo rearrangement during electrophilic addition if the initially formed carbocation can rearrange to a more stable carbocation. Rearrangement may occur by methyl or hydride shift to an adjacent carbon to form a more stable carbocation. The rearranged structure is often the major product of the reaction.

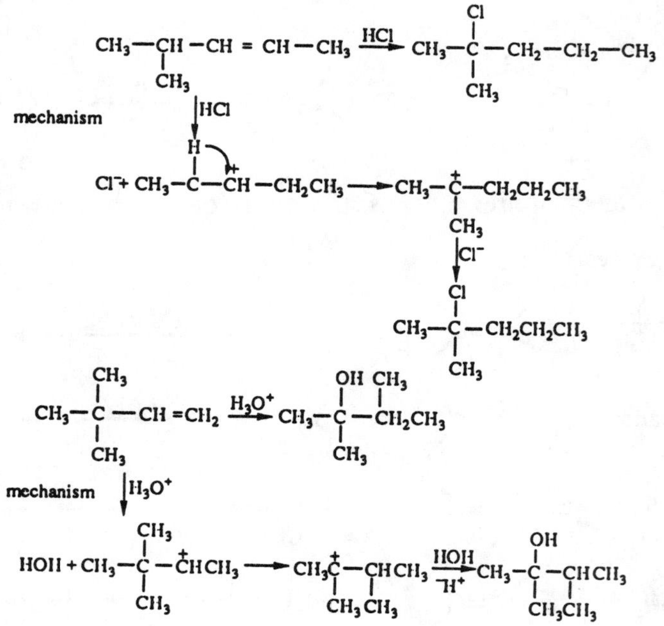

$$CH_3-\underset{CH_3}{\underset{|}{C}H}-CH=CH-CH_3 \xrightarrow{HCl} CH_3-\overset{Cl}{\overset{|}{\underset{CH_3}{\underset{|}{C}}}}-CH_2-CH_2-CH_3$$

mechanism $\downarrow$ HCl

$$Cl^- + CH_3-\overset{H}{\overset{|}{\underset{CH_3}{\underset{|}{C}}}}-\overset{+}{C}H-CH_2CH_3 \longrightarrow CH_3-\overset{+}{\underset{CH_3}{\underset{|}{C}}}-CH_2CH_2CH_3$$

$\downarrow Cl^-$

$$CH_3-\overset{Cl}{\overset{|}{\underset{CH_3}{\underset{|}{C}}}}-CH_2CH_2CH_3$$

$$CH_3-\overset{CH_3}{\overset{|}{\underset{CH_3}{\underset{|}{C}}}}-CH=CH_2 \xrightarrow{H_3O^+} CH_3-\overset{OH}{\overset{|}{\underset{CH_3}{\underset{|}{C}}}}-\overset{CH_3}{\overset{|}{C}H}CH_3$$

mechanism $\downarrow H_3O^+$

$$HOH + CH_3-\overset{CH_3}{\overset{|}{\underset{CH_3}{\underset{|}{C}}}}-\overset{+}{C}HCH_3 \longrightarrow CH_3\overset{+}{\underset{CH_3}{\underset{|}{C}}}-\underset{CH_3}{\underset{|}{C}H}CH_3 \xrightarrow[-H^+]{HOH} CH_3-\overset{OH}{\overset{|}{\underset{CH_3}{\underset{|}{C}}}}-\underset{CH_3}{\underset{|}{C}H}CH_3$$

In some additions to a double bond, both atoms or groups of the reagent add to the same side of the double bond, resulting in syn addition. When the two atoms or groups add on opposite sides, anti addition occurs.

syn addition

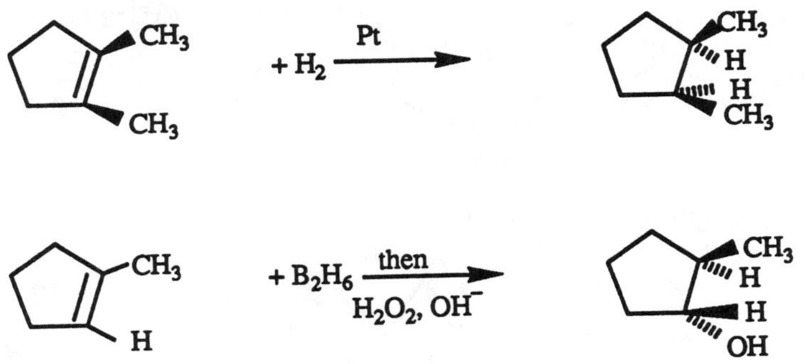

$+ H_2 \xrightarrow{Pt}$

$+ B_2H_6 \xrightarrow[H_2O_2,\ OH^-]{then}$

Anti addition

$+ Br_2 \longrightarrow$ Br^+ $\longrightarrow$

$+ Br^- Br \longrightarrow$ Br^+ $+ Br^- \longrightarrow$

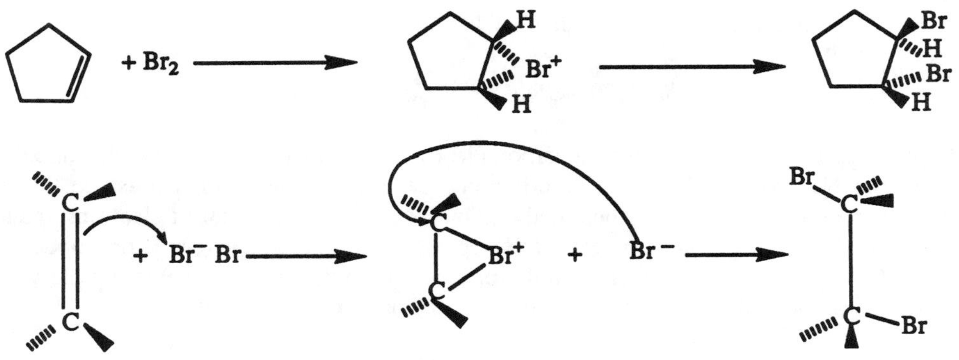

Bromonium ion

The other key feature of the double bond is its ability to stabilize carbocations, or radicals which are on adjacent carbons:

(II) carbenium ion

carbanion

radical

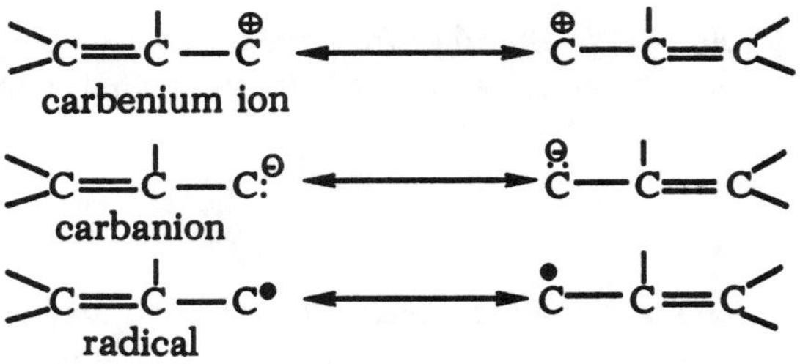

All are resonance stabilized

V. Stability of the intermediate carbocations:

Stability of the intermediate carbocations as shown in (I) (see sketch after chemical properties) above depends on the groups (G) attached which can stabilize or destabilize it. In general, groups which can share electrons by π orbital overlap (resonance) stabilize the carbenium ion (as the double bond in (II) above). In general, groups which place a positive (partial or total) charge adjacent to the carbenium ion withdraw electrons inductively (by sigma bonds) to destabilize it (see electronegativity in Section 7.21.1). (Fig. 7.79).

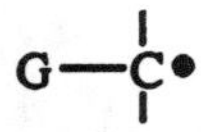

$G-\dot{C}\bullet$

G = stabilizes = O, N, benzyl, allyl, CH_3- or alkyls
benzyl ~ allyl > 3° > 2° > 1° in terms of stability

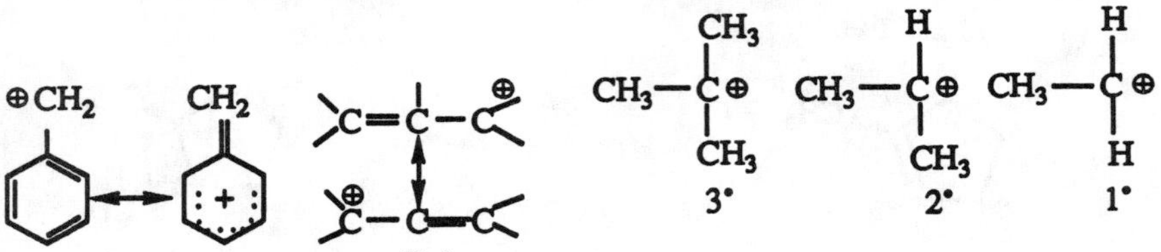

$\oplus CH_2$ — CH_2 (benzyl resonance) — allyl — $CH_3-C^{\oplus}(CH_3)_2$ (3°) — $CH_3-C^{\oplus}H(CH_3)$ (2°) — $CH_3-C^{\oplus}H_2$ (1°)

benzyl   allyl

G = destabilizes = carbonyl, alkyl halide

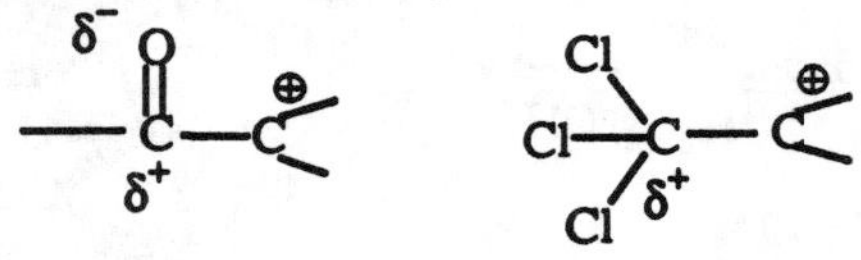

carbonyl   alkyl halide

Fig. 7.79—Stability of Carbocations

The above points are useful in predicting which carbon (1 or 2 in (I) above) will become the carbenium ion and which one the E and Nu will bond to. The intermediate carbenium ion formed must be the most stable. Markovnikov's rule is a sequel to this: the nucleophile (a molecule with a free pair of electrons and sometimes a negative charge that seeks out partially or completely positive charge species) will be bonded to the most substituted carbon (fewest hydrogens attached) in the product, or equivalently, the electrophile will be bonded to the least substituted (most hydrogens attached) carbon in the product. An example:

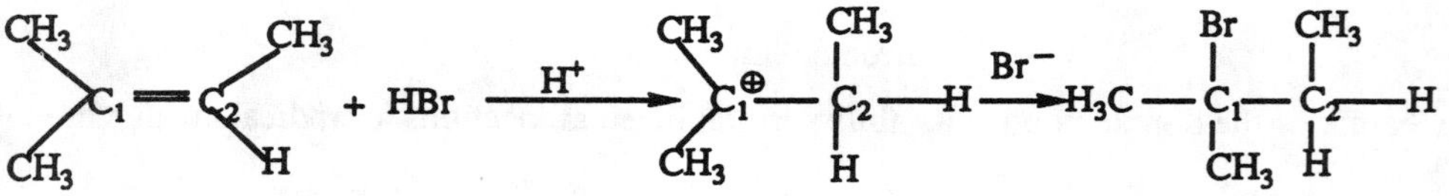

$$(CH_3)_2C_1{=}C_2(CH_3)H + HBr \xrightarrow{H^+} (CH_3)_2C_1^{\oplus}-C_2H(CH_3)-H \xrightarrow{Br^-} H_3C-C_1(Br)(CH_3)-C_2(CH_3)(H)-H$$

Ethene (ethylene) has a biological role. It is produced as fruit ripens and causes a change in the color of the skin of ripened fruit. Fruit which is picked green for shipping often is treated with ethene to give it the proper appearance.

VI. Dienes:

There are three types of dienes depending on the arrangement of the two double bonds. Dienes having double bonds separated by more than one single bond behave as if each double bond is isolated and they act independently of the other. Dienes in which the two double bonds share a common carbon atom are called allenes. Dienes having double bonds alternate with a single bond are said to be conjugated.

$RCH{=}CHCH_2CH_2CH{=}CH_2$	a 1,5-diene - double bonds are isolated
$RCH{=}C{=}CH_2$	a 1,2-diene - an allene
$RCH{=}CH{-}CH{=}CHR$	a 1,3-diene - a conjugated diene

Conjugated dienes are 2-4 Kcal/mol more stable than the corresponding isolated dienes due to their conjugation (overlap of pi orbitals of the diene) and form preferentially during elimination reactions.

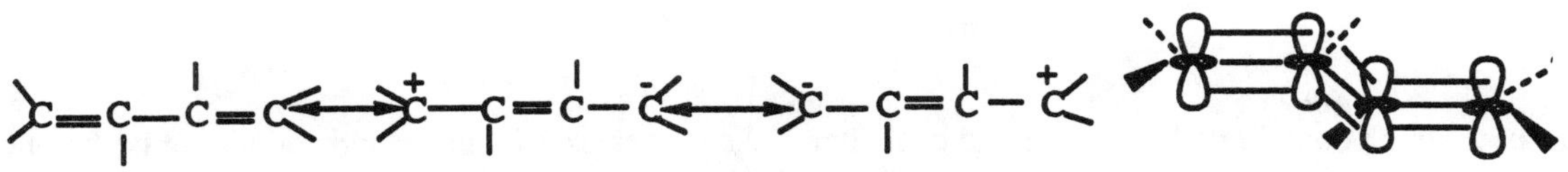

Conjugated dienes form both 1,2- and 1,4- addition products.

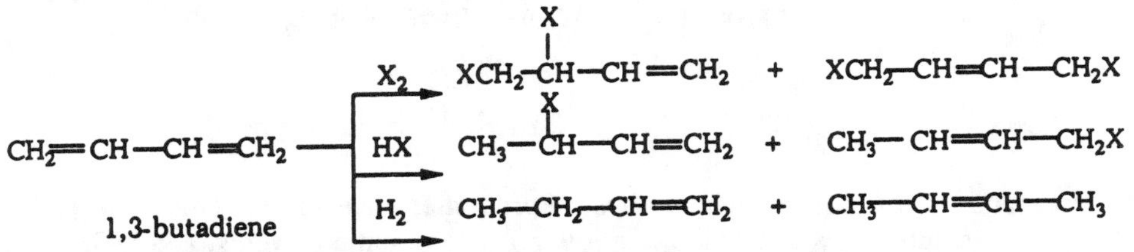

$$CH_2{=}CH{-}CH{=}CH_2 \xrightarrow{X_2} XCH_2{-}CHX{-}CH{=}CH_2 + XCH_2{-}CH{=}CH{-}CH_2X$$

$$\xrightarrow{HX} CH_3{-}CHX{-}CH{=}CH_2 + CH_3{-}CH{=}CH{-}CH_2X$$

$$\xrightarrow{H_2} CH_3{-}CH_2{-}CH{=}CH_2 + CH_3{-}CH{=}CH{-}CH_3$$

1,3-butadiene

Electrophilic addition to conjugated dienes involves the formation of an allylic carbocation. At low temperatures, the 1,2-product forms faster than the 1,4-product and is referred to as the kinetic product. At higher temperatures, the proportion of 1,4- product increases, indicating that it is the more stable or thermodynamic product.

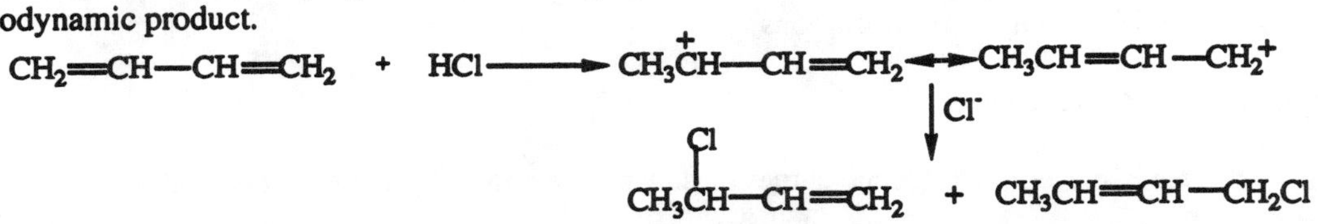

$$CH_2{=}CH{-}CH{=}CH_2 + HCl \rightarrow CH_3\overset{+}{C}H{-}CH{=}CH_2 \leftrightarrow CH_3CH{=}CH{-}CH_2^+$$

$$\xrightarrow{Cl^-} CH_3CHCl{-}CH{=}CH_2 + CH_3CH{=}CH{-}CH_2Cl$$

1, 2 - addition 1, 4 - addition

Isoprene rule: The carbon skeleton of isoprene, 2-methyl-1,3-butadiene, occurs in many compounds called terpenes which are found in plants. The basic isoprene structure occurs as a repeat unit (isoprene rule). Natural rubber also may be considered a 1,4-addition polymer of isoprene.

1,4-addition polymer of isoprene

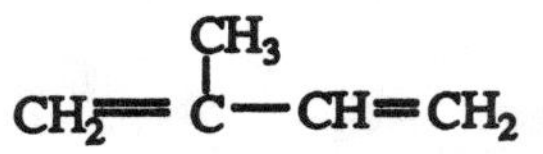

$$CH_2{=}C(CH_3){-}CH{=}CH_2$$

isoprene

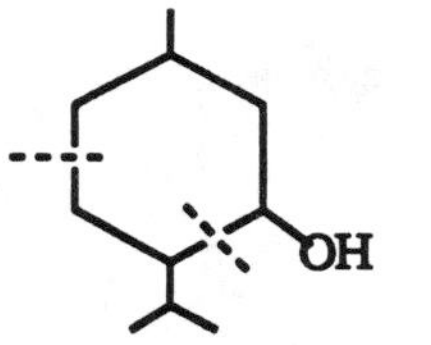

OH

Menthol

vitamin A

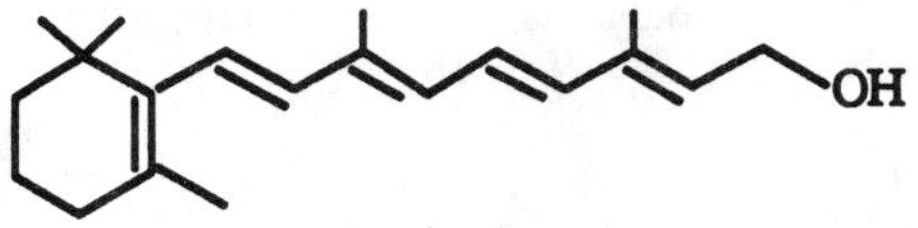

OH

VII. Alkynes:

Hydrocarbon compounds containing a carbon carbon triple bond are called alkynes. They are named in a similar fashion as alkenes by replacing the -ane name with -yne. The simplest member of the series is also known by its common name, acetylene.

$$HC{\equiv}CH$$

ethyne

(acetylene)

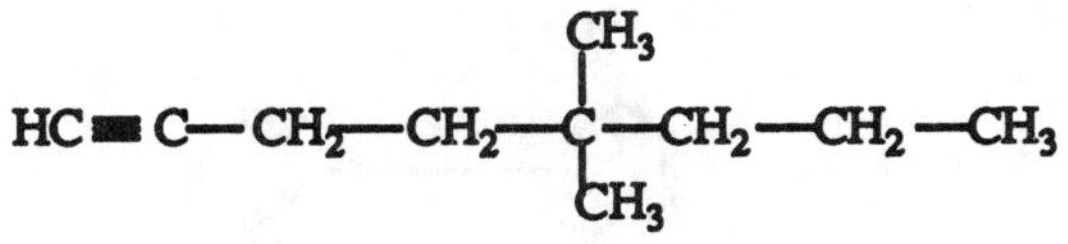

$$HC{\equiv}C{-}CH_2{-}CH_2{-}C(CH_3)_2{-}CH_2{-}CH_2{-}CH_3$$

5, 5 - dimethyl - 1 - octyne

In molecules which contain both a double and triple bond, the longest continuous chain containing both bonds is numbered to give the lowest prefix numbers with the double bond receiving the lower number if there is a choice. The -en suffix precedes the -yne suffix in the name as shown below.

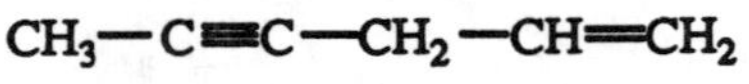

$CH_3{-}C{\equiv}C{-}CH_2{-}CH{=}CH_2$ — 1 - hexen - 4 - yne

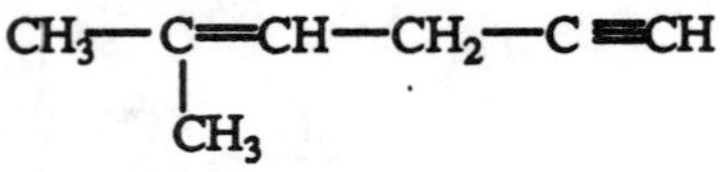

$CH_3{-}C(CH_3){=}CH{-}CH_2{-}C{\equiv}CH$ — 2-methyl-2-hexen-5-yne

Alkynes are hydrocarbons of low polarity whose physical properties are essentially the same as those of alkanes and alkenes. They are insoluble in water, soluble in low polarity organic solvents, and their boiling points are nearly the same as the corresponding alkane or alkene.

7.20.1.3 BENZENE (Aromatic Hydrocarbons)

I. Structure of aromatic compounds:

Many *monosubstituted benzenes* have special names or they can be named by the substituent attached:

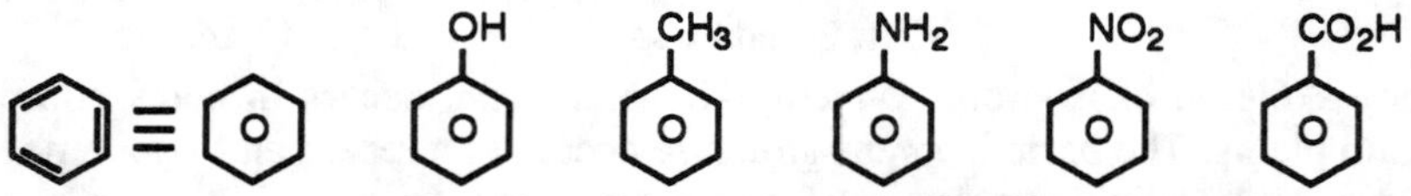

Benzene (OH) Phenol; (CH_3) Toluene; (NH_2) Aniline; (NO_2) Nitrobenzene; (CO_2H) Benzoic Acid

Disubstituted benzenes can be named as a derivative of the primary substituent with numbers or the o-p-m system:

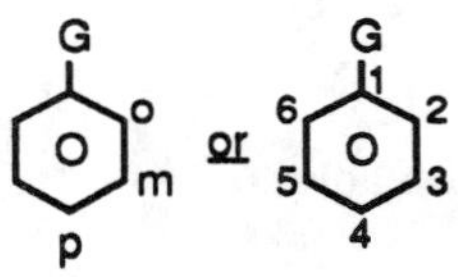

G: o, m, p or 1, 2, 3, 4, 5, 6

o = ortho
m = meta
p = para

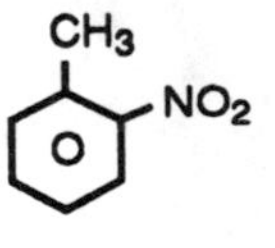

CH_3, NO_2: o-Nitrotoluene

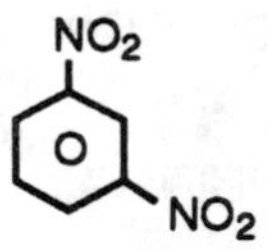

NO_2, NO_2: m-Dinitrobenzene

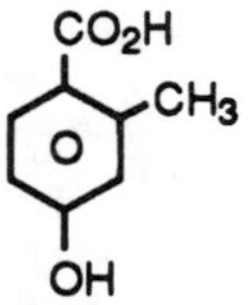

CO_2H, CH_3, OH: 2-methyl-4-Hydroxybenzoic acid

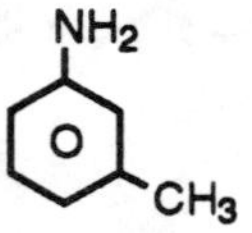

NH_2, CH_3: m-Methylaniline, or m-Aminotoluene

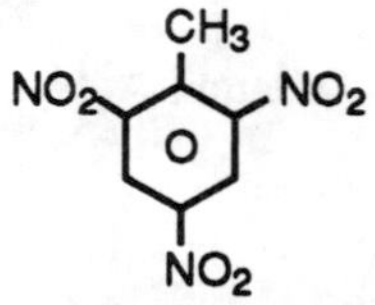

CH_3, NO_2, NO_2, NO_2: 2,4,6-Trinitrotoluene

Tri and higher substituted benzenes require the numbering system as above.

Benzene (C_6H_6) is a planar molecule in which the carbons are sp^2 hybridized. It often is represented by two resonance forms having alternate double and single bonds called Kekule' structures.

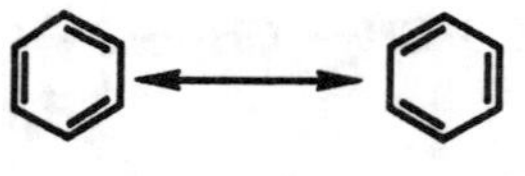

All of the carbon to carbon bonds are of equal length and the bond angles of benzene equal 120°. Since benzene is planar and has six sp^2 hybridized carbons, each carbon has a p orbital perpendicular to the plane of the ring. The six p orbitals, each containing one electron, lie close enough to overlap effectively in the lowest energy bonding molecular orbital. Because of the equal overlap of the six p orbitals, benzene is often drawn as a hexagon with a circle to represent the six delocalized pi electrons.

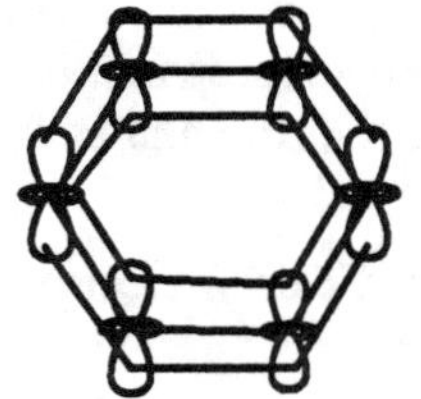

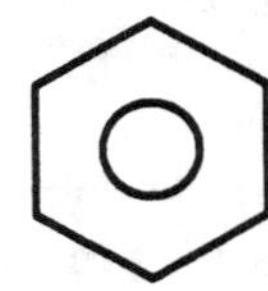

Benzene is reduced by three molar equivalents of hydrogen to cyclohexane and has a heat of hydrogenation of 49.8 Kcal/mol. Based on the heat of hydrogenation which would be expected for a compound with three double bonds, benzene is 36 Kcal/mol more stable than anticipated. That is, hydrogenation of benzene releases 36 Kcal/mol less energy than would be expected for a 1,3,5-cyclohexatriene with non-interacting double bonds. This difference in energy is referred to as the resonance energy, stabilization energy, or delocalization energy of benzene. Benzene and its derivatives are the simplest and most important representatives of a large class of aromatic compounds. Aromatic compounds are those compounds which are substantially stabilized by resonance. Some examples of benzenoid aromatic, polycyclic aromatic, and heterocyclic aromatic compounds are given below. A number of heterocyclic aromatic compounds are present in biochemical systems.

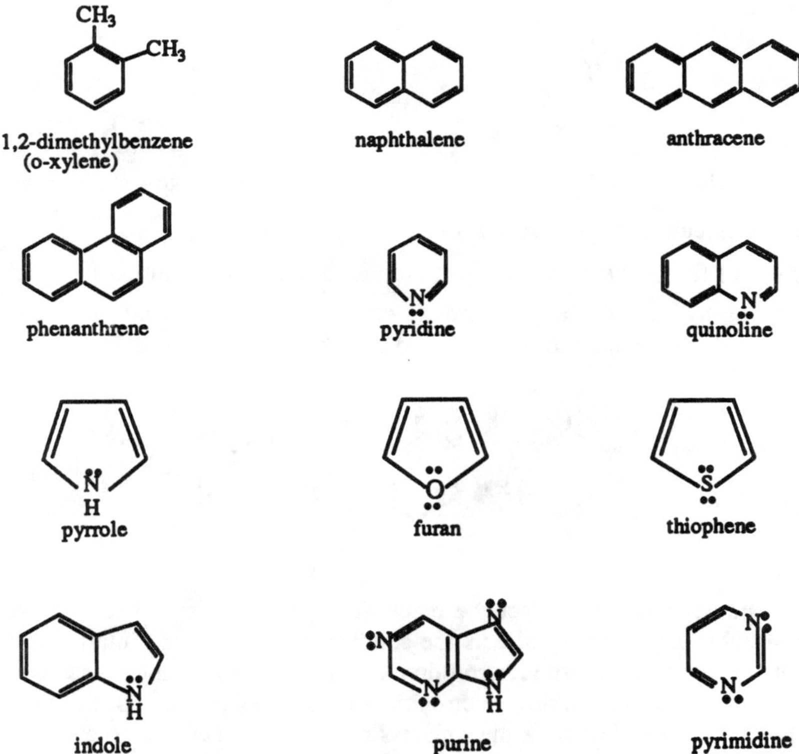

The term annulene is used for monocyclic polyenes having alternating single and double bonds (fully conjugated). The ring size of an annulene is described by a number in a bracket. Cyclobutadiene is a [4] annulene, benzene is a [6] annulene, and cyclooctatetraene is a [8] annulene. Huckel's rule states that only planar, fully conjugated, monocyclic polyenes having 4n + 2 pi electrons, where n is an integer, i.e., n = 0,1,2,3,4, . . ., should possess aromatic stability. Therefore Huckel's rule predicts that annulenes having 6, 10, 14, or 18 pi electrons should possess aromatic character providing the ring is planar.

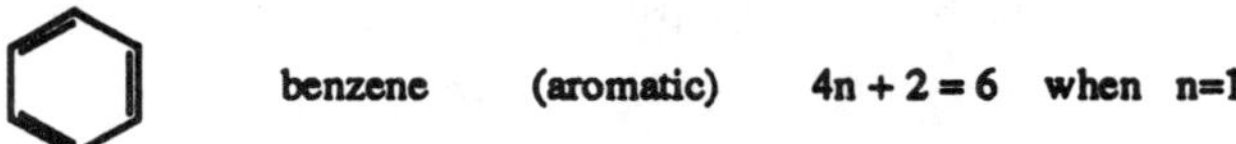

Cyclobutadiene (planar) and cyclooctatetraene (non-planar) do not meet the Huckel's criteria and do not possess aromatic character. A number of [10] and [12] annulenes have been prepared and none are aromatic. The [12] annulenes have 12 pi electrons and do not obey Huckel's rule. The [10] annulenes have the correct number of pi electrons but their rings are non-planar.

Pyrrole, furan, and pyridine are aromatic. Pyrrole has an unshared pair of electrons on the nitrogen along with 4 pi electrons in the diene portion resulting in a total of 6 pi electrons. Furan also has 6 pi electrons to constitute an aromatic system. The second unshared electron pair on oxygen are in an orbital perpendicular to the pi system of the ring and do not count when applying Huckel's rule. The lone electron pair on the pyridine nitrogen also lies in the plane perpendicular to the pi system of the ring and does not count.

Certain monocyclic anions and cations exhibit enhanced stability and are considered to be aromatic. Some examples are given below:

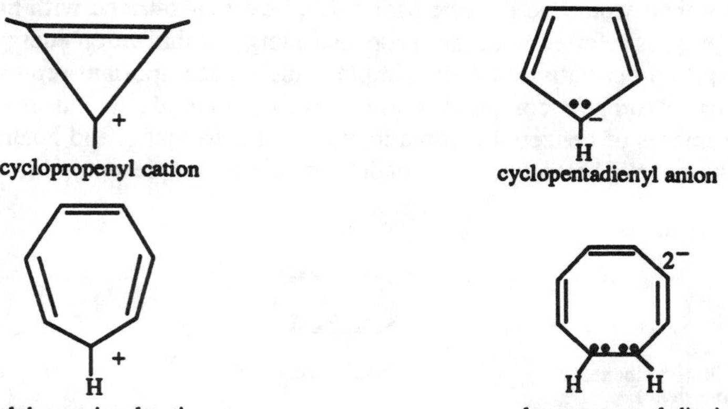

II. Aromatic Substitution (Delocalization of electrons):

The characteristic reaction of the benzene ring is electrophilic aromatic substitution in which an electrophile (E^+) is substituted for a ring hydrogen. The intermediate cation form is stabilized by charged delocalization which is especially strong at ring carbon atoms ortho and para to the entering group.

Substituents attached to the benzene ring affect the reactivity of the ring and determine the orientation of substitution. The type of substituent greatly affects the stability of the charged intermediate formed during electrophilic substitution. Groups which are electron donating make the ring more reactive than benzene to electrophilic substitution and direct the entering electrophile to the ortho and para positions. These groups are called ortho-para directors. Groups which make the ring less reactive than benzene to electrophilic substitution direct the electrophile to the meta position. These groups are called meta directors. The halogens are unique in that they deactivate the benzene ring to substitution but are ortho-para directing.

Ortho-para directors (activating): $-NH_2$, $-NHR$, $-NR_2$, $-OH$, $-OR$, $-NHCOR$, C_6H_5-, $-R$

Meta directors (deactivating): $-NO_2$, $-NR_3{}^+$, $-CF_3$, $-CN$, $-COOH$, $-COOR$, $-SO_3H$, $-CHO$, $-COR$

Ortho-para directors (deactivating): $-F$, $-Cl$, $-Br$, $-I$

Groups tend to withdraw or release electrons by resonance effects or inductive effects. Resonance effects involve delocalization of electrons to stabilize a charged species. An example of this effect is the stabilization of the charged intermediate in electrophilic substitution by an electron releasing group such as the hydroxyl group (– OH). Inductive effects depend upon the property of a substituent to release or withdraw electrons. The inductive effect of a group depends upon its electronegativity and may act through the sigma bonds of a molecule or through space. Since most elements or groups are more electronegative than hydrogen they exert an electron withdrawing effect. Groups such as, – CHO, – COR, – COOR, – COOH, – NO_2, – CF_3, and – NR_3^+ can only exert an electron withdrawing effect. Such groups as, – OH, – OR, – NH_2, – NHR, – NR_2, and the halogens may be electron releasing by resonance due to their unshared electron pairs, but electron withdrawing by inductive effects due to their electronegativity. The halogens are ortho-para directing but deactivating groups due to the fact that their electron withdrawing inductive effect reduces the electron density of the aromatic ring and thus destabilizes the cation form. The halogens direct ortho-para since they have an unshared pair of electrons which can be donated to stabilize the intermediate cation formed by ortho or para attack. For electrophilic aromatic substitution reactions, the resonance effect is usually more important than the inductive effect of a group.

o-p directors (e.g., – OH, – NH_2, – OR, – NR_2, alkyls)

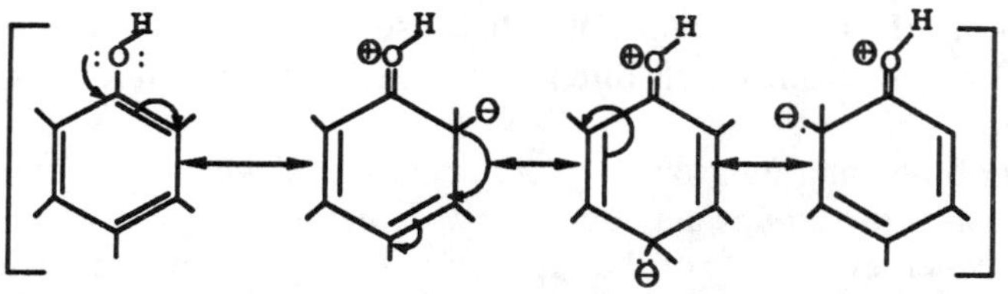

—note the electron density is at the o-p positions so the E + favors attack at o-p positions,

—with a substituent (E +) at ortho or para get good stabilization:

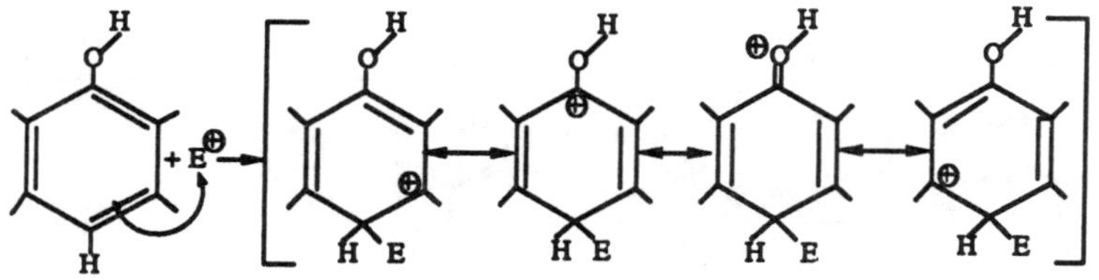

—with a substituent at meta:

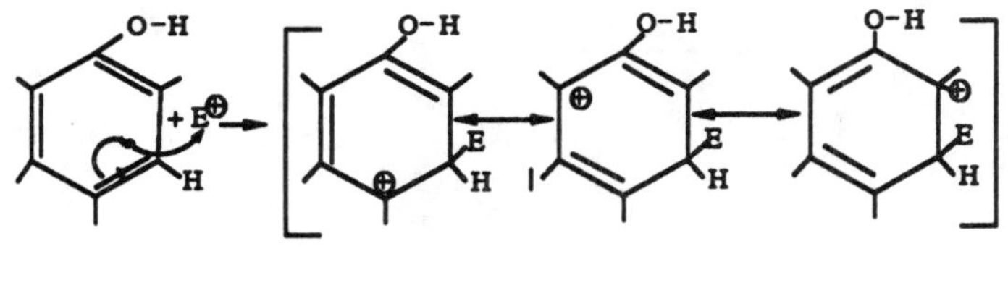

the – OH can no longer help delocalize the positive charge so the o-p is favored over the meta.

meta directors (e.g., – NO_2, – SO_2^-, – CN)

—without a substituent:

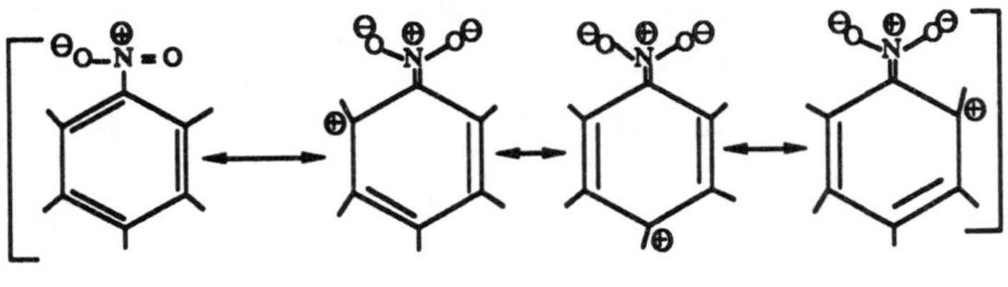

notice that + charge is put at the o-p positions so the E + favors attack at meta position

—with a substituent at meta positions:

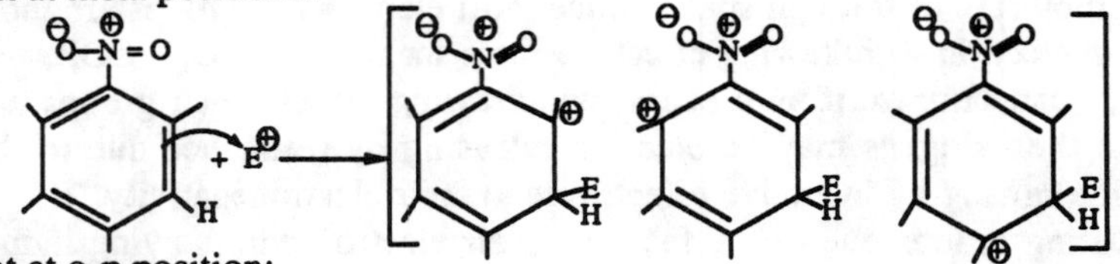

—with a substituent at o-p position:

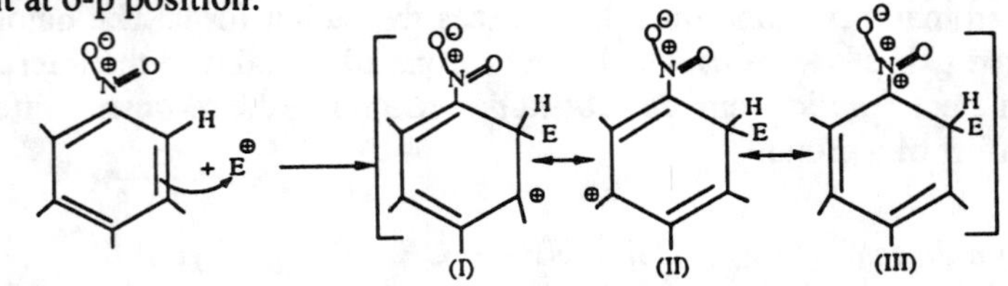

(I) (II) (III)

resonance form III is a noncontributor because of the adjacent positive charge; analogous situations exist with the other meta directors also; so, meta substitution is favored.

The problem of orientation of the entering group is more complicated when there are two substituents present on a benzene ring. In some cases the groups may be located so that the directive effect of one group reinforces that of the other. However, when the effects of the groups are in opposition it is difficult to predict the major product and a mexture of products may result. As a general rule activating ortho-para directing groups are dominant over deactivating meta directing groups or groups which are less activating. For steric reasons substitution generally does not occur between two groups which are located meta to one another.

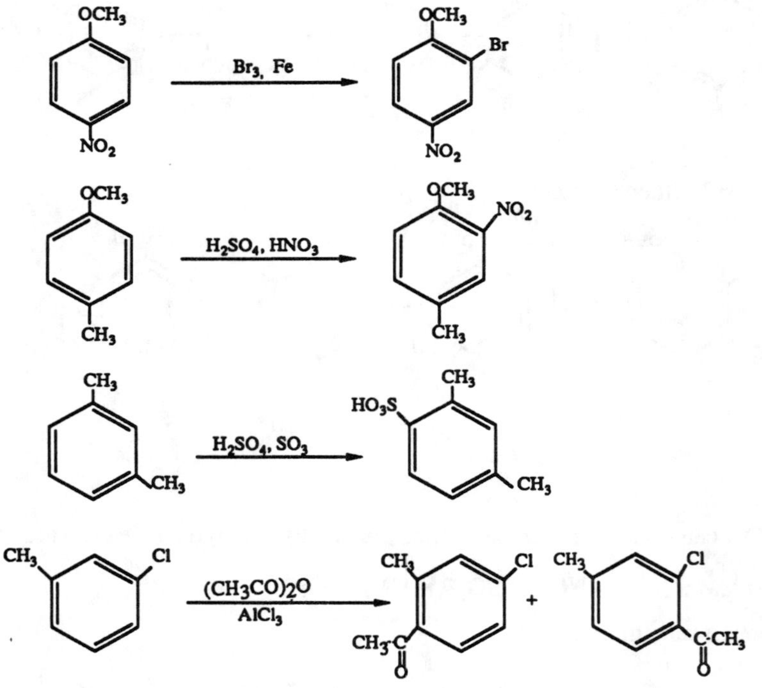

OCH_3, NO_2 — Br_3, Fe → OCH_3, Br, NO_2

OCH_3, CH_3 — H_2SO_4, HNO_3 → OCH_3, NO_2, CH_3

CH_3, CH_3 — H_2SO_4, SO_3 → CH_3, HO_3S, CH_3

CH_3, Cl — $(CH_3CO)_2O$, $AlCl_3$ → CH_3, Cl, CH_3-C(=O) + CH_3, Cl, C(=O)-CH_3

7.20.2 Questions Related to Hydrocarbons

1. Alkanes tend to have _______ boiling points because they are _______ and, hence, have _______ intermolecular forces.

   A. low, nonpolar, weak
   B. high, polar, strong
   C. low, polar, weak
   D. high, nonpolar, strong

2. Alkanes are _______ in water because they are _______.

   A. soluble, polar
   B. insoluble, polar
   C. soluble, nonpolar
   D. insoluble, nonpolar

3. Branching tends to make an alkane more _______ and this _______ the boiling point.

   A. symmetric, lowers
   B. symmetric, raises
   C. asymmetric, lowers
   D. asymmetric, raises

4. The step in which radicals react with radicals is:

   A. termination.
   B. propagation.
   C. initiation.
   D. none of these.

5. Of the following radicals, in general, the most stable is:

   A. allylic.
   B. primary.
   C. secondary.
   D. tertiary.

6. Which ring has the greatest ring strain?

   A. cyclohexane
   B. cyclopentane
   C. cyclobutane
   D. cyclopropane

7. Which of the following rings has no ring strain?

   A. cyclohexane
   B. cyclobutane
   C. cyclopropane
   D. none of the above

8. The name of the following compound is:

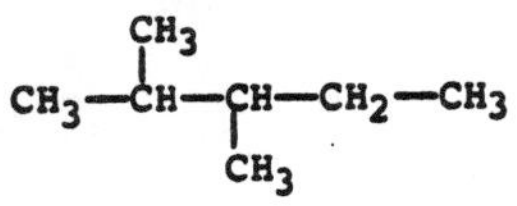

$$\begin{array}{c} CH_3 \\ CH_3-CH-CH-CH_2-CH_3 \\ CH_3 \end{array}$$

   A. 2-Isopropyl pentane.
   B. 2,3-Dimethylpentane.
   C. 3,4-Dimethyl pentane.
   D. none of the above.

9. Name the following compound:

```
                                            CH3
      CH2CH3   CH3      CH2CH2—CH
CH3—C——CH2—CH—CH                  CH3
      CH3               CH—CH3
                        CH3
```

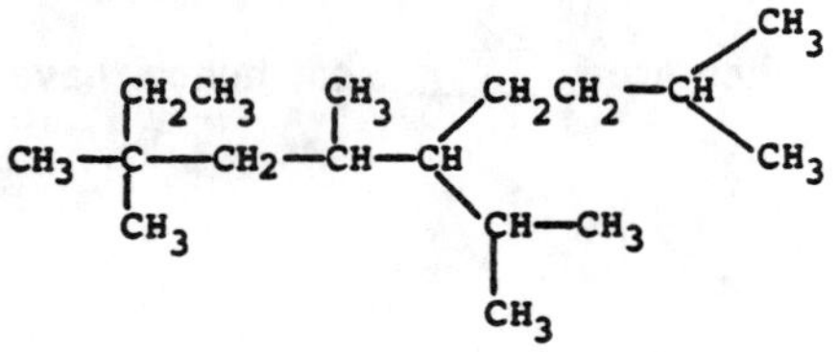

A. 2,4,8-Trimethyl-2-ethyl-5-isopropylnonane
B. diisoprene
C. 2,6,8,8-Tetramethyl-5-isopropyldecane
D. none of the above

10. Give the structure of 2,6-Dimethyl-4-ethyloctane:

```
      CH3        CH2CH3     CH3
A.  CH3—C—CH2—CH—CH2—C—CH2CH3
      CH3                   CH3

      CH3        CH2CH3     CH3
B.  CH3—CH—CH2—CH—CH2—CH— CH2CH3

      CH2CH3     CH3        CH2CH3
C.  CH3—CH—CH2—CH—CH2—CH—CH2CH3
```

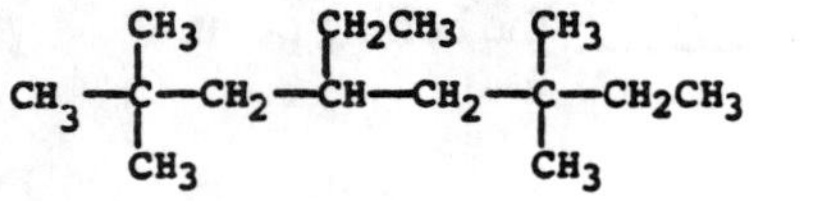

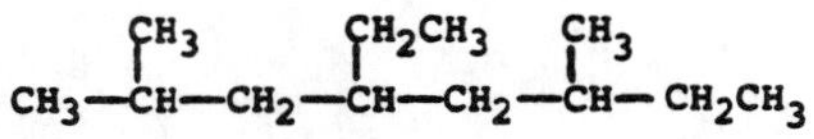

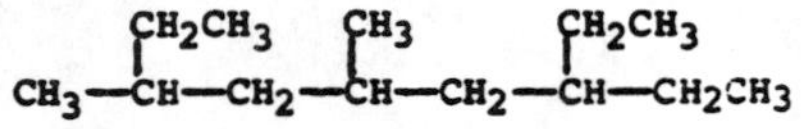

D. none of the above

11. Name the following compound:

```
        CH3
        |
        C
       / H \
  H   /     \  H
  |  /       \ |
  C ————————— C
  |           |
  H           CH2CH3
```

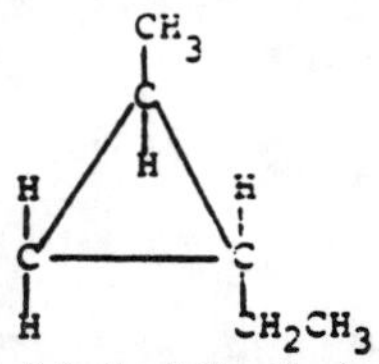

A. cis-1-Methyl-2-ethylcyclopropane
B. 2,3-Methylpentane
C. trans-Dimethylcylopropane
D. none of the above

12. What is the structure of trans-1-Ethyl-4-t-butylcyclohexane?

A. 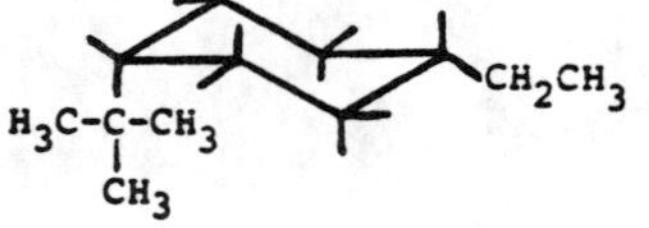 (cyclohexane chair) —CH2CH3; H3C-C-CH3 with CH3

B. (cyclohexane chair) —CH2CH3; CH3, CH3-C, CH3

C. (cyclohexane chair) —CH2CH3; CH-CH3, CH2, CH3

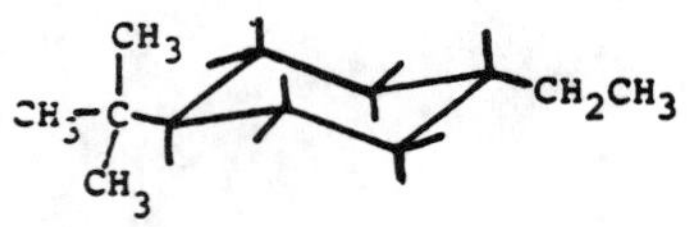

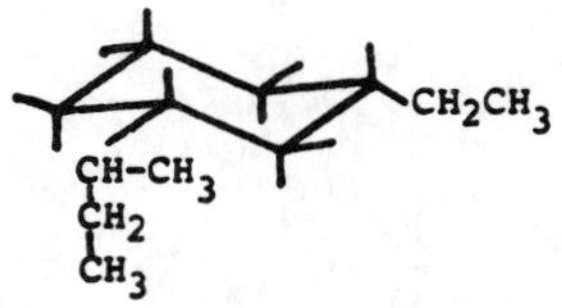

D. none of the above

13. Which compound probably has the higher boiling point?

$$CH_3{-}CH_2{-}CH_2{-}CH_2{-}CH_3 \quad \text{(I)} \qquad CH_3{-}\underset{}{\overset{CH_3}{\overset{|}{C}H}}{-}CH_2{-}CH_3 \quad \text{(II)}$$

A. I
B. II
C. both equal
D. I and II do not boil at any temperature

14. Which compound probably has the higher boiling point?

$$CH_3{-}CH_2{-}CH_3 \quad \text{(I)} \qquad CH_3{-}CH_2{-}CH_2{-}CH_2{-}CH_3 \quad \text{(II)}$$

A. I
B. II
C. both equal
D. I and II do not boil at any temperature

15. How many CO_2's are produced by the complete combustion of 3,3-Diethylhexane?

A. 10
B. 8
C. 6
D. 4

16. Which of the following radicals is the most stable?

A. 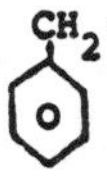 $C_6H_5{-}CH_2\cdot$ (benzene ring with $CH_2\cdot$)

B. $CH_3{-}\overset{CH_3}{\underset{CH_3}{C}}\cdot$

C. $CH_3{-}\overset{CH_3}{\underset{\cdot}{CH}}$

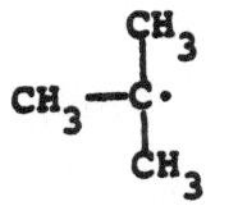

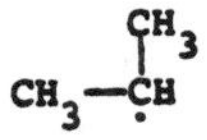

D. $CH_3\cdot$

17. The removal of which H will result in the most stable radical in the following compound?

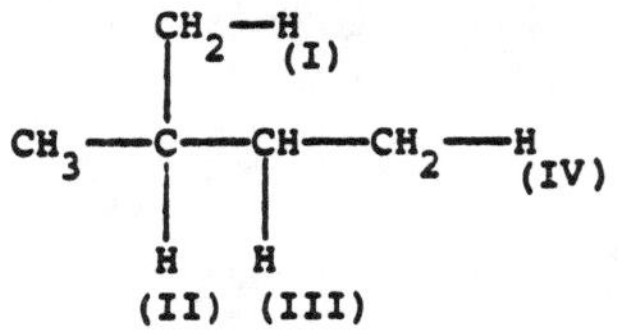

```
          CH2—H
          |     (I)
          |
CH3———C———CH———CH2———H
          |     |          (IV)
          |     |
          H     H
        (II)  (III)
```

A. I
B. II
C. III
D. IV

18. The formula for an *alkane* is C_4H_8. Therefore, this compound:

A. is a straight chain
B. is branched
C. contains a ring
D. none of these

19. The general formula for an alkene with one double bond and no rings is:

A. C_nH_{2n-2}
B. C_nH_{2n+2}
C. C_nH_n
D. C_nH_{2n}

20. Select the most stable carbenium ion:

A.

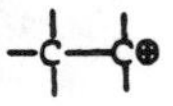

B.

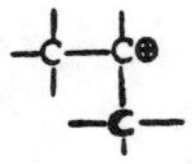

C.

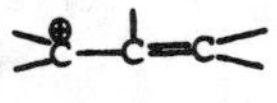

D.

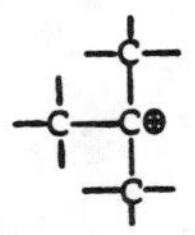

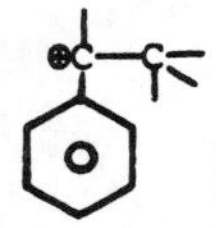

21. Select the most unstable carbenium ion:

A.

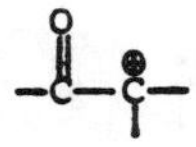

B.

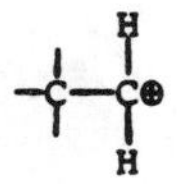

C. 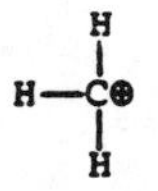 H—C⊕ (with H above and below)

D.

22. Although alkanes and alkenes are both composed of carbon and hydrogen, alkenes may show ______ due to ______.

A. hydrogen bonding, the double bond
B. less reactivity, the double bond
C. polarity, cis-trans isomerism
D. non-reactivity, high solubility

23. Name the following compound:

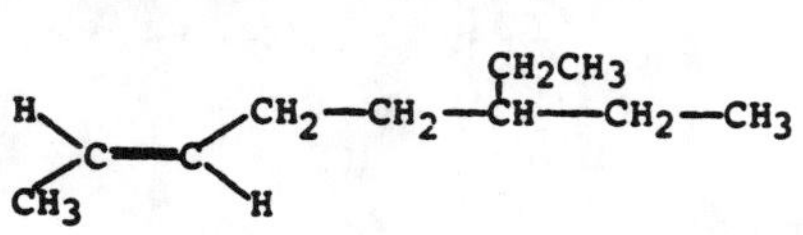

$$\mathrm{H(CH_3)C{=}C(H)\text{—}CH_2\text{—}CH_2\text{—}CH(CH_2CH_3)\text{—}CH_2\text{—}CH_3}$$

A. 2-Ethyl-trans-6-octene
B. 6-Ethyl-trans-2-octene
C. 2-Ethyl-cis-6-octene
D. 6-Ethyl-cis-2-octene

24. Give the structure for 3,4-Dimethyl-cis-2-trans-4-heptadiene:

A. 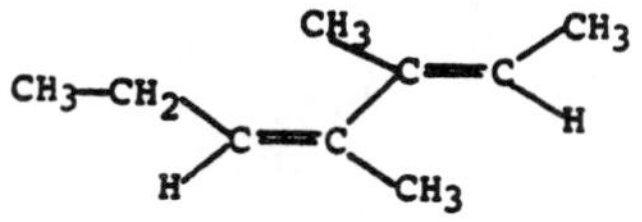 CH_3—CH_2, H, C=C, CH_3, CH_3, C=C, CH_3, H

B. CH_3, H, C=C, CH_3, H, C=C, CH_3—CH_2, CH_3

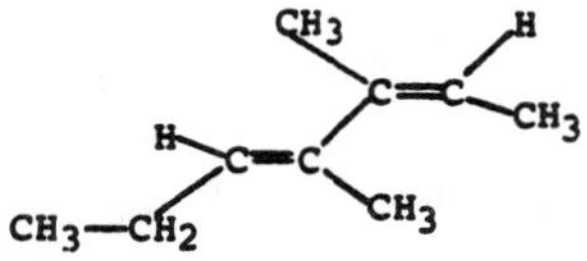

C. CH_3, CH_3-CH_2—CH, C=C, CH_2CH_3, H, CH_3

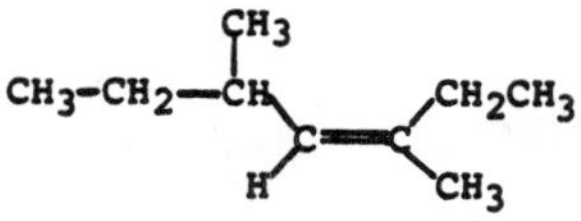

D. none of the above

25. A double bond can stabilize an adjacent carbenium ion by _______ (of) the positive charge with its _______ -bond.

A. neutralizing, π
B. neutralizing, σ
C. delocalization, π
D. delocalization, σ

26. The reaction of H^+ with the following compound will form which carbenium ion:

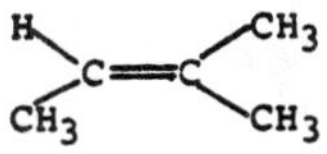

H, C=C, CH_3, CH_3, CH_3

A. H, ⊕C, H, C, CH_3, CH_3, CH_3

B. H, H, C, ⊕C, CH_3, CH_3, CH_3

C. H, C, H, C, H, CH_3, CH_3, ⊕CH_2

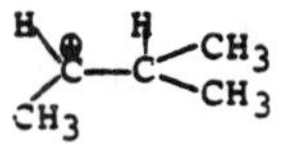

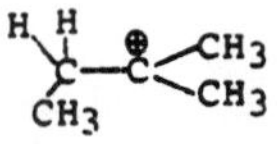

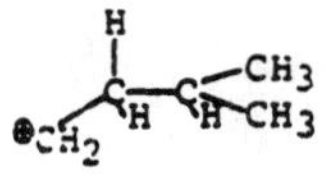

D. none of these

27. The product of the following reaction is:

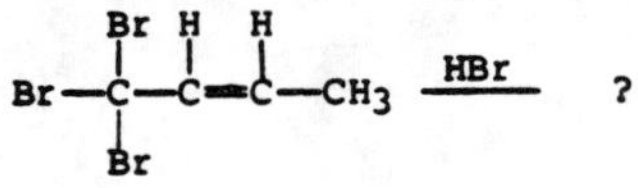

```
     Br H  H
     |  |  |
Br—C—C═C—CH3   --HBr-->   ?
     |
     Br
```

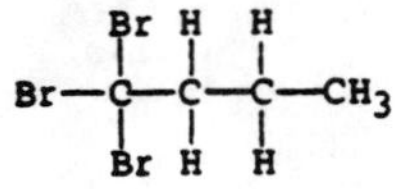

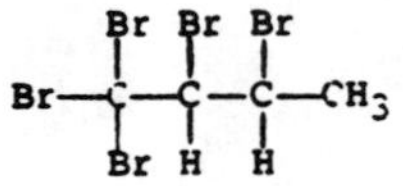

A.
```
     Br H  H
     |  |  |
Br—C—C—C—CH3
     |  |  |
     Br H  H
```

B.
```
     Br Br Br
     |  |  |
Br—C—C—C—CH3
     |  |  |
     Br H  H
```

C.
```
     Br Br H
     |  |  |
Br—C—C—C—CH3
     |  |  |
     Br H  H
```

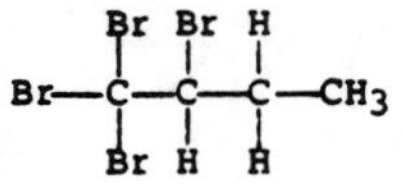

D. 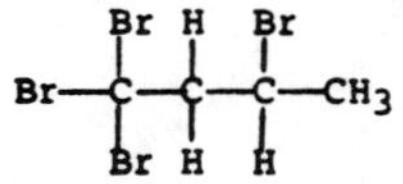
```
     Br H  Br
     |  |  |
Br—C—C—C—CH3
     |  |  |
     Br H  H
```

28. Which compound has the higher boiling point?

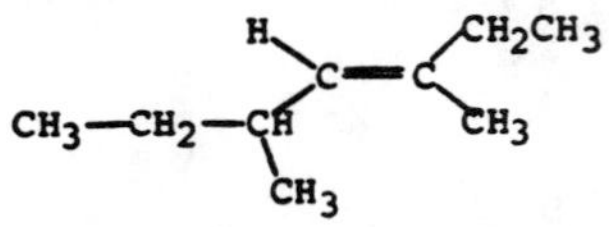

```
               H         CH2CH3                      H         CH3
                \       /                             \       /
                 C═══C                                 C═══C
                /       \                             /       \
CH3—CH2—CH            CH3            CH3CH2—CH            CH2CH3
          |                                  |
          CH3                                CH3
         (I)                                (II)
```

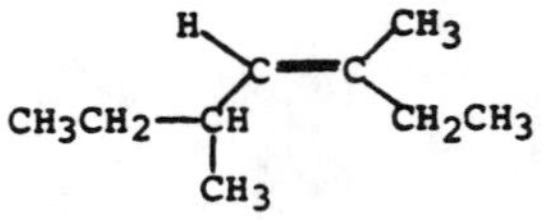

A. I
B. II
C. Both have the same boiling point.
D. I and II do not boil at any temperature.

29. Which compound has the higher dipole moment?

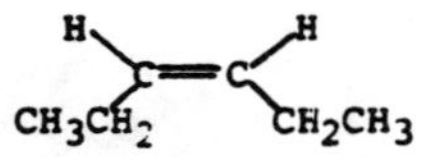

```
   H         H                  H         CH2CH3
    \       /                    \       /
     C═══C                        C═══C
    /       \                    /       \
CH3CH2       CH2CH3         CH3CH2        H
       (I)                         (II)
```

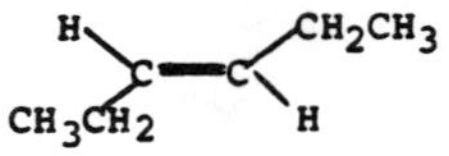

A. I
B. II
C. Both have equal dipole moments.
D. I and II have no dipole moment.

30. Hydrocarbons having two double bonds are called:

A. ethenes.
B. dienes.
C. ethynes.
D. hexenes.

31. Which of the following hydrocarbons contains a triple bond between adjacent carbon atoms?

A. alkanes
B. alkenes
C. dienes
D. alkynes

32. Name the following compound:

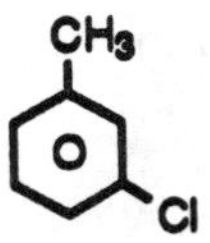

A. o-Chlorotoluene
B. p-Chloromethylbenzene
C. 1-Methyl-2-chlorobenzene
D. none of the above

33. Name the following compound:

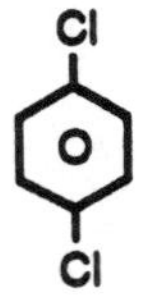

A. p-Dichlorobenzene
B. m-Dichlorobenzene
C. 1,3-Dichlorobenzene
D. none of the above

34. Give the structure of 2-Chloro-4-Iodonitrobenzene:

A. 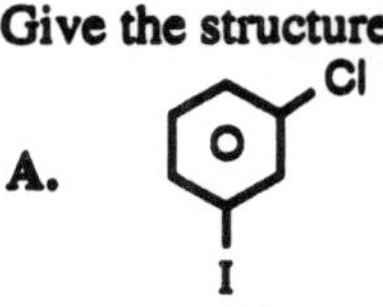

B. 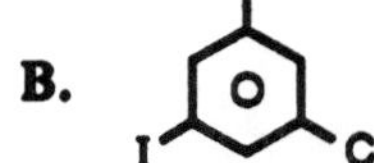

C. 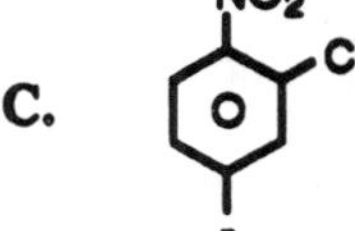

D. none of the above

35. Given the following compound, give the positions which will have the most electron density due to delocalization:

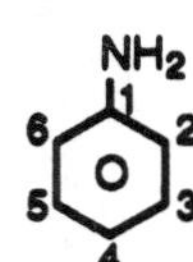

A. 1,3,5
B. 3,4,5
C. 2,5
D. none of these

36. Given the following compound, give the positions which will have the most electron density due to delocalization:

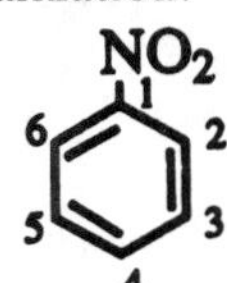

A. 3,5
B. 2,4,6
C. 3,4,5
D. none of these

37. If Br^+ is an electrophile (e.g., from $Br_2 + AlCl_3$), the most likely product of its reaction with the following compound is:

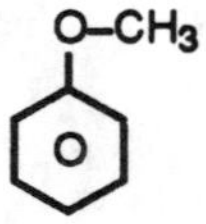

O–CH3

A. 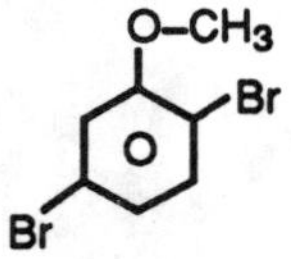 O–CH3, Br, Br

B. 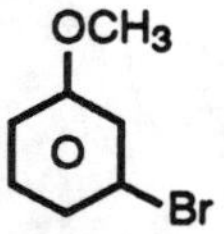 OCH3, Br

C. 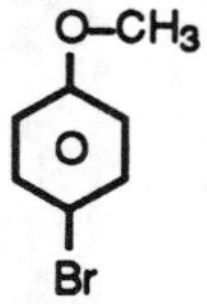 O–CH3, Br

D. none of these

38. Assume the Br^+ from #37 reacts with the following compound, the most likely product is:

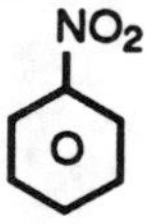

NO2

A. 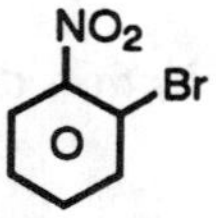 NO2, Br

B. 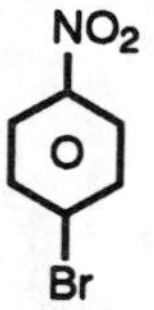 NO2, Br

C. 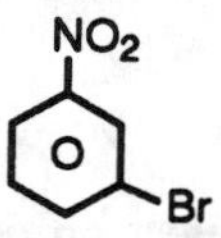 NO2, Br

D. none of these

7.20.3 Answers to Questions in Section 7.20.2

(1) A (2) D (3) A (4) A (5) A (6) D (7) A (8) B (9) C (10) B (11) D (12) B (13) A (14) B (15) A (16) A (17) B (18) C (19) D (20) C (21) A (22) C (23) B (24) B (25) C (26) B (27) D (28) B (29) A (30) B (31) D (32) D (33) A (34) C (35) D (36) A (37) C (38) C

7.20.4 Discussion of Answers to Questions in Section 7.20.2

Questions #1 to #7 Discussed in Section.

Question #8 (Answer: B) The numbering is:

$C_1-C_2(C)(C)-C_3(C)-C_4-C_5$

Question #9 (Answer: C) The numbering is:

Question #10 (Answer: B) Discussed in Section.

Question #11 (Answer: D) The correct answer is trans-1-Methyl-2-ethylcyclopropane.

Question #12 (Answer: B) Discussed in Section.

Question #13 (Answer: A) Compound (II) is more branched than (I) and has a lower predicted boiling point.

Question #14 (Answer: B) Compound (II) has the higher molecular weight and the higher predicted boiling point.

Question #15 (Answer: A) The structure is,

$CH_3-CH_2-C(CH_2-CH_3)(CH_2CH_3)-CH_2-CH_2-CH_3$

The formula is: $C_{10}H_{22}$.

The equation is: $C_{10}H_{22} + {}^{31}/{}_{2}\,O_2 \rightarrow 10\,CO_2 + 11\,H_2O$

Question #16 (Answer: A) Given in Section.

Question #17(Answer: B) The resulting radicals would be:

$CH_3-CH(\bullet CH_2)-CH_2-CH_3$ (1°) (I)	$CH_3-\dot{C}(CH_3)-CH_2-CH_3$ (3°) (II)
$CH_3-CH(CH_3)-\dot{C}H-CH_3$ (2°) (III)	$CH_3-CH(CH_3)-CH_2-\dot{C}H_2$ (1°) (IV)

Then the 3° radical (II) is the most stable.

Question #18 (Answer: C) Since the compound is an alkane, there are no double or triple bonds. One would expect C_4H_{10} for a fully saturated alkane without rings. The two missing H's (C_4H_8) suggest the presence of one ring.

Questions #19 to #22, #25, #30, #31 Discussed in Section.

Question #23 (Answer: B) The numbering is,

Question #24 (Answer: B) Discussed in Section.

Question #26(Answer: B) The only possible cations from this double bond are (A) which is 2° and (B) which is 3°. Tertiary (3°) is more stable than secondary (2°).

Question #27 (Answer: D) The mechanism is,

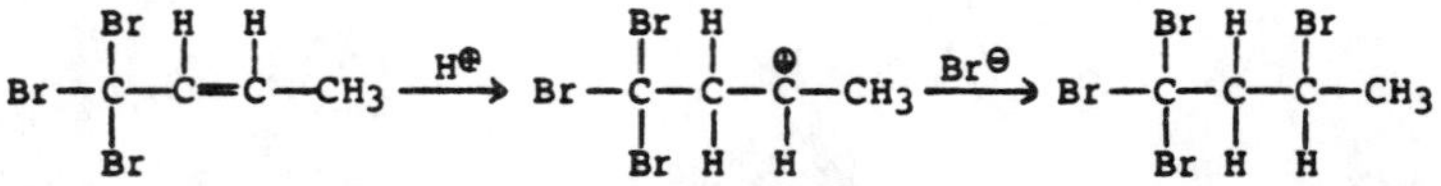

$$Br_3C-CH{=}CH-CH_3 \xrightarrow{H^{\oplus}} Br_3C-CH_2-\overset{\oplus}{C}H-CH_3 \xrightarrow{Br^{\ominus}} Br_3C-CH_2-CHBr-CH_3$$

This carbenium ion is more stable than the alternate because of the adjacent brominated carbons,

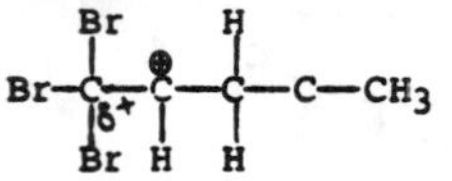

$$Br_3\overset{\delta+}{C}-\overset{\oplus}{C}H-CH_2-C-CH_3$$ (alternate; less stable)

Question #28 (Answer: B) Cis-compounds tend to have higher boiling points because of higher polarity than the corresponding trans compound.

Question #29 (Answer: A) See #10 and discussion in Section.

Question #32 (Answer: D) The correct name is m-Chlorotoluene (others also possible).

Questions #33-#36 Are adequately discussed in the Section.

Question #37 (Answer: C) The $-O-CH_3$ is an o-p director. Of the products given (C) is the most likely. This para-product is also favored over the ortho-product because of steric (bulk) consideration.

Question #38 (Answer: C) The $-NO_2$ is a meta director.

7.20.5 Advanced Concepts

- Understand three types of polymers (isotactic, syndiotactic, atactic)
- Glance over a few laboratory procedures and experimental devices: magnetic stirrer procedure and reflux condenser for two-phase mixture; Diels-Alder reaction for dienes
- Have you heard of Woodward-Hoffman rules which determine molecular orbital structures? If not, review symmetry-allowed and symmetry-forbidden concepts as they tie to the HOMO (highest occupied molecular orbital) and LUMO (lowest unoccupied molecular orbital) rules

7.21 ALCOHOLS, ALDEHYDES AND KETONES (Oxygen-Containing Compounds)

7.21.1 Introduction to Oxygen-Containing Compounds

General principles of Oxygen-Containing Compounds:

Oxygen-containing organic compounds are classified into: alcohols, aldehydes, ketones, carboxylic acids and their derivatives, ethers and phenols. Oxygen-containing compounds are covered in sections 7.21 and 7.22. General principals of oxygen-containing compounds are broadly classified into five types: hydrogen bonds and solubility; steric effects of substituents; electronic effects of substituents; acidity and basicity and other miscellaneous principles.

(i) Hydrogen bonding and solubility: The carbon atom in alcohols bonded to the OH group is called carbinol carbon. Primary and secondary alcohols have at least one H on the carbinol carbon. They oxidize to carbonyl compounds in the presence of copper at approximately 300° C. Hydrogen atom in alcohols is weakly acidic. Thiols or mercaptans which are sulfur analogs of alcohols are represented by RSH (compared to ROH for alcohols). Hydrocarbon molecules are not associated with each other through hydrogen bonds. As the length of the alkane molecular chain gets longer, the solubility of alcohols in water decreases, e.g., ethyl alcohol is *more* soluble than decyl alcohol. Most alcohol reactions have O-H bond cleavage (this cleavage forms carboxylic acid esters) and C-O bond cleavage (this cleavage forms alkyl halides). The carbonyl oxygen atom in aldehydes and ketones helps form stronger hydrogen bonds with water. Carboxylic acids, which have polar molecules, can form strong hydrogen bonds with each other and also with water. Solubility of carboxylic acids in water decreases as the length of the çarbon chain increases. Carboxylic acids and alcohols are similar in solubility characteristics. Ether molecules cannot associate with each other through hydrogen bonds but can form hydrogen bonds with water. Phenols form strong hydrogen bonds like alcohols.

(ii) Steric effects of substituents: Nucleophilic reactions are affected by steric effects especially steric hindrance. Steric hindrance is caused by arrangements of atomic or functional groups which causes hindrance at the reaction site, thus hindering rates of S_N2 reactions. The relative rate of S_N2 reactions is affected by the molecular structure and arrangement of the alkyl halide. Molecular space may be filled by various arrangements. In case the reacting part of the alkyl halide has a specific space-filling arrangement, the steric effects are dominant. Steric hindrance occurs in certain nucleophilic addition reactions (aldehydes and ketones) and in nucleophilic substitution reactions (carboxylic acid derivatives). The carbonyl carbon atom provides the reaction site or the reacting part of the molecule. Ketones with steric hindrance at the carbonyl group cannot form cyanohydrins. Aldehyde-ketone substitutions differ from carboxylic acid derivatives substitutions in that nucleophilic reactions use the addition-elimination mechanism to overcome steric hindrance.

(iii) Electronic effects of substituents: Effects of activating and deactivating substituents occur in all oxygen-containing compounds. The electronic effects include reactivity, acidity, stereoarrangements and inductive effect in carboxylic acids. Activating substituents usually increase the reaction rate whereas deactivating substituents decrease the reaction rate. The inductive effects are more pronounced in carboxylic acids. These effects are caused by electrostatic interaction of polarized substituent ring bonds, e.g., for electronegative substituents, the ring is located at the positive end of the dipole. The acidity of phenol is linked to the resonance structures which require separation of opposite charges (energy is required to separate opposite charges). Phenol has medium resonance stabilization whereas the phenoxide ion has greater resonance stabilization, e.g., the OH group in phenols behaves as an activating substituent. Bromination and sulfonation reactions are caused by the strong OH group. Carboxylic acid derivatives can be converted to acids, esters, amides and ketones due to substituent effects. Another important control mechanism is the enzyme-catalyzed reduction of acetaldehyde to ethanol by NADH (using hydride-ion transfer).

(iv) Acidity and basicity: α-hydrogen in carbonyl compounds (aldehydes and ketones) makes them acidic. The α-hydrogen is attached to a carbon atom called α-carbon. The pK_a values for α-hydrogen are around 20 (for aldehydes and ketones). Resonance stability of the anion causes this higher acidity. Tautomers which are in reversible equilibrium are keto and enol forms of isomers which are interconvertible. α, β unsaturated carbonyls react with nucleophilic reagents by simple or conjugate addition, e.g., Michael additions which are special conjugate additions. Delocalized carbanions are formed by the nucleophilic aromatic substitution mechanism (S_NAr).

(v) Miscellaneous principles: Alcohols can be synthesized from alkenes by oxymercuration-demurcuration and hydroboration-oxidation procedures. A mixture of two liquids with a boiling point (BP) either higher or lower than the BP of the ingredients is called an azeotrope. In studying permeability of biological cell membranes, the role of crown ethers and host (crown) and guest (cation) relationship should be covered. Excess acidic medium, e.g., HBr causes dialkyl ethers to cleave and form alkyl halides. Dialkyl ethers lack reactivity with bases. Ethers have weak basicity due to the O group. Carboxylate ions or anions (negatively charged) are not reactive towards nucleophilic substitution. Proton migration from α-carbon to oxygen in aldehydes and ketones with α-hydrogen forms a special isomer called enol.

7.21.1.1 ALCOHOLS

I. Nomenclature and physical properties:

See Section 7.20 for the basics of *nomenclature*. Alcohols are named by replacing the -e of the corresponding alkane with -ol for simple alcohols:

CH_4	CH_3OH	$CH_3CH_2CH_3$	$CH_3CH_2CH_2OH$
methane	methanol	propane	propanol
	(methyl alcohol)		(propyl alcohol)

For more complex alcohols, the numbering system is used and the carbon with the – OH should, in general, have the lowest number (if the compound is named as an alcohol):

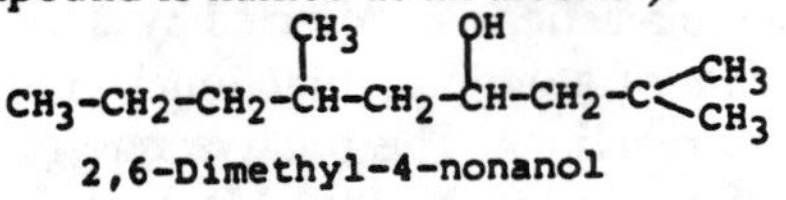

$$CH_3\text{-}CH_2\text{-}CH_2\text{-}CH(CH_3)\text{-}CH_2\text{-}CH(OH)\text{-}CH_2\text{-}C\begin{smallmatrix}CH_3\\CH_3\end{smallmatrix}$$

2,6-Dimethyl-4-nonanol

$$CH_3CH_2CH(OH)CH_2CH_3$$

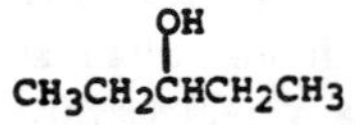

3-Pentanol

The use of sec-, iso-, and tert- are appropriate for common names only

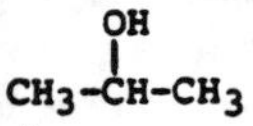

$$CH_3\text{-}CH(OH)\text{-}CH_3 \qquad CH_3\text{-}C(CH_3)_2\text{-}OH$$

isopropanol (isopropyl alcohol) — tert-butyl alcohol (tert-butanol)

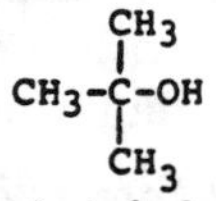

Alcohols are acidic because of the – OH group:

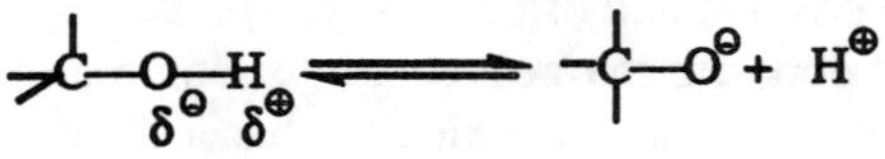

$$\geq C\text{—}\overset{\delta^{\ominus}}{O}\text{—}\overset{\delta^{\oplus}}{H} \rightleftharpoons \geq C\text{—}O^{\ominus} + H^{\oplus}$$

They are very weakly acidic, being less strong than water. As the number of carbon groups attached to the C increases, the acidity decreases:

$CH_3OH > CH_3CH_2OH$ in acidity

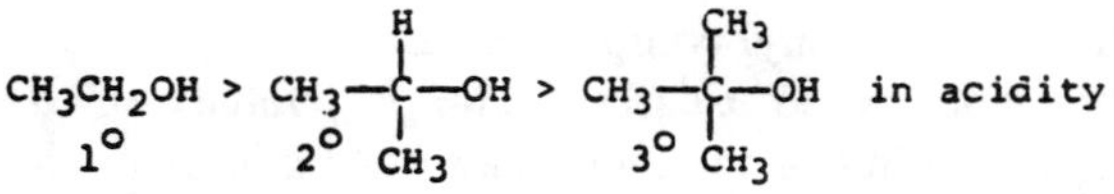

$$\underset{1^\circ}{CH_3CH_2OH} > \underset{2^\circ}{CH_3\text{—}CH(CH_3)\text{—}OH} > \underset{3^\circ}{CH_3\text{—}C(CH_3)_2\text{—}OH} \text{ in acidity}$$

See Section 7.20.1 for general comments on *physical properties* of organic compounds. The greater polarity (dipole moment) and, especially, hydrogen bonding account for the greater solubility of alcohols in water, and the higher boiling points than comparable alkanes, alkenes, aldehydes, ketones and alkyl halides. As the carbon chain gets longer this nonpolar hydrocarbon chain overshadows the – OH group and alcohols become less soluble in water.

II. Chemical Reactions:

The three major types of reactions of alcohols are dehydration, substitution, elimination, and oxidation.

Dehydration reactions: The dehydration of alcohols is catalyzed by acids and the relative ease of dehydration decreases in the order from tertiary to secondary to primary alcohols. In dehydration of tertiary and secondary alcohols an intermediate carbocation is formed and the faster reaction occurs with molecules that form the more stable carbocation. Rearrangements occur if a more stable carbocation can be formed by a methyl or hydride shift. The mechanism for dehydration is:

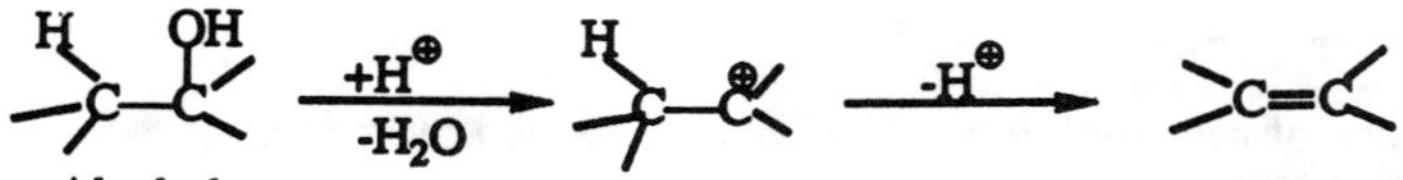

$$\underset{\text{Alcohol}}{H\text{-}C\text{-}C\text{-}OH} \xrightarrow[-H_2O]{+H^{\oplus}} H\text{-}C\text{-}C^{\oplus} \xrightarrow{-H^{\oplus}} \underset{\text{Alkene}}{>C{=}C<}$$

In general dehydration reactions occur to yield the most substituted alkene as the major product in accordance with Zaitsev's rule. Thus the alkene formed is the most stable. Note that a phenyl group (C_6H_5 –) takes preference over one or two alkyl groups.

Some examples:

$CH_3-CH(OH)-CH(CH_3)_2 \xrightarrow{H^{\oplus}} (CH_3)(H)C{=}C(CH_3)_2 > H_2C{=}C(H)-CH(CH_3)_2$

$C_6H_5-CH_2-CH(OH)-CH(CH_3)_2 \xrightarrow{H^{\oplus}} C_6H_5-CH_2-\overset{\oplus}{C}H-CH(CH_3)_2 > C_6H_5-CH_2-CH{=}C(CH_3)_2$

$CH_3-CH_2-C(OH)(CH_3)_2 > CH_3-CH(OH)-CH(CH_3)_2$ in rate of reaction

$CH_3-C(CH_3)_2-CH(OH)-CH_3 \xrightarrow{H^+} (CH_3)_2C{=}C(CH_3)_2$ (Major) $+ CH_2{=}C(CH_3)-CH(CH_3)-CH_3$ (Minor)

$CH_3CH_2CH_2CH_2OH \xrightarrow{H^+}$ trans-$CH_3CH{=}CHCH_3$ (Major) + cis-$CH_3CH{=}CHCH_3$ (Minor) + $CH_3CH_2CH{=}CH_2$ (Minor)

Alcohol substitution reactions: The substitution reactions of alcohols usually involve the replacement of the – OH by a halide (usually Cl or Br) using a variety of reagents (HCl, HBr, HI, PCl_3, $SOCl_2$). The rate of reaction between an alcohol and a hydrogen halide depends upon the structure of the alcohol and the nature of the halide. The mechanism for the reaction of secondary, tertiary, allylic, and benzylic alcohols involves the formation of a carbocation via a S_N1-type process with the protonated alcohol as substrate. Methanol and primary alcohols react by an S_N2 mechanism and require more rigorous conditions and/or the addition of acidic reagents such as $ZnCl_2$ or H_2SO_4 to promote reaction. The reactivity of the various hydrogen halides is in the order of their acidity, i.e., HI>HBr>HCl>>HF (in order of decreasing acidity and reactivity).

General mechanism:

$$ROH + HX \rightarrow ROH_2^+ + X^- \rightarrow R^+ + HOH \xrightarrow{X^-} R\text{-}X$$

Mechanism for primary alcohol

$$RCH_2OH + HX \rightarrow \overset{\delta-}{X}—\underset{R}{\underset{|}{CH_2}}—\overset{\delta+}{OH_2} \rightarrow RCH_2X + HOH$$

Some examples:

$H_2C{=}CH-CH_2-OH$ (I) $\xrightarrow{HCl}$ $H_2C{=}CH-CH_2-Cl$

$CH_3-CH_2-C(CH_3)_2-OH$ (II) $\xrightarrow{HBr}$ $CH_3-CH_2-C(CH_3)_2-Br$ (II)

$CH_3CH_2CH_2OH$ (III) $\xrightarrow[\Delta]{HCl,\ ZnCl_2}$ $CH_3CH_2CH_2-Cl$

(I) > (II)> (III) in rate of reaction.

Rearrangements may occur via carbocation intermediate.

$$(CH_3)_2CH-\overset{OH}{\overset{|}{C}H}-CH_3 + HBr \rightarrow (CH_3)_2\overset{Br}{\overset{|}{C}}-CH_2CH_3$$

Primary, secondary, allylic and benzyl alcohols react readily with $SOCl_2$, PCl_3, and PBr_3 to yield the corresponding halide.

$$ROH + SOCl_2 \rightarrow RCl + SO_2 + HCl$$

$$3ROH + PBr_3 \rightarrow 3RBr + H_3PO_3$$

Substitution reactions of alkyl halides:

Alkyl halides undergo a number of synthetically useful substitution reactions in which the halogen (the leaving group) is replaced by a nucleophile. The overall reaction is:

$$R\text{–}L + Nu^- \rightarrow R\text{–}Nu + L^-$$

Typical nucleophiles (Nu^-) include F^-, Cl^-, Br^-, I^-, CN^-, RO^-, HO^-, RS^-, HS^-, N_3^-.

nucleophilic substitution reactions can be described by two mechanisms:

S_N2—substitution nucleophilic bimolecular
S_N1—substitution nucleophilic unimolecular

The S_N2 mechanism involves a concerted attack by the nucleophile on the substrate in the rate determining step. The rate follows second-order kinetics and is dependent on the concentration of the substrate and the nucleophile. Doubling the concentration of either the substrate or the nucleophile will cause the rate to double. If both concentrations are doubled, the reaction will proceed four times faster.

$$\text{Rate} = k_2[RL][Nu^-]$$

The process involves attack of the nucleophile from the side opposite the leaving group and results in inversion of configuration. The opposite enantiomer is formed if the alkyl halide is chiral to begin with.

$$CH_3O^- + H\text{---}\overset{CH_3CH_2}{\underset{CH_3}{C}}\text{—}Br \longrightarrow \overset{\delta^-}{CH_3O}\cdots\overset{H\quad CH_2CH_3}{\underset{CH_3}{C}}\cdots\overset{\delta^+}{Br} \longrightarrow CH_3O\text{—}\overset{CH_2CH_3}{\underset{CH_3}{C}}\cdots H$$

(S) - (+) - 2 -Bromobutane *(R) - (-) - 2 -Methyoxybutane*

Steric factors are important in S_N2 reactions. The less crowded the transition state the more rapid the reaction. The order of reaction is $CH_3X > 1°RX > 2° RX > 3° RX$

Methyl halides and primary halides undergo substitution by the S_N2 process. Secondary halides may react by either mechanism depending upon the nucleophile and the solvent. In the presence of a strong nucleophile secondary halides will react by the S_N2 process whereas in the presence of a weak nucleophile in a polar solvent they may react by an S_N1 process. Tertiary halides generally do not react by an S_N2 process.

The order of reactivity of leaving groups is:

$$I^- > Br^- > Cl^- >> F^-$$

A negatively charged nucleophile is more reactive than a neutral one. $RO^- > ROH$, $RS^- > RSH$, $OH^- > ROH$.

Ordinarily, if the nucleophilic atom is the same, the more basic nucleophile is the more reactive, i.e., $RO^- > RCOO^-$.

The S_N1 mechanism is a two-step process involving formation of a carbocation. The rate is dependent only on the concentration of the substrate. Rate = $k_1[RL]$

$RL \rightarrow R^+ + L^-$ (rate determining step)
$R^+ + Nu^- \rightarrow RNu$

The S_N1 process is also favored by the use of polar solvents which stabilize the transition state leading to the carbocation. If the substrate is chiral the S_N1 reaction results in racemization (Section 7.1.1.2). In most cases racemization is not complete and more of the enantiomer having the inverted configuration is formed. In many S_N1 reactions the solvent, such as an alcohol or water, serves as the nucleophile and the reaction is termed solvolysis.

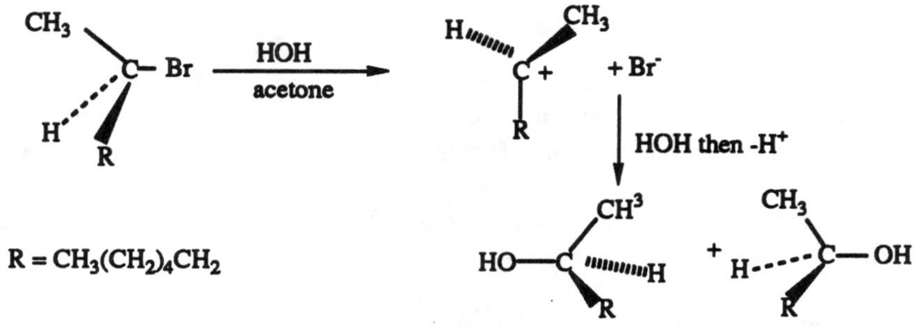

CH3 / H / R — C — Br →(HOH, acetone) H, CH3, R — C+ + Br⁻ →(HOH then -H⁺) HO—C(CH3)(H)(R) + H---C(CH3)(R)—OH

R = $CH_3(CH_2)_4CH_2$

The rate of the reaction is dependent on the stability of the carbocation formed, therefore, 3°RX > 2°RX > 1°RX > CH_3X. Generally only tertiary and secondary halides react by a S_N1 mechanism. Because the S_N1 process involves the formation of a carbocation, rearrangements may occur as shown below:

$$(CH_3)_2CHCH(Br)CH_3 \xrightarrow{\text{HOH - acetone}} (CH_3)_2C(OH)CH_2CH_3$$

The S_N1 process also is accompanied by alkene formation resulting from the loss of a proton from the common intermediate, the carbocation. This elimination process is referred to as an E_1 reaction. E_1 reactions occur under the same conditions and simultaneously with S_N1 reactions. In solvolysis reactions at lower temperatures, the S_N1 reaction is favored over the E_1 reaction. Substitution reactions of tertiary halides are not very useful as synthetic reactions since elimination occurs readily especially if the nucleophile is a moderately strong base. In the presence of strong bases, tertiary halides tend to react by the E_2 process described below.

It should be noted that vinyl halides ($>C{=}CX$) and aryl halides (C_6H_5X) are unreactive by either S_N1 or S_N2 processes.

The conversion of alcohols to alkyl halides may be considered as S_N1 or S_N2 processes depending upon the type of alcohol.

S_N1	$ROH + HX \rightarrow ROH_2^+ + X^-$
3° and 2° ROH	$ROH_2^+ \rightarrow R^+ + HOH$
	$R^+ + X^- \rightarrow RX$
S_N2	$ROH + HX \rightarrow ROH_2^+ + X^-$
Most 1° ROH & CH_3OH	$X^- + ROH_2^+ \rightarrow \overset{\delta-}{X}\text{---}R\text{---}\overset{\delta+}{OH_2} \rightarrow RX + HOH$

Elimination reactions (dehydrohalogenation reactions of alkyl halides): The treatment of an alkyl halide with a strong base such as potassium hydroxide or potassium ethoxide in ethanol on heating results in the formation of alkenes. Dehydrohalogenation reactions, also called β or 1,2-eliminations, generally occur by an E_2 mechanism. The E_2 process is a concerted second-order reaction in which the rate is dependent on the concentration of the alkyl halide and the base, rate = k[RX][base]. The reaction rate also is dependent on the nature and type of alkyl halide. The order of reactivity is:

3°RX > 2°RX > 1°RX
RI > RBr > RCl > RF

E_2 reactions occur most rapidly when the hydrogen and the halogen are in an anti-periplanar relationship as shown in the general mechanism below.

$$\text{H}-\text{C}(\ldots)-\text{C}(\text{X})(\ldots) + \text{B}^- \longrightarrow \left[\text{B}^{\delta-}\cdots\text{H}\cdots\text{C}\text{-----}\text{C}\cdots\text{X}^{\delta}\right] \longrightarrow \text{C}=\text{C} + \text{BH} + \text{X}^-$$

The reaction occurs to give the more stable alkene according to Zaitsev's rule and the trans isomer is favored over the cis isomer. Rearrangements do not occur. The use of a bulky base such as potassium t-butoxide in t-butyl alcohol favors elimination over substitution and this is especially important in the case of primary halides where S_N2 substitution competes with E_2 elimination. Tertiary halides tend to undergo elimination reactions very readily, and in the presence of strong base elimination is favored over substitution. Increased reaction temperature also favors elimination.

Some examples:

$$(CH_3)_2C(Br)CH_2CH_3 + KOCH_2CH_3 \xrightarrow{CH_3CH_2OH} \underset{\text{major}}{(CH_3)_2C=CHCH_3} + \underset{\text{minor}}{CH_2=C(CH_3)CH_2CH_3}$$

$$(CH_3)_3CBr + NaOCH_2CH_3 \longrightarrow (CH_3)_3OCH_2CH_3 + CH_2=C(CH_3)_2$$

	$(CH_3)_3OCH_2CH_3$	$CH_2=C(CH_3)_2$
25°	10%	90%
55°	0%	100%

$$CH_3CH(Br)CH_2CH_3 + (CH_3)_3COK \longrightarrow \underset{20\%}{CH_2=CHCH_2CH_3} + \underset{20\%}{\text{cis-}CH_3CH=CHCH_3} + \underset{60\%}{\text{trans-}CH_3CH=CHCH_3}$$

$$CH_3(CH_2)_{15}CH_2CH_2Br + CH_3OK \longrightarrow \underset{1\%}{CH_3(CH_2)_{15}CH=CH_2} + \underset{99\%}{CH_3(CH_2)_{16}CH_2OCH_3}$$

with $(CH_3)_3COK$ 85% + 15% $CH_3(CH_2)_{16}CH_2OC(CH_3)_3$

Oxidation reactions: Oxidation can convert alcohols to aldehydes, carboxylic acids, or ketones depending upon the structure of the alcohol, the oxidizing agent and the reaction conditions. Primary alcohols can be oxidized to aldehydes, then to carboxylic acids with potassium permanganate or acidic potassium dichromate.

Example:

$$RCH_2OH \longrightarrow RCH=O \longrightarrow RCOOH$$

$$RCH_2OH \xrightarrow{KMnO_4 \text{ or } K_2Cr_2O_7,\ H^+} RCOOH$$

Primary alcohols may be oxidized to aldehydes using chromium trioxide-pyridine complex (Collins' reagent) in an anhydrous medium such as dichloromethane or by copper oxide.

$$RCH_2OH \xrightarrow{CuO,\ \Delta} RCH=O$$

$$RCH_2OH \xrightarrow{(C_5H_5N)_2CrO_3} RCH=O$$

Secondary alcohols are readily oxidized to ketones by the same reagents, especially chromium compounds, that are used to oxidize primary alcohols. These oxidations usually stop at the ketone stage since further oxidation would require the breaking of a carbon to carbon bond.

$$RCH(OH)R^1 \xrightarrow{K_2Cr_2O_7,\ H^+} R-C(=O)-R^1$$

Note that tertiary (3°) alcohols are not oxidized under basic conditions but may be oxidized under acidic conditions by being dehydrated first and then by the double bond being oxidized.

Alcoholism: Methanol is a very toxic alcohol and its ingestion may lead to blindness and death. In the body it is oxidized to formaldehyde and then to formic acid. It is not certain whether the formaldehyde or formic acid attacks the cells of the retina and causes blindness. However it is known that the formation of formic acid can cause acidosis in the blood leading to death. Ethanol is first oxidized to acetaldehyde by an enzyme, alcohol dehydrogenase, and then to other products. One treatment of alcohol addiction involves the use of the drug disulfuram (trade name—Antabuse) which prevents further oxidation of acetaldehyde leading to its build-up in the body which causes nausea, vomiting and sweating. Taking disulfuram may cause aversion to drinking alcohol.

7.21.1.2 ALDEHYDES AND KETONES

I. Nomenclature:

See Section 7.20 for the basics of nomenclature. *Aldehydes* are generally symbolized as

$$R-\overset{O}{\overset{\|}{C}}-H.$$

and the suffix -al replaces the -e of alkanes:

$$H-\underset{H}{\overset{H}{\underset{|}{\overset{|}{C}}}}-\overset{O}{\overset{\|}{C}}-H$$

ethanal
(acetaldehyde)

$$\underset{(6)}{CH_3}-\underset{(5)}{CH_2}-\underset{(4)}{\overset{CH_3}{\overset{|}{CH}}}-\underset{(3)}{CH_2}-\underset{(2)}{CH_2}-\underset{(1)}{\overset{O}{\overset{\|}{C}}}-H$$

4-Methylhexanal
the aldehyde carbon is always #1

Ketones are generally symbolized as

$$R-\overset{O}{\overset{\|}{C}}-R'$$

and the suffix -one replaces the -e of alkanes:

$$CH_3-\overset{O}{\overset{\|}{C}}-CH_3$$

acetone <u>or</u>
2-Propanone
(the location of the $\left(\overset{O}{\overset{\|}{C}}\right)$ is always shown)

$$CH_3-CH_2-CH_2-\overset{O}{\overset{\|}{C}}-CH_2-CH_3$$

3-Hexanone <u>or</u>
Ethyl propyl ketone

II. Importance of Carbonyl Group:

The *carbonyl group* $(\overset{O}{\overset{\|}{C}})$ is the basis for the chemistry of aldehydes and ketones. The key features are:

(1) Polarity of C = O bond. The oxygen is attacked by electrophiles (E ⊕), and the carbon by nucleophiles (N: ⊖).

Both of these disrupt the double bond:

large dipole moment

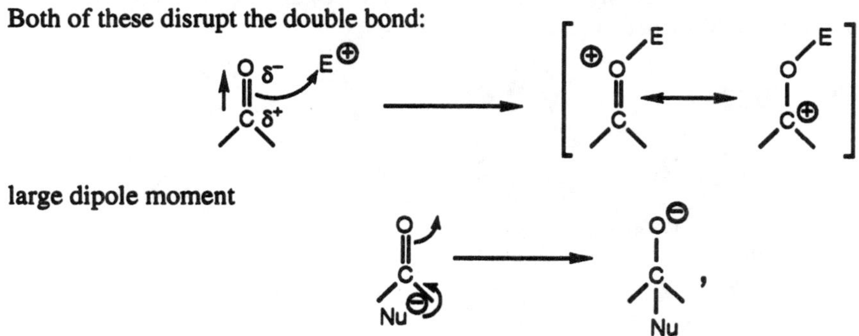

(2) The α-hydrogen is acidic and can be abstracted by bases. It is even more acidic if between two carbonyls:

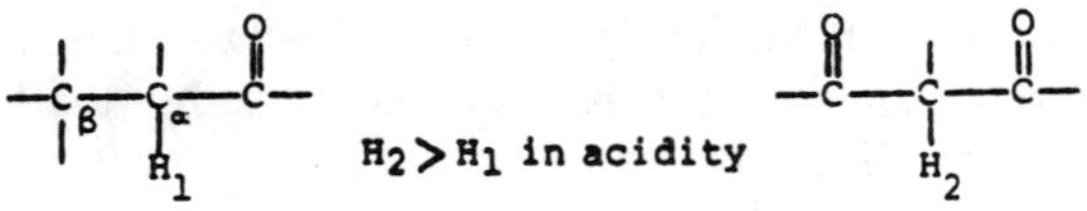

$H_2 > H_1$ in acidity

(3) The main reason for the acidity of the α-H is that the resulting α-carbanion is stabilized by resonance. This stabilization also allows for nucleophilic addition at the β-carbon in α-β unsaturated carbonyls:

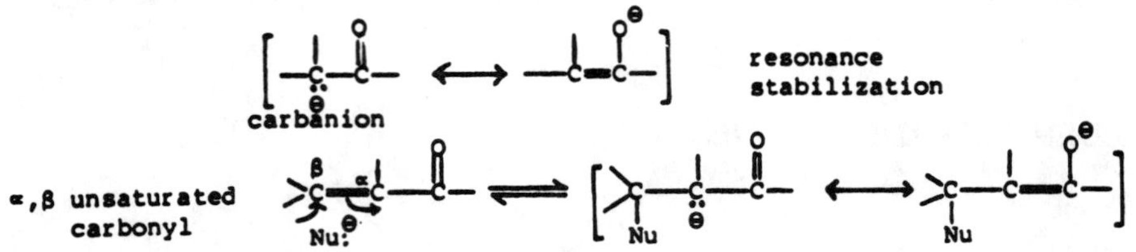

carbanion

resonance stabilization

α,β unsaturated carbonyl

(4) The carbonyl form of an aldehyde or ketone exists in equilibrium with the enol form. The enol form is a structure having a hydroxyl group attached to a double bonded carbon. This equilibrium is referred to as keto-enol tautomerism. Tautomers are compounds whose structures differ in the location of an atom, normally a proton, but which exist in equilibrium. Usually the equilibrium greatly favors the keto forms.

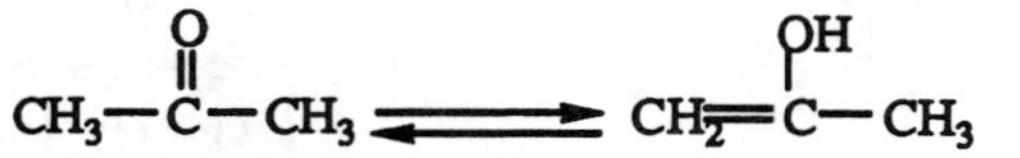

$$CH_3-C(=O)-CH_3 \rightleftharpoons CH_2=C(OH)-CH_3 \qquad K = 6 \times 10^{-9}$$

For 1,3-dicarbonyl compounds the enol form is often the major tautomer due to the stabilization provided by intramolecular hydrogen bonding and conjugation of the carbonyl group with the double bond.

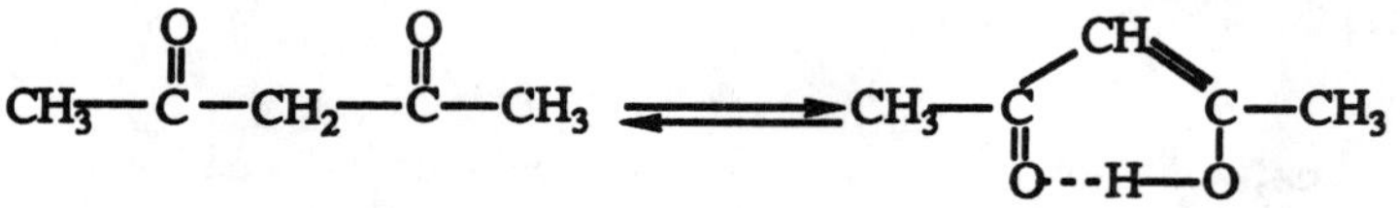

$$CH_3-C(=O)-CH_2-C(=O)-CH_3 \rightleftharpoons CH_3-C(=O \cdots H-O)-CH=C-CH_3$$

(5) The O of the carbonyl forms hydrogen bonds with H's attached to other O's or N's:

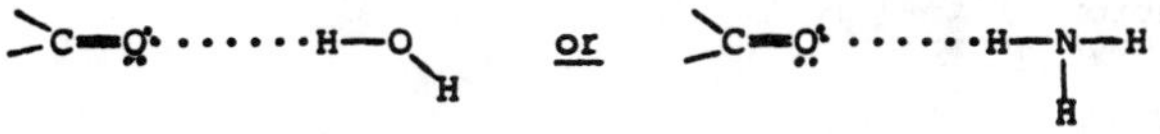

$$>C=\ddot{O}: \cdots\cdots H-O-H \quad \text{or} \quad >C=\ddot{O}: \cdots\cdots H-NH-H$$

Most of the reactions and properties of carbonyls may be understood on the basis of the above features. In general, aldehydes oxidize easier and undergo nucleophilic addition easier than ketones.

The *boiling point* of aldehydes and ketones is higher than most other polar organic molecules but less than that of alcohols and acids (each can hydrogen bond to molecules of itself). The low molecular weight aldehydes and ketones are soluble in water because they can form hydrogen bonds with it—as the molecular weights increase, they hydrocarbon part dominates and solubility decreases.

Reduction reactions of carbonyls are:

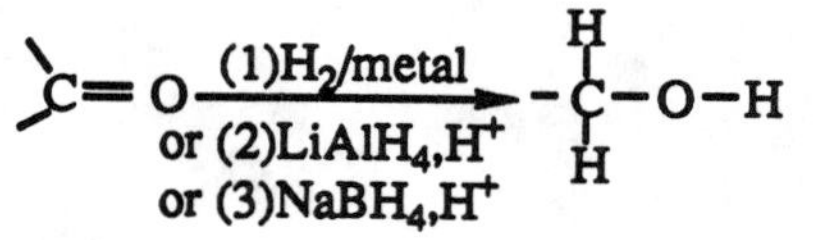

$$>C=O \xrightarrow[\text{or (2)LiAlH}_4\text{,H}^+ \text{ or (3)NaBH}_4\text{,H}^+]{(1)H_2/\text{metal}} -C(H)(H)-O-H$$

III. Oxidation reactions of Aldehydes and Ketones:

Oxidation reactions of aldehydes are:

(1) $\underset{(Ar)}{RCHO} \xrightarrow[\text{(Tollen's Reagent)}]{Ag(NH_3)_2^+\ H_2O} \underset{(Ar)}{R\text{-}CO_2H} + Ag(mirror)$

Ar = Aromatic   Benedict's Reagent is also used

(2) $\underset{(Ar)}{RCHO} \xrightarrow[\text{or}]{(1)KMnO_4} \underset{(Ar)}{RCO_2H}$

$(2)K_2Cr_2O_7$

(3) Ketones are rarely oxidized.

IV. Nucleophilic Addition Reactions:

Nucleophilic addition reactions

(1) Addition of nitrogen bases to carbonyls. The N needs two H's to add:

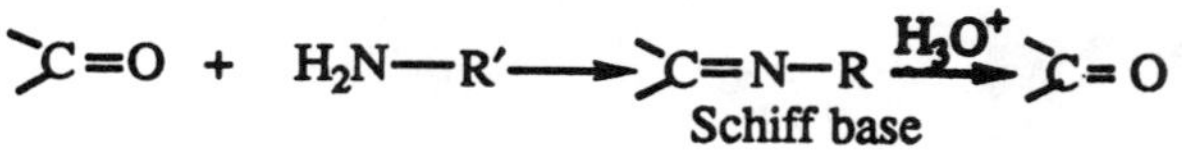

$>C=O + H_2N-R' \longrightarrow >C=N-R \xrightarrow{H_3O^+} >C=O$

Schiff base

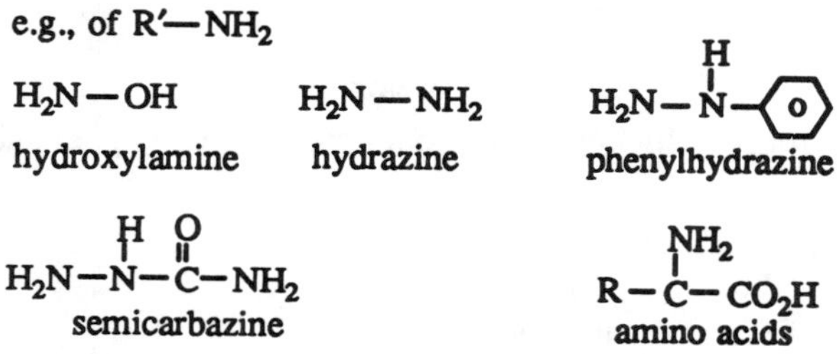

e.g., of $R'-NH_2$

H_2N-OH hydroxylamine

H_2N-NH_2 hydrazine

$H_2N-NH-C_6H_5$ phenylhydrazine

$H_2N-NH-C(=O)-NH_2$ semicarbazine

$R-CH(NH_2)-CO_2H$ amino acids

(2) Acetal (ketal) and hemiacetal (hemiketal) formation

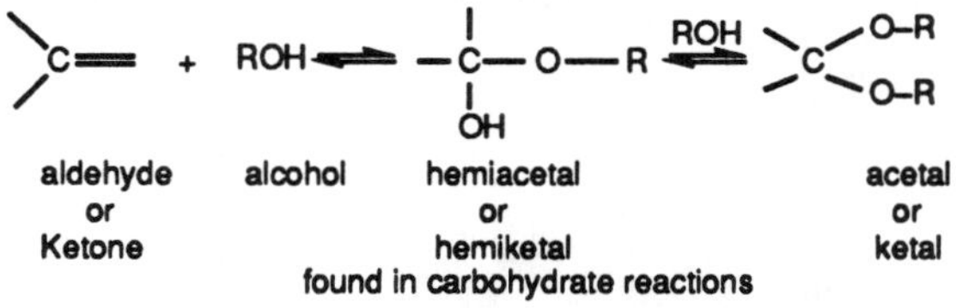

$>C= \;+\; ROH \rightleftharpoons -C(OH)-O-R \xrightleftharpoons{ROH} >C(O\text{-}R)_2$

aldehyde or Ketone; alcohol; hemiacetal or hemiketal; acetal or ketal

found in carbohydrate reactions

(3) The Aldol condensation of carbonyls. The α-H is important:

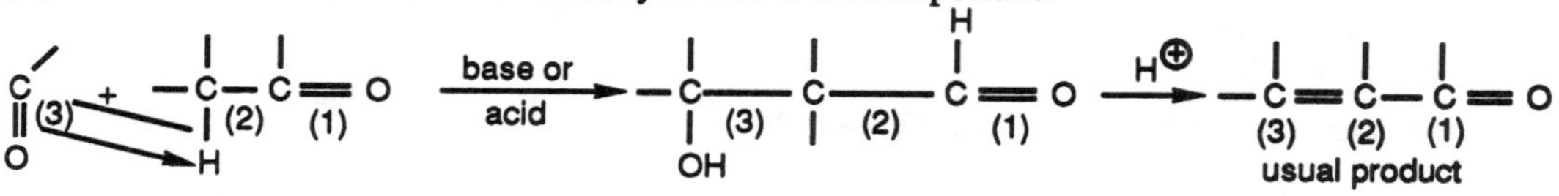

$>C=O \;(3) + H-C-C=O \;(2)\;(1) \xrightarrow[\text{acid}]{\text{base or}} -C(OH)-C(H)-C=O \;(3)\;(2)\;(1) \xrightarrow{H^{\oplus}} -C=C-C=O \;(3)\;(2)\;(1)$

usual product

(4) Nucleophilic addition to α, β-unsaturated carbonyls:

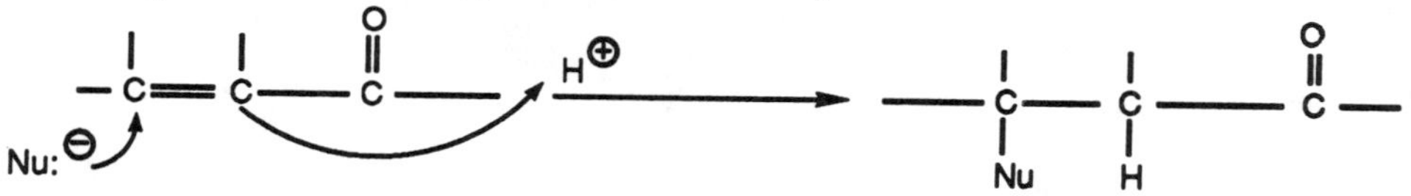

$-C=C-C(=O)- \;\; Nu:^{\ominus},\; H^{\oplus} \longrightarrow -C(Nu)-C(H)-C(=O)-$

e.g., $Nu:^{\ominus}$'s (do not have to be negative; need pair of electrons)

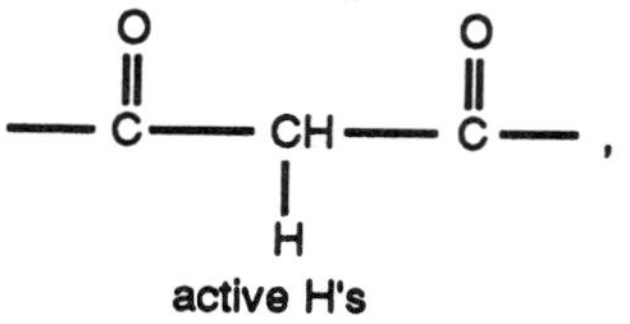

$-C(=O)-CH(H)-C(=O)-$, amines, $:CN^{\ominus}$.

active H's

7.21.2 Questions Related to Alcohols, Aldehydes and Ketones

1. Alcohols have _______ boiling points and _______ solubility in water than corresponding alkanes and alkenes which is due to _______.

   A. lower, lesser, hydrogen bonding
   B. higher, greater, hydrogen bonding
   C. lower, lesser, polarity
   D. higher, lesser, polarity

2. In the dehydration reaction of alcohols, the _______ stable double bond is formed.

   A. most
   B. least
   C. complete
   D. incomplete

3. Which of the following alcohols undergoes a substitution reaction the fastest?

   A. primary
   B. secondary
   C. allyl
   D. tertiary

4. Which of the following types of alcohols is not normally oxidizable?

   A. primary
   B. secondary
   C. tertiary
   D. all of these are oxidizable

5. Which type of alcohol probably undergoes substitution by an S_N2 mechanism?

   A. primary
   B. tertiary
   C. allyl
   D. none of these

6. Name the following alcohol:

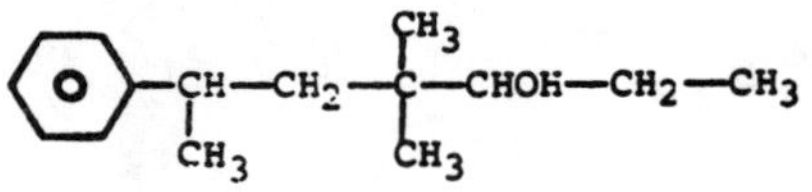

   C_6H_5—CH(CH_3)—CH_2—C(CH_3)(CH_3)—CHOH—CH_2—CH_3

   A. 2-Phenyl-4, 4-dimethyl heptanol
   B. 4,4-Dimethyl-6-phenyl-3-heptanol
   C. Phenyl-2-heptanol
   D. none of these

7. Select the strongest acid of the following:

   A. CH_3—CH(CH_3)—OH

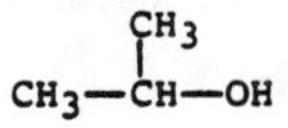

   B. CH_3—CH_2—CH(CH_3)—OH

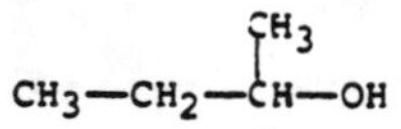

   C. CH_3—CH_2—C(CH_3)(CH_3)—OH

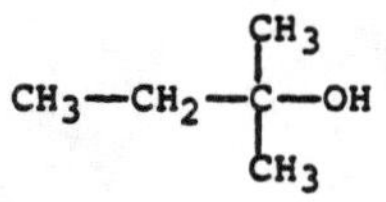

   D. CH_3—CH_2—CH_2—OH

8. Which alcohol is least soluble in water?

A. 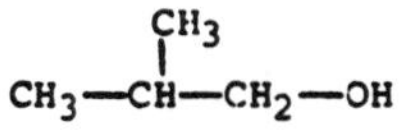 $CH_3—CH(CH_3)—CH_2—OH$

B. $CH_3—CH_2—CH_2—CH_2—CH_2—CH_2—OH$

C. $CH_3—CH_2—OH$

D. CH_3OH

9. Which alcohol will be dehydrated the fastest?

A. 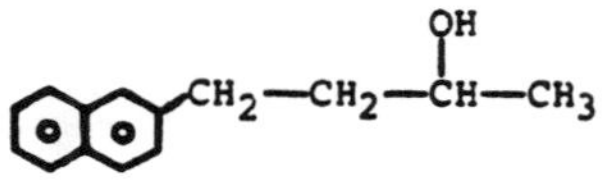 (naphthyl)$—CH_2—CH_2—CH(OH)—CH_3$

B. 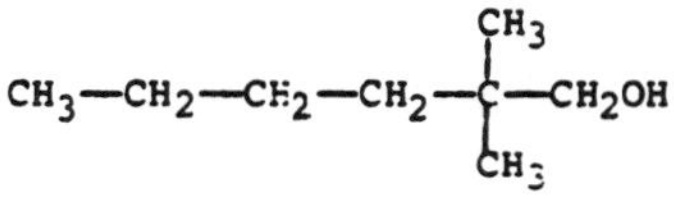 $CH_3—CH_2—CH_2—CH_2—C(CH_3)_2—CH_2OH$

C. $CH_3—CH(CH_3)—CH_2—C(CH_3)_2—OH$

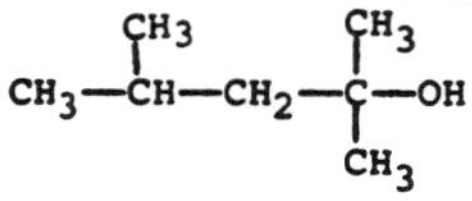

D. all at the same rate

10. What is the most likely (or greatest) product of the following reaction?

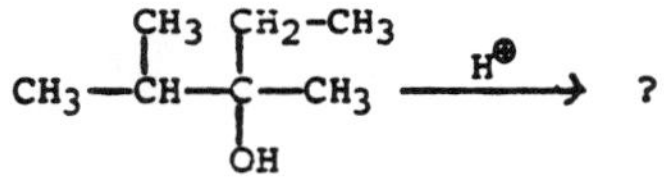

$CH_3—CH(CH_3)—C(CH_2—CH_3)(OH)—CH_3 \xrightarrow{H^{\oplus}} ?$

A. $(H_3C)_2C{=}C(CH_2—CH_3)(CH_3)$

B. $(H_3C)(CH_3)CH—C({=}CH—CH_3)(CH_3)$

C. $(H_3C)_2CH—C(CH_2—CH_3){=}CH_2$

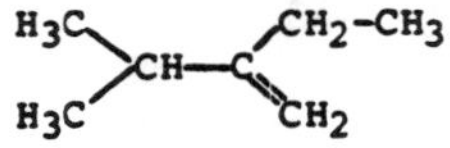

D. all are equal

11. What is the most likely product of the following reaction:

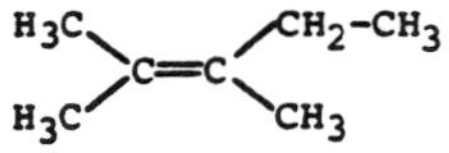

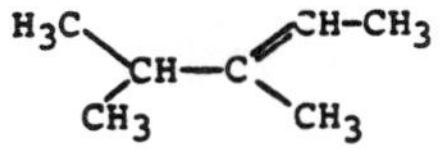

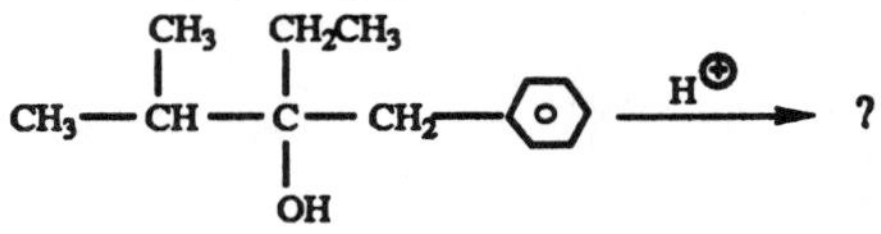

$CH_3—CH(CH_3)—C(CH_2CH_3)(OH)—CH_2—C_6H_5 \xrightarrow{H^{\oplus}} ?$

A. $(H_3C)_2C{=}C(CH_2CH_3)(CH_2—C_6H_5)$

B. $(CH_3)_2CH—C({=}CHCH_3)(CH_2—C_6H_5)$

C. $(CH_3)_2CH—C(CH_2CH_3){=}CH—C_6H_5$

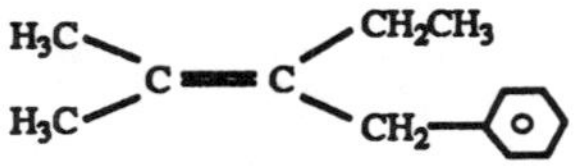

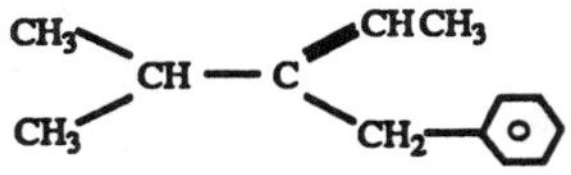

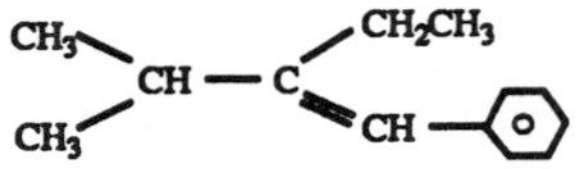

D. all are equal

12. Which alcohol will undergo the fastest reaction with HBr?

A. 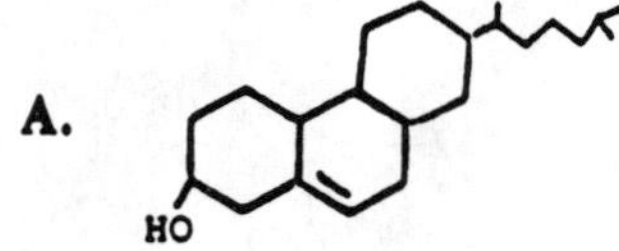

B. CH_3CH_2OH

C. 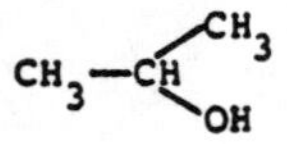 $CH_3{-}CH(CH_3)(OH)$

D. 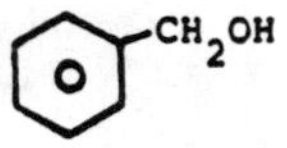 (benzene ring)$-CH_2OH$

13. The carbonyl group is ________ with the carbon being slightly ________ and the oxygen being slightly ________

A. polarized, negative, positive.
B. polarized, positive, negative.
C. polarized, positive, positive.
D. polarized, negative, negative.

14. Which hydrogen is the most acidic?

A. H_1
B. H_2
C. H_3
D. H_4

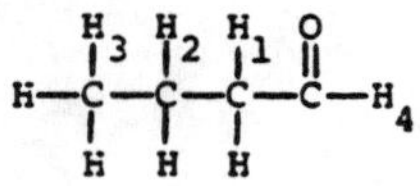

$$H{-}\overset{H_3}{\underset{H}{C}}{-}\overset{H_2}{\underset{H}{C}}{-}\overset{H_1}{\underset{H}{C}}{-}\overset{O}{\overset{\|}{C}}{-}H_4$$

15. Which of the following will undergo nucleophilic addition more easily?

A. Aldehydes
B. Alkenes
C. Both equally
D. Neither

16. Aldehydes and ketones have higher boiling points than corresponding compounds (similar carbon structures) of all the following except:

A. alkanes.
B. alkenes.
C. ethers.
D. alcohols.

17. Which of the following groups are rarely oxidized?

A. aldehydes
B. ketones
C. neither of these
D. both of these

18. Name the following compound:

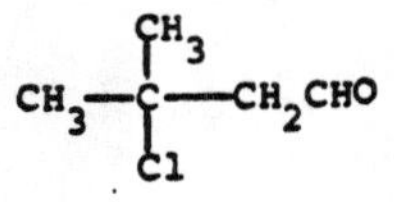

$$CH_3{-}\overset{CH_3}{\underset{Cl}{C}}{-}CH_2CHO$$

A. tert-chlorobutanal
B. tert-chlorobutyl ketone
C. hydrogen chloro-tert-butyl ketone
D. 3-chloro-3-methyl-butanal

19. Name the following compound:

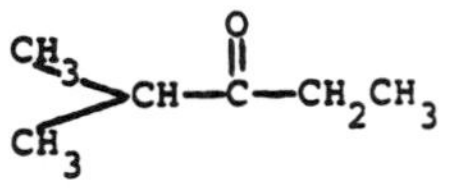

$$(CH_3)_2CH-\overset{O}{\overset{\|}{C}}-CH_2CH_3$$

A. 2-methyl-3-pentanone
B. diethyl methyl ketone
C. 2-methyl-3-butanal
D. isobutyl ethyl ketone

20. Select the product of the following reaction:

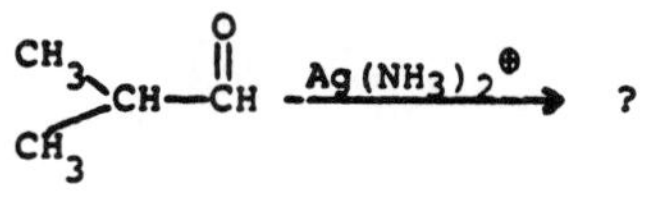

$$(CH_3)_2CH-\overset{O}{\overset{\|}{C}}H \xrightarrow{Ag(NH_3)_2^{\oplus}} ?$$

A. $(CH_3)_2CH-CH(OH)-CH(OH)-CH(CH_3)_2$

B. $(CH_3)_2CH-C(O{-}H)(H)-H$

C. $(CH_3)_2C=CH_2$

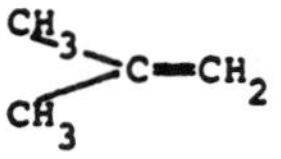

D. 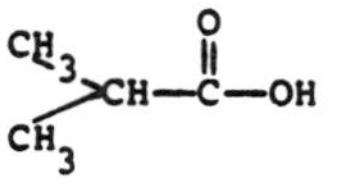 $(CH_3)_2CH-\overset{O}{\overset{\|}{C}}-OH$

21. Select the product of the following reaction:

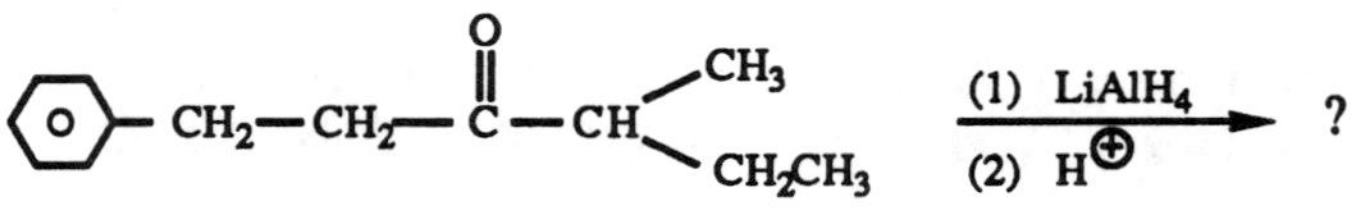

$$C_6H_5-CH_2-CH_2-\overset{O}{\overset{\|}{C}}-CH(CH_3)(CH_2CH_3) \xrightarrow[(2)\ H^{\oplus}]{(1)\ LiAlH_4} ?$$

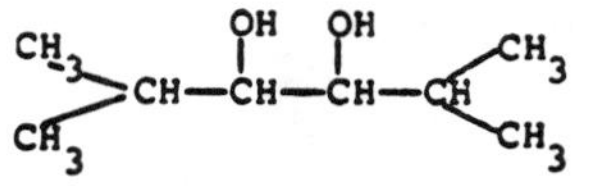

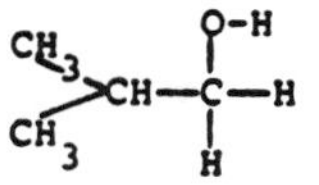

A. 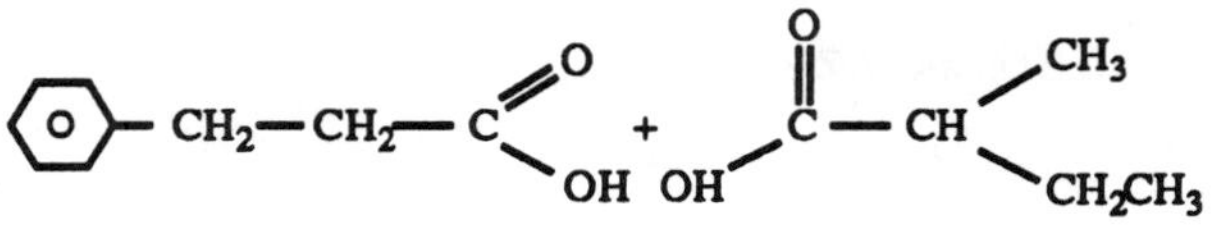 $C_6H_5-CH_2-CH_2-C(=O)OH \;+\; HO-\overset{O}{\overset{\|}{C}}-CH(CH_3)(CH_2CH_3)$

B. $C_6H_5-CH_2-CH_2-C(OH)(H)-CH(CH_3)(CH_2-CH_3)$

C. $C_6H_5-CH_2-CH_2-\overset{O}{\overset{\|}{C}}-H \;+\; H-\overset{O}{\overset{\|}{C}}-CH(CH_3)(CH_2-CH_3)$

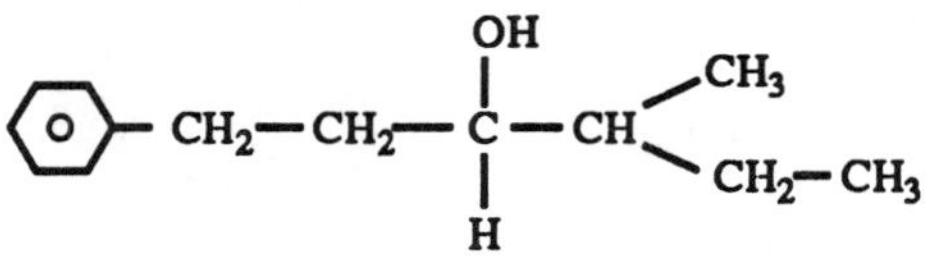

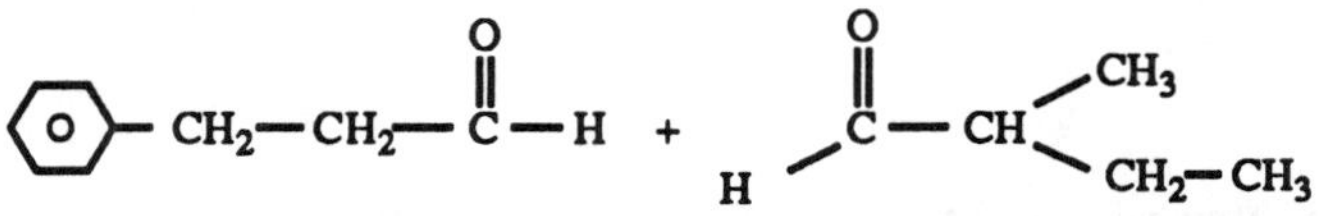

D. none of the above

22. Select the product of the following reaction:

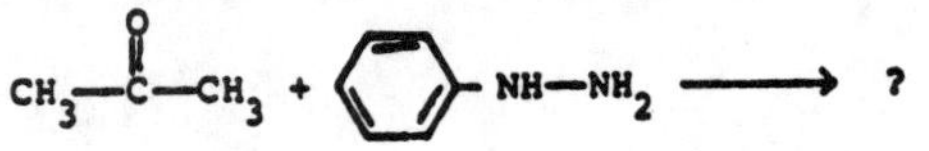

$CH_3-C(=O)-CH_3 + C_6H_5-NH-NH_2 \longrightarrow ?$

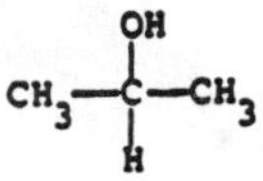

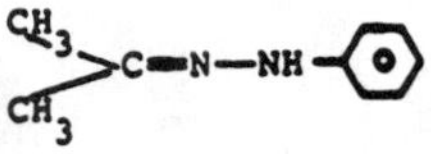

A. $CH_3-C(OH)(H)-CH_3$

B. $(CH_3)_2C=N-NH-C_6H_5$

C. $(CH_3)(H_3C)C=N(C_6H_5)NH_2$

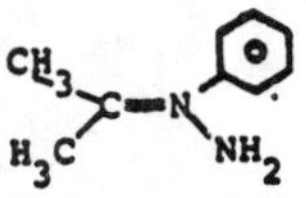

D. none of the above

23. Select the product of the following reaction:

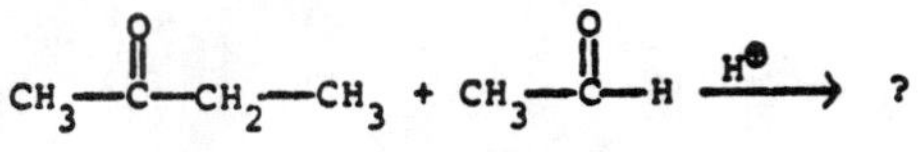

$CH_3-C(=O)-CH_2-CH_3 + CH_3-C(=O)-H \xrightarrow{H^{\oplus}} ?$

A. no reaction

B. 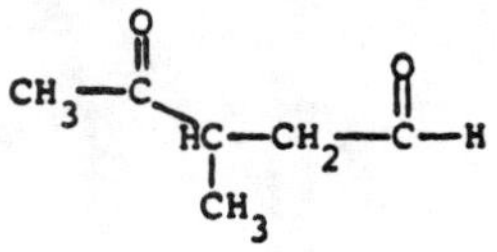 $CH_3-C(=O)-CH(CH_3)-CH_2-C(=O)-H$

C. $(CH_3)(H_3C-CH_2)C=CH-C(=O)-H$

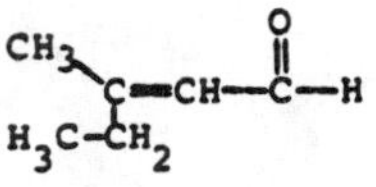

D. none of the above

7.21.3 Answers to Questions in Section 7.21.2

(1) B (2) A (3) C (4) C (5) A (6) B (7) D (8) B (9) C (10) A (11) C (12) D
(13) B (14) A (15) A (16) D (17) B (18) D (19) A (20) D (21) B (22) B (23) C

7.21.4 Discussion of Answers to Questions in Section 7.21.2

Questions #1 to #5 Discussed in Section.

Question #6 (Answer: B) The numbering is,

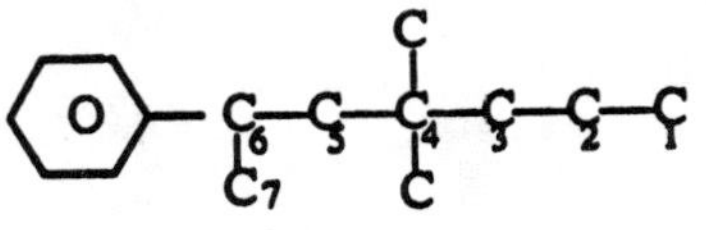

C₆H₅–C(6)(C7)–C(5)–C(4)(C)(C)–C(3)–C(2)–C(1)

Question #7 (Answer: D) Primary alcohols are stronger than similar 2° or 3° alcohols.

Question #8 (Answer: B) The longer the carbon chain, the lower the solubility in water.

Question #9 (Answer: C) Tertiary alcohols undergo dehydration faster than the 1° or 2° alcohols shown.

Question #10 (Answer: A) The most substituted double bond will be the one that is formed.

Question #11 (Answer: C) The double bond will be most stable when conjugated with the benzene ring even though it is not the most substituted.

Question #12 (Answer: D) Substitution reactions are faster for benzyl (shown) or allyl type alcohols.

Question #13 to #17 Discussed in Section.

Question #18 (Answer: D) This is an aldehyde numbered as

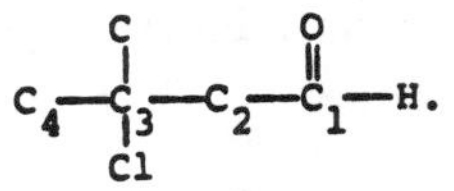

$C_4-C_3(C)(Cl)-C_2-C_1(=O)-H.$

Question #19 (Answer: A) The numbering of this ketone is

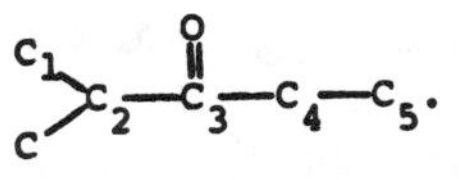

$C_1(C)>C_2-C_3(=O)-C_4-C_5.$

An alternate name is: Ethyl isopropyl ketone

Question #20 (Answer: D) This is an oxidation reaction as shown in the Section.

Question #21 (Answer: B) This is a reduction reaction as shown in the Section.

Question #22 (Answer: B) To add to the carbonyl, the N must have two H's (i.e., $-NH_2$). The N attached to the benzene ring does not complete the reaction.

Question #23 (Answer: C) There are many possible products of this reaction. The key is that the α-carbon of one carbonyl attacks the carbonyl of the other. Other possible products are:

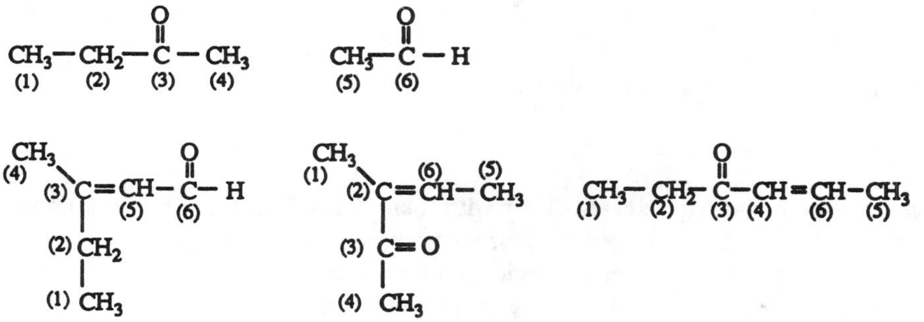

$\underset{(1)}{CH_3}-\underset{(2)}{CH_2}-\underset{(3)}{C}(=O)-\underset{(4)}{CH_3}$ $\underset{(5)}{CH_3}-\underset{(6)}{C}(=O)-H$

$\underset{(4)}{CH_3}\underset{(3)}{C}(\underset{(2)}{CH_2}-\underset{(1)}{CH_3})=\underset{(5)}{CH}-\underset{(6)}{C}(=O)-H$
(the answer given)

$\underset{(1)}{CH_3}\underset{(2)}{C}(\underset{(3)}{C}(=O)-\underset{(4)}{CH_3})=\underset{(6)}{CH}-\underset{(5)}{CH_3}$

$\underset{(1)}{CH_3}-\underset{(2)}{CH_2}-\underset{(3)}{C}(=O)-\underset{(4)}{CH}=\underset{(6)}{CH}-\underset{(5)}{CH_3}$

7.21.5 Advanced Concepts

This is a list of tools to analyze and understand alcohols, aldehydes and ketones.

- Improve review of observations linked with types and quantities and reactants and products. Identify all possible experiments to be performed. Propose any experimental modifications or new procedures to be used.
- Understand how reactions are related to basic mechanisms; how reaction rates are affected; what bonding arrangements, resonance stability structures and stereoarrangements are possible. Elucidate each mechanism in a visual format.
- Ask yourself, how can organic chemistry of medical compounds (alcohols, aldehydes and ketones) be investigated, identified and linked to the biological side effects (both microscopic and physiological).
- What biological disorders result from deficiency or abundance of medical compounds (aldehydes, alcohols and ketones), especially bioorganic molecules? e.g., protein deficiency, enzyme deficiency, etc.
- Determine how organic reaction mechanisms translate into biochemical reaction mechanisms, e.g., metabolism.

- Learn how to judge the influence of new experimental evidence on each conclusion, including experimental conditions, experimental errors and practical limitations on experiment.
- Look for hidden assumptions behind each experimental technique or procedure, theoretical explanation and practical explanation of each mechanism.
- Look for scientific reasons behind each observation (laboratory observations, untaught observations from experimental data and completely new observations).
- Determine deductive conclusions from observations in order to approve or nullify your hypotheses.

7.22 CARBOXYLIC ACIDS AND DERIVATIVES, ETHERS AND PHENOLS (Oxygen-Containing Compounds)

7.22.1 See Section 7.21.1 on "Introduction to Oxygen-Containing Compounds"

7.22.1.1 CARBOXYLIC ACIDS (Oxygen-Containing Compounds)

I. Nomenclature:

See Section 7.2 and 7.20 on general nomenclature. The -e of alkanes is replaced by -oic acid for carboxylic acids:

$CH_3–CH_2–CH_2–CH_3$
Butane

$CH_3–CH_2–CH_2–CO_2H$
(4) (3) (2) (1)
Butanoic acid

The – CO_2H carbon is always numbered #1 as above. Other rules are as before. For example:

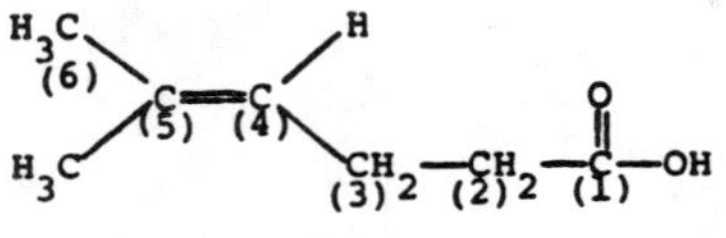

$(H_3C)(H_3C)C{=}CH–CH_2–CH_2–C({=}O)–OH$
(6) (5) (4) (3) (2) (1)

5-Methyl-4-hexenoic acid

Shown below are some common carboxylic acids along with their IUPAC names. Their common names are given in parentheses. Many acids are better known by their common names and the IUPAC nomen-clature rules are prone to accept such common names as benzoic acid as a permissible alternative to the systematic ones. Note that in naming dicarboxylic acid, the e of the alkane name is not dropped.

	$H–C({=}O)–OH$	$CH_3–C({=}O)–OH$	$C_6H_5–COOH$
IUPAC	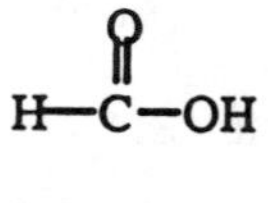 methanoic acid	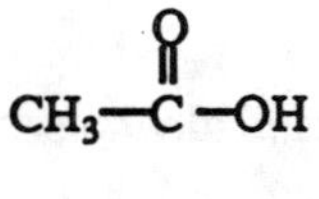 ethanoic acid	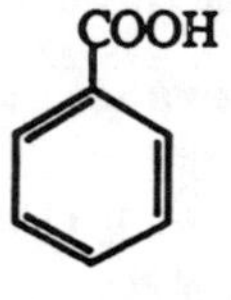 benzenecarboxylic acid
Common	(formic acid)	(acetic acid)	(benzoic acid)

	HOOC—COOH	$HOOC–CH_2–CH_2–COOH$
IUPAC	ethanedioic acid	butanedioic acid
Common	(oxalic acid)	(succinic acid)

The key functional group of these compounds is the carboxyl,

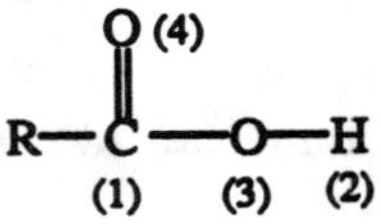

$R–C({=}O)–O–H$
O (4); C (1); O (3); H (2)

II. Properties of Carboxylic Acids:

Low molecular weight aliphatic carboxylic acids tend to be *soluble* in water due to hydrogen bonding with water; aromatic acids are not, in general, soluble. The acids are also soluble in dilute bases, NaOH or $NaHCO_3$, e.g., because of their acid properties. The *boiling points* are high because of the hydrogen bonding possible between molecules.

Carboxylic acids are the *acids* of organic chemistry. The only other compounds which approach their acid strength are substituted phenols (see Section 7.22.1.5). Organic classes of molecules by decreasing acid strength are:

$$RCO_2H > ArOH > HOH > ROH > HC = CH > NH_3 > RH$$

(substituted phenols may be stronger acids than H_2O).

The relative base strength is just the reverse. In order of decreasing base strength:

$$R\theta > NH_2\,\theta > HC = C\,\theta > RO\,\theta, > HO\theta > ArO > RCO_2\theta$$

The *relative acid strength* of carboxylic acids depends primarily on the groups attached and the distance of these groups from the carboxyl:

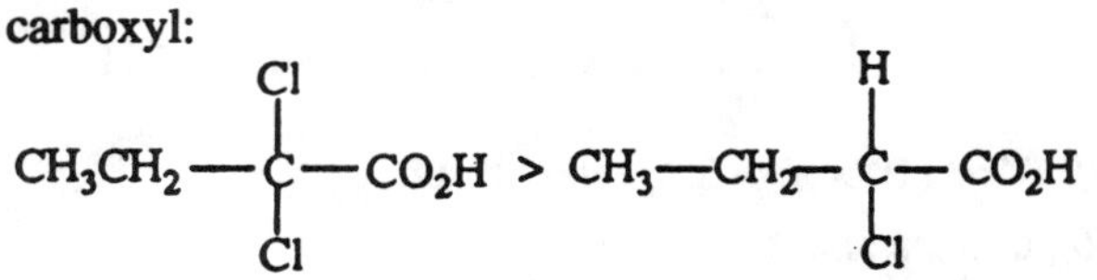

$$CH_3CH_2-CCl_2-CO_2H > CH_3-CH_2-CHCl-CO_2H \quad \text{in acid strength}$$

Cl is an electron withdrawer and stabilizes the carboxylate anion

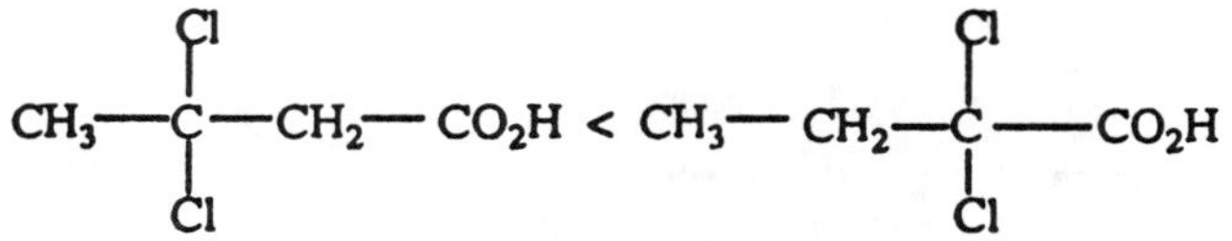

$$CH_3-CCl_2-CH_2-CO_2H < CH_3-CH_2-CCl_2-CO_2H \quad \text{in acid strength}$$

Dicarboxylic acids have two ionization constants (K_1 and K_2). The first ionization constant is larger than that for a comparable monocarboxylic acid due to the fact that there are two sites for ionization and also one carboxyl group is electron withdrawing, aiding the ionization of the other. The ionization constant of the second carboxyl group is lower since it is more difficult to remove a proton from an anion than from a neutral molecule.

CH_3-CH_2-COOH	$K = 1.3 \times 10^{-5}$	$HOOC-CH_2-COOH$	$K_1 = 1.4 \times 10^{-3}$
propanoic acid (propionic acid)		propanedicarboxylic acid (malonic acid)	$K_2 = 2 \times 10^{-6}$

III. Carboxyl Group Reactions:

Reactions of the carboxylic acids center around the four central features of the carboxyl group:

(1) The H(2) is acidic because it is weakly attached to the O(3) and because the resulting carboxylate anion is stabilized by resonance

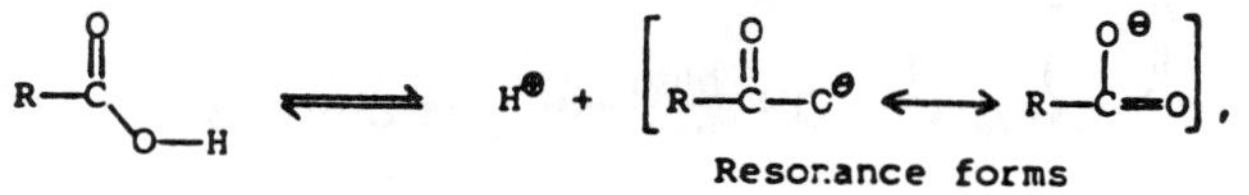

$$R-C(=O)-O-H \rightleftharpoons H^{\oplus} + \left[R-C(=O)-O^{\ominus} \longleftrightarrow R-C(-O^{\ominus})=O\right].$$

Resonance forms

(2) The carboxyl carbon (1) is very susceptible to attack by nucleophilic agents (Nu; see Section 7.23.1) because of the attached electronegative oxygens and the carbonyl oxygen (4):

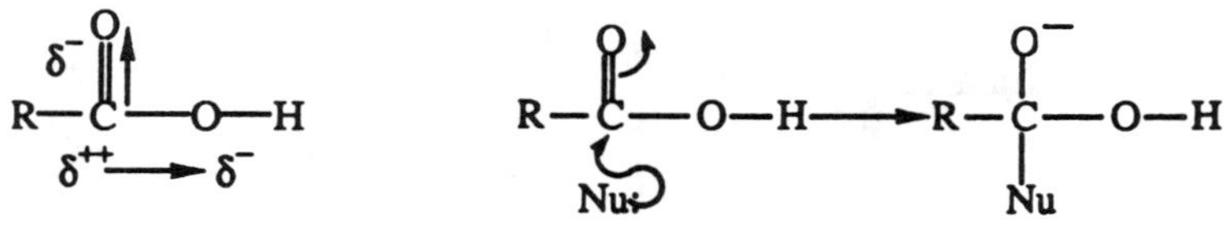

$$\overset{\delta^-}{O}{=}C(R)-O-H \quad \delta^{++} \rightarrow \delta^- \qquad R-C(=O)-O-H \xrightarrow{Nu} R-C(O^-)(Nu)-O-H$$

(3) The hydroxyl can become a good leaving group by appropriate solvent conditions (e.g., if basic) and/or by protonating if acidic solution and this also promotes nucleophilic substitution,

$$Nu:^- + R-\overset{O}{\overset{\|}{C}}-\overset{+}{O}H_2 \longrightarrow R-\overset{O}{\overset{\|}{C}}-Nu + HOH$$

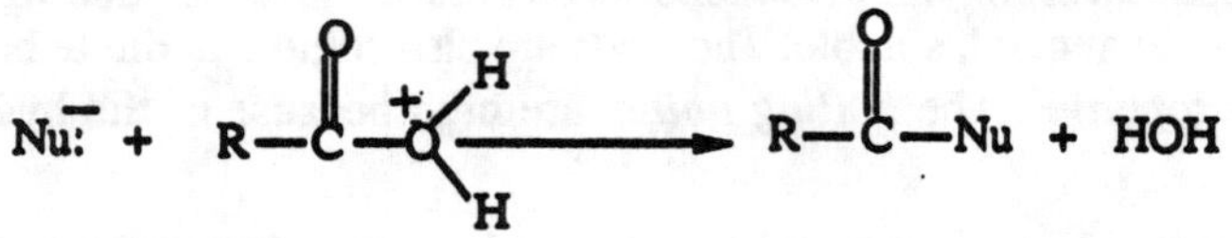

(4) Hydrogen bonding is possible between molecules (intermolecular) and/or within the same molecule (intramolecular) because of the carbonyl and hydroxyl moieties,

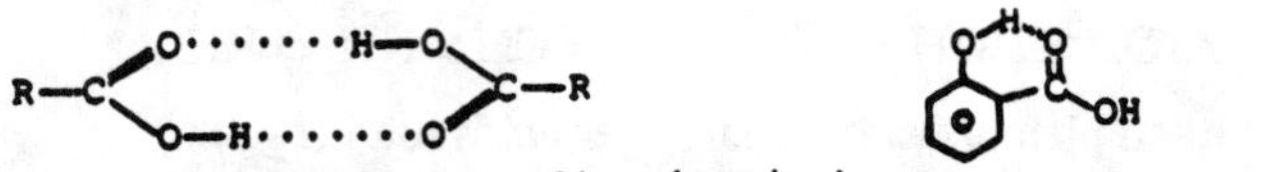

Intermolecular (dimerization) Intramolecular

Nucleophilic substitution reactions can involve a variety of nucleophiles (Nu) reacting under a variety of conditions,

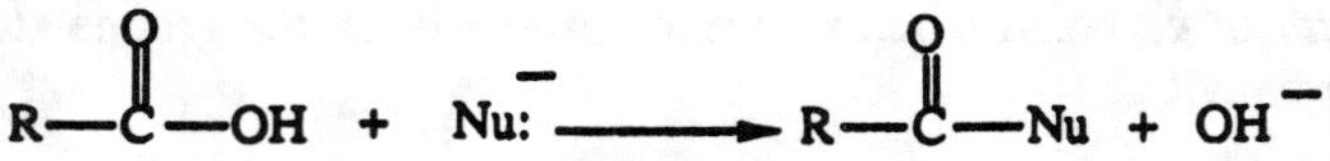

$$R-\overset{O}{\overset{\|}{C}}-OH + Nu:^- \longrightarrow R-\overset{O}{\overset{\|}{C}}-Nu + OH^-$$

Nu: = – OR′ R′ = (1° > 2° > 3°), esters result
= – NH_2, amides result
= – Cl_2 from $SOCl_2$ or PCl_3 or PCl_5, acid chlorides result

In the ester reaction,

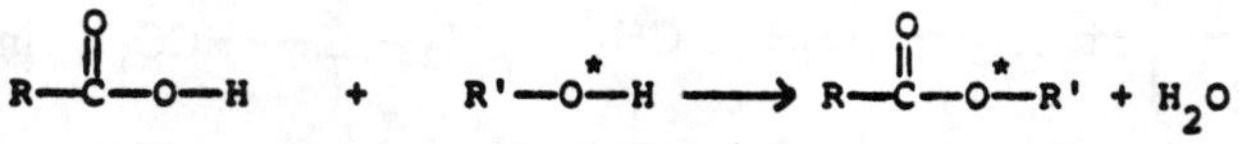

$$\underset{\text{acid}}{R-\overset{O}{\overset{\|}{C}}-O-H} + \underset{\text{alcohol}}{R'-\overset{*}{O}-H} \longrightarrow \underset{\text{ester}}{R-\overset{O}{\overset{\|}{C}}-\overset{*}{O}-R'} + H_2O$$

note the origin of the O^*

The major *reduction reaction* is with $LiAlH_4$:

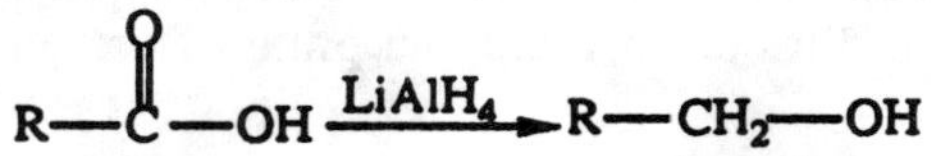

$$R-\overset{O}{\overset{\|}{C}}-OH \xrightarrow{LiAlH_4} \underset{\text{alcohol}}{R-CH_2-OH}$$

Acids can be converted to esters or amides and then reduced also.

Decarboxylation reaction involves β-diacids or β-ketoacids:

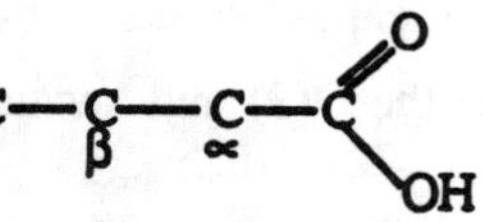

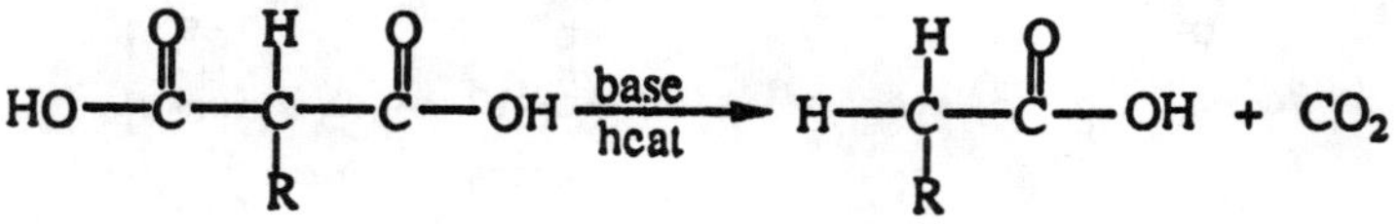

$$\underset{\delta}{C}-\underset{\beta}{C}-\underset{\alpha}{C}-C(=O)OH$$

$$HO-\overset{O}{\overset{\|}{C}}-\underset{R}{\overset{H}{C}}-\overset{O}{\overset{\|}{C}}-OH \xrightarrow[\text{heat}]{\text{base}} H-\underset{R}{\overset{H}{C}}-\overset{O}{\overset{\|}{C}}-OH + CO_2$$

β- diacid

$$R-\overset{O}{\overset{\|}{C}}-CH_2-\overset{O}{\overset{\|}{C}}-OH \xrightarrow[\text{heat}]{\text{base}} R-\overset{O}{\overset{\|}{C}}-CH_3 + CO_2$$

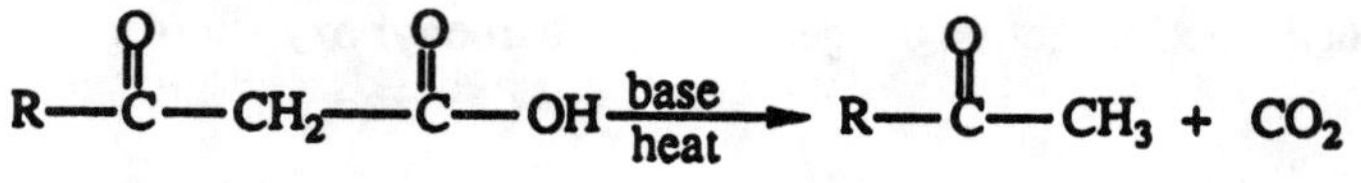

β- Ketoacid

7.22.1.2 AMIDES (Carboxylic Acid Derivatives)

See *nomenclature* of carboxylic acids (Section 7.22.1). The -oic acid (or -ic acid) is changed to -amide, e.g.:

$$\text{3-Methyl butanoic acid: } (H_3C)_2CH{-}CH_2{-}C(=O){-}OH \qquad (CH_3)_2CH{-}CH_2{-}C(=O){-}NH_2 \text{ 3-Methyl butanamide}$$

If the N is substituted, this feature is added as follows:

$$(H_3C)_2CH{-}CH_2{-}C(=O){-}N(CH_3)_2$$

N, N - Dimethyl -3- methyl butanamide

The *boiling points* of unsubstituted and monosubstituted amides are very high due to strong intermolecular hydrogen bonds. Disubstituted amides have boiling points like ketones or aldehydes (due to the carbonyl moiety). Amides have essentially no *acidity* (as compared to carboxylic acids) and no *basicity* (as compared to amines).

Amides are *formed from* carboxylic acids (or its derivatives) by,

$$R{-}C(=O){-}OH + NH_3 \text{ (or } R{-}NH_2\text{, etc.)} \xrightarrow[\Delta]{} R{-}C(=O){-}NH_2$$

Amides are susceptible to *nucleophilic substitution* at the carbonyl carbon,

$$R{-}C(=O){-}NH_2 + NuH \longrightarrow R{-}C(=O){-}Nu + NH_3$$

Amides undergo hydrolysis back to the original acid and amine under basic or acidic conditions:

$$\underset{\text{amide}}{R{-}C(=O){-}NHR} \xrightarrow[H_2O]{H^{\oplus}} \underset{\text{acid}}{R{-}C(=O){-}OH} + \underset{\text{amine}}{RNH_2}$$

$$R{-}C(=O){-}NHR \xrightarrow{OH^{\ominus}} \underset{\text{amine}}{R{-}NH_2} + \underset{\text{carboxylate}}{R{-}C(=O){-}O^{\ominus}} \xrightarrow{H^{\oplus}} \underset{\text{acid}}{R{-}C(=O){-}OH}.$$

7.22.1.3 ESTERS (Carboxylic Acid Derivatives)

The -oic acid of carboxylic acids is replaced by -oate and the carbon fragment of the ester precedes the base name:

$$\underset{\text{3-Methyl butanoic acid}}{(H_3C)_2CH{-}CH_2{-}C(=O){-}OH} \qquad \underset{\text{Ethyl-3-methyl butanoate}}{(CH_3)_2CH{-}CH_2{-}C(=O){-}O{-}CH_2CH_3}$$

Esters have no *acidity* (because no – OH) and have *boiling points* comparable to ketones and aldehydes because they have carbonyl groups but not hydrogen bonding.

Esters are formed from carboxylic acids (or derivatives) usuallv under acidic conditions.

$$\underset{\text{acid}}{R{-}C(=O){-}OH} + \underset{\text{alcohol}}{R'{-}O^{*}{-}H} \longrightarrow \underset{\text{ester}}{R{-}C(=O){-}O^{*}{-}R.}$$

Esters undergo *nucleophilic substitution* at the carbonyl carbon,

$$R-\overset{O}{\overset{\|}{C}}-O-R' + NuH \longrightarrow R-\overset{O}{\overset{\|}{C}}-Nu + R'OH \qquad Nu = \text{nucleophile}$$

Esters are *hydrolized* by acid or base back to the original acid and alcohol:

$$\underset{\text{ester}}{R-\overset{O}{\overset{\|}{C}}-OR'} \xrightarrow{H^{\oplus}} \underset{\text{acid}}{R-\overset{O}{\overset{\|}{C}}-OH} + \underset{\text{alcohol}}{R'-OH}$$

$$\underset{\text{ester}}{R-\overset{O}{\overset{\|}{C}}-OR'} \xrightarrow{NaOH} \underset{\text{carboxylate ion}}{R-\overset{O}{\overset{\|}{C}}-O^{\ominus}Na^{\oplus}} + R'OH \xrightarrow{H^{\oplus}} \underset{\text{acid}}{R-\overset{O}{\overset{\|}{C}}-OH},$$

Fats are a special class of esters of biologic importance. They are formed as follows:

$$\underset{\substack{\text{fatty acid}\\\text{(long chain acids)}}}{CH_3(CH_2)_{14}CO_2H} + \underset{\text{glycerol}}{\begin{matrix}CH_2OH\\|\\CHOH\\|\\CH_2OH\end{matrix}} \longrightarrow \underset{\substack{\text{monoglyceride}\\\text{(a fat)}}}{\begin{matrix}CH_2-O-\overset{O}{\overset{\|}{C}}-(CH_2)_{14}-CH_3\\|\\CHOH\\|\\CH_2OH\end{matrix}} \longrightarrow II \longrightarrow III.$$

More fatty acids (FA) can be added to the glycerol to form di- (II) and tri-glycerides (III). Fats may be hydrolyzed back to FA's and glycerol by base (a process called *saponification*):

$$\underset{\text{a triglyceride (a fat)}}{\begin{matrix}CH_2-O-\overset{O}{\overset{\|}{C}}-(CH_2)_{14}CH_3\\|\\CH_2-O-\overset{O}{\overset{\|}{C}}-(CH_2)_{14}CH_3\\|\\CH_2-O-\overset{O}{\overset{\|}{C}}-(CH_2)_{14}CH_3\end{matrix}} \xrightarrow{NaOH} \underset{\text{glycerol}}{\begin{matrix}CH_2OH\\|\\CHOH\\|\\CH_2OH\end{matrix}} + \underset{\text{salt of the FA}}{3\,CH_3(CH_2)_{14}CO_2^{\ominus}Na^{\oplus}}$$

7.22.1.4 ETHERS (Oxygen-Containing Compounds)

Ethers have the *general structure:* R—O—R′

R, R′ are aliphatic or aromatic but no H. Ethers are named by naming the R and R′ and following these by 'ether':

$$\underset{\substack{\text{Diethyl ether}\\\text{(or 'ether')}}}{CH_3-CH_2-O-CH_2-CH_3} \qquad \underset{\text{Methyl isopropyl ether}}{CH_3-O-CH\begin{matrix}CH_3\\CH_3\end{matrix}}$$

The *physical properties* of ethers reflect the polar oxygen and the nonpolar hydrocarbon component. There is some solubility in water due to the O hydrogen bonding with H_2O. The boiling points are less than alcohols and about the same as alkanes because there is no hydrogen bonding between the molecules of ether.

Ethers may exist in a cyclic form in which the oxygen is part of the ring. Three important cyclic ethers are shown below. The preparation, physical and chemical properties of cyclic ethers resemble in general those of their open-chain counterparts.

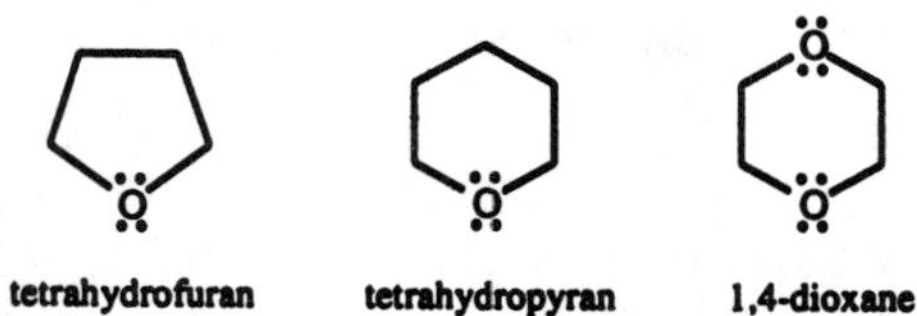

Three membered ring ethers are called epoxides or oxiranes. They are frequently known by their common names as oxides of alkenes.

epoxyethane (ethylene oxide)

epoxypropane (propylene oxide)

Because of bond angle strain, epoxides are much more reactive than are other ethers. They readily undergo acid catalyzed hydrolysis to produce diols. Epoxides also react readily with HX, hydroxide ion, alkoxide ions, and Grignard reagents.

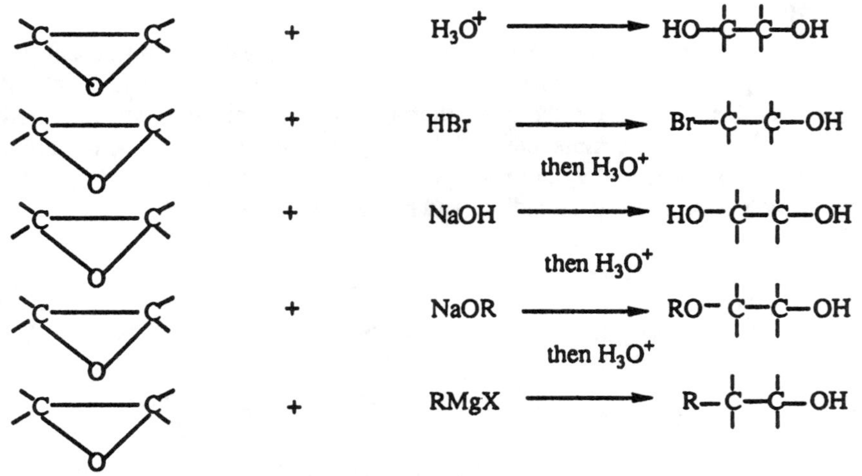

+ H_3O^+ ⟶ HO–C–C–OH

+ HBr ⟶ Br–C–C–OH

+ NaOH ⟶ then H_3O^+ HO–C–C–OH

+ NaOR ⟶ then H_3O^+ RO–C–C–OH

+ RMgX ⟶ then H_3O^+ R–C–C–OH

7.22.1.5 PHENOLS (Oxygen-Containing Compounds)

I. Nomenclature:

A phenol consists of a hydroxyl group attached to an aromatic ring. The *nomenclature* is as given in Section 7.20.1. Some phenols which have counterparts in biochemistry and medicine are:

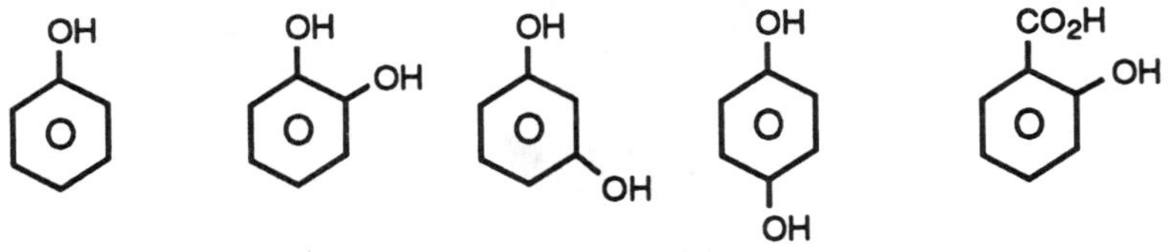

phenol cathechol resorcinol hydroquinone salicylic acid

II. Important features:

(i) Phenols are acidic due to the dissociable hydrogen on the oxygen. Phenols are more acidic than alcohols because of the electron withdrawing and resonance stabilization effects of the aromatic ring:

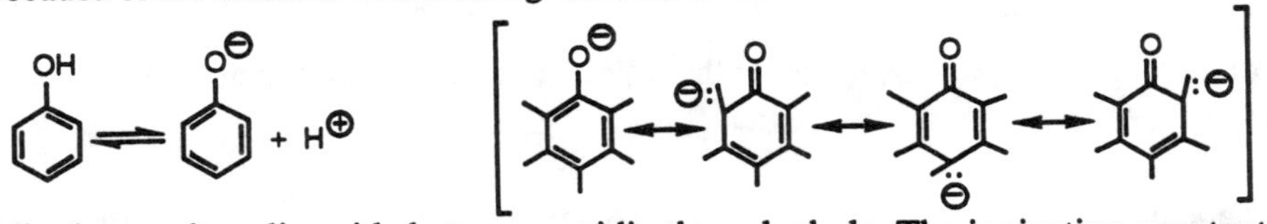

Phenols are less acidic than carboxylic acids but more acidic than alcohols. The ionization constant or acidity constant (K_a) for most phenols is about 10^{-10} ($pK_a = 10$) whereas most carboxylic acids have a K_a of approximately 10^{-5} ($pK_a = 5$). The K_a of alcohols is in the 10^{-16} to 10^{-20} range (pK_a 16-20). Note that $pK_a = -\log K_a$. These differences in acidity are of practical importance and useful in separating phenols from alcohols or carboxylic acids. Phenols will react with dilute sodium hydroxide to form the water soluble sodium phenoxide salt, but phenols do not react with dilute sodium bicarbonate. Carboxylic acids react with dilute sodium bicarbonate or sodium hydroxide to form sodium carboxylate salts whereas alcohols do not react with either sodium hydroxide or sodium bicarbonate.

The resonance forms above show that electron withdrawing meta directing groups such as $-NO_2$, $-CN$, $-COR$, $-COOH$, when placed at the o-p positions, should make the phenol more acidic. These groups can delocalize the negative charge and stabilize the phenoxide ion. Groups which can destablize (and make less acidic) the phenoxide ion are the electron donating o-p directors (see Section 7.24.1).

(ii) Phenols form intramolecular and intermolecular hydrogen bonds (see boiling point discussion below).

(iii) Phenols are powerful o-p directors.

III. Physical properties:

Physical properties are understood by considering the hydrogen bond forming capacity and the hydro-phobic nature of aromatic rings. Even phenol itself is only slightly soluble in water (due to hydrogen bonding), but most other phenols are insoluble due to the aromatic ring. Most phenols will have high boiling points, primarily due to hydrogen bonding between molecules. Within the disubstituted phenols, the ortho compounds tend to have lower boiling points because they have the potential for intramolecular hydrogen bonding whereas meta and para have intermolecular hydrogen bonding (and higher boiling points):

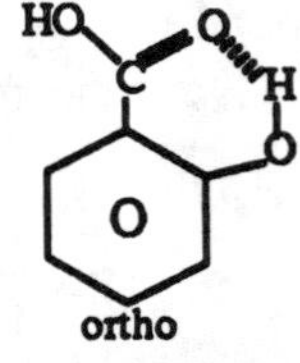

intramolecular hydrogen bonding

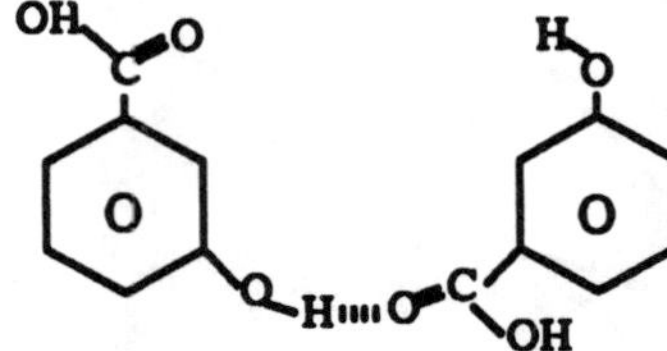

meta (or para) intermolecular hydrogen bonding

7.22.2 Questions Related to Carboxylic Acids and Derivatives, Ethers and Phenols

1. Which atom below is susceptible to nucleophilic attack?

O(III)
‖
CH_3—C—O—H
(I) (II) (IV)

A. I
B. II
C. III
D. IV

2. A high molecular weight carboxylic acid may be soluble in ________ but probably not in ________.

A. dilute acid, dilute base
B. water, dilute acid
C. water, dilute base
D. dilute base, water

3. For comparable compounds, which of the following would be most acidic?

A. water
B. alcohol
C. alkene
D. carboxylic acid

4. Name the following compound:

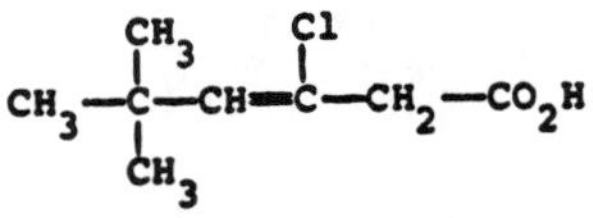

$$CH_3-\underset{CH_3}{\overset{CH_3}{\underset{|}{\overset{|}{C}}}}-CH{=}\overset{Cl}{\overset{|}{C}}-CH_2-CO_2H$$

A. 3-Chloro-5, 5-dimethylhexanoic acid
B. 3-Chloro-5, 5-dimethyl-3-hexenoic acid
C. 2,2-Dimethyl-4-chloro-3-hexenoic acid
D. none of the above

5. Select the compound that is most acidic:

A. 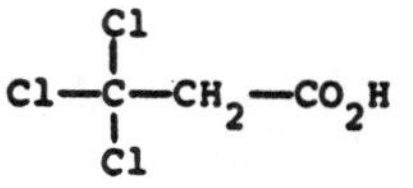 $Cl-\underset{Cl}{\overset{Cl}{\underset{|}{\overset{|}{C}}}}-CH_2-CO_2H$

B. $CH_3-CH_2-CO_2H$

C. 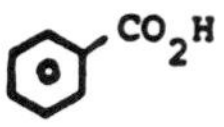 $C_6H_5-CO_2H$

D. all are equal

6. Give the product of the following reaction:

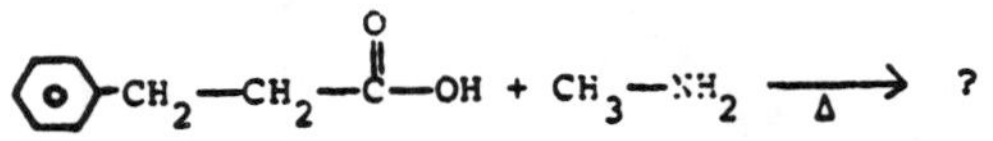

$$C_6H_5-CH_2-CH_2-\overset{O}{\overset{\|}{C}}-OH + CH_3-NH_2 \xrightarrow[\Delta]{} ?$$

A. 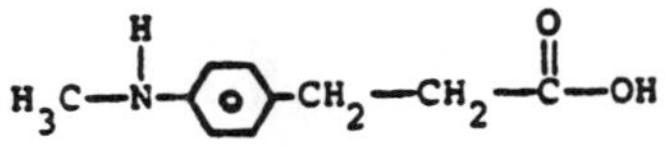 $H_3C-\overset{H}{\overset{|}{N}}-C_6H_4-CH_2-CH_2-\overset{O}{\overset{\|}{C}}-OH$

B. $C_6H_5-CH_2-CH_2-CH_2-OH$

C. $C_6H_5-CH_2-CH_2-CH_2-NH-CH_3$

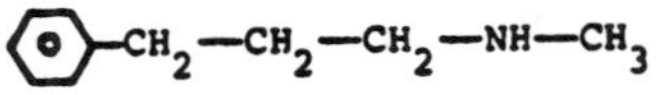

D. none of the above

7. Give the product of the following reaction:

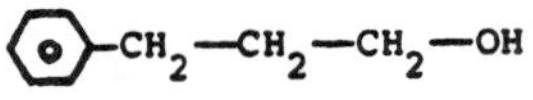

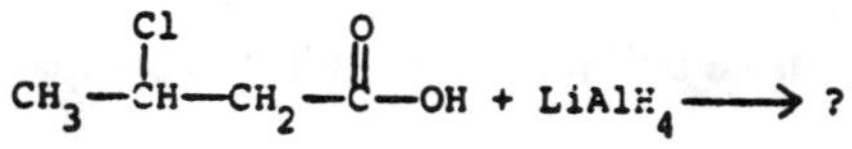

$$CH_3-\overset{Cl}{\overset{|}{C}H}-CH_2-\overset{O}{\overset{\|}{C}}-OH + LiAlH_4 \longrightarrow ?$$

A. $CH_3-\overset{Cl}{\overset{|}{C}H}-CH_2-CH_2-OH$

B. $CH_3-CH{=}CH-\overset{O}{\overset{\|}{C}}-OH$

C. $CH_3-\overset{Cl}{\overset{|}{C}H}-CH_2-\overset{O}{\overset{\|}{C}}-O^{\ominus}Li^{\oplus}$

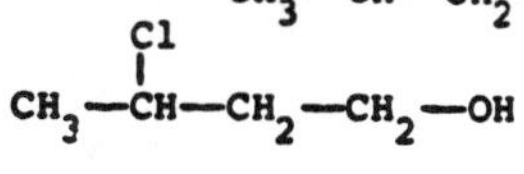

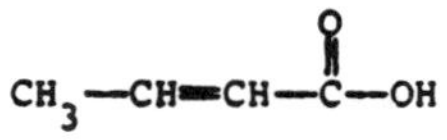

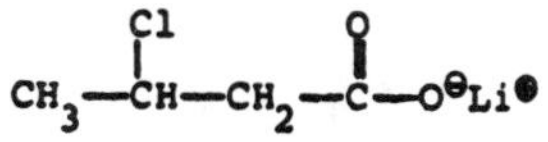

D. none of the above

8. Which of the following compounds has the potential for decarboxylation?

A. 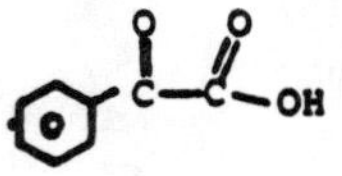 $C_6H_5-\overset{O}{\overset{\|}{C}}-\overset{O}{\overset{\|}{C}}-OH$

B. $C_6H_5-\overset{O}{\overset{\|}{C}}-CH_2-CO_2H$

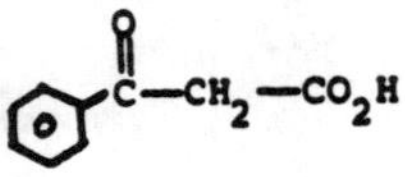

C. $CH_3-CH_2-CH\begin{cases}CO_2H \\ CH_2-CO_2H\end{cases}$

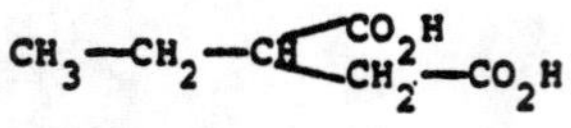

D. none of these

9. Amides have essentially no:

A. acidity.
B. basicity.
C. hydrogen bonding.
D. acidity nor basicity.

10. Fats are _______ and are made of _______ and _______.

A. esters, glycerol, fatty acids
B. amides, an amine, fatty acids
C. ethers, glycerol, fatty acids
D. none of the above

11. Saponification is the _______ of _______.

A. alkaline hydrolysis, fats
B. acidic hydrolysis, fats
C. neutral hydrolysis, amides
D. osmosis, amides

12. Name the following compound:

$(H_3C)_2C=CH-CH_2-\overset{O}{\overset{\|}{C}}-\overset{H}{\overset{|}{N}}-CH_3$

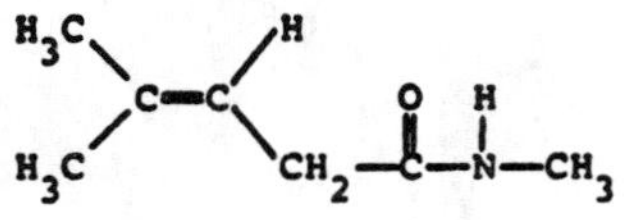

A. N-Methyl-4-Methyl-3-pentenamide
B. 2-Methyl-2-pentenamide
C. Dimethyl pentenamide
D. none of the above

13. Which of the following compounds probably has a boiling point similar to comparable molecular weight ketones or aldehydes?

A. 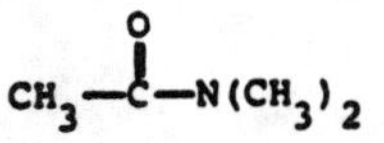 $CH_3-\overset{O}{\overset{\|}{C}}-N(CH_3)_2$

B. $CH_3-\overset{O}{\overset{\|}{C}}-\overset{H}{\overset{|}{N}}CH_3$

C. $CH-\overset{O}{\overset{\|}{C}}-NH_2$

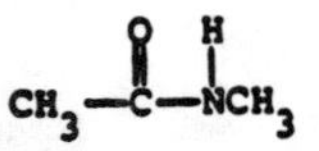

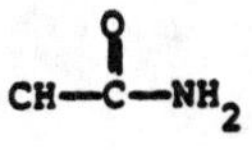

D. none of the above

14. Give the product of the following reaction:

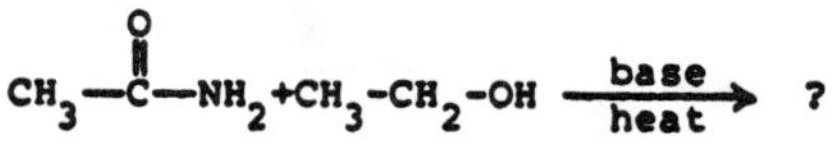

$$CH_3-\overset{O}{\overset{\|}{C}}-NH_2 + CH_3-CH_2-OH \xrightarrow[\text{heat}]{\text{base}} ?$$

A. $CH_3-CH_2-NH_2$

B. 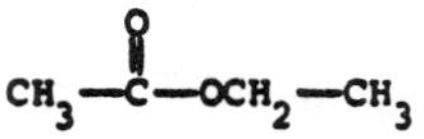 $CH_3-\overset{O}{\overset{\|}{C}}-OCH_2-CH_3$

C. $CH_3-\overset{O}{\overset{\|}{C}}-\overset{H}{\overset{|}{N}}-CH_2-CH_3$

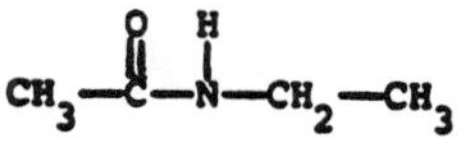

D. none of the above

15. Give the product of the following reaction:

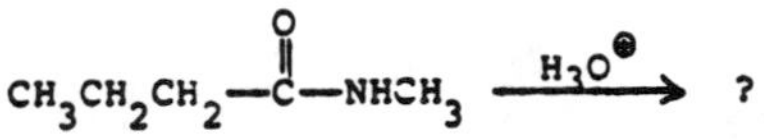

$$CH_3CH_2CH_2-\overset{O}{\overset{\|}{C}}-NHCH_3 \xrightarrow{H_3O^{\oplus}} ?$$

A. 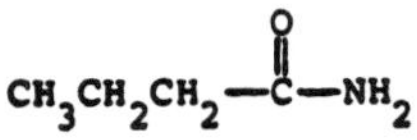 $CH_3CH_2CH_2-\overset{O}{\overset{\|}{C}}-NH_2$

B. $CH_3-CH_2CH_2-CH_2-NH_2$

C. $CH_3-CH_2CH_2-CH_2-OH$

D. none of the above

16. Name the following compound:

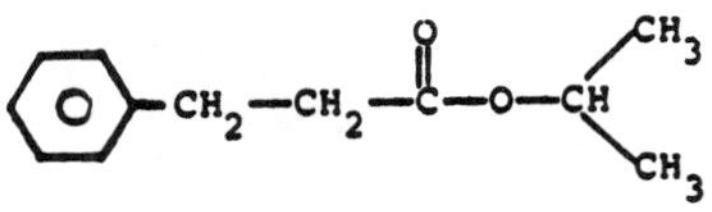

$$C_6H_5-CH_2-CH_2-\overset{O}{\overset{\|}{C}}-O-CH(CH_3)_2$$

A. Isopropyl benzoate
B. Isopropyl 3-phenyl propanoate
C. phenyl isopropyl ester
D. none of the above

17. Give the product of the following reaction:

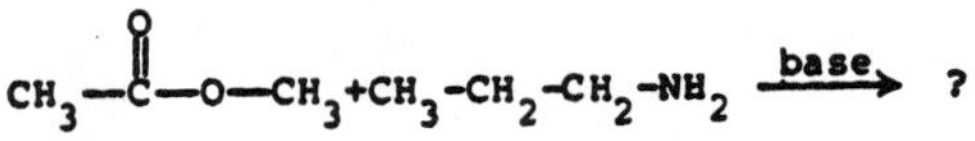

$$CH_3-\overset{O}{\overset{\|}{C}}-O-CH_3 + CH_3-CH_2-CH_2-NH_2 \xrightarrow{\text{base}} ?$$

A. 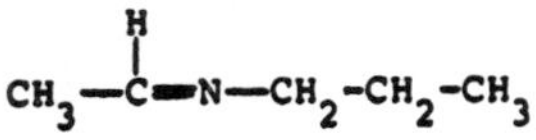 $CH_3-\overset{H}{\overset{|}{C}}=N-CH_2-CH_2-CH_3$

B. 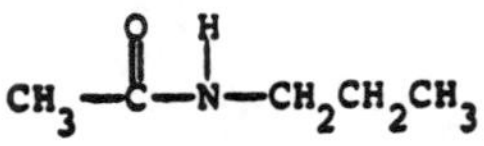 $CH_3-\overset{O}{\overset{\|}{C}}-\overset{H}{\overset{|}{N}}-CH_2CH_2CH_3$

C. $CH_3-CH_2-CH_2-OH$

D. none of the above

18. Give the product of the following reaction:

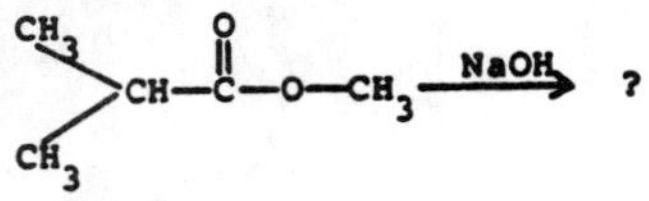

$(CH_3)_2CH-\overset{O}{\overset{||}{C}}-O-CH_3 \xrightarrow{NaOH} ?$

A. $(CH_3)_2C{=}CH_2$

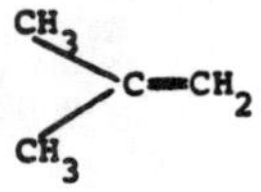

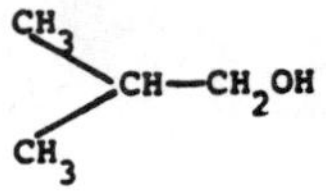

B. $(CH_3)_2CH-CH_2OH$

C. $(CH_3)_2CH-\overset{O}{\overset{||}{C}}-O^{\ominus}Na^{\oplus}$

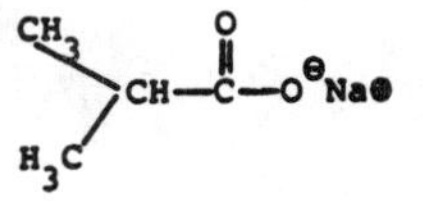

D. none of these

19. The following compound is a:

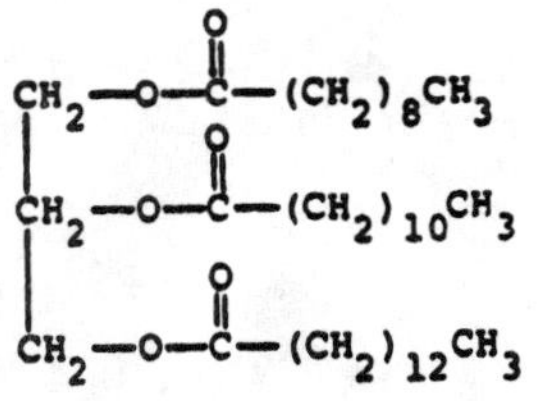

$CH_2-O-\overset{O}{\overset{||}{C}}-(CH_2)_8CH_3$
$CH_2-O-\overset{O}{\overset{||}{C}}-(CH_2)_{10}CH_3$
$CH_2-O-\overset{O}{\overset{||}{C}}-(CH_2)_{12}CH_3$

A. nucleotide
B. monosaccharide
C. amino acid
D. triglyceride

20. Name the following compound:

(benzene ring with OH and NO_2)

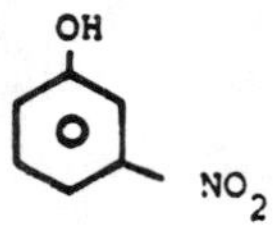

A. o,m-Hydroxynitrobenzene
B. 2-Nitrophenol
C. o-Nitrophenol
D. m-Nitrophenol

21. Which of the following is most acidic?

A. CH_3CH_2-OH

B. 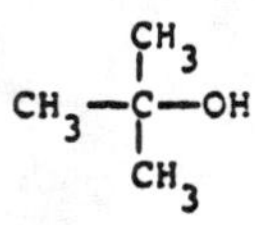 $CH_3-C(CH_3)_2-OH$

C. (benzene ring with HO and CH_3)

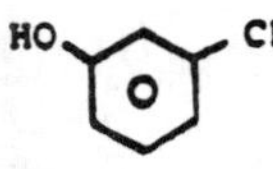

D. all are probably equal

22. Which of the following is most acidic?

A. 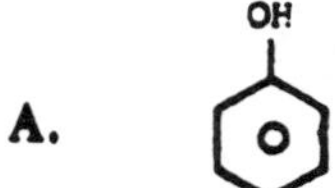

B. 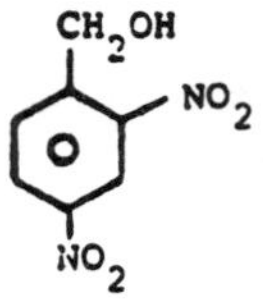 CH_2OH, NO_2, NO_2 (benzene ring)

C. 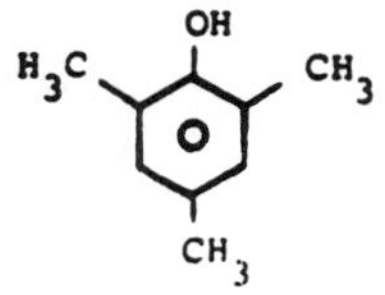 OH, H_3C, CH_3, CH_3 (benzene ring)

D. 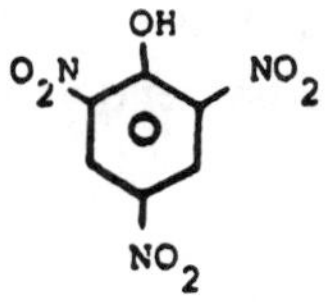 OH, O_2N, NO_2, NO_2 (benzene ring)

23. Which of the following compounds probably has the highest boiling point?

A. $CH_3(CH_2)_2-CH=CH_2$
B. CH_3-O-CH_3
C. 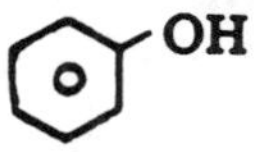 OH (benzene ring)
D. CH_3-CH_3

24. Given the following two compounds:

(I) 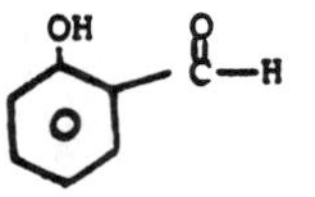 OH, $\overset{O}{\Vert}{C}-H$ (benzene ring, adjacent) and (II) 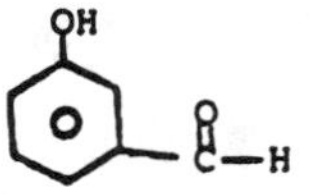 OH, $\overset{O}{\Vert}{C}-H$ (benzene ring, opposite)

compound ______ probably has the lower boiling point because there is ______ hydrogen bonding possible.

A. I, intramolecular
B. II, intramolecular
C. II, intermolecular
D. I, intermolecular

25. Rank the following compounds in order of decreasing acid strength (most acidic to least acidic):

A. 1>2>3>4
B. 2>3>4>1
C. 3>1>2>4
D. 2>4>1>3

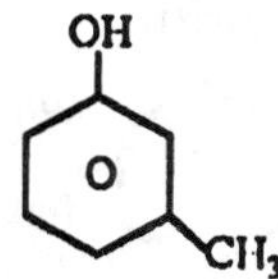

1

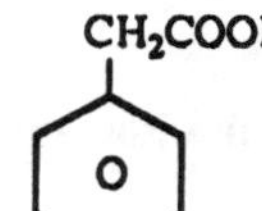

2

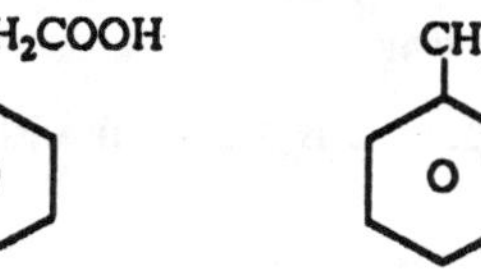

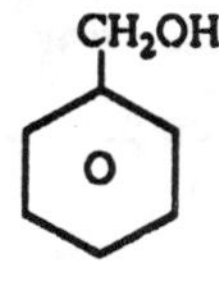

3

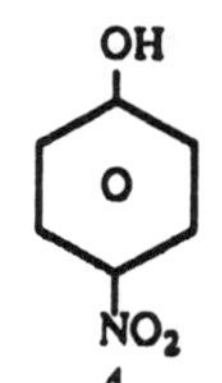

4

7.22.3 Answers to Questions in Section 7.22.2

(1) B (2) D (3) D (4) B (5) C (6) D (7) A (8) B (9) D (10) A (11) A (12) A (13) A (14) B (15) D (16) B (17) B (18) C (19) D (20) D (21) C (22) D (23) C (24) A (25) D

7.22.4 Discussion of Answers to Questions in Section 7.22.2

Questions #1 to #3 Discussed in Section.

Question #4 (Answer: B) The numbering is:

```
        C         Cl
        |         |
   C ── C ── C ══ C ── C ── CO2H
  (6)  (5)  (4)  (3)  (2)  (1)
        |
        C
```

Note how the double bond is handled.

Question #5 (Answer: C) The benzene ring withdraws electrons, and, therefore, increases the acidity. The Cl's on option (A) are one carbon from the – CO_2H and they are much less effective than a benzene ring attached to the carboxyl group.

Question #6 (Answer: D) Correct product, (O)–CH_2-CH_2-C(=O)-$NHCH_3$

Question #7 (Answer: A) Discussed in Section.

Question #8 (Answer: B) Option (B) is the only β-ketoacid (no β-diacids) given.

Question #9 to #11 Discussed in Section.

Question #12 (Answer: A) The numbering is

```
  C5
    \
     C4 ══ C3
    /        \
  C           C2 ── C1(=O) ── N ── C
```

Question #13 (Answer: A) Disubstituted amides have boiling points similar to carbonyls because there is no intermolecular hydrogen bonding.

Question #14 (Answer: B) Amides undergo nucleophilic substitution just like carboxylic acids. An ester is formed in this case.

Question #15 (Answer: D) This is hydrolysis of an amide; the products are the original acid and amine:

$$CH_3CH_2CH_2\text{–}\overset{O}{\overset{\|}{C}}\text{–}NHCH_3 \longrightarrow CH_3CH_2CH_2\overset{O}{\overset{\|}{C}}\text{–}OH + CH_3NH_2$$

Question #16 (Answer: B) The numbering is:

```
                  O
                  ‖      C
  (O)── C ── C ── C ── O ── C
        3    2    1          C
```

Question #17 (Answer: B) Esters undergo nucleophilic substitution just like carboxylic acids. An amide is the product in this reaction.

Question #18 (Answer: C) This is the alkaline hydrolysis of an ester, so a carboxylate anion results.

Question #19 (Answer: D) Refer to Section.

Question #20 (Answer: D) Name compound as a phenol with o-m-p as:

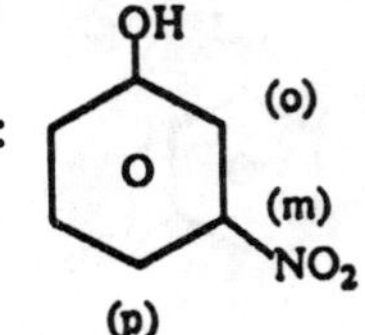

Question #21 (Answer: C) Phenols are more acidic than alcohols.

Question #22 (Answer: D) Electron withdrawing groups ($-NO_2$) at o-p positions increase the acidity of phenols.

Question #23 (Answer: C) The phenol can hydrogen bond to itself which increases the boiling point; the others cannot.

Question #24 (Answer: A) Intramolecular H-bonding is possible if the compound is ortho and this decreases the boiling point.

Question #25 (Answer: D) No. 2 is a carboxylic acid and the most acidic. No. 3 is an alcohol and the least acidic. Nos. 1 and 4 are phenols and No. 4 is the more acidic of the two phenols due to the p-NO_2.

7.22.5 Advanced Concepts

This is a list of tools to analyze and understand carboxylic acids, esters, amides, anhydrides, ethers and phenols.

- Improve review of observations linked with types and quantities of reactants and products. Identify all possible experiments to be performed. Propose any experimental modifications or new procedures to be used.
- Understand how reactions are related to basic mechanisms; how reaction rates are affected; what bonding arrangements, resonance stability structures and stereoarrangements are possible. Elucidate each mechanism in a visual format.
- Ask yourself, how can organic chemistry of medical compounds (carboxylic acids and derivates) be investigated, identified and linked to the biological side effects (both microscopic and physiological).
- What biological disorders result from deficiency or abundance of medical compounds (carboxylic acids and derivatives), especially bioorganic molecules? e.g., protein deficiency, enzyme deficiency, etc.
- Determine how organic reaction mechanisms translate into biochemical reaction mechanisms, e.g., metabolism.
- Learn how to judge the influence of new experimental evidence on each conclusion, including experimental conditions, experimental errors and practical limitations on experiment.
- Look for hidden assumptions behind each experimental technique or procedure, theoretical explanation and practical explanation of each mechanism.
- Look for scientific reasons behind each observation (laboratory observations, untaught observations from experimental data and completely new observations).
- Determine deductive conclusions from observations in order to approve or nullify your hypotheses.

7.23 AMINES (Nitrogen-Containing Compounds)

7.23.1 Introduction to Amines

Review special properties related to basicity and electronic effects of substituents, e.g. stabilization of carbocations. Review the structure of choline and acetylcholine (quaternary ammonium salt) as neurotransmitters. Understand the structure of the pyridine ring and derivatives such as NAD^+ and $NADP^+$ used in cellular metabolism. Identify the structural and mechanistic differences between histamines and antihistamines.

7.23.1.1 NOMENCLATURE AND STEREOCHEMISTRY

Amines are symbolized generally as:

$R-\ddot{N}H_2$ OR $Ar-\ddot{N}H_2$ OR $R_1-\ddot{N}(R_3)-R_2$.

R = aliphatic   Ar = aromatic

All the R's (R_1, R_2, R_3) or any combination can be carbon groups or hydrogens. If R's are carbon groups,

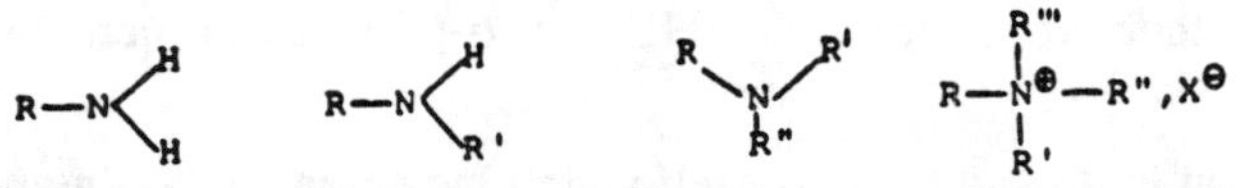

R—NH₂ (1° amine) R—NH—R' (2° amine) R—N(R')—R" (3° amine) $R-N^{\oplus}(R')(R''')-R'', X^{\ominus}$ (4° (quaternary) amine salt)

1° amine 2° amine 3° amine 4° (quaternary) amine salt

Amines may be named by locating the $-NR_2$ in a compound by numbers, e.g.,

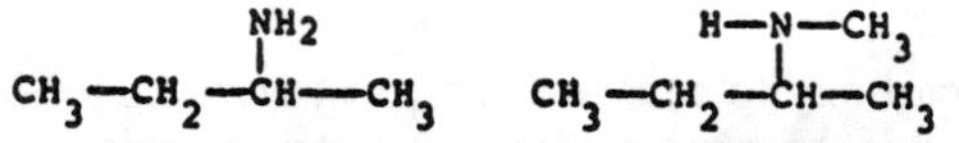

$CH_3-CH_2-CH(NH_2)-CH_3$ 2-Aminobutane

$CH_3-CH_2-CH(NH-CH_3)-CH_3$ N-Methyl-2-amino butane

Or by naming each group attached to the N,

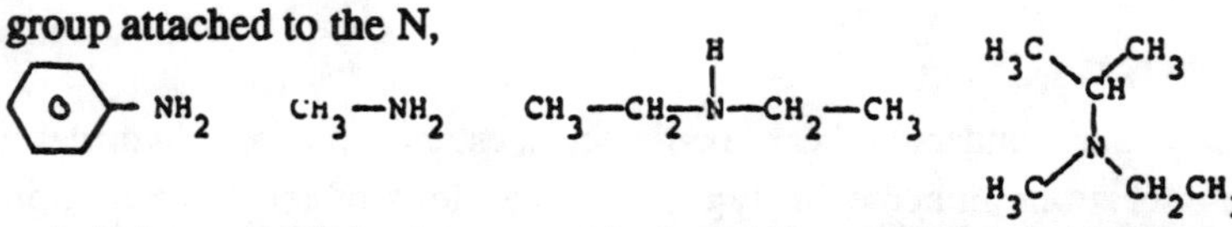

$C_6H_5-NH_2$ Aniline

CH_3-NH_2 Methylamine

$CH_3-CH_2-NH-CH_2-CH_3$ Diethylamine

$(CH_3)_2CH-N(CH_3)-CH_2CH_3$ Methylethylisopropylamine

Nearly all the chemistry of amines depends upon the free pair of electrons upon nitrogen:

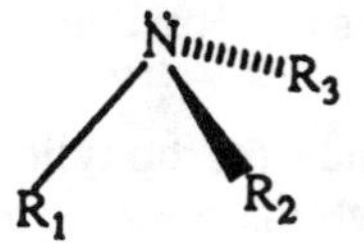

$N(R_1)(R_2)(R_3)$ R = aliphatic, aromatic or H's.

Groups that withdraw electron density (aromatics, halides, e.g.) from nitrogen decrease the availability of this electron pair. Groups that donate electron density (especially alkyls) increase the availability. The exception to this rule is the secondary amine, which is the most basic because the combination of the alkyls and the single hydrogen (provides hydrogen bonding, e.g., with water) stabilizes the ion and makes the electrons more available. The availability of the electrons is reflected in this sequence of decreasing *base strengths*:

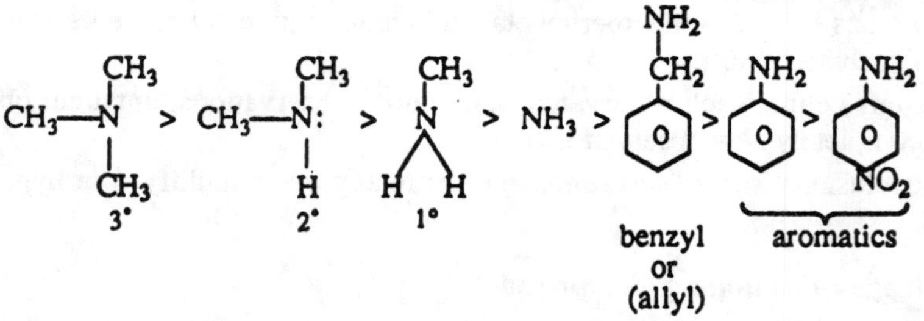

$(CH_3)_3N$ (3°) > $(CH_3)_2NH$ (2°) > CH_3NH_2 (1°) > NH_3 > $C_6H_5CH_2NH_2$ (benzyl or (allyl)) > $C_6H_5NH_2$ > $NO_2C_6H_4NH_2$ (aromatics)

The available electron pair classifies amines as Lewis bases. Amines are also nucleophiles.

7.23.1.2 IMPORTANT PROPERTIES AND REACTIONS

(1) The N can form hydrogen bonding via its electron pair with hydrogens attached to other nitrogen or oxygen atoms, and it can form hydrogen bonds from hydrogens attached to it with electron pairs of N, O, F or Cl:

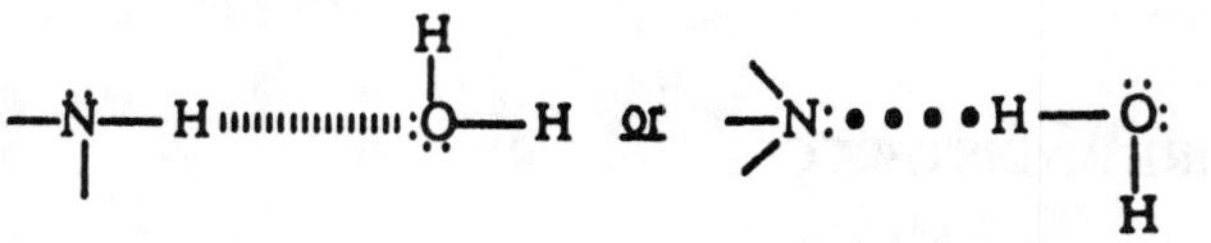

$-N-H \cdots :O(H)-H$ or $\geq N: \cdots H-\ddot{O}:-H$

Note that 1° or 2° amines can hydrogen bond with each other (intermolecularly) but 3° amines cannot (no Hs attached to the N). For this reason 1° and 2° amines have higher than expected boiling points for compounds of similar molecular weight (but lower than similar alcohols or carboxylic acids). Low molecular weight amines are also soluble in H_2O (due to H-bonding).

(2) A dipole moment is possible: $H - \underset{H}{\overset{N}{|}} - H$ ↑

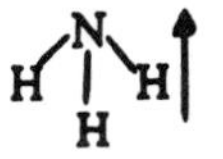

(3) Amines are ortho-para directors (Section 7.20.1.3)

(4) Remember that the key reaction of amines is the nucleophilic attack (Section 7.23.1) by it upon an electron-deficient carbon.

(5) A very important reaction of 1° and 2° amines is with carboxylic acids (or usually their derivatives) to form *amides*:

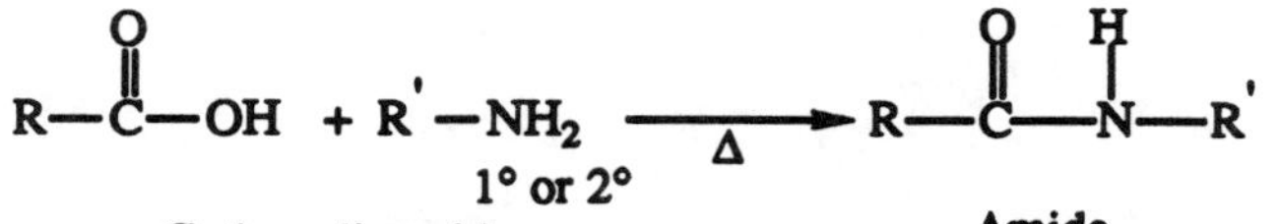

$$\underset{\substack{\text{Carboxylic acid}\\ \text{(or Acyl chloride)}}}{R-\overset{O}{\overset{\|}{C}}-OH} + \underset{1° \text{ or } 2°}{R'-NH_2} \xrightarrow[\Delta]{} \underset{\text{Amide}}{R-\overset{O}{\overset{\|}{C}}-\overset{H}{\overset{|}{N}}-R'}$$

This is the reaction important in protein synthesis.

(6) Another common reaction of amines is *alkylation* of amines by alkyl halides:

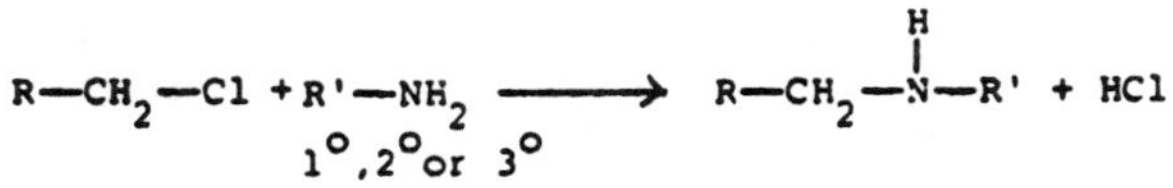

$$R-CH_2-Cl + \underset{1°,2° \text{or } 3°}{R'-NH_2} \longrightarrow R-CH_2-\overset{H}{\overset{|}{N}}-R' + HCl$$

Both amide formation and alkylation make use of the nucleophilic character of the electrons on nitrogen.

7.23.2 Questions Related to Amines

1. Name the following compound:

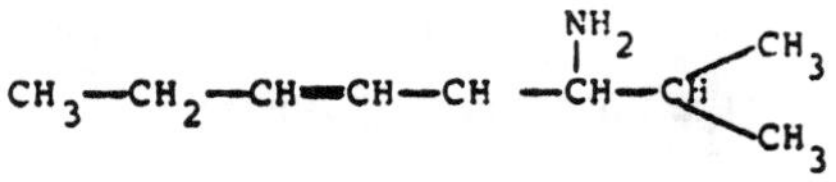

$$CH_3-CH_2-CH{=}CH-CH-\overset{NH_2}{\overset{|}{CH}}-CH(CH_3)_2$$

A. 6-Amino-7-methyl-3-octene
B. Isononenyl amine
C. 2-Methyl-3-aminooctene
D. none of the above

2. Give the structure of Isopropyl diethyl amine:

A. 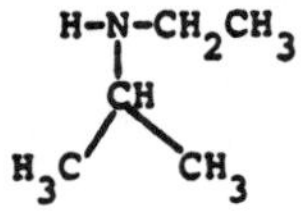 $H-N(CH_2CH_3)-CH(CH_3)_2$ [H‑N‑CH₂CH₃ on CH bearing H_3C and CH_3]

B. 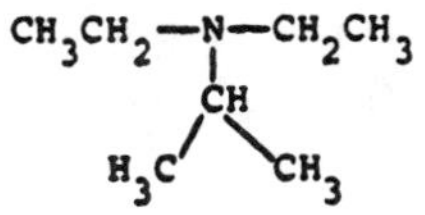 $CH_3CH_2-N(CH_2CH_3)-CH(CH_3)_2$

C. 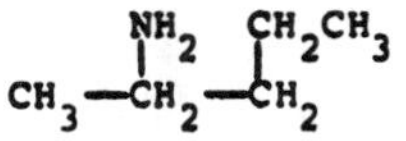 $CH_3-\overset{NH_2}{\overset{|}{CH_2}}-\overset{CH_2CH_3}{\overset{|}{CH_2}}$

D. none of the above

3. Which compound has the greatest base strength?

A. CH_3-NH_2

B. 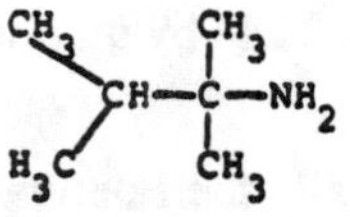 $(CH_3)_2CH-C(CH_3)_2-NH_2$

C. $CH_3CH_2CH_2-N(CH_3)-CH_3$

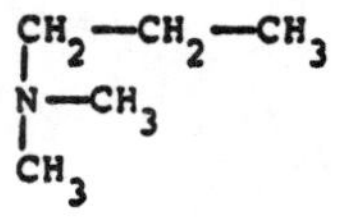

D. all are equal

4. Which compound has the greatest base strength?

A. 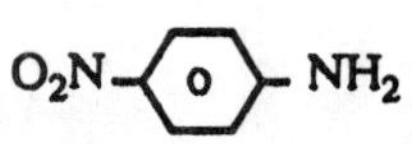 $O_2N-C_6H_4-NH_2$

B. $NC-C_6H_3(CN)-NH_2$

C. $H_3C-C_6H_4-NH_2$

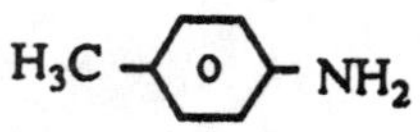

D. none of the above

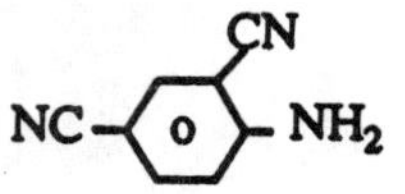

5. Which of the following compounds probably has the lowest boiling point?

A. 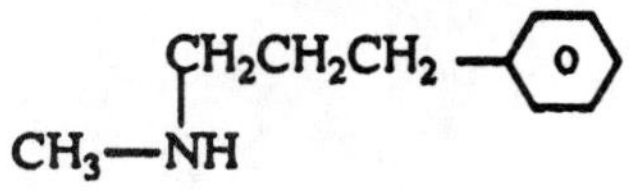 $CH_3-NH-CH_2CH_2CH_2-C_6H_5$

B. $C_6H_5-(CH_2)_3-NH_2$

C. $C_6H_5-CH_2-N(CH_2CH_3)-CH_3$

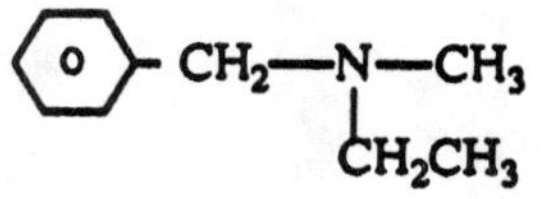

D. all are equal

6. Give the product of the following reaction:

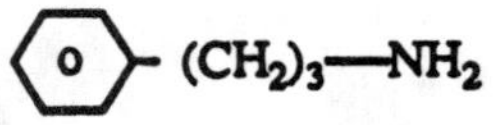

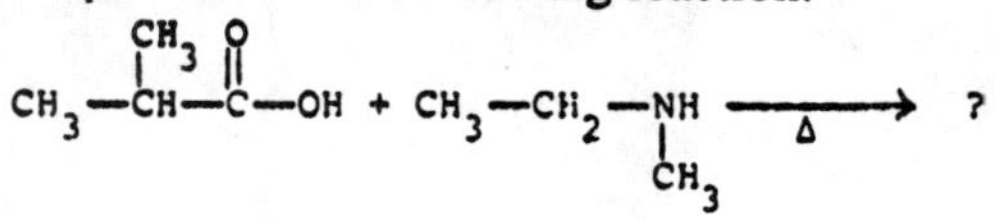

$$CH_3-CH(CH_3)-C(=O)-OH + CH_3-CH_2-NH(CH_3) \xrightarrow{\Delta} ?$$

A. 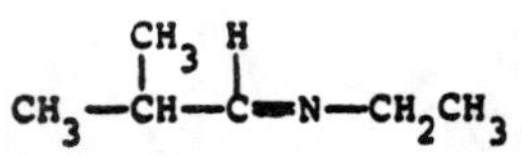 $CH_3-CH(CH_3)-C(H)=N-CH_2CH_3$

B. 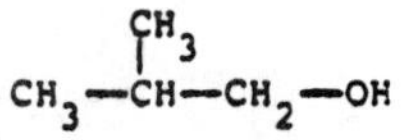 $CH_3-CH(CH_3)-CH_2-OH$

C. 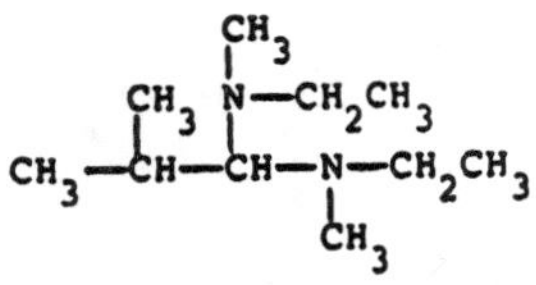 $CH_3-CH(CH_3)-CH(N(CH_3)CH_2CH_3)-N(CH_3)-CH_2CH_3$

D. 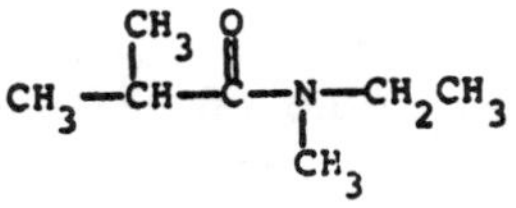 $CH_3-CH(CH_3)-C(=O)-N(CH_3)-CH_2CH_3$

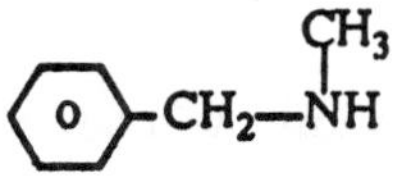

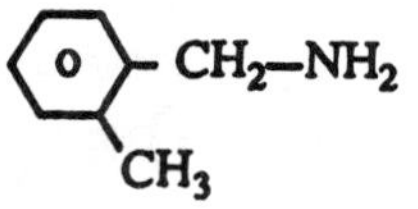

7. Give the product of the following reaction:

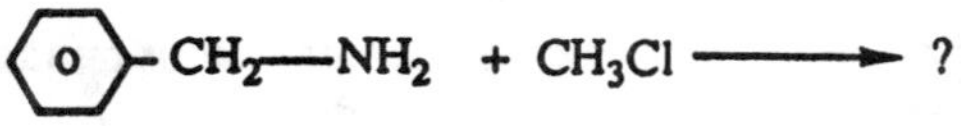

$$C_6H_5-CH_2-NH_2 + CH_3Cl \longrightarrow ?$$

A. $C_6H_5-CH_2-NH(CH_3)$

B. $CH_3-C_6H_4-CH_2-NH_2$ (ring CH_3 ortho)

C. $Cl-C_6H_4-CH_2-NH_2$ (ring Cl ortho)

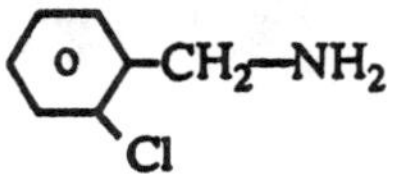

D. none of the above

7.23.3 Answers to Questions in Section 7.23.2

(1) A (2) B (3) C (4) C (5) C (6) D (7) A

7.23.4 Discussion of Answers to Questions in Section 7.23.2

Question #1 (Answer: A) The compound is named as an alkene and the amino group is considered to be a substituent (it could have been named as an amine also). The numbering is,

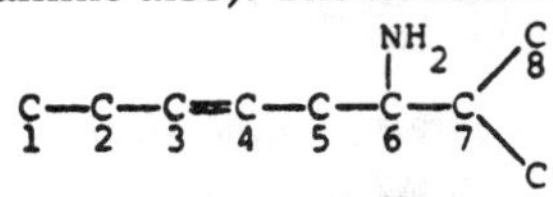

$$\underset{1}{C}-\underset{2}{C}-\underset{3}{C}=\underset{4}{C}-\underset{5}{C}-\underset{6}{C}(NH_2)-\underset{7}{C}(\underset{8}{C})-C$$

Question #2 (Answer: B) Review the structure of methyl-ethylisopropylamine given in the section.

Question #3 (Answer: C) Tertiary amines (option C) have greater base strength than primary (A or B) or secondary amines.

Question #4 (Answer: C) Aromatic amines have low base strength in general, but electron withdrawing groups (– CN, – NO_2) placed ortho/para decreases it even more. Electron donating groups (– CH_3) placed o/p can increase base strength.

Question #5 (Answer: C) Tertiary amines have lower boiling points than 1° and 2° because there is no intermolecular hydrogen bonding.

Question #6 (Answer: D) This is the amide forming reaction.

Question #7 (Answer: A) This is the alkylation reaction.

7.23.5 Advanced Concepts

This is a list of tools to analyze and understand amines.

- Improve review of observations linked with types and quantities of reactants and products. Identify all possible experiments to be performed. Propose any experimental modifications or new procedures to be used.
- Understand how reactions are related to basic mechanisms; how reaction rates are affected; what bonding arrangements, resonance stability structures and stereoarrangements are possible. Elucidate each mechanism in a visual format.
- Ask yourself, how can organic chemistry of medical compounds (amines and alkaloids) be investigated, identified and linked to the biological side effects (both microscopic and physiological).
- What biological disorders result from deficiency or abundance of medical compounds (amines and alkaloids), especially bioorganic molecules? e.g., protein deficiency, enzyme deficiency, etc.
- Determine how organic reaction mechanisms translate into biochemical reaction mechanisms, e.g., metabolism.
- Learn how to judge the influence of new experimental evidence on each conclusion, including experimental conditions, experimental errors and practical limitations on experiment.
- Look for hidden assumptions behind each experimental technique or procedure, theoretical explanation and practical explanation of each mechanism.
- Look for scientific reasons behind each observation (laboratory observations, untaught observations from experimental data and completely new observations).
- Determine deductive conclusions from observations in order to approve or nullify your hypotheses.

7.24 SEPARATIONS AND PURIFICATIONS

7.24.1 Introduction to Separations and Purifications

Understand *all* physical and chemical design features of basic instruments and equipment used in separation and purification of organic mixtures. Compare the laboratory and industrial methods with special attention to working mechanisms and analytical procedures.

7.24.1.1 SOLVENT EXTRACTION

Solvent extraction is a means of purifying a compound by partitioning it between two immiscible liquids in such a fashion that the compound of interest is held strongly in one solvent preferentially over other solutes. Quantitatively, the preference of a solute for a given solvent A in preference to another solvent B may be expressed as its partition coefficient defined below:

$$K_{A/B} = [\text{solute}]_A / [\text{solute}]_B = (\text{grams solute/volume of A})/(\text{grams solute/volume of B})$$

For example, if 1.20 g of a substance is partitioned between 50.0 ml CH_2Cl_2 and 50.0 ml of H_2O and it is determined that 0.95 g are in CH_2Cl_2 and 0.25 g are in H_2O, the partition coefficient is calculated as:

$$K_{CH_2Cl_2/H_2O} = (0.95\ \text{g}/50.0\ \text{ml})/(0.25\ \text{g}/50.0\ \text{ml}).$$

The higher the value of the partition coefficient, the more soluble the compound is in one solvent compared to the other.

It is often useful to take advantage of differences in the acid-base properties of solutes and separate them on that basis. Chemical reactions ionize functional groups in organic molecules and render them soluble in water. Compounds containing very acidic protons (i.e., carboxylic acids) are extracted readily from organic solvents such as dichloromethane into aqueous solutions of a weak base such as $NaHCO_3$. Compounds containing less acidic protons (i.e., phenols) are extracted from dichloromethane by stronger aqueous bases such as NaOH. Compounds that are moderately basic (i.e., amines) are extracted from dichloromethane by aqueous hydrochloric acid. Very weakly basic compounds (i.e., alcohols, alkenes, carbonyl compounds) are extracted by concentrated H_2SO_4. Once the compound of interest has been obtained in the aqueous medium to the virtual exclusion of other compounds, the aqueous solution can be brought to neutral pH and back extracted into an organic solvent. The separation and purification of a mixture of toluene, benzoic acid, phenol, and aniline will illustrate the concept (Fig. 7.80).

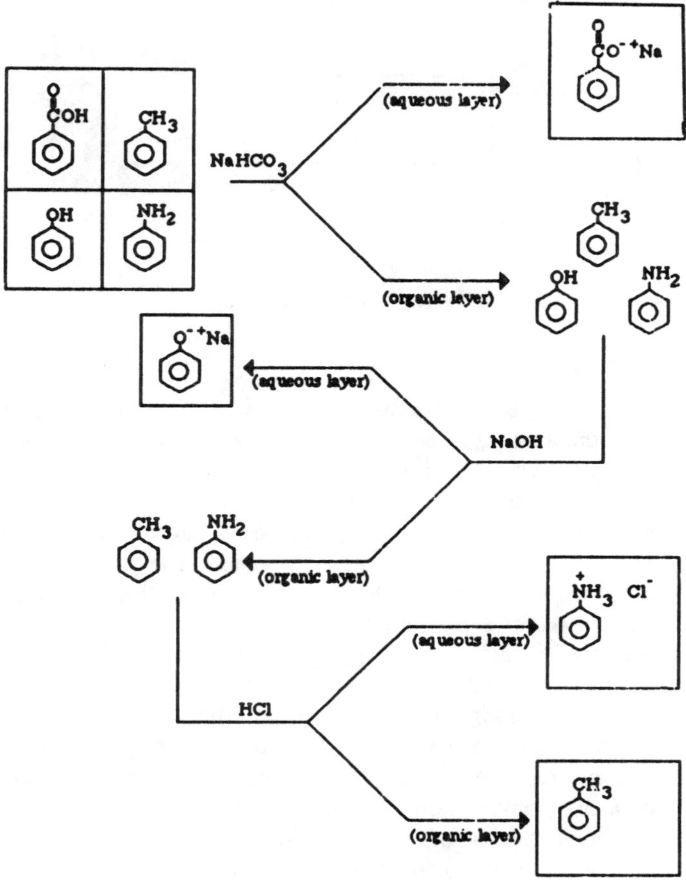

Fig. 7.80—Separation of Benzoic Acid, Toluene, Phenol, and Aniline by Solvent Extraction

7.24.1.2 CHROMATOGRAPHY

Chromatography, as a technique for separation and purification, is quite similar to solvent extraction. Chromatographic separations may be viewed as continuous partitions between a mobile phase and a stationary phase. Compounds with different partition coefficients between the mobile and stationary phase are separated because they move at different rates. The greater a compound favors the mobile phase, the faster it will move. The greater the difference in partition coefficients between compounds, the greater the difference in their respective velocities, and the easier their separation. The old generalization "like dissolves like" is applicable to chromatographic separations too.

Gas-liquid-chromatography (glc), or as it is more commonly called, gas chromatography (gc), permits the quantitative separation of mixtures of compounds that can be vaporized. The "gas" refers to either helium or nitrogen gas as the mobile phase in this separation technique. The "liquid" refers to a high molecular weight liquid such as octadecane coated on an inert solid support such as finely ground firebrick as the stationary phase. The stationary phase is packed into glass or metal tubing called a column. A typical gas chromatograph is shown in Fig. 7.81.

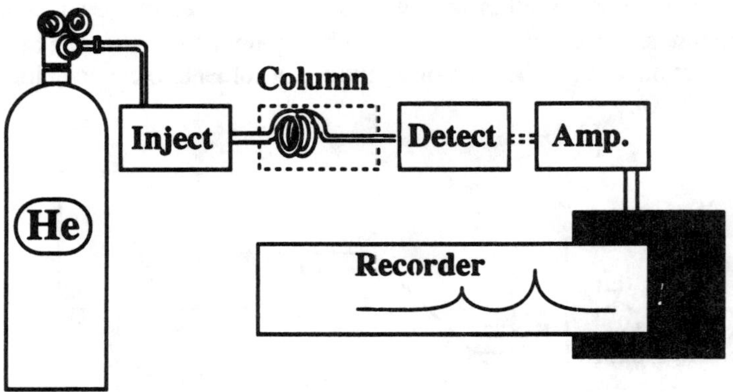

Fig. 7.81—A Typical Gas Chromatograph

I. Gas chromatography:

Gas chromatography is frequently employed to establish the purity of a sample, identify components in the sample, and quantitatively measure the amount of each component present in the sample. It is also possible to employ gas chromatography for preparative separation of milligram quantities of reaction mixtures. A solution containing the sample to be separated and analyzed is introduced via microliter syringe into an injector port that instantaneously vaporizes the entire sample. The vapor thus produced is partitioned between the high molecular weight liquid stationary phase and the helium or nitrogen mobile phase. The greater affinity a component has for the stationary phase, the longer it will be retained in the stationary phase. The larger the difference in affinity for the stationary phase the components of a mixture have, the easier is their separation. Identification of compounds is made on the basis of the retention time of authentic compounds, the length of time it takes from injection until a component exits the column and is detected. As a rule, in addition to the affinity considerations, the higher a compound's boiling point, the longer its retention time. The detector drives a strip-chart recorder producing triangles whose area is proportion to the amount of material passing the detector. Quantitative data can be obtained from calibration curves based on known amounts of authentic material. The free radical chlorination of cyclohexane produces a combination of unreacted cyclohexane, chlorocyclohexane, and some isomeric dichlorocyclohexanes. The presence of each compound can be detected and its concentration determined if authentic samples of each compound are available for comparison and calibration.

II. Thin layer chromatography (tlc):

Thin layer chromatography (tlc) is useful for the rapid separation of small quantities of materials. Such separations are valuable for the determination of purity of a sample, identification of components of a mixture, and for establishing conditions for the separation and purification of larger quantities of material using a buret packed with silica gel or alumina. It is possible to employ tlc for preparative separations of milligram quantities of compounds. Thin layer chromatography is not generally used for quantitative analyses. The most common stationary phase is a plastic sheet coated with silica gel or alumina cut into small strips called plates. Both silica gel and alumina are polar since they contain -O-H groups. A non-polar solvent, such as hexane, is employed as the mobile phase or it is mixed with a polar solvent, such as dichloromethane or diethyl ether, to adjust the polarity of the mobile phase for the best separation. A non-polar mobile phase will have minimal electrostatic interaction with the stationary phase so compounds will separate according to their polarity—the most polar compound will move slowest in the mobile phase while the least polar compound will travel fastest. A more polar mobile phase will interact with the polar stationary phase and hasten the movement of all compounds since the stationary phase interacts with the solvent to a greater extent than the sample due to the greater abundance of the solvent. A few microliters of a solution of the mixture to be separated is spotted near the bottom of a tlc plate. The plate is placed in a covered breaker or jar containing the mobile phase. The mobile phase rises on the plate by capillary action carrying with it components of the mixture to be separated. Fig. 7.82 shows schematically the separation of a three component mixture on a silica gel plate. Compound **a** is the most polar component and **c** is the least polar component and **b** is of intermediate polarity. Identification of the components is made on the basis of the ratio of the distance moved by a given spot to the distance traveled by the solvent (mobile phase).

$$R_f = \frac{\text{distance spot "A" moves from the origin}}{\text{distance solvent "S" moves from origin}} = A / S$$

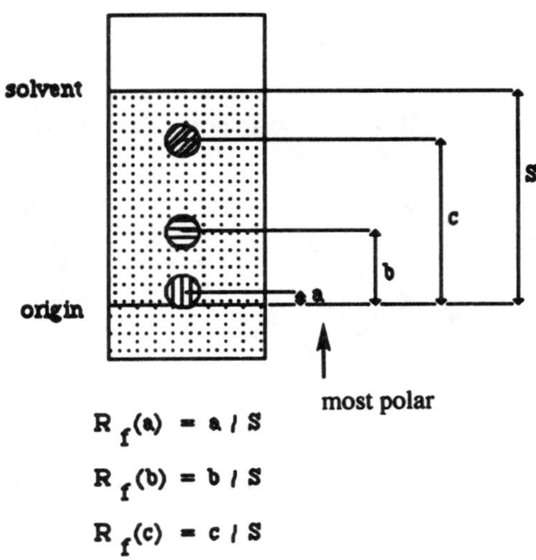

Fig. 7.82—tlc Separation of a Three Component Mixture

Such R_f values are, by definition, equal to or less than unity. It is often convenient to spot authentic samples on the same plate as an unknown to measure their R_f values under identical conditions. The basis for the separation of fluorene from fluorenone on silica gel is shown in Fig. 7.83. Fluorene, a non-polar compound, has an R_f value close to 1.00 while the polar fluorenone has an R_f of nearly half that using silica gel as a stationary phase and hexane as the mobile phase. For the separation of large quantities of fluorene from fluorenone a solvent or solvent mixture is selected by tlc. For the separation of fluorene and fluorenone, hexane provides two readily distinguishable, separated spots. A buret is filled with a suspension of silica gel in hexane, excess hexane is drained off, and the stopcock of the buret is closed. The mixture to be separated is introduced as a concentrated solution at the top of the buret and the stopcock is open.

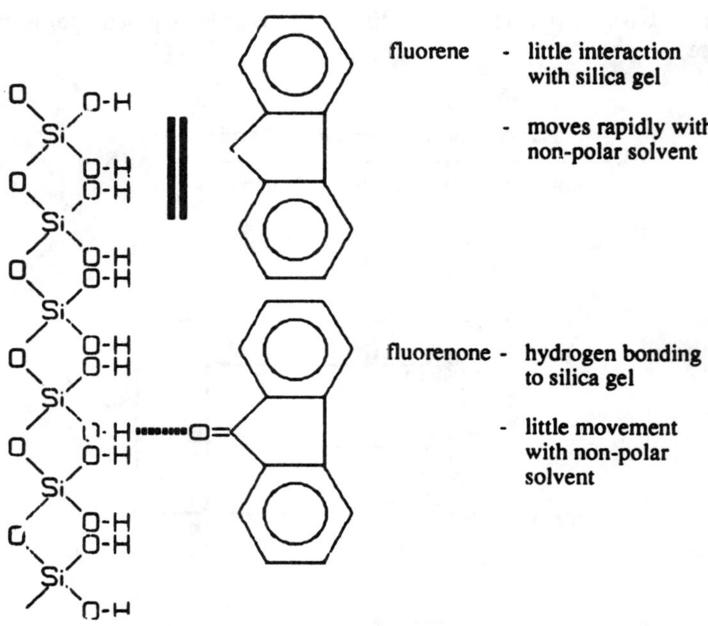

Fig. 7.83—Silica Gel Interaction with Fluorene and Fluorenone

Additional hexane must be added to the buret to replace the mobile phase that flows out. As the hexane moves down the buret it carries with it the fluorene, leaving the fluorenone near the top of the silica gel. Once the non-polar fluorene has eluted, dichloromethane is used as the mobile phase to chase out the polar fluorenone. Fig. 7.84 illustrates this separation schematically.

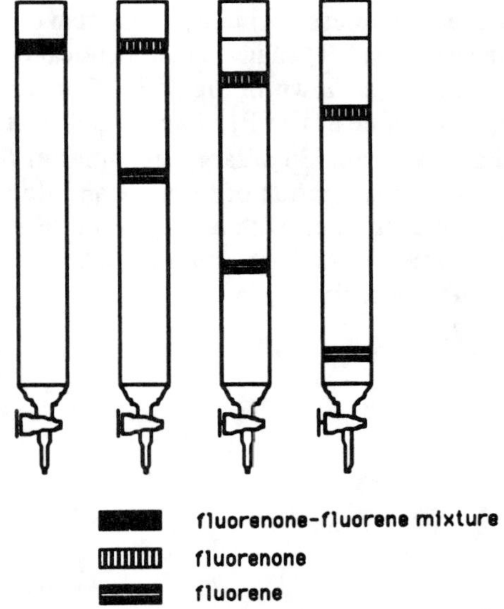

Fig. 7.84—Column Chromatographic Separation of Fluorene and Fluorenone

7.24.1.3 DISTILLATION

Distillation is a means of purifying a liquid by vaporizing it, separating its vapor from that of impurities and/or other compounds, and finally condensing the purified vapor back to a liquid and collecting it in a separate container.

Every liquid has molecules above it in the vapor phase. Heating the liquid increases the kinetic energy of the molecules in the liquid state to the point where they are no longer attracted to other molecules of the liquid and therefore pass into the gas or vapor phase. This, in turn, increases the partial pressure of vapor above the liquid. At the temperature where the partial pressure of vapor above the liquid equals ambient pressure, the liquid boils. The actual temperature required to boil a liquid depends on the presence or absence of factors that hold molecules of liquid near each other. Such factors include van der Waals forces, dipolar electrostatic attractions, and hydrogen bonding.

The distillation process can be viewed as a series of vaporizations and condensations that enrich the vapor in the more volatile compound. In an equimolar mixture of two liquids A and B, if A is the more volatile substance, the vapor above the A/B mixture is richer in A than B. That vapor is condensed back to a liquid, now enriched in A. The vapor above this enriched liquid is even richer in A, the more volatile compound. Each vaporization-condensation cycle is termed a "theoretical plate." In research and academic laboratories this "theoretical plate" has no physical being (i.e., it is really theoretical.) In industrial distillations each theoretical plate corresponds to a distinctly different heating-condensing apparatus. Liquids with widely different boiling points require few theoretical plates to achieve a vapor that is practically pure in the low boiling, more volatile compound. Similarly, two liquids whose boiling points are close together require several vaporization-condensation cycles to obtain a vapor that contains only one compound because the enrichment of each step is smaller. Figure 7.85 shows an idealized graph of the vapor and liquid compositions for mixtures of A and B where A is the more volatile liquid. Point **a** represents the starting point of 0.5 mole fraction A in the liquid phase. Point **b** represents the composition of the vapor above the liquid in A at the same temperature. Note that the vapor has a greater mole fraction of A than does the liquid (about 0.85 mole fraction A in the vapor phase). Point **c** represents the vapor from point **b** condensed to a liquid with the same 0.85 mole fraction A. The path from point **a** to **b** to **c** represents one theoretical plate. The figure shows that two theoretical plates are needed to produce a vapor of nearly pure A. A third plate would be required to complete the process. From a practical standpoint, the number of theoretical plates in a research or academic laboratory distillation may be increased by increasing the surface area available for condensations. Experimentally this is accomplished by packing the fractionating column with glass beads, ceramic "saddles," or copper wool.

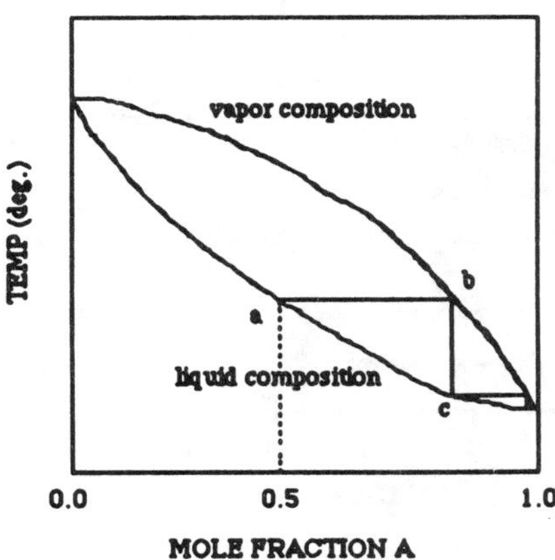

Fig. 7.85—Liquid and Vapor Composition of an Ideal Two Component Mixture as a Function of Temperature

The illustration in Fig. 7.86 shows the apparatus for the distillation of a mixture of ethyl acetate (B.P. = 78°C) and toluene (B.P. = 111°C). Note that the vapor about to distill is virtually free of toluene while the vapor closer to the distilling flask contains increasingly higher amounts of that compound.

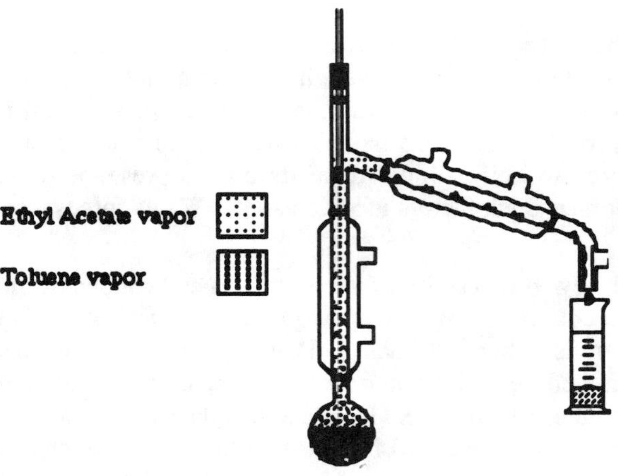

Fig. 7.86—Distillation of Ethyl Acetate and Toluene

As each pure material is distilled, the temperature will remain constant at the boiling point for the compound distilling. An idealized graph of temperature as a function of volume for the fractional distillation of a mixture of ethyl acetate (B.P. = 78°C) and toluene B.P. = 111°C) is shown in Fig. 7.87. Four regions or fractions on the graph may be discerned. There is an initial fraction where the temperature rises from room temperature (25°) to the boiling point of ethyl acetate. The liquid collected during that region is termed "fore-run." Although the liquid collected in this fore-run is largely ethyl acetate, it is not pure and should not be combined with the fraction that will contain the pure material. Experimentally, the fore-run is usually small in volume. The second fraction that is observed is where the temperature remains constant at 78°, the boiling point of pure ethyl acetate. This is collected in a separate container as a pure liquid. The third fraction is observed as the temperature rises from 78° to 111°, the boiling point of toluene. This fraction contains both ethyl acetate and toluene. Accordingly, it should be collected in a different container. The fourth fraction boils at a constant 111° and is pure toluene.

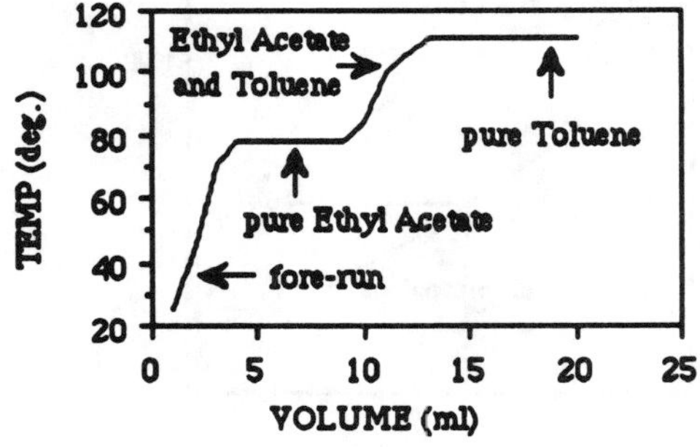

Fig. 7.87—Variation of Temperature with Volume during the Distillation of Ethyl Acetate and Toluene

7.24.1.4 RECRYSTALLIZATION

Recrystallization is a technique for the purification of a solid by breaking down the crystal lattice structure of the solid by dissolving it in a suitable solvent and then allowing the crystal lattice to form again. A saturated solution of an impure solid is prepared at an elevated temperature. When the solution cools, it becomes supersaturated with respect to the compound of interest and crystals of that compound will form. The more slowly the solution cools, the larger will be the resulting crystals. The original impurities are excluded from the crystals that form for two reasons: 1) the solution is not supersaturated with respect to the impurities (i.e., they remain dissolved), and 2) the impurities do not easily fit into the growing crystal lattice structure. Once the solution has deposited all the crystals that it will yield, the crystals are filtered from the solution, washed with cold solvent, and dried. If the recrystallization has indeed improved the purity of the solid sample, its melting point should increase over that recorded for the initial material and it should melt over a narrower temperature range.

A good choice of solvent is crucial to the success of a recrystallization. The following criteria should be met:

1) The solvent should not react chemically with the sample.
2) The solvent should dissolve the sample poorly at room temperature and dissolve it well at steam bath temperature.
3) The solvent should dissolve impurities known to be present even at sub-ambient temperatures.
4) The solvent should be reasonably easy to evaporate from the purified sample.

Water, methanol, ethyl acetate, dichloromethane, hexane, and toluene were tested as potential solvents for the recrystallization of a solid with the following results, where s = soluble, s_h = soluble in hot solution and i = insoluble:

water: i methanol: s_h ethyl acetate: s dichloromethane: s hexane: s toluene: s

Based on the second criterion, methanol would be the solvent of choice to purify the solid by recrystallization assuming that the other criteria are also met by methanol. Ethyl acetate, dichloromethane, hexane, and toluene dissolved the sample at room temperature. In order to induce crystallization, the volume of solution would have to be substantially reduced to obtain any crystals on cooling. Water failed to dissolve the sample in the first place, so it is an unacceptable recrystallizing solvent for this solute.

Fractional crystallization can be used to separate a mixture of two solids if a solvent can be found that dissolves one compound readily even cold and dissolves the other only when it is hot. A typical example is the separation of trans-cinnamic acid from urea. The problem is more interesting since both melt at nominally 132°. The mixture has a melting point considerably less than that.

The following observations on solubility are typical:

compound	water	methanol	ethyl acetate	dichloromethane	hexane	toluene
cinnamic acid	s_h	s	s	s	s	s
urea	s	s	i	i	i	i

From this data, it can be seen that a mixture of cinnamic acid and urea dissolved in hot water would yield crystals of cinnamic acid on cooling. Urea will remain dissolved in the cold water. The crystals thus obtained should melt close to 132°. Proof of the crystal's identity as tans-cinnamic acid can be obtained by a mixed melting point with authentic trans-cinnamic acid.

7.24.2 Questions Related to Separations and Purifications; Chromatography

1. In order for two compounds to be separated by $NaHCO_3$ extraction, they must have:

A. different dipole moments.
B. different acid-base properties.
C. different boiling points.
D. different molecular weights.

2. Which pair of compounds could be separated *most readily* by solvent extraction?

A. aminocyclohexane and chlorocyclohexane
B. cyclohexanol and cyclohexanone
C. phenol and p-cresol
D. butanoic acid and 2-methylpropanoic acid

3. Carboxylic acids are generally separated as their methyl esters in gas chromatography. Why are the carboxylic acids themselves difficult to separate by this technique?

A. Carboxylic acids all have the same nominal polarity.
B. Carboxylic acids are insoluble in most organic solvents while their methyl esters are soluble.
C. Carboxylic acids decompose readily in a gas chromatographic column.
D. Carboxylic acids do not vaporize readily but their methyl esters do so easily.

4. Which pair of compounds would be separated *most readily* on silica gel by thin layer chromatography?

A. 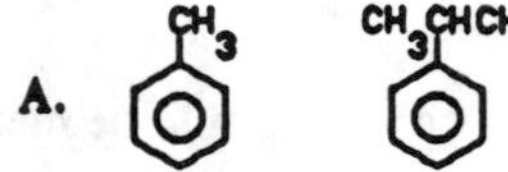

B. 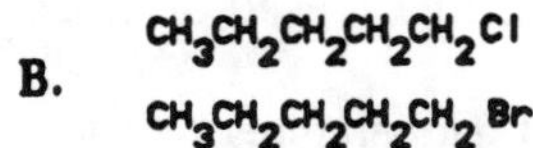

C. 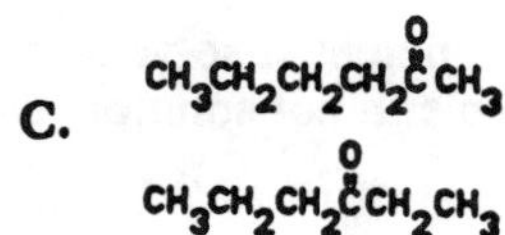

D. 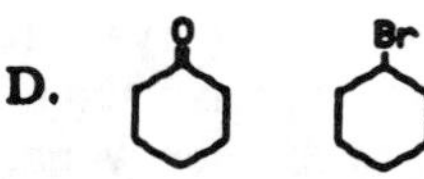

5. Fractionating columns in distillations are frequently packed with glass beads, ceramic saddles, or copper wool in order to:

A. increase the condensation of the vapor in the fractionating column.
B. decrease the rate at which pure liquid distills.
C. maintain a constant temperature in the fractionating column.
D. provide a surface on which impurities may be absorbed and removed.

6. According to the temperature vs. volume graph of the distillation below, how many compounds were present in the initial mixture?

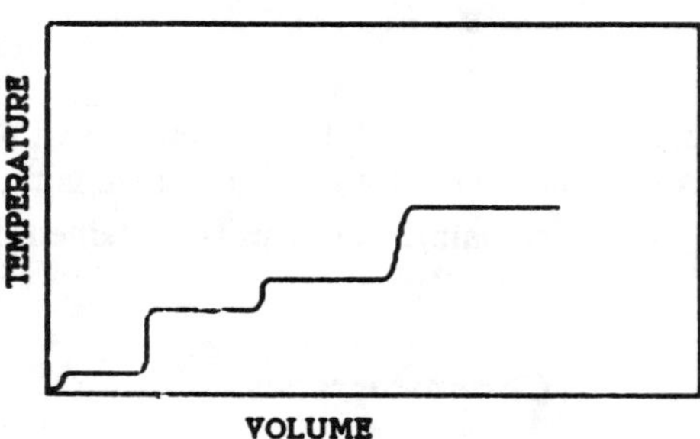

A. one
B. two
C. three
D. four

7. An impure solid gives the following solubility test results where i = insoluble s = soluble s_h = soluble when the solvent is hot:

water: i methanol: i hexane: s_h dichloromethane: s.

Which solvent would be most appropriate to attempt the recrystallization of this impure solid?

A. water
B. methanol
C. hexane
D. dichloromethane

8. Impurities are removed in the recrystallization process because of the following factors:

   I. Impurities do not "fit" into a growing crystal lattice.
   II. Impurities lower the melting point of the compound.
   III. Impurities remain dissolved in the solvent employed.

   A. I only
   B. I and II
   C. I and III
   D. I, II, and III

7.24.3 Answers to Questions in Section 7.24.2

(1) B (2) A (3) D (4) D (5) A (6) D (7) C (8) C

7.24.4 Discussion of Answers to Questions in Section 7.24.2

Question #1 (Answer: B) Separation by solvent extraction requires different acidity/basicity. Sodium bicarbonate is a weak base. In order for it to serve as the basis of a separation, one compound must be capable of reacting with $NaHCO_3$ while the other does not.

Question #2 (Answer: A) Separation by solvent extraction requires different acidity/basicity. This is an application of the same principle as question #1 using HCl. An amine can be protonated and therefore water solubilized leaving behind the alkyl halide. The remaining pairs of compounds are not readily distinguishable by their acid/base properties.

Question #3 (Answer: D) By definition compounds to be separated by gas chromatography must be capable of being vaporized. Carboxylic acids form hydrogen bonded dimers that keep their vapor pressure low. Hydrogen bonded dimers do not form from the methyl esters.

Question #4 (Answer: D) Thin layer chromatography separates compounds on the basis of polarity. A ketone and an alkyl halide have different polarities while the other compounds are similar in theirs.

Question #5 (Answer: A) Distillation is a series of vaporizations and condensations. The efficiency of the distillation is improved if more condensations take place in the fractionating column.

Question #6 (Answer: D) A pure compound distills at constant temperature. There are four regions where temperature remains constant so four compounds were initially present.

Question #7 (Answer: C) The best solvent for recrystallization on the basis of solubility tests is the one that needs to be heated for the solute to dissolve. In that manner, obtaining pure crystals will be easy: cool the solution below room temperature.

Question #8 (Answer: C) Crystals grow in highly ordered patterns into which impurities do not fit unless the impurities look very much like the compound of interest. With a properly chosen solvent, the impurities should remain in solution as the pure crystals form.

7.24.5 Advanced Concepts

This is a list of tools to analyze and understand separations and purifications.

- Improve review of observations linked with types and quantities of reactants and products. Identify all possible experiments to be performed. Propose any experimental modifications or new procedures to be used.
- Learn how to judge the influence of new experimental evidence on each conclusion, including experimental conditions, experimental errors and practical limitations on experiment.
- Look for hidden assumptions behind each experimental technique or procedure, theoretical explanation and practical explanation of each mechanism.

- Look for scientific reasons behind each observation (laboratory observations, untaught observations from experimental data and completely new observations).
- Determine deductive conclusions from observations in order to approve or nullify your hypotheses.

7.25 USE OF SPECTROSCOPY IN STRUCTURAL IDENTIFICATION

7.25.1 Introduction to Use of Spectroscopy in Structural Identification

Review laboratory and commercial spectroscopic techniques and identify differences. Understand the mechanical and electrical design, working and accuracy of various types of spectrometers.

7.25.1.1 INFRARED SPECTROSCOPY

Infrared spectroscopy, sometimes called "vibrational spectroscopy," is useful for identification of functional groups present in a molecule. Bonds that vibrate in a manner that changes the net dipole moment of the molecule absorb infrared radiation according to Hooke's law for the vibration of a spring (see Section 5.20.1). In the case of carbon dioxide, there are four possible vibrational modes: symmetrical stretching, unsymmetrical stretching, in-plane bending, and out-of-plane bending. These are shown schematically in Figure 7.88 below. The symmetrical stretching vibration does *not* alter the net dipole moment of the compound as the vector sum of the dipoles is still zero. Accordingly, this vibrational mode of carbon dioxide is not "ir active."

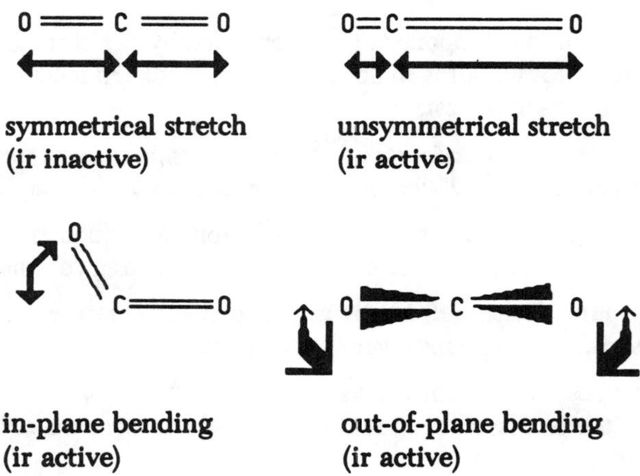

Figure 7.88—Vibrational Modes of Carbon Dioxide

Frequencies are given in wavenumbers (cm^{-1}) which is really the reciprocal of wavelength or in microns (μm) which is also a unit of wavelength. The two frequency units may be interconverted by the following formulae; $v = 1/\lambda$ (λ in cm) $= 10{,}000/\lambda$ (λ in μm). Texts and lab manuals give extensive correlation tables of frequencies and functional groups. A concise summary of important functional groups and their characteristic frequencies is given below. The frequencies listed are not absolute, as structural features of different compounds will shift the vibrational frequencies of the functionality.

Common Characteristic Group Absorptions

frequency (cm^{-1})	functionality	comments
3500 (broad)	OH, NH	hydrogen bonding causes broadness of the peak
3000	CH	virtually every organic compound has this
2200	alkyne, nitrile	
1715	C = O	exact frequency will vary with the type of C = O
1600	C = C	
1500-600		(fingerprint region—each compound has a unique pattern)
1100	C-O	useful to identify esters and ethers
600-800	aromatic C-H	one peak = o or p disubstituted; two peaks = mono substituted or m disubstituted

7.25.1.2 PROTON MAGNETIC RESONANCE SPECTROSCOPY

Proton magnetic resonance spectroscopy measures the number and types of different protons in a compound. Certain nuclei rotate on an axis and precess about that axis in much the same manner that the earth rotates and precesses on its axis. This rotation and precession sets up a magnetic moment of the nucleus—it can be aligned with or against an externally applied magnetic field. Alignment in the same direction as the external field is easier, just as it is easier to swim downstream than upstream. The difference in energy required for each magnetic orientation is measured by radio frequency radiation according to the equation $\Delta E = h\nu$. A plot of radiation absorbed as a function of frequency provides information about the local magnetic environment of the nuclei examined. Protons are one of a number of such nuclei that rotate. It is important to note that in proton magnetic resonance spectroscopy (pmr) only protons are observed. The presence of carbon can only be inferred. Equally important is the fact that substitution of deuterium (D) = H_1^2 for a type of proton H_1^1 will render that type of proton invisible.

I. Diastereotopic and Enantiotopic Protons:

The number of different signals depends on the number of magnetically different protons that are present in a molecule. Fig. 7.89 shows some different compounds and an indication of the number of magnetically different protons on each. There are two means by which protons can be considered "identical"—by symmetry or by being geminal (twins on the same carbon atom). The four protons of methane are all geminal and so only one signal is observed. Similarly, all six protons of ethane are identical by symmetry. But the two methyl groups of methyl ethanoate (methyl acetate) are *not* identical. One methyl group is attached to a carbonyl carbon while the other is attached to an oxygen. Each methyl group is then in a different magnetic environment. Propane is symmetrical about carbon-2 and so has two magnetically different types of protons. Propene offers the chance to make a careless error in selecting the number of magnetically different protons present. There are four. Protons (c) and (d) are *not* identical. Proton (c) is cis to a methyl group while proton (d) is trans to the methyl group. Again, this gives a different magnetic environment to these protons. In an analogous fashion, protons (c) and (d) of 1,2-dimethylcyclopropane are *not* identical. Here (d) is cis to two methyl groups while (c) is cis to two protons. Different magnetic environments. (S)-2-bromobutane is a more difficult case. Protons (c) and (d) here are again superficially the same, but in fact they are *not*. They are called "diastereotopic" protons. Replacing each of these protons with some other group will give diastereomers—easily distinguished by chemical and physical properties. Proton (d) will "feel" the effects of the bromine atom of carbon-2 more than will proton (c) in the configuration shown. Each is in a magnetically different environment. If replacement of each of two suspected identical protons with another group yields enantiomers, the protons are called "enantiotopic" and are magnetically indistinguishable.

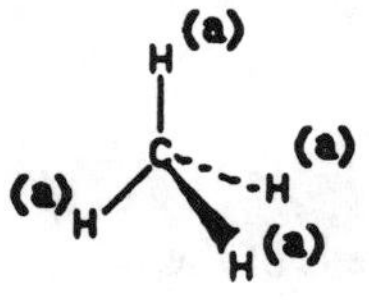

CH_3CH_3 (a)(a)

$CH_3\overset{O}{\overset{\|}{C}}OCH_3$ (a) (b)

methane
four identical protons

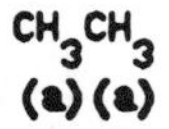

ethane
six identical protons

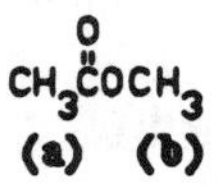

methyl ethanoate
two types of methyl protons

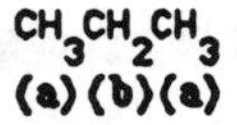

$CH_3CH_2CH_3$ (a)(b)(a)

propane
two types of protons

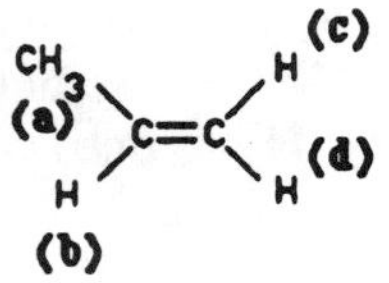

1-propene
four types of protons

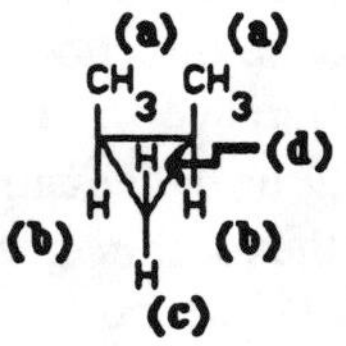

cis-1, 2-dimethylcyclopropane
four types of protons

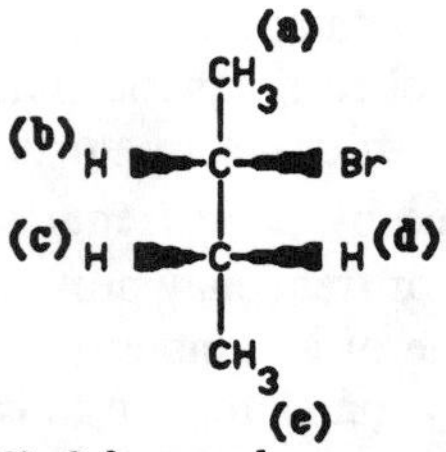

(S)-2-bromobutane
five types of protons

Fig. 7.89—Magnetically Different Protons

II. Chemical Shifts for Protons:

The chemical shift of a proton resonance is the difference in frequency between a signal absorbed by a sample and the frequency at which tetramethylsilane (TMS), a common reference material, absorbs radiation in the same instrument. This difference is expressed in a δ scale in units of parts per million (ppm). TMS is a good reference standard since its resonance frequency is different from most other types of protons, it is chemically inert, it has 12 identical protons so it gives a very strong signal, and it is easy to remove from the sample after the spectrum is recorded (B.P. = 26° – 28°). Protons that absorb at lower frequencies than TMS are said to be "shielded" from the external magnetic field since less energy is required to meet the resonance condition $\Delta E = h\nu$. Some instruments maintain a constant radio frequency and use an electromagnet to vary the strength of the magnetic field applied. The same "shielded" protons resonate upfield of TMS, that is to say at higher magnetic field strength than TMS. Such shielding stems from a local magnetic flux that opposes the external field. Protons may also be "deshielded" or shifted downfield of TMS by local magnetic flux that reinforces the applied field. [18]-annulene provides a compound with examples of both phenomena. Protons on the inside of the ring are shielded by a magnetic field that opposes the applied external field while the outside protons are deshielded by the same field. This field that shields and deshields is induced by the ring current that flows in the aromatic [18]-annulene ring. Its flux opposes the external applied field for the inside protons and it reinforces the external applied field for the outside protons. Fig. 7.90 illustrates this schematically.

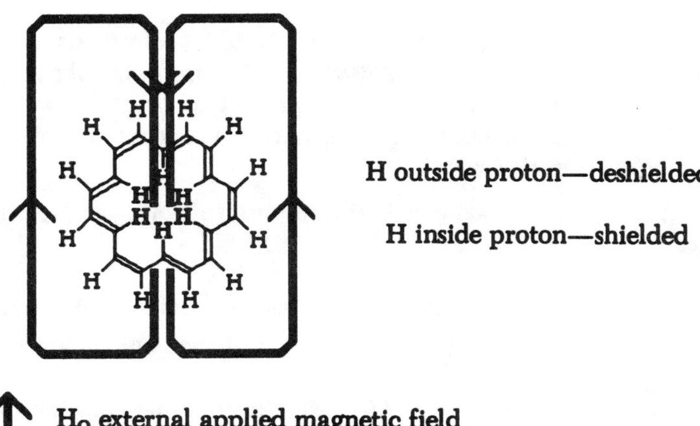

Fig. 7.90—[18]-annulene Showing Shielding and De-shielding

Protons along the perimeter of an aromatic ring are then de-shielded (shifted to higher δ). Protons attached to carbons bearing an electronegative element, such as O or Cl are also de-shielded from their customary resonance frequency in the absence of the electronegative element. The electron density near such electronegative elements is greater, so higher magnetic field strength is required to achieve the resonance condition. The chemical shift of a proton gives information about its magnetic environment. Textbooks and lab manuals provide detailed tables of chemical shifts for a variety of different types of protons. While such tables may be helpful in predicting the chemical shift of a given type of proton, they are not as crucial to structure determination given the spectrum. For that purpose, there are only three chemical shift values that need to be memorized:

Chemical Shift (δ ppm)	proton type
7	aromatic C-**H**
9	aldehyde RCHO
11	carboxylic acid RCO_2**H**

III. Spin-Spin Splitting of Protons:

It is sometimes useful to note that methyl protons (CH_3) give a typical resonance near δ 1 ppm and methylene protons (CH_2) generally give a resonance in the range δ 2-3 ppm. The fine structure or multiplicity of the signal (splitting pattern) provides a great deal of information about the protons in the vicinity of the one at resonance. This is because protons will "couple" with protons one carbon atom away. The magnetic environment of a proton is slightly altered by the magnetic orientation of those nearby protons. The fine structure or multiplicity is defined as follows:

Multiplicity of pmr signal = 1 + (total number of protons on adjacent carbon atoms)

The fine structure of pmr signals is symmetric and in relative ratios that are defined by Pascal's triangle (the coefficients for the binomial expansion of $[a + b]^n$). This is shown below:

singlet (1 let)	1
doublet (2 let)	1 1
triplet (3 let)	1 2 1
quartet (4 tet)	1 3 3 1
quintet (5 tet)	1 4 6 4 1

Thus a triplet consists of three peaks of relative intensity 1:2:1 and is indicative of a proton with a total of two protons on the adjacent carbon atoms. The term multiplet (m let) is used when the relative intensity of the first peak is too small to detect and accurately count. Aromatic protons are described as a singlet, broad singlet, or multiplet depending on the specific compound. The chemical shift is more useful than multiplicity in the identification of the presence of aromatic rings.

If there are other spinning nuclei, for example F-19, protons will also couple with that nucleus so that multiplicity then becomes:

Multiplicity of pmr signal = 1 + (total number of protons on adjacent carbon atoms)
+ number of F-19 atoms on the same carbon

The proton spectrum of cumene shown in Fig. 7.91 will illustrate the splitting of adjacent protons. The multiplicity of the two identical methyl groups is one plus the number of protons on the adjacent carbon atoms. There is only one proton on that "adjacent" carbon so the methyl protons appear as a doublet. In the same manner the methine proton (CH) appears as a septet because there are six protons on the adjacent carbons. The benzene ring appears as a singlet because in this case, the o, m, and p protons are very nearly, though not exactly, alike.

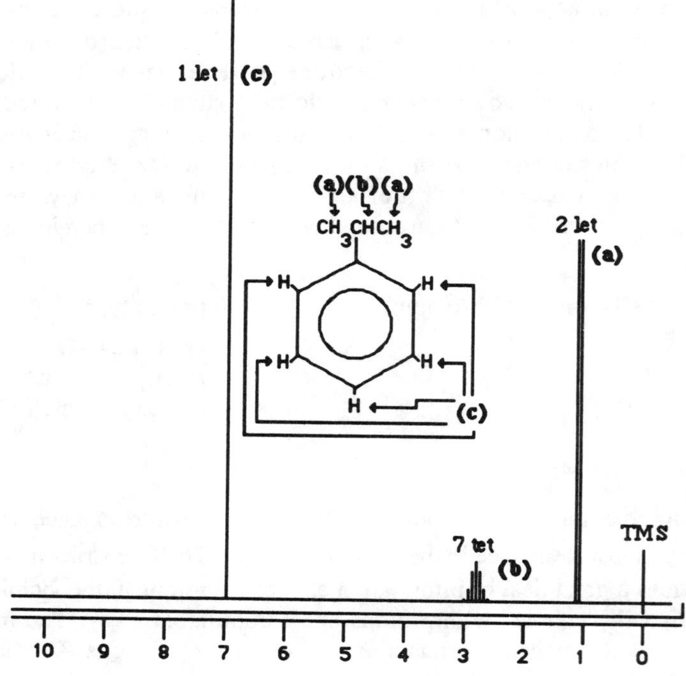

Fig. 7.91—PMR Spectrum of Cumene

There are two splitting patterns that are especially important.

3 let and 4 tet ethyl group
2 let and 7 tet iso-propyl group

In order to count the protons that give a signal, the area under each peak is electronically determined by charging a capacitor and plotting the charge on that capacitor as a function of the frequency scanned. The change in capacitor charge plotted on the y axis is proportional to the number of protons at a given resonance position. A ratio is established between the total integration distance and the total number of protons in the structure and that ratio is employed to determine the number of protons on signal. The spectrum in Fig. 7.92 below for a compound of formula C_8H_{10} (ethyl benzene) will illustrate the use of this methodology.

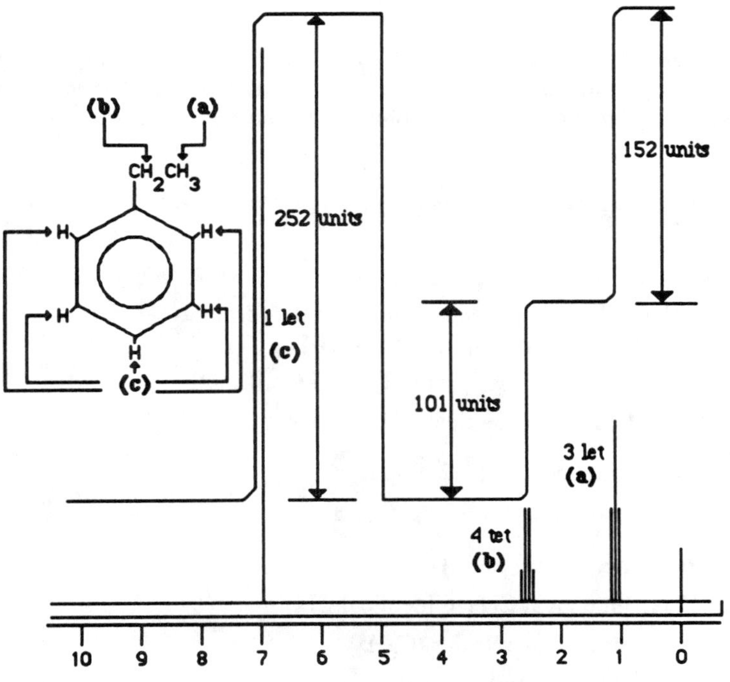

Fig. 7.92—PMR Spectrum of Ethylbenzene

The total integral distance is 505 units. A proportion is then set up as:

total integral distance/total protons in molecule = integral distance of one signal/protons giving rise to the signal.

That translates into the following for the triplet: 505 units/10H = 152 units/xH

Solving for x gives 3.01 protons which is close enough to 3 to be correctly identified with a set of methyl protons.

7.25.1.3 SYSTEMATIC APPROACH TO SPECTROSCOPY PROBLEMS

Following is a systematic means of approaching a typical spectroscopy problem where a molecular formula, proton magnetic resonance spectrum, and infrared spectrum are presented and an organic structure consistent with the data presented is demanded. It is like putting together a jigsaw puzzle, but first the individual pieces must be shaped.

1. Examine the molecular formula provided.
   a. What is its index of hydrogen deficiency (IHD)?

      This tells the sum of the rings and pi bonds that must be accommodated in the structure.
      The infrared spectrum can help locate the type of pi bond(s) present. An index of hydrogen deficiency of four is required for a benzene ring.

      Its value is conveniently calculated as shown: IHD = (A-V)/2

      A = number of electrons needed for acyclic, single bonded structure
      = 6*N + 2 (N = number of non-hydrogen atoms)

      V = number of valence electrons in a formula
      (Remember to add one electron for each unit negative charge and subtract one electron for each unit positive charge.)

   b. What atoms are present that should appear in the infrared spectrum? (O,N)
   c. What atoms are present that will not appear in the infrared spectrum? (Cl,Br)

2. Check the infrared spectrum for functional groups. Most do not contain protons and will, therefore, be transparent to proton magnet resonance spectroscopy. If the ir shows *both* OH and C = O, consider the possibility of a carboxylic acid. This should be obvious in the pmr spectrum with a chemical shift of about δ11 ppm.

3. Look at the pmr spectrum for evidence of aromatics (δ 7 ppm), aldehyde (δ 9 ppm), or carboxylic acid (δ 11 ppm).

4. Make pmr assignments on the basis of the number of protons shown for a given signal.

(1 H)	**CH**, NH, OH depending on elements present in the formula (check the ir spectrum for OH or NH)	
(2 H)	**CH_2** or 2 identical CH, or 2 identical NH, or 2 identical OH	
(3 H)	**CH_3** or 3 identical CH, or 3 identical NH, or 3 identical OH	
(4 H)	**2 identical CH_2,** 4 identical CH δ 2-4 ppm **disubstituted aromatic** (C_6H_4) δ 7 ppm	depending on chemical shift
(5 H)	**monosubstituted aromatic** (C_6H_5)	
(6 H)	**2 identical CH_3,** 3 identical CH_2, 6 identical CH	
(8 H)	**2 identical disubstituted aromatics** (C_6H_4), 4 identical CH_2, 8 identical CH	
(9 H)	**3 identical CH_3**	
(10 H)	**2 identical monosubstituted aromatics** (C_6H_5)	

Some of the possible choices (CH_3 or 3 identical CH, or 3 identical NH, or 3 identical OH) may be eliminated on the basis of the element not being present or by requiring more carbon atoms than are indicated in the molecular formula. The more likely possibility is in boldface.

5. Verify that all elements present in the compound are pieces of a jigsaw puzzle. Add up the atoms that are identified in the puzzle pieces and subtract from the given molecular formula. The result is a formula of what is still missing. If needed, an educated guess can be made on the manner in which the missing atoms are arranged.

6. Put the puzzle together following the splitting pattern dictated by the proton spectrum. Remember that the multiplicity is one plus the number of hydrogen atoms on the next carbon. Recall also that the combination of triplet and quartet is indicative of an ethyl group and that a doublet and septet shows the presence of an iso-propyl group.

7. Verify that this trial structure is consistent with *all* the data given.

   Some problems may not provide all the clues cited here. When that happens, improvise—but be systematic about it. Always verify that the trial structure fits ALL the data given.

7.25.1.4 SAMPLE SPECTRAL INTERPRETATION PROBLEM SOLUTION

What structure is consistent with the following data?

$C_7H_{12}O_4$ pmr spectrum:	3 let δ 1.25 ppm	(6H)	(a)
	1 let δ 3.35	(2H)	(b)
	4 tet δ 4.20	(4H)	(c)

ir spectrum: 1754 cm^{-1} and 1042 cm^{-1}

1. Calculate the **I**ndex of **H**ydrogen **D**eficiency (IHD)

Valance electrons:

$$\begin{array}{rcl} C & = & 7 \times 4 = 28 \\ H & = & 12 \times 1 = 12 \\ \underline{O} & \underline{=} & \underline{4 \times 6 = 24} \\ V & = & \text{valence e- } = 64 \end{array}$$

Electrons needed for acyclic, singled bonded compound:

A = 6*N + 2 (N = number of non-hydrogen atoms)
A = 6* (11) + 2
A = 68

Index of Hydrogen Deficiency calculation

IHD = (A – V)/2
= (68 – 64)/2
= 2

The compound has a combination of two rings and pi bonds. This can be accommodated as two pi bonds, one ring and one pi bond, or two rings. A benzene ring is out of the question since it requires an IHD of four.

2. Check the infrared spectrum. There are four oxygen atoms present. Are they present as alcohols, ethers, aldehydes, ketones, carboxylic acids, or esters? The peak at 1754 cm^{-1} is indicative of C = O. The peak at 1042 cm^{-1} may be a C-O of an ether or an ester. The absence of a broad peak near 3500 cm^{-1} rules out the possibility of an alcohol or carboxylic acid.

3. The pmr spectrum shows no peaks that may be assigned as aromatic, aldehydic, or carboxylic acid on the basis of their chemical shift. A benzene ring had been eliminated as a possibility in step 1.

4. The triplet of six protons is most likely due to two identical methyl groups. The singlet of two protons is probably a methylene (CH_2) group. The quartet of four protons is reasonably assigned as two identical methylenes (CH_2) different from the one that gives the singlet.

5. On the basis of the previous steps, the following pieces of a jigsaw puzzle are indicated:

CH_3	CH_3	CH_2	CH_2	CH_2	C = O
(a)	**(a)**	**(b)**	**(c)**	**(c)**	**(ir)**

This accounts for $C_6H_{12}O$ of a molecule of $C_7H_{12}O_4$. That leaves CO_3 unaccounted for by subtraction. The pieces of the puzzle also reveal only one pi bond. The calculation in step 1 showed that a combination of two rings and pi bonds are needed to satisfy the molecular formula. The deduced fragments show little inclination to form a ring, so there is a good chance that a second pi bond between a "missing" carbon and oxygen is appropriate. The same frequency in the ir spectrum that indicated the first carbonyl group indicate this one as well. The remaining "CO_3" is then formulated as C = O, -O-, -O-. The fragments that make up the $C_7H_{12}O_4$ are then:

CH_3	CH_3	CH_2	CH_2	CH_2	C = O	C = O	-O-	-O-
(a)	**(a)**	**(b)**	**(c)**	**(c)**	**(ir)**	**(5.)**	**(5.)**	**(5.)**

6. It is usually convenient to start at a terminal group such as CH_3 to combine the fragments. The methyl group identified as (a) appears as a triplet, so there are two protons on the next carbon atom (i.e., a CH_2). The CH_2 identified as (b) cannot be next to (a) because (b) is a singlet—there are no protons on the adjacent carbon. Thus CH_2 (c) is adjacent to CH_3 (a). The multiplicity of CH_2 (c) is a quartet, indicating three adjacent protons. Remember that a triplet and a quartet signify an ethyl group. There are no protons attached to the atom next to the CH_2(c). Bear in mind that there are two such identical ethyl groups. For them to be identical, they must have symmetry about a central atom and/or be geminal on that atom. There are two means by which that can be arranged. Fig. 7.93 illustrates both these possibilities.

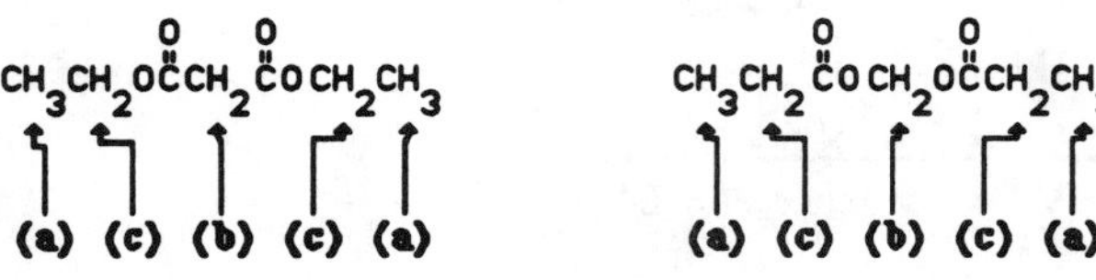

Fig. 7.93—Potential Structures for Sample Spectroscopy Problem

The selection of a "best" response from between these two possibilities becomes a bit more of a challenge. There are often occasions when more than one structure will give the same functional groups and splitting patterns. When this happens, then the exact chemical shifts in the pmr become important. In the structure on the left, diethyl malonate, the chemical shift of the (c) protons (quartet) are expected to be shifted downfield (higher δ) than the typical CH_2 resonance by virtue of the electronegativity of the oxygen attached to it. Likewise, for the structure on the right, (O-formylethoxy) methyl propanoate (commonly called methylene propionate), the chemical shift of the (b) protons (singlet) would be shifted downfield (higher δ) than the typical CH_2 resonance by virtue of the electronegativity of they oxygen attached to it. The observed chemical shift of the quartet (δ4.20) is well downfield from that expected of a typical CH_2 resonance (δ2-3). The singlet (δ3.35) is in a "normal" CH_2 position, indicating no electronegative atoms are influencing it. The decision is then made to select diethyl malonate as the best trial structure for the spectral data provided.

7. It is still important to ascertain that the trial structure is indeed consistent with the information given. In this instance the question in fact was formulated from spectral data of diethyl malonate, the structure on the left.

7.25.2 Questions Related to Use of Spectroscopy in Structural Identification

1. In the structure below, how many magnetically different protons are present?

$CH_3CH_2CHCH_2CH_3$ (with CH_2CH_3 attached to the CH)

- **A.** three
- **B.** four
- **C.** five
- **D.** seven

2. Which pair of compounds *cannot* be readily distinguished by infrared spectroscopy?

A.

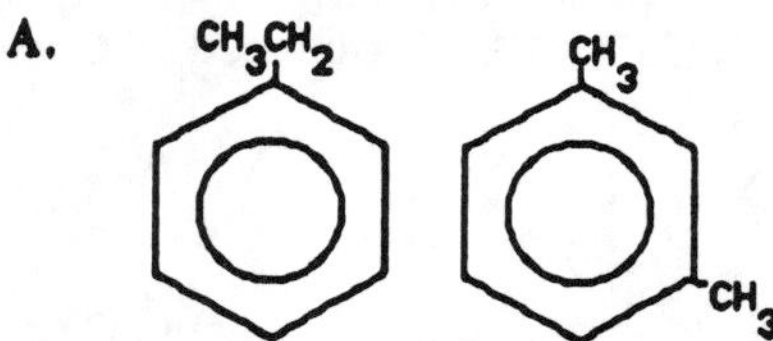

B. $CH_3CH_2CH_2CH_2\overset{O}{\overset{\|}{C}}CH_3$

$CH_3CH_2CH_2CH_2CH_2CH_2OH$

C. $CH_3CH_2CH_2CH_2\overset{O}{\overset{\|}{C}}OH$

$CH_3CH_2CH_2CH{=}CHCH_2CH_3$

D. $CH_3CH_2CH_2CH_2CH_2CH_2Cl$

$CH_3CH_2CH_2CH_2CH_2CH_2OH$

3. In the molecule below, in the proton magnetic resonance spectrum the indicated protons should appear as a:

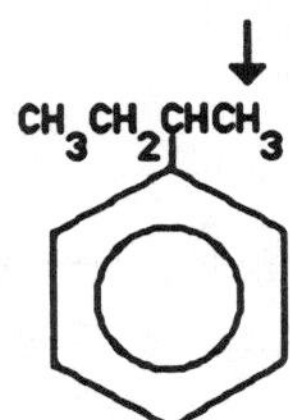

A. singlet
B. doublet
C. triplet
D. quartet

4. A compound of formula C_5H_{12} is studied by proton magnetic resonance spectroscopy. The total integral distance was measured as 144 mm. One signal gave an integral distance of 72 mm. How many protons give that signal?

A. two
B. three
C. six
D. nine

5. The signals below represent magnetic resonance signals. Which one is a quartet?

A.

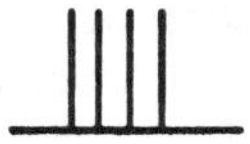

B.

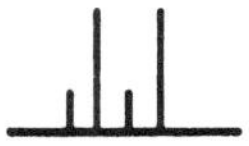

C.

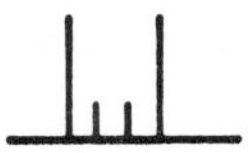

D.

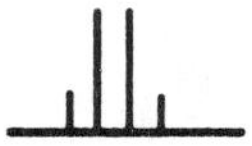

6. A broad peak in the 3500-3000 cm^{-1} region of the infrared spectrum is due to:

A. O-H vibrations damped by hydrogen bonding.
B. C = C vibrations damped by hydrogen bonding.
C. C = O vibrations damped by hydrogen bonding.
D. aromatic ring vibrations.

7. In the compound shown below, which of the indicated protons will give their resonance signal farthest downfield (highest δ)?

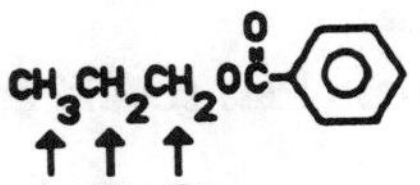

$CH_3CH_2CH_2O\overset{O}{\overset{\|}{C}}-C_6H_5$

↑ ↑ ↑
A. B. C.

D. All protons will have the same nominal chemical shift.

8. In the proton magnetic resonance spectrum, a singlet that corresponds to one proton disappears on addition of D_2O. This disappearance is due to the fact that:

A. deuterium exchanges with *all* protons.
B. deuterium exchanges with *acidic* protons.
C. deuterium causes instrument malfunctions.
D. the deuterium signal is much stronger than the proton signal.

9. How many magnetically different protons are present in the molecule below?

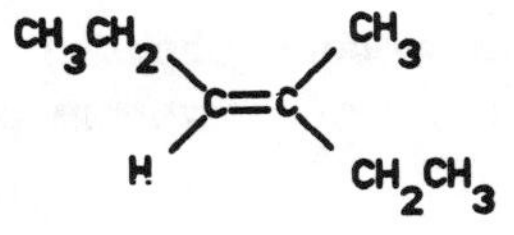

$(CH_3CH_2)(H)C{=}C(CH_3)(CH_2CH_3)$

A. three
B. four
C. five
D. six

10. An unknown compound has been determined to be either cis-1,2-dimethylcyclopropane or its trans isomer. The magnetic resonance spectrum of the compound revealed four magnetically different types of protons. Which isomer is the unknown?

A. trans
B. cis
C. mixture of both
D. cannot tell

11. An unknown molecule has been found to contain oxygen. From the infrared spectrum shown below it is clear that the oxygen is present as which functional group?

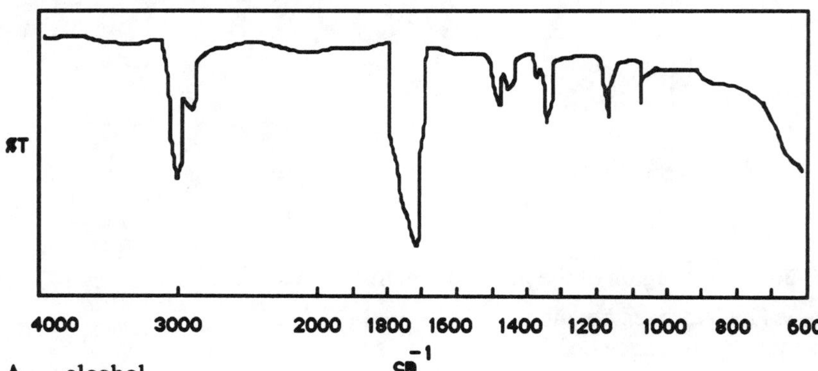

A. alcohol
B. carboxylic acid
C. ether
D. ketone

12. Which structure is consistent with the spectral data below for $C_4H_8O_3$?

3 let δ 1.27 (3H)
4 tet δ 3.66 (2H) ir: 2500-3000 cm^{-1} broad
1 let δ 4.13 (2H) 1715 cm^{-1}
1 let δ 10.95 (1H)

A. $CH_3C(=O)CH_2OCH_2OH$

B. $CH_3CH(CH_3)C(=O)OH$

C. $CH_3CH_2OCH_2C(=O)OH$

D. $CH_3OCH(CH_2OH)OCH_3$

7.25.3 Answers to Questions in Section 7.25.2

(1) A (2) A (3) B (4) C (5) D (6) A (7) C (8) B (9) D (10) B (11) D (12) C

7.25.4 Discussion of Answers to Questions in Section 7.25.2

Question #1 (Answer: A) There are three identical ethyl groups (two types of protons) and one methine (CH) proton. Thus there are three different types of protons present.

Question #2 (Answer: A) Mono-substituted benzenes and meta di-substituted benzenes *both* give two major peaks in the 600-800 cm^{-1} region of the infrared spectrum.

Question #3 (Answer: B) The multiplicity of a proton magnetic resonance signal is one plus the number of protons on adjacent carbons. In this case, there is one carbon adjacent to the terminal methyl group and it has but one proton. The multiplicity is (1 + 1) = 2 = doublet.

Question #4 (Answer: C) A ratio of total integration distance : total protons = signal distance : signal protons is set up. 144 mm / 12 H = 72 mm / x. Solving for x gives six protons.

Question #5 (Answer: D) Magnetic resonance signals are symmetrical and follow Pascal's triangle for their relative intensity. The correct ratio for a quartet is 1:3:3:1.

Question #6 (Answer: A) Peak broadening in the ir spectrum is due to hydrogen bonding. Of the choices listed, alcohols are the only functionality capable of hydrogen bonding to other like molecules.

Question #7 (Answer: C) Protons on carbons bonded to electronegative elements or electron withdrawing groups will have their resonance condition shed to higher δ (downfield).

Question #8 (Answer: B) Deuterium exchange for protons will cause a pmr signal to disappear. In order for such an exchange to take place, the proton must first be removed and then replaced. That can only happen with D_2O when the proton is acidic (alcohols, carboxylic acids, etc.).

Question #9 (Answer: D) The two ethyl groups here are *not* identical. One is cis to a methyl group while the other is cis to a proton. Each will have a slightly different magnetic environment.

Question #10 (Answer: B) The trans isomer has three magnetically different types of protons while the cis isomer has four.

Question #11 (Answer: D) The peak near 1700 cm^{-1} is characteristic of C = O.

Question #12 (Answer: C) The triplet and quartet are characteristic of an ethyl group. The singlet of two protons corresponds to a CH_2 with no protons on atoms on either side of it. A singlet at δ10.95 is due to a carboxylic acid, a functionality confirmed in the infrared spectrum.

7.25.5 Advanced Concepts

This is a list of tools to analyze and understand use of spectroscopy in structural identification.

- Improve review of observations linked with types and quantities of reactants and products. Identify all possible experiments to be performed. Propose any experimental modifications or new procedures to be used.
- Understand how reactions are related to basic mechanisms; how reaction rates are affected; what bonding arrangements, resonance stability structures and stereoarrangements are possible. Elucidate each mechanism in a visual format.
- Learn how to judge the influence of new experimental evidence on each conclusion, including experimental conditions, experimental errors and practical limitations on experiment.
- Look for hidden assumptions behind each experimental technique or procedure, theoretical explanation and practical explanation of each mechanism.
- Look for scientific reasons behind each observation (laboratory observations, untaught observations from experimental data and completely new observations).
- Determine deductive conclusions from observations in order to approve or nullify your hypotheses.

7.26 REFERENCES

Biological Science, 4th or latest ed. William T. Keeton and James L. Gould. New York: W. W. Norton & Co., Inc.

Experimental Organic Chemistry, 2nd or latest ed. H. Dupont Durst and George W. Gokel. New York: McGraw Hill Book Co.

Macroscale and Microscale Organic Experiments, 1989, Kenneth L. Williamson. Lexington, Mass: D.C. Heath and Company.

Organic Chemistry, 2nd or latest ed. G. M. Loudon. Redwood City, Calif.: Benjamin-Cummings Publishing Co.

Organic Chemistry, 5th or latest ed. R. T. Morrison and R. N. Boyd. Needham Heights, Mass.: Allyn & Bacon, Inc.

Organic Chemistry, 4th or latest ed. T. W. Solomons. New York: John Wiley & Sons, Inc.

The Organic Chem Lab Survival Manual: A Student's Guide to Techniques, 2nd ed. James W. Zubrick. New York: John Wiley and Sons.

Chapter 8:

Test-Taking Strategies and Practice Passages

Review test-taking strategies in this chapter at an early stage of your MCAT preparation. As a student you most certainly use test-taking strategies at school and at work, but you may not be as familiar with the new MCAT passage-linked test items. Techniques are provided for working passage-based problems during MCAT preparation. An Error Analysis Chart is also included here in section 8.4 to help you identify any weaknesses in your test-taking skills and to suggest ways to address them constructively.

This chapter is organized to provide strategies that can be applied during the test, as well as study strategies that can lead to improved test performance. These topics include:

- using principles of logic in passages and test items
- remembering definitions of scientific terms and concepts
- learning how to work with multiple-choice test items
- using error analysis
- working at a certain speed without sacrificing accuracy
- learning how to cope with stress and anxiety
- learning how to eliminate wrong answers and guessing
- remembering things to be done before, during and after the test

8.1 STRATEGY #1: USING LOGIC TO IMPROVE TEST-TAKING SKILLS

A central component to good test-taking is the ability to understand and use logic and to recognize logical connectors immediately. We use logical reasoning to understand what we read and to organize our thoughts when we write. In national standardized tests in particular, form and syntax are governed by the rules and language of logic. Logical reasoning governs our understanding of test questions in terms of what is being asked and how to choose an answer. (Further discussion of logical reasoning and its applications in problem solving is included in chapter 4.)

8.1.1 Using Deductive and Inductive Reasoning

Learn to recognize whether a question asks you to use deductive or inductive reasoning. This will help to clarify the question and assist you in working through the problem. As you read the descriptions below, pay attention to the processing differences involved in the two types of reasoning.

Deductive Reasoning

In the deductive reasoning form you are provided with statements that lead to a particular conclusion. If the reasons are accurate or confirmed by facts, the conclusion must follow. For example, evaluate this statement: *Bacteria contain protoplasm.*

Protoplasm is found in cells of all living organisms.
Bacteria are living organisms.

Bacteria contain protoplasm.

Your job during the test is to evaluate the accuracy of the supporting evidence. If you can say that the supporting evidence is true, you can also accept the conclusion as well. The above example is a syllogism and is in the structure of an argument. Laid out in this form it is easy to evaluate. In a test, however, the information is rarely if ever given to you in this format. The more common test question format is:

Which of the following statements are false?

A. Bacteria do not contain protoplasm.
B. Bacteria consist of prokaryotic cells.
C. Bacteria cannot be seen with the naked eye.
D. Bacteria do not have circulatory systems.

This format may make it less clear how deductive logic can help you in a test situation. However, in order to evaluate these statements, you must reconstruct the supporting evidence in your mind. In order to determine whether statement A is true, you would recall that protoplasm is found in cells of all living organisms and, from what you know about bacteria in general, you know they are living organisms. Hence, bacteria contain protoplasm. Therefore, statement A is correct. Now you construct the syllogism for statements B, C, and D.

Inductive Reasoning

In inductive reasoning, your task is to evaluate the level of probability under which the conclusion does follow. In written text, you can tell by the syntax whether a sentence is a conclusion suggested or a conclusion confirmed. That is, if the sentence is a conclusion suggested, it will contain the conditional verbs such as *may, seem, can,* etc., or adverbs such as *probably, primarily, most likely, most nearly,* etc. In logic, these conditional verbs and/or adverbs signify to you, the reader, that you are to read the sentence according to the rules of inductive logic, that is, the conclusion is to be judged according to probability.

This is different from a deductively phrased statement in which you are to judge the information according to logical validity. Remember that logical validity states that if the premises are true, then the conclusion must also be true. Perhaps an example will help.

> You ask me to dinner at your house, and I say, "I may come." This is a very different statement from saying, "I will come." The first statement is to be read as, "I may" or "I may not," and you have to judge whether to expect me or not on the basis of probability. On the other hand, if I say, "I will come," I mean, "all other things being equal, I will be there."

Many students are uncomfortable with inductively phrased questions and their conclusions because they are based on probability. For everyone, in real life and the MCAT, probability causes trouble in at least two related ways. First, in an inductively phrased multiple-choice question, there can be more than one possible right answer, but one will be more probable than the other. Second, probability involves a sliding scale of certainty. For example:

Consider a brown paper bag that contains 10 blue marbles, 3 green marbles, and 4 yellow marbles. If one marble is pulled out at random, what is its more probable color? Blue, of course. But now 5 orange marbles and 8 white marbles are added to the bag. Again, one marble is selected at random. What is the most probable color of this second marble?

The answer is still blue simply because there are more blue marbles than any other one color, but the probability is less. As different colored marbles are added, "blue" will remain the correct answer as long as there are more blue marbles than any other color. But the answer "blue" will feel less and less certain to you until only the deliberate application of the rules of probability will help you to answer. As the probability lessens, you will no longer feel as certain as to which answer is correct.

Students who try to be clever have an additional difficulty. They tend to look for the obscure (but possible) answer rather than choosing the probable answer that seems too easy. This can be corrected if you understand that the syntax of the question stem tells you that you must make your answer selection based on probability rather than possibility or certainty.

Question Formats Used to Test Logical Reasoning

The following test question formats are familiar ones to persons who have taken the "old" and the "new" MCATs. The first, the keyed choice, was on the old MCAT, and the multiple and multiple-multiple choice are used in the 1991 MCAT. They will be explained further in this chapter.

Keyed Choice (Old MCAT)	**Multiple-Choice**	**Multiple-Multiple Choice**
A. (Response 1) B. (Response 2) C. (Response 3)	A. (Response 1) B. (Response 2) C. (Response 3) D. (Response 4)	I. (Premise 1) II. (Premise 2) III. (Premise 3)
1. (A premise is placed here to be compared with one of the responses above)		A. (Response 1) B. (Response 2) C. (Response 3) D. (Response 4)

8.1.2 Applying Logic to Double Questions/Double Answers

The pre-1991 or "old" MCAT used two types of choices for test items: keyed choice and multiple choice. The 1991 or "new" MCAT uses only multiple choice or multiple-multiple choice. The keyed choice items are an excellent tool to learn logical reasoning and to apply true-false logic to a statement. These keyed choice items are included for two basic reasons:

1. to sharpen your logic (using "supported or true", "contradicted or false", or "neither supported nor contradicted" statements) in reading passages and test items.
2. both the new and the old MCAT have always included a certain percentage of double level multiple-multiple choice items. Three premises (identified with I, II, and III) are given, and the multiple choice questions include a combination of these premises to be true or false. Medical students often call them K-type questions. The second reason to keep keyed choice items is to train you how to evaluate a premise (true or false) before selecting the correct answer.

A double question is one that contains more than one logical proposition. An example of a sentence with more than one logical proposition is:

"Breathing involves the pumping of air into and out of the lungs of terrestrial animals as well as the pumping of water over the gills of fish."

The logic that is used in working with double questions and answers is basically the same as that used for single propositions; that is, in working with single propositions you must evaluate **each** proposition. Here is an example of the responses in a "keyed choice" question:

A. **supported or true,** according to the passage; (Response 1)
B. **contradicted or false,** according to the passage; (Response 2)
C. **neither supported nor contradicted, or irrelevant,** according to the passage. (Response 3)

Premise: **1.** Fish do not use gills for breathing.

To evaluate the information in a double question/double answer test item, you must first learn to recognize when sentences contain more than one logical proposition and then divide the statement into its separate propositions. Each one can then be evaluated separately according to the above criteria. These are included to give you more experience with items and the responses that accompany them.

Rules for Answering Double Questions/Double Answers

Most students read for facts and can judge whether a fact in a test question is true. However, determining whether a fact is supported or contradicted, or irrelevant is often problematic, since students are generally not taught to evaluate this type of information. Yet choosing the correct answer in multiple-choice questions often depends on being able to evaluate facts.

In working with a double question/double answer format, judge each part separately and write above each one which criterion applies: **A** (supported or true), **B** (contradicted or false), or **C** (neither supported nor contradicted, or irrelevant). Once you have done this, construct an equation and apply the following rules:

Rule 1: supported + supported = supported; true + true = true (A and A gives A).

Rule 2: contradicted + contradicted = contradicted; false + false = false (B and B gives B).

Rule 3: two propositions, neither supported nor contradicted, taken together = a statement that is neither supported nor contradicted (C and C gives C).

Also consider the following additional but less obvious rules:

Rule 4. two propositions, one of which is supported and one of which is nether supported nor contradicted = statement that as a whole is neither supported nor contradicted (A and C gives B).

Rule 5: two propositions, one of which is supported or true and one of which is contradicted or false = statement as a whole that is contradicted or false (A and B gives B).

Rule 6: a statement that contains two propositions, one of which is false and one of which is neither supported nor contradicted = statement that as a whole is contradicted or false (B and C gives B).

Remember that in double questions, both propositions must be satisfied or supported by the answer. In test items with double answers, both propositions contained in the answer must be supported or true as well.

8.2 STRATEGY #2: STUDYING DEFINITIONS DURING MCAT REVIEW

Make entries in your vocabulary notebook and review them regularly. This will reinforce your working vocabulary significantly. This is necessary for the MCAT because difficult words and technical terminology can cause trouble. The three principal ways the test maker assesses your ability to handle definitions of technical or difficult words in MCAT problems or passages is by asking you to:

- distinguish between unfamiliar technical terms that are closely related.
- distinguish between words that sound alike.
- demonstrate your understanding of the issues involved in defining a concept in an extended definition.

Distinguishing Between Closely Related Terms

On some problems or passages, you are likely to be presented with an unfamiliar topic or an advanced concept. The passage will resemble an introduction with a presentation of basic technical terminology. To answer the questions, you might be asked to distinguish between related subgroups within the topic area. For example, you might be asked to distinguish between different kinds of immune disorders presented in the passage. Students often have difficulty reading this kind of passage for one of the following reasons:

- lack of precision in distinguishing one term from another,
- anxiety related to the time it takes to understand such unfamiliar material,
- failure to have an available strategy for dealing with the difficulty.

When reading and answering questions, learn to recognize whether the form of the passage is definitional. This provides insight into the purpose of the passage and alerts you to what you will likely be asked to do in answering the questions. As you read, it is helpful to make a note (such as "def") in the margin wherever you have identified a definition.

Distinguishing Between Words that Sound Alike

If "affect" and "effect" caused you trouble in high school English, the distinction between "astronomy" and "astrology" may be likely to cause confusion on the MCAT, and the terms "afferent" and "efferent" will undoubtedly cause you some difficulty in medical school and on the National Medical Board Examinations. You can counter this by a specific strategy for dealing with terms that are confusing simply because of acoustic similarities.

While you are studying, collect words that you typically confuse with each other. Write them on index cards and practice them often. Develop mnemonics to help distinguish between them. For example, you can associate "exit" and "efferent." A more complex mnemonic for distinguishing between "afferent" and "efferent" would be SAME and DAVE. SAME reminds you that sensory and afferent go together, as do motor and efferent; DAVE reminds you that dorsal and afferent belong together, as do ventral and efferent. Words with similar sounding but different prefixes almost always cause trouble: homogeneous vs. heterogeneous, intercellular vs. intracellular, etc. Learn to anticipate tricky comparison/contrast questions and keep a list for frequent review.

Understanding Extended Definitions Used in Passages

You may have problems with MCAT passages that present an extended definition of a word. The word can be a technical term that requires a thorough extended discussion, e.g., "psychosis." Note that unlike passages that introduce totally new but rather specific terminology, extended definition passages often deal with a broad term that you might find somewhat familiar, but which you understand imprecisely. Often, a purpose of the extended definition passage can be to refute a commonly held definition in favor of the author's own view.

You may find extended definition passages difficult either because you fail to recognize the "argument" aspect of the discussion or because you answer the questions based on your own view, which is not necessarily that of the author. Remember that all definitions are open to examination and modification. For example, astronomers are currently debating the precise definition of "planet" because new data seem to require a revised one. This means that you must read with an open mind and be especially careful to focus on what the author says without mixing in your own biases.

8.3 STRATEGY #3: USING QUESTION ANALYSIS TO IMPROVE PERFORMANCE

Another consideration in improving your test-taking performance is the use of systematic strategies such as question analysis. Regardless of the test, you can become a more confident test-taker by learning the item types, question formats and responses used in constructing tests. The ability to apply systematic strategies during a test is helpful because it is more time-efficient and minimizes the kinds of careless mistakes that can result from an inconsistent approach.

The MCAT uses a conventional multiple-choice format with questions based on passages that call for careful reading, idea organization and critical thinking. This section reviews multiple-choice and keyed-choice questions and suggests strategies you can develop for answering each type.

8.3.1 Conventional Multiple-Choice Questions and Question Analysis Strategy

The conventional multiple-choice question is composed of a stem and a set of four answer choices. For example, the stem of the question might read: "The main topic of this passage is the . . .", and the answer choices are the responses **A, B, C, D.**

Multiple-choice items appear to be constructed in much the same way on tests from high school level SATs right through the National Medical Board Examinations for medical students. The test-maker puts the correct answer in one of the slots. Then the trickiest, and most difficult WRONG answer is added. This most difficult wrong answer tends to be very close to the right answer—which is why it is called the "almost-right" response. The test-maker knows that the closer the "almost-right" answer is to the correct answer, the more difficulty you will have distinguishing one from the other. For example, if the question stem says, "All of the following are functions of the liver EXCEPT . . .", the exception might be a function of the spleen, one that the test maker knows students tend to relate incorrectly to the liver.

Because there tends to be at least two seemingly right answers, the student who leaps for a single, correct answer can be easily misled. For example, under the pressure of the real MCAT you might be easily tempted to choose the first answer choice that seems correct, but that answer may turn out to be the "almost-right" answer or what the test maker calls "the most likely distractor." *You need to read all the answer choices carefully. If you do not see at least two "correct" or "nearly correct" answers (that is, if you do not see what the test maker thought was difficult), you may be responding too superficially.*

<u>The Importance of Strategy</u>

The MCAT tests examinees by posing a variety of questions about mixed-content areas over a long period of time (5-plus hours). Taking the MCAT is, therefore, more like running a marathon than a sprint. When running a sprint, the contestant simply runs as fast as possible from starting gun to finish line. In running a marathon, the contestant develops an overall plan with appropriate strategies for each part of the race well in advance. The runner then practices until the targeted actions for the actual race are deliberate yet automatic. In preparing for and taking the MCAT, you will do best if you have an overall plan and specific, well-practiced strategies for each test section.

When you have decided on strategies for answering multiple-choice questions, you will find that it is less risky and time-consuming to use these strategies consistently until they become habit. Here are three basic rules:

1. Read all of the options presented before eliminating any of them.
2. Reject a clearly wrong answer by putting a slash through the identifying letter.
3. Identify most likely answer choices and consider them carefully to assure best possible choice.

A word of warning! In many ways, much of a student's classroom training runs counter to the deliberate, careful strategies suggested here for best performance on multiple-choice items. Consider that as early as junior high school, many students are already competing not only to get the right answers, but also to get them faster than everyone else. This focus on speed encourages students to rely on rote memory and intuition leaps rather than rewarding those who carefully work their way to the correct answer. To benefit from the strategy recommended here, you will need to practice consistently until you can respond automatically. On the day of the test, then, you can concentrate on content and your search for correct answers.

Since answer choices require a certain amount of thought, you may be concerned about how you will be able to find time during the MCAT examination to worry about test-taking strategies. However, effective strategies not only lead to right answers, but are time-efficient as well.

8.3.2 Question Analysis Strategy

For most readers, recall of information from the passage or problem is usually insufficient to pick the best answer on the MCAT Verbal Reasoning test section. In using a question analysis strategy, however, you **read the question stem first** so that you know what to look for and then you search the passage for the sentence (usually only one) that gives the answer.

You know when you have found the right sentence in the passage because of the number of important words (primarily significant nouns) that it has in common with the question. For example, if the question asks, "In what historical period was U.S. population growth the lowest?," you can scan the passage for "population growth" and "lowest." The passage sentence that provides the answer might read: "This was the lowest rate of population growth recorded until the 'Great Depression' when the net growth rate fell to 7 per 1,000 population during the 1930–1935 period."

At first, you may find the question analysis strategy awkward and time-consuming. After all, it is unlikely you have read this way before. However, practice will increase your accuracy and ensure that you have enough time to complete this section of the test. To develop your skill using the question analysis strategy, follow these steps:

1. Skim the passage using the first and last sentence in each paragraph *only.*
2. Read the question stem first, but do not spend time reading all the answer options.
3. Underline the significant words in the question stem, primarily the nouns and active verbs.
4. Scan the selection, marking as you go and looking for words and sentences that match those you underlined in the stem. Words in the passage may appear in a different order than they appear in the question.
5. Put the number of the question in the margin where you found the information in the passage.
6. Steps 1 through 4 can be learned quickly, but after you narrow your choices, slow down to evaluate them carefully.
7. Answer the question carefully, working back and forth between passage and question. Pay special attention to the remaining words in the sentence, especially to the precise meaning of conjunctions and qualifiers such as adverbs, adjectives and restrictive phrases.

Practice this strategy with the passages in this chapter. Remember to pick out the significant nouns and verbs in the question stem and passage. Note when you begin to anticipate where the difficulty lies in choosing the right answer. Continue practicing until you feel that you have developed the efficiency needed to be effective.

<u>Modified Question Analysis Strategy</u>

Many students, even with continued practice, find the Question Analysis Strategy difficult to use. They find that while they have located specific places to look for designated words and phrases, they do not have a sense of the overall development of the topic. This makes it difficult to work with questions that involve interpretation, inference, or application. If this is your problem, then you might want to try modifying the question analysis strategy. Begin working with a passage by doing the following:

1. **Skim the text quickly** to find the main idea of the passage. The main idea statement is typically located in the first or last sentence of the first paragraph, or at the end of the last paragraph.
2. **Skim the remaining paragraphs** to determine the main idea of each paragraph. Again look at the first or last sentence in each paragraph to find the main idea statement.
3. **Watch for key words** that indicate the topic's pattern of development. Examples of key words include: *but, consequently, only, in addition, similar to,* etc.
4. **Return to the question analysis strategy**, using the seven steps described above.

Work with both the question analysis strategy and the modified question analysis strategy to determine which is best for you. Evaluate your performance, checking your speed and accuracy for each method. Once you have determined the best approach, **do not go back and forth between the two methods.**

8.3.3 Keyed-Choice Questions and Question Analysis Strategy

Keyed-choice questions may or may not be included in the MCAT at this time, but you should become familiar with this item style. It will provide an excellent alternative thinking approach. Keyed-choice questions may be less familiar to you than conventional multiple-choice questions, but they are used in various tests including the former MCAT subtests. Keyed-choice options require you to decide how a given statement is related to the passage. In other words, in keyed-choice questions you are asked to evaluate the statements according to the following:

A. Statement **is supported** by the information in the passage.
B. Statement **is contradicted** by the information in the passage.
C. Statement **is neither supported nor contradicted** by the information in the passage.

The key from which you are to select an answer can be quickly coded as follows:

A. support
B. contradict
C. neither

As with multiple-choice questions, use the question analysis strategy to reduce reading time. Most students quickly learn to do keyed-choice questions rapidly and accurately using the question analysis strategy. When answering this type of question, remember to:

1. **Read the question statement first**, noting whether it is a double question and whether it is inductively or deductively phrased.

2. **Underline the significant nouns** in the question statement.

3. **Scan the passage,** marking it up while looking for the passage statement that shares as many significant words as possible with the question statement.

4. **Find the passage statement**, putting the number of the question in the margin and considering the similarities and differences.

5. After completing the first four steps, **carefully select the BEST answer** from the key, paying special attention to the qualifier words, including restrictive phrases.

8.4 STRATEGY #4: USING ERROR ANALYSIS TO IMPROVE TEST PERFORMANCE

Learning to analyze error patterns is a key element to improvement in all parts of the MCAT. Since the errors we make tend to repeat over and over again, it is essential to know our error patterns to begin developing corrective strategies.

8.4.1 Error Analysis Procedure

Read the error analysis procedure below, then complete the Error Analysis Chart that follows in section 8.4.2. Fill in the chart by recording the errors you make in the practice passages at the end of this chapter. Error analysis is a very useful part of your MCAT preparation. The more completely and thoughtfully you approach this task, the more benefit you will receive. By analyzing your errors on a regular basis, you will not only be able to identify problems, but monitor your progress as well. In evaluating your test-taking performance, consider the following:

1. Passage content familiarity. Note whether the content was drawn from the social sciences, natural sciences, humanities or medicine, according to the *MCAT Student Manual* topics. Review Appendix A in this book to develop familiarity with passage format.

2. Passage type. Examine passage types this chapter, chapter 2, and in Appendix A. Check those that you believe give you the most trouble:

   ___ cause/effect
   ___ comparison/contrast
   ___ reasons
   ___ time order
   ___ definition
   ___ classification
   ___ spatial or graphic orientation
   ___ process

3. Pattern of organization. Determine whether errors more frequently involve:

   ___ experimental data
   ___ experimental procedures and designs
   ___ basic information understanding
   ___ analysis
   ___ research methodologies

4. Question type. Note whether the question type was:

   ___ multiple choice: single level with only A, B, C , D; or double level* I, II, III with A, B, C, D.
   ___ keyed choice: support, contradict or neither.

   *Double level multiple-choice questions are called multiple-multiple choice, or K-type questions.

5. Reason for choosing the wrong answer. Determine the reason for an error by comparing your answer choice with the correct answer.

___ Was your error due to carelessness in choosing the best answer?
___ Did you have trouble with inductively phrased questions?
___ Did you have difficulty sorting out main ideas from details?
___ Did you ignore the negative stem?
___ Did you begin to feel pressured for time?
___ Did you not study the right information?
___ Did the passage mislead you?
___ Did you answer a different question than was asked?

6. Analyze your errors for patterns. After recording your experience on the Error Analysis Form, analyze your performance by searching for error patterns in the data. A tally of the frequency of various errors in each column will suffice. This provides important information to use in trying to eliminate repetitive errors.

8.4.2 Common Error Patterns and Solutions

Identify error patterns to enable you to anticipate problems. Be aware of your usual pitfalls. This method allows you to deliberately apply strategies to eliminate them. You may have your own pattern of error, but there are a number of common errors to which you will want to pay particular attention as you analyze your error patterns.

1. Basic Comprehension Problems

General Reading Skills

PROBLEM: You find that you continue to make frequent errors, even though you are practicing to build accuracy.

SOLUTION: Take time to work on basic reading skills. A speed reading course will not help, since these courses typically do not concentrate on increasing comprehension. One of the best ways to improve comprehension is to read more. Many students limit their reading only to materials related to their course work. Consequently they feel insecure when asked to read in other topic areas. While reading your textbooks is important, spend at least 30 minutes or more each day reading for pleasure. This provides you with exposure to a wider range of writing styles and formats and stimulates your reading flexibility and rate.

Careless or Hasty Reading of the Passage

PROBLEM: You find that you are able to identify the correct sentence in the passage, but are still failing to get the correct answer. The problem may be due to superficial reading.

SOLUTION: Finding the correct passage sentence is only the first step. Once you have found the passage, read it critically to be sure that you understand what was stated. The passage should be read as **evidence** and you, as the reader, are the detective looking for very precise clues.

Inattentive Reading of the Question

PROBLEM: You are making errors due to careless reading of the question rather than lack of content information. Typical errors that fall into this category: not reading the question through to completion; overlooking important qualifiers (such as "some" or "not"); inattention to comparison/contrast factors in the passage and questions; failing to recognize that a question has more than one proposition.

SOLUTION: Go back to labeling the important parts of the question or proposition when you are doing practice questions, and strive to be more active in the strategies you use.

Language Difficulties

PROBLEM: You have word comprehension problems involving synonyms because you are inaccurate in how you classify terms. For example, "dog" and "German shepherd" are not synonymous because a German shepherd is only one kind of canine.

SOLUTIONS: The discussion of synonyms is actually a discussion of the relationship between two terms under consideration. Using outlines or Venn diagrams can help to sort out relationships between two words. (See chapter 2, section 2.2.3, under "Visual Imaging or Mapping.")

2. Reasoning Problems

Analytical Reading Errors

PROBLEM: You are not accustomed to the precise, problem solving approach of reading analytically. You read for facts and fail to apply reasoning strategies to develop a more in-depth understanding of the material.

SOLUTION: Do some additional practice in this area. There are a number of excellent books on the art of problem solving that offer strategy suggestions and practice exercises. Review chapter 4 to reinforce your knowledge and use the suggested book references.

Reasoning Pattern Identification

PROBLEM: You have difficulty with inductively phrased questions. You either fail to recognize that you are dealing with probability, or, if recognized, you do not apply effective reasoning skills.

SOLUTION: Reread the discussion on inductive reasoning in Section 8.1.1 above. Compare inductively phrased questions with deductively phrased questions. Do you see why they are written inductively? Do you see how inductive phrasing allows for more than one possible answer? **Inductive phrasing is a clue that you should choose the best or most likely answer**.

Proportional Reasoning

PROBLEM: You have trouble with questions that include the words "increase" or "decrease," especially when proportional reasoning is required to understand the passage or determine the correct answer.

SOLUTION: Use arrows and make a chart in the margin. This helps you visualize what is happening and facilitates choosing the right answer.

3. Problems Related to Question Format

Keyed-choice Question

PROBLEM: Your trouble on this type of question is related to distinguishing between choice **B** (contradicted) and choice **C** (neither supported nor contradicted).

SOLUTION: If you notice that you pick **B** when it should be **C** and vice versa, place the **question** statement into the passage next to the **passage** statement you have identified. If it fits logically but is not stated in the passage as a true fact, then the answer is **C** (neither supported nor contradicted). On the other hand, if you put the question statement into the passage and it does not logically fit, the answer is **B** (contradicted). Look back over the practice passages with keyed-choice questions and compare questions where the answer is either **B** or **C**.

Questions with Negative Stems

PROBLEM: You have more trouble with the presence of negative words in a question or answer. Since we are **unaccustomed** to reading for what is **not** true of the exception, this type of question may require extra concentration.

SOLUTION: When you see an item with a negative stem, circle the negative word as a reminder. Consider each answer and decide whether it is true or false, then put a "T" or "F" next to each one. If you are not sure, put down a "?T" or "?F". After you have evaluated all the information, make your choice. When working with this type of question, be sure that you do not fall back into thinking about what **is** rather than what **is not.**

Double Questions

PROBLEM: You have trouble with questions with more than one proposition or answers with more than one variable. Errors may be due either to failure to recognize that more than one proposition is involved, or failure to evaluate all pieces of information.

SOLUTION: Identify each proposition and **number** them. Then methodically evaluate each proposition to be sure that each one satisfies all of the conditions given.

4. Variations in Degree of Concentration

Interest Level in the Topic

PROBLEM: You find yourself losing interest in passages that are not interesting to you and you have trouble concentrating. This is natural, but it can affect your performance in a negative way.

SOLUTION: To maintain your concentration, try to approach each passage and its attendant set of questions as though they were an enclosed puzzle. The Verbal Reasoning section on the MCAT presents nine of these puzzles, each of which requires about 9 minutes of concentrated effort.

Length of the Task

PROBLEM: You find it difficult to maintain concentration for more than 30 minutes at a time. Given the length of each MCAT test section, this could have a negative effect on your test performance. The MCAT is a long exam requiring stamina. Stamina is developed over time and is both physical and mental. During the examination you will find that when the mind begins to tire, it takes a break of its own accord. This can happen in at least two ways: either you begin to think about something else (washing the car on the weekend, for example) or you begin to read a single question over and over again.

SOLUTION: As a first step to improving your concentration, eliminate **unconscious** breaks when you are studying. Take a deliberate break as soon as you need it. Work with a clock in front of you. Deliberately change what you are doing by standing, stretching, or moving around for 2 to 5 minutes. When you go back to studying, try to concentrate just a little longer before your next break. You build slowly to increase speed for the MCAT! Increase your concentration in the same systematic way. Practice doing this so that you will be able to work productively, taking only controlled breaks. If you do this, you will be taking the test rather than letting the test take you. Take full-length practice tests under exact time limits to build endurance.

Anxiety Factors

PROBLEM: You find that a high level of anxiety on a test affects your level of concentration. It is serious enough to affect your performance. How do you respond to pressure? Does the first question make your mind go fuzzy, or does anxiety rise as time passes and you are suddenly aware that you are never going to finish in allotted time unless you speed up?

SOLUTION: If your anxiety tends to increase at the beginning of the test as soon as you see a difficult question, do not answer it. Move on until you find a question you can answer with confidence. Then go back to the question(s) you skipped and carefully match the numbers. If pacing is your problem, try to get pacing under control **before** you take the MCAT. Learn the techniques for keeping track of your pace. Speeding up under pressure tends to increase the number of careless errors. Speeding up because you are aware of the time is a confidence-builder and puts you in control. You do **not** get extra points just for answering every question on the test. However, you may lose points if you do not attempt to answer. Appropriate pacing assures that an answer is recorded for each question.

5. Your Personal Profile

As you work the various practice exercises in this book, enter your errors on the chart and analyze the data for continued error patterns. You may find that you develop a different profile across subtest areas that will then guide further preparation efforts. Remember that an important part of improving your performance is developing greater self-awareness of your personal test-taking skills and your ability to appropriately modify them.

The chart form that follows is divided into eight columns. Beginning with the item number, the column heads include: Content Area, Passage Type, Pattern Type, Question Type, Reasoning Process, Item Type, Reason for Error.

An introduction to the error analysis procedure is given above in section 8.4.1, which explains the segments in greater detail. Below are examples of the column heads.

ERROR ANALYSIS CHART

Item No.	Content Area	Passage Type	Pattern Type	Question Type	Reasoning Process	Item Type	Reason for Error
	Social Sciences Natural Sciences Humanities Medicine Biological Sciences Physical Sciences	Description Argument Data Interpretation Information Presentation Research Hypothesis Experimental/Instrumental	Cause/Effect Definitions Comparison/Contrast Classification Reasons Spatial/Graphic Time Order Process	Multiple choice Keyed choice Multiple-multiple choice	Inductive Deductive Other patterns Proportional Analogical Comparative Visual Multiple	Main Idea Detail Inference Application Prediction Definition Explicit Implicit	Careless/Hasty reading Inattention Language Definitions Logical Process Question Format Interest Level Lack of sufficient background

8.5 STRATEGY #5: DETERMINING YOUR MCAT TEST-TAKING SPEED

Test-wiseness means that you are in charge during the test day. You have learned the mechanics of handling test questions, you know how to pace yourself, mark the test booklet as you work, keep your place on your answer sheet, and so on. You are comfortable with the MCAT test item format. You have developed your skills for accuracy even if you are not yet working at MCAT speed. You have reviewed the natural science sections, concentrating to master weak areas while maintaining your mastery of strong areas. You are now able to concentrate for two-hour segments, including short, structured breaks.

If you have disciplined yourself to prepare for the MCAT, and if your accuracy level is satisfactory on all sections of the MCAT practice tests, you are now ready to develop your test-taking speed. The actual MCAT takes 5 hours and 45 minutes. The following chart provides information on the timing requirements for each test section.

8.5.1 Test Day Schedule: MCAT Timing Requirements by List of Tasks

Time management for the MCAT includes finishing the following tasks within 5 hours and 45 minutes. Your test-taking speed is a function of these tasks. A time range for each task is provided, giving you a goal to complete each task within the time range.

Task 1: **Passage skimming, reading, and classification.** There are a total of 30 passages and you are expected to finish Task 1 in 60 to 90 minutes. Speed for Task 1 = 2 to 3 minutes per passage.

Task 2: **Underlining key words and marking passages** (including maps, etc.). All 30 passages will take 15 to 25 minutes of your total time.

- Verbal Reasoning will take *more* time to mark up than either the Physical or Biological Sciences sections because of the amount of reading material. This includes 9 Verbal Reasoning passages to be marked in 5 to 9 minutes.
- speed for Verbal Reasoning task = 30 to 60 seconds per passage.
- the sciences have 20 or 21 shorter passages (most are shorter than Verbal Reasoning) to be marked in 10 to 12 minutes.
- speed for Physical and Biological Sciences task = 25 to 35 seconds per passage.

Task 3: **Writing essays in 60 minutes.** For details see chapter 6.

Task 4: **Answering independent questions.** There is a total of 30 independent questions in Biological and Physical Sciences. These will take about 20 to 30 minutes (an average of 40 to 60 seconds per item).

Task 5: **Answering passage-based questions.** There is a total of 189 questions in Verbal Reasoning, Physical and Biological Sciences. You can expect to spend about 189 minutes on this task, which is the major task on the MCAT. Pacing is especially important for this task.

Task 6: **Marking your answer sheet.** You may be able to avoid marking errors on your answer sheet if you mark after you have completed the passages and questions. Do this by circling the correct responses in your answer booklet as you work and then spend about 5 minutes to fill the ovals on the answer sheet. This prevents you from skipping questions and marking on the wrong lines. Skipping an answer accidentally can mean all following answers will be wrong. Practice on this to get acquainted with the columns and ovals on the answer sheet. One caution: keep track of your time so that you allow time for the answer sheet marking.

<u>MCAT Timing Requirements by Task</u>

Task 1 = 60 to 90 minutes	Task 2 = 15 to 21 minutes	Task 3 = 60 minutes or less
Task 4 = 20 to 30 minutes	Task 5 = 189 minutes or less	Task 6 = 15 to 20 minutes

You are allowed a total of 345 minutes for the entire test. If you add up the time we have shown for tasks 1 through 6 you would need from 359 to as much as 410 minutes. That means you need to cut your time in the areas **where you can best afford it** by 15 to 20 percent. Learning what takes **you** the most time will help you meet your goal to complete the test. With this kind of practice, you will soon notice an ability to work faster with a constant level of accuracy. Remember, there are no extra points given simply for finishing a subtest. Gauge yourself for the best speed/accuracy ratio to achieve the highest score.

Your speed will vary from section to section. Within each subtest, some questions take longer than others. You will not spend an equal amount of time on each item within a given subtest, but you will take less time on those that are "easy," saving time for more difficult items. Since there are no extra points for answering the hardest questions, you will get every point possible by working the easiest questions first and finishing with the more difficult.

Separate subscores are given for each section. This means equal effort for each area. Whether or not you like one science better than another, you will develop a disciplined approach producing effective effort regardless of the area. The pressure of real testing situations tends to make you revert to past behaviors. Keep your discipline in place for the entire time.

8.5.2 Speed and Accuracy Relationship

Faulty Pacing

PROBLEM: Misunderstanding the relationship between speed and accuracy. Managing time during the MCAT is a complex matter. Figuring out how many minutes per question on average that you have for each section of the test does not help, simply because the test-maker does not expect you to spend the same amount of time on each question.

SOLUTION: The test-maker carefully balances relatively quick-to-answer questions with those that take longer. As a sophisticated test-taker, you need to develop a sense for determining both types so that you can appropriately judge your time and set a reasonable pace.

Low Accuracy-Speed Ratio

PROBLEM: Working too slowly on tests. In the classroom, this may not affect the final score. However, on a test where time is an issue, too much speed can lower your score (and contribute to errors) and too slow a speed means too few items are completed which lowers your score.

SOLUTION: The best way to monitor this problem is to evaluate your pace when working practice tests. You may find that your current rate is appropriate, but if it needs modification, do it early in the preparation process so that you have a comfortable rate of speed/accuracy the day of the MCAT.

8.5.3 Practical Exercises to Build Speed

Begin approximately six weeks before the exam date to work seriously on speed. Work with a clock in front of you. Start with a passage or two having 7 or 8 questions each. Work first for accuracy, noting how much time it takes to reach an accuracy level that satisfies you. On the next set of practice items, push yourself to work just a little faster. If your accuracy level stays the same, work just a little bit faster on the next practice set. At the point where your accuracy level begins to suffer, work at that speed to bring the accuracy level back up. Increase your speed only when the accuracy level meets your standards. Work in this way on passages from each subtest area.

Look for short-cuts as you work to build your test-taking speed. For example, don't work too hard on calculating something where a quick estimate will let you eliminate several wrong answer possibilities quickly. Continually look for the more efficient way to approach a problem and don't become overly stubborn about answering a question that simply takes up too much time.

Practice independent questions frequently, since there are 30 on the test with 15 in each science subtest. This way you are ready for them when they appear on the test and it may be a way to gain some more time for the more complex passage-based items.

8.6 STRATEGY # 6: LEARNING TO COPE WITH INITIAL STRESS

Stress often builds quickly when you worry about material you don't understand and when errors increase as you study and practice test problems. The pressure of correcting errors and learning new materials can easily confuse you. Chapter 2 has good advice on avoiding most of the stress from this kind of situation.

To relieve stress take one MCAT topic that bothers you and go to the library. Study that topic from three or four references. This "library distraction" will increase your confidence when you return to regular study. Since you cannot learn or know everything, selective study of topics is more useful than memorizing too many details. Or meet with a study partner when stress builds up; this interaction can help you "let off steam" as well as help to clarify your MCAT concerns from your partner. Try going to your science laboratory to review various lab procedures by "hands on" work with your partner. Finally, mastering the topic will be greatly satisfying.

8.7 STRATEGY # 7: USING INTUITION, NOT GUESSWORK

It is good advice to avoid guessing. Do not give up and move into a guess mode as soon as something looks unfamiliar or difficult. In the face of uncertainty, put more reliance on your intuition and less on random guessing. Talk to yourself about what you know about a problem topic, even if it seems only tangentially related. This process often triggers associations that did not immediately come to mind and it will often give you enough information to answer the question correctly. If you remain uncertain after brainstorming about what you know, use common sense to make your decision. Lean toward the answer that makes the best impression on you at that point. If guessing cannot be avoided entirely, you will at least be in a position to make an educated guess, which improves your chances of answering the question correctly.

8.8 STRATEGY #8: PLANNING THREE WEEKS BEFORE THE TEST

Take the full length simulated MCAT from AAMC about three or four Saturdays before the actual test. The Association of American Medical Colleges provides actual tests that may be purchased from Betz Publishing Company. Use the actual *MCAT Practice Test I* or *MCAT Practice Test II.* The results enable you to determine your readiness for the MCAT and guide you in spending your time most profitably for the last few weeks of study. During the last few weeks, practice on the following skills for reinforcement.

1. Try to predict test questions while studying.
2. Read test instructions/directions carefully.
3. Read questions carefully and identify key terms.
4. Attempt to define key terms in a question before working through the question.
5. Determine the intent of the test item without over-interpretation.
6. Evaluate all information before choosing an answer.
7. Use a problem solving strategy rather than guessing.
8. Apply consistent logic to answers or responses within a test question.
9. Be flexible and follow multiple paths to problem solutions.
10. Distinguish between fact and opinion provided in the passage.
11. Rely on reasoning rather than personal feelings and/or impressions.
12. Determine similarities and differences among concepts and details.
13. Draw diagrams or write equations, when appropriate, to develop perception and to clarify ideas.
14. Test answers for relevancy to a problem.

If you can get others to participate in the simulation with you, so much the better. But remember, even if you do it on your own, the closer you simulate the real thing the more benefit you will derive from the experience. Carefully follow the time limits in the MCAT test booklet and make your environment as much like a real test site as possible.

You will benefit from a careful analysis of the results. Score one point for each correct answer. There is no penalty for incorrect or unanswered items. Total your correct answers to produce your raw score. You may then compute your percent right score by dividing your raw score by the number of items in that subtest. If there are fifty questions and you answered thirty-five correctly, your percent correct is 70. Next tabulate your converted or scaled score against our simulated MCAT Scoring Chart. This scoring chart should in **no** case be interpreted as part of the actual AAMC scoring system. The MCAT Scoring Chart was developed for test materials in this book only. The scoring chart serves only as a guide to check your performance on a relative basis with past test-takers. Actual tests vary from one to the other depending on how difficult they are, how well the test conditions are simulated, your personal disposition on the day of the test, and other factors. Use this simplified chart below to develop familiarity with the scoring process and to evaluate the status of your preparation.

Important: Use this chart to estimate your scores with BETZ Prep simulated Tests or any other simulated MCAT. In order to obtain free information about BETZ Prep call us at 1-800-634-4365.

AAMC MCAT SCORING CHART

Verbal Reasoning Section

Raw Score	Scaled Score	Percentile Rank
65	15	>99
62-64	14	94-98
60-61	13	87-93
58-59	12	80-86
56-57	11	71-79
53-55	10	64-70
51-52	9	55-63
46-50	8	47-54
41-45	7	33-46
36-40	6	23-32
31-35	5	17-22
26-30	4	10-16
24-25	3	8-9
21-23	2	4-7
0-20	1	0-3

Raw Score Statistics*
Mean = 49.5, Std.Dev. = 10.9
AAMC Statistics 1991-95
Mean Score = 7.79
Standard Deviation = 2.45

Physical Sciences Section

Raw Score	Scaled Score	Percentile Rank
75-77	15	>99.5
68-74	14	98-99
61-67	13	94-97
56-60	12	91-93
51-55	11	82-90
48-50	10	70-81
46-47	9	60-69
44-45	8	45-59
41-43	7	32-44
36-40	6	20-31
31-35	5	15-19
26-30	4	10-14
21-25	3	7-9
11-20	2	3-6
0-10	1	0-2

Raw Score Statistics
Mean = 44.2, Std.Dev. = 12.3
AAMC Statistics 1991-95
Mean Score = 7.87
Standard Deviation = 2.31

Biological Sciences Section

Raw Score	Scaled Score	Percentile Rank
75-77	15	>99.5
71-74	14	98-99
66-70	13	94-97
61-65	12	91-93
56-60	11	82-90
53-55	10	66-81
51-52	9	52-65
46-50	8	38-51
41-45	7	25-37
36-40	6	15-24
31-35	5	10-14
26-30	4	7-9
21-25	3	4-6
11-20	2	2-3
0-10	1	0-1

Raw Score Statistics
Mean = 48.4, Std.Dev = 12.8
AAMC Statistics 1991-95
Mean Score = 7.94
Standard Deviation = 2.40

On the Writing Sample the median score was the letter O. On the average the scores varied between the letters M and Q.

The AAMC Statistics and this Scoring Chart are based on actual AAMC reports prepared from April 1991 to April 1995 based on a total population of 267,740 students.

*The AAMC statistics show that the actual MCAT scores during April 1991 had the same mean for all sections and the standard deviations were almost the same for all sections, which makes it harder for the average student to compare performance in various parts of the MCAT. Use this chart to estimate your scores when using any practice test materials.

There is no advantage to taking the actual MCAT only to learn that you are not yet ready for it. You may take the MCAT as many times as you wish but all your scores will be forwarded to the schools where you apply.

Be rigorous in maintaining your MCAT daily schedule. Use the time limits of a real MCAT testing day as a guide. This includes the time you get up, what you do when you wake up, appropriate diet, and the time you go to sleep. You may not be at your best on a test starting in the morning if you have maintained a night-study schedule up until the test day.

8.9 STRATEGY #9: PLANNING THE LAST WEEK BEFORE THE TEST

If possible on the Saturday before the actual MCAT, drive to the testing location at the same time as on the day the MCAT is given. Pay attention to route, traffic, parking, etc. Locate the testing room, bathroom, snack bar. Over-preparation is a good antidote to anxiety.

Schedule review sessions that emphasize short-term memory tasks. The rest of your MCAT study time should be spent working item sets from each section under timed conditions. During these final sessions, simulate real test situations as closely as possible. For example, do not allow yourself to spend too much time solving one problem. In a good simulation, the adrenaline should be flowing just enough so you feel the stress, but not enough to make you anxious.

In these final practice sessions, stick to the strategies you have practiced. Be deliberate. Consider carefully and mark the answer clues in the question. Cross out wrong answers. Work with a watch in front of you that you intend to bring to the real test day. It should have a large, clear face and a minute hand. Work without calculators, since such use is not allowed. You know by now that accuracy and speed are a trade-off. Know beforehand what speed on each subtest gives you the highest level of accuracy.

8.10 STRATEGY #10: PLANNING THE TEST DAY

Prepare in Advance What You Will Take With You

This includes your watch, three or four well-sharpened pencils with erasers, and snacks such as small boxes of raisins. Remember to eat a good breakfast. Research at the Johns Hopkins medical center shows that protein at breakfast is particularly important for problem solving activities. Get up in time to eat your breakfast calmly.

Go to the Testing Room in Time to Settle In

1. Once the test starts, you may want to note in the margins of your test booklet certain short-term memory items.
2. Remember to stick to your strategies throughout the test. Do not be distracted by what others are doing around you. Periodically, make sure your mark on the answer sheet corresponds to the number of the question you are answering, or follow the suggestion above to mark your answer sheet from marks you make in the test book.
3. If your mind goes blank on the first item, go on to the next one. Continue until you find one you can answer. Then go back. Once begun, keep to the pace that allows you the highest level of accuracy.
4. Do not omit any items. For those you honestly do not know, fill in your predetermined guess answer. There is no penalty for wrong answers.
5. During breaks, do not talk to other test takers. Keep your energies focused on the test.
6. Stay in control of your time and energy. Remember, you are taking the test, do not let the test take you.

Summary of Test-Taking Rules

Read instructions carefully. Make sure that you understand the directions. You do not want to miss a question that you knew because you failed to note a detail in the directions.

Scan test for question types and plan strategy. Certain types of questions take more time than others. Negative stemmed questions, questions on particularly complex material, and multiple-multiple questions require a little more thought and processing time, so you need to budget your time accordingly. If you are worried about being able to finish on time, then leave those questions for last. Plan to answer all questions. Since all of the questions are equally weighted, it is better to answer more questions than labor over getting just a few correct.

Read the stem of the question carefully. Be particularly careful to notice qualifying words, such as *almost, usually, characteristically, decrease, except, not,* as well as word prefixes that change the meaning, such as *un-, dis-, in-, pre-, post-*. If you read the qualifiers, but tend to forget them when thinking through the question, underline or circle them. Remember to go back and double check your answer against the words you have highlighted as being important.

Interpret questions at face value. Test questions, especially professionally constructed ones, are not intended to be trick questions, so do not read an intent into the question that is not stated. Interpret the question as straightforwardly as possible.

Avoid liberal guessing. Do not give up and move into a guess mode as soon as something looks unfamiliar or difficult. In the face of uncertainty, talk to yourself about what you do know, even if it seems only tangentially related. This process often triggers associations that did not immediately come to mind and may give you enough information to answer the question. If you remain uncertain after brainstorming about what you know, use common sense to try to make a decision. If guessing cannot be avoided, you will at least be in a position to make an educated guess that will increase your chances of answering correctly.

Maintain consistent logic. Make sure that your answer rationale does not contain contradictory information. On questions where several answers may be correct, evaluate each answer choice individually for accuracy, but then look at whether your combination of information is in agreement. Evaluate each answer separately without bias.

Resolve vagueness or ambiguity. It is very difficult to make a decision when you are uncertain of what a word or phrase means. In this situation, determine exactly which word or phrase is unclear, and try to define it according to what you think it might be. Then use that definition to solve the problem. Although there is always the chance that your definition may not be accurate enough for you to arrive at the correct answer, more often than not, you will be able to come close enough to the correct definition to answer the question correctly.

Read all information provided, even when you see an immediate answer. Do not allow yourself to respond solely on the basis of familiarity. This can cause you to read carelessly and not pay attention to the context in which the words are used. You may find that what you had anticipated to be there, in fact, was not there.

Anticipate what the answer should include before reading the answer choices. Give thought to what you think the answer should include. If you look at the answer choices immediately after reading the question, you run the risk of narrowing the field of information that you use to solve the problem to what is directly in front of you. Trying to work with as much information as you can is especially important when you have a degree of uncertainty about the answer.

Use True/False strategy on multiple-choice questions. As a general guideline, you should stay with your first answer choice. Do not go back and forth between two uncertain choices. Only change answers if you come up with new information, or find that you misread part of the question.

Transfer answers in a batch to the answer sheet. Mark your answers on the test booklet as you work with the questions. Periodically stop and transfer a block of answers to the answer sheet. This will save you time and reduce the risk of transfer errors.

Pace yourself to answer all questions. Do not spend long periods of time with a single question. If you are not sure, pick an answer and move on. Circle the number so that, if you have time at the end, you can look at it again. Watch your time. Set interim checkpoints for where you want to be on the test at a given time. Then try to pace yourself accordingly.

<u>After the Test</u>
If you feel sick during the exam or realize that you are not adequately prepared, you can void your test. If you do this, you will not receive scores (the proctor will record your decision in your presence). Similarly, unsatisfactory scores will not be recorded against your name.

When the test is finished, do not compare what you remember answering with what someone else remembers answering. It is unreliable at best and often depressing. Be good to yourself!

Both preparation and luck have a part in any event that is going to occur at a specific time. If you have not performed as well as you should, you may take the test again. Start early on a routine that allows you to analyze weaknesses and get your new preparation program under way. Special strategies for working with MCAT passages in the physical and biological sciences are presented in Appendix A.

8.11 PRACTICE EXERCISES WITH PASSAGES AND TEST ITEMS

A variety of question formats have been used here to provide you with practice examples for the MCAT. Also included are other question formats that may not appear on the MCAT but which test your knowledge of integrative thinking. Twenty-two passages with accompanying questions are included. Use chapter 4 and chapter 8 skills along with Appendix A to work these practice exercises. Passages 21 and 22 are slightly more difficult than the actual MCAT passages.

<u>A Final Note</u>
Because of the recent major changes in the MCAT, chapter 8 should be reviewed thoroughly to help you master some of the new technological, perceptive, and analytical skills that are blended with test-taking skills in the MCAT.

Learning to work with text-based, text-linked, and text-extension items is an important strategy to master for the MCAT to perform well on it. In working with all passages try to understand the differences between text-based, text-linked, or text-extension items.

- Text: usually refers to information provided in tables, graphs, research descriptions or experimental analysis, instrumental working or design.
- Text-based items: basically these are comprehension items.
- Text-linked items: remotely or tangentially connected to the topics in the text.
- Text-extension items: includes new information in the test item to be linked to the text presented in the passage.

Appendix A gives details on the nature of MCAT passages used by the Association of American Medical Colleges.

Passage 1 - (Questions 1–6)
Verbal Reasoning

Paul was diagnosed as having cystic fibrosis at five years of age. As a youngster, he was watched over and guarded by adults who were oriented to the possibility of imminent death. He was usually avoided by peers and potential friends who would "take a step back" upon learning that he had a serious illness. Teachers from grade school through college were reluctant to make demands or encourage long-range tasks which might prove stressful or be abruptly terminated by death.

The attitudes of others toward illness and death were always difficult for him to deal with. Rather than confront people and ask for clarification of their ideas about his situation, he would withdraw. He became hesitant to involve himself with others because of his anxieties about exposing his feeling regarding the implications of his grave medical problems.

Several times in his life, Paul had felt that psychiatric help would be quite useful in learning to cope with his everyday problems of living. He was unsuccessful in pursuing his idea because he was uncertain whether his vague depression and anxieties were appropriate to take to a psychiatrist. Even when seen by a counselor in college, he found it difficult to describe his needs and guide the therapist toward his areas of discomfort. The therapist, in turn, tended to be more concerned about his illness, following the pattern of seeing him primarily as a sick person.

A doctor friend helped Paul change his self-image from a seriously ill person to a man with a serious illness, a shift of attitude which proved successful in all areas of his life. He was able to broaden his horizons and to persevere in looking for a job. He had graduated from college with a business degree, but interviewers had only to hear that he had a chronic illness to refuse his application. With support from his doctor friend, he finally was hired in a managerial capacity with a major distribution and retail firm. His drive to success carried him quite rapidly into additional areas of responsibility. Having given up a death orientation, Paul decided to marry. Although he denies neither the threat of death or the reality of being alive, his newfound confidence and strength in dealing with himself and others has led to a more productive, rewarding life.

(Multiple choice)

1. Which of the following phrases best describes the central idea of the passage?

A. Changing one's life style
B. Coping with mental illness
C. Adjusting to life's demands
D. Learning to live with serious illness

2. The college counselor's primary concern for Paul was:

A. his future career.
B. his imminent death.
C. his physical illness.
D. his emotional health.

3. Which adjective best describes people's attitude toward Paul during his childhood?

A. Authoritarian
B. Compassionate
C. Hostile
D. Protective

4. Why did Paul not seek psychiatric help?

A. He considered his illness only a physical disorder.
B. He refused to talk with others about his emotional distress.
C. He doubted the suitability of psychiatric help for solving his coping problems.
D. He felt inhibited when talking with medically trained people about his inner feelings.

5. Paul's success in dealing with his illness was due to:

A. his desire to get well.
B. his change in mental attitude.
C. his having completed a college degree.
D. his strict adherence to medical treatments.

6. From information in the passage, one can infer that:

A. cystic fibrosis cannot be cured.
B. cystic fibrosis can be inherited.
C. cystic fibrosis is difficult to diagnose.
D. cystic fibrosis is an emotionally disabling disease.

Passage 2 - (Questions 7–11)
Verbal Reasoning

Senate Joint Resolution One: This Resolution proposes an Amendment to the Constitution of the United States to abolish the antiquated electoral college and undemocratic "unit vote" system and substitute direct popular election of the President and Vice-president. The proposed amendment provides, further, in the unlikely event no candidate receives 40 percent of the popular vote, the President and Vice-president will be elected in a runoff election between two pairs of candidates receiving the highest number of votes.

Senator Smith's Speech: "Under our present electoral system, a member of the losing party carries no long-term liability. Losing neither invites insidious discrimination, nor endangers the security of one's liberty. Among the losers may be a person representing a geographic area or an ethnic, religious, social, or economic group. Most Americans are inclined to forget that they are members of some minority group and this group, potentially, might become a vulnerable minority. The power of minorities comes from the skill with which they are able to join forces with other minorities. Indeed, a minority group which fails to align itself with other minorities finds its political power greatly diminished. One of the chief virtues of the electoral college system is that it not only encourages such alliances, it virtually requires them. It builds moderate majorities, while protecting the interests of all minorities that are willing to compromise."

Senator Brown's Speech: "Perhaps the one aspect of the electoral-college system which carries the greatest burden for ethnic or racial minorities is the "unit rule." This system awards all of a state's electoral votes to the candidate who wins a majority of the popular vote. It carries real potential to erase the views of the minority voter, while magnifying the strength of the majority voter. I have considered the argument that a direct election would deprive my constituents of an advantage they now possess under the electoral system. The "one-man, one-vote" rule has effectively franchised black Americans and other minority group members in voting for Congress. In a similar way, the direct election of the President will effectively enfranchise black Americans and other minority and ethnic groups. It will ensure that their vote will count in those states where it is currently ineffectual. It will mean that the people will vote for President as a citizen of the United States rather than merely as a citizen of a state. It will allow the vote of each person, black or white, to carry equal weight."

(Multiple choice)

7. The "unit vote" system refers to which of the following:

   A. all the electoral votes of a state are committed to one candidate.
   B. the Republican votes go to the Republican candidate and the Democratic votes to the Democratic candidate.
   C. each candidate receives a "unit" or a proportion of the vote based upon the state population.
   D. only Senate votes count since each state has two senators to encourage fairness.

8. In the event that neither presidential candidate receives 40% of the vote under the current system, how would the President and Vice-president be elected?

   A. By a runoff election between the two pairs of candidates
   B. Popular vote of the people
   C. By naming the President from one party and the Vice-president from another party
   D. Passage does not stipulate a process

(Keyed choice)

The following statements are related to the passage. Based on the information given, select:

A. if the statement **is supported** by the passage
B. if the statement **is contradicted** by the passage
C. if the statement **is neither supported nor contradicted** by the passage

9. Senator Smith asserts that the electoral college provides protection for individuals within religious groups.

10. Senator Brown indicates that election of the President should be similar to the election of state officials.

11. Each speaker believes his proposal will enfranchise minority and ethnic groups.

Passage 3 - (Questions 12–16)
Verbal Reasoning

The three components of population growth are births, deaths, and net migration. The birth rate in the United States has varied in importance in the determination of overall population trends in different periods in our nation's history. For the 50 years between the Civil War and World War I, changes in the birth and death rates generally paralleled each other. This produced a rather smooth, declining rate of natural increase (birth rate minus death rate) during this period. As a result, the net growth rate (natural increase plus net migration) was heavily influenced by changes in the rate of net migration rather than by birth or death rates during the late 1800s and early 1900s.

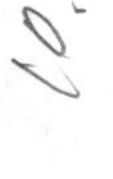

Low migration rates, combined with the influenza epidemic of 1918, resulted in a net growth rate of 10.5 per 1,000 population for the 1915–1920 period. This was the lowest rate of population growth recorded until the "Great Depression" when the net growth rate fell to 7 per 1,000 population during the 1930–1935 period. The Immigration Act of 1924, which established immigration quotas based on national origin, substantially reduced the number of immigrants to about 1 per 1,000 population per year. The fairly constant net migration rate and death rate since the 1920s have made the birth rate the primary factor in the determination of population growth patterns for the last 50 years.

Increases in the birth rate (from 7.0 to 15.6 per 1,000) contributed to the doubling of the net rate of population growth between the 1930–1935 and 1945–1950 periods. However, a decline occurred in the net annual growth rate from 1.7 percent in the 1950–1955 period to less than 1 percent in the 1970–1975 period. This decline was almost entirely due to corresponding declines in the birth rate (from 24.8 to 15.9 per 1,000).

(Multiple choice)

12. Changes in the rate of population increase in the 1930–1935 period and the 1945–1950 period were due to:

    A. declining death rate.
    B. increases in birth rates.
    C. a relaxation of immigration laws.
    D. a declining death rate.

13. What factor most influenced the net population growth in the U.S. during the late 1800s and early 1900s?

    A. Lower death rates
    B. An epidemic-free period
    C. An increased immigration rate
    D. More accurate recording of births

14. In what historical period was the U.S. population growth the lowest?

    A. During World War II
    B. In the depression years
    C. Following the 1918 influenza epidemic
    D. After passage of the Immigration Act

15. If the most recent census count found that the birth rate had been miscalculated in the country, the most important effect would be:

    A. the number of deaths would be higher.
    B. the ratio between births and deaths would change.
    C. the new numbers would be used to determine population growth.
    D. the census count would be retaken.

16. The main topic of this passage is the:

    A. rationale for demographic studies.
    B. effects of birth declines on population.
    C. population declines in the United States.
    D. net population growth in the United States.

Passage 4 - (Questions 17–22)
Verbal Reasoning

The following comments are from an interview with a recent winner of the Nobel Prize in Physiology/Medicine. His work revealed the overall structure of the antibody molecule.

"Since getting the Nobel Prize, I've been asked to do a lot of talking to nonscientists about research. It's a frustrating thing. Scientists, and certainly I'm included, forget about how abstract what we do is. How getting that structure depends on feeling about Avogadro's Number more or less the way I feel about the ends of my fingers. That's because after living with it for ten years, I think I understand it. Maybe that's all understanding is—a terrific familiarity.

"Scientific research proceeds by a process of self-correction and linearization. It falsified the actual events of discovery. Later, it's hard to remember that it really didn't happen that way, that you were blundering around, and something happened. You said "ah-so!", and you looked back and regularized it, thereby wiping out the serendipitous nature of the experience.

"We can now see the relationship of one class of antibodies to the other, and the relationship of structure to function. The whole genetic language in immunology emerged as a result of this. It became quite clear in a very nice 'why-didn't-I-think-of-it?' way. The initial impact of such an organizing principle is always astonishing, and then it becomes a habit. We accept it as dogs accept automobiles—they were here forever.

"It's interesting that there is a kind of conviction that leads to any major discovery, but the person who has that conviction hardly knows that the result is going to come out so neatly. What he has is the feeling of 'Well, this is the most important thing.' That's all he has.

"I remember reading a book by Simone de Beauvoir that had to do with growing old. She commented in an anecdotal way about scientists and artist, and how artists, as they grow older, seem to be able—if they are really great—to just churn it out. That just isn't true in science, by and large. And there are deep reasons why. First of all, it's not fair to compare a painting with a long, analytical effort that involves a communal enterprise. Second, that effort to try to remove the arbitrary from what you're doing sure does slow you down! You can have a million, beautiful ideas—if only they would be accepted. With the artist—all due credit to his tradition—they are. So maybe it's that, or maybe it's some other deep factor that we don't understand. If you have an impatient nature, as I think I do, it can be pretty hard to hang in there. And once you have hung in there, and understand that there is no other choice, it takes an awful lot of promise to convince you to take another 15 years of your life to do it.

"I wonder, in fact, whether structure work is the only thing where that's true. It may really be true in some sense about all scientific experimental enterprise. There is a kind of logistic sense, a quartermastering sense, that good scientists will have. They'll tell you 'Well, I don't know how to work it, or make it go, but I can tell you it's going to take five years'."

(Multiple choice)

17. The main topic of this passage is:

- **A.** the discovery of the structure of the antibody molecule.
- **B.** the impact of organizing principles on a science.
- **C.** the demands of a scientific research on a scientist.
- **D.** the relationship of structure to function in science.

18. According to the author, explaining research to the lay person is frustrating because:

- **A.** much of science depends on intuition.
- **B.** it is a very long and time-consuming process.
- **C.** real comprehension only comes by close contact.
- **D.** interpretation of the results involves complex numbers and mathematics.

19. According to the passage, all of the following might accompany or characterize a major scientific discovery EXCEPT:

- **A.** sudden insight.
- **B.** the ability to see new relationships.
- **C.** conviction of the importance of the work.
- **D.** accurate initial perception of the outcome.

20. Which of the following is NOT implied or stated in the passage comparing artists and scientists?

A. A scientist must prove his ideas
B. They have different standards for "greatness"
C. Some artists continue productively in old age
D. They have different traditions of "acceptance"

21. The passage indicates that a good scientist needs:

A. organization.
B. a good memory.
C. language abilities.
D. a quartermastering sense.

22. The writer perceives scientific research to be all of the following EXCEPT:

A. anecdotal.
B. abstract.
C. analytic.
D. serendipitous.

Passage 5 - (Questions 23–28)
Verbal Reasoning

From the earliest medical records to the present, physicians and laymen have postulated an association between diet and the development of cancer. This has proved a fertile area for a wide range of speculation extending from food faddists to epidemiologists. An objective approach views diet composition and practices in food preparation as possible environmental factors which may influence tumor development.

There are large demographic differences in the prevalence of gastric cancer. Japan, Chile, Austria, Finland, and Iceland have rates (predominantly in males) four or more times those of U.S. Caucasians. In the U.S. and Europe, higher rates are noted for gastric as well as esophageal cancer among low income groups.

Certain ethnic groups in the U.S. appear to have increased risk. Studies of dietary practices in patients with gastric cancer have yielded few or no significant differences from control groups. An association with alcohol intake has been suggested and denied. The increased use of laxatives or mineral oil in affected individuals has been noted. It has been suggested, but remains unproved, that the high incidence of this tumor in Iceland is related to the large intake of smoked food in association with a low intake of vitamin C. It has been pointed out that Japanese prefer talc-dusted rice and that the talc may contain asbestos. The latter is implicated in the development of gastrointestinal cancer, especially gastric cancer. It is postulated that the asbestos-contaminated talc on rice is the carcinogen or cocarcinogen responsible for the high incidence of stomach cancer in Japan.

Death rates for carcinoma of the large bowel (colonic cancer) have a strong negative correlation with those of gastric cancer, the one being common where the other is rare. In the U.S. and England, colonic cancer is second only to lung cancer in numbers of deaths. It has been suggested that cancer of the colon in New Yorkers is associated with a high fat intake. In Japan where colonic cancer is uncommon, fat intake is about 12% of calories and mostly of the unsaturated type compared to the 40 to 44% figure in the United States.

Japanese immigrants, and especially their children born in the U.S., have a much higher incidence of this disease than those in Japan. The same has been noted for Puerto Ricans living in Puerto Rico and on the mainland of the United States.

Japanese with colonic cancer have a higher socioeconomic status than those with rectal cancer and tend to eat diets with more calories in the form of fats and fresh fruit. Czechs have approximately twice the U.S. rate for intestinal cancer. Their dietary intake is appreciably lower in animal-derived protein and fat and in vitamins. While their caloric intake is the same, it is derived more from vegetable sources than is the American diet. Contrary to the observations with carcinoma of the esophagus and stomach, the incidence of colonic cancer in the U.S. does not vary appreciably with color or socioeconomic status.

(Keyed choice)
Use the following options in answering the questions below. For any question, you may select more than one option.

A. gastric cancer
B. colonic cancer
C. esophageal cancer
D. intestinal cancer

23. The second more prevalent cause of death in the United States and England is associated with which cancer? B

24. Which cancer(s) is/are associated with dietary intake which is low in animal-derived proteins and fat, and in vitamins? D

25. Which cancer(s) is/are linked with low income groups in the United States? A, C

26. Which cancer(s) is/are related to talc-dusted rice? A, D

27. Which cancer(s) is/are not associated with income group in the United States? B

28. Which cancer(s) is/are linked to smoked fish? A

Passage 6 - (Questions 29–34)
Physical Sciences
Solubility of NaCl in H_2O: 100 g NaCl Placed in 1 Liter of H_2O

Temperature	No. of grams dissolved			
	Lab A	Lab B	Lab C	Lab D
10°C	5	4	6	4
20°C	15	16	8	15
30°C	16	15	15	17
40°C	23	25	24	23
50°C	40	40	38	41
60°C	45	45	47	46
70°C	50	52	50	50
80°C	60	58	60	60
90°C	70	73	71	69
100°C	80	81	80	81

(Keyed choice)
Based on the information given, select:

A. If the statement **is supported** by the information given.
B. If the statement **is contradicted** by the information given.
C. If the statement **is neither supported nor contradicted** by the information given.

29. Solubility of NaCl in H_2O goes up with temperature in the range 10°C to 100°C. A ✓

30. If 100 g of NaCl are placed in a 1 liter container of water at 50°C, approximately 40g of the NaCl will dissolve. A ✓

31. There is substantial error in Lab C's 20°C reading. A ✓

32. If the water in this experiment were at 120°C virtually all of the salt would dissolve. C

33. At 75°C approximately 55 grams of salt would dissolve. A ✓

34. Variability in the number of grams of NaCl dissolved at each temperature is the result of measurement error in the temperature readings. C ✓

Passage 7 - (Questions 35–41)
Biological Sciences

The effects of two drugs on the quality of sleep in four patients was measured over an eight-night period (four nights for each drug) by means of eight-hour continuous EEG, EOG, and EMG tracings. From these tracings, the percent of time in each of four sleeping stages (Stage I, somnolence; to Stage IV, deep sleep) and in REM state were determined. Additionally, nurse observers recorded in minutes for each patient the amount of "sleep" and "wake" time and the number of times each patient awakened during the sleeping period.

To establish baseline data from which to make comparisons, the tracings and observations were made for one eight-hour sleep period without either drug having been administered. Baseline data showed the average sleep time to be 432 minutes. Percentages by stages were I, 4 percent; II, 60 percent; III, 8 percent; IV, 4 percent; and the REM stage, 23 percent. Patients awakened six times during the night and averaged 48 minutes of "wake" time.

Drug A

Patients awakened an average of four times during the night for an average total of 2-4 minutes of "wake" time. Average "sleep" time was 455 minutes. Percentage of "sleep" time in the four sleep stages were: I, 4 percent; II, 63 percent; III, 9 percent; and IV, 10 percent. Fourteen percent of the "sleep" time was in the REM stage. Morning drowsiness or "hangover" was observed in one of the patients.

Drug B

Patients awakened an average of five times during the night for an average total of 21 minutes of "wake" time. Percentage of "sleep" time in the four stages were: I, 4 percent; II, 56 percent; III, 9 percent; and IV, 3 percent. Twenty-eight percent of the sleep time was in the REM stage. Average sleep time was 458 minutes. All four patients reported morning "hangover."

(Keyed choice)
The following statements are related to the passage. Based on the information given in the passage, select:

A. if true of Drug A, but **not** true of Drug B.
B. if true of Drug B, but **not** true of Drug A.
C. if true of **both** Drug A and Drug B.
D. if **neither** Drug A **nor** Drug B.

35. Most of the sleeping time was in the REM stage.

36. Reduced morning "hangover" was reported.

37. Less than one-fifth of the sleep time was in the REM stage.

38. Stage II sleep accounted for most of the "sleep" time.

39. Patients awakened frequently during the night.

40. Tracings showed reduced sleep time in Stage IV.

41. Somnolence was not affected.

Passage 8 - (Questions 42–46)
Biological Sciences

Percentage of Regular Smokers Among Male Teenagers in the U.S.

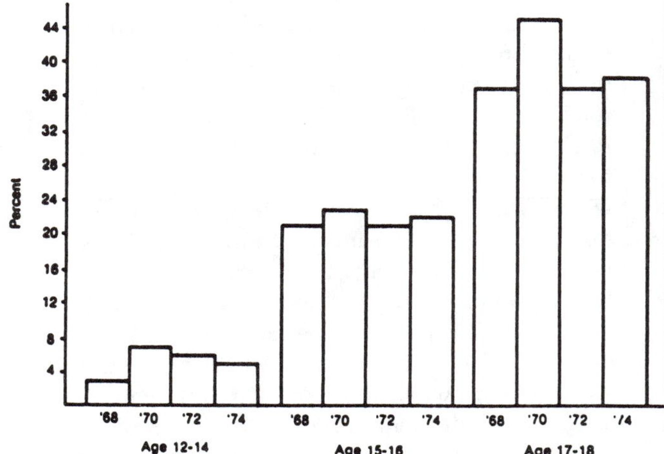

(Keyed choice)
Based on the information given, select:

- **A.** if the first item is larger than the second.
- **B.** if the second item is larger than the first.
- **C.** if they are equal.
- **D.** if the difference cannot be evaluated on the basis of the information provided.

42. 1. Percentage of 17–18 year olds in the U.S. who were regular smokers in 1974.
2. Percentage of 17–18 year olds in the U.S. who were regular smokers in 1970.

43. 1. Number of 12–14 year old males in the U.S. who were regular smokers in 1970.
2. Number of 12–14 year old males in the U.S. who were regular smokers in 1974.

44. 1. Percentage of 12–14 year old males in the U.S. who were regular smokers in 1972.
2. Percentage of 15–16 year old males in the U.S. who were regular smokers in 1972.

45. If a similar graph were given for females, could one answer question 42?

1. Yes, the answer is ________________.
2. No.

46. If the percentages were exactly the same for females as for males, could one answer question 42?

1. Yes, the answer is ________________.
2. No.

Passage 9 - (Questions 47–51)
Biological Sciences

The "lampbrush" giant chromosome is found in developing female sex cells of certain amphibians. Fortunately, these chromosomes are large enough and refractile enough so that they can be examined unfixed and unstained with the phase contrast microscope. Consequently, their observed structure is that which they actually possess in life, free from the artifacts of preparation. Close examination reveals that they consist of a thin, central strand from which the bristle-like projections arise. The bristle-like projections are, in actuality, loops. The central strand seems to be thickened where the loops join it. These areas of thickening with their attached loops are called chromomeres.

Another type of giant chromosome is found in the salivary glands of certain two-winged insects of the Diptera order. These chromosomes are quite different from the amphibian lampbrush. Although they are cylindrical, they look like ribbons across which are light and dark bands of varying widths. The insects in which these giant chromosomes occur breed and develop rapidly and are easily raised in the laboratory.

While the chromosomes of most species are only visible during cell division, it has been shown that the giant chromosomes of insects and amphibians are actually interphase chromosomes. Thus, they make possible the observation of chromosomes in their normal functioning condition, rather than in the much-contracted and metabolically inactive state that they assume during mitosis.

In cases of the insects, the chromosomes are few in number, easily differentiated from one another, and the pattern of the bands can be defined. It was not long, therefore, before geneticists realized the possibility of not only associating certain genes with specific chromosomes, but possibly determining their locations within the individual chromosomes.

Now, after a great deal of painstaking work, the sites of many genes are known. It appears that each band is the locale of a gene or a group of closely related genes. In this way, the gene, which was originally a purely conceptual idea of a unit of heredity, has been given a physical embodiment.

(Multiple choice)

47. The main topic of this passage is the:

- **A.** characteristics of giant chromosomes.
- **B.** difference in chromosomal structures.
- **C.** location of gene sites in chromosomes.
- **D.** use of giant chromosomes in general genetic studies.

48. What appearance, under a microscope, would differentiate the giant chromosome in developing female sex glands of amphibians from those in the salivary glands of Diptera insects?

- **A.** Activity patterns
- **B.** Color and size
- **C.** Ribbon-like bands
- **D.** Brush-like appearance

49. All of the following are characteristics of the chromosomes of the Diptera insect EXCEPT for the:

- **A.** cylindrical shape.
- **B.** bands of varying widths.
- **C.** bristle-like projections.
- **D.** fewer chromosomes.

50. From the information in the passage, one can infer that:

- **A.** chromosomal structure determines genetic structure.
- **B.** giant chromosomes are present only in amphibians and insects.
- **C.** chromosomal development in salivary glands is more rapid than in sex cells.
- **D.** more can be learned about chromosomes during interphase than during mitosis.

51. Studies of the structure of giant chromosomes are important because these studies have provided:

- **A.** a mapping scheme for locating genes.
- **B.** further proof of the gene-hereditary link.
- **C.** additional knowledge of genetic construct.
- **D.** supportive evidence for genetic construct.

Passage 10 - (Questions 52–59)
Biological Sciences

Prior to the emergence of HMO health plans, less than 50% of the U.S. population received regular health examinations. In 1973 eye care edged out chest x-rays in every age bracket. Women tended to seek preventive examinations more frequently than men and pap smears were obtained by roughly two out of every three females. Thus it is likely that the statistics for males were even lower than those indicated in the chart below, where data for the two genders have been lumped together. Since eye exams in the total population were more widely sought than chest x-rays, but less common than pap smears in the female population, it is possible that males avoided tests that might force them to consider their mortality while females under the age of 65 preferentially sought out information most likely to prolong their lives. Nevertheless it is difficult to escape the conclusion that for most Americans sight is more precious than life.

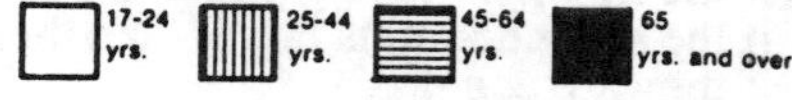

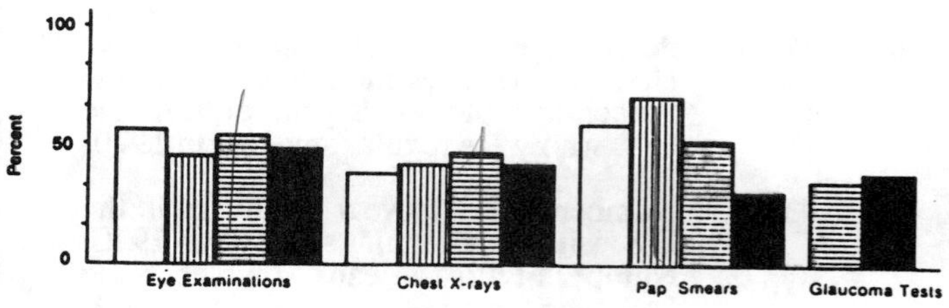

Percentage of Population with Selected Preventive Care Examinations (Studied period = 2 years)

(Subjective Questions 52, 53)

52. The article implies that HMO plans encourage preventive examinations; what evidence does it give to support this claim?

53. In only one case is the bar for eye examination higher than that for pap smears; why then does the author conclude that Americans act as though sight were more precious than life?

(Keyed choice Questions 54–57)
Based on the information given, select:

A. if the first item is larger than the second.
B. if the second item is larger than the first.
C. if they are equal.
D. If the difference cannot be evaluated on the basis of the information given.

54. 1. Number of 45–64 year olds who had received an eye examination in the studied period.
2. Number of 45–64 year olds who had received a chest x-ray in the studied period. A

55. 1. Number of 45–64 year olds who had received a pap smear in the studied period.
2. Number of 45–64 year olds who had received a chest x-ray in the studied period. A

56. 1. Number of 45–64 year olds who had received a chest x-ray in the studied period.
2. Number of 45–64 year olds who had received a chest x-ray **and** a glaucoma test in the studied period. B

57. 1. Number of 17–24 year olds who had received an eye examination in the studied period.
2. Number of 45–64 year olds who had received a chest x-ray in the studied period. A

(Subjective Questions 58, 59)

58. Can one draw any conclusions about the importance for health on any of the examinations in this graph or the popular knowledge about their importance?

59. Does this graph support the claim that the pap smear is considered a more important test for a 25–44 year old woman than for a woman 65 or older?

Passage 11 - (Questions 60–64)
Biological Sciences

Reptiles have little brain matter in excess of the necessary minimum for the preservation of life. Their tiny brains manage to persuade them to eat, to reproduce, and to defend themselves. Improvement of the reptilian brain came about either through evolutional brain enlargement or through the encephalization process.

Triconodon, an early mammal that lived among the dinosaurs about 150 million years ago, is the first animal to have a significantly encephalized brain. Most evolutional brain enlargement is merely the result of the entire animal growing bigger. Encephalization refers to the special process wherein the brain expands more rapidly than would be expected from the growth of the rest of the body.

To learn more about the mysterious encephalization process, cerebral paleontologists spend much of their lives peering into fossil skulls. Their basic tool is the endocast, or mold of the inside of the cranium. In many animals, the brain is wedged tightly inside the head. Negative impressions of the wiggling convolutions of the brain are quite clearly imprinted on the inside of the skull. Sometimes, natural processes fill the interior of a fossil skull with dirt or sand that turns to rock, providing a natural endocast. More frequently, paleontologists produce their own endocasts from latex. Either way, the endocast provides a clear, positive model of the surface of the animal's brain.

Besides studying skeletal remains, paleontologists also apply a technique known as allometric analysis to estimate total body size. They then calculate the expected brain volume of the animal had it not been encephalized. By measuring the volume of the brain endocast, they are then able to determine the degree of brain encephalization that is expressed as an "encephalization quotient," or EQ. The EQ expresses the relationship between the actual brain volume and the expected brain volume had average encephalization occurred.

One paleontologist had estimated that Triconodon possessed about four times the brain volume (in proportion to body weight) of its reptilian contemporaries. Others have estimated the degree of encephalization as ranging from between 1.6 and 7 times that of other reptiles.

(Multiple Choice)

60. Allometric analysis is used to estimate the:

- **A.** total body size.
- **B.** total brain volume.
- **C.** degree of encephalization.
- **D.** ratio of body weight to brain size.

61. An endocast can be defined as:

- **A.** fossilized animal skull.
- **B.** mold of skeletal remains.
- **C.** model of the brain's surface.
- **D.** latex cast of the brain's convolutions.

62. How did Triconodon differ from other mammals 150 million years ago?

- **A.** Its life span increased.
- **B.** Its reproduction process changed.
- **C.** It underwent evolutional brain enlargement.
- **D.** Its brain volume, relative to size, was greater.

63. When average encephalization occurs, the term "EQ" refers to:

- **A.** an estimate of total body size.
- **B.** an evolutionary enlarged brain.
- **C.** the degree of brain encephalization.
- **D.** the relationship between actual and expected brain volume.

64. Which of the following could you conclude from information in the passage?

- **A.** Paleontologists study ancient forms of life.
- **B.** To conduct his studies, the paleontologist needs only simple, crude tools.
- **C.** Triconodon was more intelligent than other mammals living 150 million years ago.
- **D.** The process of encephalization occurred frequently in prehistoric times.

Passage 12 - (Questions 65–70)
Biological Sciences

Number of Person-years of life gained to age 70 in the U.S.
(By eliminating causes of death during 1970)

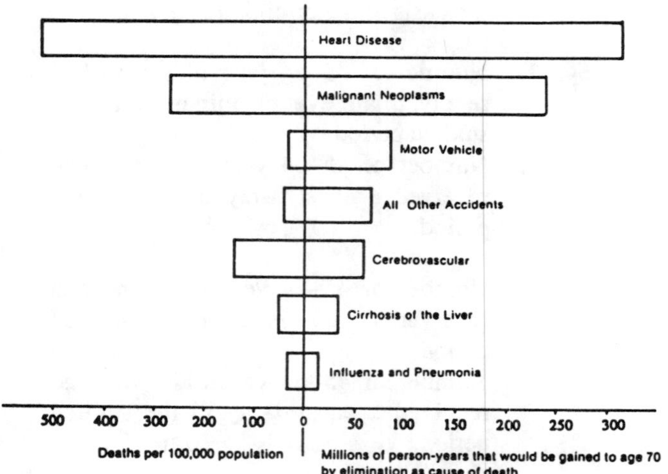

(Subjective)

65. Which accounts for more deaths per year in the U.S., influenza and pneumonia or cirrhosis of the liver?

66. The elimination of which would provide more person-years gained to age 70, cirrhosis of the liver or influenza and pneumonia?

67. If the death rate for people under 70 by heart disease was 300 per 100,000 population and the population under 70 totaled 180,000,000 in 1970, what was the average age of heart disease-induced death for people under 70?

68. Can one say how many person-years to age 70 would be gained if the number of motor vehicle accidents were cut to 10 per 100,000 population? If so, how many? If not, why not?

69. If the rate of deaths from malignant neoplasms was cut to 100 per 100,000 population with the cut made proportional to the incidence of deaths across the age range, can one say about how many person-years would be gained to age 70? If so, how many? If not, why not?

70. Cerebrovascular diseases cause far more deaths per year than do automobile accidents. Yet elimination of automobile accidents would add more person-years to the life span than would elimination of cerebrovascular disease. How is this possible?

Passage 13 - (Questions 71–74)
Biological Sciences

In the breathing process known as external respiration, oxygen is taken from the environment and carbon dioxide is returned to it. In plants and small animals, exchange of gases by diffusion is sufficient; in fish, the exchange occurs as water passes through the gills; in man, exchange occurs as air is pumped in and out of the lungs that are composed of pinkish-gray, spongy tissue. In man, the right lung is a little larger than the left and has three sections or lobes, whereas the left lung has two lobes, with the heart taking up some of the room on the left side of the chest.

Air inhaled from the nose passes through the nasal cavity, the pharynx, and the trachea (or windpipe) into the two main air passages of the lung called bronchi, one of which goes to the right and one to the left lung. The bronchi branch into bronchioles, smaller and smaller passages that carry air to all parts of the lung. Several different kinds of cells line the air passages in the lungs: some produce mucus that covers the surface of the bronchial tube, while others have tiny hair-like projections, called cilia, that sweep phlegm up toward the throat, helping to cleanse the lungs of impurities in the air.

The bronchioles contain millions of alveoli, or air sacs, which are surrounded by an intercommunicating network of many capillaries, the smallest blood vessels of the body. Oxygen from the inhaled air passes the thin membrane that separates the air sac from the blood in the capillaries. The oxygen is picked up by the red blood cells that carry it through the bloodstream to all cells of the body. Carbon dioxide, a product of the body's metabolic process, is passed from the blood into the alveoli and eliminated when air is expelled from the lungs. The air that enters and leaves the lungs during normal breathing (about 500 cm^3 in man) is called tidal air.

(Multiple Choice)

71. All of the following are probably true of the bronchi EXCEPT:

A. each bronchus is lined with cells that produce mucus to trap dust and other impurities in the air.
B. in all vertebrates, including man, one bronchus carries air to the left, and one to the right lung.
C. carbon dioxide, a product of a chemical process involving the breakdown of compound organic molecules to simpler molecules, is eliminated through the bronchi.
D. in man, air is carried through the trachea to the bronchi, the bronchioles, and then to the alveoli, in inspiration.

72. According to the passage, phlegm:

A. is produced by the bronchioles.
B. is synonymous with mucus that is produced by cells lining the bronchi in the respiratory system of man.
C. is normally found in the alveoli of air-breathing vertebrates.
D. is moved by cilia up through the trachea as part of the body's mechanism for cleansing the lungs.

73. It can be inferred that all of the following are true of respiration EXCEPT:

A. it can involve both inspiration and expiration.
B. it supplies oxygen and removes carbon dioxide.
C. it involves the pumping of air into and out of the lungs of terrestrial animals, as well as the pumping of water over the gills of fish.
D. It involves the pumping of air into and out of the lungs of terrestrial animals, but not the diffusion of oxygen in protozoa and lower invertebrates.

74. By inference, from the passage, which of the following is probably FALSE?

A. About 500 cm^3 of air is the maximum capacity of the lungs in man.
B. Years of inhaling dirty air or cigarette smoke can damage the lungs in man.
C. One could expect that the rate of lung disease would be higher in urban than in rural areas.
D. Respiration usually involves an exchange of gases with the environment.

Passage 14 - (Questions 75-81)
Biological Sciences

Inclusion of Osmium Tetroxide in Diet of Laboratory Animals

Group	Amount of chemical g/day	No. dead after two weeks	No. dead after four weeks
50 rats	0	5	7
50 rats	10	12	38
30 rabbits	0	3	4
30 rabbits	10	5	7
30 rabbits	20	15	25
70 monkeys	0	1	3
70 monkeys	10	1	4
70 monkeys	30	7	15
70 monkeys	40	18	45

(Keyed choice)
From the information in the table, select:

- **A.** if the statement is true or probably true.
- **B.** if the information in the table is not sufficient to indicate whether there is any degree of truth or falsity in the statement.
- **C.** if the statement is false or probably false.

75. The number of rabbits that died during the experiment is greater than the number of rats that died during the experiment.

76. The number of rabbits that died during weeks 3 and 4 is greater than the number of rats that died during weeks 3 and 4.

77. The percentage of rats living after week 2 that died during weeks 3 and 4 is greater than the percentage of monkeys that died during the experiment.

78. Many more monkeys were studied than rats and rabbits because the metabolism of a monkey is closer to that of a human being.

79. The percentage of rats (given 10 g/day of chemical) that died is higher than the percentage of monkeys (given 40 g/day of chemical) that died because 10 g is a higher percentage of a rat's weight than 40 g is of a monkey's weight.

80. There was less problem with disease in the monkey cages than there was in the rat cages.

81. It does not hurt a rabbit to consume 20 g/day of osmium tetroxide.

Passage 15 - (Questions 82–86)
Biological Sciences

Genes are carried on chromosomes, threadlike structures found in the nucleus of every cell in the body. Each chromosome carries thousands of different genes that determine physical and chemical characteristics, such as eye color, stature, facial features, as well as many health conditions. Geneticists estimate that every person carries as many as seven to eight genes that could be associated with serious health problems. Although the specific gene responsible and the chromosome that carries the gene have not been identified, it is estimated that one of every 20 persons in the United States, or about 10 million people, carry a gene for Cystic Fibrosis, a hereditary health problem.

Inheriting a single gene for Cystic Fibrosis (CF) causes no special health problems. Every parent of a child with Cystic Fibrosis, however, is a "carrier" of a single CF gene. "Carriers" show no symptoms themselves, and there is no test at this time to determine a person's "carrier" status. Even when both parents are carriers of the CF gene, their children will not automatically have CF. Only one-half of the father's sperm and one-half of the mother's eggs will carry the CF gene. Both reproductive cells must carry the CF gene in order for the child to have CF. When only one of the reproductive cells carries the CF gene, the child will be a carrier. There is also the chance that neither reproductive cell would carry the CF gene, and the child would neither demonstrate the symptoms nor be a carrier.

While the exact incidence varies in reported studies, an estimated one out of every 1,600 Caucasian babies is born with CF in the United States. CF occurs much less frequently among Black and Oriental populations. At the present time, there is no medical procedure that can detect CF in an unborn child, and there is no medication or procedure that can prevent CF when a child inherits two CF genes. The sweat test, the most reliable method of diagnosing CF, can detect whether a child has CF, but it can't distinguish between a carrier and an individual without a CF gene.

(Multiple Choice)

82. If both parents are members of the general population, and neither has any family history of CF, the risk that their child will inherit CF is:

A. about 1 in 40.
B. about 1 in 400.
C. about 1 in 1,600.
D. cannot be determined from the information given.

83. If the sister of a person with CF has a normal sweat test, she would:

A. have a 1 in 40 chance of having CF.
B. have no chance of having a child with CF.
C. be certain to have a child with CF if she has children.
D. have a 2 out of 3 chance of being a carrier for CF.

84. If both parents are known "carriers" for the CF gene, the chance that their child will have CF is:

A. 100 percent.
B. 1 in 4.
C. 1 in 6.
D. 75 percent.

85. According to the text, a "carrier" is someone who:

A. has the symptoms of the disease.
B. is not infected, although he or she can transmit the disease to others.
C. does not have the disease, and therefore, cannot transmit it to others.
D. can transmit the disease, although he or she demonstrates no symptoms him or herself.

86. Cystic Fibrosis is a hereditary disease that can be detected by:

A. amniocentesis for the unborn.
B. a sweat test for both carriers and the diseased.
C. a sweat test for the diseased, but not for the carriers.
D. all of the above.

Passage 16 - (Questions 87–91)
Biological Sciences

Age (yrs.)	Patient A Pulse*	Patient A Weight (lbs)	Patient B Pulse*	Patient B Weight (lbs)	Patient C Pulse*	Patient C Weight (lbs)	Patient D Pulse*	Patient D Weight (lbs)
15	68	140	70	110	72	120	76	130
20	68	180	72	140	72	150	76	160
25	72	190	76	145	72	150	76	165
30	72	190	82	150	72	150	78	166
35	76	190	84	155	72	155	74	168
40	76	195	84	165	74	157	76	166
45	76	190	86	170	72	155	76	170
50	76	193	82	170	74	156	78	170
55	74	193	86	174	76	156	76	171
60	78	191	88	176	74	158	78	168
65	76	190	88	175	74	154	74	169
70	78	194	90	174	74	155	76	176
75	80	196	90	176	74	156	78	171
80	78	195	90	178	74	155	80	172

Pulse rate, weight for four male patients

(Keyed choice)
From the information in the table, select:

A. if the statement is true or probably true.
B. if the information in the table is not sufficient to indicate whether there is any degree of truth or falsity in the statement.
C. if the statement is false or probably false.

87. In this sample, increasing age increases the pulse rate significantly.

88. In this sample, increasing obesity increases the pulse rate significantly.

89. There is a correlation between weight and pulse rate in this sample.

90. If patient B had reduced his weight to 145 lbs. when in his fifties, his pulse rate would have gone down to the mid 70s.

91. What attention should we pay to ages 15 and 20 in considering the obesity of the patients? (Do not answer with A, B, or C.)

Passage 17 - (Questions 92–95)
Biological Sciences

The immune system is an enormously complex network of specialized organs and cells that has evolved to defend the body against attacks by "foreign" invaders. The success of this system in defending the body depends on an incredibly elaborate and dynamic regulatory-communication network. Millions and millions of cells, organized into sets and subsets, pass information back and forth like clouds of bees swarming around a hive. The result is a sensitive system of checks and balances that produces an immune response that is prompt, appropriate, effective, and self-limiting. Antigens are one key component of this system.

An antigen is any substance—any of the millions of "non-self" molecules—that can trigger an immune response because the body recognizes it as foreign. When functioning properly, the immune system can successfully fight off infections caused by agents such as bacteria and viruses by bringing to bear a sophisticated array of weapons. When it malfunctions, however, it can unleash an enormous variety of diseases from allergy to arthritis to cancer.

The most common types of allergic reactions—hay fever, some kinds of asthma, and hives—are produced when the immune system responds to a false alarm. In a susceptible person, a normally harmless substance, such as grass pollen or house dust, for example, is perceived as a threat and is attacked. Such allergic reactions are related to the antibody known as immunoglobulin E. Like other antibodies, each IgE antibody is antigen (or allergen) species-specific, that is, one reacts against oak pollen, another against ragweed, etc.

An immune deficiency disease results when the immune system lacks one or more essential components. Immune deficiency diseases can be inherited, acquired through illness, or produced as an inadvertent side effect of certain drug treatments. Immune responsiveness can also be depressed by blood transfusions, malnutrition, and stress. A defect in even one small component of the complex immune system can have far-reaching effects.

When cells of the immune system proliferate uncontrollably, the result is cancer. Leukemias, which are caused by the proliferation of white blood cells or leukocytes, are examples of such immunoproliferative disorders. Moreover, the cells of the immune system must maintain a delicate balance if the system is to work properly. If suppressor T cells are sluggish, for example, B cells may over-produce antibody; the same is true if helper T cells are overactive. Diseases associated with a deficiency in suppressor T cells include rheumatoid arthritis, multiple sclerosis, and some anemias.

(Multiple Choice)

92. Severe allergic eczema is associated with a deficiency in suppressor T cells. This disease is most likely the result of:

A. an immunoproliferative disorder.
B. a disorder of the immune regulation system.
C. an immune response to a false alarm related to the antibody immunoglobulin E.
D. an autoimmune response.

93. In this passage, the author primarily:

A. described the complex immune system.
B. provides a definition and some examples of autoimmune disease.
C. introduces some of the disorders of the immune system.
D. focuses on immunoproliferative disorder.

94. Sometimes the immune system's recognition apparatus goes awry, and the body begins to manufacture antibodies directed at the body's own components—cell-components, or specific organs. According to the passage, when this happens, it could result in:

A. an immunoproliferative disorder.
B. an immune complex disease.
C. an immune deficiency disease.
D. none of the above.

95. According to the passage, it can be inferred that:

A. a child born with defects in the B cell component, and who is unable to produce antibodies as a result, is probably suffering from an immune disease.
B. a person with AIDS, a disease characterized by very low levels of helper T cells, but normal levels of suppressor T cells, is probably suffering from an immune deficiency disease.
C. an infant who lacks T cells and whose thymus is either missing, or small and abnormal, is probably suffering from an immune deficiency disease.
D. probably all of the above are suffering from an immune deficiency disease.

Passage 18 - (Questions 96–106)
Biological Sciences

A manufacturer wants to market its product as a cure for cancer. Focus group research has revealed that people will not believe claims for a product that is aimed at more than three different kinds of cancer. The sales department is convinced that a product for women can be sold at a price that will produce twice the profit of a male-oriented elixir. But market data suggests that 45% of the male population are potential purchasers while only 1/5 of the female population is likely to buy. The legal department has advised that government action to halt sales will be more rapid if more than one product is sold.

Cancer Incidence/Deaths by Site and Gender in the U.S.:

Cancer Incidence by Site and Gender*

Male	Cancer Type	Female
1%	Skin	1%
5%	Oral	2%
22%	Lung	6%
---	Breast	26%
14%	Colon and Rectum	15%
12%	Other Digestive	9%
17%	Prostate	---
---	Ovary	5%
---	Uterus	14%
9%	Urinary	4%
8%	Leukemia and Lymphomas	7%
12%	All Other	11%

*Excluding non-melanoma skin cancer and carcinoma *in situ* of uterine cervix.

Cancer Deaths by Site and Gender

Male	Cancer Type	Female
1%	Skin	1%
3%	Oral	1%
33%	Lung	11%
---	Breast	20%
12%	Colon and Rectum	15%
15%	Other Digestive	14%
10%	Prostate	---
---	Ovary	6%
---	Uterus	7%
5%	Urinary	3%
8%	Leukemia and Lymphomas	9%
12%	All Other	13%

You may assume that total cancer incidence is approximately equal for men and women. Percentages are to the nearest 1%.

(Keyed choice Questions 96–101)
From the information above, select:

- **A.** if the statement is true or probably true.
- **B.** if the information given is not sufficient to indicate whether there is any degree of truth or falsity in the statement.
- **C.** if the statement is false or probably false.

96. More women get lung cancer than men.

97. More women get cancer of the colon and rectum than men do.

98. More men die of prostate cancer than women die of urinary cancer.

99. A man with lung cancer is more likely to die than a woman with lung cancer.

(For questions 100–101 assume that 30% of male urinary tract cancers diagnosed are cancers of the bladder.)

100. There are more men with bladder cancers than men with oral cancer.

101. More men die of bladder cancer than of skin cancer.

(Subjective Questions 102–106)

102. What three cancers would produce the largest market for a male-oriented product?

103. What three cancers would produce the largest market for a female-oriented product?

104. Which product type, male or female, would be more likely to produce the larger total profit?

105. Which product type, male or female, would have the higher total number of deaths associated with it?

106. Which product type, male or female, would have the higher percentage death rate?

Passage 19 - (Questions 107–113)
Biological Sciences

The first studies of the mental effects of the adrenocorticotropic hormones (ACTH) showed that a learned response was maintained longer in rats treated with ACTH than in untreated rats. Later it was shown that with their pituitaries removed (hypophysectomized), these rats were much less capable of learning responses than intact animals. Further, when hypophysectomized animals were given ACTH, their learning disturbance was partially eliminated. Thus the pituitary seemed to be involved in brain function.

Later, scientists studied the influence of ACTH and hypophysectomy on the learning of conditioned avoidance behavior in rats. These studies confirmed that ACTH was indeed involved in learning. The 39 amino acids that make up the ACTH molecule were broken down into fragments.

The behavioral effect of ACTH was shown to be contained in only four amino acids, those numbering 4 to 7 in the ACTH sequence. These simple sequences of amino acids were known collectively as short-chain polypeptides. The ACTH 4 to 7 fragment, or the more common fragment, 4 to 10, and a similar sequence of amino acids from another hormone, called alpha-MSH, have now been studied in human volunteers. Alpha-MSH mediates the control of skin color in frogs, but its effect on man seems to be on behavior. These simple peptides, when administered to humans, produced decreased anxiety and generally influenced the occipital electroencephalogram (EEG) towards a pattern consistent with increased attention.

How these peptides influence the brain is still largely a mystery. However, scientists have noted a clear decrease in the levels of ribonucleic acid (RNA) and of protein synthesis in the brains of hypophysectomized rats. This disturbance in protein synthesis was limited to a small fraction of rapidly turning over protein, and when ACTH was given to these animals, the rate of protein synthesis was restored almost to that of normal animals. This suggests that the rapidly turning over proteins are involved in learning behaviors, and peptides exert an influence on these proteins.

(Multiple Choice)
Based upon the information given in the passage, select:

- **A.** if the item is associated with **A** only.
- **B.** if the item is associated with **B** only.
- **C.** if the item is associated with **A** and **B**.
- **D.** if the item is associated with **neither A nor B.**

107. Mental changes can be induced by ACTH and adrenocortical hormones when they are:

- **A.** excessive.
- **B.** deficient.
- **C.** both **A** and **B.**
- **D.** neither **A** nor **B.**

108. Treating hypophysectomized rats with ACTH resulted in:

- **A.** increasing their intelligence quotients (IQ).
- **B.** deficient intelligence quotients (IQ).
- **C.** both **A** and **B.**
- **D.** neither **A** nor **B.**

109. Removal of the pituitary gland causes rats to exhibit:

- **A.** aggressive behavior.
- **B.** impaired muscular control.
- **C.** both **A** and **B.**
- **D.** neither **A** nor **B.**

110. Studies of the 4 - 10 ACTH fragment have shown that it can affect man's:

- **A.** learning.
- **B.** behavior.
- **C.** both **A** and **B.**
- **D.** neither **A** nor **B.**

111. The effect of alpha-MSH on humans has been shown to:

- **A.** decrease anxiety.
- **B.** control skin color.
- **C.** both **A** and **B.**
- **D.** neither **A** nor **B.**

112. Human subjects have been used in studies of the effect of:

- **A.** ACTH 4 - 10.
- **B.** alpha-MSH.
- **C.** both **A** and **B.**
- **D.** neither **A** nor **B.**

113. Studies have shown that ACTH is related to protein synthesis in:

- **A.** rats.
- **B.** humans.
- **C.** both **A** and **B.**
- **D.** neither **A** nor **B.**

Passage 20 - (Questions 114–123)
Biological Sciences

The Bread Spread Company decides to conduct a series of experiments to show that its product is effective in reducing cholesterol levels. Three experiments were run under the conditions given:

Experiment 1—Group 1 was fed a diet of bread and water with 1 oz of spread allowed per day. Group 2 was fed only french fries and milk shakes.

Experiment 2—Group 3 ate a normal diet, but the company's spread was substituted for butter. Group 4 also ate a normal diet but with butter instead of the spread.

Experiment 3—Group 5 consisted of company employees. No attempt was made to control their diet, but they were allowed to take home as much product as they wished. Group 6 consisted only of the company researcher, who never ate any of the company's product at all.

Average Cholesterol Level (mg/100 ml) for Each Group

Group No.	1	2	3	4	5	6
Avg.Age:	21 yrs	48 yrs	65 yrs	22 yrs	33 yrs	57 yrs
Avg.Wgt:	95 lbs.	165 lbs	195 lbs	110 lbs	150 lbs	190 lbs
	female	female	female	female	male	male
Fri., 3/4	194	222	234	201	215	230
Mon., 3/7	195	220	235	199	220	235
Tue., 3/8	201	227	246	206	230	245
Wed. 3/9	201	229	246	204	230	235
Thur., 3/10	200	228	247	202	225	230
Fri., 3/11	201	230	246	200	220	235
Mon., 3/14	198	231	245	194	210	240
Tue., 3/15	199	231	246	192	215	235
Wed., 3/16	198	230	244	194	210	235
Thur., 3/17	197	228	242	196	205	230
Fri., 3/18	198	227	241	197	205	235
Average	198	228	243	199	217	235

(Keyed Choice)
Based on the information given, select:

- **A.** if the statement is **supported** by the information given.
- **B.** if the statement is **contradicted** by the information given.
- **C.** if the statement is **neither supported nor contradicted** by the information given.

(Keyed Choice Questions 114–120)

114. The jump in average cholesterol level seen in all participants between March 7 and March 8 must have been caused by the accidental inclusion of some hidden saturated fat in their diets.

115. Group 1's average cholesterol level on Sunday, March 13 is probably about 199 mg/100 ml.

116. Group 2's average cholesterol level on Sunday, March 27 is probably approximately 228 mg/100 ml.

117. There is evidence that obesity causes higher cholesterol levels.

118. Group 4's cholesterol level will rise as they grow older.

119. For the people in these experiments, cholesterol level is not related to age.

120. On the average, 50-70% of a person's cholesterol is ester, so Group 4's cholesterol ester level is probably about 124 mg/100 ml on Tuesday, March 8.

(Subjective Questions 121, 122)

121. Which groups provide data which might bear on the hypothesis that two weeks of eating Bread Spread will have little or no effect on cholesterol level?

122. Which two groups would make the best comparison to test the hypothesis that Bread Spread, as part of a modified diet, can reduce cholesterol levels?

(Multiple Choice)

123. In the experiment described in the previous question, no significant difference is found between the two groups. What change would be most likely to expose a significant difference if there is indeed one?

- **A.** Increase the size of each sample
- **B.** Increase the length of time over which the experiment is conducted
- **C.** Reduce the variance of weight and age in each group
- **D.** Control for possible sex differences between the two populations sampled

Passage 21 - (Questions 124–130)
Physical Sciences

Alzheimer's disease and Parkinson's disease can be treated slowly by transporting drugs to the brain and spinal cord. Drugs can be taken orally, by intravenous methods or by small pumps that can be implanted in the patient. Pumps are small instruments that deliver drugs at a certain flow rate and under a certain pressure. Pumps are controlled manually or electronically. At body temperatures of around 98° F a Freon gas pump may be easily used. The Freon in the pump exerts pressure to push liquid medication from the reservoir into a catheter leading to the brain.

An implantable pump consists of a battery, a peristaltic pump, a drug reservoir and a self-sealing septum. The peristaltic pump can be controlled to function continuously by electronic means. Successive waves of involuntary contraction pass through the pump and the medication is forced outward.

In a patient with Parkinson's disease, medications A_1 and B_1 were tried for various periods. Medication A_1 was pumped at 250 mg/min through a catheter diameter of 0.2 cm. The equations used to check constant infusion are as follows:

Steady Infusion Rate (SIR) = $C_m V_{cl}$ ------ (a)

Time to reach 50% conc. = $t_{1,2} = \frac{0.69}{K}$ ------ (b)

Clearance constant, $K = \frac{V_{cl}}{V_d}$

where,

SIR = Steady Infusion Rate (mg/min)
C_m = Medication concentration (mg/L)
V_{cl} = Clearance rate (L/min)
$t_{1,}$ = Half time for concentration to reach 50% (min)
K = Clearance constant (min)
V_d = Discharge volume (mL)

The time for medication A_1 to fall to 50% of its concentration was 11 hours and 40 minutes. The total discharge volume was approximately 20,000 mL. Medication B_1 was pumped at 1,000 mg/min through a catheter diameter of 0.5 cm. The time for medication B_1 to fall to 50% of its concentration was 38 hours. The total discharge volume was approximately twice that of Medication A_1. The patient was more satisfied with medication B_1 because of the 38 hours time gap before a new dose was pumped. The physician was more concerned about the effect of medication A_1 as being stronger in its after effects. Assume that the density and temperature of drug A_1 and drug B_1 are the same as water at 20° C.

(Multiple Choice)

124. Calculate the approximate velocity ratio of drug A_1 to drug B_1 through their respective catheters.

A. 4:1
B. 2.5:1
C. 1.6:1
D. 0.3:1

125. The patient with Parkinson's disease monitors the time for dosage electronically. The nurse accidentally gives the patient medication A_1, then medication B_1, and then medication A_1. The total time from medication A_1 to medication B_1 is 16 hours and between the second and the third dosage is 30 hours. Based on this information and the half-times of both drugs, which of the following statements are valid?

I. It will take approximately 92 hours for medications A_1 and B_1 to reach almost zero level from the time the first dosage was given.
II. Ten hours after the second dosage is given, the patient may have 86% B_1 and almost zero level A_1.
III. In the 48th hour after the first dosage the patient has only 50% or less of Medication A_1.

A. I only
B. II only
C. I and II only
D. II and III only

126. The clearance rate for medication B_1 is different than the clearance rate for medication A_1 by:

A. Less than 10L/min.
B. More than 10L/min.
C. Less than 11L/hr.
D. More than 11L/hr.

127. The concentration C_m of medication A_1 that was used to prepare the dosage reservoir was calculated by the lab technician to be:

A. 1.250 mg
B. 12.7000 mg
C. 125.000 mg
D. 1,000.000 mg

128. Which of the following claims cannot be scientifically supported from the information provided in the passage *except:*

A. A peristaltic pump can be only used for Parkinson's disease treatment.
B. Medication A_1 takes longer to eliminate from the bloodstream of the Parkinson's disease patient.
C. Medication B_1 is very weak in treating Parkinson's disease.
D. Either medication A_1 or medication B_1 can be pumped to the brain, depending on the conditions of the patient.

129. After reading the passage above, the following *assumptions* seem to be true:

I. An implantable pump is more convenient than other devices to transport medication.
II. The flow through the catheter tube is turbulent.
III. The infusion of medication can be maintained at a steady rate.

A. I only
B. I and II only
C. I and III only
D. I, II, and III

130. A small plastic bead blocks the medication transport in catheter B_1. The diameter of the unblocked tube is 0.2 cm, the same as for catheter A_1. This will change some flow variables in catheter B_1. Which of the following options are false?

I. The liquid pressure in the catheter tube B_1 will suddenly drop.
II. The velocity of the fluid in catheter B_1 will suddenly rise.
III. The drug in catheter B_1 will separate from the liquid and cause more blockage.

A. I and II
B. II only
C. II and III
D. III only

Passage 22 - (Questions 131–136)
Biological Sciences

Blood is pumped in the human fetus before birth and the heart continues working until you die. The heart *cannot* stop from pumping blood at any time in a living human. The heart is an important organ of your body. It is made up of cardiac muscle. There are two types of muscle: voluntary and involuntary. The cardiac muscle has a different structure than involuntary muscles in your body. Heart diseases that may be fatal are heart attack, heart stroke, ventricular fibrillation, congestive heart failure, and atrial fibrillation (rare).

The muscles of the heart must contract synchronously in order to pump blood properly. During atrial fibrillation there is a synchronous contraction of the atrial muscles. The atria may contract up to seven times faster than the ventricles. In general there is a 12 to 15 percent loss of pumping efficiency. The symptoms of atrial fibrillation may be shortness of breath and fatigue during exercise such as jogging. According to the American Heart Association, there are almost 2 million Americans with signs of atrial fibrillation. Hypertension, heart rheumatism, and arteriosclerosis may be causes of atrial fibrillation. Various factors such as alcohol, caffeine, fatigue, and tension can trigger atrial fibrillation. Running on a hot summer day and drinking a large volume of cold water right after exercise may lead to atrial fibrillation. To stop atrial fibrillation, drugs such as digoxin and procainamide are administered in varying doses until they become effective. Procainamide may cause inflammation of the pericardium.

For a resting adult, the heart beat is approximately 70 to 80 beats per minute. The atrial contractions are somewhat coordinated even during atrial flutter—heart beat is between 200 to 350 beats per minute. The atria pump almost no blood during this state. During atrial fibrillation, an electrocardiogram will show no P waves (on the P-Q-R-S-T cycle). Ventricular fibrillation is more dangerous than atrial fibrillation. The ECG shows dominant disorder in the Q-R-S part. Electrical defibrillation is the best way to stop ventricular fibrillation. During atrial or ventricular fibrillation, the atria and the ventricles, respectively, become almost ineffective in pumping blood to various parts of the body.

(Multiple Choice)

131. Rapid atrial contractions mean:

A. excessive blood flow occurs in the sinoatrial node.
B. less blood is pushed out of the upper chambers.
C. pumping efficiency can increase due to intake of large volumes of caffeine.
D. electrical defibrillation is producing excessive heart beat.

132. Atrial flutter and ventricular fibrillation are related *except:*

I. ventricular fibrillation occurs at 155 beats per minute and causes the Q-R-S wave to be disoriented.
II. digoxin is not useful for ventricular fibrillation or atrial flutter.
III. atrial flutter occurs around 200 beats per minute and causes the P wave to be disoriented.

A. I and III.
B. I and II.
C. III only.
D. I, II, and III.

133. Following is a correct blood flow sequence through the heart:

A. left atrium, aorta, right atrium, right ventricle, left ventricle.
B. aorta, right ventricle, right atrium, left ventricle, left atrium.
C. right atrium, right ventricle, left atrium, left ventricle, aorta.
D. left ventricle, aorta, right ventricle, right atrium, left atrium.

134. The following facts pertain to atrial fibrillation and not ventricular fibrillation *except:*

A. This type of fibrillation is only stopped by electric defibrillation.
B. This type of fibrillation is usually prevented by digoxin and procainamide.
C. Shortness of breath and fatigue during exercise can cause this type of fibrillation.
D. Enough blood is not pumped by the atria during this type of fibrillation.

135. The refractory period of a cardiac muscle cell is approximately 250 milliseconds. Sinoatrial node is a small bunch of special cardiac muscle cells. The cell membranes of the sinoatrial node are more permeable to Na^+ ions. The Na^+ ions decrease the membrane potential. The $Na^+ - K^+$ pump is always working in the sinoatrial node cells. As stated by the Frank-Starling law, the force of contraction inside the heart increases when the cardiac muscle is stretched.

Based on the above additional information and the passage, the following conclusion is valid:

A. Doubling the refractory period of a cardiac muscle would double the force of contraction in the sinoatrial node.
B. The $Na^+ - K^+$ pump causes the force of contraction in the sinoatrial node.
C. Atrial fibrillation leads to stretching of the cardiac muscle.
D. Doubling the refractory period of a cardiac muscle would double the force of contraction in the sinoatrial node.

136. Which of the following would lead to congestive heart failure?

A. The renal system excretes large volumes of fluid.
B. The blood volume in the human body decreases.
C. The activities of the sympathetic system to the heart increase.
D. The pericardium is inflamed and causes blood leakage.

ANSWER KEY

Directions: Check your answers against the summary listing. If you cannot determine why your answer is incorrect, read the additional answer explanation provided in "Expanded Explanatory Solutions."

Passage 1
1. D
2. C
3. D
4. C
5. B
6. A

Passage 2
7. A
8. D
9. A
10. B
11. A

Passage 3
12. B
13. C
14. B
15. C
16. D

Passage 4
17. C
18. C
19. D
20. B
21. D
22. A

Passage 5
23. B
24. D
25. A, C
26. A, D
27. B
28. A

Passage 6
29. A
30. A
31. A
32. C
33. A
34. C

Passage 7
35. D
36. A
37. A
38. C
39. D
40. B
41. C

Passage 8
42. D
43. D
44. B
45. 2
46. 1, B

Passage 9
47. A
48. D
49. C
50. D
51. D

Passage 10
52. None
53. (See explanation)
54. A
55. A
56. A
57. D
58. No
59. Yes

Passage 11
60. A
61. C
62. D
63. D
64. A

Passage 12
65. Cirrhosis
66. Cirrhosis
67. Cannot say
68. No
69. 150 million person yrs
70. (See explanation)

Passage 13
71. B
72. D
73. D
74. A

Passage 14
75. C
76. C
77. A
78. B
79. B
80. B
81. C

Passage 15
82. D
83. D
84. B
85. D
86. C

Passage 16
87. C
88. A
89. A
90. B
91. (Little attention)

Passage 17
92. B
93. C
94. D
95. B

Passage 18
96. C
97. B
98. B
99. B
100. C
101. B
102. (Lung, prostate, colon)
103. (Breast, colon, uterine)
104. Male
105. Male
106. Male

Passage 19
107. C
108. D
109. D
110. B
111. A
112. C
113. A

Passage 20
114. C
115. A
116. C
117. C
118. C
119. B
120. C
121. 1,3
122. 1,4
123 B

Passage 21
124. C
125. C
126. A
127. B
128. D
129. D
130. D

Passage 22
131. A
132. B
133. C
134. A
135. D
136. C

EXPLANATORY EXPANDED SOLUTIONS

Passage 1 - Verbal Reasoning

No.	Key	
1.	D	Choices **A**, **B**, and **C** do not mention the central fact of the passage—Paul's illness.
2.	C	The last sentence in the third paragraph indicates that the counselor's primary concern was Paul's illness.
3.	D	The second and fourth sentences in the paragraph state that Paul was "watched over," "guarded" and denied tasks "which might prove stressful."
4.	C	This choice is a restatement of the reasons given by Paul in the second sentence in paragraph three.
5.	B	The first sentence in the fourth paragraph indicates Paul's success was due to a "change in his self-image."
6.	A	No information is given in the passage to support the conclusion of choices **B** and **C.** Although cystic fibrosis may require therapy for emotional issues, the disease may not be "emotionally disabling." The passage supports Choice A—that cystic fibrosis is an incurable, terminal illness.

Passage 2 - Verbal Reasoning

7.	A	"Unit rule" is defined under Senator Brown's speech as awarding all of the state's electoral votes to the candidate with the highest popular vote.
8.	D	The discussion about how the election would be conducted if neither candidate received a 40% vote relates to the proposed amendment. The question, however, focuses on the current system for which there is no information provided.
9.	A	Senator Smith discusses how the electoral system "virtually requires" that minority groups band together into alliances. These groups encompass persons from geographic areas, ethnic, religious, social, or economic groups.
10.	B	Senator Brown discusses how votes will count in states where presently the power of minority votes can be diminished in the "winner take all" approach. He does not compare it to the election procedures for state officials.
11.	A	The Senators present quite different views on how the election of a President should be handled. However, each feels that his/her way is the most advantageous.

Passage 3 - Verbal Reasoning

12.	B	You will find the answer to this question in the first sentence in the last paragraph.
13.	C	Once you have found the right time period in the passage, the key words in the stem are "most influenced." The last sentence in the first paragraph indicates that migration was the primary influencing factor.
14.	B	In order to answer this question correctly, you need to read the second sentence of the second paragraph all the way through (otherwise you might choose **D**) and rephrase the information found therein. Marginal notes indicating growth or decline (perhaps in the form of arrows up or down) would have helped you find this information more quickly.

15. **C** A is incorrect since births would not affect the number of people dying. There is no support for **D. B** and **C** are both true answers, but the stem asks for the "most important effect" which would be the impact of the numbers in determining trends.

16. **D** If you look carefully at choices **A** and **B**, you will see that they deal with specifics—demographic studies, birth rate, and immigration. Choices **C** and **D** are more general—population decline versus population growth. Choosing the correct answer was a matter of deciding between two statements expressing opposite ideas.

Passage 4 - Verbal Reasoning

17. **C** Only choice **C** can serve as a thesis or summary of the passage as a whole. Choices **A, B,** and **D** apply to single paragraphs, but not to the whole (too narrow). Choice **A** comes from the introductory or background material (too broad).

18. **C** Although all of the choices may be true about scientific research in general, choice **C** is a paraphrase of the specific conclusions found in the paragraph about talking to nonscientists about research.

19. **D** Choice **D** in this negative-stemmed question is false. The last sentence in paragraph three and the first sentence in paragraph five indicate that, at the outset, scientists have no clear idea of the results of their research.

20. **B** This is another negative-stemmed question. Choice **C** is directly stated in paragraph six. Choices **A** and **D** are implied in that the scientist must "remove the arbitrary" from his work. Choice **B** is neither stated nor implied, since no comparison was made between scientists and artists on the criteria for "greatness."

21. **D** This fairly easy question is answered in the third sentence of the last paragraph.

22. **A** Yet another negative-stemmed question. All of these words are found in the passage, but "anecdotal" refers not to scientific research but to Simone de Beauvoir's book.

Passage 5 - Verbal Reasoning

23. **B** The answer is stated in the second sentence of the fourth paragraph.

24. **D** The answer is in the discussion about the Czechs in the last paragraph.

25. **A, C** Information is provided in the last sentence of paragraph two.

26. **A, D** Paragraph three indicates that two areas of the body are involved, both the stomach and the intestines. The passage states that gastro-intestinal cancer as well as gastric cancer are related to the talc-dusted rice.

27. **B** The answer is found in the last sentence of the passage.

28. **A** In paragraph three, sentence four, there is a relationship stated between "this tumor" and cancer related to smoked fish. The paragraph must be studied for the antecedent to "this tumor", which is found in the second sentence of the paragraph.

Passage 6 - Physical Sciences

29. **A** Supported. Except for the 10° C increase in temperature from 20° to 30° for Lab B, the data for all four labs show an increased NaCl solubility in H_2O (no. of grams dissolved/liter of H_2O) with every 10° C increase of temperature in the range 10° C to 100° C.

30. **A** Supported. Using the data of all four labs at 50° C, the average number of grams of NaCl that will dissolve in 1 liter of H_2O is 40 g (the numerical average = 39.75) with the range in the data being 3 g. Since this range is so small, it is reasonable to expect that approximately 40 g of NaCl will dissolve.

31. **A** Supported. At all temperatures except 20° C, the range in the data of the four labs is between 1 g and 4 g (most often being 2 g) whereas at 20° C the range is 8 g, or 1 g if Lab C's result, which is 7 g outside this 1 g range, is not included. Thus, excluding Lab C's 20° C reading, the data indicate an allowable random error of no more than 4 g at each of the temperatures that measurements of NaCl's solubility were taken. Therefore, the data support the statement that Lab C's 20° reading is 7-8 g from the other 20° C reading because of a substantial error in it.

32. **C** Neither supported nor contradicted. The data between 70° C and 100° C show, on average, a 1 g increase in dissolved NaCl for a 1° increase in temperature which, if extrapolated to 120° C, would show that virtually all 100 g of salt would dissolve at 120° C. Nevertheless, we are not justified in assuming that this 1 to 1 linear relationship would continue above 100° C where our data stop. Anyway, if this experiment were done near normal atmospheric pressure, the water would start to evaporate at about 100° C (we would also have to start to take into account boiling point elevation caused by the dissolved salt).

33. **A** Supported. The data show that between 10° C and 100° C the amount of dissolved NaCl increases with temperature, there being roughly a 1 g increase for a 1° C increase between 70° C and 100° C. This justifies interpolating between 70° C and 80° C to get a good prediction of how much salt would dissolve at 75° C. The interpolated reading for 75° C is the average of the readings at 70° C and 80° C. Thus, all four labs predict that approximately 55 g of NaCl would dissolve at 75° C.

34. **C** Neither supported nor contradicted. We have not been told the magnitudes of the error in the measurements used to collect these data. Measurement error in the volume of water and in the number of grams of NaCl dissolved itself could also contribute to this variability.

Passage 7 - Biological Sciences

35. **D** The data indicate that neither drug showed the majority of the sleep time in the REM stage.

36. **A** Only one patient (Drug A) versus four patients (Drug B) reported "hangover."

37. **A** The passages indicated 14 percent of the sleep time (Drug A) and 28 percent of sleep time (Drug B) was spent in the REM stage. Thus, only Drug A had less than 20 percent in this stage.

38. **C** In the data for both drugs, the majority of time was spent in Stage II. Drug A had 63 percent; Drug B had 56 percent.

39. **D** Patients awakened on average less frequently with Drug A (4 times) and Drug B (5 times) than during the baseline period (6 times).

40. **B** Stage IV sleep comprised 3 percent (Drug B) versus 10 percent (Drug A) of total sleeping time.

41. **C** Stage I, somnolence, accounted for 4 percent of total sleep time in baseline, Drug A, and Drug B conditions.

Passage 8 - Biological Sciences

42. **D** The data in the histogram are for male teenagers only: so, it is not sufficient for evaluating the difference between the percentage of 17–18 year olds, both male and female, who were regular smokers in 1974 and the same percentage in 1970.

43. D To evaluate the difference between (1) and (2), we would also need to know the numbers of 12–14 year old males in the U.S. in 1970 and 1974 respectively or, at least, the relative magnitudes of these two numbers. The percentages in the histogram are not sufficient.

44. B (1) % of 12–14 year old males in the U.S. who were regular smokers in 1972 = about 6% (2) % of 15-16 year old males in the U.S. who were regular smokers in 1972 = about 21%

45. No Even if we were given a similar percentage histogram for females, we could not, in general, determine the percentages of 17–18 year olds in the U.S. who were smokers in 1974 and 1970 without knowing the relative numbers of 17–18 year old males and females in both 1974 and 1970. This is because

percentages of 17–18 year olds who were regular smokers +

$$\frac{\text{(no. of 17–18 yr old males)(\% 17–18 yr old male smokers) + (no. of 17–18 yr old females)(\% 17–18 yr old female smokers)}}{\text{no. of 17–18 yr old males + no. of 17–18 yr old females}}$$

46. Yes, B As can be seen from the equation in (45) above, if the percentages were exactly the same for females as for males, the percentage of 17-18 year olds as a whole who were regular smokers would be equal to the percentage of 17–18 year old males (or females) who were regular smokers. Thus, from the histogram:

(1) % of 17–18 year olds in the U.S. who were regular smokers in 1974 = about 38%
(2) % of 17–18 year olds in the U.S. who were regular smokers in 1970 = about 45%

Passage 9 - Biological Sciences

47. A The passage is about giant chromosomes. Not only are the two types described physically, but also their characteristic actions during cell division are described. The word "giant" in answer choice **A** should have been a clue to choosing **A** as the correct answer. In a textbook-type passage such as this one, the passage tends to be primarily "about" the noun that is repeated most often.

48. D From the question stem, you should have been looking in the passage for "female sex cells of amphibians." The first sentence in the passage gives you the answer if you associate the term "lamp-brush" with "brush-like appearance."

49. C The significant nouns in the question stem are "characteristics" and "Diptera insect." Some readers have difficulty switching their focus from amphibians in question 48 to Diptera insects in question 49.

The second difficulty posed is that this question has a negative stem. Readers often miss negative-stemmed questions because they have difficulty reversing their thinking from looking for a true choice to looking for one that is false. You can significantly lower your MCAT score, particularly in the biological sciences, simply by failing to use a specific strategy to deal with the following three small words: **not, except,** and **false.**

50. D An inference question asks you to read the passage for supporting evidence, but the conclusion you draw will only be probable, not certain. Choice **D** is an inference you can draw from the statement in the third paragraph. One statement indicates that chromosomes of insects and amphibians are interphase chromosomes; the following statement implies that interphase is more active than other states. Later statements imply that more can be learned during active than during inactive states.

51. D The answer to this question can be found in the last sentence. "Supporting evidence" is a rephrasing or synonym for "physical embodiment"; similarly, "genetic construct" is a rephrasing or synonym for that "which was originally a purely conceptual idea of a unit of heredity."

Passage 10 - Biological Sciences

52. **None** No evidence in support of this claim is given in the article.

53. **-** The percentage of population seeking pap smears involves females only, while the percentage given for eye exams includes both genders, a group roughly twice as large. The author's conclusion seems to be based on the percentage of eye exams for the total population studied vs. the percentage of pap smears for female participants only.

(Below, note that within a single age group, comparing percentages is equivalent to comparing numbers)

54. **A** (1) Percentage of 45–64 year olds who received eye examinations greater than 50%
(2) Percentage of 45–64 year olds who had chest X-rays less than 50%

55. **A** (1) Percentage of 45–64 year olds who had pap smears about 50%
(2) Percentage of 45–64 year olds who had chest X-rays less than 50%

56. **A** (Note that since a greater percentage of 45–64 year olds had chest X-rays than had glaucoma tests, the percentage who had both cannot be greater than the percentage who had glaucoma tests.)

(1) Percentage of 45–64 year olds who had chest X-rays greater than 33%
(2) Percentage of 45–64 year olds who had both chest X-rays and glaucoma tests at most about 33%

57. **D** Without knowing both the number of 17–24 year olds and the number of 45–64 year olds (i.e., in this question the two numbers being compared are not from the same age group), the percentages in the histogram cannot be used to compute the numbers in (1) and (2) for comparison.

58. **No** Value judgement conclusions of this sort, e.g., the importance of preventive examinations for health, cannot be drawn from frequency data of the sort in the histogram for this problem. Popular knowledge and opinion are irrelevant in considering such conclusions.

59. **Yes** Given the claim that the pap smear is considered a more important test for a 25–44 year old woman than for a woman 65 or older, the information in the graph—that about 75% of 25–44 year old women had received a pap smear while less than 33% of women 65 or older had—supports this claim. Note that the question asks if the data support the claim, not the truth or falsity of the claim to be concluded from the data.

Passage 11 - Biological Sciences

60. **A** This question asks for a definition of "allometric analysis." If you noted definitions as you read, you should have had little difficulty in spotting the correct choice. It's an exact statement from the text.

61. **C** This also asks for a definition, this time from the last sentence, third paragraph, which reads "a clear, positive model of the surface of the animal's brain." Thus, an endocast is not a mold "of skeletal remains"—a restricting phrase, but rather a model "of the animal's brain."

62. **D** To answer this question, you have to relate the information given in the second paragraph about the Triconodon's brain with information in the last paragraph about its extraordinarily increased volume.

63. **D** Yet another definition question, this one asks about information found in the last two sentences in paragraph four. Your marginal notes should have helped you to find this answer in the passage very quickly.

64. **A** Each of the four statements could be a conclusion (inductive phrasing), except there are minor errors (something false or not true) about all but one of these choices. This question requires the test-taker to read each statement in terms of true, false, or don't know. Remember, in order for the answer to be true, all parts of it must be true.

Look at choices **B, C,** and **D.** Do you see the false part of each? Look particularly at the choice **B**. It is false because of the word "crude." Paleontologist's tools are "basic," according to the passage, but not "crude." The words "crude" and "basic" are not synonyms.

Passage 12 - Biological Sciences

In case it is not clear, for each cause of death we have been given two pieces of data for the U.S. in 1970: the deaths per 100,000 population for each cause of death and the number of person-years that would be gained to age 70 by the elimination of each cause of death. The latter quantity means, for example, all 45-year old people who would previously have died of heart disease would each contribute 25 person-years that would be gained to age 70 in the U.S. by the elimination of heart disease as a cause of death.

65. **Cirrhosis of the liver.** Directly from the left-hand bar graph, cirrhosis of the liver is responsible for about 50 deaths per 100,000 population, while influenza and pneumonia are responsible for only about 33 deaths per 100,000 population.

66. **Cirrhosis of the liver.** Directly from the right-hand bar graph, elimination of cirrhosis of the liver as a cause of death would gain to age 70 about 33 million person-years, while the elimination of influenza and pneumonia would gain only about 15 million person-years.

67. **Cannot say.** In order to determine the average age of heart disease-induced death for people under 70, we would have to solve the equation: average age of heart disease induced death in people under 70 =

$$\frac{\text{number of person-years gained to age 70 by the elimination of 1970 heart disease deaths}}{\text{total number of deaths caused by heart disease in 1970}}$$

With the information given, we can determine the denominator but not the numerator of the fraction in this equation. We have not been told what part of the total number of person-years gained to age 70 by the elimination of heart disease as a cause of death in 1970 would be gained in 1970, separate from what would be gained in subsequent years because it was eliminated as a cause of death in 1970. This quantity is the numerator we would have to be able to determine in order to solve the equation above.

68. **No** We have not been told how this cut (from about 33 down to 10 per 100,000 population) in death rate due to motor vehicle accidents was distributed across the age range and therefore cannot calculate how many person-years to age 70 would be gained. For example, if we had been told that this cut in death rate was made proportional to the incidence of motor vehicle accident deaths across the age range, we could have done this calculation—see (69) below.

69. **150 million person-years.** Since the cut in death rate was made proportional to the incidence of malignant neoplasm deaths across the age range, the proportional drop in death rate is equal to the proportional gain in person-years to age 70 by the partial elimination of malignant neoplasm deaths. Reading from the bar graphs for malignant neoplasms, there are about 267 deaths per 100,000 population and about 240 million person-years to be gained to age 70 by its total elimination as a cause of death. The cut in death rate to 100 is then equivalent to a 167/267 = 5/8 reduction in death rate. Therefore, the number of person-years to be gained to age 70 is about (5/8) x 240 million = 150 million person-years.

70. Motor vehicle accidents are more likely to happen to young people, thus each death removes many more potential years of life than does cerebrovascular death, which most likely happens to an elderly person with many fewer years of life left. (Deaths of persons over 70 will remove zero years from the statistic shown on the graph.)

Passage 13 - Biological Sciences

71. B Did you remember to use a true and false strategy? Did you remember to check your answer carefully because of the negative stem? The false answer is **B** because "all vertebrates" include exceptions, e.g., fish, which have gills rather than lungs.

72. D Bronchial cells may produce mucus—but not phlegm, so **A** is not correct. Phlegm is not synonymous with mucus, so **B** is not correct. Phlegm is not normally found in the alveoli, so the answer is not **C**. Answer **D** is correct because it exactly parallels the last sentence of the second paragraph.

73. D According to the passage, **A, B,** and **C** are all true. The first half of **D** is true, but the second half is false; thus, **D** is the exception and, therefore, the correct answer.

74. A The volume $500cm^3$ is the normal capacity of lungs in man according to the passage; by inference, then maximum capacity would be more than $500cm^3$.

Passage 14 - Biological Sciences

75. C False. The number of rabbits that were dead after four weeks (= 36) is less than the number of rats that were dead after four weeks (= 45).

76. C False. The number of rabbits that died during weeks 3 and 4 (= 36 - 23 = 13) is less than the number of rats that died during weeks 3 and 4 (= 45 - 17 = 28).

77. A True. The percentage of rats living after week 2 that died during weeks 3 and 5 = (28/83) x 100 = 34%; this is greater than the percentage of monkeys that were dead after four weeks which = (67/280) x 100 = 24%.

78. B Information insufficient. In considering this statement, the data in the table are irrelevant. While more monkeys were studied than rats or rabbits, we have not been given any rationale for the respective numbers of each animal used in this experiment.

79. B Information insufficient. Even though it is true that the percentage of 10 g/day rats dead after four weeks (= 76%) is higher than the percentage of 40 g/day monkeys dead after four weeks (= 64%), we cannot tell if this explanation is true or false. One reason is that, because of the data on the 0 g/day animals, not all the 10 g/day rats and 40 g/day monkeys that died necessarily did so from ingestion of osmium tetroxide. If we subtract out the % of 0 g/day animals that died, for example, the percentages become 62% and 60%, instead of 76% and 64%. Another reason is that we do not know, in fact, that the monkeys used weighed more than four times the rats used in this experiment. Basically, evaluating this statement is way beyond the information we have been given.

80. B Information insufficient. This is only a possible explanation for the fact that the percentage of 0 g/day monkeys that died during this experiment (= 4%) is less than the percentage of 0 g/day rats that died during it (= 14%).

81. C Probably false. The percentage of 20 g/day rabbits that died during this experiment (= 83%) is considerably greater than the percentage of 0 g/day rabbits that died during it (= 13%).

Passage 15 - Biological Sciences

82. **D** Although the first sentence of the third paragraph provides references to "one out of 1,600 Caucasian babies," the answer to the question, as posed, cannot be determined from the information given.

83. **D** The passage continually makes a distinction between those who have the disease and those who are carriers. According to the passage, the sweat test provides certain identification only for those who actually have the disease. It does not identify carriers from non-carriers, so the sister's chance of being a carrier is determined by the genetic chance only; that is, the sweat test is irrelevant. We know that both parents carried CF genes; therefore, the sister's chance of being a carrier herself is 2 out of 3—as explicated at the end of paragraph 2.

84. **B** The CF gene is recessive. Using a Mendelian box (Punnett Square) provides the answer:

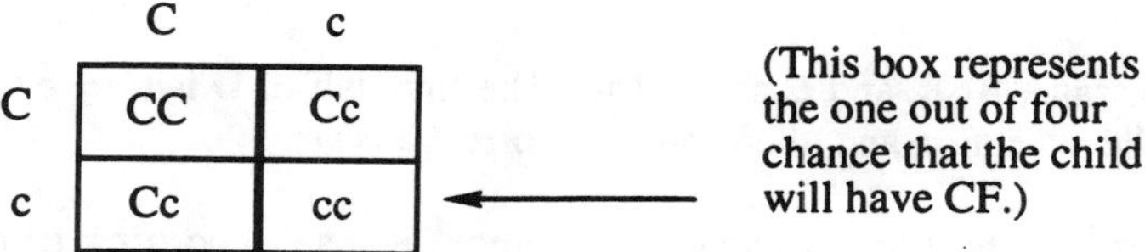

85. **D** This answer can be derived from the second paragraph in the text.

86. **C** The passage states that there is no test for the unborn, therefore, both **A** and **D** are wrong. The passage directly contradicts **B**. Answer **C** is supported in the third paragraph.

Passage 16 - Biological Sciences

87. **C** False. The scope of the data allows us to consider the dependence of pulse rate on the patients' ages and/or weights. In order to evaluate the relationship between age and pulse rate, we have to look for data in the table where the weight of a patient is essentially constant, so that any dependence of pulse rate on weight is eliminated. Consequently, we have to select our data that meet this criterion; moreover, it would be time wasted to answer this question by looking carefully at **all** the data. Clearly, patient C's data are the best place to start since his weight varies very little; since his pulse rate also varies very little, his data suggest that there is little, if any, dependence of pulse rate on age. In an attempt to be more methodical, we can, for example, select out the following data:

Patient A (wt = 190 lb)		Patient B (wt = 170 lb)		Patient C (wt = 155 lb)		Patient D (wt = 166 lb)	
Age	Pulse	Age	Pulse	Age	Pulse	Age	Pulse
25	72	45	86	35	72	30	78
30	72	50	82	45	72	40	76
35	76			70	74		
45	76	(wt = 174 lb)		80	74	(wt = 168 lb)	
65	76	55	86			35	74
		70	90	(wt = 156 lb)		60	78
				50	74		
				55	76		
				75	74		

Observing how the pulse rate varies with increased age in the data above, especially in that for patients **A** and **C,** we can conclude that it is false that increasing age increases the pulse rate significantly.

88. **A** Probably true. Analogous to what was done in answering (87), we have to eliminate or account for the effects of age on pulse rate before we can determine the relationship between weight and pulse rate. Since the nature of the data is such that we cannot look for pulse rate vs. weight data on each patient where age is "constant," we have to account for the effects of age on pulse rate before the relationship between it and weight can be considered. This has already been done in (87) where it was concluded that there is little, if any, dependence of pulse rate on age. Thus, we can look at each patient's pulse rate vs. weight data, ignoring the age associated with each data point (pulse rate/weight pair). The data for patients A, C, and D, between the ages of 25 and 80, show modest increases in weight which are paralleled by small increases in pulse rate. These data suggest a positive correlation between weight and pulse rate, but are not conclusive in themselves because of the small magnitudes involved. The data for patient B are much more definitive because they show a strong positive correlation between weight and pulse rate, especially in the data for ages 20 to 45 where a steady increase in weight from 140 to 170 lb. is paralleled by an increase in pulse rate from 72 to 86. Therefore, we can conclude that, in this sample, it is probably true that increasing obesity increases the pulse rate significantly.

89. **A** True. This is basically the same question as (88) which, in answering, we already took note of the positive correlation between weight and pulse rate in this sample, especially in the data of patient B.

90. **B** Information insufficient. In answering (87) and (88), we concluded that increasing obesity, but not increasing age, increases pulse rate significantly in this sample. With this in mind, the data might seem to suggest that this statement is true. However, it is not necessarily true because we did not actually conclude nor do the data actually show that decreasing obesity decreases pulse rate. In other words, the data do not cover the case of what happens to pulse rate when obesity is decreased significantly, so we cannot predict what would have happened to patient B's pulse rate if he had drastically reduced his weight in his mid 50s.

91. **(Little attention).** The age range of 15 to 20 is a period of significant physical growth for many individuals. Any weight gain in this period can reflect increased obesity and/or physical growth. The data do not allow us to separate these components of the age 15 to 20 weight gains.

Passage 17 - Biological Sciences

92. **B** Answer **D** is not discussed; answers **A** and **C** can be eliminated from the text. Answer **B** is the best answer choice—which is what is asked for by the inductive phrasing "most likely" in the question stem.

93. **C** Answer **A** is too broad; answers **B** and **D** are too narrow. Answer **C** is the best choice.

94. **D** All of the answers **A** through **C** can be eliminated. What is described would most likely be an autoimmune disease that is not described in this passage.

95. **B** Answer choice **B** appears to best fit the requirements for an immune deficiency disease as described in the passage.

Passage 18 - Biological Sciences

96. **C** False. We are told that we can assume that the total cancer incidence is approximately equal for men and women. Thus, if one sex has a considerably higher percentage incidence of a particular kind of cancer than the other sex, then it follows directly that more individuals of that sex get that kind of cancer than the other sex. Since the percentage incidence of lung cancer in women is 6% while that in men is 22%, more men than women get lung cancer.

97. **B** Information insufficient. Reading directly from the cancer incidence table, the percentage incidence of colon and rectum cancers in women (= 15%) is greater than in men (= 14%). However, since these percentages are rounded to the nearest 1%, their respective true percentages may be very close. We have assumed that the total cancer incidence is **approximately**, not exactly, equal in men and women. Thus, our knowledge of the total cancer incidences in men and women is not exact enough to judge this question as true or false.

98. **B** Information insufficient. We have not been told anything about the total cancer deaths for each sex; the percentages in the cancer deaths table are insufficient by themselves for answering this question. It is not reasonable to extend the assumption that total cancer incidence is approximately equal for men and women to an assumption that their respective total cancer deaths are also approximately equal.

99. **B** Information insufficient. In order to answer this question, using the lung cancer percentages in the cancer incidence table, we would have to be told the respective lung cancer death rates for men and women, or, using the lung cancer percentages in the cancer deaths table, the relative numbers of men and women who die from lung cancer.

100. **C** False. Using the assumption that total cancer incidence is approximately equal for men and women, the 30% of 9% = 2.7% incidences of bladder cancers in men is less than the 5% incidences of oral cancers.

101. **B** Information insufficient. We have been told that 30% of urinary cancers diagnosed in men are due to bladder cancer, *not* that 30% of urinary cancer deaths in men are due to bladder cancer. Hence, we cannot determine the percentage of cancer deaths in men that are due to bladder cancer for comparison with the percentage that are due to skin cancer.

102. - Find the three most common male cancers.

103. - Find the three most common female cancers.

104. **(Male)** This problem involves pulling information from many sources. Under the second table we are told that the total cancer incidence for males and females is approximately equal. This means that 1% of male cancers represents about the same number of people as 1% of female cancers. From table 1 we find the top three cancers account for 53% of the male total and 55% of the female. If T = total number of male cancers (and also the total number of female), then the possible male market is 0.53T, but only 45% of these men are likely to buy. Thus the market is 0.45 x 0.53T = 0.24T. For females, the market is 0.2 x 0.55T = .11T. The female market may generate twice the profit per sale, but it is less than half the size of the male market.

105. **(Male)** We must look at table 2 to find the rates of death. For men, the death rates are 33% lung, 10% prostate, and 12% colon. But each of these cancers make up a different fraction of the men likely to buy the product. We can work out the number of deaths in each group and add them together.

For males: .33 x .22T + .1 x .17T + .12 x .14T = .1T
For females: .2 x .26T + .15 x .15T + .07 x .14T = .08T

The incidences of death are higher for men than for women; furthermore, we expect to sell to more than twice as many men as women, so the total deaths will be higher for the males than it would be for the females. The legal department will probably argue for selling the less profitable product.

106. **(Male)** This answer was calculated in the answer to question (105).

Passage 19 - Biological Sciences

107. **C** This first paragraph indicates that either excess or deficient ACTH will induce mental changes.

108. D Paragraph two states that the ACTH treatment caused the "learning disturbance" of hypophysectomized rats to be partly eliminated. This would not necessarily include IQ or discrimination. IQ, or intelligence quotient, would be considered "innate." Pay special attention to distinctions between what a person is born with as opposed to what he learns. The ability to discriminate is not discussed.

109. D Removal of the pituitary gland caused a decreased capability of learning responses, not a loss of either aggression or muscular control.

110. B Paragraph three states that alpha-MSH seems to affect man's behavior, not his learning. Inductive language in the paragraph is reflected in the question.

111. A Choice **A** is applied to humans in the last sentence of paragraph three. Choice **B** applies to frogs.

112. C The sixth sentence of paragraph three states that both ACTH 4-10 and alpha-MSH have been used with humans.

113. A The last paragraph only cites research studies done on hypophysectomized rats. No reports are given involving human beings.

Passage 20 - Biological Sciences

114. C Neither supported nor contradicted. The data in the table tell us only that a jump in cholesterol level occurred in all groups, not that, in addition, a particular cause (s) was responsible. The data presented in this table can only show the changes in cholesterol levels, not the reasons for these changes.

115. A Supported. Because Group 1's cholesterol level varies slowly and smoothly (at most 1 mg/100 ml per day for consecutive days shown) between 3/8 and 3/18, we can interpolate, using data for 3/11 and 3/14, to get the probable average cholesterol level for 3/13. On 3/11 the cholesterol level = 201, while on 3/14 it = 198. There are three days between 3/11 and 3/14, so the cholesterol level probably decreases about (201 - 198)/3 = 1 per day. Thus, the cholesterol level on 3/13 is approximately 201 - 2 = 199 mg/100 ml.)

116. C Neither supported nor contradicted. The table shows that the cholesterol levels fluctuate considerably with no particular pattern; so there is no reason to assume that any group's level will be near any particular value (including the average) at any particular time, unless measurements made around that time show levels around that value. In short, unless we know the level's value by having actually measured it, to put a probable value on it a situation has to exist, as in (115) above, where it can be interpolated. Sunday, 3/27, is more than a week after the last recorded value and so we have nothing to go by, i.e., we cannot interpolate it.

117. C Neither supported nor contradicted. The heavier people in this sample do have higher cholesterol levels, but there is insufficient evidence that their weights actually cause the higher cholesterol levels. The data in support of this statement are obscured because the higher levels might just as well be caused by age.

118. C Neither supported nor contradicted. Although it appears that the older people in this sample have higher cholesterol levels, we cannot conclude that the levels for any particular person will rise as s/he gets older. In order to prove this statement, a "longitudinal" study would be needed (several measurements on the same patient over a period of time) rather than a "snapshot" study (measurements on several patients all at one time) as we have here.

119. B Contradicted. For both the men and women in this study, the cholesterol levels go up steadily with age (this is seen most clearly by plotting cholesterol levels vs. age).

120. C Neither supported nor contradicted. The 50 - 70% range in a person's cholesterol ester level translates into a 103 - 144 mg/100 ml range in cholesterol level for Group 4 on 3/8. This is much too large a range to be described as "about 124 mg/100 ml," there is nothing to tell us that the real value is probably in the middle of this range.

121. 1, 3 Groups 1, 3 and 5 all had access to Bread Spread, but Group 5 may have chosen not to eat it; so Groups 1 and 3 might be useful in such a study.

122. 1, 4 Group 1 has the diet most drastically modified so as to reduce cholesterol. Group 2 diet was modified to increase cholesterol, so this is not a fair comparison; but Group 4 may be a good comparison. Groups 1 and 4 are also similar in age and weight.

123. B The question requires the use of the general knowledge that cholesterol levels may not change much in two weeks (March 4 - 18). Answer **A** is a possibility, but increasing sample size (and we have no idea of the original size) does not tend to increase the size of a small effect. Answers **C** and **D** are not linked to the question.

Passage 21 - Physical Sciences

This passage deals with fluid flow equations through thin tubes. It presents information on transport of drugs by pumps and requires fundamental problem solving activities in Physics. Concepts related to estimation, proportional reasoning and appraising the strength of experimental evidence are tested through various items.

124. C This question requires use of proportional reasoning and also definition of fluid velocity applied to flow through catheters. Velocity of a fluid = Flow Rate/Cross Sectional Area. In this case, the density of both liquids is the same. It would be easier to solve the problem in two parts, one for drug A_1 and one for drug B_1. Note: 1 = mL = 1 cm^3 approximately. Assume that 1 mg = 1 mL for both fluids.

Drug A_1	Drug B_1
D = Diameter = 0.2 cm	D = Diameter = 0.5 cm
$A_1 = A = \frac{\pi}{4}D^2 = \frac{\pi}{4}(.2)^2 = 0.03\ cm^2$	$A_2 = A = \text{Area} = \frac{\pi}{4}D^2 = \frac{\pi}{4}(.5) = .196$
Infusion discharge rate = 250 mg/min	Infusion discharge rate = 1000 mg/min
$\text{Velocity} = \frac{\text{Infusion rate}}{\text{Area}} = \frac{250}{0.03}$	$\text{Velocity} = \frac{\text{Infusion rate}}{\text{Area}} = \frac{1000}{0.196}$

Velocity ration = V_{A1}/V_{B1} = 8,333/5,000 ≅ 1.6

A quicker way would be to use proportional reasoning as

$$\frac{V_{A_1}}{V_{B_1}} = \frac{IR_{A_1}}{A_1} \cdot \frac{A_1}{IR_{B_1}}$$

$$= \frac{IR_{A_1}}{IR_{B_1}} \frac{(D_2)^2}{(D_1)^2}$$

$$= \frac{IR_{A_1}}{IR_{B_1}} \left(\frac{D_1}{D_2}\right)^2$$

$$= \frac{250}{1000}\left(\frac{0.5}{0.2}\right)^2 = \frac{250}{1000}\frac{(0.25)}{(0.04)} \cong 1.6$$

125. C This problem tests your deductive logic. Arrangement of information in a chronological form is the first step. To save time, draw a time line from 0 hours to 100 hours and study the concentration variations of A_1 and B_1. The total time elapsed between dosage 1 and the last dosage is 16 + 30 = 46 hours. Drug A_1 is administered at that point. B_1 takes 39 hours to fall down to 50% concentration, whereas A_1 takes only approximately 12 hours to fall to 50% concentration. Drug B_1 is given at the 16th hour. It will take 38 hours to drop B_1 concentration to 50% and another 38 hours to drop B_1 to almost zero. Hence, 16 + 38 + 38 = 92 hours are required (at least) before the effect of B_1 is gone. The second dosage is given after 16 hours from the first dosage, and 10 hours from that would be 10 + 16 = 26 hours. Drug A_1 takes 11.5 + 11.5 hours to drop to almost 0%. Ten hours after B_1 is given, the concentration of B_1 may have dropped by $\frac{10}{38}$ (50) ≅ 12%. Hence, at 26 hours the concentration of A_1 is almost zero, whereas B_1 is around 86%. The third dosage is given at 16 + 30 = 46 hours from the start. The 48th hour is only 2 hours from the start. The 48th hour is only 2 hours after the new dosage for A_1 has been given. Hence, A_1 cannot drop to even 50%. Choices **I** and **II** are correct but **III** is incorrect.

126. A This question tests correct use of equations to determine "clearance rate" and comparative reasoning to determine the difference in clearance rates.

Drug A_1	Drug B_1
$V_d = 20{,}000$ mL	$V_d = 40{,}000$ mL
$t_{1/2} = 11$ hrs - 40 mins = 700 min	$t_{1/2} = 38$ hrs = 2,280 min
$K_{A_1} = \frac{0.69}{t_{1/2}} = \frac{.69}{700}$	$K_{B_1} = \frac{0.69}{t_{1/2}} = \frac{.69}{2280}$
$V_{cl} = KV_d = \frac{.69\ (20{,}000)}{700}$	$V_{cl} = KV_d = \frac{.69\ (40{,}000)}{2280}$
= 19.7 L/min	= 12.1 L/min

The difference in the clearance rates is approximately 19.7 – 12.1 = 7.6 L/min.

127. B This question requires understanding of infusion rate and its relation to C_m. As shown in the passage, equation (a), S.I.R. is directly proportional to C_m. The clearance rate for drug A_1 was calculated earlier as 19.7 L/min. C_m can be found from the following equation,

$$C_m = \frac{\text{S.I.R.}}{V_{cl}} = \frac{250\ \text{mg/min}}{19.7\ \text{L/min}}$$
$$\cong 12.7\ \text{mg/L}$$

128. D This is a double negative question. The best way to solve such problems would be to find the scientifically supported claims, the "not" and the "except" cancel each other out. This question tests verbal reasoning skills **II (E)** and **III(A)**. Starting with choice **A**, the word only is incorrect, hence eliminate choice **A**. The time for medication A_1 to leave the bloodstream is *not* explicitly mentioned in the passage, but using a proportional model 2(11.5) ≅ 23 hours is approximately the time to clear A_1 through your bloodstream. Twenty-three hours is much faster than 38 hours to eliminate 50% of drug B_1. Hence, choice **B** is eliminated. The effectiveness of medication A_1 or B_1 was never brought up in the passage. Choice **D** is correct and it is the central idea of the experimental information. Both A_1 and B_1 are suitable; one is slower in responding than the other.

129. D This question checks your ability to sift through information and look for hidden assumptions. Assumption **I** is explained in the introductory paragraph and the writer justifies small pumps as better control instruments to deliver medication. Assumption **II** is harder to find in the paragraph. With velocities as high as 8,000 cm/min, a Reynold's number of 2000 is easy to achieve. Turbulent flow occurs at Reynold's number of 2000 or more, hence Assumption **II** is valid. Steady infusion rate is justified by equation (a) and the word "constant" in the third paragraph. All *three* assumptions are correct.

130. D This question is supposed to test your verbal and scientific reasoning by incorporating new information and arriving at conclusions as shown in verbal reasoning skills **IV(A)** and **IV(C)**. To avoid any verbal reading mishaps, answer the question looking for "true" options. The false options will become more apparent. Decreasing the diameter of a tube decreases the cross sectional area or flow area. From the continuity principle, when area decreases, the corresponding velocity increases. According to Bernoulli's equation, as velocity increases, the dynamic pressure drops. Hence option **I** and option **II** are correct. Option **III** presents a concept that the drug and the liquid mixture will separate. A liquid drug is a compound whereas the chemical components cannot be separated by a physical jam in the tube. Hence option **III** is incorrect or false.

Passage 22 - Biological Sciences

This passage explains the causes, diagnosis, and physiological effects of atrial fibrillation. It also explains various concepts connected with atrial flutter and ventricular fibrillation. It is an "information presentation" passage.

131. A This question is a direct inference from the second paragraph. It is a test of verbal comprehension (**I-D**). Atrial contractions at a rate faster than normal would cause excessive blood intake in the right atrium. This makes choice **A** correct. Upper chambers implying atria will not push or force wording the blood *out* to any location is ambiguous. Caffeine increases heart beat but cannot be related to pumping efficiency of the heart. The amount of caffeine is not mentioned in the passage. Defibrillation means to stop the fast beating of the atria. The answer is contradictory in choice **D**.

132. B This question tests comparative reasoning skills and distinguishes supported and unsupported information (**II-E**). Each of the statements has to be checked as a supporting claim for atrial flutter and ventricular fibrillation information according to the passage. Option **I** specifies 155 beats per minute for ventricular fibrillation that is *never* mentioned in the passage. Choice **I** is a correct response to the question. Option **II** explains digoxin and its usefulness to ventricular fibrillation/atrial flutter. *Useful* is a general term that makes option **II** correct and *except* makes it incorrect. Digoxin aids in stopping the fibrillation. Option **III** is not correct because of *except*. Options **I** and **II** are hence the correct options leading to **B** as the correct answer.

133. C This question brings new information in addition to the passage. It can be solved with the correct diagram of blood flow through the heart. As mentioned in the Flower's guide, the correct flow is identified from the right atrium to the right ventricle, then the left atrium, left ventricle, and finally the flow through the aorta.

134. A The test item stem should be read carefully and rephrased to make it easier. Careful reading of test items show which facts do *not* relate to atrial fibrillation (or in other words *do* relate to ventricular fibrillation). Verbal reasoning skills **III-A** and **III-D** are used in this question. Electric defibrillation is a quicker way to stop fibrillation and is used for ventricular fibrillation, which is extremely dangerous. Choice **A** is the correct response. Ventricular or atrial fibrillation cannot *be* prevented by using medications. The passage does stress that atrial fibrillation may be treated by digoxin and procainamide and is usually effective. In the second paragraph atrial fibrillation is symptomized by shortness of breath and exercise fatigue. The last paragraph explains that atria pump almost *no* blood during atrial fibrillation. The body does not receive enough blood during ventricular fibrillation.

135. D This question brings a new piece of information. Include that in the analysis. It involves an active search for each response in the passage. The sinoatrial node is introduced in the item paragraph. The refractory period of the cardiac muscle is *never* related to the force of contraction. Hence, **A** is incorrect. The $Na^+ - K^+$ pump does *not* cause the SA node force of contraction but it keeps the SA node actively working. Hence choice **B** is wrong. Stretching of the cardiac muscle is *not* correlated to atrial fibrillation. Knowledge is also being tested here, the student should understand the mechanics of stretching of the cardiac muscle. The force of contraction of the heart is supplied by ventricular contractions and, according to the Frank-Starling law, the excessive stretching of the ventricle may lead to less ventricular contraction. The ventricle is already so stretched, it cannot exert enough force on the blood during ventricular contraction.

136. C This question requires you to project your abilities beyond the passage. It is a multiple skill question focusing on how conclusions from the passage can be modified to coincide with additional information (**IV-C**). This question also integrates your physiological reasoning that involves synthesis of concepts that link the nervous and the circulatory system. Choice **A** is designed to check if you understand renal fluid volumes related to atrial fibrillation and then congestive heart failure. Define "Congestive heart failure" as symptoms leading to poor pumping by the heart. Cholesterol deposits may lead to less blood flow to the brain cells. Less oxygen than is required by the body is supplied by the blood pumped from the heart. Hence, choice **A** is not related to the congestive heart failure symptoms, less blood is pumped to various far-reaching parts. Hence choice **B** is incorrect. The kidneys and other organs retain blood and other fluids. The sympathetic part of the nerves has to increase the heart activity because of poor cardiovascular problems. The cardiac muscle strength is increased through the increased action of sympathetic nerves. The pericardium inflammation is related to drugs such as procainamide, but not to congestive heart failure. Hence, choice **C** is correct and choice **D** is false.

Appendix A

AN INTERPRETATION OF PASSAGES FROM AAMC PRACTICE TESTS AND MATERIALS*

A.1 INTRODUCTION

This research report presents an analytical summary of scientific content and strategies mentioned in AAMC MCAT practice tests and other materials, including the MCAT videotape.

You are provided a quick content analysis of *all* the physical and biological science passages found in MCAT materials. Science review and practice with AAMC materials will become more useful and efficient once you familiarize yourself with the science concepts related to these passages. The passages are also interpreted and classified using the author's experiences with students and faculty.

The importance of the MCAT passages related to developing good problem solving strategies is discussed in detail. It will help you to become a better passage analyst. Use this appendix during your review to make your MCAT preparation more structured and highly efficient. Interpretation of passage-based knowledge and data is required to monitor scientific problem-solving activities. The main purpose of this report is to guide you in using the practice materials from AAMC with a better understanding of the ways to interpret passages as you review science content and problem solving in your textbooks and lab reports.

A.2 AAMC PUBLICATIONS CURRENTLY AVAILABLE

AAMC has published four sets of practice materials for the new MCAT. This report is based on an analysis of the AAMC publications listed below. Details concerning new passages and their impact on the overall understanding of the MCAT format have been fully explained in section A.5. Publications are available from AAMC or Betz Publishing Company, Inc.

1. *MCAT Student Manual,* © 1993, with *Practice Test I* included .... 126 pages in manual
97 pages in test

2. *MCAT Practice Test II* (reprint of April 1991 exam), © 1991 .... 99 pages in test
MCAT Practice Items, © 1991. One booklet: Verbal Reasoning/Writing 81 pages
One booklet: Physical/Biological Sciences 111 pages

3. *Preparing for the MCAT,* © 1991. Video (VHS) .... 25 minutes

4. *MCAT Practice Test III,* © 1995. .... 134 pages in test

All practice tests and materials have been actually tested and used in previous MCATs given by AAMC. A brief introduction to each of these products is given here so that you can determine the ones most useful to you at various stages of your MCAT preparation.

The *MCAT Student Manual* and *Practice Test I* were published in November 1990 and reprinted in 1993. The *MCAT Student Manual* is an excellent starting point for MCAT study, giving detailed outlines and descriptions for the four subtests. The items in *Practice Test I* were actually tested during the experimental phase of the new MCAT. *Practice Test I* may be used as a "pretest" or diagnostic test in your review program. At this writing, there is no plan to produce a revision of this set in the foreseeable future.

Practice Test II is the full-length MCAT administered nation-wide in April 1991. It has been released to the public for a practice test. It is accompanied by *MCAT Practice Items*, two booklets containing many practice passages and items in all four subject areas of the exam. The *MCAT Practice Items* booklets should be used

* This statistical content interpretation of passages in physical and biological sciences was done by Aftab Hassan, Ph.D., MCAT Educational Researcher. All opinions are those of the researcher, and Betz Publishing Company, Inc. does *not* consider those views to be theirs in whole or in part.

during your review of course outlines, class notes, and your textbooks. *Practice Test II* should be used as a diagnostic instrument to assess your weaknesses.

Practice Test III was released by AAMC in February 1995. It is the most current and most valid instrument in the AAMC series. The practice test presents actual questions used for the MCAT in the past. Questions are classified as easy, moderate, and difficult; and graphs are presented so students can determine their weaknesses. This test should definitely be used as a "posttest" to determine your level of preparedness for the actual MCAT.

The MCAT video should be watched with a copy of the student manual at your side. Take quick notes because the video presents quite a few graphic illustrations of problem types and medical equipment covered on the test. The MCAT video presents all subtests of the MCAT. It gives you a quick overview of verbal reasoning strategies and writing sample strategies to be used during your review and practice sessions. The video does not present a comprehensive model for problem solving in biological or physical sciences. It clarifies the structure of the new MCAT passages, illustrating various types of passages and how to interpret information from them. The video is a good illustrative supplement to the *MCAT Student Manual.* The video and the manual are deficient in presenting a model for passage analysis or a model to learn mathematics concepts required for the science subtests. Summaries of parts of the video have been interpreted in the following sections. This will help you understand it better, and it will also help students who are unable to watch the video.

A.2.1 Problem Solving and Passage Interpretation According to the AAMC Video

Problem solving in sciences on the new MCAT is measured through the following techniques:

1. Passage interpretation, recall of concepts.
2. Comprehension with emphasis on determining probable causes and evaluating design.
3. Interpretation of data.
4. Application of science concepts to various problems.
5. Evaluation of arguments and information provided.

The general methods for data presentation on the MCAT include tables, charts, graphs, and diagrams of instruments. These usually can be observed in laboratory exercises, laboratory work plans and analysis, and literature from medical technology companies. The video also suggests that in order to find more passages and to help you with problem solving, you should do the following:

(a) Talk to instructors and ask them questions.
(b) Read selected parts of basic science textbooks.
(c) Read scientific journals and learn how to interpret graphs.
(d) Perform work in laboratories that includes research, planning, and analysis of experiments in physical and biological sciences.

A.2.2 Experimental and Medical Equipment According to the AAMC Video

- Pressure gauges, manometers, pressure transducers
- CATSCAN machine, Dynamic Spatial Reconstruction (DSR) machine
- X-rays used in graphic analysis as obtained in radiology with lighted background
- Human skeleton (3D) model, heart model, advanced microscopes
- Surgery room equipment—overhead flood lights, blood pressure monitors, EEG/EKG monitors, pulse rate monitors
- Small flashlight used by nurse to check a baby's eye in pediatrics
- Electron microscope used in neurosurgery
- Dissection tools for use during surgery
- Chemistry laboratory equipment—including volume measuring flasks, cylinders, etc.
- Instruments as used in chemical separations and purifications laboratory—showing complex network of distillation, pressure measuring devices

ASK YOURSELF—TIP FOR THE MCAT:

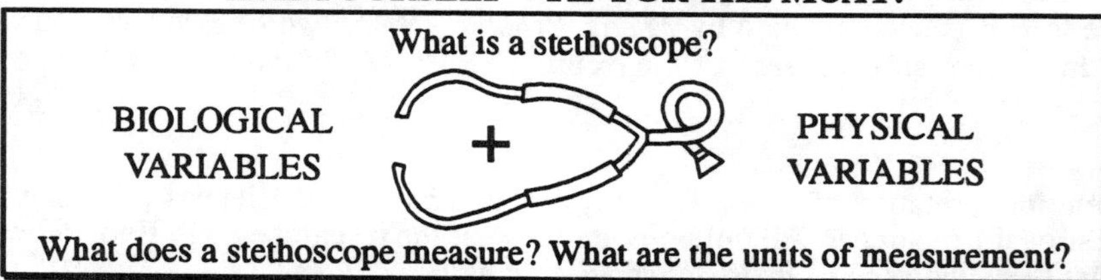

A.2.3 Writing Sample According to the AAMC Video

You are given a claim with more than one interpretation-—it could be a statement of opinion, philosophy, or policy. You are supposed to write a first-draft composition that addresses and completes the following tasks:

1. Develop a central idea
2. Synthesize concepts and ideas
3. Present ideas cohesively and logically
4. Write clearly (syntax, grammar, and punctuation)

Your evaluation will be based on the following, using the designations shown in Roman numerals here:

I. Explain or interpret the statement (not factually supported)
II. Concrete example to judge if statement is contradictory
III. Resolve the conflict (compare judgmental value of statement)

Evaluation of I, II, and III will determine your MCAT score. The depth, clarity, and precision presented in I, II, and III will be measured.

Scoring Sheet

J	K	L	M	N	O	P	Q	R	S	T
0–1	2–3	...	...	...	...	...	...	94–95	96–97	98–99

Percentile Ranks

A.2.4 Verbal Reasoning Strategies According to the AAMC Video

The MCAT video proposes three basic strategies to improve verbal reasoning:

Strategy 1. Skim the passage, including reading the first paragraph and then the first sentence of each paragraph. Some paragraphs may be incomplete (they may be excerpts from the original publication). This should take about 30 seconds.

Strategy 2. Read the statements of all questions or test items quickly and check to see if they relate to the passage you skimmed earlier. This should take between 30 and 45 seconds.

Strategy 3. Take about 2 to 3 minutes to read each passage (using underlining or marking) with reference to each test item. This gives you more focus on where and how to find answers to each test item.

In order to understand each passage really well, use the following techniques:

(a) Each passage presents a written discourse or argument; the writer mentioned at the bottom of each passage takes a position to persuade the reader. The reader should uncover that argument.

(b) Verbal reasoning skills include your learning of argument development, argument types. These are usually taught in undergraduate logic and philosophy courses. Study course outlines for various classes being offered on your campus.

A.3 WHAT IS AN MCAT SCIENTIFIC PASSAGE?

A scientific passage represents a written description of a medically related situation. The MCAT scientific passages describe the situation in a few short narrative paragraphs and are supplemented with or without data. The data appear in one of the following forms: diagrams, charts, tables, or laboratory graphs. A careful review of the AAMC practice materials reveals that each passage serves as a brief exposure to fairly advanced medical problems. It serves only as a linkage device or a mental bridge to connect various undergraduate courses to the medical field. The questions following each passage *cannot* and *should not* be answered using the information in the passage alone. The passage may touch upon advanced medical concepts only tangentially, and the questions following the passage are either partially or totally unrelated to the advanced concepts. Students should not look for answers in the passage.

To understand the nature of MCAT science passages look at each passage as a source of current, advanced medical concepts (instruments used in medicine, experimental methods used in medicine, applications of medical technology, difficult medical terminology). Each passage is an excerpt or a small unit of medically related information. Each passage is *not* complete as provided. Information contained within each passage is rarely sufficient to answer questions following it. More information is sometimes provided in the questions, which should be integrated with the passage before answering the question.

As suggested by AAMC's *MCAT Student Manual* and the MCAT video presentation, scientific passages are fairly easy to find, starting with your college textbooks, laboratory manuals, and workbooks. For your own skills development, we advise you to select long and difficult paragraphs from textbook chapters not studied in class. These provide you with the basic training to relate to passages and also acquaint you with unfamiliar topics and concepts. More extensive training in passage reading and analysis should be done at the library. Look for encyclopedias, scientific journals, and magazines. Literature sources, including catalogs from medical technology organizations, pharmaceutical manufacturers, hospital equipment and research companies also include medical passages of a type to be found on the MCAT.

A.3.1 Understanding the Nature of MCAT Scientific Passages

Physical and Biological Sciences subtests on the new MCAT are each composed of three basic testing elements:

i. ten or eleven passages (about 250 words each), made up of approximately 2500 to 2700 total words with supporting graphical information.
ii. a total of 62 test items with four responses each (multiple-choice), including new information in the form of graphs, diagrams, or statements.
iii. a total of 15 independent questions or science problems with four responses each (multiple-choice), including new information in the form of graphs, diagrams, or statements.

On the actual testing day, you are required to do the reading and problem solving of these three elements (and mark your answers on the answer sheet) within 100 minutes. Given an average of 1 minute per test item would take 77 minutes of your time for elements (ii) and (iii). This leaves you with approximately 23 minutes to read and understand 10 or 11 passages. Each passage and the information related to the passage have to be fully understood in approximately 2 minutes. It is important for you to understand the nature of each passage before answering the questions following it. In order to capture the gist of the passage and be ready to use the information given in the passage, the following tips will help you:

1. Learn to classify the passage by format (there are four formats mentioned in the *MCAT Student Manual).*

2. Learn to classify the subject matter of the passage as biology, inorganic or general chemistry, organic chemistry, physics, or a mixture of various subjects.

3. Learn to classify the key words and medical vocabulary to associate with MCAT concepts. e.g., DNA virus, genetic engineering, thermoneutral zone, radioactive DNA label, anomers, bone stress and strain, microphysiology, Doppler stethoscopes, mutant viral inhibitors.

4. Learn to classify arguments or statements in the passage by basic scientific reasoning and problem-solving skills such as hypothesis–conclusion, analysis of a complex chart, evaluating design and methods presented, and cause–effect analysis.

5. Learn to classify the passage, based on your medical experiences collected through hospital visits, emergency room visits, reviewing medical literature, talking with friends or relatives with medical problems, discussing topics with your physician or dentist, and other relevant experiences. This helps you find medical applications or look for medical clues in the passage. These medical experiences can be broken down into:

   i. observing medical instrumentation.
   ii. observing and evaluating medical experimentation.
   iii. observing and evaluating clinical methods or procedures.
   iv. classifying medical descriptions in physiology, microbiology, biochemistry, molecular biology, histology, or immunology.

6. Learn to classify the passage as it relates to each question—using associative reasoning to link various parts of the passage to various questions. This step is the most difficult and most efficient in solving the problems given in each passage.

A.3.2 Frequency Analyses of Passage Content (AAMC Practice Materials)

For research purposes, this analysis of the physical and biological sciences passages is based on a solitary reading of the passages. The solitary reading lets you divorce passages from the questions and provides the opportunity to see how the words and charts in each passage impact the reader. Most key words, concepts, and medical applications of each passage were considered in this analysis. The questions were *not* seen, read, or used in any other way to bias the analysis. This chart will show you how the practice tests (approximately 7) and materials provided by AAMC relate to the *MCAT Student Manual* course outlines. This analysis shows you the selective topics that were presented and discussed in the passages. There were 69 passages in physical sciences and 71 passages in biological sciences that were analyzed. Frequency analyses were completed for all topics presented in the AAMC practice materials.

It was found that some topics appeared more frequently than some others; e.g., phase and phase equilibria. It was also noticed that in physical sciences the physics and general chemistry tested in each passage included one concept or topic from each subject. The passages included quite a few instrumental designs and workings. By contrast, in the biological sciences the biology and organic chemistry tested in each passage sometimes included four to five concepts or topics from biology with only one concept in organic chemistry. The test items were more intense and more concepts were mixed within biology than in traditional organic chemistry. The biological sciences passages included quite a few descriptions of experimental projects or research projects with multiple experiments (two or three experiments) in each passage.

The topical frequency analyses demonstrated that the passage-selectors and test-makers had inherent bias in their selections. The *MCAT Student Manual* does mention that medically important materials will be tested. The passage frequency analysis indicates that medically related content is selected more often than traditional undergraduate topics. Students should realize that the MCAT linkage to medicine is quite apparent in the new test format. The passages do test your skills in orientation to medical knowledge, familiarity with current medical practices and medical terminology and, above all, your problem-solving abilities as a medical novice. The idea is to see how a newcomer in medical school will apply current knowledge of biology, chemistry, and physics in solving problems. Advanced medical school courses such as biochemistry, microbiology, and human physiology are used to construct some questions.

A.3.2.1 Passage Format and Types (*MCAT Student Manual* and Practice Tests)

According to the *MCAT Student Manual,* four types of passages are used in the physical and biological sciences subtests on the MCAT. They are as follows:

1. Information-presentation passages:
   - a. Source: Textbook or journal articles
   - b. Structure: Assume background knowledge
     - + New information
     - + New *uses* of basic information
   - c. Skills tested: Comprehension, application
2. Problem-solving passages:
   - a. Source: Chemistry or physics situations (descriptive) from traditional science textbooks
   - b. Structure: Probable causes of situations
     - + Events
     - + Phenomena
     - + Problem-solving methods
   - c. Skills tested: Determining probable causes using scientific theories, selecting appropriate methods to solve
3. Research-study passages:
   - a. Source: Research studies (microbiology, histology, genetics research studies, or lab reports)
   - b. Structure: Background rationale (whole or part)
     - + Research methods
     - + Research study results
     - + Understanding of underlying research
   - c. Skills tested: Understanding experimental designs and methods, evaluating methods relating to conclusions of the experiment

4. Persuasive-argument passages:

a. Source: Newspaper articles, *Scientific American* magazine/*Discover* magazine, dialogue between scientists in a meeting or conference

b. Structure: Checking for validity of persuasive arguments
+ Looking at pieces of evidence
+ Understanding methodologies
+ Interpreting particular perspectives on biochemical/biomedical products

c. Skills tested: Comprehending arguments, convincing the reader that particular conclusions from arguments are correct, specific methods or evidence are appropriate to evaluate the validity of the arguments

A.3.2.2 Passage-Related Comments According to AAMC

In addition to the four passage types, the *MCAT Student Manual* describes the passages in other ways, including:

- reading selections from the social and natural sciences and the humanities (Verbal Reasoning Test),
- brief informational passages (Physical and Biological Sciences subtests),
  -- passages may include data presented in graphs, tables, or figures, and some of the questions related to these passages may require you to interpret the data,
- although passages may discuss advanced-level topics, the questions accompanying the passages will not require knowledge of these topics.

A.3.2.3 Scientific Content-Related Comments According to AAMC

Another set of comments on the content of the physical sciences and biological sciences subtest as noted from the *MCAT Student Manual* is:

Because the content outline focuses primarily on areas necessary to preparing for the study of medicine, it may differ in several important ways from the content of your introductory courses:

1. Some topics, which are important to the discipline as a whole and normally covered in undergraduate courses, have been omitted from the MCAT because they are not as relevant to the study of medicine as are the topics included.
2. The organization of the topics in the outline may differ from that of the topics presented in your courses.
3. Some of the topics included in the outline may not have been emphasized in your school's introductory undergraduate courses.

Following is a complete list of all topics for physical and biological sciences as given in the AAMC *MCAT Student Manual* :

Physical Sciences

I. Stoichiometry
II. Electronic Structure and the Periodic Table
III. Bonding
IV. Phases and Phase Equilibria
V. Solution Chemistry
VI. Acids and Bases
VII. Thermodynamics and Thermochemistry
VIII. Rate Processes in Chemical Reactions: Kinetics and Equilibrium
IX. Electrochemistry
X. Translational Motion
XI. Force and Motion, Gravitation
XII. Equilibrium and Momentum
XIII. Work and Energy
XIV. Wave Characteristics and Periodic Motion
XV. Sound
XVI. Fluids and Solids
XVII. Electrostatics and Electromagnetism
XVIII. Electric Circuits
XIX. Light and Geometrical Optics
XX. Atomic and Nuclear Structure

Biological Sciences

I. Molecular Biology
II. Microbiology
III. Generalized Eukaryotic Cell
IV. Specialized Eukaryotic Cells and Tissues
V. Nervous and Endocrine Systems
VI. Circulatory, Lymphatic, and Immune Systems
VII. Digestive and Excretory Systems
VIII. Muscle and Skeletal Systems
IX. Respiratory and Skin Systems
X. Reproductive System and Development
XI. Genetics and Evolution
XII. Biological Molecules
XIII. Oxygen-containing Compounds
XIV. Amines
XV. Hydrocarbons
XVI. Molecular Structure of Organic Compounds
XVII. Separations and Purifications
XVIII. Use of Spectroscopy in Structural Identification

A.3.2.4 Total Number of AAMC Items and Passages

The following chart provides the total number of passages and items in *all* AAMC publications released through June 1995.

AAMC Guidelines		**6–10 items per passage**	**4–8 items per passage**		**4–8 items per passage**
Solved Problems	**Name of Publication**	**Verbal Reasoning**	**Physical Sciences**	**Writing Sample**	**Biological Sciences**
Solved/ answer	MSM	P = 4 I = 28 I/P = 7	P = 7 I = 26 I/P = 3.7	T = 2 R = 4	P = 6 I = 28 I/P = 4.7
NS/answer	MPT I	P = 9 I = 65 I/P = 7.2	P = 10 I = 62 I/P = 6.2	T = 2 R = 0	P = 10 I = 62 I/P = 6.2
NS/answer	MPT II	P = 9 I = 65 I/P = 7.2	P = 11 I = 62 I/P = 5.6	T = 2 R = 0	P = 11 I = 62 I/P = 5.6
NS/answer	MPT III	P = 9 I = 65 I/P = 7.2	P = 11 I = 62 I/P = 5.6	T = 2 R = 12*	P = 11 I = 62 I/P = 5.6
NS/answer	MPI	P = 31 I = 263 I/P = 8.5	P = 30 I = 199 I/P = 6.6	T = 2 R = 0	P = 33 I = 223 I/P = 6.8
Total number of passages and items released in all AAMC publications		P = 62 I = 486 I/P = 7.8	P = 69 I = 411 I/P = 6.0	T = 0 R = 16	P = 71 I = 437 I/P = 6.2

Index and Comments to Table on AAMC Items and Passages

- P = Passages
- I = Items
- T = Topics
- R = Sample responses from students

- Total Independent Questions: (from all publications) 51 in physical sciences; 52 in biological sciences
- Number of tests:
  - Verbal Reasoning: 6.9 tests
  - Physical Sciences: 6.2 to 6.9 tests (based on 10 or 11 passages)
  - Writing Sample: 4 tests
  - Biological Sciences: 6.5 to 7.1 tests (based on 10 or 11 passages)

- It was observed that independent questions are given in three places within each of the subtests provided. On the average, four passages and items are given first, then independent questions, then four more passages and items followed with independent questions, etc., as follows:

  4 passages, 5 independent questions; 4 passages, 5 independent questions; 3 passages, 5 independent questions (one possible arrangement).

- **Solved/answer:** the number of problems and items with answers given and explanatory solutions provided
- **NS/answer:** the number of problems and items in which answers are given but no explanatory solutions provided
- **Name of publication:**
  - MSM = *MCAT Student Manual* (AAMC)
  - MPT I = *MCAT Practice Test I* (AAMC)
  - MPT II = *MCAT Practice Test II* (AAMC)
  - MPT III = *MCAT Practice Test III* (AAMC)
  - MPI = *MCAT Practice Items* (AAMC)

* 12 responses include 6 essays for MPT III and 6 essays on the other topics.

A.4 FUNCTIONAL CLASSIFICATION OF AAMC SCIENCE PASSAGES

The science content and current technical information presented in each passage provide a better functional classification of each passage. The functional classification will help you link various passages to textbooks, journals, manuals, or laboratory research reports. Following is a list with interpretation of each functional class:

i. **DESC** refers to "descriptive." These passages are basic information passages describing a scientific process, including instruments, in a narrative style.

ii. **GR.DESC** refers to "graphic description." These passages usually have a brief narrative accompanied with charts, tables, line graphs from experimental/theoretical studies, diagrams showing a part of a process or system, or a set of equations or a cycle in biology or chemistry. **GR.EXPT** refers to graphical and experimental data.

iii. **EXPT** refers to "experimental." These passages include one or more experiments carried out to compare various laboratory results by changing a variable or function in a process. Some experimental passages present unusual research experiments to verify one or more hypotheses in biology or physiology.

iv. **INST** refers to "instrumental." These passages describe a piece of equipment, a laboratory machine, or a household appliance, and usually describe the working, design, and operational pros and cons of the instrument. Some instruments are used in biophysics labs or biochemical labs, and one reason for using them on the MCAT is to check a student's evaluation skills and mechanical ability. Some instruments discussed in passages are used only in medical diagnosis and research. **MED.INSTR** refers to "medical instrument."

v. **DEVI** refers to a "device." These passages usually illustrate a nonconventional laboratory device created by a scientist to check a concept or to verify a theory. A device is different from medical machines or instruments. Most devices are laboratory tools or simple mechanisms created to manually demonstrate a principle in science.

Tables I through IV illustrate comparisons between the "AAMC classification of passages" and the "functional classification of passages." Charts A and B provide a systematic breakdown of *all* physical and biological sciences passages. All AAMC publications were included in this analysis.

AAMC CLASSIFICATION COMPARED TO FUNCTIONAL CLASSIFICATION

Table I: Physical Sciences (69 Passages)

	DESC.	GR. DESC	INST.	LAB DEV.	EXPT.	MED. INST.	GR. EXPT.	Only Sketches
Information Passages (18)	12	3	3	—	—	—	—	—
Problem Solving Passages (19)	2	4	6	1	6	—	—	—
Research Study Passages (19)	—	2	4	1	11	—	1	—
Persuasive Argument Passages (13)	10	1	—	—	1	1	—	—
TOTAL = 69	24	10	13	2	18	1	1	0

Table II: Biological Sciences (71 Passages)

	DESC.	GR. DESC	INST.	LAB DEV.	EXPT.	MED. INST.	GR. EXPT.	Only Sketches
Information Passages (19)	17	2	—	—	—	—	—	—
Problem-Solving Passages (19)	5	8	—	—	4	—	1	1
Research Study Passages (22)	1	2	—	1	18	—	—	—
Persuasive Argument Passages (11)	7	2	—	—	2	—	—	—
TOTAL = 71	30	14	0	1	24	0	1	1

AAMC CLASSIFICATION COMPARED TO FUNCTIONAL CLASSIFICATION

Table III: Combined MCAT Sciences (140 Passages)

Passage Types	DESC	GR. DESC	INST.	LAB DEV	EXPT	MED. INST	GR. EXPT	Only Sketches	TOTAL
Information Passages (27%)	29	5	3	0	0	0	0	0	37
Problem Solving Passages (27%)	7	12	6	1	10	0	1	1	38
Research Study Passages (29%)	1	4	4	2	29	0	1	0	41
Persuasive Argument Passages (17%)	17	3	0	0	3	1	0	0	24
TOTAL	54	24	13	3	42	1	2	1	140
Total	**39%**	**17%**	**9%**	**2%**	**30%**	**1%**	**1%**	**1%**	**= 100%**

Table IV(A): Summary of Total Percentages (Tables I, II, and III)

Physical Sciences — AAMC Breakdown		Biological Sciences — AAMC Breakdown	
• Information passages	26%	• Information passages	27%
• Problem-Solving passages	28%	• Problem-Solving passages	27%
• Persuasive Argument passages	19%	• Persuasive Argument passages	15%
• Research Study passages	27%	• Research Study passages	31%

Table IV(B): Summary of Total Percentages (Tables I, II, and III)

Physical Sciences — Functional Breakdown		Biological Sciences — Functional Breakdown	
• Descriptive (narrative)	35%	• Descriptive (narrative)	43%
• Descriptive and graphs (line)	15%	• Descriptive and graphs (line)	20%
• Instrument design and function	19%	• Instrument design and function	0%
• Laboratory device	3%	• Laboratory device	1%
• Experimental (multiple)	26%	• Experimental (multiple)	34%
• Medical Instrumentation design and function	1%	• Medical Instrumentation design and function	0%
• Experiments and graphs (line)	1%	• Experiments and graphs (line)	1%
• Sketches and figures (no description)	0%	• Sketches and figures (no description)	1%
Note: According to the percentage breakdown, the functional classification of passages does show a better correlation to materials found in textbooks, course outlines, and research publications.			

IMPORTANT FOR ALL MCAT STUDENTS:

In Physical Sciences, work *more* on understanding graphs drawn in physics and chemistry labs; design and operation of laboratory equipment as it applies to physics and general chemistry concepts. Understand and review lab experiments.	In Biological Sciences, read and analyze *more* research articles in journals on biology, organic and molecular biochemistry, physiology; understand how several variables are shown in tables and graphs to accept and reject research hypotheses.

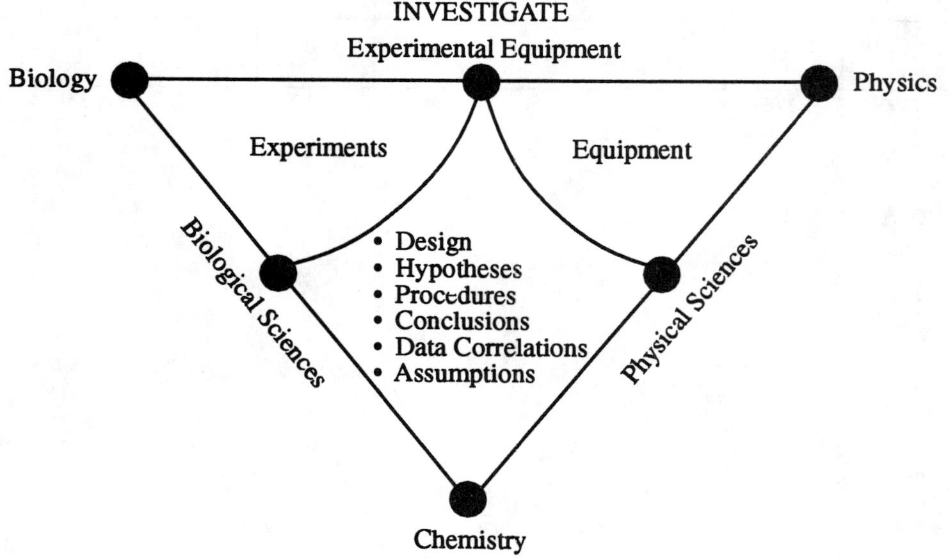

CHART A **PHYSICAL SCIENCES** **CHART A**

Information Passages (26%)

AAMC Topic		
XX.D	α, β, γ radioactive decay	(DESC)
IV.C	Physical/chemical allotropes of sulfur	(DESC)
IV.C	Phases of water, BP & FP, density	(DESC)
XI.E, F	Dynamic forces on projectiles	(DESC)
XX.D	Excited states/energy levels of electrons	(DESC)
XVII.B	EM waves, fields, antenna, $E = hf$	(DESC)
IX.A	Electrochemistry, ligands, trans. elements	(DESC)
VII.A, XVIII.C	Water-heater circuit diagram, calorimeter	(INST)
XVI.A	Aerofoil design, fuel, wings, lift, drag	(DESC)
X.F, XI.E	Projectile motion, Coriolis force, 2 projectiles	(DESC)
III.B	Molecular formulas & bonds for acids and bases	(DESC)
III.B, IV.B	Water molecules, bonds, amphoteric compounds	(DESC)
V.A, IX.A	Solvent extraction of quinine, Pb^{+2}, Zn^{+2} separation	(GR.DESC)
XVI.A, XVIII.B	Lub. oil tank design with electric heaters, drain plug	(INST)
XII.A, XIII	Exercise bike design, base metabolic rate	(INST)

Research Study Passages (27%)

AAMC Topic		
XIX.B,C; XVII.A	Retroreflecting arrays, pinhole beam splitter	(INST)
VII.A	Exothermic reactions (three experiments)	(EXPT)
VII.A, XVIII.C	Water heater, immersion type, Ohm's law, calorimeter	(INST)
XIII.C, D; XIV.B, XVII.B	Spring stiffness, oscillations, mag. potential energy	(EXPT)
XVI.A	H_2O + glycerine flow in pipe, viscosity, density	(EXPT)
X.E,F; XIII.D	Tennis balls, rebound height, microphone, projectiles	(EXPT)
XIV.B, XVII.B	Mag. dipole moment, harmonic oscillator, 2 magnets	(EXPT)
VIII.B, D, G; V.B	Esterification, equilibrium shift, molar ratio	(GR.DESC)
IV.A	Mol. wt of 2 unknown gases, effusion, vac. pump	(GR.INST)
V.B, IV.B	Vol., temperature & solubility of KNO_3 data table	(EXPT)
IV.B, C	Four reactions with alum, crystal prep. temperature	(EXPT)
IV.A	Measuring gas constant R with chemical reaction	(DEVI)
VI.A, B; V.B	Adsorption of dye by eggs, vinegar, pH, 3 expts.	(GR.EXPT)
XVI.A, V.B	Gasoline separation, glass fibers, select. adsorption	(INST)
I.H, III.B	$CaCO_3$ decomposition chemistry, 4 experiments	(EXPT)
V.B	Solubility products & properties of nitrates, Pb^{+2}	(EXPT)

Problem Solving Passages (28%)

AAMC Topic		
XVII.B, XIII	Electromagnetic railgun	(INST)
XVI.A	Open liquid tank with three spheres/floats	(INST)
VIII.D, G	Activation energy, reactants/products	(EXPT)
VI.B, IV.A	Titrations, gas laws, reactions	(INST)
XI.E, XX.E	Fluorescent lamp, electron acceleration	(INST)
XI.F, G	Dynamics on inclined plane with friction	(DEVI)
XVI.A, XV.B, D	Doppler stethoscopes, ultrasound imaging of organs	(MED.INST)
XII.B, XIV.B	Pendula in series, colliding pendula, elas./plas.	(EXPT)
VII.A, VI.A	Styrofoam calorimeter, acid–base reactions	(EXPT)
VII.A, IX.A	ΔG equations, constants, electrochemical reactions	(DESC)
VII.B	Steam engine, refrigerator working & efficiency	(GR.DESC)
XVIII.C, E; XVII.A	IC, silicon wafer, plasma etcher, electric field	(GR.DESC)
IV.A	Two methods to find N_2 density in laboratory	(EXPT)
XIV.B	Simple pendulum characteristics, $T = K\sqrt{\frac{L}{g}}$	(EXPT)
XVI.A	Raft design to travel in a river	(DESC)

Persuasive Argument Passages (19%)

AAMC Topic		
VI.B, I.H	Ammonia titration and preparation methods	(EXPT)
V.A, B; I.H, III.B	Soaps, hardness of H_2O and its removal	(DESC)
XX.C	Natural nuclear reactor, fission reactions	(DESC)
VI.A, III.B, V.B	Rainwater acidity, pH < 4, etc.	(DESC)
XV.A, D; XVI.A	Ultrasonic diagnosis, Doppler blood velocity	(MED.INST)
XIX.C, D	Hubble telescope, optical detectors, mirror	(DESC)
XII.A, B; XIII.F	Seatbelts, collision design, airbags, safety	(DESC)
XVIII.B, XIV.A, XVII.B	Circuit breaker design, EM waves	(DESC)
XI.E, XIII.F, XIX.C	Space stations in orbit, solar cells, biological needs	(DESC)
VI.A, V.B	Buffered solutions, pH – pK_a equations, blood buffer	(DESC)
VIII.B, D, E	Reaction pathways, two chemists' analysis	(DESC)
VIII.E, I.H, II.B	$O_3 \rightarrow O_2$ reactions, 5 series of reactions	(GR.DESC)

CHART B

BIOLOGICAL SCIENCES

CHART B

Information Passages (27%)

AAMC Topic		
IV.C, I.B, VI.A	Oxyhemoglobin/PO_2 graphs, ligands, genetics	(GR.DESC)
XIII.A, D	Bimolecular rate constants, nucleophiles, S_N2	(DESC)
VI.A, IX.A	Carbaminohemoglobin, haldane, respiration (ext/int)	(DESC)
X.A, C; XI.A	Ectopic pregnancy, HCG, tubal pregnancy	(DESC)
IX.B, XI.B	Human sweating, salt regulation, other species	(DESC)
I.B, XI.A	Mol. genetics of inherited human vision, red/green	(DESC)
XII.A, III.D	Signal peptides, signal recog. particle, ER/SPR	(DESC)
VI.C, II.A, I.B	Antigenic shifts on virulence, influenza	(DESC)
II.A,B; IV.B, VIII.A	Tetanus infection, spore germination	(DESC)
II.A, B, C; I.B, XII.A	African sleeping sickness, various surf glycoproteins	(DESC)
XI.B, I.B, III.D, E	Cystic fibrosis, molecular hybrids, DNA/RNA test	(DESC)
III.C, VI.A, IV.B	Hypovolemic shock, hemorrhage, Na^+/K^+ pump	(DESC)
VIII.B, III.D	Stress/strain in bones, bone fracture, osteoblasts	(DESC)
VII.A, B; XII.A	Rabbits, cows, cecum, rumen, omasum, digest	(DESC)
VIII.A, IV.B	Vertebrate smooth muscle (unitary or multi unit)	(DESC)
II.A, I.B	Vaccinia, AIDS virus, virus fighting infection	(DESC)
III.D, E; III.C	Mitotic spindle, kinetochore microtubules, etc.	(GR.DESC)

Research Study Passages (31%)

III.C, IV.B, VI.A	Na^+ pump, erythrocytes bathing, ATP	(EXPT)
I.A, XII.B	Photosynthesis cycle, Calvin cycle, biochem reaction	(GR.DESC)
II.A	Bacteriology of aerobic genus implants, stains	(EXPT)
I.A, X.A, V.C	Nonshivering thermogenesis, pineal gland, reproduc.	(EXPT)
XIII.A,B,C,F;XVII.D	Soluble/insoluble organic compounds, complex charts	(GR.DESC)
VIII.B, V.C	Osteoclasts, PTH binding, Ca^{++}, UV light, calcitonin	(EXPT)
X.A, I.B, XI.A	RNA/radioact. protein, haploid cells, fungus mutation	(EXPT)
II.A, I.B, III.E	Ames test for mutagens/carcinogens in air	(EXPT)
XVIII.B,A; XVII.A,C	Antifungal chemical, separations 10 steps	(EXPT)
XIII.D, XII.C	Iodonium ion, unsaturated fats, three-step study	(EXPT)
XVII.B, XII.A	Protein separation by gel and ion-exchange chromatog	(EXPT)
XIII.D, A; XIV.C	Expt. alkyl halides produced from alcohols	(EXPT)
I.B,XII.A	Guanosine, adenosine, synthesis to produce compound	(EXPT)
II.A, VI.A, C	Potomac horse fever, rickettsias, blood serum study	(EXPT)
I.B, II.A	DNA repair using bacteriophage assay, lab data	(EXPT)
XV.B, XVI.C	Butene isomers, reaction mechanisms and kinetics	(EXPT)
XVIII.A, XVII.A	^{1}HNMR and IR spectra and separation experiments	(EXPT)

Problem Solving Passages (27%)

AAMC Topic		
XV.B, XVI.C	Conjugated dienes, electrophilic addition	(DESC)
I.A, XII.A	Proposed catalytic hydrolysis steps, chymotrypsin	(7 Figs.)
VI.A, IV.B, III.D	Basophilic/acidophilic cardiac muscle cells	(DESC)
I.A, II.A, XII.C	Biokinetic microbial activity in sludge	(GR.DESC)
III.C, VII.B	Vasopressin, osmolarity, ADH, plasma, kidneys	(DESC)
I.A, V.C	Alcohol dehydrogenase, drinking, Krebs cycle	(DESC)
XII.A, B, C; I.B	Biotin, biotinidase deficiency, biotin cycle	(GR.DESC)
II.A, I.B	λ bacteriophage, lytic, lysogenic, excision	(GR.DESC)
VI.C, V.C	Radioimmunoassay graph, assayed antigen, radio-label	(GR.DESC)
II.A, XII.B	Complex graphs, growth kinetics of bacteria, lactose	(GR.EXPT)
X.C, II.B, I.B	Binary fission reproduction, co-stimulation, buffer	(EXPT)
I.A, XII.A	Angiotensinogen, pK_a, histidine, ACE enzyme	(GR.DESC)
XVII.A, D; XVI.C	Albuterol synthesis in lab, asthma, org. properties	(EXPT)
XII.B, XIII.B	Hydrolysis of glycosides, temperature-rate table	(EXPT)
III.C, X.C	How bird eggs breathe, chorioallantois, diffusion	(DESC)
IX.B, VI.A	Oxygen consumption/temperature in various animals	(GR.DESC)
XI.A, B; IV.A; V.A	Synaptic transmission of nerve impulse, synapsin	(GR.DESC)
XII.A, I.A, X.A	ACTH, reprod enzyme chart, adrenocortical hyperplasias	(GR.DESC)

Persuasive Argument Passages (15%)

VI.C, II.A, I.B	AIDS, AZT, T-lymphocytes, cancer cells	(DESC)
XVI.C, XVIII.A	React. mechanisms, organic, IR spectra, kinetics	(EXPT)
VI.C, XI.A	Factor VIII, hemophilia, genetic linkage	(DESC)
III.C, D; II.A	Crawling cells, force mechanism types	(DESC)
IV.B, VIII.B	Ca^{++} in contraction of smooth muscle, myosin, MLCK	(DESC)
XIII.D, A; XIV.C	Alklyation of carbanion, 3 products, BuLi/KH	(EXPT)
XIII.C, XII.C	Phosphoglycerides, esters, properties and structure	(DESC)

A.5 OBSERVATIONS AND CONCLUSIONS CONCERNING SCIENTIFIC PASSAGES

1. The charts and tables shown in the previous section indicate that in addition to descriptive passages (with and without graphs or tables), experimental research, instrument design and operation, and laboratory devices are *more* significant in testing sciences on the current MCAT.
2. All "instrumental" passages include a schematic diagram to show working of instrument/machine and also a paragraph describing the working of the instrument/machine. (Most instruments are not labeled to show parts; also simple experiments with instruments are sometimes used.)
3. All "experimental" passages with multiple experiments are written to develop a general understanding of an existing or new research hypothesis, and data tables or continuous line graphs are given to illustrate observed values. Formulas or equations used may also be stated. The test items test the validity and application of a hypothesis to form conclusions.
4. Test items with functional graphs (such as P.E./disp. graph, viscosity vs. temperature, speed vs. mass) are to test the student's ability to decipher the underlying functional relationship or to draw various functions and provide their graphical interpretation (activation energy, etc.).
5. All "procedural" passages include a set of logical statements written in a compact style with some mix of textbook knowledge and some methodologies. These fall into the "Persuasive Argument" type of passages.
6. Some instrumental or experimental passages are designed to include "nontraditional" comparisons between experimental variables, instrument design and working, and hypothetical analysis of two or more similar instruments. Sometimes these passages are used to test problem-solving abilities of the student.
7. Some functional charts shown on the MCAT need to be divided into categories as shown in the *MCAT Student Manual* (especially in math concepts or problem-solving concepts), and students should be told how to read them for manageable use on the MCAT—descriptive charts, not numerical charts—logical process charts.
8. The *MCAT Student Manual* does *not* provide a description of "Components of a Passage" and how to relate knowledge to the passage to solve various problems (narrative, graphs, charts, tables, chemical reactions, equations, instrumental sketches, implied verbal reasoning, etc.).
9. Based on a review of passages both in physical and biological sciences, the AAMC has used quite a few resources, which may include:
   - Medical encyclopedia
   - Fluid/solid properties in physics labs
   - Anatomy/physiology lab
   - Engineering mechanics laboratories
   - Bioengineering/biophysics books
   - Technology Review magazine
   - Chemical Engineering books
   - Medical English books
   - English technical books
   - Medical Instrumentation books
   - Engineer-in-training books
   - Microbiology/Histology books (medical technician)
   - Wastewater/Water Supply books
   - Electrical Appliance books with technology understanding
   - A complete AAMC cited bibliography is included in section A.6.
10. The AAMC materials do *not* provide enhanced strategies on "how to relate passages to the MCAT," i.e., how to find physics, chemistry, and biology-related concepts in passages (both instrumental and experimental). The publications do not present examples of passages to show "scientific concept extraction and application techniques." The explanatory solutions are the only application tools.
11. The student should focus on developing a glossary covering technological terms and their usage (find one in a book store).
12. The student should be fully aware of how unusual or irrelevant material can creep into passage construction.
13. Descriptive passages—Biological Sciences have one or two paragraphs of textbook information accompanied by a schematic diagram, chemical equation or reactions, or any other illustration found in college textbooks. These passages are traditional in describing scientific information found in college textbooks, manuals, and study guides.
14. Look for more experimental passages in laboratory reports, laboratory manuals, and research reports. Understand the physical design of experimental equipment, laboratory standards/assumptions, conclusions, and experimental testing leading to verification of scientific hypotheses.

A.6 MCAT BIBLIOGRAPHY CITED IN AAMC PUBLICATIONS AND MATERIALS

Source of Passages used in MCAT Verbal Reasoning

1-VR Adapted from Curtis B. Gans, "How to Take the Big Money Out of Politics." © 1985 by *The Washington Monthly.*

2-VR Adapted from Larry McMurtry, *In a Narrow Grave: Essays on Texas.* © 1968 by Larry McMurtry.

3-VR From Lawrence H. Fuchs, *Hawaii Pono: A Social History.* © 1961 by Lawrence H. Fuchs.

4-VR From Paul R. Ehrlich and Anne H. Ehrlich, "Population, Plenty, and Poverty." © 1988 by the National Geographic Society.

5-VR From Stephen W. Hawking, *A Brief History of Time: From the Big Bang to Black Holes.* © 1988 by Stephen W. Hawking.

6-VR From David Elkind, *Miseducation: Preschoolers at Risk.* ©1987 by David Elkind.

7-VR From James MacGregor Burns, J. W. Peltason, and Thomas E. Cronin, *Government by the People.* © 1989 by Prentice-Hall, Inc.

8-VR From Jacob Bronowski, "The Reach of Imagination." © 1978 by MacMillan Publishing Co., Inc.

9-VR From Stephen Jay Gould, *The Mismeasure of Man.* © by Stephen Jay Gould.

10-VR From Ronald G. Walters, *American Reformers: 1815–1860.* © 1978 by Ronald G. Walters.

11-VR From Luciano Berti, *Florence: The City and Its Art.* © 1979 by Luciano Berti.

12-VR Adapted from Daphne Merkin, "The Plight of Reading: In Search of the New Fiction." © 1984 by P.R., Inc.

13-VR From Northrop Frye, "The Keys to Dreamland," *The Conscious Reader.* © 1978 by Macmillan Publishing Co., Inc.

14-VR From B.F. Skinner, *Reflections on Behaviorism and Society.* © 1978 by Prentice-Hall, Inc.

15-VR From C. L. Duddington, *Evolution and Design in the Plant Kingdom.* © 1969 by C. L. Duddington.

16-VR Adapted from Freeman J. Dyson, "Disturbing the Universe." © 1979 by Freeman J. Dyson.

17-VR From Barbara W. Tuckman, *The First Salute.* © 1988 by Barbara W. Tuckman.

18-VR Adapted from R. Z. Sheppard, "A Time for Heroes, Not Saints." © 1988 by Time, Inc.

19-VR Adapted from Eliot Marshall, "Mountain Sheep Experts Draw Hunters' Fire." © 1990 by the American Association for the Advancement of Science.

20-VR From Theodore Roszak, *Where the Wasteland Ends.* © 1972 by the Atlantic Monthly Company.

21-VR Adapted from Eville Gorham, "What to Do about Acid Rain." © 1987 by The Dushkin Publishing Group, Inc.

22-VR Adapted from William K. Hartmann, "Birth of the Moon." © 1989 by the American Museum of Natural History.

23-VR From Kurt Baier, *The Moral Point of View: A Rational Basis of Ethics.* © 1965 by Random House, Inc.

24-VR Adapted from René Wellek and Austin Warren, *Theory of Literature.* © 1977 by René Wellek and Austin Warren.

25-VR Adapted from "Opossums and Career Women." © 1990 by The Economist Newspaper Ltd.

26-VR Adapted from the Solar System Exploration Committee of the NASA Advisory Council, 1990, *Planetary Exploration Through the Year 2000: An Augmented Program.*

27-VR From John Naisbitt, *Megatrends: Ten New Directions Transforming Our Lives.* © 1984 by Warner Books.

28-VR Adapted from Phyllis Culham, "Authenticity Not Authority for Feminists: A Modest, Existentialist Proposal." © 1990 by the American Philosophical Association.

29-VR From John P. Reganold, Robert I. Papendick, and James F. Parr, "Sustainable Agriculture." © 1990 by Scientific American, Inc.

30-VR Adapted from John Allen Paulos, *Innumeracy: Mathematical Illiteracy and Its Consequences.* © 1988 by John Allen Paulos.

31-VR From G. Calvin Mackenzie, *American Government Politics and Public Policy.* © 1986 by Random House, Inc.

32-VR Adapted from Bruce Stutz, "Hurricanes of the Arctic Nights." © 1986 by the American Museum of Natural History.

33-VR Adapted from August W. Staub, "Toys, Adults, Frivolity, Understanding, and the Demise of Serious Art Education." © 1990 by the Helen Dwight Reid Educational Foundation.

34-VR Adapted from R. Monastersky, "Rise of Tibet and Rockies Set Ice-Age Stage." © 1989 by Science Service, Inc.

35-VR From John Hay, *The Immortal Wilderness.* © 1987 by John Hay.

36-VR From G. E. Moore, *Ethics.* © 1971 by the Oxford University Press.

37-VR Adapted from Carl G. Jung, *The Spirit in Man, Art, and Literature* (Translated by R. F. Hull). © 1966 by the Bollingen Foundation.

38-VR Adapted from Richard Dawkins, *The Blind Watchmaker.* © 1987 by Richard Dawkins.

39-VR Adapted from W. John O'Brien, et al. "Search Strategies of Foraging Animals." © 1990 by Sima Xi, The Scientific Research Society, Inc.

40-VR Adapted from Walter Gropius, *Apollo in the Democracy: The Cultural Obligation of the Architect.* © 1968 by McGraw-Hill, Inc.

41-VR From David Attenborough, *Life on Earth: A Natural History.* © 1979 by David Attenborough Productions Ltd.

42-VR Adapted from Phil Brown, *Perspectives in Medical Sociology.* © 1989 by Wadsworth, Inc.

43-VR Adapted from Laurence Perrine, *Sound and Sense: An Introduction to Poetry.* © 1977 by Harcourt Brace Jovanovich, Inc.

44-VR From John Stuart Mill, "On Liberty." © 1938 by Oxford University Press, Inc.

45-VR Adapted from Peter A. Rona, "Metal Factories of the Deep Sea." © 1987 by the American Museum of Natural History.

46-VR Adapted from Frederick P. Brooks, Jr., "No Silver Bullet: Essence and Accidents of Software Engineering." © 1986 by IFIP.

47-VR Adapted from Herbert P. Ginsburg and Sylvia Opper, *Piaget's Theory of Intellectual Development.* © 1988 by Prentice-Hall.

Sources for Passages used in MCAT Biological and Physical Sciences

1-BS Adapted from Hermann Rahn, Amos Ar, and Charles V. Paganelli, "How Bird Eggs Breathe." © 1979 by Scientific American, Inc.

2-BS Table adapted from Sod-Moriah, Uriel A., Ella Magai, Jacob Kaplanski, Nissan Hirschman, and Isaac Nir, "The Role of the Pineal Gland in Thermoregulation in Male Hamsters." © 1983 by Pergamon Press, Inc.

3-BS Adapted from Thomas H. Lowry and Kathleen Schueller Richardson, *Mechanism and Theory in Organic Chemistry.* © 1976 by Thomas H. Lowry and Kathleen Schueller Richardson.

4-BS Figures adapted from Peter Flessel, Yi Y. Wang, Kuo-In Chang, and Jerome J. Wesolowski, *Ames Testing for Mutagens and Carcinogens in Air.* © 1987 by the Division of Chemical Education, American Chemical Society.

5-BS Table adapted from Jeremy Nathans, Thomas P. Piantanida, Roger L. Eddy, Thomas B. Shows, and David S. Hogness, "Molecular genetics of inherited variation in human color vision." © 1986 by the American Association for the Advancement of Science.

6-BS Tables adapted from Albert L. Lehninger, *Principles of Biochemistry.* © 1982 by Worth Publishers, Inc.

7-BS Figure adapted from Vicky L. McKinley and J. Robie Vestal, "Biokinetic Analyses of Adaptation and Succession: Microbial Activity in Composting Municipal Sewage Sludge." © 1984 by the American Society for Microbiology.

8-BS Figure from B. Wolf, et al., "Newborn Screening for Biotinidase Deficiency." © 1986 by Alan R. Liss, Inc.

9-BS Figure adapted from Werner Arber, "A Beginner's Guide to Lambda Biology." © 1983 by Cold Spring Harbor Laboratory.

10-BS Figure adapted from J. Richard McIntosh and Kent L. McDonald, "The Mitotic Spindle." © 1989 by Scientific American, Inc.

11-BS "Human Physiology—The Mechanisms of Body Function." © 1980 by Arthur Vander, James Sherman, and Dorothy Luciano.

12-BS *Textbook of Medical Physiology.* © 1981, 1986, by Arthur Guyton.

Other Sources from Which MCAT Passages Might Be Drawn

1. Books on agriculture, ethics, China, architecture, finance
2. *Journal of American Medical Education*
3. Medical Center progress reports
4. *Academic Medicine*
5. *The New England Journal of Medicine*
6. *U.S.A. Today* (newspaper)—debate section
7. *The Washington Post* (newspaper)—editorial section
8. *Directory,* American Medical Education (AAMC publication)
9. *The Wall Street Journal*
10. *Newsweek*
11. *The New Yorker*
12. *U.S. News and World Report*
13. *Science*
14. *Abacus* magazine
15. Design and decorating magazines
16. *The Constitution and American Education*, 2nd ed. A. A. Morris. St. Paul: West Publishing Co.
17. *Personal Finance—Principles and Case Problems,* 7th ed., © 1990. J. B. Cohen. R. D. Irwin, Inc.